Maternal-Newborn

Nursing Care

Mary Ann Towle, RN, MEd, MSN
Faculty
Boise State University
Boise, Idaho

PEARSON
Prentice
Hall

Upper Saddle River, New Jersey 07458

Library of Congress Cataloging-in-Publication Data

Towle, Mary Ann.
    Maternal-newborn nursing care / Mary Ann Towle.
        p. ; cm.
    Includes bibliographical references and index.
    ISBN-13: 978-0-13-113730-1
    ISBN-10: 0-13-113730-1
    1. Maternity nursing.
    [DNLM: 1. Neonatal Nursing—methods. 2. Nursing,
    Practical—methods. WY 157.3 T742m 2009] I. Title.
    RG951.T693 2009
    618.2'0231—dc22   2007043077

Publisher: Julie Levin Alexander
Assistant to Publisher: Regina Bruno
Editor-in-Chief: Maura Connor
Senior Acquisitions Editor: Kelly Trakalo
Development Editor: Rachel Bedard
Editorial Assistant: JulieAnn Oliveros
Media Product Manager: John Jordan
Director of Marketing: Karen Allman
Senior Marketing Manager: Francisco Del Castillo
Marketing Coordinator: Michael Sirinides
Managing Editor, Production: Patrick Walsh
Production Liaison: Yagnesh Jani
Production Editor: Trish Finley, GGS Book Services
Media Project Manager: Stephen Hartner
Manufacturing Manager/Buyer: Ilene Sanford
Composition: GGS Book Services
Printer/Binder: Quebecor World Color/Versailles
Senior Design Coordinator: Maria Guglielmo-Walsh
Cover Designer: Mary Siener
Cover Illustration: Daisies and Bee Background and Image, Photographer: Richard Woldendorp; Dahlia (close-up), PNC/Getty Images Inc.; Lotus Lily, Jeremy Woodhouse/Getty Images Inc.; Siberian Blue Dianthus (close-up), Medio Images/Getty Images Inc.; Lily Pad with Bloom, Eyewire/Getty Images Inc.; Pink Flower Field, Creatas Images/Jupiter Images; Poppy Behind Rainy Window, Steve Satushek/Jupiter Images.
Cover Printer: Phoenix Color Corporation

Pearson Education LTD.
Pearson Education Australia PTY, Limited
Pearson Education Singapore, Pte. Ltd
Pearson Education North Asia Ltd
Pearson Education Canada, Ltd.
Pearson Educación de Mexico, S.A. de C.V.
Pearson Education—Japan
Pearson Education Malaysia, Pte. Ltd
Pearson Education, Upper Saddle River, New Jersey

Notice: Care has been taken to confirm the accuracy of information presented in this book. The authors, editors, and the publisher, however, cannot accept any responsibility for errors or omissions or for consequences from application of the information in this book and make no warranty, express or implied, with respect to its contents.

The authors and publisher have exerted every effort to ensure that drug selections and dosages set forth in this text are in accord with current recommendations and practice at time of publication. However, in view of ongoing research, changes in government regulations, and the constant flow of information relating to drug therapy and reactions, the reader is urged to check the package inserts of all drugs for any change in indications or dosage and for added warning and precautions. This is particularly important when the recommended agent is a new and/or infrequently employed drug.

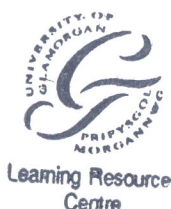

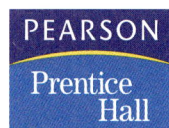

PEARSON
Prentice Hall

10 9 8 7 6 5 4 3 2 1
ISBN-13: 978-0-13-113730-1
ISBN: 0-13-113730-1

Student Success is built-in from the start...

Practical and vocational nurses from around the country told us that they needed two things to succeed as students in order to achieve their LPN/LVN licenses. First, they needed books that explain what the LPN/LVN needs to know and do. Second, they needed a variety of excellent review materials to reinforce their learning. *Maternal-Newborn Nursing Care* contains power-packed, built-in support to ensure your success throughout your LPN/LVN education.

As you start each chapter—

Brief Outlines preview what the chapter will cover for quick access and review.

Learning Outcomes identify what you can expect to learn from each chapter and help you focus your reading.

MediaLinks call your attention to the additional learning tools that are available on the CD-ROM and Companion Website that accompany your textbook, including:

Prentice Hall Nursing MediaLink CD-ROM

- Learning Outcomes
- Audio Glossary—key terms, definitions, and pronunciations
- NCLEX-PN® Review Questions
- Animations & Videos—difficult concepts brought to life

Companion Website

- Learning Outcomes
- Chapter Outlines
- Audio Glossary
- NCLEX-PN® Review Questions
- Key Term Review—matching questions and crossword puzzles to help with new terminology and definitions.
- Case Studies—scenarios and critical-thinking questions
- Challenge Your Knowledge—visual critical thinking questions
- WebLinks—content-related hyperlinks
- Nursing Tools—handy reference materials

Chapter 14

Care During Normal Labor and Birth

BRIEF Outline

Theories About the Beginning of Labor
Signs of Impending Labor
Admission to the Birthing Facility
Variables Affecting Labor

Pain in Labor
Stages of Labor
Delivery Room Care of the Neonate
Nursing Care

NURSING CARE PLAN CHART: Planning for Client with Premature Rupture of Membranes
HEALTH PROMOTION ISSUE: Client Wanting Second Labor to Be Better Than First
NURSING PROCESS CARE PLAN: Woman in Active Stage One Labor
CRITICAL THINKING CARE MAP: Caring for a Woman in Precipitous Labor

LEARNING Outcomes

After completing this chapter, you will be able to:
1. Define key terms.
2. Describe variables affecting labor and birth.
3. Differentiate the stages of labor.
4. Discuss the mechanisms of labor.
5. Identify nursing diagnoses and nursing interventions to assist in the labor process.
6. Provide appropriate care for a client during labor and birth.
7. Describe delivery room care of the neonate.

MediaLink
Preeclampsia

MediaLink Tabs MediaLink Tabs prompt you to explore videos, animations, and activities on the Student CD-ROM and Companion Website.

Makes need-to-know information easy to find and use!

Maternal-Newborn Nursing Care contains color-coded boxes and tables with important information for you to remember.

BOX 14-4 | CULTURAL PULSE POINTS

Expression of Pain During Labor

Pain response varies from culture to culture, and pain caused by labor and birth is no different. Some women are very stoic and labor quietly; this is frequently true with African American women. Others are notoriously loud. Many cultures feel that women must experience pain and discomfort during labor (e.g., Mexican, Iranian, and Filipinos). In fact, very difficult labor usually results in lavish gifts for Iranian women.

Mexican women are frequently heard repeating "*aye yie yie*" throughout labor. Interestingly, repeating "*aye yie yie*" in succession requires long, slow deep brea... described as "Mexican Lamaze." This phr... expression of pain but rather is a cultura... of pain relief.

Cultural Pulse Points boxes provide insight into populations and situations nurses may meet.

BOX 11-1 | COMPLEMENTARY THERAPIES

Cabbage Leaves for Treatment of Breast Engorgement

If the client does not feel relief from the suggestions provided in the text, suggest that the woman try using a few cabbage leaves. An enzyme found in green cabbage leaves has been effective in decreasing the swelling and increasing milk flow in breastfeeding mothers. Instructions for use of cabbage leaves follow:

- Wash and dry crisp, cold green cabbage leaves.
- Gently bend the leaves to release some of the natural juice.
- Apply a cabbage leaf directly to the skin for approximately 1 hour; then try feeding the baby or expressing milk.
- Reapply cabbage leaves 3 to 4 times a day. (Additional times may lead to a decrease of the wo...
- Discontinue use immediately if skin rash... is very rare.)

Client Teaching and Nutrition Therapy and Complementary Therapies boxes help you prepare for your role as educators in health care settings.

BOX 12-1 | LIFESPAN CONSIDERATIONS

Teen in Labor

- Teens often have greater need for emotional support. Emotional needs are often more complex than those of an adult woman.
- Adequate pain control must be provided. Teens need teaching prior to labor about the progression of pain in labor.
- Age, preparation, and family support will all affect the quality of the labor experience.
- Teen may want to have a friend come for labor support. (Friend may compete with teen's partner or parent for position; this problem occurs at a time that the young mother is most vulnerable; this needs to be discussed in prenatal class.)
- Peer support programs are effective in prenatal education programs.
- Teens' attitude of immortality and narcissism may make it difficult to address potential complications. ("Of course my body can give birth! Why shouldn't it?" This is part of the "it can't happen to me" way of thinking that is typical of this age group.)
- Any procedure (vaginal exam, epidural, IV lines, cesarean) may be terrifying to a teen. Be honest but gentle in providing an explanation prior to the procedure.
- Teens may be skeptical about relaxation and breathing techniques. They may want to prepare a tape or CD of their own music to use for relaxation during labor. (The nurse educator may prepare a tape or CD of music with phrases about deep breathing interspersed and provide it to the prenatal class.)

Lifespan Considerations boxes provide perspective on adapting nursing interventions to different developmental levels.

BOX 13-4 | ASSESSMENT

Preeclampsia and Eclampsia

Mild Preeclampsia

- Blood pressure of 30 mmHg systolic or 15 mmHg diastolic above the client's normal blood pressure reading *or* BP reading of 140/90
- Possible edema in hands and face
- Weight gain of more than 1 pound per week
- Possible urine output reduction
- Urine may show 1+ protein on a dipstick
- Hyper reflexes
- Complaints of headache, blurred vision, scotoma (spots before eyes), irritability, epigastric pain

Severe Preeclampsia

- Blood pressure increases to 160/110 or higher
- Generalized edema in hands, face, sacrum, lower extremities, and abdomen
- Possible weight gain of 2 or more pounds in a few days to a week
- Urine protein 2+ or more on a dipstick
- Urine output reduced, possibly less than 500 mL in 24 hours

Eclampsia

- Grand mal seizures
- Possible coma
- Initiation of contractions (The seizure activity may induce uterine contractions, but the comatose client may be unable to let anyone know.)
- Death

Assessment box summarizes data collected during assessment, common risk factors, and manifestations you might observe.

TABLE 14-5

Pharmacology: Systemic Pain Medications Used During Labor

DRUG (GENERIC AND COMMON BRAND NAME)	USUAL ROUTE/DOSE	CLASSIFICATION AND PURPOSE	SELECTED SIDE EFFECTS AND NURSING CONSIDERATIONS	DON'T GIVE IF
Butorphanol tartrate (Stadol)	1–2 mg IV every 3–4 hours	Opioid analgesic for pain	Respiratory depression, dizziness, euphoria	In second stage of labor
Meperidine HCL (Demerol)	2.5–15 mg IV every 3–4 hours	Opioid analgesic for pain	Respiratory depression, sedation	In second stage of labor *or* if allergic to drug
Naloxone (Narcan)	0.4–2 mg IV may repeat every 2–3 minutes to total of 10 mg	Narcotic antagonist for relief of respiratory depression in substance abuse	Respiratory depression may recur when Narcan wears off; monitor respiratory status carefully	Total of 10 mg has been given without improvement, *or* if you suspect narcotic overdose

Pharmacology Tables reinforce selected common medications nurses will encounter in practice. Additional boxes and tables offer information on key topics.

Nursing Care Checklists provide handy summaries of important nursing interventions.

Clinical Alerts call your attention to clinical roles and responsibilities for heightened awareness, monitoring, and/or reporting.

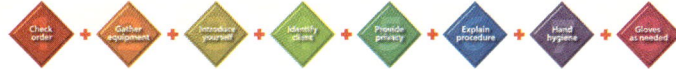

Procedures give you step-by-step instructions and rationales for nursing actions. Special icons in the procedures reinforce essential preliminary steps in client care. "Live" documentation at the end of each procedure demonstrates samples of good record-keeping.

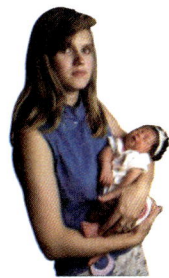

Health Promotion Issues examine topical issues and show you how to move from problems to solutions as you care for clients.

Learn to prioritize nursing actions and deliver safe, effective nursing care as part of the health care team!

Nursing Care is presented in the five-step nursing process format, but emphasizing the scope of practice for the LPN/LVN. Rationales after nursing actions explain why interventions are important and support evidence-based nursing process.

Critical Thinking Questions allow you to apply your new knowledge to a specific client.

NURSING CARE PLAN CHART
Planning for Adolescent Single Parent

GOAL	INTERVENTION	RATIONALE	EXPECTED OUTCOME
1. Risk for Impaired Parenting related to developmental stage			
Client will effectively bond with her newborn and will provide attentive, loving direct care to the baby to meet the neonate's physical, developmental, psychosocial, and spiritual needs.	Provide anticipatory guidance and parent education.	Adolescent mothers (especially the youngest) generally lack the developmental maturity necessary to put aside self-centeredness and to focus on the many needs of a newborn.	Client will demonstrate personal interest in her newborn, shown by active participation in the neonate's daily care routine (feeding, bathing, diapering, etc.).
		Adolescent mothers may put more emphasis on their personal relationships with members of the opposite sex than on their own offspring.	Client will anticipate and respond appropriately to the newborn's cues (e.g., she will attempt to comfort the crying baby, to check for a soiled diaper, etc.).
	Provide emotional support. Help the mother learn ways to be responsible for herself and the baby.	Guidance, support, and facilitation are ways to meet the adolescent's own developmental needs, enabling the client to focus on her child.	
		Adolescent mothers generally know less about newborns' needs and the basics of child care than mature women do. They tend to be less sensitive to, and less accepting of, the newborn's behavior.	
	Promote attachment. Encourage the mother to hold, look at, and talk to her child.	Impaired bonding has been linked to the development of mental illness in the child.	
2. Situational Low Self-Esteem related to unexpected pregnancy			
Client will demonstrate improved self-esteem and a positive self-concept. Client will avoid development of mental disorders associated with poor self-esteem, such as major depression.	Provide emotional support and active listening. Help the mother become more self-aware. Help her clarify what her values are.	In highly developed nations, adolescent pregnancy is generally discouraged. In many cultures, pregnancy outside of marriage is considered taboo. Single adolescent parents may feel guilt and shame regarding their sexual behavior. Social stigma contributes to poor self-concept. Adolescent parents may experience social isolation, as the demands of parenting consume time and energy, taking them away from normal peer interac-	Client will verbalize a self-affirming, yet realistic self-perception. Client will demonstrate continued interest in her environment and activity in her social network. Client will avoid negative self-talk indicative of a poor self-image. Client will engage in personal goal setting and will list three key goals she wants to meet in the next 3 months (e.g., "I will

Nursing Care Plan Charts help you reinforce the progression from client goals to nursing interventions to client outcomes.

Nursing Process Care Plans illustrate nursing care in a "real-life" scenario.

NURSING CARE

PRIORITIES IN NURSING CARE

The priorities of nursing care for the high-risk newborn are similar to those for the normal newborn. However, the method in which the needs are met may be different.

- Maintaining the airway, breathing, and circulation
- Maintaining body temperature
- Providing nutrition
- Ensuring elimination
- Teaching parents to provide care for their newborn.

ASSESSING

The high-risk newborn requires a more frequent and in-depth assessment than the normal newborn. The high-risk newborn may have equipment such as a heart monitor, a mechanical ventilator, or a feeding tube. The nurse must ensure that the equipment is functioning properly. The high-risk newborn may have had surgery to correct a congenital anomaly, or he or she may have infections or other conditions that require assessment and monitoring. Parents and family members require assessment information and support in the care of their high-risk newborn.

Priorities in Nursing Care focus your thinking on key assessments and interventions.

Comprehensive reviews at the end of the chapter...

Key Terms by Topic link important new vocabulary to its content area in the chapter.

Key Points summarize need-to-know concepts from the chapter.

EXPLORE MediaLink encourages you to use the Prentice Hall Nursing MediaLink CD-ROM and Companion Website for a multi-modal review, regardless of your learning style.

For Further Study shows where related content areas are cross-referenced throughout the book.

Chapter Review

KEY TERMS by Topic

Use the audio glossary feature of either the CD-ROM or the Companion Website to hear the correct pronunciation of the following key terms.

Signs of Impending Labor
lightening, Braxton Hicks contractions, false labor, effacement, dilatation, bloody show, spontaneous rupture of membranes, ballotable, prolapsed umbilical cord, premature rupture of membranes

Admission to the Birthing Facility
clonus

Variables Affecting Labor
5 Ps affecting labor, passage, cephalopelvic disproportion, station, passenger, fetal

attitude, fetal lie, transverse lie, fetal presentation, cephalic presentation, vertex presentation, occiput, mentum, sinciput, breech, fetal position, sutures, fontanels, molding, contractions, frequency, duration, intensity, Ferguson's reflex

Schultze mechanism, Duncan mechanism, fourth stage of labor, fundus, postpartal chills

Delivery Room Care of the Neonate
Apgar score

Nursing Care
effleurage

Pain in Labor
natural childbirth, regional blocks

Stages of Labor
labor, first stage of labor, dilatation stage, latent phase, active phase, amniotomy, second stage of labor, crowning, episiotomy, mechanism of labor, cardinal movements, engagement, descent, flexion, internal rotation, extension, restitution, external rotation, expulsion, third stage of labor,

KEY Points

- Labor progresses in a planned sequence of events.
- Nursing care during labor involves providing comfort measures for the mother and monitoring the well-being of the infant.
- The mother should be taught relaxation techniques before labor begins.
- The husband or a significant other can be useful in helping the mother relax and remain in control during labor.
- To determine if labor is progressing in a normal pattern, the nurse must understand the stages of labor and the mechanism by which the infant maneuvers its way through the birth canal.
- The nurse must be constantly on the alert to see whether labor is progressing normally. If it is not, the care provider must be notified at once.
- The LPN/LVN assists the RN by attaching monitoring equipment, assisting with relaxation techniques, preparing the delivery room, assisting with the birth, and monitoring client during recovery.

EXPLORE MediaLink

Additional interactive resources for this chapter can be found on the Companion Website at www.prenhall.com/towle. Click on Chapter 14 and "Begin" to select the activities for this chapter.

For chapter-related NCLEX-style questions and an audio glossary, access the accompanying CD-ROM in this book.

Animations
Second stage labor
Delivery of infant
Leopold's maneuver
Placenta cord blood

FOR FURTHER Study

See Chapter 3 for additional information on cord blood banking.

Figure 8-4 shows the two types of placental expulsion.

A full discussion on breastfeeding and nutrition is found in Chapter 11.

For more about complications of pregnancy, see Chapter 13.

For information about complications of labor and birth, see Chapter 15.

For steps in performing fundal massage, see Procedure 16-1.

See Chapter 17 for care of the normal newborn.

Critical Thinking Care Map

Caring for a Woman in Precipitous Labor
NCLEX-PN® Focus Area: Physiologic Integrity: Basic Care and Comfort

Case Study: 0630 Alyce, a 22-year-old, gravida 2, para 1, is admitted in transition. She states she woke up in labor and her water broke on the way to the hospital. She is obviously uncomfortable and is having difficulty keeping relaxed. States last labor lasted 6 hours.

Nursing Diagnosis: Pain related to increasing frequency and intensity of contractions

COLLECT DATA

Subjective _____ Objective _____

Data Collected
(use only those that apply)

- Cervix 9 cm dilated, 100% effaced
- Station +2
- BP 142/80
- Contractions every 5 minutes, lasting 90 seconds
- Obviously uncomfortable, moaning
- Having difficulty maintaining control
- Fetal heart rate 110
- Clear fluid draining from vagina

Nursing Interventions
(use only those that apply; list in priority order)

- Oxygen at 10 L per mask.
- Administer pain medication IV.
- Encourage to breathe with each contraction.
- Provide popsicles, ice chips, and nonbig material as distraction.
- Position on left side.
- Prepare sterile field for birth.

Would you report this? Yes/No

If yes, to: _____

Nursing Care

_____

How would you document this? _____

Compare your documentation to the sample provided in Appendix I.

NCLEX-PN® Exam Preparation

TEST-TAKING TIP: If you see words such as, "earlier," "observe," or "check" in the stem, the question is referring to the assessment phase of the nursing process. The answer should be consistent with that first phase of the nursing process as well.

1. The nurse is preparing an expectant mother for a positive prenatal visit. This client asks you to review the hormonal theory of labor with her. When you are finished reviewing you will evaluate that she understands the hormonal theory of labor if she says fetal production of which of the following hormones increases as the fetus matures and when sufficient starts a chain of hormonal events that causes labor?
   1. cortisol
   2. oxytocin
   3. progesterone
   4. estrogen

2. When gathering data on a client who has experienced "lightening," the client would most likely claim which of the following?
   1. "I can breathe much better."
   2. "My ankles are less swollen."
   3. "I don't have to urinate as often now."
   4. "My lower back pain has been relieved."

3. The student nurse observing a birth hears the obstetrician and the circulating nurse talking about the fetus being "vertex." The student realizes that the fetal part presenting first is which of the following body parts?
   1. forehead
   2. face
   3. buttocks
   4. occiput

4. A client in labor complains of feeling faint and the nurse turns her on her side. What effect will the side-lying position have on the laboring client's contractions?
   1. little or no effect at all
   2. increase in the frequency
   3. increase in the intensity
   4. will stop the contractions

5. A client is 3 cm dilated, excited about labor, and having contractions every 3 to 5 minutes. This phase is best described as:
   1. active phase, second stage
   2. latent phase, first stage
   3. transition phase, second stage
   4. active phase, first stage

6. The nurse explains the phases and stages of labor to first-time expectant parents. The nurse realizes the client understands

when she describes the average length of active phase for a primigravida as lasting which of the following lengths of time?
   1. 18–30 hours
   2. 12–24 hours
   3. 8–10 hours
   4. 4–6 hours

7. A client is in labor has no family or friends to support her during the labor process so you are supporting her. The physician says the cervix is 8 cm dilated. The client's contractions are strong and she gets irritable with you and tells you not to touch her. Which of the following actions would be appropriate? Choose all that apply.
   1. Ask for another nurse to support the client.
   2. Tell the client to be cooperative and do as you say.
   3. Teach simple relaxation and breathing techniques.
   4. Ask the client to actively push with each contraction.
   5. Offer the client warm socks to her lower back.
   6. Re-position the client for comfort.

8. You hear the obstetrician, working with a laboring client, say that engagement has occurred. You realize this means which of the following things?
   1. The fetus has now become ballotable.
   2. Presenting part has entered the true pelvis.
   3. Presenting part is just above the ischial spines.
   4. There is now otherwise crowning.

9. You are caring for a client in the fourth stage of labor. At the end of 1 hour, you find the client has saturated two perineal pads. Which of the following actions would be most important?
   1. Notify the primary nurse immediately.
   2. Assure the client that this is normal.
   3. Put the client on the bedpan to void.
   4. Start a count of the pads and chart it.

10. The nurse is monitoring a client in the fourth stage of labor. Which of the following are appropriate nursing interventions? (Select all that apply.)
   1. Assess vaginal flow for amount and character.
   2. Take maternal vital signs every hour for 4 hours.
   3. Provide the mother with a cooling bath.
   4. Check the fundus for position and firmness.
   5. Provide the mother with warm blankets.

Answers for NCLEX-PN® Review and Critical Thinking questions appear in Appendix I.

Critical Thinking Care Maps prepare you for success on NCLEX-PN®, in clinical, and on-the-job with a focused review of a client problem, including:

- NCLEX-PN® Focus Area
- Case Study
- Nursing Diagnosis
- Data Collection
- Reporting
- Nursing Care
- Documentation

NCLEX-PN® Exam Preparation includes:

- A Test-taking Tip with a focused study hint
- NCLEX-PN® -style questions for review and test practice, with questions in both traditional and alternative formats. Answers are found in Appendix I.

Prepare for your career as an LPN/LVN...

After each unit in this book, use the **Thinking Strategically About** ... pages as an opportunity to reflect on the topics you have just read in the context of important themes across the LPN/LVN curriculum. Short scenarios and project ideas spotlight the unit's content from a variety of angles. Review of concepts enables you to approach unit topics from a more integrated perspective.

Thinking Strategically About...

You are an LPN/LVN employed in an obstetrician's office. Your responsibilities are to collect and record data on each client, to prepare the client for examination by the obstetrician, and to assist the RN in providing instruction. The following three clients have been taken to examination rooms, and vital signs have been taken.

- Joyce, a 21-year-old married woman, comes for a routine prenatal checkup. She is 18 weeks pregnant with her first child.
- Hilda, a 24-year-old married woman, comes for an unscheduled checkup. She is 34 weeks pregnant with twins. She reports headache, blurred vision, and decreased urine output. She has swelling in her hands and feet that does not resolve at night.
- Anna, a 17-year-old single woman, comes for an initial office visit. She reports a positive at-home pregnancy test. She lives with her parents while she finishes high school. She has not told them about the pregnancy.

CRITICAL THINKING
- What questions should you ask Hilda to add the intellectual standard of *precision* to your assessment of her?
- What questions should you ask Anna to add the intellectual standard of *relevance* to your data about her past health history?

COLLABORATIVE CARE
- What agency should Anna be referred to that will provide support for young single pregnant women?

MANAGEMENT OF CARE AND PRIORITIES IN NURSING CARE
- In what order will you visit these clients?
- What is your rationale for prioritizing care?

DELEGATING
- What part of care of the client in an office or clinic can the LPN/LVN perform?

COMMUNICATION AND CLIENT TEACHING
- What routine teaching should be provided to Joyce at this point of her pregnancy?
- If the obstetrician admits Hilda to the hospital, what information should be communicated to the hospital nurse?

DOCUMENTING AND REPORTING
- What information from Anna's health history should be documented and reported to the RN?

CULTURAL CARE STRATEGIES
- If Hilda is of Hispanic origin, how will her cultural impact her care?

Critical Thinking questions highlight specific challenges you will face as a new nurse and assist you to provide the best possible care.

Collaborative Care challenges you to think about the different health care settings and to envision the many health care workers who may participate in a client's care.

Delegating helps you determine which nursing interventions may be delegated to assistive personnel.

Management of Care highlights specific nursing interventions appropriate to the care of the client.

Communication and **Client Teaching** focus on communication methods and educational strategies necessary to teach the client and the family.

Time Management and **Priorities in Nursing Care** help you organize care and focus on the most important aspects of care first.

Documenting and Reporting helps you practice what and how to document and when to report your findings.

Cultural Care Strategies build your confidence by providing information and scenarios to familiarize you with cultural patterns and differences.

Maternal-Newborn Nursing Care will be a key resource as you progress through your nursing courses and become a nurse.

The nature of nursing—grow with it!

To my God and my church family who provide me with spiritual energy to face life challenges.

Mary Ann

Preface

Maternal-Newborn Nursing Care is written to provide you, the LPN/LVN student, with a foundation for providing safe, effective nursing care of mothers and newborn infants. Although the traditional role of the LPN/LVN has been in acute and long-term care, nursing practice has moved out of the hospital and into a variety of settings within the community. This shift has resulted in a more interdisciplinary approach to client care. The task of defining the role of the LPN/LVN in community-based nursing practice is in its early stages. The education of the LPN/LVN level of nurse is extremely important in this time of transition. LPNs and LVNs will need to be competent, confident, and articulate in providing compassionate care in a variety of settings. They must understand the meaning of signs and symptoms, and they need to distinguish between normal and abnormal findings. Because the LPN/LVN will practice with a varying degree of supervision, *Maternal-Newborn Nursing Care* addresses the LPN/LVN scope of practice, roles, and collaborative relationships with the registered nurse and other health care professionals.

Organization

Maternal-Newborn Nursing Care is divided into six units. Unit I focuses on community-based nursing practice. This unit helps you make decisions, delegate activities, and provide care within the legal scope of practice for an LPN/LVN. You will learn how to assist the registered nurse in health promotion activities, in working with families, and in client teaching in a variety of client settings, including the home.

Unit II focuses on human reproduction and reproductive health issues. Emphasis is placed on health promotion and activities that encourage reproductive health. You will learn to recognize symptoms of reproductive health issues and take appropriate actions.

Unit III focuses on the care of the woman during pregnancy. You will be introduced to the complexities of fetal development. You will learn to assess the developing fetus within the role of the LPN/LVN and to assist the RN and primary care provider in conducting diagnostic exams related to fetal well-being. You will learn to care for the mother during uncomplicated pregnancy and to assist the RN when common complications occur.

Unit IV focuses on care of the woman during the birthing process. You will learn to assist the RN in caring for the uncomplicated and complicated labor and birth, including cesarean section.

In Unit V, you will learn to care for the new mother. She will need adequate knowledge in order to provide a healthy environment for her new family. It is important for her to receive effective teaching to promote her healing and the health of her family.

Finally, in Unit VI you will learn to care for the normal newborn and to provide instruction to the new mother regarding home care of her infant. You will also learn how to assist the RN in care of the high-risk newborn.

Features

Throughout each chapter you will find consistent features to facilitate and reinforce your learning.

- Each chapter begins with **Learning Outcomes** to help you focus your learning.

- A **Nursing Care** section demonstrates the nursing process format and includes references to the role of the LPN/LVN in a variety of settings. Because time management and prioritizing tasks are such an important part of your day, this section begins with **Priorities in Nursing Care**, a summary of the areas on which you must focus in order to provide quality nursing care. Nursing interventions are followed by rationales, to reinforce your understanding of why selected nursing actions are performed.

- **Case Studies** and **Critical Thinking** exercises are designed to bring the concepts to life and to engage you in problem solving in situations you might encounter at work.

- **Health Promotion Issues** explore current issues in health care and provide a step-by-step solution for managing them.

- **Pharmacology** tables occur within clinical chapters to reinforce some of the most common medications you will administer.

- **Key Terms** and **Key Points** are reviewed at the end of each chapter.

- **NCLEX-PN®** **Review Questions** help you practice your test-taking skills.

- **Appendices** contain invaluable reference material including newborn rating scales, normal laboratory values, and answers to Critical Thinking and NCLEX-PN® Review Questions.

Acknowledgments

A project such as this requires the contributions of many people. Without LPN/LVN students, there would not be a need for this book. Students have been the inspiration and motivation for the work. Their enthusiasm for learning

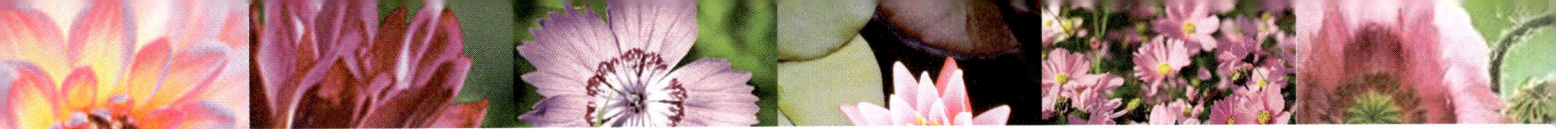

stimulates and challenges us to provide a quality textbook. It is my hope that this text will enhance students' knowledge and understanding of the care of mothers and newborns and will prepare students for success. I want to thank my students—past, present, and future—from whom I have gained so much.

Many nursing professionals gave invaluable time and expertise to this project. The contributors provided knowledge and writing skills in selected features of the book. Reviewers used their skill as educators to help maintain quality. They gave ongoing assistance in deciding what students need to know and how to express ideas for optimal learning. Contributors and reviewers for *Maternal-Newborn Nursing Care* are shown in a listing that follows this preface.

Health care is a team effort. This textbook is no different. Many intelligent individuals contributed their expertise to this work. Kelly Trakalo, Senior Acquisitions Editor, was an active supporter of the book's goals throughout.

My developmental editor, Rachel Bedard, was my supporter, my challenger, my cheerleader and, most importantly, my friend. When my energy was drained, she provided inspiration; when deadlines came too soon, she provided encouragement; and when units were completed, she celebrated with me. Through weekly conversations, she helped me to remain focused and not let the day-to-day challenges of life prevent me from accomplishing this goal. This book is what it is because of Rachel, and I thank her from the bottom of my heart.

Other important people in the production of this book were Yagnesh Jani (production editor); JulieAnn Oliveros (editorial assistant); Patrick Walsh (managing production editor); Ilene Sanford (manufacturing manager); Trish Finley (GGS project manager) and the GGS staff; Mary Siener and Maria Guglielmo-Walsh (design); John Jordan and Stephen Hartner (media); Teresa Himpsl (editorial assistant); and Francisco Del Castillo and Michael Sirinides (marketing). My thanks to all of you!

Finally I want to thank my colleagues, my friends, and my family for their support and encouragement. To all of you I am most grateful!

Nursing is an exciting, ever-changing profession. Advances in the medical management of clients have resulted in shorter length of stay in acute care hospitals and more clients being cared for in the home. Providing care in the home is a new challenge for many nurses and a new role for the LPN/LVN. To meet this challenge, the LPN/LVN must be more knowledgeable than ever before and be able to think critically in a variety of situations. With this text, I hope to prepare the LPN/LVN for these challenges.

About the Author

Mary Ann Towle, RN, MEd, MSN

Mary Ann Towle "always wanted to be a nurse" but teaching science in high school also seemed appealing. After graduating from Idaho State University with a Baccalaureate Degree in Nursing, she moved to Boise, Idaho, where she accepted a position at St. Luke's Medical Center. Mary Ann felt confident with her entry-level knowledge but was unsure of herself when it came to performing nursing procedures. Several LPNs helped her gain the necessary skills and confidence. Within a few months, she was working in the Coronary Intensive Care Unit as the evening charge nurse.

While Mary Ann enjoyed the direct client care of the CICU, she felt something was missing in her career. She taught a few in-service programs and workshops to nurses as well as to Respiratory Therapy students from Boise State University. After three years, an opportunity became available to teach in the LPN program at Boise State University. Mary Ann jumped at the chance to combine her love for nursing and her desire to teach.

All faculty in the Vocational-Technical Education programs were required to take education classes in order to improve their teaching performance. With a husband and two young children to care for and while teaching full time, Mary Ann attended classes two or three nights a week. After five years, she completed a Master of Education degree with a specialty in Vocational Education. A proponent of life-long learning, Mary Ann returned to school once her family was grown and completed a Master of Science degree in Nursing. Having taught the entire curriculum, Mary Ann sees herself as a generalist with experience in maternity, pediatrics, medical-surgical nursing, and geriatrics.

It has been 31 years since Mary Ann began her career as a nursing instructor at Boise State University. She has been recognized by the American Vocational Association as Vocational Teacher of the Year at the state and regional levels and as first runner-up at the national level. Mary Ann is the co-author of several other articles and nursing textbooks.

Mary Ann is a strong advocate for the LPN/LVN. She works to advance their education and scope of practice within the health care community. She feels that by reducing the stress involved in learning, providing positive feedback, and role modeling, she can help all students develop into quality nurses who can think critically and function in any situation.

Contributor Team

Chapter Contributor

Jeanne Hately, RN, MSN, PhD
President, Professional Nurse Consultants, LLC
Aurora, CO

Supplement Contributors

Student CD-ROM

Ann L. Bianchi, RN, MSN, ICCE, ICD
Clinical Assistant Professor
University of Alabama
Huntsville, AL

Companion Website (www.prenhall.com/towle)

Ann L. Bianchi, RN, MSN, ICCE, ICD
Clinical Assistant Professor
University of Alabama
Huntsville, AL

Terrilynn Quillen, RN MSN
Department of Environments for Health
Community Health Nursing
Indiana University School of Nursing
Faith Community Nurse
New Life in Christ Ministries
Indiana, IN

Instructor's Resource Manual and Instructor's Resource CD-ROM

Debra S. McKinney, MSN, MBA/HCM, BSN, RN
Nursing Educational Consultant
Warrenton, VA

We would also like to thank contributors to the *Maternal-Child Nursing Care* supplements whose work formed the backbone of this work.

Janice Ankenmann-Hill, RN, MSN, CCRN, FNP
Faculty
Napa Valley College
Napa, CA

Laura L. Brown, RN, MSN, CPN
Nursing Instructor
Asheville-Buncombe Technical Community College
Asheville, NC

Kim Cooper, RN, MSN
Instructor
Ivy Tech Community College
Terre Haute, IN

Cheryl DeGraw, RN, MSN, CRNP
Faculty/Course Coordinator
Florence-Darlington Technical College
Florence, SC

Jane Headland, RNC, MSN
Nursing Instructor
Asheville-Buncombe Technical Community College
Asheville, NC

Virginia Lester, RN, MSN
Assistant Professor
Angelo State University
San Angelo, TX

Jan Weust, RN, MSN
Instructor
Ivy Tech Community College
Terre Haute, IN

Julie Anne Will, RN, MSN
Instructor
Ivy Tech Community College
Terre Haute, IN

Reviewer Panel

Marjorie L. Archer, MS, RNC, WHCNP
Vocational Nursing Coordinator
North Central Texas College
Gainesville, TX

Jill Becker, RN, MSN
Assistant Professor of Nursing
Northern Essex Community College
Lawrence, MA

Marti Burton, RN, BS
Instructor and Curriculum Designer/Developer
Canadian Valley Technology Center
El Reno, OK

Rebecca Cappo, RN, MSN
Coordinator
Lenape LPN Program
Ford City, PA

Traudel Cline, RN, MSN
Nursing Instructor
Milwaukee Area Technical College
Milwaukee, WI

Mary Davis, RN, MSN
Nursing Faculty
Valdosta Technical College
Valdosta, GA

Shari Gholson, MSN, RN
Associate Professor
West Kentucky Community and Technical College
Paducah, KY

Julie Hansen, RN, BSN, MA
LPN Program Instructor
Southeast Technical Institute
Sioux Falls, SD

Jeanne Hately, RN, MSN, PhD
President, Professional Nurse Consultants, LLC
Aurora, CO

Michelle Helderman, RN, MSN
Nursing Instructor
Ivy Tech Community College
Terre Haute, IN

Susie Huyer, MSN, RN
Nursing Education Consultants
Chantilly, VA

Julie Kay, RN, BSN, MSN
Nursing Instructor
San Joaquin Delta College
Stockton, CA

Kimberly McDonnell, RN
NICU Nurse
Lancaster General Hospital
Respiratory Home Care Nurse
Lancaster, PA

Jeffrey C. McManemy, PhD, APRN, BC
Associate Professor/Program Coordinator
St. Louis Community College
at Florissant Valley
St. Louis, MO

Mary Pat Norrell, RNC, BSN, MS
Professor, Nursing Department
Ivy Tech Community College of Indiana
Seymour, IN

Deborah Andreas Ostdiek, RNC, BSN
PN Instructor
Western Nebraska Community College
Scottsbluff, NE

Noel Piano, RN, MS
Instructor/Coordinator
Lafayette School of Practical Nursing
Williamsburg, VA

Becki Quick, RN, BA, MAC
Director of Nursing VN Program
Maric College San Diego
San Diego, CA

LuAnn Reicks, RNBC, BS, MSN
Professor/PN Coordinator
Iowa Central Community College
Fort Dodge, IA

Betty Kehl Richardson, PhD, RN CS Psych-MH, BC
Professor Emeritus
Austin Community College
Private Practice Marriage and Family Therapy
Austin, TX

Russlyn St. John, RN, MSN
Coordinator, Practical Nursing
St. Charles Community College
St. Peters, MO

Contents

Contents   **xix**

Introduction to Maternal-Newborn Nursing

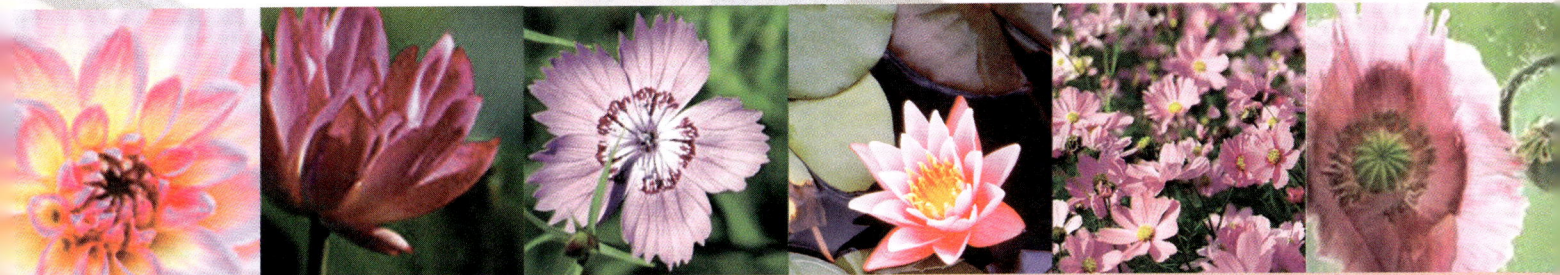

Chapter 1

The LPN/LVN in Maternal-Newborn Nursing

NURSING PROCESS CARE PLAN:
Caring for a Family That Desires Alternative Therapies

HEALTH PROMOTION ISSUE:
Male Circumcision Without Anesthesia

BRIEF Outline

History of Maternity Nursing

Developments in Nursing

Nursing Process in Maternal-Newborn Nursing

Research-Based Nursing Practice

Community-Based Nursing Practice

Roles of the LPN/LVN in Community Care

Employment Opportunities for LPNs/LVNs in Community-Based Nursing

LEARNING Outcomes

After completing this chapter, you will be able to:

1. Define key terms.
2. Relate the history of maternal-newborn nursing to current trends.
3. Describe the benefit of research on nursing practice.
4. Describe community-based nursing practice.
5. Describe LPN/LVN roles in maternal-newborn nursing.

What is **maternal-newborn nursing?** Maternal-newborn nursing (also called obstetric nursing) is the care of women during pregnancy, childbirth, and postpartum, and the care of the child from birth through the first 6 weeks of life.

History of Maternity Nursing

Throughout history, women learned about pregnancy through interaction with female family members in the home. In the early 1900s in the United States, more than 90% of births were in the home. These births were attended by female family or close friends, or sometimes by midwives without formal training.

From 1900 to the early 1950s, medical science made dramatic changes (Table 1-1 ■). The standard for childbirth shifted from care provided by untrained personnel to care provided by physicians. Hospitals were built, and health care increasingly moved from the home environment to the hospital setting. Improvements in anesthesia led to more common use of spinal blocks and inhaled medications that

TABLE 1-1
Interesting Names and Events in Maternal-Newborn Care

DATE	NAME AND/OR EVENT	IMPORTANCE TO OR EFFECT ON MATERNAL-NEWBORN CARE
2nd Century AD	Soranus	Known as the father of obstetrics. Developed the Podalic version procedure in which the fetus is rotated to a breeched position (was important in delivering the second twin).
16th Century AD	Fallopius	Fallopius, an Italian anatomist, identified the tubes that carry eggs from the ovary to the uterus; hence, fallopian tubes.
1796	Edward Jenner	His experiments mark the beginning of immunology. He infected people with cowpox to make them immune to small pox. This procedure involves injecting less harmful microbes to stimulate immunity to a more dangerous microbe. His contribution both enabled control of this dreaded disease and established the science of immunization.
1802	Pediatric hospitals	The first children's hospital was established in Paris, France. In 1855, the United States established its first children's hospital, known as The Children's Hospital of Philadelphia (still in existence today).
1807	Samuel Bard	Wrote the first American textbook for midwives.
1842	Oliver Wendell Holmes	Published a paper on the contagious nature of puerperal fever, which increased the survival rate of the mother and child during childbirth.
1853	New York City Children's Aids Society	This society was the first founded in the United States to care for homeless children.
1861	Ignaz Semmelweis	Pioneer in the use of antisepsis, he required medical students to wash their hands with chlorinated lime solution between examinations. He also proved puerperal fever is a form of septicemia. He theorized that the relationship between the incidences of puerperal fever was higher when examination of the new mother was done by doctors working on cadavers. This was not an accepted theory until 1890. He wrote *The Causes, Understanding and Prevention of Childbed Fever*.
1860s	Louis Pasteur	He confirmed that puerperal fever was caused by bacteria, "germ theory of disease." Established that simple handwashing is an important means of preventing the spread of infection.
1867	Joseph Lister	He adopted the use of carbolic acid as an antiseptic agent in the prevention of infections. This form of sterilization introduced the era of antiseptic surgery, and dramatically reduced mortality rate following surgery.

(continued)

TABLE 1-1

Interesting Names and Events in Maternal-Newborn Care (continued)

DATE	NAME AND/OR EVENT	IMPORTANCE TO OR EFFECT ON MATERNAL-NEWBORN CARE
1884	Karl Sigismund Franz Credé	Developed the method of placing drops of an antiseptic solution of silver nitrate in the eyes of the newborn to prevent blindness caused by gonorrhea.
1888	Arthur Jacobi	Recognized as the "Father of Pediatrics." He established pediatric units in several New York hospitals and was instrumental in the formation of the American Pediatric Society. He also initiated the boiling of milk to lower the incidence of diarrhea in children.
1896	Incubators	These were first developed in 1896 by a German physician. In 1903 the incubator was brought to the United States by Dr. Martin A. Couney, the "incubator doctor." He set up incubators at Coney Island as part of the carnival's exhibition. He also toured the country with his display, including the World's Fair in 1933. He reportedly saved 6,500 of the 8,000 babies who used his incubators. However, it was not until the 1940s that incubators were used in hospitals.
1912	Children's Bureau	Creation of this bureau marked the beginning of modern child-welfare programs and public recognition of children's special needs. Focused on infant and maternal mortality. Mandated birth registration in all states. It established the hot lunch school program in 1930.
1920	"Twilight Sleep"	This form of anesthesia was a major influence in a women's choice to deliver in a hospital. Morphine and scopolamine were used to ease the pain; it also gave physicians more control over the birthing process. This in turn led to an increase in hospital births.
1921	Sheppard Tower Act	Provides funds for state-managed programs for maternity care. It also provides federal grants-in-aid to states to promote better care for mothers and dependent children.
1930	White House Conference on Children and Youth, development of Children's Charter	Issued statements related to the needs of children in the areas of education, health, welfare, and protection.
1930	American Academy of Pediatrics	Dr. Clifford Grulee, Dr. Isaac Abt, and Dr. William Lucas were key figures in the founding of the American Academy of Pediatrics, whose goals are to develop the scope and field of pediatrics, and to have a positive influence on the life and health of its clients.
1931	School of the Association for the Promotion and Standardization of Midwifery	Provided formal education for midwives.
1932–1970	Neonate stimulation and maternal deprivation	Joseph Brennamen was the first to recognize the relationship between an infant's poor health and the lack of stimulation the infant received in the maternity wards. Over the years many physicians have studied mother–infant bonding and the effects of a long-term stay in the hospital on children. Today, hospitals have modified their policies of visitation to reflect these findings.
1939	Mary Breckinridge	Opened the Frontier School of Midwifery. After a family nursing curriculum was added to the school's program in 1970, the name was changed to the Frontier School of Midwifery and Family Nursing.
1955	American College of Nurse-Midwifery (later renamed the American College of Nurse-Midwives)	Instituted to develop and support educational programs, sponsor research, develop professional relationships, and participate in the international organization of midwives.
1956	La Leche League	Breastfeeding rates in the United States had dropped close to 20% when the first meeting of LLL was held. Their first publication was a loose-leaf edition of *The Womanly Art of Breastfeeding*.

DATE	NAME AND/OR EVENT	IMPORTANCE TO OR EFFECT ON MATERNAL-NEWBORN CARE
1960	Lamaze childbirth method	The Lamaze organization, currently known as Lamaze International, Inc., promoted the philosophy that childbirth is a natural event that women are equipped to handle. They consider the ideal birthing experience to be awake, aware, supported by family and friends, and with no maternal–infant separation.
1962	Child Protection Laws	Laws that require the reporting of incidents of child abuse. All states are required to have such laws.
1974	Women, Infants, and Children (WIC)	Program provides supplemental food and education to lower-income children under the age of 5, and women who are pregnant, postpartum, or breastfeeding.
1975	Amniocentesis	Test that allows physicians to diagnose congenital or inherited diseases before childbirth. A new, less invasive procedure (called *chorionic villus sampling*) is now available for genetic screening.
1979	International Year of the Child	Focused attention to the critical needs of the world's children. Its stated mission was to consider how to provide food globally to children in need.
1980s	Artificial insemination	Initiated as a means of fertilization. Many couples now resort to various methods of in-vitro fertilization ("test-tube" babies) or transplantation of fertilized ova from one womb to another.
1992	Office of Alternative Medicine (OAM) within the National Department of Health	Agency developed to promote research and publicize information on complementary and alternative therapies. Emphasizes prevention, wellness, and a holistic approach to health care.
1996	Newborns' and Mothers' Health Protection Act	Provides for a postpartum stay of 48 hours following a vaginal birth and 96 hours for a cesarean birth.
2002	Best Pharmaceutical for Children Act (BPCA)	Established a drug program that identifies drugs and clinical studies that are needed for children.
2003	Human Genome Map	Completion of 99% of human genome map has led to enhanced diagnosis of genetic disorders. The use of gene transfer therapy in curing some genetic conditions is a new and expanding field.

produced a "twilight sleep" for painless deliveries. This was seen as a tremendous advance in the care of women in labor.

However, in the 1960s through the 1980s, data were gathered showing some negative effects of this type of anesthesia. Mothers under anesthesia were unable to push effectively, leading to the use of forceps to deliver the infant. Large doses of medication caused respiratory distress in the neonate. The number of caesarean deliveries in hospitals increased dramatically. Eventually, questions were raised about whether births were occurring at the convenience of physicians or of mothers.

The result of research was that women began taking charge of the birthing process as much as possible. Prenatal classes formed to teach women about pregnancy, nutrition, and childbirth. In an attempt to have the safety of hospital deliveries in a "homelike" environment, birthing suites were built to allow the woman to labor, deliver, and recover in the same room. The husband, and sometimes other family members, may be present at the birth. Epidural anesthesia has replaced spinal block anesthesia, allowing for a painless delivery with fewer adverse effects.

As hospitals became the main setting for childbirth, maternity nursing emerged as a specialty. The Nurses Association of the American College of Obstetricians and Gynecologists (NAACOG), later renamed the Association of Women's Health, Obstetric and Neonatal Nurses (AWHONN), was formed to improve the health of women and newborn infants. Together with the American Nurses Association, AWHONN works to improve the education of nurses engaged in obstetric-gynecologic care.

Today, many couples are postponing childbirth to pursue a career. As a result, they may come to parenting with greater risk of complications or fetal anomalies than they would have had if they had gotten pregnant in early adulthood. For example, the risk of having a child with Down syndrome is increased when parents are older than 40. Older parents, though highly motivated to have a child, may find that the changes and discomforts of pregnancy place a greater strain on overall wellness than would have been the case a decade or two earlier in their lives. At the same time, changes in the health care system have resulted in shorter hospital stays than previous generations of women experienced. Instead of having a week of bed rest after delivery, women are now expected to return to the home 2 or 3 days after the birth.

Nurses in this type of environment must be knowledgeable about the physiology of pregnancy and about family dynamics. They must be alert to potential difficulties as the pregnancy progresses. They must be prepared to provide client teaching at every available opportunity. They must be able to recognize and work with a variety of family dynamics in order to promote the health of both mother and child.

Parents today are involved in every aspect of the birthing process. They are less likely to be viewed as **patients** (with its suggestion of people who are ill, who need care, and who may rely on others to make decisions for them). They are more often seen as **consumers** (purchasers of a service) and as **clients** (active participants in a process who obtain assistance from specialists). We use the word *clients* throughout this book.

Developments in Nursing

Like maternity care, nursing has changed dramatically since it began. In Florence Nightingale's time, nursing involved providing for the sick person's activities of daily living. Nurses would do cooking, cleaning, stoking the coal stove, and trimming the wicks on the kerosene lamps. The nurse worked for the doctor, assisting as requested and doing assigned tasks. There was no expectation that the nurse would function independently.

Today, nursing is described as a knowledge-based process discipline where the licensed nurse's specialized education, professional judgment, and discretion are essential for quality nursing care (National Council of State Boards of Nursing [NCSBN], 1995). The American Nurses Association (ANA) defines nursing practice as "the nursing diagnosis and treatment of human response to actual or potential health problems" (ANA, 1980, p. 9). The ANA (1991) further identifies four essential features of nursing practice.

- Attention to the full range of human experiences and responses to health and illness without restriction to a problem-focused orientation.
- Integration of **objective data** (data that can be observed and measured by the senses or by mechanical instruments) with **subjective data** (knowledge gained from an understanding of the client or group's subjective personal experience).
- Application of scientific knowledge to the process of diagnosis and treatment.

- Provision of a caring relationship that facilitates health and healing.

Until the mid-20th century, nursing care followed the medical model, focusing on the treatment of illness. The nurse worked "for" and depended on the doctor's medical orders, and this was reflected in the way they talked about people who came for treatment. It was quite common for nurses and hospital staff to refer to "the appendectomy in room 225" or "the C-section in room 20." Medical advances, such as the development of antibiotics and laparoscopic surgery, had a tremendous impact on the medical care of individuals, but they did little to change nursing practice.

Although many areas of medicine have continued to become more specialized, nursing has become **holistic** (inclusive of the physical, psychological, and spiritual aspects of the person). Through the work of nursing theorists such as Jean Watson, Martha Rogers, and others, nursing has come to recognize that health and illness are more than simple physical states. Instead, they reflect the whole person, the person's level of development, mental status, physical health, coping ability, and more.

Furthermore, especially in maternity nursing, the client is no longer just the individual. Instead "the client" refers to the entire family (Figure 1-1 ■). The nurse who obtains the vital signs of an infant is also actively involved in helping the parent promote the infant's health. This is done by observing parenting skills and by providing teaching to the parent to create positive effects for the child.

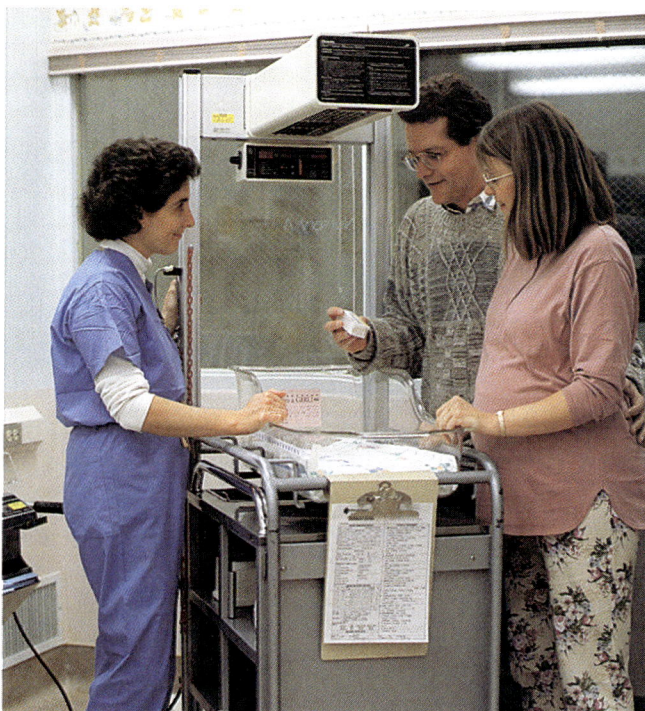

Figure 1-1. ■ One of the most important roles in maternal-newborn nursing is client education.

Nursing Process in Maternal-Newborn Nursing

The nurse must use a systematic approach (the nursing process) when planning and implementing nursing care. The licensed practical or vocational nurse (LPN/LVN) participates in every aspect of the nursing process. The depth of involvement depends on:

1. The particular state's nurse practice acts.
2. The policies of the facility where the nurse works.
3. The nurse's skills and experiences.

ASSESSING

The nursing process is a continuous, unbroken process (Figure 1-2 ■). During assessment, LPNs/LVNs collect and analyze data from the client and family. They are not required to analyze and synthesize data as much as the registered nurse (RN) does. Still, it is LPNs/LVNs at the bedside who monitor changes in the client, compare the data with given normal ranges, and decide whether findings should be reported. Critical thinking is an important aspect of quality care that the nurse will employ in every phase of the nursing process (see Chapter 2 ⊕ for an in-depth discussion of critical thinking).

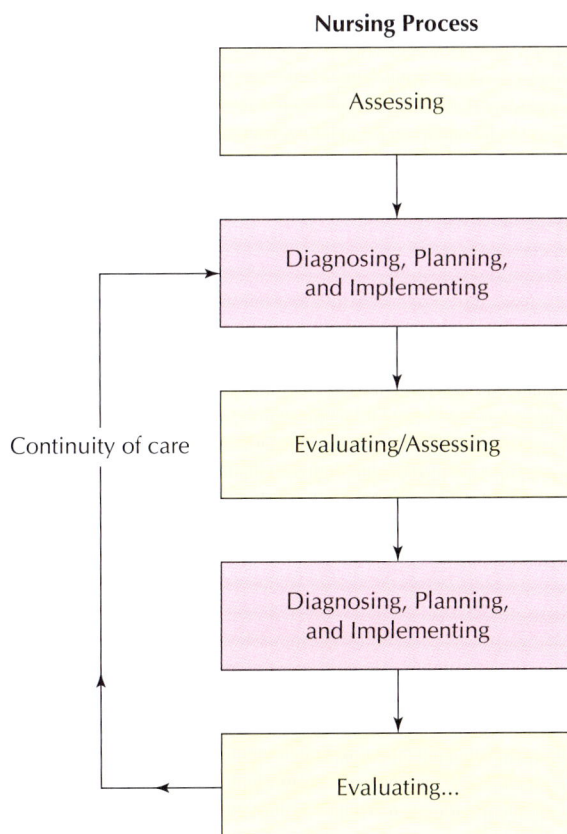

Nursing Process

Figure 1-2. ■ Nursing process model.

DIAGNOSING AND PLANNING

In defining nursing as a distinct profession, it is important to identify actions the nurse performs independently of physicians or other members of the health care team. Names for client conditions that nurses are qualified and trained to treat independently (called **nursing diagnoses**) have been defined and developed by the North American Nursing Diagnosis Association (NANDA, 2008). When a NANDA label such as Pain is identified, an experienced nurse immediately knows the desired **outcome** (the client goal that relates to a specific nursing diagnosis). When Pain is identified as the nursing diagnosis, the desired outcome for the client would be reduction in pain to tolerable levels. The experienced nurse can also name several possible nursing actions to assist the client toward an improvement in health. These nursing actions (called **interventions**) include administration of prescribed analgesics, nonpharmacologic comfort measures such as a bath or backrub, or distractions such as soft music or a favorite TV program.

In some states, the LPN/LVN assists the RN in writing and updating the nursing diagnoses and nursing **care plan.** The care plan (an organized and prioritized plan) addresses the nursing diagnoses and helps the client reach measurable, identified outcomes (or goals). For example, for a client with a pain measuring 9 on a scale of 1 to 10, a client outcome might be to reduce the client's sensation of pain to 5 or lower to allow rest.

Regardless of whether planning is a shared role with the RN, the LPN/LVN must understand the difference between the nursing diagnoses and the medical diagnoses and follow both the nursing and the medical plan of care.

Nursing Versus Medical Diagnoses

Medical diagnoses are statements about a disease process or disorder. For example, a client may have a medical diagnosis of urinary tract infection. Because of this medical diagnosis, the client may be in pain, be dehydrated, and have perineal odor. In this instance, the NANDA diagnoses would include Pain, Deficient Fluid Volume, and Infection. These are the conditions of the client that the nurse is trained and licensed to treat independently.

IMPLEMENTING

The nurse would follow the doctor's order by administering antibiotics, giving pain medication when needed, and documenting them promptly. The nurse would also use diversion to help the client focus on something other than the pain. Turning and positioning the client, providing adequate nutrition and fluids, and ensuring adequate elimination are examples of nursing orders in this situation.

In implementing the nursing and medical plan of care, the LPN/LVN stays within the rules and regulations of the state board of nursing related to scope of practice. The amount of independence the LPN/LVN has in performing nursing care varies not only from state to state but also from one health care agency to another. For example, in some states the LPN/LVN can administer medication by the intravenous route into a central venous catheter. In other states, this route of medication administration is reserved for the RN. In a large, acute-care hospital, the LPN/LVN may be expected to provide direct client care to four to six clients. In a long-term care facility, this same nurse might assume the responsibility of "charge nurse" for an entire unit. (In the charge nurse role, the LPN/LVN would supervise the care, instead of providing the care.)

EVALUATING

Once nursing actions have been carried out, the responsibility of the nurse is to evaluate those actions and determine whether they are moving the client toward identified goals. Data collected from ongoing assessments are compared with expected outcomes and with decisions made about care. In the case mentioned above, the nurse would return to evaluate (and document) how well the medication has worked. If the client says the pain is reduced to 4 and he feels sleepy, the goal has been met. If the client is moaning and still reports pain at 9, the goal has not been met. The LPN/LVN would report this to the team leader or charge nurse. This report could lead to a medical solution (e.g., a change in medication) or to a nursing solution (e.g., increased use of nonpharmacologic methods to help reduce pain).

LPNs and LVNs will work with a variety of care plans and care pathways, depending on the facility. This book illustrates Nursing Process Care Plans in each chapter to provide realistic examples of situations in which LPNs and LVNs must make decisions. Questions following the care plans will help students practice necessary thought processes that will be part of everyday nursing practice. The following is a sample.

NURSING PROCESS CARE PLAN
Caring for a Family That Desires Alternative Therapies

A family brings their 6-week-old son to the pediatrician's office. The child is gaining weight appropriately. He is breastfed and has adequate output. The nurse discusses immunizations with the family. The mother and father express concern about the safety of immunizations. They have done some reading on the Internet that led them to believe that a child could be healthy without immunizations.

There are no other children in the home. The mother reports allergies, and the father smokes regularly in the home.

Assessment
- Believe child could be healthy without immunizations
- Stated resource is the Internet
- Unaware of the need for immunizations, especially in a high-risk environment (family history of allergies and smoking in the home)

Nursing Diagnosis
- Deficient **K**nowledge related to misinterpretation of information

Expected Outcome
- Parents will demonstrate adequate knowledge about immunizations prior to giving informed consent.

Planning and Implementation
- Assess the parent's ability to learn. *If the parents had learning disabilities, it would be important for the nurse to know prior to developing a teaching plan.*
- Clarify the knowledge the parents have about immunizations. *The nurse needs to understand what information should be confirmed and what should be corrected.*
- Collaborate with the RN and the physician prior to developing a teaching plan for these clients. *This situation will be handled best with a team approach.*
- Design an environment conducive to learning to present the teaching plan. *To maximize learning, the family should be comfortable and the area should be free of distractions.*
- Present information about the effects of disease for which immunizations are available. *It is important for the parents to understand the symptoms, treatments, and long-term effects of the diseases.*
- Present information about methods of immunizations and the side effects related to each. Include rates of occurrence. *Clear, concise, accurate information about the immunizations will give the parents an understanding of immunizations.*
- Encourage feedback and document understanding. *The nurse can assess learning better when the parents provide verbal feedback.*
- Provide the parents with printed literature. *This provides a way to reinforce the teaching the nurse has given.*

Evaluation.
Verbal and written information provided to family. Father expressed surprise that items on Internet might not be reliable. Internet address to Centers for Disease Control and Prevention (CDC) site is offered, so parents could pursue reliable sources and statistics. Mother had wondered whether her allergies might affect her child. Both agreed to consider the possibility of immunizing child at the 6-month visit.

Critical Thinking in the Nursing Process

1. Describe the alternative thinking of those who do not want to immunize their children.
2. Review the history of the polio vaccine.
3. How might you show support to a family who chooses not to immunize their child?

Note: Discussion of Critical Thinking questions appears in Appendix I.

Research-Based Nursing Practice

Nurses are educated to ask questions and to observe. Observations that begin to form a pattern are often the basis for nursing research. Research gives direction to nursing practice. When research indicates a need for change in current practice, the prudent nurse alters the way he or she provides care. Over time these changes can have a tremendous impact on the quality of health.

As medical science made dramatic improvements early in the 20th century, researchers began to note differences between care of adults and care of children. For example, as care improved and children survived illnesses that had once been fatal, children spent long periods of time recovering in hospitals. However, they did not thrive in that environment. Research studies determined that children recover faster in their own family homes than in institutional settings. Today, children remain in the hospital until their condition stabilizes and are discharged at any time of the day or night.

Nurses in the hospital environment must be knowledgeable about the physiology of pediatric disorders and about family dynamics. They need to be ready to provide client teaching at every available opportunity and to work with a variety of family dynamics to promote the health of the child and the family. They must be alert to potential complications and alterations in the healing process.

MORTALITY

The health of mothers and infants is of critical importance in assessing the current health status of a population and in predicting the health of the next generation. **Mortality** describes the number of deaths over a given period of time for a given population. For example, infant mortality rate is the number of deaths per 1,000 live births during the first year of life. The disparity in mortality rates among different races, areas of the country, or parts of the world is significant in reflecting the general health of the population. The infant mortality rate of 5.7 for White infants and 13.5 for Black infants, as well as other data about the circumstances of the mother, documents the lower health status of Black families in the United States. This information can be used when seeking funding to provide prenatal care to Black women in poverty-stricken areas or when identifying target groups for prenatal teaching. Infant mortality rates for the United States are illustrated in Table 1-2 ■.

Maternal mortality in the United States has declined from 363.9 in 100,000 live births in 1940 to 8 in 100,000 live births today, according to the Centers for Disease Control. The incidence stands at 7 to 8 deaths per 100,000 live births, a 98% decline from 1940 (Table 1-3 ■). It is estimated that perhaps half these deaths would be preventable with improved prenatal care. Some factors that may interfere with reduction in the maternal death rate are access to and use of health care services, differences in pregnancy-related morbidity, and the content and quality of care.

TABLE 1-2

Infant, Neonatal, and Postneonatal Deaths and Mortality Rates by Origin of Mother: United States, 2004

HISPANIC ORIGIN AND RACE OF MOTHER	LIVE BIRTHS	NUMBER OF DEATHS			MORTALITY RATE PER 1,000 LIVE BIRTHS		
		INFANT	NEONATAL	POSTNEONATAL	INFANT	NEONATAL	POSTNEONATAL
All origins[1]	4,090,007	27,936	18,593	9,343	6.79	4.52	2.27
Total Hispanic	912,331	5,151	3,573	1,579	5.65	3.92	1.73
Non-Hispanic White	2,321,921	13,228	8,797	4,431	5.70	3.79	1.91
Non-Hispanic Black	576,047	7,836	5,335	2,501	13.60	9.26	4.34
Not stated	28,609	448	368	80	N/A	N/A	N/A

N/A: Category not applicable.

[1]Origin of mother not stated included in "All origins" but not distributed among origins.

Notes: Infant deaths are weighted so numbers may not exactly add to totals due to rounding. Neonatal is less than 28 days and postneonatal is 28 days to less than 1 year.

Source: National Vital Statistics Report, Vol. 54, No. 16, May 3, 2006.

TABLE 1-3

Maternal Mortality for Complications of Pregnancy, Childbirth, and the Puerperium, According to Race and Age: United States, Selected Years 1950–1999

RACE, HISPANIC ORIGIN, AND AGE	1950[1]	1960[1]	1970	1980	1990	1995	1996	1997	1998	1999[2]
NUMBER OF DEATHS										
All persons	2,960	1,579	803	334	343	277	294	327	281	391
White	1,873	936	445	193	177	129	159	179	158	214
Black	1,041	624	342	127	153	133	121	125	104	154
American Indian or Alaska Native	N/A	N/A	N/A	3	4	1	6	2	2	5
Asian or Pacific Islander	N/A	N/A	N/A	11	9	14	8	21	17	18
Hispanic[3]	N/A	N/A	N/A	N/A	47	43	39	57	42	67
White, non-Hispanic[3]	N/A	N/A	N/A	N/A	125	84	114	121	116	149
DEATHS PER 100,000 LIVE BIRTHS										
All ages, age adjusted	73.7	32.1	21.5	9.4	7.6	6.3	6.4	7.6	6.1	8.3
All ages, crude	83.3	37.1	21.5	9.2	8.2	7.1	7.6	8.4	7.1	9.9
Under 20 years	70.7	22.7	18.9	7.6	7.5	3.9	N/A*	5.7	N/A*	6.6
20–24 years	47.6	20.7	13.0	5.8	6.1	5.7	5.0	6.6	5.0	6.2
25–29 years	63.5	29.8	17.0	7.7	6.0	6.0	6.6	7.9	6.7	8.2
30–34 years	107.7	50.3	31.6	13.6	9.5	7.3	7.6	8.3	7.5	10.1
35 years and over[4]	222.0	104.3	81.9	36.3	20.7	15.9	19.0	16.1	14.5	23.0

N/A: Data not available.

*Based on fewer than 20 deaths.

[1]Includes deaths of persons who were not residents of the 50 states and the District of Columbia.

[2]Starting with 1999 data, changes have been made in the classification and coding of maternal deaths under ICD-10. The large increase in the number of maternal deaths between 1998 and 1999 is due to changes associated with ICD-10.

[3]Excludes data from states lacking an Hispanic-origin item on their death and birth certificates.

[4]Rates computed by relating deaths of women 35 years and over to live births to women 35–49 years.

Source: National Center for Health Statistics. Health, *United States,* 2002. Hyattsville, MD.

Sudden Infant Death Syndrome

The leading causes of infant mortality are congenital anomalies, sudden infant death syndrome (SIDS), and low birth weight. Research into causes and prevention of these problems affects the nursing care provided to infants, parents, families, and communities. For example, until the mid-1990s, parents were taught to position infants on their abdomens to sleep. It was believed that if an infant vomited during sleep, this position would enable the infant to clear the airway and prevent aspiration. Through research led by the American Academy of Pediatrics, it was determined that infants positioned on their side or back during sleep had fewer incidents of SIDS (American Academy of Pediatrics, 2005). This information has changed not only the nursing

care of infants, but also the teaching that nurses provide to parents (see Chapter 18).

MORBIDITY

Morbidity is the prevalence of a specific disease or disorder in the population at a specific period of time. Data are collected from physician office visits, hospital admissions, and interviews. The data may not reflect the general population, but they do reflect those who are accessing health care in a given area. It is important, therefore, to look at trends rather than one-time numbers.

Childhood morbidity rate varies according to the age of the child. By studying the common causes of childhood illness or injury, plans for prevention can be made. For example, at one time polio was a leading cause of illness, disability, and death. However, through immunization against polio, this illness is being eradicated.

Falls from playground equipment are a leading cause of injury in the preschool child. Knowing this, nurses can focus on parent teaching toward prevention. They can try to influence the design and selection of playground equipment. They can also encourage community leaders to provide safe places for children to play.

The nurse must use every opportunity to improve health care. This is done through teaching clients and families, conducting research to document quality of care (either via formal study or informal data collecting), and assisting in the revision of facility's standards-of-practice policies. The Health Promotion Issue on pages 12 and 13 shows how observations and information gathered during the nursing process can lead to improvements in care of the mother and the child. The issue of circumcisions is presented here as an example of how data can be used to initiate change. Further information about circumcision is presented in Chapter 17 .

Community-Based Nursing Practice

Community-based nursing is a response to the changes in health care. The philosophy of community-based nursing is that care should be provided to individuals, families, and groups wherever they are, including where they live, work, play, pray, or attend school (Zotti, Brown, & Stotts, 1996).

In recent years, there has been a tremendous debate over health care reform. Policy makers have pressed for a cost-effective health care system. This cost consciousness has resulted in decreases in the average length of stay for inpatient care. Along with clients being discharged "sicker," there has been greater emphasis on the impact of lifestyle choices on individual health and illness prevention.

Community-based care is vital to bringing health promotion initiatives to underserved populations. The "Issue and Trends" portion of *Healthy People 2010* indicates that effective community-based programs would have the following characteristics (U.S. Department of Health and Human Services, 2000):

■ Community participation with representation from at least three of the following areas:
  • Government
  • Education
  • Business
  • Faith organizations
  • Health care

  • Media
  • Voluntary organizations
  • Public
■ Community assessment of the community's health problems, resources, perceptions, and priorities for action. (The community decides together what problem areas should be addressed. It is not told what its problems are by an outside agency.)
■ Measurable objectives addressing at least one of the following:
  • Health outcomes
  • Risk factors
  • Public awareness
  • Services and protection
■ Monitoring and evaluation processes to determine whether goals have been reached.
■ Interventions that target several areas for change and that are culturally relevant. Interventions would address the community at several levels:
  • Individual (e.g., racial or ethnic, age, or socioeconomic group)
  • Organizational (e.g., schools, workplaces, faith communities)
  • Environmental (e.g., local policies and regulations)
AND
■ Interventions would include multiple approaches to change:
  • Education
  • Community organization
  • Regulatory and environmental reform

In an effort to implement these guidelines, neighborhood health care clinics have become common. Education programs are being produced to teach children the effect of lifestyle choices on their health. Greater effort is being placed on providing care to those with limited financial resources. These advances have caused a necessary change in the way nursing care is provided.

In response to political debates, the ANA and the National League for Nurses composed *Nursing's Agenda for Health Care Reform* (also known as *Nursing's Agenda*). *Nursing's Agenda* for reform is "to provide primary health care services to households and individuals in convenient, familiar places" (ANA 1991, p. 1). The "convenient, familiar places" are homes, schools, work sites, churches, and neighborhood clinics.

LEVELS OF CARE
Community-based nursing encompasses primary, secondary, and tertiary care.

• **Primary care** includes prevention activities such as immunizations, well-child checkups, routine physical examinations, and use of infant car seats. Its purpose is to maintain health and prevent illness or injury from occurring.

(*Text continues on p. 14.*)

HEALTH PROMOTION ISSUE

MALE CIRCUMCISION WITHOUT ANESTHESIA

The staff in the newborn nursery has become increasingly concerned that their male clients are not given anesthesia during circumcision because they have observed painful reactions to the procedure. Parents are questioning more frequently why their children are not given anything for pain relief. Also, two of the nurses attended a national nursing convention where they learned that providing anesthesia during circumcision is common practice in many hospitals nationwide. At the monthly unit meeting, these nurses address their concerns to the unit manager.

DISCUSSION

The debate lingers: Is there pain associated with newborn circumcision? If so, how can we be sure? Pain can be assessed by looking at the behavioral parameters and physiologic parameters. Several assessment tools have been developed to assist health care practitioners in assessing pain in the newborn. These include the Neonatal

Infant Pain Scale (NIPS); the CRying, Increased vital signs, Expression, and Sleeplessness scale (CRIES); and Pain Assessment In Neonates (PAIN). Each scale measures criteria associated with pain and awards a score indicating pain or lack of pain.

Behavioral parameters associated with pain in the newborn include furrowing of the brow, tightly closed eyes, a quivering chin, a high-pitched cry, increased motor movements, and withdrawal from painful stimulus. Physiologic symptoms indicating pain include tachycardia, tachypnea, hypertension, and sweating of the palms.

Pain Relief Options for Newborns

The American Academy of Pediatrics suggests that health care practitioners provide pain relief in the newborn during circumcision in the form of environmental, nonpharmacologic, or pharmacologic measures.

- Environmental measures would include decreasing the stimuli in the setting where the circumcision is performed. Music, increased room temperature, a soft surface, and dimmed lighting are environmental measures for pain relief.
- Nonpharmacologic measures include nonnutritive sucking on either a pacifier or the breast of the mother who has not begun to lactate. Nonnutritive sucking provides analgesia only during the period of sucking. Nutritive sucking in the form of breastfeeding has also been found to provide pain relief to the newborn. Nutritive sucking or ingestion of sucrose has been found to provide analgesia. Sucrose

can be supplied to the infant via a specially designed pacifier, nasogastric tube, or drops placed directly on the tongue.

- Pharmacologic measures for pain relief in the newborn include administration of acetaminophen preoperatively and postoperatively. Application of eutectic mixture of local anesthetic (EMLA) cream administered 60 minutes before the circumcision will give the newborn up to 3 hours of pain relief. Nerve blocks can also provide the newborn with pain relief during circumcision.

What Is Evidence-Based Practice (EBP)?

EBP can be defined as use of current research to make decisions about client care. If a clinical procedure is not based on research, it is based on a commonly accepted tradition. Health care practitioners have the responsibility of providing the best care possible. This care must be based on scientific data. Evidence-based care provides benefits to the nurse, physicians, client, and administration.

Implementing Research into Practice

These eight steps have been suggested by Gennaro, Hodnett, and Kearney (2001).

1. Review the current literature related to the clinical issue.
2. Resolve to move forward only when you have gathered enough data to provide a rationale for the proposed change in practice.
3. Present your findings creatively. Use graphs, charts, posters, etc.

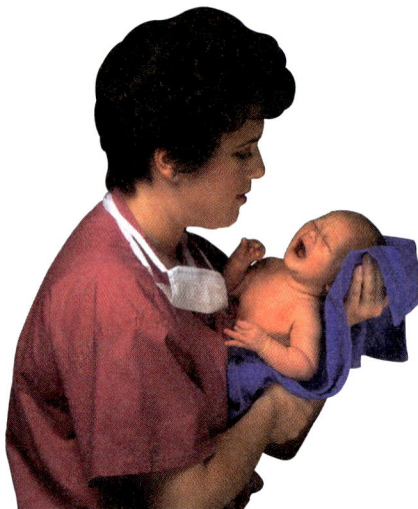

4. Include in your presentation a detailed clinical practice guideline. Develop a timeline for implementation.
5. Present a plan for evaluating client outcomes as they relate to the change in practice. Include how and when data will be reported.
6. Invite to the presentation each practitioner and administrator who might be affected by this change in practice. Discussing the idea with the opposition as well as with supporters is crucial for the plan to succeed.
7. Realize that small measures may need to be implemented prior to a full-blown change in policy.
8. Publish positive client outcomes and successful changes in practice in order to inspire others.

PLANNING AND IMPLEMENTATION

During the unit meeting, the nursing supervisor selected staff members and formed a committee to research the issue of pain relief during circumcision. The committee consisted of the two staff members who had recently attended the convention (one LPN and one RN), one pediatrician, one obstetrician, the nursing supervisor, and a parent who volunteers regularly in the nursery. Following is an outline of the committee's work.

1. They performed a literature search using the databases Cumulative Index to Nursing and Allied Health Literature (CINAHL) and MedLine. Key words used in the search were *pain, analgesia, anesthesia, newborn*, and *circumcision*.
2. Each committee member was responsible for outlining several research articles. Once in summary form, each article was reviewed by each member of the committee.
3. The information was developed into a PowerPoint presentation depicting the risks and benefits of using pain relief for newborn circumcision.
4. The committee also contacted several hospitals who had policies for using analgesia and anesthesia for newborn circumcision. After reviewing these policies, the committee developed a proposed policy for their own institution based on the literature review.
5. The committee also developed a cost analysis and client outcome evaluation method for implementing this change in practice.
6. All nursing staff, pediatricians and family physicians, obstetricians, nursing administration, and hospital administration were invited to hear the presentation of the literature review and proposed policy change.
7. After the presentation, it was decided that nonpharmacologic pain relief methods would be implemented immediately. Pharmacologic pain relief methods would be reviewed carefully by each obstetrician. Obstetricians would meet with the committee in 6 months to discuss which pharmacologic method they would implement.
8. The committee planned to compare CRIES pain assessment scores in three situations:
   a. Prior to implementation of pain relief during circumcision
   b. Following implementation of nonpharmacologic pain relief methods
   c. Following implementation of pharmacologic pain relief methods

They planned to publish the results of this research.

SELF-REFLECTION

Have you ever heard this rationale for a procedure: "Because we've always done it that way"? What procedures or nursing interventions do you perform routinely without considering whether there is adequate research to support it? Could client safety be compromised because of your belief? Develop an action plan to review the literature as it related to this procedure. Develop a plan, if necessary, for changing your unit's policy and procedure for this procedure.

SUGGESTED RESOURCES

Brady-Fryer, B., Wiebe, N., & Landeer, J. (2004). Pain relief for neonatal circumcision. *The Cochrane Library*, 4.

Clifford, P.A., String, M., Christensen, H., & Mountain, D. (2004). Pain assessment and intervention for term newborns. *Journal of Midwifery and Women's Health, 49*(6), 514–519.

Gennaro, S., Hodnett, E., & Kearney, M. (2001). Making evidence-based practice a reality in your institutions: Evaluating the evidence and using the evidence to change clinical practice. *The American Journal of Maternal/Child Nursing, 26*(5), 236–250.

Henry, P.R., Haubold, K., & Dobrzykowski, T. (2004). Pain in the healthy full-term neonate: Efficacy and safety of interventions. *Newborn Infant Nursing Review, 4*(2), 126–130.

Razums, I., Dalton, M., & Wilson, D. (2004). Practice applications of research. Pain management for newborn circumcision. *Pediatric Nursing, 30*(5), 414–417.

- **Secondary care** refers to relatively serious or complicated care. Historically, this care was provided in acute-care hospitals, but with new techniques and procedures, much of this has been moved to community settings, including outpatient centers and home care. The purpose of secondary care is to help the client return to health after an acute disorder or disease. An example of this level of care would be care of a client after an appendectomy.

- **Tertiary care** is the management of chronic, terminal, complicated, long-term health care problems such as osteoporosis or chronic obstructive pulmonary diseases (COPD). This level of care is frequently delivered in hospitals and community settings, including rehabilitation centers and home care. Its purpose is to help the client return to or maintain the highest possible level of functioning and to adapt as necessary to the changes the condition requires.

CULTURALLY PROFICIENT CARE

For more than three decades, nurses have placed increased emphasis on understanding and responding to unique aspects of diverse groups of clients. At first, ethnicity was equated with culture and was identified on admission paperwork. Slowly, the term *culture awareness* was used to describe knowledge of the similarities and differences among cultures. Unfortunately, many nurses focused on clients' differences instead of their similarities. The quality of nursing care did not change.

Since the 1990s, the nursing profession has been talking about **cultural competence,** or a set of skills, knowledge, and attitudes that include:

- Awareness and acceptance of differences.
- Awareness of one's own cultural values.
- Understanding of the dynamics of difference.
- Development of cultural knowledge.
- Ability to adapt practice skills to fit the cultural context of the client or patient.

When these components become second nature to the nurse, **cultural proficiency** has been obtained (Ramont, Niedringhaus, & Towle, 2006).

The United States as a nation is becoming more supportive of its variety of cultures. Colleges and universities are requiring that educational programs provide courses addressing cultural differences. Health care institutions are adapting to provide a better environment for people from many different backgrounds. Being bilingual or multilingual is becoming a requirement for employment in some areas. Box 1-1 ■ illustrates some ways that health care institutions are working to provide culturally proficient care. Each chapter of this text contains further information about culture and culturally proficient nursing care.

BOX 1-1	CULTURAL PULSE POINTS

Ways Institutions Can Respond to Cultural Diversity

- Hiring interpreters when there is a sizable non-English-speaking population in an area
- Posting "Se habla español" signs at hospitals and clinics where Spanish is spoken
- Providing teaching materials that are visual, not just written
- Offering options on hospital menus for special diets (kosher, vegetarian, etc.)
- Opening neighborhood clinics that cater directly to non-English-speaking populations
- Purchasing toys for children's hospitals that reflect a variety of racial and ethnic backgrounds

Roles of the LPN/LVN in Community Care

COLLABORATING WITH THE INTERDISCIPLINARY TEAM

For families to receive quality health care, nurses cannot practice in isolation. As health care moves from the acute-care setting into community locations, the members of the health care team must have a better understanding of how each role affects the quality of care provided. It is essential for members of the health care team, in partnership with the family, to collaborate and be in consultation with one another (Figure 1-3 ■). The health care team consists of physicians, social workers, psychologists, respiratory care professionals, physical therapy professionals, dietitians, and pharmacists, as well as nurses with a variety of educational backgrounds. Auxiliary workers, unlicensed assistive personnel, and family members may be trained to perform selected tasks. As a result, nurses

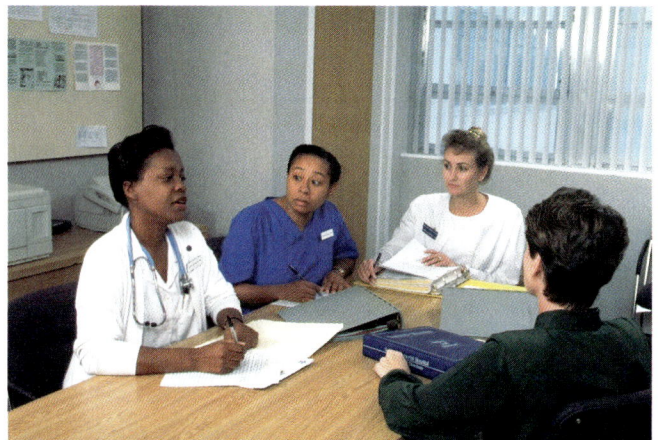

Figure 1-3. ■ Interdisciplinary team with LPN/LVN. (Pearson Education/PH College.)

collaborate with a wide variety of individuals in delivering professional care.

To provide nursing care outside the acute-care setting, nurses used to need a bachelor's degree. Today, though, LPNs and LVNs have many opportunities in community-based nursing practice. With the move to community-based nursing practice, nursing roles are being redefined. The role of the LPN/LVN is no exception. Because the scope of practice for the LPN/LVN is more varied from state to state than that of the RN, the role of this nurse in community-based nursing practice is varied as well. Collaborative efforts with other health team workers are always based on the state's nurse practice acts, facility policy, and individual LPN/LVN capabilities.

PARTICIPATING IN THE NURSING PROCESS

In an acute-care setting, the LPN/LVN assists the RN and physician to provide direct client care. In most cases, this involves assisting in all aspects of the nursing process.

In community-based nursing practice, the LPN/LVN performs the same functions as in the acute-care facility. In this case, though, the client and the client's family are the recipients of care. The LPN/LVN is responsible for keeping the RN informed of changes in the client or the family.

Communication and collaboration with other nurses and health care team members might be by telephone or electronic device instead of face to face. For example, an LPN/LVN might be providing care to a new mother in the home. The nurse may notice that a surgical incision site has become red and inflamed and is draining purulent fluid, and that the mother's temperature is elevated. The LPN/LVN would instruct the mother and possibly other family members in the care of the wound and in the disposal of contaminated dressings. The LPN/LVN would then contact the nursing supervisor and provide input to revise the plan of care to include more frequent nursing assessments and dressing changes. The physician would be notified and appropriate medications obtained. The pharmacist might provide instructions about medication use and side effects.

PROBLEM SOLVING

Problem solving is a complex process that is at the heart of nursing. The LPN/LVN must collect data, evaluate the importance of the information to the safety of the client, and take appropriate action. The nurse uses a variety of cognitive skills in the problem-solving process. The nurse must be able to collect data, think rapidly, and make timely decisions. To do this, the nurse uses inductive and deductive reasoning, critical thinking, and decision-making skills. The problem-solving process including critical thinking and decision making is discussed in Chapter 2 .

PRIORITIZING AND IMPLEMENTING CARE

Prioritizing care is something the LPN/LVN must do constantly. The most critical aspects of care must be initiated first. They include the ABCs of nursing (ensuring that the client has an open Airway, is Breathing, and has adequate Circulation). The next priority is to make the client safe and comfortable.

Nurses follow the established priorities in care plans. However, a change in the client's condition may cause the nurse to shift priorities suddenly in response. For example, the LPN/LVN assigned to care for a first-day postoperative client may be planning to bathe the client and then get her out of bed. While bathing the legs, the nurse notices a large, hard, red area behind the knee. The client states that the area hurts. The nurse does not get the client out of bed because determining the cause of the hard, red area has a higher priority at that moment in time. If the cause is a blood clot, moving the client could cause the clot to move, resulting in life-threatening complications.

The LPN/LVN also establishes priorities when planning and implementing care for several clients at a time. The nurse must make priority decisions about each individual client and then about care of all the clients. For example, the nurse must decide which client to assess first, which one to bathe first, and so on. Although each situation is different, Table 1-4 ■ identifies general guidelines that can help with priority setting.

DELEGATING

In today's health care environment, nurses have an increased responsibility to provide care to the individual client, to support the family, to develop health promotion activities, and to work to improve the health of entire communities. As a result, there is an increasing use of unlicensed assistive personnel (UAP) in direct client care activities. To maintain quality care, it is critical for the nurse to understand **delegation** (transferring to a competent individual the authority or right to perform selected nursing tasks in a selected situation). The nurse retains the accountability for the delegation. Delegation is discussed in more detail in Chapter 2 .

HEALTH PROMOTION TEACHING

A major role of LPNs and LVNs is client teaching. The U.S. Department of Health and Human Services (1991) developed a systematic approach to health with its set of goals called *Healthy People 2000*. In this publication, goals and objectives were identified to assist individuals, communities, and the nation to move toward improved health. Its update, *Healthy People 2010* (U.S. Department of Health and Human Services, 2000), continues the effort to educate the public about ways they can positively affect their own health.

TABLE 1-4

Priority-Setting Guidelines

PRIORITY ACTIVITY	RATIONALE
1. Check sickest client or the one at most risk first. Assess ABC (airway/breathing/circulation), pain/safety. Check operation of all equipment.	The condition of this client may change rapidly, and he or she may not be able to call for help.
2. Check remainder of assigned clients in order of highest risk.	Ensures all clients are safe.
3. Return to complete assessments on each client.	Detailed assessments are needed to determine client problems and condition.
4. Update a written time line identifying what each client needs and at what time.	A written time line will provide a visual view of what will need to be completed at each time. The nurse can then decide what has priority at that time.
5. Administer medications within 30 minutes of scheduled time.	Medication administration is a high priority.
6. Review lab values and diagnostic study results as available.	Lab values/diagnostic study results may need to be called to the doctor. Some values may affect the administration of medication.
7. Provide all treatments, assessments, and basic care as ordered/scheduled.	Treatments generally have a higher priority than bathing, but the nurse may be able to do several things at one time.

More and more people are recognizing the benefits of staying healthy. Health promotion activities emphasize nutrition, exercise, and stress reduction. Nurses often provide information about complementary or alternative therapies that can support a client's efforts to achieve or maintain health. Box 1-2 ■ lists some complementary

BOX 1-2   COMPLEMENTARY THERAPIES

Selected Complementary and Alternative Therapies

- **Homeopathy**   A healing system that uses a small amount of a substance to produce the same symptom as the disorder. It stimulates the body's system to increase its immune response.
- **Naturopathy**   Natural medicines are used in the prevention and treatment of a disease. Naturopathy often employs a variety of approaches to solve a problem (e.g., changes in diet, increased ingestion of some vitamins, changes in activity).
- **Traditional Chinese Medicine**   Trigger points in acupressure and acupuncture, and breathing movements in T'ai chi or Qi Gong, are used to achieve a balance of energy and promote well-being and harmony throughout the body.
- **Reiki (ray-key)**   Japanese energy healing employs a light laying on of hands from head to throat, heart, abdomen, knees, and feet. It is often used with people who have cancer or chronic health problems.
- **Mind-based Therapies**   Guided imagery, hypnosis, visualization, biofeedback, music therapy, meditation, prayer, and chanting all help in the reduction of stress and can be helpful in the relief of chronic pain and some addictions. These therapies can also be combined with exercise forms of therapies such as yoga that use meditation, exercise, and diaphragmatic breathing to induce a relaxation response.

- **Massage Therapy and Therapeutic Touch**   Touch in the form of massage and reflexology is used to relax muscles, improve blood flow, and stimulate the immune system.
- **Chiropractic**   Manipulation to correct misalignment of the vertebrae can reduce the stress of pregnancy on the lower back. Client should be cautioned to use a fully qualified chiropractor.
- **Hydrotherapy**   Relaxation is achieved through the use of water. It is often used during labor and delivery in the form of a relaxing shower or to deliver the baby underwater. Cold compresses, hot compresses, and sweat baths are also types of hydrotherapy.
- **Herbal Therapies**   Plants have been used for medicinal purposes for thousands of years. Herbal therapies are often used to treat specific symptoms, such as to reduce menopausal symptoms. *Note:* A pregnant client should be aware that certain herbs can cause a miscarriage or have other toxic effects. (See Box 10-2 🔗.)
- **Aromatherapy**   Aromatherapy uses scented oils for relaxation and a psychological response. It is believed that different aromas can influence heart rate and blood pressure. The oils can also be used on the skin during massage therapy. *Note:* Because of little or no regulation of essential oils, pregnant women should be advised not to use them during pregnancy.

therapies that are commonly seen today. Related topics (such as immunizations, infection control, and identifying risk factors) are directed toward illness prevention. Nurses are instrumental in health promotion and illness prevention by providing health teaching to individuals and groups. Teaching is an important role of the LPN/LVN. Health promotion activities are presented throughout the text.

Employment Opportunities for LPNs/LVNs in Community-Based Nursing

Because of the acute nature of labor and birth and the potential complexity of care during labor, employment opportunities for the LPN/LVN tend to be limited more to postpartum and well-infant care. Employment opportunities for the LPN/LVN have increased as more neighborhood clinics have opened. In some states, employment opportunities are also increasing in immunization clinics, home health, and school nursing. Because LPNs/LVNs are unable to practice in an independent role in maternity care, the employing agency should have clear policies identifying the RN or doctor who is responsible for directing and reviewing their work.

Note: The reference and resource listings for this and all chapters are compiled at the back of the book.

Chapter Review

KEY TERMS by Topic

Use the audio glossary feature of either the CD-ROM or the Companion Website to hear the correct pronunciation of the following key terms.

Introduction
maternal-newborn nursing

History of Maternity Nursing
patients, consumers, clients

Developments in Nursing
objective data, subjective data, holistic

Nursing Process in Maternal-Newborn Nursing
nursing diagnoses, outcome, interventions, care plan, medical diagnoses

Research-Based Nursing Practice
mortality, morbidity

Community-Based Nursing Practice
community-based nursing, primary care, secondary care, tertiary care, cultural competence, cultural proficiency

Roles of the LPN/LVN in Community Care
delegation

KEY Points

- Nursing care of mothers and newborns is evolving to include the entire family.
- The nursing process guides the care planning process.
- Community-based nursing practice is the provision of nursing care wherever the client lives, works, plays, or prays.
- Nursing includes health promotion and illness prevention activities as well as assistance in the medical management of illness.
- The terms *client*, *patient*, and *consumer* all refer to the recipient of health care services. The term *client* indicates the person is actively involved in health care decisions.
- Being able to set priorities is essential in providing safe care.
- The state nurse practice act governs nursing practice. Facility policy regulates nursing practice within the specific clinical setting.

FOR FURTHER Study

See Chapter 2 for an in-depth discussion of critical thinking and delegation processes.

Further information about circumcision is presented in Chapter 17.

See Chapter 18 for discussion of SIDS.

EXPLORE MediaLink

Additional interactive resources for this chapter can be found on the Companion Website at www.prenhall.com/towle. Click on Chapter 1 and "Begin" to select the activities for this chapter.

For chapter-related NCLEX®-style questions and an audio glossary, access the accompanying CD-ROM in this book.

1 The nurse understands that primary nursing care is best identified as:
  1. providing nutritional counseling to a pregnant woman who is at risk for gestational diabetes.
  2. administering magnesium sulfate for treatment of preterm labor.
  3. assisting a woman with diabetes to adapt her medication now that she is pregnant.
  4. teaching the parents of a child with jaundice how to use a BiliBlanket.

2 The nurse understands that tertiary nursing care is best identified as:
  1. obtaining a sterile urinary specimen for the purpose of determining the effectiveness of antibiotic therapy.
  2. immunizing a 3-year-old child for influenza.
  3. monitoring hematocrit each trimester during pregnancy.
  4. administering tracheostomy care to a 4-year-old with a permanent tracheostomy.

3 The LPN/LVN has many roles in the acute-care setting. Choose all of the following that apply to these roles.
  1. administering PO medications
  2. supervising unlicensed assistive personnel
  3. collecting data
  4. monitoring lab values
  5. developing a nursing diagnosis based on assessment data

4 Four women are sharing thoughts on childbirth. Which of the following statements by one of the women is reflective of someone from the 1920s?
  1. "Two days after I gave birth I went home to care for my family."
  2. "The birthing suite allowed me to give birth and recover in the same room."
  3. "I want to continue my career before I have my first child."
  4. "I don't remember too much after they gave me scopolamine."

5 Which of the following comments by an LPN/LVN demonstrates that people under the care of an LPN/LVN are viewed as active participants in their own care?
  1. "My patient in room 212 would like something for pain."
  2. "My client would like to speak with the doctor now."
  3. "Don't worry, the doctor will be able to make decisions for you."
  4. "I will help the person in the next room feed her baby."

6 The nurse is concerned about a particular health issue for a client and has been given approval to research the issue to document if a change in practice is necessary. List the following steps for implementing research into practice in the correct order.

  1. Develop a plan to evaluate client outcomes.
  2. Create a presentation presenting the risks and benefits to support a change in practice.
  3. Document approved changes to the clinical guidelines.
  4. Invite practitioners and administrators to discuss the proposed new practice guidelines.
  5. Review current literature.
  6. Publish positive client outcomes relating to the new clinical practice guidelines.
  7. Develop clinical practice guidelines and a time frame for possible implementation.
  8. Gather data that provides rationales for a proposed change in practice.

7 The nurse has requested the LPN/LVN to assist her during a home visit. Which of the following agencies should the LPN/LVN refer to before collaborating with the nurse during a home visit?
  1. Individual state's nurse practice act
  2. Association of Women's Health, Obstetric and Neonatal Nurses
  3. Nurse's Association of the American College of Obstetricians and Gynecologists
  4. American Nurses Association

8 The LPN/LVN has been assigned to care for the following clients. Based on the morning report, which client should the LPN/LVN assess first?
  1. a 1-hour old newborn with acrocyanosis
  2. a 24-hour postpartum client needing assistance with newborn care
  3. a post C-section client complaining of pain and tenderness behind her knee when walking
  4. a 12-hour postpartum client complaining of sore nipples

9 During a home visit with a breastfeeding mother, the LPN/LVN assesses swelling and erythema in the right outer quadrant of the breast. Which of the following health care team members should the LPN/LVN contact first?
  1. unlicensed assistive personnel
  2. nursing supervisor
  3. breastfeeding mother's significant other
  4. pediatrician

10 Which of the following tasks reflects the LPN/LVN role for maternal-newborn nursing care?
  1. establishes a nursing diagnosis for a client recovering from a C-section
  2. independently plans care for clients in the home setting
  3. teaches the client how to bathe a newborn
  4. prescribes an antibiotic for a client with bladder infection

Answers for NCLEX-PN® Review and Critical Thinking questions appear in Appendix I.

Chapter 2

Critical Thinking in Maternal-Newborn Nursing

LEARNING Outcomes

After completing this chapter, you will be able to:

1. Define key terms.
2. Discuss the critical thinking process and standards that define it.
3. Identify the elements of thought.
4. Discuss the intellectual traits that result from critical thinking.
5. Describe decision making and prioritizing as they relate to nursing scope of practice.
6. Describe the delegation process related to nursing scope of practice.

MEDLINE database, the two most common databases of medical, nursing, and allied health literature. Some health care facilities do not allow access to the Internet in the workplace for fear the technology will be misused. Hospital libraries, if they exist, usually have limited hours and may not be readily available to the nursing staff.

Once professional literature is obtained, nurses may not be prepared to evaluate the validity of the content. More nurses are familiar with the Internet and the World Wide Web as sources of information than the CINAHL and MEDLINE search engines. One problem with Internet searches is the uncertain reliability of the information received.

PLANNING AND IMPLEMENTATION

Nurses must make time in their busy schedules to read professional literature to remain up-to-date. Ideally, time and resources will be available in the workplace. If that is not the case, the nurse

must read during his or her personal time. Performing literature searches using educational technology is an essential skill the nurse must acquire. Colleges and universities, technology assistants, and other resources are available to teach the nurse these skills.

The nurse uses critical thinking skills to read critically. At times, professional journal articles need to be read several times to ensure complete understanding. The first reading is used just to rephrase the author's words into your words. Writing down this paraphrasing helps in capturing the text's essential meaning. If the paraphrasing lacks clarity, depth, breadth, logic, and fairness, the article should be read again. The nurse should be able to identify the question or problem being addressed, understand the assumptions and the implications being made, and describe the concepts (ideas) and conclusions.

After the nurse has reviewed the literature, further data may need to be collected in the form of research. (This was true in the research case presented in Chapter 1 of

this text.) Once data are collected, they should be shared with other nurses through professional journal articles. The nurse uses best-practice evidence when writing the client's care plan, providing direct client care, supervising unlicensed personnel, and collaborating with other nurses in revising facility policy.

The LPN/LVN must critically read evidence-based practice to learn and remain up-to-date with research findings. As the LPN/LVN identifies best-practice evidence that contraindicates the care provided in his or her facility, the nurse should share the research with the supervising RN and with other nurses.

SELF-REFLECTION

When reading a journal article, do you accept the concepts at face value, or do you try to apply concepts of critical thinking to better understand the issue? What can you do to get a deeper understanding from your reading? How can you apply critical thinking concepts to other aspects of your life?

SUGGESTED RESOURCES

Estabrooks, C. (1998). Will evidence-based nursing practice make practice perfect? *Canadian Journal of Nursing Research, 30*(1), 15–36.

Spratley, E., Johnson, A., Sochalski, J., Fritz, M., & Spenser, W. (2001). *The registered nurse population March 2000: Findings from the National Sample*

Survey of Registered Nurses. Rockville, MD: U.S. Department of Health and Human Services.

Pravikoff, D., Ranner, A., & Pierce, S. (2005). Readiness of U.S. nurses for evidence-based practice. *American Journal of Nursing, 105*(9), 40–51.

reasoning is the process of making specific statements from a generalized concept. For example, the nurse reads in the chart that this same client has been vomiting much of her food and liquid for 2 weeks. The nurse knows that vomiting can cause dehydration. From this generalized information, the nurse can deduce that the client's mucous membranes will be dry, the urinary output will be low, and the urine will be dark amber. The nurse will expect these findings in the client. The use of evidence-based thinking and research to improve nursing practice is illustrated further in the Health Promotion Issue that starts on page 22.

The nurse must look at the information and determine the **significance** (importance) to the client's health at this point in time. By asking, "Is this the most important problem to consider?" the nurse sets priorities in providing care. In the case previously mentioned, dehydration is very significant because it will affect the health of both mother and fetus.

Elements of Thought

To do critical thinking, it helps to identify the different elements of thought (Box 2-2 ■). All critical thinking has a **purpose** (an end, aim, or result), which should be stated

---

BOX 2-2

Elements of Thought

Our thoughts include all of the following components:

- Purpose of our thinking
- Question at issue
- Available information
- Point of view
- Interpretation and inference
- Concepts
- Assumptions
- Implications and consequences

Source: Paul, R., & Elder, L. (2006). *The miniature guide to critical thinking concepts & tools.* Dillon Beach, CA: Foundation for Critical Thinking.

---

clearly and specifically. In nursing, each step of the nursing process contains at least one purpose. For example, the purpose of assessment is to collect and analyze data to determine the client's health status. The nurse must determine the accuracy and precision of the data, and then determine its relevance to the client's condition.

All critical thinking is an attempt to figure out something or settle some problem or question. The problem should be stated clearly and precisely. In many instances in nursing, the problem may be the client's presenting health issue. The problem may be broken down into several underlying subproblems. For example, when a client is short of breath, has an increased respiratory rate, has wheezy lung sounds, and has a nonproductive cough, the nurse would determine that the client has an alteration in respiratory function (the problem). However, underlying problems are bronchial constriction (which causes the wheezing) and inability to clear the airway (which results in nonproductive cough). The nurse states the problem in terms of nursing diagnoses (in this case, "Ineffective Breathing Pattern" and "Ineffective Airway Clearance" [NANDA, 2008]).

The critical thinker bases decisions on accurate, complete, and relevant **information** (knowledge gained through research or observation). The nurse would ask, "What information am I using to reach this conclusion?" "What more information do I need?" and "What experience do I have that supports my conclusion?" At times, it is important for the critical thinker to consider different **points of view** (perspectives). By asking, "Is there another point of view I should consider?" the critical thinker maintains an open mind to other alternatives or actions.

Before taking action, the critical thinker would explore **interpretations** (ways of clarifying the meaning), **inferences** (deductions), and **assumptions** (ideas taken for granted). The

results would be used to reach informed **conclusions** (decisions based on prior thought). By asking questions such as, "Is there another way to interpret this information?" "What am I taking for granted?" and "Are these inferences consistent with the data?" the nurse can reach accurate conclusions.

The critical thinker uses **concepts** (theories, laws, and principles) from many disciplines to further understand the problem and address possible solutions. For example, the nurse uses gas laws identified by the chemist to understand the transport of oxygen from room air to the blood. Principles of microbiology are used in infection control practices. The nurse applies education theory when providing infant care instruction to new mothers.

The critical thinker explores the **implications** (consequences) of actions or decisions. By asking, "If someone accepted my position, what would be the implications?" or "What would be the consequences of this action?" the critical thinker develops sound judgment.

These elements of thought are an important part of the nursing process, because the nurse must reach accurate conclusions about the client's health problem, about which interventions to try first, and about the effectiveness of treatments. Learning to apply these elements of thought and standards of critical thinking to the care of clients takes practice. The nursing student may be asked to demonstrate critical thinking through written care plans, examinations, and clinical performance. Each chapter of this book will provide the student with exercises to improve critical thinking skills applicable to the mother and newborn infant.

Critical Thinking Care Maps

This text provides an interactive tool for practicing critical thinking. At the end of each chapter of this book, critical thinking exercises are presented in the form of a Critical Thinking Care Map. The care map presents a clinical situation related to the content of the chapter. It identifies the NCLEX-PN® focus area related to the case study to help the student think in terms of the categories needed for licensure. An **NCLEX-PN® Focus Area** is 1 of 11 areas of client needs around which the NCLEX-PN® test is constructed. The care map then identifies one appropriate NANDA nursing diagnosis for the client. A list of data is shown. Some of it is relevant to the identified nursing diagnosis. Some of it is not. The student selects and organizes the relevant information under the subjective and objective data headings. Irrelevant data are omitted.

The student then decides if any of the information needs to be reported. Are any ranges outside of normal? Is there an acceptable explanation for the data outside the normal range? For example, if a client is receiving an IV infusion to correct hypercalcemia, it would not be necessary to report the calcium imbalance unless the condition was not improving with therapy, or unless it appeared that the client's calcium level was decreasing.

The student needs to decide who should get the report. For example, the nurse might report to the team leader or charge nurse if a postsurgical client complains that pain medications are not effective. However, if a client complains of pain 4 days after cesarean section, and the client also has bright red bleeding from the wound site, the nurse would immediately inform the surgeon of the possibility of a *wound dehiscence* (separation of the wound.)

The next step in the care map is for the student to select relevant interventions. Again, the student would select *only* those interventions that relate to the nursing diagnosis identified for this exercise. Other interventions, even though they might be suitable for the client, would not be chosen from the list provided.

Finally, the student practices documenting pertinent information. The date, the time, the pertinent data, the intervention performed, the results of the nursing actions, and the nurse's signature are all essential elements of narrative notes in the client chart. Sample documentations for the Critical Thinking Care Maps and the answers to the questions posed in the exercise are provided in Appendix I. A sample Critical Thinking Care Map is provided on page 26.

Essential Intellectual Traits or Values

As with any skill, critical thinking develops with practice. However, critical thinking is especially valuable because it can improve virtually every area of one's life. As one thinks about thinking and gains strength in these skills, it is helpful to keep in mind what the *best* critical thinking would be. These standards of excellence in critical thinking (also called essential intellectual traits for critical thinking) are provided, with examples, in Box 2-3 ■. **Intellectual humility** is having a consciousness that one's knowledge base, prejudices, biases, and point of view have limitations. It implies the lack of boastfulness, arrogance, and conceit. **Intellectual courage** is facing and fairly addressing ideas, beliefs, or viewpoints that might, on a superficial level, seem absurd or false, or toward which we might have negative emotions. Through intellectual courage, we may come to have a deeper understanding of others, their ideas or beliefs, and the environment in which they live. **Intellectual empathy** is

---

BOX 2-3	

Essential Intellectual Traits

When critical thinking is occurring, certain positive intellectual traits surface. (The sentences next to each intellectual trait provide a way of rephrasing the traits in everyday terms.)

Intellectual humility—I know that I do not know everything.

Intellectual courage—I dare to consider other points of view.

Intellectual empathy—I try to learn about and understand others.

Intellectual autonomy—I can think something even if people do not agree with me.

Intellectual integrity—I hold myself to the same standard as I hold others.

Intellectual perseverance—I will continue to think until I understand.

Fair-mindedness—I treat all viewpoints equally before deciding.

Confidence in reason—I trust the solution that results from logical thinking.

---

imagining oneself in the place of others in order to better understand them. It requires consciously ignoring one's own perceptions, long-standing ideas, or beliefs. At times, we need to remember occasions when we were wrong despite strong feelings that we were right and understand that this might be the present case. **Intellectual autonomy** is having a rational control over one's ideas and beliefs. The critical thinker learns to think for himself or herself, to question when it is rational to question, and to conform when it is rational to conform. **Intellectual integrity** is being true and consistent with intellectual standards, holding oneself to the same standards of proof as one holds those with opposing views, and honestly admitting when one is inconsistent in one's thoughts and actions. **Intellectual perseverance** is persistence in the attempt to understand. It is having the consciousness to use intellectual insights, principles, and truths, when distractions, obstacles, and confusion over unsettled questions lead to frustrations over an extended period of time. **Fair-mindedness** is consciously treating all points of view equally, without reference to one's own points of view. By applying the intellectual standards to the elements of thought, over time one develops **confidence in reason** (trust in the outcome of logical thought). By encouraging people to think for themselves, to draw reasonable conclusions, and to persuade each other with reason, the interests of humankind will best be served (Paul & Elder, 2006).

This line provides an appropriate nursing diagnosis.

This line provides the appropriate NCLEX-PN® focus area.

This information is provided to give you basic information about the client.

Critical Thinking Care Map

Caring for a Client with Pregnancy-Induced Hypertension
NCLEX-PN® Focus Area: Physiologic Integrity

Case Study: Sophia Williams, a 20-year-old black woman, is 8 months pregnant with her first child. She comes to the clinic complaining of blurred vision, severe headache, and swelling in her hands and feet. Her blood pressure is 162/98. She has gained 3 pounds in the last 2 weeks and has 2 + protein in her urine.

Nursing Diagnosis: Ineffective Tissue/Organ Perfusion related to hypertension

COLLECT DATA

Subjective _____   Objective _____

Would you report this? Yes/No
If yes, to: _____

Nursing Care
_____

How would you document this? _____

Compare your documentation to the sample provided in Appendix I.

Data Collected
(use only those that apply)

- Unemployed
- Unmarried
- Lives alone
- Family not supportive
- VS:T 98.8, P 92, R 24, BP 162/98
- 3-pound weight gain
- 2 + protein in urine
- Diet 2,500 calorie, low sodium prescribed at first prenatal visit
- Client states, "I eat a lot of potato chips and olives."
- Prenatal vitamins daily
- Blurred vision
- Headache
- Swelling

Nursing Interventions
(use only those that apply; list in priority order)

- Teach client to do nonstressful exercise such as walking.
- Discuss treatment options.
- Teach relaxation techniques used in labor.
- Discuss with client reasons for not following diet.
- Recognize racial/ethnic influence on hypertension.
- Teach client to have frequent rest periods lying on side.
- Determine client's previous knowledge related to diagnosis.
- Teach use and side effects of any new medications.

Carefully consider the data. What statements and data collected would support this nursing diagnosis? What data are subjective, and what data are objective? What data are not relevant?

Subjective data: Severe headache, blurred vision, "I eat a lot of potato chips and olives."

Objective data: VS:T 98.8, P 92, R 24, BP 162/98; 3-pound weight gain; 2+ protein in urine; swelling; 2,500-calorie, low-sodium diet prescribed at first prenatal visit

Irrelevant data: Unemployed, unmarried, lives alone, family not supportive

Think about the data you have collected. Are any of the data abnormal? Would they indicate pathology that could have a negative impact on the client's health? Would it be important to report this information? If so, to what person? **Yes, report headache, blurred vision, edema, proteinuria, and blood pressure reading to physician.**

This question allows you to practice your documentation. It is not necessary to document all the data or interventions for this exercise. For example, the assessment documentation might be:

(date, time) Client seen in clinic with c/o severe headache, blurred vision, and swelling in hands and feet. States, "I have been eating a lot of potato chips and olives." BP 162/98. 2 + protein in urine. Weight up 2 lb since last visit. M. Fowler, LPN

Consider the client's deficient knowledge about the medical condition and its consequences. Make a decision about which interventions are relevant and which are not. Place relevant interventions in priority order.

Relevant interventions: Recognize racial/ethnic influence on hypertension. Determine client's previous knowledge related to diagnosis. Discuss with client reasons for not following diet. Teach client to do nonstressful exercise such as walking. Teach client to have frequent rest periods lying on side. Teach use and side effects of any new medications.

Irrelevant interventions: Discuss treatment options. Teach relaxation techniques used in labor.

DECISION MAKING AND DELEGATION

Decision Making

LPNs/LVNs are faced with daily decisions about performing specific acts. Sometimes they will be asked to perform acts or tasks outside of the usual routine, and they need to decide whether or not to perform them. New graduates or inexperienced nurses who are learning the routine might find decision making challenging. LPNs/LVNs working in community agencies may face more decisions than nurses working in a structured environment, such as an acute or long-term care agency. In all cases, however, the nurse will be held to the standards of reasonable and prudent care.

LPNs/LVNs have guidelines to follow when making decisions about performance of specific acts. Box 2-4 ■ provides these guidelines. By specifically identifying the act and collecting data through client assessment, the nurse has a clear picture of what needs to be done. Once the nurse understands the act and the client's condition, a series of questions should be answered.

1. Is the act expressly permitted or prohibited by the nurse practice act, Board of Nursing rules, or Board of Nursing position statements? The registered nurse and LPN/LVN need to be familiar with the state nurse practice act and the Board of Nursing rules and regulations. Copies of these documents can be obtained by contacting the state board of nursing or, in most states, by accessing its Internet website. If the act is prohibited by law, the LPN/LVN must inform a nursing supervisor or physician.

2. Is the act expressly permitted or prohibited by agency policy? A review of the agency policy book reveals whether the act is sanctioned by the agency. Agency policy can be more restrictive than the Board of Nursing rule, but it cannot be more lenient. If the nurse performs an act against agency policy and the client outcome is not positive, the nurse might not be supported by the agency.

3. Once it is determined that the act may be performed per the above standards, the nurse needs to examine her or his own competence to perform the act. Is the act something that was taught in the nursing education program, and does he or she possess current clinical skills? Even if the act was taught in the basic nursing education program, if the nurse has not performed the act for a long time, it may not be wise to proceed unassisted or unsupervised. It is expected that even an experienced nurse would need assistance when confronted with an unfamiliar act.

As advances are made in health care, new techniques will be found and new equipment will be produced. Before performing a new procedure the nurse should ask, "Is the act consistent with positive and conclusive data in nursing literature and supported by research? Have I been trained in performing this procedure, and if so is documentation of that training on file?" Most agencies provide in-service programs where new equipment and techniques are demonstrated and supervised practice is offered. Documentation of completion of these programs becomes part of the continuing education file.

When these questions are answered, the correct decision about performing the act will become clear (Figure 2-1 ■).

Delegation

The shift to community-based nursing has resulted in increased responsibility for nurses to provide care to the individual client, support the family, develop health promotion activities, and work to improve the health of entire communities. Consequently, there has been an increase in the use of unlicensed assistive personnel in direct client care activities. To maintain quality care, it is critical the nurse understands the delegation process. **Delegation** is transferring to a competent individual the authority or right to perform selected nursing tasks in selected situations. To help the nurse make wise decisions regarding delegating tasks, the National Council of State Boards of Nursing published a list of premises or explanatory statements. These premises are listed in Box 2-5 ■.

BOX 2-4

Decision-Making Guidelines

- What specifically is the act that needs to be performed?
- Is the act expressly permitted or prohibited by the state nurse practice act, Board of Nursing rules, or Board of Nursing position statements?
- Is the act expressly permitted or prohibited by agency policy?
- Is the act something that was taught in your basic nursing education program, and do you possess current clinical skills?
- Is the act consistent with positive and conclusive data in nursing literature and supported by research?
- Can you document successful completion of additional education that includes instruction and supervised clinical practice?

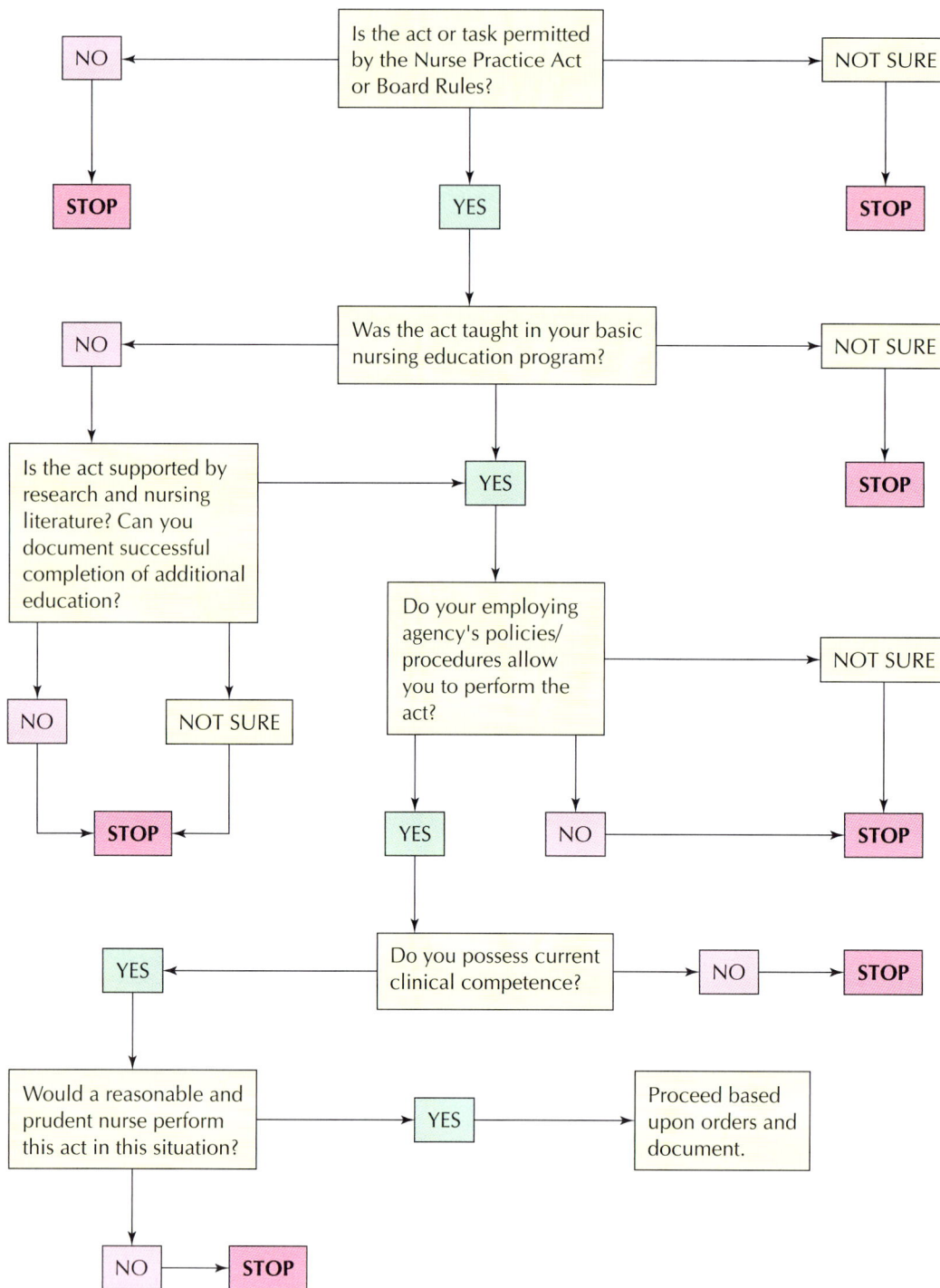

Figure 2-1. ■ Decision-making model.

Every decision related to delegation of nursing tasks must be based on the fundamental principle of protecting the health, safety, and welfare of the public. State Boards of Nursing have established through the nurse practice act the standards of delegation. Because the scope of practice varies from state to state, it is important for the LPN/LVN to read and follow the state nurse practice act. Five rules of delegation are presented in Box 2-6 ■ as a basis for understanding the role of the LPN/LVN in community-based nursing practice.

When delegating, the nurse retains the accountability for the delegation. Key words in the definition must be further described. A **competent individual** is a person who has received training, including instruction and clinical practice, to perform certain tasks and can demonstrate safe performance. Before care is delegated to an unlicensed

BOX 2-5

National Council of State Boards of Nursing Premises for Delegating Tasks

The following premises constitute the basis for the delegation decision-making process.

1. All decisions related to delegation of nursing tasks must be based on the fundamental principle of protection of the health, safety, and welfare of the public.
2. Boards of Nursing are responsible for the regulation of nursing. Provision of any care which constitutes nursing or any activity represented as nursing is a regulatory responsibility of Boards of Nursing.
3. Boards of Nursing should articulate clear principles for delegation, augmented by clearly defined guidelines for delegation decisions.
4. A licensed nurse must have ultimate responsibility and accountability for the management and provision of nursing.
5. A licensed nurse must be actively involved in and be accountable for all managerial decisions, policy making, and practices related to the delegation of nursing care.
6. There is a need and a place for competent, appropriately supervised, unlicensed assistive personnel in the delivery of affordable, quality health care. However, it must be remembered that unlicensed assistive personnel are equipped to assist—not replace—the nurse.
7. Nursing is a knowledge-based process discipline and cannot be reduced solely to a list of tasks. The licensed nurse's specialized education, professional judgment, and discretion are essential for quality nursing care.
8. While nursing tasks may be delegated, the licensed nurse's generalist knowledge of client care indicates that the practice-pervasive functions of assessment, evaluation, and nursing judgment must not be delegated.
9. A task delegated to an unlicensed assistive personnel cannot be redelegated by the unlicensed assistive person.
10. Consumers have a right to health care that meets legal standards of care. Thus, when a nursing task is delegated, the task must be performed in accord with established standards of practice, policies, and procedures.
11. The licensed nurse determines and is accountable for the appropriateness of delegated nursing tasks. Inappropriate delegation by the nurse and/or unauthorized performance of nursing tasks by unlicensed assistive personnel may lead to legal action against the licensed nurse and/or unlicensed assistive personnel.

Source: National Council of State Boards of Nursing, Incorporated. (1995). *Delegation: concepts and decision-making process.* Chicago: National Council of State Boards of Nursing.

BOX 2-6

Five Rules of Delegation

- RIGHT TASK: One that is delegated for a specific client
- RIGHT CIRCUMSTANCES: Appropriate client setting, available resources, and other relevant factors considered
- RIGHT PERSON: *Right person* is delegating the right task to the *right person* to be performed on the *right person*
- RIGHT DIRECTION/COMMUNICATION: Clear, concise description of the task, including its objective, limits, and expectations
- RIGHT SUPERVISION: Appropriate monitoring, evaluation, intervention as needed, and feedback

assistive person, the nurse must verify that the unlicensed person is competent to perform the task. Many health care agencies hire only unlicensed assistive personnel who have completed a certified nursing assistant course and are listed on the state registry. In this case, the nurse needs to observe the certified nursing assistant (CNA) perform the desired tasks in order to evaluate his or her competence. If the unlicensed assistive person has not completed formal instruction, the nurse must provide instruction and clinical supervision prior to allowing the unlicensed person to provide care independently. In either case, periodic evaluation

of the unlicensed person's competence is necessary to ensure the health and safety of clients.

The nursing task being delegated must be selected based on client assessment, the individual situation, and the skill of the individual unlicensed person (Figure 2-2 ■). For example, assisting a client in ambulating might be delegated if the client's condition is stable, but if the client has been in bed for some time, has been unstable, or has just had surgery, then it might not be wise to delegate this task to an unlicensed person. In addition, the nurse must keep in mind that "while nursing tasks may be delegated, the licensed nurse's generalist knowledge of client care indicates that the practice-pervasive functions of assessment, evaluation, and nursing judgment must not be delegated" (National Council of State Boards of Nursing, 1995, p. 3). Therefore, if the purpose is to assess the client's stability or progress, the task should not be delegated. For example, if the client's strength needs to be evaluated to determine if the client is ready for discharge or able to care for himself, the ambulation should not be delegated.

Once the nurse decides to delegate specific tasks to a competent unlicensed person, the nurse must give specific directions including what is to be done, the expected outcome of the task, possible complications, and the actions

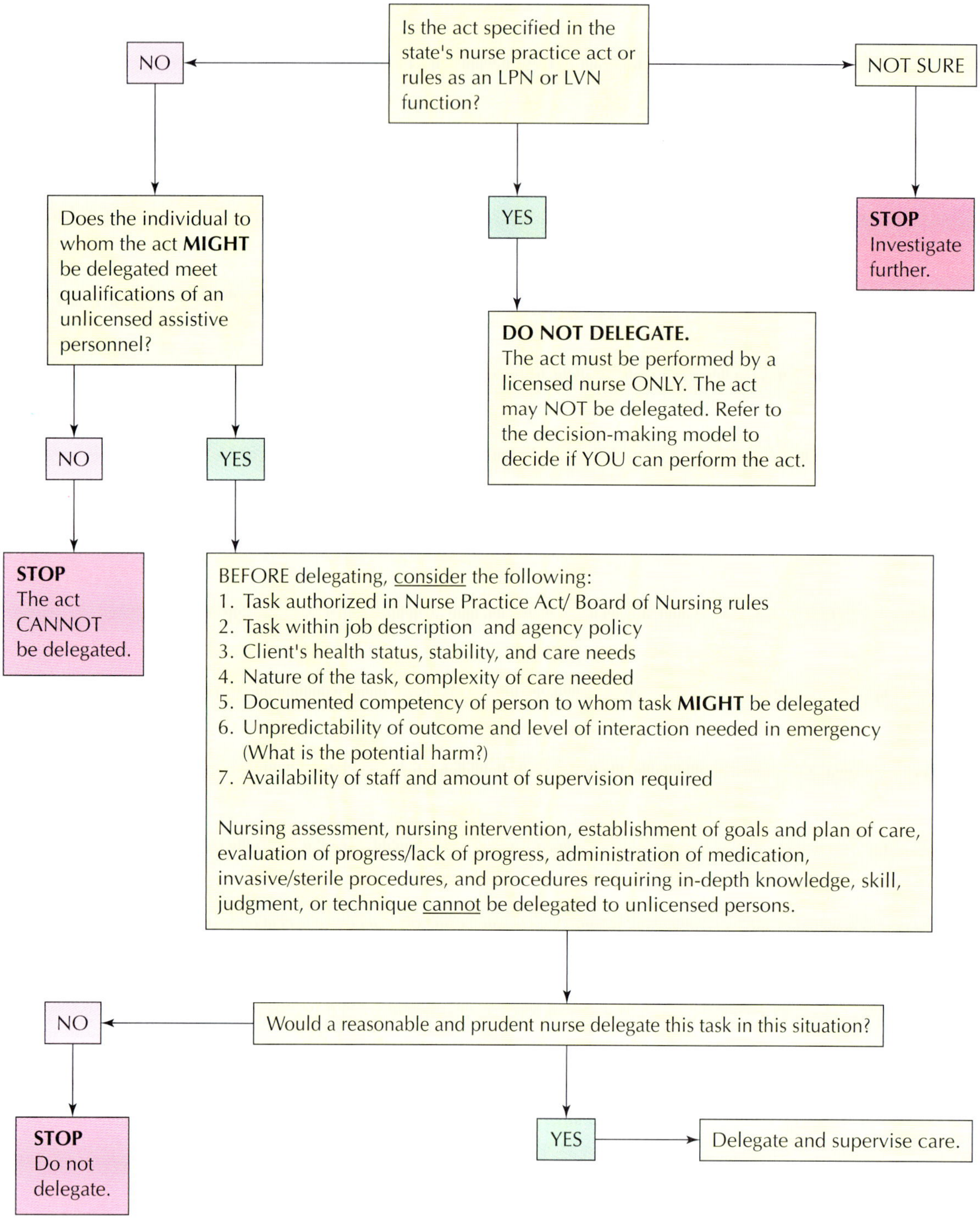

Is the act specified in the state's nurse practice act or rules as an LPN or LVN function?

NO

NOT SURE

Does the individual to whom the act **MIGHT** be delegated meet qualifications of an unlicensed assistive personnel?

YES

STOP Investigate further.

DO NOT DELEGATE. The act must be performed by a licensed nurse ONLY. The act may NOT be delegated. Refer to the decision-making model to decide if YOU can perform the act.

NO

YES

STOP The act CANNOT be delegated.

BEFORE delegating, consider the following:
1. Task authorized in Nurse Practice Act/ Board of Nursing rules
2. Task within job description and agency policy
3. Client's health status, stability, and care needs
4. Nature of the task, complexity of care needed
5. Documented competency of person to whom task **MIGHT** be delegated
6. Unpredictability of outcome and level of interaction needed in emergency (What is the potential harm?)
7. Availability of staff and amount of supervision required

Nursing assessment, nursing intervention, establishment of goals and plan of care, evaluation of progress/lack of progress, administration of medication, invasive/sterile procedures, and procedures requiring in-depth knowledge, skill, judgment, or technique cannot be delegated to unlicensed persons.

NO

Would a reasonable and prudent nurse delegate this task in this situation?

STOP Do not delegate.

YES

Delegate and supervise care.

Figure 2-2. ■ Delegation model.

to take if a complication occurs. In some circumstances such as acute care where the licensed nurse is readily available, the directions may be given verbally with close supervision by the LPN/LVN. In other circumstances such as home care where the LPN/LVN is not readily available but may be reached by telephone, both verbal and written directions should be given. For example, if the unlicensed person will be assisting the home-bound elderly client

with administering ear drops, the licensed nurse should provide the unlicensed person with written directions on how to administer ear drops, the name of the medication, the reason for the medication, the dose, the side effects, and the actions to take in case of emergency. The licensed nurse should visit the client with the unlicensed person and observe the unlicensed person administering the medication.

Once the unlicensed person has accepted the delegation, he or she may not redelegate the task to someone else. For example, if the LPN/LVN delegates the obtaining of a blood sugar measurement by finger stick, and for some reason the unlicensed assistive person cannot complete the task, the unlicensed assistive person should inform the LPN/LVN instead of asking another unlicensed assistive person to do the task. Because it is the responsibility of the LPN/LVN to determine the competence of the individual performing delegated tasks, the unlicensed assistive person is not qualified to delegate nursing care.

LPNs/LVNs are accountable for the outcome of the tasks they delegate. Therefore, the LPN/LVN must provide supervision to the unlicensed assistive personnel to whom the tasks have been delegated. Supervision means to give direc-tions and inspect the tasks performed. The LPN/LVN must provide appropriate monitoring of the unlicensed assistive person's work to evaluate the performance and provide feed-back as needed. If the unlicensed assistive person is not per-forming to an acceptable standard of care, the LPN/LVN needs to make provisions for review of instructions, further education, clinical practice, and reevaluation. This process might involve other LPNs/LVNs such as agency nurse educa-tors, or it might be the responsibility of the individual LPN/LVN. In either case, documentation of the evaluation, education, clinical practice, and reevaluation must become part of the unlicensed assistive person's employment file.

Note: The reference and resource listings for this and all chapters have been compiled at the back of the book.

Chapter Review

KEY TERMS by Topic

Use the audio glossary feature of either the CD-ROM or the Companion Website to hear the correct pronunciation of the following key terms.

Critical Thinking
critical thinking

Intellectual Standards
intellectual standards, clarity, accuracy, precision, relevance, depth, breadth, fairness, reasoning, logical, inductive reasoning, deductive reasoning, significance

Elements of Thought
purpose, information, points of view, interpretations, inferences, assumptions, conclusions, concepts, implications

Critical Thinking Care Maps
NCLEX-PN® Focus Area

Essential Intellectual Traits or Values
intellectual humility, intellectual courage, intellectual empathy, intellectual autonomy, intellectual integrity, intellectual perseverance, fair-mindedness, confidence in reason

Delegation
delegation, competent individual

KEY Points

- Critical thinking is done to improve our ability to understand situations more fully. It provides ways to overcome the limits each person has, resulting from our unique experience, upbringing, and education.

- Critical thinking does not mean that we give up what we believe. It means that we respect and value the experiences and thinking of others without having to think the same way.

- Critical thinking explores options to find the best possible outcome.

- LPNs and LVNs must use critical thinking for their increasing responsibilities in the workplace.

- Making decisions, setting priorities, and delegating tasks are just some of the ways that LPNs/LVNs use critical thinking.

- The person who does the delegating is always responsible for the results.

- Delegated jobs should not be redelegated.

- A delegated job is not complete until evaluation and follow-up have occurred.

EXPLORE MediaLink

Additional interactive resources for this chapter can be found on the Companion Website at www.prenhall.com/towle. Click on Chapter 2 and "Begin" to select the activities for this chapter.

For chapter-related NCLEX®-style questions and an audio glossary, access the accompanying CD-ROM in this book.

FOR FURTHER Study

Nursing process is reviewed briefly in Chapter 1. Hyperbilirubinemia is discussed in detail in Chapter 18.

Critical Thinking Care Map

Caring for a Client with Hyperbilirubinemia*
NCLEX-PN® Focus Area: Physiologic Integrity

Case Study: Andrew, a 4-day-old infant, was discharged from the hospital following a diagnosis of hyperbilirubinemia (physiologic jaundice). His pediatrician ordered that he spend time each day wrapped in a *BiliBlanket* (a fiber-optic phototherapy blanket designed to provide light therapy and to keep the baby warm). An LPN was assigned to make a home visit to reassess the infant. On the first home visit, the LPN found that the parents were accurately using the BiliBlanket. The baby's urine output was only four wet diapers a day. She also noted that his mucous membranes were dry and that he was lethargic. The mother stated that Andrew was rarely hungry and drank about 5 ounces of formula every 5 to 6 hours.

Nursing Diagnosis: Deficient Fluid Volume related to inadequate fluid intake and exposure to BiliBlanket

COLLECT DATA

Subjective

_____

_____

_____

_____

_____

_____

Objective

_____

_____

_____

_____

_____

_____

Would you report this? Yes/No

If yes, to: _____

Nursing Care

_____

_____

_____

_____

_____

_____

_____

_____

_____

How would you document this?_____

_____

_____

_____

Compare your documentation to the sample provided in Appendix I.

Data Collected
(use only those that apply)

- Decreased urine output (four diapers daily when typical should be six to eight)
- Dry mucous membranes
- Father states Andrew smiled yesterday
- Umbilical cord drying
- Lethargy
- Decreased oral intake
- Mother states infant rarely hungry
- Intake of 5 ounces every 5 to 6 hours

Nursing Interventions
(use only those that apply; list in priority order)

- Contact the registered nurse to report findings.
- Encourage parents to also place infant in the sunlight several times a day.
- Teach parents the importance of adequate fluid intake during the use of the BiliBlanket.
- Teach parents symptoms of dehydration.
- Obtain vital signs every 1 to 2 hours.
- Closely monitor vital signs.
- Obtain a daily electroencephalogram (EEG).
- Provide fluid replacement per order.
- Teach parents to obtain and record vital signs.

*This care map gives students the chance to apply critical thinking concepts and prior knowledge in a real situation. Hyperbilirubinemia is discussed in detail in Chapter 18.

NCLEX-PN® Exam Preparation

1 An LPN/LVN has recently graduated from nursing school and has a first job in labor and delivery. The LPN/LVN is alone in a client's room when the physician says, "I want you to apply a fetal scalp electrode." Which decision below is appropriate for the LPN/LVN to make?

1. Apply the fetal scalp electrode as the LPN/LVN had seen the RN do yesterday.
2. Read the policy and procedure for applying the fetal scalp electrode and then go ahead with the procedure.
3. Contact the RN and ask the RN to complete the physician's order.
4. Tell the physician, "I do not know how to perform that procedure. Ask someone else."

2 The LPN/LVN appropriately applies the five rules of delegation. When she or he evaluates the care given by the unlicensed assistive personnel, which of the following rules is being applied?

1. right task
2. right circumstances
3. right direction
4. right supervision

3 The LPN/LVN needs to delegate a finger-stick blood sugar (FSBS) on a client who is hospitalized for management of diabetes mellitus. Which of the following is an appropriate individual to perform this skill?

1. unlicensed assistive personnel in his or her first week on the job
2. unit secretary who is also a diabetic
3. client's husband
4. certified nursing assistant with 5 years of experience

4 The LPN/LVN has been delegated the skill of blood glucose testing. The client's blood sugar is found to be elevated. Which of the following scenarios is appropriate nursing care?

1. Ask the client's husband to administer the insulin.
2. Ask the UAP to give the insulin and then notify the LPN/LVN.
3. The LPN/LVN notifies the RN and works collaboratively to administer the insulin.
4. The UAP notifies the physician about the client's blood sugar.

5 The LPN/LVN determines that the CNA instructed the client to obtain a 24-hour urine specimen by adding the first voided urine to the container. Which nursing action, in a supervisory role, is appropriate?

1. Praise the CNA.
2. Review the procedure with the CNA.

3. Recommend that the CNA be reassigned to another unit.
4. Recommend that the CNA receive a raise.

6 A client calls complaining of a backache. The LPN/LVN gathers the following assessment: estimated date of birth, length of time the client has experienced the pain, use of relief measures. Which of the following intellectual standards is the LPN/LVN using in this situation?

1. relevance
2. clarity
3. accuracy
4. precision

7 The nurse uses _____ reasoning to determine that a client who says she has a full bladder may experience a boggy uterus, heavy lochia flow, and passage of large clots. (Fill in the blank.)

8 The LPN/LVN reviews the fetal monitor strip of a laboring client and considers the consequences of each possible nursing action prior to implementing care. Which of the following elements of thought is the LPN/LVN using in this situation?

1. points of view
2. assumptions
3. implications of actions
4. concepts

9 Which of the following statements by the LPN/LVN demonstrate the intellectual standard that refers to clarity? Select all that apply.

1. "Could you be more specific about the type of pain you have?"
2. "How would you describe the sensation you feel?"
3. "Give me an example of how it feels."
4. "Are there any related factors that might contribute to your pain?"
5. "Tell me more about your pain."

10 The LPN/LVN has received an order to hang IV fluids using the new IV pump. After evaluating the situation, the LPN/LVN may decide not to proceed because:

1. an unlicensed assistive personnel can hang the fluids.
2. proper training has not been completed by the LPN/LVN.
3. only RNs can hang IV fluids.
4. certified nursing assistants can hang IV fluids.

Answers for NCLEX-PN® Review and Critical Thinking questions appear in Appendix I.

Chapter 3

Legal and Ethical Issues in Maternal-Newborn Nursing

BRIEF Outline

Federal Programs Affecting
Maternal-Newborn Care

Legal and Ethical Issues
Affecting Adolescent Birth
Control and Pregnancy

Legal and Ethical Issues
Affecting the Mother

Role of the LPN/LVN

Nursing Care

LEARNING Outcomes

After completing this chapter, you will be able to:

1. Define key terms.
2. Describe federal initiatives to protect women and newborns.
3. Describe parents' rights as they relate to the care of adolescents and newborns.
4. Describe client rights as they relate to adolescents.
5. Name situations in which the nurse must legally report to public agencies.
6. Describe common legal and ethical issues that can affect the mother, newborn, and family.
7. Describe the role of the LPN/LVN in legal and ethical issues.

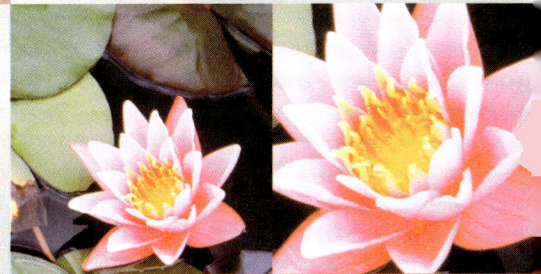

HEALTH PROMOTION ISSUE:
Sexually Transmitted Infection
Education

NURSING PROCESS CARE PLAN:
Client with Preterm Labor

CRITICAL THINKING CARE MAP:
Caring for a Client Desiring
Pregnancy Termination

Maternal care, like other areas of nursing, may sometimes present nurses with challenges to their worldview and their values. While most pregnancies progress without incident and end in the delivery of a healthy newborn, some couples are faced with difficult decisions regarding infertility, maintaining a pregnancy, terminating a pregnancy, and caring for a sick or disabled newborn. **Legal** (required by law) and **ethical** (values and ideas that shape a sense of right and wrong) issues surrounding these decisions are not just confined to the pregnancy. For example, when fertilized eggs are stored for future use, decisions regarding the use, study, or disposition of these eggs may not occur for years. A pregnant woman may experience legal or ethical issues with other children in the family. The stress involved in these situations may impact the pregnancy.

Nurses may be required to help families make legal and ethical decisions. Most health care agencies have policies to guide the nurse in these situations. Nurses may disagree with state or federal laws or agency policies but still be required to uphold them. They may also disagree with a client's ethics. It is certain that every nurse will someday face a situation in which his or her personal standards of right and wrong are challenged. The challenge may come from a client, a supervisor, a facility regulation, or a state or federal law. Also, the nurse may encounter situations in which there is no "right" decision because all solutions involve some negative outcomes. At these times, the nurse will need to act professionally and without bias to support the client and family and help them come to a decision. Because legal and ethical issues that involve the pregnant woman may also affect the fetus, the newborn, older children, and the family, this chapter will provide guidelines for the LPN/LVN in providing care in these situations.

Federal Programs Affecting Maternal-Newborn Care

Since the early 1900s, groups, such as the White House Conference on Children and Youth, have met at the national level to discuss and make recommendations to improve health. In response to these recommendations, the U.S. government established programs such as Medicaid's Early and Periodic Screening, Diagnosis, and Treatment (EPSDT) and the Women, Infants, and Children (WIC) program (Table 3-1 ■). Because the health of the child is affected by the health of his or her mother before, during, and shortly after birth, funding for such programs as WIC provides health assessment and nutritious foods at a decreased cost for the mother, infant, and young children.

HEALTHY PEOPLE 2000 AND HEALTHY PEOPLE 2010

In 1990, the U.S. Department of Health and Human Services (USDHHS) released *Healthy People 2000: National Health Promotion and Disease Prevention Objectives.* This document presented an opportunity for Americans to take responsibility for their health. It recommended access to health care for all, particularly the most vulnerable. Figure 3-1 ■ illustrates factors from the most recent *Healthy People 2010* that determine an individual's health (USDHHS, 2000).

Some of the objectives in the *Healthy People 2000* document that related to maternal health included the following:

- Reducing disparities in key maternal and infant health indicators so that all could have access to quality care
- Understanding issues related to preconception, prenatal, and obstetric care
- Preventing birth defects and developmental disabilities
- Reducing teen pregnancy

TABLE 3-1

Federal Programs Affecting Women and Children

ACRONYM OF FEDERAL PROGRAM	FULL NAME OF FEDERAL PROGRAM
EPSDT	Early and Periodic Screening, Diagnosis, and Treatment
ICHP	Innovative Community Health Programs
SCHIP	State Children's Health Insurance Program
VFC	Vaccination Funding for Children
WIC	Women, Infants, and Children

Healthy People 2010 **Leading Health Indicators**

- Physical Activity
- Overweight and Obesity
- Tobacco Use
- Substance Abuse
- Responsible Sexual Behavior
- Mental Health
- Injury and Violence
- Environmental Quality
- Immunization
- Access to Health Care

Figure 3-1. ■ *Healthy People 2010* identifies objectives for each health indicator (USDHHS, 2000).

The U.S. Department of Health and Human Services updates goals and objectives for health care every 10 years. *Healthy People 2010* contains 467 objectives divided into 28 focus areas, one of which is Maternal, Infant, and Child Health. Important topics within the maternal-infant focus area are as follows:

- Reducing infant and maternal mortality
- Increasing the proportion of women who receive early and adequate prenatal care
- Increasing the percentage of healthy full-term infants who are put down to sleep on their backs
- Reducing the occurrence of developmental disabilities
- Increasing abstinence from alcohol, cigarettes, and illicit drugs among pregnant women (USDHHS, 2000)

Achieving maternal-infant objectives involves both research and teaching. The government publishes weekly reports on various topic areas of *Healthy People 2010*. Current information about *Healthy People 2010* is available on the Internet.

Legal and Ethical Issues Affecting Adolescent Birth Control and Pregnancy

Even when laws and programs ensure health care for an adolescent, legal and ethical issues will still exist. For example, can a 15-year-old obtain birth control without parental consent? A 16-year-old girl is pregnant and wants an abortion. Because she is a minor, does she need parental consent? If she delivers, can she make decisions about the health care of the infant? At what age can a minor make decisions to accept or refuse treatment? Although answers to these questions might differ from state to state, the nurse should understand and practice within the state regulations and obtain legal advice for complex issues.

PARENTS' RIGHTS

In most situations, parents or legal guardians have the authority to make decisions for their minor children. This authority would include decisions for the treatment of the newborn as well as the pregnant adolescent. There are a few exceptions:

- If the parent(s) is (are) incapacitated and cannot make a decision
- If there is actual or suspected abuse or neglect
- If the parent's choice does not permit lifesaving procedures for the newborn or pregnant teen

Even though the nurse may not agree with the parent's decision about treatment, nursing care must be provided in an unbiased manner. The LPN/LVN should report all concerns to the supervising RN. Legal counsel might be necessary to settle disputes.

Usually it is the parent or legal guardian who gives **informed consent** (written approval for a treatment or procedure, following explanation of pros and cons by the physician or other professional who is performing the procedure). Procedure 3-1 ■ reviews important steps and rationales for witnessing informed consent.

Legal and Ethical Issues Affecting the Mother

The "Patient's Bill of Rights," a fundamental document of health care, is illustrated in Box 3-1 ■. These rights, with some modifications, apply both to the adult and to the teenage client. For example, the pregnant 13-year-old may not be able to understand the diagnosis and treatment of a disorder affecting the pregnancy in order to provide an informed consent, yet she should still be included in the process. Explanations in age-appropriate language should be given, and every attempt should be made to acquire her cooperation. It is important to give adolescents as much control as possible over what happens to them by including them in decisions about their welfare.

It is reasonable to expect parents and adolescents to participate in health care in the following ways:

- By providing accurate and complete information about health issues
- By increasing their knowledge about diagnosis and treatment
- By being responsible for their own actions
- By reporting changes in client condition
- By keeping appointments
- By meeting financial obligations for health care

There are many ethical and legal issues that affect the mother. These issues do not have easy answers, and they are addressed here for discussion purposes only. Each person's situation will be different, and at times, the courts will make the final decisions. The nurse must be able to look at each situation with an open mind and provide the necessary care for the mother, newborn, and family. Box 3-2 ■ reviews steps in making ethical decisions. Nurses who frequently work with these families must become familiar with the state and federal laws governing these situations.

ASSISTED REPRODUCTION

For a variety of reasons, some couples who try to have children are unable to conceive. Some of these couples use their ova and sperm for *in vitro* fertilization. Others use the ova and/or sperm

MediaLink Issues for Minors

PROCEDURE 3-1 **Witnessing Informed Consent**

Purpose

■ To document informed consent (agreement by a client, client's parent, or guardian to accept a course of treatment or procedure after complete information has been provided by the health care provider).

Equipment

■ Copy of the agency informed consent form
■ Black pen

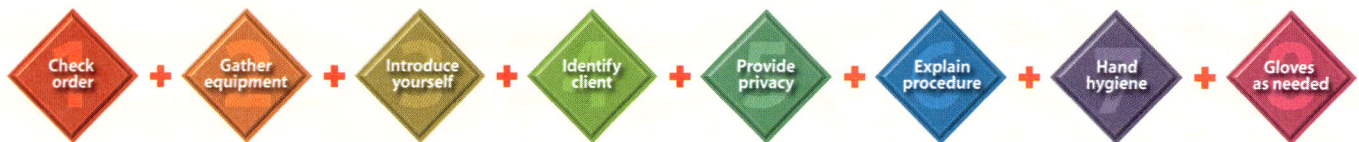

Check order + Gather equipment + Introduce yourself + Identify client + Provide privacy + Explain procedure + Hand hygiene + Gloves as needed

Interventions and Rationales

1. Perform preparatory steps (see icon bar above).

2. Stamp the agency informed consent form with the client's addressograph plate. *The addressograph information identifies the form as a part of the legal record.*

3. Complete all information requested on the form. Note: The informed consent form may be computer generated in some facilities. Complete the information requested before printing out the form. *Ensures complete, accurate information is obtained.*

4. Write the procedure for which consent is being given in the space provided. Use proper medical terminology with no abbreviations. Include "right" or "left" as appropriate (e.g., "Right inguinal herniorrhaphy" not "fix R inguinal hernia"). *For accuracy in communication, the legal record must contain appropriate medical terminology and identification of appropriate body part when more than one exists.*

5. Listen to the information the primary care provider gives to the client, client's parent, or guardian. *When you witness an informed consent, you are witnessing the exchange between the primary care provider and the client, client's parent, or guardian. You are establishing that they really did understand (were informed).*

6. Have the client or client's parent or guardian sign the form. The nurse should sign as a witness. Note: Some schools of nursing do not allow student nurses to serve as witness for informed consent. *Signatures document that information was provided and the client, client's parent, or guardian understood and agreed to the procedure.*

7. If the primary care provider is not present and you did not hear the information provided, ask the client, client's parent, or guardian to tell you what they were told. Ask if they have any questions. If they have accurate information and no questions, have them sign the consent form. Sign on the witness line with the statement "witnessing signature only" written under your signature. *Because you did not hear the information provided by the physician, you cannot witness that interaction. If they have accurate information and no questions, you can be reasonably assured they have been informed. When you write "witnessing signature only," you are not held accountable for the information.*

8. If the information they tell you is incorrect or they have questions, do not have the consent signed. Instead, notify the primary care provider. *It is the responsibility of the primary care provider to obtain informed consent. If more teaching is needed, the primary care provider should provide it.*

9. Place the signed informed consent form in the client's chart. *The informed consent form is part of the legal record and should be kept with the client's chart.*

SAMPLE DOCUMENTATION

(date/time) Dr. R. Jones talked with parents about need to repair right inguinal hernia, including benefits, risks to the newborn, and possible complications. Informed consent form for right inguinal herniorrhaphy signed and witnessed. L. Lopez, LPN

BOX 3-1

Patient's Bill of Rights

A Patient's* Bill of Rights was first adopted by the American Hospital Association (AHA) in 1973. The Bill of Rights below incorporates the AHA update as well as Bill of Rights information from the American Academy of Pain Management and the National Institutes of Health.

Bill of Rights

These rights can be exercised on the client's behalf by a designated surrogate or proxy decision maker if the client* lacks decision-making capacity, is legally incompetent, or is a minor.

1. The client has the right to considerate and respectful care.
2. The client has the right to and is encouraged to obtain from physicians and other direct care givers relevant, current, and understandable information about diagnosis, treatment, and prognosis. Except in emergencies when the client lacks decision-making capacity and the need for treatment is urgent, the client is entitled to the opportunity to discuss and request information related to specific procedures and treatments, the risks involved, the possible length of recuperation, and the medically reasonable alternatives and their accompanying risks and benefits.

   Clients have the right to know the identity of physicians, nurses, and others involved in their care, as well as when those involved are students, residents, or other trainees. The client also has the right to know the immediate and long-term financial implications of treatment choices insofar as they are known.
3. The client has the right to make decisions about the plan of care prior to and during the course of treatment and to refuse recommended treatment or plan of care to the extent permitted by law and hospital policy and to be informed of the medical consequences of this action. In case of such refusal, the client is entitled to other appropriate care and services that the hospital provides or transfers to another hospital. The hospital should notify the client of any policy that might affect client choice within the institution.
4. The client has the right to have an advance directive (such as a living will, health care proxy, or durable power of attorney for health care) concerning treatment or designating a surrogate decision maker with the expectation that the hospital will honor the intent of that directive to the extent permitted by law and hospital policy.

   Health care institutions must advise clients of their rights under state law and hospital policy to make informed medical choices, ask if the client has an advance directive, and include that information in client records. The client has the right to timely information about hospital policy that may limit its ability to implement fully a legally valid advance directive.
5. The client has the right to have every consideration of privacy. Case discussion, consultation, examination, and treatment should be conducted as to protect each client's privacy.
6. The client has the right to expect that all communications and records pertaining to his/her care will be treated as confidential by the hospital, except in cases of suspected abuse or public health hazard when reporting is permitted or required by law. The client has the right to expect that

the hospital will emphasize the confidentiality of this information when it releases it to any other parties entitled to review information in these records.

7. The client has the right to review the records pertaining to his/her medical care and have information explained or interpreted as necessary, except when restricted by law.
8. The client has the right to expect that, within its capacity and policies, a hospital will make reasonable response to request of a client for appropriate and medically indicated care and services. The hospital must provide evaluation, services, and/or referral, as indicated by urgency of the case. When medically appropriate and legally permissible, or when a client has so requested, a client may be transferred to another facility. The institution to which the client is to be transferred must first have accepted the client for transfer. The client must also have the benefit of complete information and explanation concerning the need for, risks, benefits, and alternatives to such a transfer.
9. The client has the right to ask and be informed of the existence of business relationships among the hospital facility, educational institutions, other health care providers, or payers that may influence the client's treatment and care.
10. The client has the right to consent to or decline to participate in proposed research studies or human experimentation affecting care and treatment or requiring direct client involvement, and to have those studies fully explained prior to consent. A client who declines to participate in research or experimentation is entitled to the most effective care that the hospital can otherwise provide.
11. The client has the right to expect reasonable continuity of care when appropriate and to be informed by physicians and other caregivers of available and realistic client care options when hospital care is no longer appropriate.
12. The client has the right to be informed of hospital policies and practices that relate to client care, treatment, and responsibilities. The client has the right to be informed of available resources for resolving disputes, grievances, and conflicts such as ethics committees, client representatives, or other mechanisms available in the institution. The client has the right to be informed of the hospital's charges for services and available payment methods.
13. The client has the privilege to examine and receive an explanation of the bill.
14. The client has the right to expect that medical information about him or her discovered at the Clinical Center, as well as an account of his or her medical program there, will be communicated to the referring physician.
15. The client has the right, at any time during the medical program, to designate additional physicians or organizations to receive medical updates. The client should inform the Outpatient Department staff of these additions.

Note: This book uses the word *client* instead of *patient* to indicate that the person is an active participant in the process of achieving or maintaining health.

Data from: American Hospital Association, Chicago, IL; American Academy of Pain Management, Sonora, CA; National Institutes of Health, Washington, DC.

BOX 3-2	NURSING CARE CHECKLIST

Steps in Making Ethical Decisions

☑ **Step 1: Review the situation to determine:**
1. Health problems—physical, spiritual, mental, psychosocial
2. Decision/actions needed immediately and in near future
3. Key individuals potentially affected by the decision/action and outcomes
4. Any potential human rights violations in the situation

☑ **Step 2: Gather additional information to clarify and understand:**
1. Legal constraints, if any
2. Limited time to thoroughly explore
3. Decision capacity of individual(s)
4. Institutional policies that affect choices in situation
5. Values inherent in choice of information

☑ **Step 3: Identify the ethical issues or concerns in the situation:**
1. Ethical components/concerns of situation and decision/action
2. Explore historical roots of each
3. Identify current philosophical/religious positions on each issue
4. Discuss societal/cultural views on each issue

☑ **Step 4: Define personal and professional moral positions on ethical concerns:**
1. Review personal biases/constraints on issues raised
2. Understand personal values affected by situation/ethical issues raised
3. Review professional codes of ethics (moral behavior) for guidance
4. Identify any conflicting loyalties and/or obligations of professionals and family in the situation
5. Think about your level of moral development operant in the situation
6. Identify the virtues needed for professional action

☑ **Step 5: Identify moral positions of key individuals in the situation:**
1. Think about levels of moral development operant in each participant
2. Identify any communication gaps or misunderstandings

3. Provide guidance in clarifying varying levels of moral development

☑ **Step 6: Identify value conflicts, if any:**
1. Provide guidance in identifying potential conflicts, interests, competing values
2. Work toward possible resolution of conflict based on respect for differences
3. Seek consultation if needed to resolve key conflicts

☑ **Step 7: Determine who should make needed decision:**
1. Clarify your role in the situation
2. Who "owns" the problem/decision?
3. Who stands to lose or gain the most from the decision/action?
4. Is the decision to be made by a single individual or group?

☑ **Step 8: Identify the range of actions with anticipated outcomes of each:**
1. Determine the moral justification for each potential action
2. Identify the ethical theory that supports each action
3. Apply concepts of beneficence and fairness to each potential action
4. Attach outcomes to each potential action and determine best outcome
5. Are additional actions/decisions required as a result of each action?

☑ **Step 9: Decide on a course of action and carry it out:**
1. Understand why a given action was chosen
2. Help all involved understand these reasons
3. Establish a time frame for review of the decision/action and expected outcomes
4. Determine who can best carry out the chosen action/decision

☑ **Step 10: Evaluate/review outcomes of decisions/actions:**
1. Determine whether expected outcomes occurred
2. Is a new decision or action needed?
3. Was the decision process fair and complete?
4. What was the response to the action by each key individual?
5. What did you learn from this situation?

Source: Adapted from Thompson, J. B., & Thompson, H. O. (1981). *Ethics in nursing.* New York: Macmillan. Copyright Joyce Thompson. Used with permission. Updated July 2006.

---

from donors. Some couples adopt infants from other mothers. Some couples choose to have a surrogate mother carry the fetus and give the infant to the couple after delivery.

Many ethical and legal questions arise from situations seen today. What are the rights and responsibilities of the ova/sperm donors? What are the rights and responsibilities of the surrogate mother? What if the surrogate mother chooses not to give the infant to the couple after birth? If more than one infant is produced, must the couple assume responsibility of all the infants? If the infant born from ova/sperm donation or surrogacy has birth defects, who is

financially responsible for this child? Does the child have the right to know the birth mother and father and to develop a relationship with them?

NONTRADITIONAL PARENTS

Regulations that placed adopted children only in traditional family settings no longer apply. Blended families (see Chapter 4 ⬯) can adopt. Single parents who show they have the means to support a child may also adopt.

It is becoming more common for same-sex couples to want to marry and raise children. Gay men might request to adopt a child or donate sperm to have a child carried by a surrogate mother. Gay women could have one (or both) partners inseminated and carry the pregnancy. Because few states recognize same-sex marriages, which partner is legally responsible for the child? If the partners separate, who retains legal custody of the child?

PREGNANCY AFTER RAPE

Many women are sexually assaulted every year. The rapist could be a stranger, a friend, or a relative. At times, pregnancy results from these crimes. If the woman seeks health care immediately, measures may be taken to prevent pregnancy. However, even with medical care, pregnancy could result. The woman could choose to abort the pregnancy, adopt the child to another person, or keep the infant. Regardless of whether she chooses to keep the child, some ethical and legal questions exist. For example, if she keeps the child and the rapist is identified by DNA testing, can he be forced to pay child support? What rights would he have as the biologic father?

ABORTION

At times a pregnancy will end before the due date. While medically, termination of pregnancy is termed **abortion,** a spontaneous occurrence is more commonly called a **miscarriage.** The term *abortion* most often refers to the planned termination of pregnancy. The legalization of abortions has resulted in great debate. Each state has laws pertaining to the stage of pregnancy at which an abortion can be performed. Legal and ethical questions are also under discussion. For example, if a woman desires an abortion, does the father need to give consent? What are the rights of the grandparents? Do parents of minors, including the parents of the minor father, have any rights and responsibilities? Abortion is discussed further in Chapter 7 🔗.

BARRIER-BREAKING TECHNOLOGIES

Increased capability with DNA testing and therapy has raised a host of ethical issues. Stem cell therapy can be viewed as a huge medical breakthrough, similar to the discovery of penicillin in the last century. It may have potential to correct heart defects, cure inherited diseases such as sickle cell anemia, and prevent degenerative diseases such as Parkinson's. However, it can also be viewed as the intrusion of humans into the very process of life. When more genes and gene markers are identified, it may be possible to know with near certainty that a baby will be born with a crippling condition. What effect will it have if insurance companies refuse to cover the needs of this child? What controls will there be to ensure quality of life for those who cannot afford advanced and expensive gene therapy?

Parents may now be presented with the option of "banking" their child's umbilical cord blood after birth. The frozen stem cells from the cord could be used in later years if the child needed therapy, such as for leukemia. However, it is not clear who owns the blood. Would the parent have the right to sell this cord blood for cash? Would the hospital have the right to keep the blood and use it to help others who have an immediate need for it? Could a child sue a parent or a facility because his or her cord blood was disposed of without his or her consent?

Fetal research is another broad area of ethical conflict. Some believe that unused embryos from *in vitro* fertilization should be used to aid research. Others believe equally strongly that these embryos are alive and that no human has the right to terminate that life. Advances in neonatal care and equipment only further the controversy, as neonates survive from increasingly premature stages of development.

Medical advances can also raise ethical issues from the maternal side. Consider the case of the pregnant dying woman who asked to be maintained on life support to bring her child to term. Is it right to maintain life support on someone who is brain dead? Does the family have the right to demand life support? Is it right to stop life support, knowing that the fetus will not survive? What might the effects be on an infant if most of its development has occurred inside a cadaver? These and other questions will become more common as technology continues to advance.

ADOLESCENT RIGHTS

There are some exceptions to parents giving informed consent. Some states have a **mature minor act** (an act that permits adolescents age 14 or 15 to make decisions about their treatment). In some cases, self-supporting adolescents are emancipated by court decision. Such minors, including minors who marry, are called **emancipated minors.** They are responsible for their own health care decisions and expenses.

PRIVACY AND CONFIDENTIALITY

The newborn or adolescent has as much right to privacy and confidentiality as an adult. On the physical level, privacy means screening from view: closing curtains and draping the client to prevent a third party from seeing the body or body parts. At the legal level, privacy also means keeping the client's chart screened from a third party. **Confidentiality** means keeping secret any privileged information.

For an infant, this right may not pose a problem. The nurse protects the infant's privacy by screening him or her from view during procedures and by keeping the medical record secure. The parent's confidentiality is also maintained.

With an adolescent, maintaining confidentiality may cause some conflict for the nurse. For example, an adolescent may request treatment for a sexually transmitted disease, birth control, pregnancy, or drug and alcohol treatment without notifying the parents. If the nurse breeches confidentiality and informs the parents, the client may lose trust in the nurse and possibly in the entire health care system. However, if the parents learn about the health problem from another source, they may accuse the nurse of withholding information from them. As parents, they may have the right to access their dependent teen's medical record. The nurse should check facility policy and ask the nursing supervisor about guidelines for handling this situation.

REPORTABLE SITUATIONS

In certain instances, the decision about reporting the health concern of an infant or adolescent is made by law.

- If the infant or adolescent has a **reportable disease** (a disease that poses a public health hazard), the health care provider must file a report with the appropriate agency (usually the public health department).
- Suspected cases of abuse or neglect must be reported to state law enforcement officers (local police, child protection services, and the department of health and human services).
- Threats to injure oneself must be reported to the supervisor in charge. This must be done even if an adolescent asks the nurse to "promise" not to tell anyone. In this case, the nurse would tell the adolescent that the nurse's job requires him or her to report anything that might cause harm to a client.

It is important for the nurse to be clear with clients about the limits of confidentiality and the mandatory reporting requirements.

Reportable diseases may include, but are not limited to, sexually transmitted infections, some food-borne infections, and some viral or airborne infections such as measles, whooping cough, and tuberculosis. The LPN/LVN might contact the health care provider or report the condition directly to the local health department. Infections must be reported immediately so that investigation, diagnosis, and treatment of others can be made in a timely manner. The nurse would be provided with reporting forms either from the employing agency or from the health department. Documentation should also be included in the client chart.

Suspicion of Abuse

Every state has abuse laws that define different types of abuse and the agency to which abuse issues should be directed. Any professional who reasonably suspects that abuse has occurred is required to report the suspicion to the local authorities. The practical or vocational nurse should follow facility policy and always be careful to ensure privacy during the interview. Questions should be referred to the registered nurse.

Reports of suspected abuse that are made in good faith are not liable for countersuits. However, professionals who fail to report suspicions may be held responsible by the courts. The nurse must record detailed information in the client's chart and complete any report forms provided by the investigating agency.

clinical ALERT

Reports of abuse must be made immediately in order to protect the client from further harm. The client *should not be left alone.* In some cases, a client is admitted to the hospital for "observation" while authorities are notified and an investigation is conducted.

PATIENT SELF-DETERMINATION ACT

The federal Patient Self-Determination Act requires health care institutions to inform clients of their rights to treatment, including advanced directives or "living wills" (Figure 3-2 ■). Nurses frequently discuss these issues with adult clients and families. They might need to discuss them with an adolescent and their parents.

While it is unusual for a pregnant teen to have a terminal disorder, there are some circumstances where this may be the case. For example, an adolescent with a malignant brain tumor could become pregnant. A pregnant adolescent may be involved in an accident resulting in irreversible brain damage. When it becomes apparent a teenage child will not recover, an open discussion about treatment and terminal care should take place. This discussion should involve key decision makers in the family. It should also involve the adolescent as appropriate in the situation.

"Do not resuscitate" orders for a pregnant woman, newborn, or adolescent can raise a more emotional response than the same order for an older adult. Conflict over resuscitation can arise between members of the family. For example, some family members may want to continue life support for a pregnant woman until the fetus can be delivered. Conflict can develop when the adolescent wants to stop treatment but the parent(s) is (are) not ready to allow the child to die. Conflict can arise if one parent wishes to stop treatment of the terminally ill newborn, and the other parent wants to continue treatment. It is important for the nurse to use effective therapeutic communication in all situations, including group meetings, to help resolve the conflict.

Role of the LPN/LVN

LPNs and LVNs are not ultimately responsible for resolving legal or ethical issues. However, they need to have a basic understanding of the issues in order to be supportive of the client, the family, and other health care professionals. The

POWER OF ATTORNEY FOR HEALTH CARE

(1) **DESIGNATION OF AGENT:** I designate the following individual as my agent to make health care decisions for me: _____

_____
(Name of individual you choose as agent)

_____
(address) (city) (state) (zip code)

_____
(home phone) (work phone)

OPTIONAL: If I revoke my agent's authority or if my agent is not willing, able, or reasonably available to make a health-care decision for me, I designate as my first alternate agent:

_____
(Name of individual you choose as first alternate agent)

_____
(address) (city) (state) (zip code)

_____
(home phone) (work phone)

OPTIONAL: If I revoke the authority of my agent and first alternate agent or if neither is willing, able, or reasonably available to make a health care decision for me, I designate as my second alternate agent:

_____
(Name of individual you choose as second alternate agent)

_____
(address) (city) (state) (zip code)

_____
(home phone) (work phone)

(2) **AGENT'S AUTHORITY:** My agent is authorized to make all health care decisions for me, including decisions to provide, withhold, or withdraw artificial nutrition and hydration, and all other forms of health care to keep me alive, **except** as I state here:

(3) **WHEN AGENT'S AUTHORITY BECOMES EFFECTIVE:** My agent's authority becomes effective when my primary physician determines that I am unable to make my own health care decisions unless I mark the following box. If I mark this box [ ], my agent's authority to make health care decisions for me takes effect immediately.

(4) **AGENT'S OBLIGATION:** My agent shall make health care decisions for me in accordance with this power of attorney for health care, any instructions I give below, and my other wishes to the extent known to my agent. To the extent my wishes are unknown, my agent shall make health care decisions for me in accordance with what my agent determines to be in my best interest. In determining my best interest, my agent shall consider my personal values to the extent known to my agent.

(5) **AGENT'S POSTDEATH AUTHORITY:** My agent is authorized to make anatomical gifts, authorize an autopsy, and direct disposition of my remains, except as I state here or elsewhere in this form:

INSTRUCTIONS FOR HEALTH CARE
Strike any wording you do not want.

(6) **END-OF-LIFE DECISIONS:** I direct that my health care providers and others involved in my care provide, withhold, or withdraw treatment in accordance with the choice I have marked below: **(Initial only one box)**
[ ] (a) **Choice NOT To Prolong Life**
I do not want my life to be prolonged if (1) I have an incurable and irreversible condition that will result in my death within a relatively short time, (2) I become unconscious and, to a reasonable degree of medical certainty, I will not regain consciousness, or (3) the likely risks and burdens of treatment would outweigh the expected benefits, **OR**
[ ] (b) **Choice To Prolong Life**
I want my life to be prolonged as long as possible within the limits of generally accepted health care standards.

(7) **RELIEF FROM PAIN:** Except as I state in the following space, I direct that treatment for alleviation of pain or discomfort should be provided at all times even if it hastens my death:

DONATION OF ORGANS AT DEATH
(8) Upon my death: (mark applicable box)
[ ] (a) I give any needed organs, tissues, or parts,
OR
[ ] (b) I give the following organs, tissues, or parts only: _____
[ ] (c) My gift is for the following purposes:
(strike any of the following you do not want)
(1) Transplant
(2) Therapy
(3) Research
(4) Education

(9) **EFFECT OF COPY:** A copy of this form has the same effect as the original.

(10) **SIGNATURE:** Sign and date the form here:

_____	_____
(date)	(sign your name)
_____	_____
(address)	(print your name)
_____	_____
(city)	(state)

(11) **WITNESSES:** This advance health care directive will not be valid for making health care decisions unless it is either: (1) signed by two (2) qualified adult witnesses who are personally known to you and who are present when you sign or acknowledge your signature; or (2) acknowledged before a notary public.

Figure 3-2. ■ A sample power of attorney for health care plus organ donor form.

BOX 3-3

Code of Ethics for the LPN/LVN

The LPN/LVN shall:
- Consider as a basic obligation the conservation of life and the prevention of disease.
- Promote and protect the physical, mental, emotional, and spiritual health of the client and his/her family.
- Fulfill all duties faithfully and efficiently.
- Function within established legal guidelines.
- Accept personal responsibility for his/her acts, and seek to merit the respect and confidence of all members of the health team.
- Hold in confidence all matters coming to his/her knowledge, in the practice of his/her profession, and in no way at no time violate this confidence.
- Give conscientious service and charge just remuneration.
- Learn and respect the religious and cultural beliefs of his/her client and of all people.
- Meet the obligation to the client by keeping abreast of current trends in health care through reading and continuing education.
- As a citizen of the United States of America, uphold the laws of the land and seek to promote legislation that will meet the health needs of its people.

Source: Reprinted by permission of the National Association of Practical Nurse Education and Service.

BOX 3-4   NURSING CARE CHECKLIST

Accurate Documentation

When documenting, remember the following guidelines:

- ☑ Make documentations correct and accurate.
- ☑ Show the timing and the sequence of actions.
- ☑ Identify the dose, route, and time of medications.
- ☑ Indicate equipment or materials used.
- ☑ Use accepted terminology and abbreviations.
- ☑ Label late entries and continued notes on charts. Provide facts, not opinions.

Note the two examples below. The underlined portions of Example 2 make the second documentation much more accurate and measurable than the first.

Example 1

(date) 0830 Routine prenatal clinic visit. BP 118/64, wt. 142 lbs. Urine negative for protein. Teaching about signs of labor done. M. Penn, LVN

Example 2

(date) 0830 Routine prenatal clinic appointment *at* 34 wks gestation. BP 118/64, wt 142 lbs, up 3 lbs in past month. FHR 152. Urine clear, pale yellow, negative for glucose and protein. 1+ edema in ankles. States she is tired of being pregnant and can't wait for labor to begin. States she doesn't know what to expect with labor. Verbal and written instructions regarding signs of labor provided. M. Penn LVN

health care team discussing legal and ethical issues will need to use critical thinking skills (discussed in Chapter 2 ⚭). The LPN/LVN must practice ethically in all situations. The Code of Ethics for LPNs/LVNs is shown in Box 3-3 ∎.

FOLLOWING SCOPE AND STANDARDS OF PRACTICE

In maternal-newborn nursing, as in any other area, the nurse must know and abide by the scope and standards of practice. Familiarity with a procedure does not give the nurse the right to perform it. State practice acts and facility policies provide the framework for nursing practice. The facility's policies can be more restrictive than state nurse practice acts; however, they cannot be more lenient.

PROVIDING TESTIMONY

When the courts decide legal issues, the LPN/LVN may be required to provide documentation or testimony. Therefore, it is critical for the nurse to provide accurate and complete documentation of the care provided, the client response, and family interactions. Box 3-4 ∎ illustrates the principles and importance of accurate documentation. If the nurse is called to provide testimony in court, professional grooming and behavior will be required. The nurse should answer questions honestly, without bias. The nurse should not try

to protect other health care personnel, but should relate facts as they occurred.

DO NO HARM

Practical and vocational nurses often witness parents struggling with treatment options. Because newborns are not capable of making decisions that affect them, ethical issues in pediatrics are more complex. The underlying principle is to "do no harm." Sometimes consultation with other health care professionals is necessary to determine whether responsibility is limited to care of the infant or includes the wishes of the parents.

ETHICS COMMITTEES

Health care institutions generally have ethics committees that make treatment recommendations or decisions. LPNs and LVNs may be asked to serve on these committees (see Health Promotion Issue on pages 46 and 47). Work on ethics committees would require the nurse to increase his or her knowledge in several areas such as:

- The specific health care problem
- The makeup of the family
- The religious and cultural beliefs of the family

- State and local statutes that relate to the legal and ethical choice of the client

Through group decision by nonfamily members, an unbiased, objective decision can be made.

COMPLEMENTARY THERAPIES

There is a movement toward integrating complementary therapies into health care. Research into the use and safety of complementary and alternative treatments has grown dramatically in recent years. The use of complementary therapies raises some legal and ethical issues. What standards are used to ensure public safety in placebo-controlled clinical trials? What are the legal and ethical responsibilities when health care professionals administer controversial complementary therapy instead of conventional treatment? The LPN/LVN may be involved in this clinical research by assisting with the administration of the complementary therapy and collecting data. It is important for the LPN/LVN to understand the purpose of the research and the legal and ethical responsibilities for reporting adverse client reactions.

REFERRAL TO SUPPORT GROUPS

There are also many community agencies and groups to support the family. Some of these agencies are federally funded, whereas others are privately funded. The LPN/LVN should be aware of community support groups that can help families cope with pediatric issues. For example, local churches or hospice may be the site of support groups for parents of terminally ill infants.

SUPPORT GROUPS FOR STAFF

Many facilities have staff support groups to assist nurses and other health care workers to adjust to difficult situations in neonatal intensive care units and in pediatric care. For example, when a premature infant has received care at the same hospital for several months, the staff may become attached to both client and family. If the baby dies, the staff may need time and a safe place away from work to share their feelings of loss. They may also experience feelings of failure because the baby died despite their care.

NURSING CARE

PRIORITIES IN NURSING CARE

When providing nursing care to a client who has legal or ethical issues, the priorities are therapeutic listening, critical thinking, and awareness of the law. Using skills such as reflecting, open-ended questions, and silence, the nurse can support the client and family to explore their reactions to the situation, whether it is an unplanned pregnancy or the death of an infant. The nurse can practice critical thinking by teaching the family about treatment options and by helping them to shape questions to ask the care provider. In situations such as suspected abuse, the nurse will also know that the law requires a report to social services.

ASSESSING

The data the nurse gathers in legal and ethical situations will likely relate to psychosocial factors. Does the newborn cry constantly and exhibit signs of stress? Does the family argue in the visitors' lounge about treatment decisions for their newborn with spina bifida? Has the teenager been yelling at the staff since she heard the diagnosis of pregnancy? The nurse would document these findings in objective, nonjudgmental terms. In situations that have legal or ethical difficulties, the LPN/LVN would collaborate with other members of the health care team to see that client needs were met.

DIAGNOSING, PLANNING, AND IMPLEMENTING

Some common nursing diagnoses in legal and ethical client situations are:

- Deficient **K**nowledge related to [details, such as beginning pregnancy].
- Interrupted **F**amily Processes related to [details, such as learning an infant was born with cerebral palsy].
- **G**rieving related to [details of terminal illness of the infant].
- Risk for **I**njury related to physical abuse.
- Risk for **V**iolence (parent) related to inability to manage anger.

The expected outcomes for these clients and their families might include:

- Client/family will express a clearer understanding of the condition and treatment options.
- Client/family will confer with social services to establish a plan of care and to obtain referrals.

Nursing interventions for clients with legal and ethical issues are based on the particular situation. The following interventions may apply:

- Always practice within the limits of the nurse practice acts of your state and the guidelines of your facility. *It is your responsibility to learn the laws of the state in which you practice and the guidelines (which may be more strict) of your workplace.*

HEALTH PROMOTION ISSUE

SEXUALLY TRANSMITTED INFECTION EDUCATION

STI Prevention & Treatment

MediaLink

The nurse works for a family planning clinic and has provided sex education in the public school system for 11th graders for the past 5 years. Recently, the state regulations for sex education have changed and her curriculum needs to be revised. She now needs to promote abstinence and provide information about contraception. She will also need to include detailed information about sexually transmitted infections (STIs). She needs to understand her state laws, as well as neighboring state laws, related to consent to care in pregnancy, contraception, abortion, and STI treatment. She seeks the assistance of her nurse manager on this project.

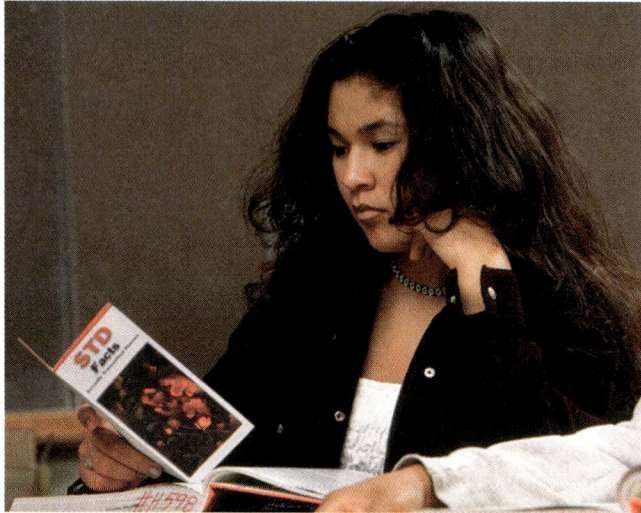

DISCUSSION

There is a great need to approach the issue of teenage pregnancy and teenage STI prevalence. In the United States, more than 800,000 women under the age of 20 become pregnant every year. Nine million teenagers will acquire an STI each year. Although these rates seem staggering, they are down for the first time in many years. Data seem to support the promotion of abstinence in sex education and the increased use of condoms as effective in this decline.

Although the decline is encouraging within our own nation, when compared to other nations American teens still get pregnant more often, have more abor-

tions, and get more STIs. Data from the Alan Guttmacher Institute suggest that American teens do not have more sex than teens in other nations, but they are less likely to use effective contraception and have more sexual partners. The other countries with lower pregnancy, abortion, and STI rates are more accepting of teenage sex but strongly condemn teenage parenthood. These countries also provide greater access to contraception and have more developed sex education programs, including STI prevention.

Sex education curricula should include comprehensive information about physical and emotional changes of adolescence, pregnancy and conception, the emotional effects of sexual intercourse, decision making related to sexual intercourse, the risks of sexual

intercourse to include pregnancy and STIs, and contraception control methods including abstinence. Each state has particular regulations that must be followed related to the content taught in sex education programs.

States regulate whether sex education and HIV/STI prevention is mandated in the school setting. The content is also regulated. For sex education and HIV/STI prevention alike, abstinence and contraception may be stressed, covered, or not allowed. Each state also regulates the parental role in sex education as it relates to consent. The regulation may require consent, not require consent, or allow the parent who is religiously or morally opposed to sex education for their children to ask that their children be placed in another class.

- Become familiar with the laws of your state as they relate to health care. *It will be useful for you as a professional to know more about legal or ethical situations you may encounter in your job.*
- Think about your own values, and imagine positive ways of responding to those whose values are different from your own. Never advise clients to choose one option over

another. *Your job is to provide quality care, no matter what the client decides. Your own decisions and choices must be left aside.*
- Uphold client confidentiality. *Violation of HIPAA regulations can lead to severe penalties. Your standing as a professional and the trust of your clients and colleagues depend on your integrity.*

PLANNING AND IMPLEMENTATION

The LPN and her nurse manager decide that a committee needs to be developed to redesign this curriculum. The committee members are a teacher in the public school system, a physician, a certified nurse-midwife, the LPN and her nurse manager, and several parents from the community.

The community carefully reviews the existing curriculum for age and development appropriateness. They also review the teaching methods for applicability to all learning styles. They take care to include the state regulations for abstinence.

It is decided that all content should be presented in a nonjudgmental, risk–benefit manner. The nature of this content requires students to make life decisions that may be at times life altering. Therefore, a course will be presented prior to this one on how to make sound decisions. The LPN can then incorporate those methods into the content on sex education and HIV/STI prevention.

Audiovisual (AV) aids are discussed in the committee. All posters, videos, and slides are reviewed for age appropriateness and content. AV aids chosen include images of teenagers of this era that are simple and easy to understand. There was much discussion about the use of graphic, realistic images of STIs. Some committee members were concerned that the images would be ignored due to the graphic nature. Other committee members rationalized that these images presented a reality that discussion alone could not afford. The committee decided that the benefits of these slides were important and that the LPN should use her judgment regarding the appropriateness from class to class.

There also was some discussion among the committee members about whether the class should include males and females or should separate them into different sections. There was discussion about whether the female LPN would be as effective with the male students. It was decided that separate classes would be best and that they would hire a male nurse to teach the male students. These decisions were made to encourage students to discuss the issues presented.

The committee was pleased with the final product. They have expanded the curriculum and added a section with a new male instructor. Long-term evaluations will be conducted to determine the effectiveness of this program.

SELF-REFLECTION

What are your personal beliefs about teenage sexuality and pregnancy? Where did you learn information regarding sex during your teenage years? What information do you wish you had during that time frame? Was there any education or support system that would have influenced your sexual behavior during adolescence?

Why do you think the rates of teenage sexuality and pregnancy in America are so high? Do you think the promotion of abstinence in sex education is a good idea? Why or why not? Should school clinics distribute contraceptive devices to students? What is the parent's responsibility? Devise a plan you believe would be effective in decreasing the teenage pregnancy rate. Approach a school system and offer to present this program in the school system.

SUGGESTED RESOURCES

Centers for Disease Control. (2005). National surveillance data for Chlamydia, gonorrhea, and syphilis. *Trends in Reportable Sexually Transmitted Diseases in the United States, 2005.* The Centers for Disease Control website offers several downloads related to STI prevention, including slides containing realistic images of STIs.

Guttmacher Institute. An overview of minors' consent laws. Guttmacher Institute State Policies in Brief. (April 2007). Accessed online. The Guttmacher website provides information concerning state policies and requirements for minors related to pregnancy, contraception, abortion, and STIs.

- Use other members of the health care team as a resource when you are unsure of an answer or correct action. Do not try to answer what you do not know. *Your facility will have a person or persons trained to answer difficult legal questions, or will have referrals to qualified people in the community.*
- Practice culturally sensitive nursing care (Box 3-5 ■). *Most communication occurs through nonverbal "language." By paying attention to cues and showing genuine concern for clients, nurses can provide culturally proficient, individualized care.*
- Always provide quality nursing care using the "six rights and three checks" of medication administration (Box 3-6 ■). *The most common reason for lawsuits is improper administration of medications. Be careful and consistent in order to ensure client safety.*

Ethical Issues

The following situations relate to cultural issues and ethical issues. They have the potential to affect the nurse–client relationship.

- A woman from the Middle East might not want to have a male nurse do postpartum care because of the cultural rule that no one but her husband see her unclothed.

- A Korean mother may be upset when she must consent to emergency surgery without discussing the decision with her husband.

- An African American woman may be offended by being asked to be quiet during a visit with friends who come to celebrate her new baby.

- A Hispanic woman may avoid breastfeeding in the hospital because of the chance of being seen with her breasts exposed.

- A young Vietnamese mother may be reluctant to ask for pain medication after a cesarean delivery.

- An Irish Catholic family may reject therapeutic abortion, even if the pregnancy puts the mother's life at risk.

Think about your own reactions to these situations. What are some of the ways you could help clients make decisions without expressing your personal point of view?

| BOX 3-6 | |

Six Rights and Three Checks for Administering Medication

The most common reason for legal action against a nurse can be avoided by remembering and practicing these safety measures:

Six Rights	Three Checks
Right Client	Compare the drug to the Medication Administration Record (MAR) when removing the drug from the drawer.
Right Drug	
Right Dose	
Right Route	Compare the drug to the MAR when pouring it into the cup.
Right Time	Compare the drug to the MAR when returning the container to the drawer.
Right Documentation	

Source: Adapted from Ramont, R. P., & Niedringhaus, D. M. (2008). *Fundamental nursing care* (2nd ed.). Upper Saddle River, NJ: Prentice Hall, p. 639.

- Be prompt and accurate in reporting any incidents. Remember that the nurse who delegates a task is responsible for the successful completion of that task. Figure 3-3 ■ shows an incident report form. *Prompt reporting can prevent further problems from occurring and supports quality care for the client.*

EVALUATING

In evaluating legal and ethical issues, the nurse would collect data about whether the specific interventions were effective. For example, the client's questions have been answered sufficiently for the time. The parents state that they have met with social workers. The nurse would ensure that reports and referrals have been made, and that written materials have been provided if possible. The nurse would also note any conclusions about treatment the family has reached.

NURSING PROCESS CARE PLAN
Client with Preterm Labor

Jean, a 17-year-old girl, is admitted to the obstetric unit with a diagnosis of preterm labor. Jean has been treated for preterm labor for 3½ weeks. Labor had stopped for 4 days but has started again. The doctor feels labor will progress to delivery of a 24-week fetus. Survival of the fetus is questionable, and the pediatrician believes no resuscitation should be attempted. Jean and her boyfriend have been arguing about what to do. Jean's parents are present, but they want Jean to make decisions about the baby since she and the baby's father are not married.

Assessment

The following data should be collected as soon as possible after admission:

- Strength and character of all relationships
- Knowledge of preterm labor, treatment of preterm infants, survival rates of 24-week fetuses
- Jean's feeling about the fetus and treatment
- Boyfriend's feelings about the fetus and treatment

Nursing Diagnosis

The following important nursing diagnosis (among others) is established for this client:

- Dysfunctional Family Processes related to preterm labor and care of preterm infant

Expected Outcomes

The family will:

- Develop methods of communication and problem solving related to care of the baby.
- Come to an agreement concerning the baby's treatment that is satisfying for all parties.

Planning and Implementation

- Provide opportunities for the family and the client to express feelings and expectations both privately and collectively. *Therapeutic communication will enhance family dynamics and facilitate decision making.*

CONFIDENTIAL REPORT OF UNUSUAL OCCURRENCE
NOT a part of the Medical Record - Please forward to RISK MANAGEMENT

I. (COMPLETE IF ADDRESSOGRAPH UNAVAILABLE)

CLIENT/VISITOR _____ PHYSICIAN _____

MEDICAL RECORD # _____ DATE OF BIRTH _____

ADDRESSOGRAPH

II. DATE OF OCCURRENCE _____ TIME OF OCCURRENCE _____ LOCATION (ROOM OR FLOOR) _____

NAME OF M.D. NOTIFIED _____ CLIENT AWARE OF OCCURRENCE: YES___NO___ FAMILY AWARE OF OCCURRENCE: YES___NO___

REPORT COMPLETED BY _____ OTHERS FAMILIAR WITH OCCURRENCE _____

III. ADMITTING DIAGNOSIS _____

CLIENT CONDITION PRIOR TO OCCURRENCE: ALERT _____ ASLEEP _____ ANESTHETIZED _____ DISORIENTED _____ OTHER _____

IF SEDATIVE/NARCOTICS/DIURETICS GIVEN IN LAST 12 HOURS (WHERE APPLICABLE) PLEASE COMPLETE: (MED, DOSE, TIME)

IV. EVENT

FALLS
- 100 Unobserved Fall
- 101 Assisted to Floor
- 102 Fell from Bed
- 103 Fell from Table/Equipment
- 104 Fell in Bathroom
- 105 Walking/Standing/Slip & Fall
- 106 Sitting Commode/Wheelchair
- 107 Restrained Prior to Fall
- 108 Restrained After Fall
- 109 Bed Rails Up (1 2 3 4)
- 110 Bed Rails Down (1 2 3 4)
- 112 Visitor Fall
- 113 Outpatient Fall
- 119 Other_____

BURNS
- 120 Electrical/Chemical Burn
- 121 Spill
- 122 Fire
- 129 Other_____

ALTERCATION/COMPLAINTS
- 130 Pt/Family/Employee/Visitor
- 131 Complaint-Waiting Time
- 132 Complaint-Billing Services
- 133 Complaint-Food Services
- 134 Complaint-Housekeeping/Ancillary
- 135 Complaint-Nursing
- 136 Complaint-Medical Staff
- 137 Complaint-Security
- 139 Other_____

MISCELLANEOUS
- 140 Suicide/Attempt
- 141 Left AMA/Elopement
- 142 Equipment-Struck/Failure
- 143 Property Loss/Damage
- 144 Unexpected Death
- 145 Non-Compliant Smoking
- 148 Development of Pressure Ulcer
- 149 Other_____

MEDICATIONS   Drug_____
- 150 Order (Computer Entry)
- 151 Wrong Time
- 152 Wrong Dosage
- 153 Wrong Route
- 154 Wrong Drug
- 155 Wrong Patient
- 156 Omission
- 157 Adverse Drug Reaction
- 158 Prescribing Error
- 159 Other_____

INTRAVENOUS Sol._____
- 160 Infiltration
- 161 Wrong Rate
- 162 Wrong Solution
- 163 Wrong Time
- 164 Order (Computer Entry)
- 165 Infected Site/Phlebitis
- 169 Other_____

BLOOD TRANSFUSION
- 170 Allergic/Adverse Reaction
- 171 Delay in Administration
- 172 Incorrect Flow Rate
- 173 Infiltration
- 174 Omitted/Client Refusal
- 175 Wrong Amount
- 176 Wrong/Omitted Filter
- 177 Wrong Component
- 178 Biological Product Deviation
- 179 Other_____

PATHOLOGY
- 180 Reference Laboratory Error
- 181 Lost/Mishandled Specimen
- 182 Specimen Collection Error
- 183 Cytology/Biopsy Discrepancy
- 184 Biopsy/Resection Discrepancy
- 185 Autopsy Suggests Serious Clinical Discrepancy
- 186 Frozen Section/Pathological Discrepancy
- 187 Error Performing Test/Error Reporting Results
- 188 Delayed Draw
- 189 Hematoma Following Draw
- 190 Other_____

OR/PACU/OPS/WOR
- 200 Removal Foreign Body
- 210 Incorrect Count-Sponge/Needle/Instr
- 202 X-rays Taken/Deferred
- 203 Arrest
- 204 Wrong Pt/Side/Site/Procedure
- 205 OPS Pt Admitted Post-Op
- 206 Unplanned Organ Repair/Removal
- 207 Lac/Tear/Puncture-Organ/Body Part
- 208 Canceled Surg-Prep/Equipment Problem
- 209 Unplanned Return to OR
- 210 Surgery Delayed
- 211 Consent Incorrect/Incomplete/Not Done
- 212 Reddened Area
- 213 Unsterile Situation
- 214 Specimen Problem
- 215 Eye Irritation/Injury
- 216 Post Arterial Hematoma
- 217 Improper Discharge
- 219 Other_____

ANESTHESIA
- 220 Unexpected Arrest
- 221 Canceled Surgery After Induction
- 222 Injury/Death Post Induction
- 223 Tooth/Face/Lip/Mandible Damage
- 224 CNS Injury/Brain Damage
- 225 Unplanned Transfer to Special Care Unit
- 226 Aspiration
- 229 Other_____

EMERGENCY DEPARTMENT
- 230 Arrives DOA After Discharge/Seen in ED within Past 7 Days
- 231 Seen for Complication Post Treatment/Procedure from Prev. Hospitalization
- 232 Left AMA
- 239 Other_____

OB/GYN/INFANT CARE
- 240 Delivery Occurred Outside L&D Area
- 241 Mother Transferred to ICU
- 241 Unplanned Return to Surgery
- 243 Stirrup Related Injury
- 244 Delivery Unattended by any Physician
- 245 Blood Loss > 1500 cc
- 246 Cord Blood Gas pH <7.0
- 247 Cardiac/Respiratory Arrest
- 248 Infant Seizures in Delivery Room
- 249 Apgar Score 5 or Less at 5 Minutes
- 250 Unusual Condition - Child
- 251 Infant Injury-skull fx/paralysis/palsy
- 252 Transfer From NB Nursery to ISC/NICU
- 253 Instrumented Delivery-Injury
- 259 Other_____

ADULT/PEDIATRIC CARE
- 260 Unexpected Tx – Higher Care Level
- 261 Significant Neurosensory/Functional Deficit/Intractable Pain not Present upon Admit
- 262 Acute MI/CVA within 48 hours of Surgery/Procedure
- 263 Death within 48 hours of Surgery/Procedure
- 264 Nosocomial Infection Prolonging Stay or Complicating Pt's Condition > 5 days
- 265 Client Found Unresponsive
- 266 Self Extubation
- 267 Arrest – Code Team Activation
- 268 Soft Tissue Injury
- 269 Other_____

TESTS/TREATMENTS
- 270 Wrong Client
- 271 Wrong Test/Treatment
- 272 Treatment Delayed
- 273 MD Ordered-Not Done
- 274 Complication Resulting in Injury
- 275 Computer Entry
- 276 Infection Control issue
- 279 Other_____

RADIOLOGY/RAD ONC/IMAGING
- 280 Complication Requiring Surgical Correction
- 281 New Onset Nerve Deficit
- 282 Reaction to Contrast Agent
- 283 Overexposure to Radiation
- 284 Cardiac/Respiratory Arrest
- 285 Treatment Delayed Worsening Condition
- 286 Unplanned Repeat Diagnostic Procedure
- 287 Monitored Inadequately
- 288 X-ray Inaccurately Read
- 289 Equipment Failure
- 290 Lack of Prep-Cancel Procedure
- 291 Wrong Pt/Side/Site/Prodedure
- 299 Other_____

V. OUTCOME

SEVERITY OF OUTCOME
- 350 **No Injury/Unaffected**
- *351 **Minor Injury**
- *352 **Major Injury/Consequential**

*_SPECIFY INJURY BELOW –

GENERAL
- 300 Delay in Therapy
- 301 Embolism
- 302 Reaction/Toxic Effect
- 303 Death
- 304 Prolonged Hospital Stay
- 305 Neurological Sensory
- 306 Decubitus
- 307 Arrest/CPR
- 309 Other_____

OBSTETRICAL
- 310 Unusually Low Apgar
- 311 Fetal Injury
- 312 Fetal Death
- 313 Maternal Injury
- 314 Maternal Death
- 319 Other_____

SKELETAL
- 320 Fracture
- 321 Dislocation
- 322 Teeth
- 323 Sprain
- 329 Other_____

TISSUE
- 330 Hematoma/Contusion
- 331 Necrosis
- 332 Laceration
- 333 Fistula
- 334 Dehiscence
- 335 Abrasion/Blister
- 336 Swelling
- 337 Reddened Area/Ecchymosis
- 338 Skin Tear
- 339 Other_____

VI. BRIEF COMMENTS IF NECESSARY _____

1004952 (9/01)

Figure 3-3. ■ An incident report form.

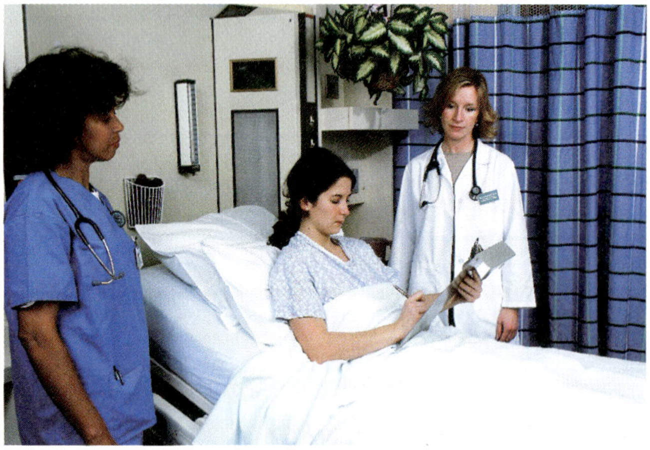

Figure 3-4. ■ Obtaining informed consent is the responsibility of the person performing the procedure. The nurse may be asked to witness the consent signature.

- Promote understanding and empathy among family members and client. *Understanding of feelings, concerns, and viewpoints will promote respect and trust.*
- Encourage family members to set appropriate goals as they work through the decision-making process. *Goal establishment helps the family with organization and provides a framework for decision making.*
- Ask questions to be sure client and family understand procedures for which they must give written consent. Obtain answers to questions if necessary, or report the need for more information. Witness informed consent (Figure 3-4 ■). *If client and family cannot answer questions, they might not really be informed. By asking questions, the nurse can document that they are informed about the procedure.*
- Provide referrals as necessary. *These provide the family with information and assistance as they work through the issues.*

Evaluation

The nurse would review client outcomes to determine whether they have been met. The nurse might also assess the following: Have the client and family members verbalized their fears? Do client and family members verbalize appropriate goals for health care? Have client and family members been in contact with support groups/agencies?

Critical Thinking in the Nursing Process

1. Explore Jean's legal right in your state to refuse treatment for the baby.
2. If other family members are unaware of the situation, what should the nurse do?
3. What type of resources would be helpful to Jean and her family?

Note: Discussion of Critical Thinking questions appears in Appendix I.

Note: The references and resources for this and all chapters have been compiled at the back of the book.

Chapter Review

KEY TERMS by Topic

Use the audio glossary feature of either the CD-ROM or the Companion Website to hear the correct pronunciation of the following key terms.

Introduction
legal, ethical

Legal and Ethical Issues Affecting Adolescent Birth Control and Pregnancy
informed consent

Legal and Ethical Issues Affecting the Mother
abortion, miscarriage, mature minor act, emancipated minors, confidentiality, reportable disease

KEY Points

- Nurses should be familiar with the agencies and groups in their community.
- The infant is guaranteed the same rights as any other client, but it is often the parent who will make decisions about treatment(s).
- Conflicts may arise when the wishes of the pregnant teen are different from the wishes of the parent(s). LPNs and LVNs may seek assistance from the shift supervisor or from legal counsel.
- If any client has a health problem that puts the community at risk, or if abuse or neglect is suspected, the nurse must notify the appropriate public health or law enforcement agency.

EXPLORE MediaLink

Additional interactive resources for this chapter can be found on the Companion Website at www.prenhall.com/towle. Click on Chapter 3 and "Begin" to select the activities for this chapter.

For chapter-related NCLEX®-style questions and an audio glossary, access the accompanying CD-ROM in this book.

FOR FURTHER Study

Critical thinking skills are discussed in Chapter 2.

For a full discussion about care of the family, see Chapter 4.

Abortion is discussed further in Chapter 7.

Loss of a child is discussed in Chapter 13.

Critical Thinking Care Map

Caring for a Client Desiring Pregnancy Termination

NCLEX-PN® Focus Area: Safe and Effective Care Environment: Coordinated Care

Case Study: SV is a 15-year-old female who is 12 weeks pregnant. Her parents are unaware of her pregnancy. SV states she just does not know what to do. There is no way she can raise a baby, but she does not think abortion is right for her either. She is crying inconsolably.

Nursing Diagnosis: Hopelessness related to unanticipated pregnancy

COLLECT DATA

Subjective	Objective
_____	_____
_____	_____
_____	_____
_____	_____
_____	_____
_____	_____
_____	_____

Would you report this? Yes/No

If yes, to: _____

Nursing Care

_____
_____
_____
_____
_____
_____
_____
_____
_____
_____

How would you document this? _____
_____
_____
_____

Compare your documentation to the sample provided in Appendix I.

Data Collected
(use only those that apply)

- Crying
- States lack of sleep times 3 days
- LMP 2-3-05
- Reports breast tenderness and nausea
- 24-hour diet recall: six soft drinks
- No eye contact with nurse
- Current weight: 135 pounds
- States unable to care for a baby
- States family incapable of financially supporting another family member
- Urine dipstick negative for protein and glucose
- Reproductive history: no previous pregnancies
- "My boyfriend says I have to abort the baby or he won't have anything to do with me."
- Concerned father will be physically abusive if he finds out she is pregnant

Nursing Interventions
(use only those that apply; list in priority order)

- Teach client breathing exercises for labor.
- Explore options available to this client and the pros and cons of each.
- Encourage client to express feelings and concerns openly.
- Discuss importance of prenatal care.
- Teach client signs and symptoms of early pregnancy.
- Encourage client to explore personal strengths.
- Encourage client to engage parents in decision-making process.
- Encourage client to register for childbirth classes and a tour of the birth facility.
- Address client in a nonjudgmental fashion.
- Explore client's past successes in difficult circumstances.

NCLEX-PN® Exam Preparation

1 A pregnant 14-year-old girl is seen in the clinic with complaints of burning on urination. The nurse notices two large bruises on her inner thigh. Her stepfather states she fell on the bar of her brother's bicycle. The LPN/LVN should:
   1. believe the stepfather.
   2. call the police.
   3. keep the stepfather's comment confidential.
   4. report the information to the RN.

2 A newborn is diagnosed with hemophilia and requires a blood transfusion. His mother agrees, but his father refuses because of religious beliefs. The nurse should:
   1. side with the mother to save the newborn's life.
   2. side with the father because the man is the head of the household.
   3. provide care for the newborn without taking sides.
   4. refuse to provide care for the newborn until the parents resolve the conflict.

3 Which of the following is NOT a breech of confidentiality?
   1. The nurse talks with her neighbor about a client's terminal condition and the parent's conflict over how to resolve it.
   2. The nurse leaves the client chart open on the counter in the hall.
   3. The nurse talks with the hospital chaplain about the parents' conflict over end-of-life decisions for their child.
   4. An off-duty nurse from the adult unit, a friend of a terminally ill client, reads the client's chart.

4 A 13-year-old girl confides in the nurse that she is sexually active with several partners who are 15 to 17 years old and states she does not want her parents to know. She states she cannot get pregnant because she only has sex during her menstrual period. The most appropriate nursing response would be to:
   1. call her parents.
   2. provide instruction on use of condoms and contraceptives.
   3. tell her she is breaking the law and you will not help her.
   4. ask her the names of her partners so you can call the authorities.

5 A premature newborn is failing despite advanced technological care. His family asks the nurse what to do in planning for the infant's death. The best nursing response would be:
   1. "It would be best not to tell the mother until the baby is in the final stages."
   2. "I will notify the charge nurse and set up a meeting with the entire family and the doctor."
   3. " We only keep babies on life support for 2 days."
   4. "We will let you know when it is time to make funeral arrangements."

6 A mother: "I understand this hospital does lots of research. I don't want you experimenting on my baby or giving her experimental drugs." The best nursing response should be:
   1. "I don't know which drugs are experimental and which are sugar."
   2. "You must sign a consent to participate in research studies, so you can be assured no experimental treatment would be done without your knowledge and permission."
   3. "Only the doctor knows when experiments are being done. You need to talk with him."
   4. "You are wrong; only prisoners are used for experiments."

7 The nurse understands that which of the following are appropriate expectations for clients and families regarding their participation in health care decisions? Choose all that apply.
   1. Complete and accurate health information will be provided to health care personnel.
   2. Families and clients have a responsibility to seek information regarding their medical condition and required treatments.
   3. Health care personnel have the sole responsibility to ensure that families and clients understand their medical condition and required treatments.
   4. Health care personnel are responsible to ensure that families and clients keep all appointments.
   5. Families and clients are financially responsible for health care.

8 The newborn nursery nurse is concerned about privacy issues in the nursery. Which of the following would be of most concern to her?
   1. Crib cards are visible to the public through the nursery windows.
   2. Client charts stay in the nursery instead of on the crib when infant is taken to mother's room.
   3. Procedures such as circumcisions are performed in a closed procedure room.
   4. Consent forms are signed by parents prior to releasing information to hospital website.

9 Parents are debating whether to "bank" their child's cord blood for further use. The mother states "I understand the hospital will store the blood here but we want to make decisions about the use of the cord blood." The nurse understands this is an ethical issue because:
   1. ownership of the cord blood is uncertain.
   2. hospitals do not have any rights concerning human issues.
   3. the child has the right to sell the cord blood.
   4. parents can overrule decisions on all cord blood issues.

10 The nurse is caring for a 15-year-old pregnant female who recently married her 16-year-old boyfriend. The nurse knows the couple is responsible for their own health care decisions because they are considered _____ by the court.

Answers for NCLEX-PN® Review and Critical Thinking questions appear in Appendix I.

Introduction to Nursing Care of the Family

BRIEF Outline

The Family Unit

Theoretical Framework for Working with Families

Roles and Functions of the Family

Family Assessment Techniques and Tools

LPN/LVN Role in Family Care

Family Under Stress

Nursing Care

LEARNING Outcomes

After completing this chapter, you will be able to:
1. Define key terms.
2. Describe the characteristics of family systems.
3. Describe the normal changes a family undergoes over time.
4. Describe the effect of cultural and religious beliefs on family functioning.
5. Describe family assessment techniques such as genogram and ecomap.
6. Identify the role of the LPN/LVN in family assessment and care.
7. Describe the characteristics of a family under stress.
8. Apply the nursing process to care of the family.

When planning care for the individual client, the LPN/LVN must also consider the needs of the family. This is most obvious in the areas of maternal/infant care, pediatrics, geriatrics, and mental health. Individuals rarely live alone or in isolation. The quality of the interactions and relationships between the individual and others is important to the health of the individual. **Family-centered care** is treatment to a designated client with recognition that the family system or unit may also need intervention. The practical/vocational nurse must have a basic understanding of how a family functions and how to assess that functioning. The LPN/LVN must be able to identify characteristics of families under stress and understand when to seek assistance and guidance from the supervising registered nurse.

The Family Unit

What is a **family?** The classic definition of family is two or more people related by blood or marriage who reside together. In recent years, the definition has been broadened to two or more individuals who come together for the purpose of nurturing. The structure of families traditionally is linked to the relationship between parent and child, between spouses, or both.

NUCLEAR FAMILY

The traditional family type is the **nuclear family,** consisting of parents and biologic offspring. At one time, the majority of nuclear families in America were made up of a married father and mother with two to four children. The father was the breadwinner, working 9 A.M. to 5 P.M. to provide for his family. The mother remained at home, caring for the children and completing the household chores. Today, this traditional nuclear family makes up only 23% of American family units (U.S. Census Bureau, 2000), and more than half of mothers live in single-parent households.

EXTENDED FAMILY

The **extended family** was traditionally described as a network of relatives including grandparents, aunt, uncles, and cousins who lived within a 50-mile radius and took an active role in the emotional support of the family. Today, the makeup of the family is changing. For reasons of employment, income, or living conditions, nuclear families have moved away from extended families. Some individuals now include close friends as part of their extended family unit. Individuals may even consider pets as vital family members. It is important to remember that the family, not the nurse or society, identifies its members (Figure 4-1 ■).

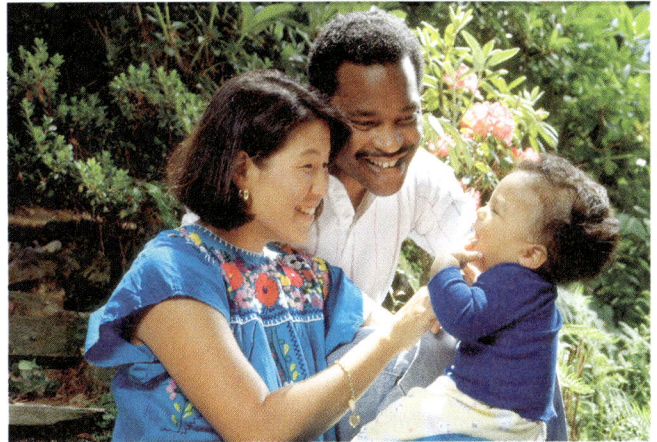

A

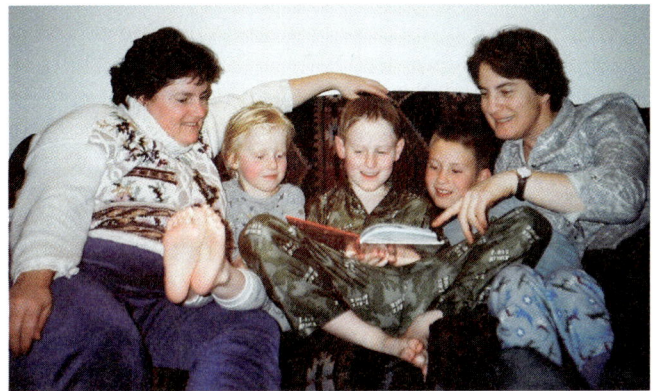

B

Figure 4-1. ■ **(A)** Families come in many different sizes, racial or gender mixtures, and types. **(B)** Evidence indicates that children raised in a homosexual family are at no greater developmental or dysfunctional risk than children raised in a heterosexual family (Ariel & McPherson, 2000). *(A. Lawrence Migdale/Lawrence Migdale/Pix.)*

The dividing of the family structure is believed by many social scientists to be the cause of the breakdown of American society. This book does not address global issues of family functioning. Instead, the functioning of the family in neighborhoods or communities is the focus.

SINGLE-PARENT FAMILY

Today, we see many types of families. With the high divorce rate and an increasing number of unwed mothers, single-parent families are becoming more commonplace. In a **single-parent family,** either a mother or a father raises the children alone. There may be support from extended family, but the second parent does not play an active role. At times, conflict can arise over custody, visitation rights, or restraining orders. The nurse has the responsibility of ensuring the child's safety. Social workers and law enforcement officers may be needed if conflicts could endanger the child.

MediaLink   Defining Family

OTHER FRAMEWORKS FOR FAMILY

The rise in the divorce rate since the mid-1950s has meant that a majority of children do not spend their developing years in nuclear families. In a **binuclear family,** both parents share custody of the children, and the children move between two households. Conflicts can arise between the parents about different rules and methods of discipline at each house. When parents remarry, they find themselves in a **stepfamily** situation; the new marriage creates family relationships between people who were previously in different families.

The term **blended family** describes a situation in which one or both adults have had a previous relationship and children from that relationship (Figure 4-2 ■). Blending of families can cause major changes for children in the midst of other developmental challenges. Often, the blending of families brings greater financial and emotional stability to a family, as well as "ready-made" siblings. The struggle to become a larger functioning family can encourage tolerance and understanding. Occasionally, however, the blending of families results in child abuse (when new parents and children clash) or in sexual abuse (by the stepparent, a stepbrother, or stepsister). The nurse needs to be aware of the potential for these situations.

Guardians, foster care, and adoptions provide a family for almost 2 million children in this country. There is also an increase in the number of families in which grandparents are raising their grandchildren.

Interracial families are an ever-growing part of family groupings. In 2000, nearly 7 million Americans of all ages were identified as more than one race.

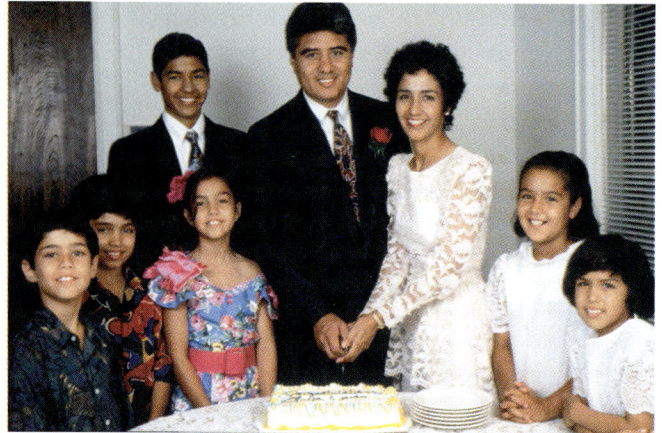

Figure 4-2. ■ Blended families are a regular part of U.S. culture in the 21st century. (Photo Edit, Inc.)

Unmarried partners with or without children form a **cohabitating family.** In the 2000 census in the United States, the number of these families had increased 72% in the previous decade (including same-sex and heterosexual couples).

Many women, whether married or single, are entering pregnancy near the middle or the end of their childbearing years. These older-parent families must consider the challenges of raising children when the parents may develop health issues related to the aging process. Some of the issues that are involved in pregnancy at advanced maternal age are discussed in the Nursing Care Plan Chart starting on this page.

The final family type is the **communal family.** This family includes several adults and children, who may or

NURSING CARE PLAN CHART

Planning for Client of Advanced Maternal Age (Over Age 35)

GOAL	INTERVENTION	RATIONALE	EXPECTED OUTCOME
1. Deficient Knowledge related to advanced maternal age			
The client or couple will obtain information about risks to mother and fetus associated with advanced maternal age.	Provide written information on major risks including diabetes, hypertension, preeclampsia, placental abnormalities, cesarean delivery, premature birth, stillbirth, or offspring with genetic abnormalities, such as Down syndrome.	*Written information allows clients to review information at home.*	Client or couple will verbalize understanding of the health risks of pregnancy over age 35.
	Explain contents of written materials.	*Verbal instruction meets the needs of auditory learners.*	Client or couple will list six major disease risks associated with pregnancy over age 35.

GOAL	INTERVENTION	RATIONALE	EXPECTED OUTCOME
2. Risk for Unstable <u>B</u>lood Glucose related to altered body processes during pregnancy			
Client will be regularly screened for risk of gestational diabetes. Serum glucose level will be monitored during each prenatal visit to the health care provider.	Obtain blood and urine specimens from the client per agency protocol. Share any "stat" results with the client or couple; explain significance of the results. Inform clients who have elevated serum glucose or glucose / ketones present in the urine of the need for further testing and/or treatment. Explain anticipated treatment plan as ordered by the physician or nurse-midwife.	*Elevated blood sugar is the hallmark symptom of diabetes. Insulin resistance has been identified as a risk factor for developing cardiovascular disease as well as preeclampsia.* *Treatment of gestational diabetes depends on the client's blood glucose pattern. Some clients may achieve balance in blood glucose by dietary restriction alone; other clients may need pharmacologic intervention(s).*	Client or couple will state understanding of the impact of test results on the client's own as well as the fetus's well-being. Client or couple will agree to participate in regular screening as advised.
3. Risk for Imbalanced <u>N</u>utrition: More than Body Requirements			
Client's pattern of weight gain per trimester and total number of pounds gained over the course of the entire pregnancy will remain within normal limits.	Provide client or couple with written information on healthy diet, exercise, and weight gain patterns during pregnancy. Discuss the benefits of a healthy diet low in saturated fats and concentrated sweets. Warn clients about the danger of attempting to *lose* weight during pregnancy. Discuss the need for regular physical exercise. Refer client or couple to a registered dietitian. Refer client or couple to visit the U.S. Food and Drug Administration website to learn more about nutrition.	*Middle-age women are at increased risk of natural weight gain due to the effects of aging and perimenopause.* *Maternal obesity is associated with complications such as cesarean delivery, stillbirth, and congenital disorders of the fetus.* *Women over 35 are at increased risk of developing hyperlipidemia, another compound risk factor associated with diabetes and maternal hypertension.* *Older women also have an increased risk of delivering a premature and/or low birth weight neonate.* *Exercise is necessary to avoid excessive weight gain and to maintain cardiovascular health.* *Clients will benefit from further nutritional counseling, especially when dramatic dietary and lifestyle changes are necessary.*	Client or couple will demonstrate understanding of healthy diet and exercise by identifying key features of the U.S.D.A. nutritional pyramid and the servings required daily to maintain a healthy weight during pregnancy. Client's weight gain will be within normal limits throughout pregnancy.

may not be related, who live in the same household. In this type of family, family decisions and responsibilities are shared. A communal family should not be confused with a **cult family,** a group in which a leader makes all decisions and controls the actions of those who live there.

Theoretical Framework for Working with Families

As stated in Chapter 1 ⚭ of this book, theory guides nursing practice. As part of community-based nursing practice, family theories and culture theories are used to determine the health of the family unit. This section briefly examines several theories that are beneficial in understanding and assessing the family functioning.

FAMILY SYSTEMS THEORY

The *general systems theory* was developed by Ludwig von Bertalanffy in 1936. He felt that several disciplines had parallel characteristics that would allow researchers to identify laws and principles that would apply to many systems. With a common framework, researchers could better communicate their findings and build on each others' work. The understanding of systems has evolved to the point that many concepts are part of everyday language. For example, we understand what is meant by health care system, body system, information system, and banking system. A **system** is defined as an organized group of entities that can perform a particular function in the face of change from within or without. The **family system,** therefore, is a group of individuals (as defined by its members) who establish a relationship for the benefit of nurturing, supporting, educating, and providing for the needs of each individual.

In **family systems theory** (a set of concepts to describe the functioning of families in the larger society), the family system maintains a flexible boundary with the world. A **boundary** is an imaginary border beyond which the members of the system come in contact with others outside the system. Boundary maintenance is healthy when the family can adjust the boundary to the needs of its members. For example, at times the family allows friends to visit, have dinner, and interact with the family members. At other times, friends are not allowed to participate in family business. The family chooses when to allow friends into the interaction and when to keep them out.

How well the family changes when faced with problems is called **adaptability.** A family that has an open boundary is able to adapt to problems by accepting new ideas. It can reach out for help from available resources. The family that has a closed boundary resists input and has more difficulty adapting to change. When illness occurs, a closed family's stress increases because it is forced to allow health care providers to participate in family decisions. Even when the family as a whole is not closed, the nurse needs to understand that some family members may need time to adjust to help from an "outsider."

FAMILY DEVELOPMENT THEORY

Family development theory describes the changes the family undergoes over time. Family restructuring will occur several times over the parents' life span. People

have children and form a family knowing that, in time, the children will leave the home. The family unit changes with the addition of each child, the death of grandparents or parents, and the departure of grown children. The flexibility of boundaries with each of these events is expected, although stressful. The maturing of the family unit brings strength through adaptation. The mature family may be better prepared to make decisions than the young family. Therefore, it may need less assistance from the nurse.

For the individual to have a healthy development, the family must progress through predictable stages of a family life cycle. Table 4-1 ■ provides a snapshot of stages in the family life cycle. By being familiar with each stage of development, the practical or vocational nurse can assess the family more accurately and report areas of concern.

CULTURE THEORY

Cultural and religious beliefs have an impact on the interaction of family members. It is vital for the nurse to have an understanding of these beliefs and the importance the family places on them. **Culture** is a style of behavior patterns, beliefs, and *products of human work* (e.g., art, music, literature, architecture) within a given community or population. Patterns of behavior include dress, language, and patterns of person-to-person interaction. Beliefs include **religion,** the belief in a superhuman power recognized as creator or governor of the universe, and other ideas accepted as true or factual.

An understanding of cultural background can give clues to assessment and implementation of care. The nurse must be careful not to engage in **stereotyping** (expectation that all members of a group will think and behave the same). This kind of generalized thinking is not appropriate.

Ethnicity is identity based on common ancestry, race, religion, and culture. Ethnicity is deeply rooted in the family and is transmitted by family values. For example, food preparation and family recipes are handed down from generation to generation. Religious beliefs influence food preparation and avoidance. The specific combination of seasoning, cooking, and presenting the food is part of the family's ethnicity.

Race should not be confused with ethnicity. **Race** is defined by biologic deviations shown in physical features, such as skin color, hair texture, and facial features. People of one race can have different cultures and ethnicity. For example, the Black race living in the African rain forest differs in culture and ethnicity from the Black race living in the southern United States.

TABLE 4-1

Stages of Family Development

STAGE	FAMILY TASKS	FAMILY ROLES	PARENTAL TASKS AND CLIENT TEACHING
I. Beginning family (no children)	■ Learn to live together ■ Relate harmoniously to three families (families of origin and newly established family) ■ Engage in family planning (whether to have children) ■ Develop satisfactory sexual and marital roles	Husband Wife Parent of adults In-laws	**Tasks:** Partners establish patterns of communication and problem solving. Roles at work and home are set. **Teaching:** Nurses should use every opportunity to encourage open, healthy communication techniques. For example, this formula can be used for discussing conflicts: "When _____ [something happens], I feel _____ because _____." It is much easier to problem-solve with a statement like, "When the kitchen counter gets left messy, I feel frustrated because I have to clear a place to make my sandwich," than with a blaming statement like this, "You always leave messes around so that I'll have to clean them up!"
II. Early childbearing (birth of first child until infant reaches 30 months of age)	■ Develop a stable family unit with new parent roles ■ Reconcile conflicting developmental tasks of family members ■ Facilitate development needs of family members to strengthen the family unit ■ Accept new child's (children's) personality	Husband Wife Parent Child In-law Parent of adults Grandparent	**Tasks:** Bonding with the child. Learning to understand the child's cues. Supervising safety and development. Adjusting roles to fit new responsibilities. **Teaching:** Teach all caregivers (parents, siblings, grandparents) methods of holding, feeding, cleaning, and dressing. Identify actions, reflexes, appearance, and behavior that can be expected at each stage. Encourage a calm but watchful response to exploration.
III. Families with preschool children (firstborn 2½ to 5 years)	■ Allow child to explore environment ■ Establish privacy, housing, and adequate space ■ Involve husband-father in more household responsibilities ■ Allow preschooler to assume responsibilities of self-care ■ Socialize children ■ Integrate new family members ■ Separate from children as they enter school	Husband Wife Parent Child In-law Parent of adult Grandparent Sibling	**Tasks:** Accepting child's beginning independence. Supporting learning. Establishing behavioral norms. **Teaching:** Provide information about limit setting, "time-out" sessions, usual attention span of children (e.g., some suggest 1 minute of time-out per year of life as a guide). Stress the value of consistent expectations. Encourage "play groups" that can provide support for both the child and the parent. Support the parents as primary decision makers for their children.

(continued)

TABLE 4-1

Stages of Family Development (continued)

STAGE	FAMILY TASKS	FAMILY ROLES	PARENTAL TASKS AND CLIENT TEACHING
IV. Family with school-age children (firstborn 6 to 13 years)	■ Promote school achievement of children ■ Maintain satisfying marital relationship ■ Promote open communication in family ■ Accept approaching adolescence	Husband Wife Parent Child In-law Parent of adult Grandparent Sibling	**Tasks:** Letting children participate consistently in group settings for education and socialization. **Teaching:** Teach that children need to learn from positive and negative experiences. The parents' role is not to ensure that the child always "feels good," but to help the child learn how to deal with life's ups and downs. The parent should guide but should not make all decisions for the child. Grandparents can often provide useful support and perspective.
V. Families with teenagers	■ Maintain satisfying marital relationships while handling parental responsibilities ■ Maintain family ethical and moral standards while teens are searching for their own beliefs and values ■ Allow children to experiment with independence ■ Begin to become involved in care of aging parents	Husband Wife Parent Child In-law Parent of adult Grandparent Sibling Adolescent	**Tasks:** Recognizing the importance of peers. Allowing the child to make independent decisions and to accept the consequences of his or her actions. **Teaching:** Humor and empathy may be valuable when discussing changes in teens. Emphasize that teens are beginning to view the world through their own eyes, not as they have been taught to see it. Teach that some rejection of parental habits or life choices is normal and not always permanent.
VI. Launching center families (first child through last child leaving home)	■ Expand the family circle to include new members by marriage ■ Accept new couple's own lifestyle and values ■ Devote time to activities and relationships other than with children ■ Reestablish the wife-husband roles as children achieve independence ■ Assist aging and ill parents of husband and/or wife	Husband Wife Parent Child In-law Parent of adult Grandparent Sibling Young adult	**Tasks:** Assisting children to leave the parental home. Adapting to and incorporating people children choose as mates. Readjusting life in the home to fewer people. Parents beginning to take on some care of older generation. **Teaching:** Support parents in considering life problems from a broader perspective and in beginning to plan for their future without children in the home and with needier parents.
VII. Families of middle years ("empty nest" period through retirement)	■ Maintain a sense of well-being psychologically and physiologically by living in a healthy environment ■ Attain and enjoy a career or other creative accomplishments by cultivating leisure-time activities and interests	Husband Wife Parent Child In-law Parent of adult Grandparent Grandchild Sibling	**Tasks:** Finding mutually acceptable ways to keep connected with grown children. Being caring listeners while respecting that children will solve their own problems. Assisting grandparents to adapt to changes of old age or to death of spouse.

TABLE 4-1

Stages of Family Development (continued)

STAGE	FAMILY TASKS	FAMILY ROLES	PARENTAL TASKS AND CLIENT TEACHING
	■ Sustain satisfying and meaningful relationships with aging parents and children ■ Adopt new role of grandparent ■ Sometimes provide housing and/or support for a grown child who returns home	Young adult Great-grandparent	**Teaching:** Support parents to separate from grown children and to explore their own interests. Encourage parents to seek information about activities they can enjoy independently of their children.
VIII. Families in retirement and old age (begins with retirement of one or both spouses, continues through loss of one spouse to death, and terminates with death of other spouse)	■ Maintain satisfying living and extended family relationships ■ Maintain marital relationship ■ Adjust to reduced income ■ Adjust to loss of spouse, family member, or friend	Husband Wife Parent Child In-law Parent of adult Grandparent of adult Grandchild Sibling Great-grandparent	**Tasks:** Welcoming grandchildren. Accepting children's lifestyle and choices. Accepting the loss of loved ones. **Teaching:** Encourage participation to create a bond with grandchildren. Encourage acceptance of differences and a focus on positive aspects of child or situation. Provide information on activities and support groups to keep the survivor from becoming isolated in his or her loss.

MediaLink What Is Cultural Competence?

Cultural family groups are an important consideration in planning and implementing family-centered care. In the United States, there are four main cultural groups: Rasa Latina, Asian Pacific, American Black, and Caucasian. Box 4-1 ■ provides some insight into these cultural groups. Detailed descriptions of all cultural and religious beliefs is not possible within this chapter. However, it is important for the nurse to become familiar with the cultural and religious beliefs of families in the immediate community. Family roles, views, and expectations may vary widely among these groups.

Culture theory describes factors of culture that should be considered when working with families. These factors include:

■ Communication
■ Space
■ Time
■ Role

Communication

Communication can be problematic when the nurse is working with families of a different cultural background. We know that communication includes verbal language and dialect. Yet, more of what we "mean" is expressed nonverbally through touch, gestures, eye contact, and volume of speech than through words themselves. (Consider the rolled-up eyes and sarcastic tone a teenager might use with the words "thanks a lot!" when a parent will not let him use the family car.) The words "thanks a lot" have a very positive meaning. When the nonverbal rolling of eyes and tone of voice are added to the communication, the result has a negative meaning.

Expression and interpretation of communication vary from culture to culture. For example, a person who is raised in a family with Japanese ancestry might not be comfortable speaking loudly or requesting more analgesics, even when in pain. In contrast, a person from a Mediterranean culture might be quite vocal, both about the pain and about the need for more medication. The nurse who cares for these clients must be able to perceive the differences in the ways they communicate. Otherwise, the nurse might miss the needs of the first client and feel "yelled at" by the second.

clinical ALERT

Nursing measures that comfort one person may seem intrusive or wrong to another. The best way for you to know what the client wants is to ask.

BOX 4-1   CULTURAL PULSE POINTS

Major Cultural Groups and Traits

Rasa Latina Group

Rasa Latina families are those whose native language is Spanish and whose religion, most commonly, is Catholic. The family is led by a male head of the household, who is strong but distant, especially with father–son relationships. Mothers and daughters have a very close relationship. In the traditional family, the mother's role is to care for the home and children and to teach daughters to do the same. The Rasa Latina family functions in the here and now. Customs, ethnic foods, and music are important and they are passed on, especially during celebrations. The family may follow native health care practices rather than seeking medical care. This is frequently related to lack of access to medical care. Health care professionals frequently become frustrated with Rasa Latina mothers who are reluctant to make health care decisions, especially for their children. Before she can make a decision, the Rasa Latina woman must often discuss it with the head of the household. (Note: Modern Rasa Latina women are changing. Many are seeking education and job training. Attempts to increase their independence may cause resentment and family disruptions.)

Asian Pacific (or Pacific Rim) Group

The Asian Pacific or Pacific Rim group includes Japanese, Chinese, Vietnamese, Filipinos, Pacific Islanders, etc. These cultures do not have a common language or religion. The one common thread with this culture is the fact that they are not time limited. When Asian Pacific individuals speak of family, they are including many generations of ancestors. The family is a continuation of those who have gone before. An individual who brings shame on himself or herself brings shame on the entire family. Many times a young Asian female who becomes pregnant prior to marriage may be reluctant to confide in her family because of the disgrace she perceives she has brought on her family. When young people marry, they do not form a new family. Instead, the young wife is absorbed into the family of the new husband. Although the westernization of young Asian individuals has precipitated change, many families continue to arrange marriages. Health practices may involve Eastern medical treatment with the acceptance of some alternative medical practices in this country. Asians are more comfortable using Western medicine along with the native health care practices. In the Asian Pacific family, the father is the head of the household. His main responsibility is providing for the family. Traditionally, he leaves all household and childbearing responsibilities to the wife. An Asian Pacific mother would seek medical care for the children and herself, and make decisions in this area independently.

American Black Group

The American Black (or African American) family is traditionally a matriarchal family. This is a result of husbands and fathers being separated from the family during the slavery period in the United States. Today, there continues to be an alarming number of fatherless Black American families. This is especially true in lower socioeconomic areas. Middle-class Black American families are frequently two-parent families. Many of them also are two-income families. Black American children often have the advantage of care by extended family members. Children contribute to the household early on by learning to do chores. They often seek employment as soon as they are of age. Family, as well as the church, is the center of the Black American family social support system. Health-seeking behaviors in the lower socioeconomic area continue to be a problem. Access is difficult, and many Black American children are without a primary health care provider. In many urban areas, hospital emergency rooms have become the primary provider for Black children. This fact is frightening when it is noted that the highest infant mortality rates in this country are in three of our largest urban areas (Philadelphia, Detroit, and Washington, DC).

Caucasian Group

The Caucasian family in the United States has changed dramatically since the mid-1970s. Once the middle-class family was provided for by the husband and father, and the mother was the homemaker and primary caregiver for the children. Now, a second income is often required, and child care is provided outside the home. Caucasian women are better educated than other groups and often seek a career. Women are no longer completely dependent on the status of their husbands. For Caucasians, the "American dream" includes not only a house and one or more cars, but also health care. Good health care is viewed as a right by middle-class White families. They also believe that health care should be paid for by their employer and that they should have a choice in who delivers the care. Caucasian workers may turn down a career opportunity because of benefits that do not equal those of the present job. The White American family differs from other family groups in that individual needs frequently take precedence over the needs of the family.

Source: Ramont, R. R., Niedringhaus, D. M., & Towle, M. A. (2006). *Comprehensive nursing care.* Upper Saddle River NJ: Prentice Hall, p. 457.

Space

Personal space and feelings of territory are developed in a cultural setting. Although the environment can have an impact on personal space, the need to have some personal space is consistent. For example, the person living in a two-room apartment with ten other people still has a need for a small area in which to keep belongings. Personal space also includes the area around the individual. Invading personal space or moving someone's personal belongings decreases a sense of security and causes stress.

Time

The element of time varies greatly among cultures. Members of a cultural group may be past, present, or future oriented. Those who focus on the past generally work to maintain traditions. They may have difficulty setting goals. Those who focus on the present may also have difficulty setting goals and may not save for the future. Those who focus on the future will put off rewards and work today to accomplish future goals.

The importance each member of the family places on time can have a great effect on health care decisions. For example, the family who is focused on the past may not bring a child to the clinic for immunizations to prevent future illness. The family who is focused on the present may be late to an office visit because a good friend dropped by. The family who is working for future goals may have difficulty dealing with a family crisis that causes them to move away from their set plans.

Role

The **family role** (expectations or behaviors associated with position in the family, such as mother, father, grandparent, child) is affected by the family's culture. Distinct roles based on gender may be stressed by the culture and are taught to the children. For example, in some cultures the husband makes all decisions for each family. When pregnancy occurs, the husband would decide between breastfeeding or bottle-feeding. These roles may conflict with the health care provider's expectation that clients will make decisions for themselves.

The LPN/LVN must be observant of the family's environment, take clues offered by family interactions, and ask direct questions to identify specific aspects of the family's culture and religious beliefs. By being aware of the family's culture and religion, care planning and implementation can better meet the needs of the client and the family.

Roles and Functions of the Family

The functions of the family are to:

- Provide economic support for other family members.
- Satisfy emotional needs for love and security.
- Provide a sense of place and position in society.

Roles play an important part in healthy family functioning. Clear roles within a family are directly connected to the family's ability to deal with day-to-day life.

Individual members occupy specific roles. As family members mature, they take on new roles. Children grow, mature, leave home, marry, and become parents. Parents become grandparents. A person's role is always expanding or changing, depending on age and family stage. Family expectations are closely connected to roles. Parents are expected to teach, discipline, and provide for their children. Children are expected to cooperate with and respect their parents.

Parenting styles play an important part in family expectations. Two important factors to consider when analyzing parenting styles are:

- **Demandingness,** which relates to the demands that parents make on the children, their expectations for mature behavior, the discipline and supervision they provide, and their willingness to confront behavioral problems.
- **Responsiveness,** which relates to how much parents foster individuality, self-assertion, and self-regulation, and how responsive they are to special needs and demands.

Table 4-2 ■ lists types and descriptions of some parenting styles.

TABLE 4-2

Parenting Styles

STYLE	CONTROL	WARMTH	DESCRIPTION
Authoritative	High	High	Give-and-take communication; clear expectations for behavior. Children are mature, resilient, and achievement oriented. "We can talk about it."
Authoritarian	High	Low	Highly directive, value obedience. Children show lower internalization of prosocial values and ego development. "Because I said so."
Permissive	Low	High	Parents make few demands, allow children to regulate self, and avoid confrontation of behavior. "Do whatever you want."

Family Assessment Techniques and Tools

ASSESSMENT OF RELATIONSHIPS

Each family member is continually growing and developing. The stage of growth and development of these members needs to be identified and recorded so appropriate care can be given. Infants must meet milestones such as sitting and crawling in order to be prepared for walking. Adolescents are striving for independence, and as a result they may not understand or follow their parent's requests to "be home early." Grandparents, who are becoming self-actualized, take pride in watching their children become parents.

Family assessment is an ongoing process of examining the relationships and functioning of family members. These relationships need to be identified in order to understand the individual family.

The first step in family assessment is to ask the client to identify the members of the family and their relationships to each other. To do this, a genogram is often used. A **genogram** is a diagram of relationships among family members. Figure 4-3 ■ illustrates an uncomplicated genogram. Symbols are used to represent family members. For example, a square is used for males, and a circle is used for females. The client is identified by a double circle or square. Small marks inside the circle or square represent

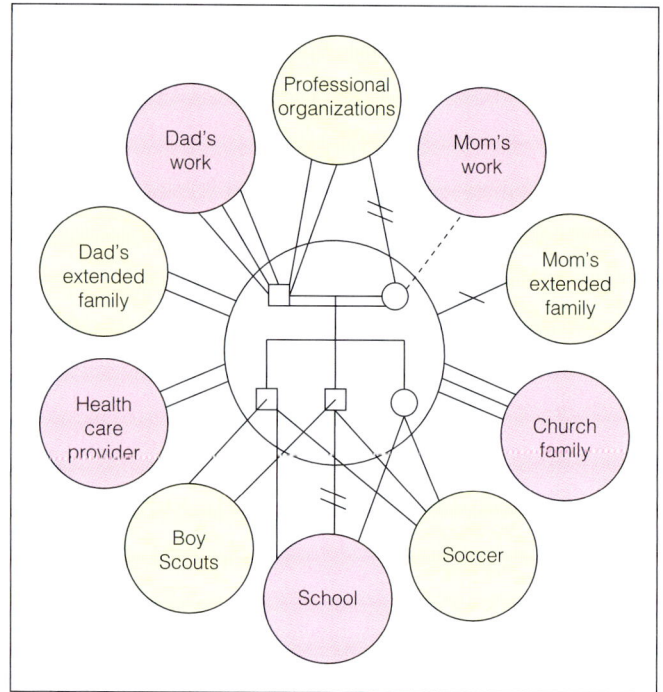

Figure 4-4. ■ Ecomap.

deceased members. Straight lines are used to identify the relationships. Slash marks represent broken relationships, such as separation and divorce. A dotted line is drawn around all members living in the same household. As more information is learned about the family members, it is added to the genogram.

The second step in family assessment is to develop an **ecomap.** An ecomap provides a diagram of family member interactions with the immediate environment. Figure 4-4 ■ shows an uncomplicated ecomap. The family is located in the center with significant people, organizations, and agencies placed in circles around the family. Different lines are used to show relationships between family members and those outside influences. Straight lines represent strong relationships, dotted lines represent tenuous relationships, and slashed lines represent stressful or conflicted relationships.

ASSESSMENT OF THE ENVIRONMENT

Assessment of the family would not be complete without an assessment of the family's environment. A complete environmental assessment is necessary in a community-based approach to nursing care. The practical or vocational nurse assists the RN with the environmental assessment. Only general topics are discussed here.

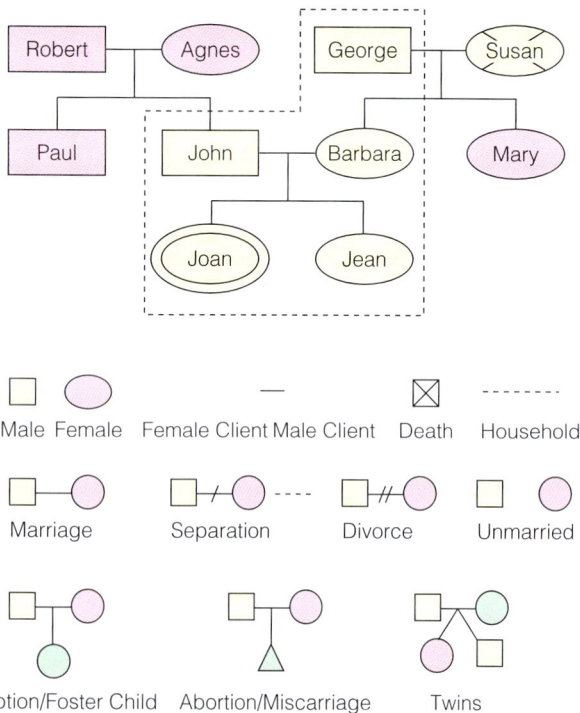

Figure 4-3. ■ Genogram.

When assessing the home, the following should be considered.

Dwelling Type	Own:	Rent:
House	Apartment	# Bedrooms
Year constructed _____ (Note: older homes may contain lead-based paint)		

Condition of Exterior			
Paint/Siding	Intact	Detached	Flaking/peeling
Yard	Clean/trimmed	Unkempt	Fenced
Hazards	Sand box	Play equipment	Swimming pool

Condition of Interior			
Paint	Intact	Flaking	Notes:
Furnishings	Safe	Notes:	
Floors/stairs/railing	Safe	Notes:	
Heating/cooling	Adequate	Notes:	
Lighting	Adequate	Notes:	
Telephone access	Adequate	Notes:	
Water supply	Hot/cold	Notes:	
Cleanliness/sanitation	Good	Vermin infestation	Notes:
Pets	Clean	Sanitation	Notes:
Kitchen	Clean	Water	Sanitation
	Refrigeration	Cooking facilities	Notes:
Bathroom	Clean	Shower/tub	Toilet function
	Towels	Soap	Safety rails
Bedrooms	Adequate #	Clean	Private

SAFETY ISSUES	Medication storage	Toxic substance storage	Toys
Notes:	Electric cords	Smoke/fire detector	Hobby supplies

Figure 4-5. ■ Home assessment tool.

Assessing the home is essential in planning care for children. Figure 4-5 ■ suggests some questions to use in assessing the home. Key areas to assess are:

■ The condition of housing, both inside and outside.
■ The availability of sanitary conditions, running water, toilet facilities, and garbage disposal.
■ The kitchen area, including cooking and refrigeration facilities.
■ Sleeping arrangements for each member of the family.
■ Presence or absence of safety hazards.

Certain aspects of the neighborhood or community must also be assessed. Figure 4-6 ■ offers sample questions used to assess the neighborhood. The major topics to examine here are:

■ Availability of shopping for clothes and groceries.
■ Location of schools and churches.
■ Availability of health care, including doctors' offices, clinics, and hospitals.
■ Opportunities for employment.

In assessing the neighborhood or community, the following should be considered.

Type of neighborhood	Rural	Suburban	Urban	Inner-city
Types of buildings	Residential	Agrarian	Industrial	Combined
Condition of buildings	Excellent	Good	Poor	Unsafe
Condition of streets	Paved Unpaved	Curbs	Sidewalks	Kept up Deteriorating
Traffic	Congested	Stop signs/ lights	Public transportation	
Environmental hazards	Soil	Air	Water	Noise
Population	Young families	Older families	Sparsely populated	Densely populated
Facilities available	Market Shopping	Church	School	Parks & playgrounds
Health care facilities	Doctor office Clinics	Hospital Long-term care	Home health	Other
Distance from home to health care facility				

Figure 4-6. ■ Neighborhood or community assessment form.

The gathering of data in family assessment is quite time consuming. Relationships between family members and the environment change. Although the nurse might think the family is stable with working, healthy relationships, outside stressors can threaten the stability of the relationships.

The nurse will use active listening and therapeutic communication to obtain assessment data. At times, the nurse talks with individual members. At other times, group meetings are best in order to see family interaction. The nurse must always keep an open mind and a nonjudgmental attitude. The nurse's role is not to take sides or show preference to individuals, but rather to facilitate a move toward healthy relationships.

ASSESSMENT OF POTENTIAL ABUSE

The nurse, working with families, must be alert for signs of possible family violence. Family violence includes spousal abuse, child abuse and neglect, and elder abuse. While in the home, children learn behaviors they will practice as adults. In homes where spousal or child abuse occurs, children grow up believing that this behavior is acceptable, and the cycle continues. Abusive parents may have a knowledge deficit about the needs of their children and how to meet these needs best. Abusive parents are often without a support system. They may be alone, angry, in crisis, or have unrealistic expectations.

Indicators of abuse may include the following:

■ Changes in appointments with the health care provider (increased appointments with vague somatic complaints or missed appointments)
■ Depression, attempted suicide, self-directed abuse
■ Severe anxiety, insomnia, violent nightmares
■ Alcohol and/or drug abuse
■ Unexplained bruising or other injuries

Questions that need to be addressed during family assessment are included in Box 4-2 ■. As you recall (see Chapter 3 ⬭), if the nurse suspects abuse or neglect, a report must be filed with law enforcement agencies. The LPN/LVN must also notify the supervising RN or health care provider. Complete documentation of the nurse's observations must be made in the client record.

Abuse in Women or Children

Actions Suggestive of Abuse in Adults
1. Inappropriate laughing
2. Crying
3. No eye contact (may be usual in some cultures)
4. Searching eye contact (look of "fear")
5. Comments about emotional abuse (of self or of "friend")

Questions for Pregnant Women
1. Are you in a relationship with a person who hurts you?
2. Does the person threaten to abuse you?
3. Has the person hit, slapped, kicked, or hurt you since you have been pregnant?
4. If yes, has the abuse increased since you became pregnant?
5. Do you know where you can go for help?

Actions Suggestive of Abuse in Children
1. Failure to thrive
2. Poor hygiene, unclean, inappropriate dress
3. Frequent injuries, unexplained injuries and bruising
4. Dull, inactive, passive behavior
5. Begging or stealing food
6. Frequent absences from school, poor or declining grades
7. Drug and/or alcohol abuse
8. Vandalism, shoplifting

Questions for Children
1. Has someone hurt you?
2. Did they hit, slap, kick, or hurt you in some other way?
3. Are you left alone?
4. Has someone touched you in your "private parts"?
5. How did you get this bruise (and other injuries)?

home, and there may be no end to the parents' financial care of the child. Dealing with such stress can strengthen family ties and promote a healthy family unit, or it can cause additional stress and lead to a breakdown in family unity.

When family unity is severely disrupted, divorce is the most likely outcome. Divorce has become a common stressor for families; it involves all family and extended family members. Although divorce is no longer considered a stigma, it is a difficult transition that causes stress and that can adversely affect the health of family members. The LPN/LVN helps identify signs of the unhealthy family unit and communicates this information to the caregiver in charge.

In most instances, parents use the same or similar strategies to reduce stress that their parents used. Healthy families tend to work together to reduce stress, whereas unhealthy families tend to become defensive and blame others for their problems. If individuals learn healthy strategies, they will use effective communication and problem-solving techniques to reduce stress and promote emotional stability. Unhealthy families, using ineffective communication and problem solving, place blame on others for their problems, causing those individuals to feel unwanted, unloved, and worthless. These negative feelings tend to block communication and lead to additional stress. Box 4-3 ■ lists some signs of an unhealthy family that should be reported to the charge nurse. The Health Promotion Issue on pages 68 and 69 describes nursing care for one client's concerns.

LPN/LVN Role in Family Care

The LPN's or LVN's role is to assist with data collection, report findings, and implement the written plan of care. For example, the practical or vocational nurse can assist in collecting information about family members and can diagram relationships on a genogram and ecomap. When interacting with family members, the nurse identifies healthy functioning patterns as well as characteristics of stress, documents this information, and reports observations to the registered nurse.

Family Under Stress

Many factors can put stress on the family unit. Financial problems, drug and alcohol use, extramarital relationships, and chronic illness of family members are but a few. Chronic illness of family members places a huge, long-term burden on a family and requires many adjustments. The child who is chronically ill may never leave

Signs of an Unhealthy Family
The following signs of an unhealthy family should be reported to the registered nurse:
- Denial of problem(s)
- Active overt exploitation/scapegoating
- Use of threat
- Abandonment
- Drug or alcohol abuse
- Violence including
  - Spouse abuse
  - Child abuse
  - Sibling abuse
  - Elder abuse
  - Parent abuse
  - Gay/lesbian abuse

HEALTH PROMOTION ISSUE

WOMAN AT RISK FOR PREMATURE LABOR

Peggy James, a 26-year-old, African American, gravida 2, para 1, is seen in the obstetrician's office for her initial obstetric assessment. Ms. James's obstetric history reveals her last child was born 3 years ago at 32 weeks. This child was low birth weight and had difficulty with respiratory distress syndrome (RDS). He was hospitalized for 6 weeks. Peggy wants to avoid a premature baby this time if possible.

Ms. James's assessment further reveals that the client is married. She did not finish high school and works 50 to 60 mandatory hours each week in a local factory where she stands on her feet for most of the day. She smokes one pack of cigarettes per day and does not drink alcohol or use illegal substances. Her prepregnancy weight is appropriate for her height. Her 24-hour diet recall reveals protein and calcium deficits.

DISCUSSION

What Is Prematurity?

Prematurity is a live birth prior to the completion of 37 weeks of pregnancy. When considering prematurity, low birth weight must also be considered. Low birth weight is defined as an infant who weighs less than 2,500 grams regardless of gestational age. The extremely low birth weight (ELBW) infant weighs less than 800 grams at birth regardless of gestational age.

In the United States, more than 476,000 infants (one in eight babies) are born prematurely each year. Approximately 10% of these infants die and about 25% will have a significant health problem. These health problems include respiratory distress syndrome (RDS), intraventricular hemorrhage (IVH), and necrotizing enterocolitis (NEC). The babies may also deal with lifelong complications such as respiratory illnesses, poor vision, poor hearing, cerebral palsy, and a host of developmental deficits.

Why Does Prematurity Occur?

According to Moos (2004), 25% of the cases of prematurity are due to iatrogenic causes. For example, elective inductions may be performed based on inaccurate dating of the pregnancy. Twenty-five percent of the cases are due to premature rupture of membranes. The remaining 50% are due to idiopathic causes or spontaneous labor.

Researchers have studied this problem and have determined two methods for predicting preterm birth. These methods are fetal fibronectin (fFN) testing and transvaginal ultrasonographic assessment of cervical length. These tests have proven to be effective in determining which clients are unlikely to deliver prematurely, not which clients will deliver prematurely.

The fFN test measures the presence of fFN in a cervical mucous specimen. The fFN, a glycoprotein, is found between gestational weeks 16 and 20 and then again prior to birth. To obtain the appropriate specimen, a sterile speculum examination is performed, and a sample of vaginal and cervical fluids is obtained. The rapid fFN test provides results in 1 hour; the standard test provides results in 24 hours. This test is not used in a woman whose cervix is dilated more than 3 centimeters, has rupture of membranes (ROM), has had a vaginal examination in the last 24 hours, has a cervical cerclage, has placenta previa, has vaginal bleeding, or has had sexual intercourse in the last 24 hours.

Transvaginal ultrasonographic assessment of cervical length measures cervical length and width as well as the funneling or dilatation of the internal cervical os. Between 30% and 40% of clients with a shortened cervix give birth prematurely.

Who Is at Risk for Premature Labor and Birth?

The following factors place a client at great risk for giving birth prematurely:

- African American ethnicity
- Age less than 17 or more than 34 years
- Low socioeconomic status
- Single-parent status
- Low educational level
- History of premature labor or birth
- Multiple abortions
- Parity 0 or more than 4
- Preexisting diabetes or hypertension
- Multiple gestation
- Infections
- Incompetent cervix
- Placental irregularities such as placenta previa or abruptio placentae
- Anemia
- Premature rupture of membranes (PROM)
- Exposure to toxins such as cigarette smoke, diethylstilbestrol (DES), alcohol, other illicit drugs, air pollution
- Poor nutritional status
- Domestic violence
- Lack of prenatal care
- Stress
- Long work hours (Moos, 2004)

Premature labor can be prevented through prenatal education, smoking and alcohol cessation programs, assessment for domestic violence, continuous prenatal care, improved nutritional status, avoidance of the use of illicit drugs, stress reduction, and prompt notification of signs and symptoms of premature labor.

PLANNING AND IMPLEMENTATION

It is important for the nurse to identify Ms. James's risks for prematurity. These would include her race, her history of a premature birth, low educational level, long work hours, stress, smoking, and poor nutritional status.

Ms. James most likely understands the risk of prematurity to her unborn child, but she may not understand how she can prevent it from recurring. The nurse can assist her in developing a plan for stress reduction. They should explore the option of changing her work assignment so it is not as physically taxing. If possible, she should reduce her hours or break them up and implement rest periods throughout the day.

The nurse should discuss with Ms. James the importance of smoking cessation. Referral to a program with identified success and regular follow-up would be of assistance. The nurse can assist Ms. James in improving her nutritional status and discuss with her sources of protein and calcium. She can assist her in meal and snack planning. If she needs financial assistance, the nurse should make the appropriate referrals.

Finally, the nurse must ensure that Ms. James is familiar with the symptoms of premature labor and understands the importance of seeking prompt medical attention if the symptoms occur. These symptoms include uterine contractions occurring every 10 minutes or more frequently, a low dull backache, stomach cramps that may or may not be accompanied by diarrhea, pelvic pressure, and increased vaginal discharge or fluid leaking from the vagina.

SELF-REFLECTION

Carefully consider your knowledge of the effects of prematurity. Do you consider this to be a problem related to only a specific population? Do you recognize the need to provide all pregnant women with teaching about the effects of prematurity and ways to prevent it? What type of community education could you provide for the nonpregnant woman to increase awareness of the problem of prematurity?

SUGGESTED RESOURCES

For the Nurse

Bernhardt, J., & Dorman, K. (2004). Pre-term birth risk assessment tools: Exploring fetal fibronectin and cervical length for validating risk. *Lifelines*, 8(1), 38–45.

Moos, M. (2004). Understanding prematurity: Sorting fact from fiction. *Lifelines*, 8(1), 33–37.

For the Client

Sears, J., Sears, M., & Sears, R. (2004). *The premature baby book: Everything you need to know about your premature baby from birth to age one*. New York: Little, Brown Publishers.

NURSING CARE

PRIORITIES IN NURSING CARE

When caring for individuals, remember to include family members as well. Focus your care on establishing a therapeutic relationship based on trust. Be careful to develop a nonthreatening, nonjudgmental attitude when family values and behaviors differ from yours. Use positive, supportive words of encouragement and provide a list of resources for family support.

ASSESSING

The practical or vocational nurse follows state nurse practice acts and facility policies to help the RN or care provider collect the individual's data and identify signs of healthy and unhealthy family units. LPNs and LVNs document and report findings to the registered nurse. They implement the plan of care to help the family achieve a healthier level of functioning.

DIAGNOSING, PLANNING, AND IMPLEMENTING

Families cope with health events together throughout their lives. They may be excitedly awaiting the birth of their first child. They may be trying to decide whether a family member should have surgery, chemotherapy, and/or radiation for cancer. They may be exhausted from years of caring for a chronically ill child or spouse.

Certain NANDA diagnoses that relate particularly to families are the following:

- **C**aregiver Role Strain
- **C**ompromised, Disabled, or Readiness for Enhanced Family **C**oping
- Interrupted or Readiness for Enhanced **F**amily Process
- Impaired or Readiness for Enhanced **P**arenting
- Parental **R**ole Conflict
- Ineffective **T**herapeutic Regimen Management: Family

Client outcomes for these diagnoses would address the particulars of the family situation. For example, a family with a chronically ill child with a worsening condition of cystic fibrosis may have a nursing diagnosis of Caregiver Role Strain. The nurse would be sure to inform the family of all groups and services that might be able to provide some support for the primary caregivers. In a new family in which the mother has just had a cesarean delivery, the nursing plan might indicate that the father is eager to learn to help (Readiness for Enhanced Parenting). The nurse could demonstrate diaper care and burping techniques to the father so the mother could get more rest.

Situations with Compromised Family Coping are more challenging for the nurse because they often involve working with family members who are in conflict. The movement from unhealthy to healthy functioning takes time and patience. Once the plan of care is established, all health care providers must be consistent in their approach to individual family members. For example, the nurse may observe a mother who continually tells a child he is "a brat" and "nothing but trouble." The nurse could suggest that the child might listen better if the parent focused on his good attributes and if the parent was specific and matter of fact when correcting undesirable behaviors. The LPN/LVN, working with families in the care of the maternal or pediatric client, has the opportunity and responsibility to promote a healthier family unit.

Nursing interventions could include the following:

- Provide instructions (on topics specific to the situation). *An important role of LPNs and LVNs is teaching and reinforcing the teaching of others. In stressful situations such as health crises, it is useful to repeat or explain information that has been given. This may allow the family to ask questions about the disorder or about treatment options. If nurses do not know the answer, they can either obtain it and tell the family or refer the family to the appropriate professional.*
- Provide a list of support groups and agencies. *Continuity of care includes having information about follow-up after leaving the facility.*
- Support the family in decision-making processes. *The nurse provides information, answers questions, encourages the family to explore options, and shows respect for family processes and decisions.*
- Observe family relationships, watching for signs of abuse. *Thankfully, abuse is not common. However, the nurse must be vigilant in noting injuries or actions that suggest abuse may have occurred.*

clinical ALERT

Signs of abuse or neglect must be reported to law enforcement agencies.

EVALUATING

Working from the care plan laid out for the family, the LPN/LVN would ask questions to determine whether desired outcomes had been met. Progress and unmet outcomes are documented and reported as necessary. The nurse would report any suspicions of abuse to the appropriate agency (see Chapter 3 ⚭).

DISCHARGE CONSIDERATIONS

The nurse should ensure that the client and family are prepared for discharge. The new mother must be given instruction in both self-care and infant care. The parents (or care providers) will need home care instructions specific to the care of the individual child. Printed information should include:

- Use, action, and side effects of medication.
- Use and care of any equipment.
- Signs of complications that need to be reported to the health care provider.
- The date and time of follow-up appointments.
- Name, address, and phone number of any referral agency (WIC, abuse shelters, counseling services, etc.).

Documentation of client and family understanding of instructions should be included in the client chart.

NURSING PROCESS CARE PLAN
Stressful Family Situation

Jean, a 5-year-old girl, was injured in an automobile accident on June 10. She sustained a ruptured spleen, a compound fracture of her left arm, and a traumatic amputation of the left leg. Her parents and baby sister were also in the accident but received only minor injuries. The nurse is preparing the client for discharge.

Assessment
The following data should be collected:

- Family knowledge of extent of traumatic event
- Family knowledge of care necessary for family member
- Coping mechanisms used by the family

- Support systems available to the family
- Resources available to the family

Nursing Diagnosis
The following important nursing diagnosis (among others) is established for this client:

- Compromised Family Coping related to traumatic event

Expected Outcome
- Family members will identify the effect of the traumatic event on the family unit and identify resources to assist with coping.

Planning and Implementation
- Assess past family coping to include strengths and weaknesses.
  Past coping is a predictor of future coping.
- Identify symptoms of family stress to include fatigue, insomnia, and depression.
  Stress symptoms would further compromise family coping.
- Identify support system and outside resources available to the family.
  Support and resources assist with coping. Family coping is compromised by lack of support and resources.
- Assist the family in developing a plan for coping with the traumatic event.
  The nurse provides suggestions and resources and then supports the family's decisions in coping with the traumatic event.
- Offer assistance in contacting resources if accepted by the family.
  Following periods of illness or trauma, families usually require outside assistance in managing these events.

Evaluation
Parents were instructed in care of the wound and given written information about signs of infection or other reasons to contact the physician. Follow-up visits were scheduled. Parents were provided with referrals for physical therapy, occupational therapy, and an amputees' support group. Parents reported that their church would provide dinners for the family for the first 2 weeks.

Critical Thinking in the Nursing Process
1. What information would be important to include in an ecomap for this family?

2. In assessing the family home, what areas would be most important?
3. What community or neighborhood resources should be assessed and included in Jean's care?

Note: Discussion of Critical Thinking questions appears in Appendix I.

Note: The reference and resource listings for this and all chapters have been compiled at the back of the book.

Chapter Review

🔊 KEY TERMS by Topic

Use the audio glossary feature of either the CD-ROM or the Companion Website to hear the correct pronunciation of the following key terms.

Introduction
family-centered care

The Family Unit
family, nuclear family, extended family, single-parent family, binuclear family, stepfamily, blended family, cohabitating family, communal family, cult family

Theoretical Framework for Working with Families
system, family system, family systems theory, boundary, adaptability, family development theory, culture, religion, stereotyping, ethnicity, race, culture theory, family role

Roles and Functions of the Family
demandingness, responsiveness

Family Assessment Techniques and Tools
family assessment, genogram, ecomap

KEY Points

- The LPN or LVN who works with families in an acute-care setting or home/community setting must be alert for signs of healthy and unhealthy family functioning.
- Tools such as a genogram and ecomap are useful in assessing the family.
- Cultural and religious beliefs affect the functioning of the family members.
- By understanding the characteristics of family systems, the nurse can more accurately assess family functioning.
- The family develops and changes over time.
- Identifying the characteristics of the family under stress enables the nurse to make appropriate referrals.

For chapter-related NCLEX®-style questions and an audio glossary, access the accompanying CD-ROM in this book.

Animations
What Is Cultural Competence?

Defining Family

🔗 FOR FURTHER Study

For a discussion of community-based nursing practice, see Chapter 1.

For information about reporting abuse, see Chapter 3.

🌐 EXPLORE MediaLink

Additional interactive resources for this chapter can be found on the Companion Website at www.prenhall.com/towle. Click on Chapter 4 and "Begin" to select the activities for this chapter.

Critical Thinking Care Map

Caring for a Child Following Divorce of the Parents
NCLEX-PN® Focus Area: Health Promotion and Maintenance

Case Study: Ms. Jacobs brings her 7-year-old son, Sam, to the pediatrician's office. She reports that he is not eating, sleeps frequently, complains of a stomachache daily, and refuses to go to school. Ms. Jacobs reports that she and her husband have recently finalized their divorce. She and her ex-husband are finding it difficult to be civil to one another. Sam is living with her but sees his father weekly, sometimes spending several nights at his father's house. His father has a girlfriend who also spends the night.

Nursing Diagnosis: Interrupted Family Processes related to parents' recent divorce

COLLECT DATA

Subjective	Objective
_____	_____
_____	_____
_____	_____
_____	_____
_____	_____
_____	_____
_____	_____

Would you report this? Yes/No

If yes, to: _____

Nursing Care

_____
_____
_____
_____
_____
_____
_____
_____
_____
_____
_____

How would you document this? _____
_____
_____
_____

Compare your documentation to the sample provided in Appendix I.

Data Collected
(use only those that apply)

- Weight 35 pounds
- Bowel sounds active in all four quadrants
- No masses or tenderness noted following light abdominal palpation
- Complaint of daily stomachache
- Sleeping 10 hours plus a 2.5-hour nap daily
- Refuses to go to school
- Parents recently divorced
- Parental relationship strained
- Some days spent with mother, some spent with father
- Father has new female relationship
- Pulse 55 bpm
- Sam's responses barely audible
- Dark circles under eyes

Nursing Interventions
(use only those that apply; list in priority order)

- Assist the family in setting realistic goals
- Encourage the use of stimulation to keep Sam awake during the day
- Refer to community resources as needed
- Encourage Sam and his mother to express concerns and fears
- Explore negative feelings of anger, worry, sorrow, etc.
- Evaluate family strengths and weaknesses
- Administer antidepressant as ordered
- Encourage each family member to try to understand the other's feelings

NCLEX-PN® Exam Preparation

1 A family's 6-month-old son has been diagnosed with cystic fibrosis. In assessing the dynamic of this family, the nurse completes a genogram. This assessment tool is useful in:

1. understanding the family member's relationships in the community.
2. understanding the relationships of family members.
3. identifying the genetic link for cystic fibrosis.
4. identifying the physical characteristics of family members.

2 A family of five is new to the area. They have come to the health clinic for an introductory visit. To understand each family member's relationship to the community, the nurse would complete the assessment tool called a _____.

3 A Chinese family is in the United States as tourists when their 10-year-old daughter develops appendicitis and requires emergency surgery. The emergency room nurse notes that the child's mother never makes eye contact with the doctor. The nurse should:

1. request that the woman look at the doctor when spoken to.
2. understand the behavior is consistent with her culture.
3. ignore the mother and ask the doctor to speak with the father.
4. determine that this behavior could indicate guilt over child abuse, and contact social services.

4 A pediatric client is discharged following an acute episode of muscular dystrophy. You have been asked by the RN to make a home visit and collect data for an environmental assessment. Choose the following assessments that would be appropriate.

1. lawn maintenance
2. condition of the floors
3. exterior color
4. number of televisions and their locations
5. availability of hot and cold water

5 A young child has leukemia. The mother says to you, "I just need to pray with my minister in order to make my child well." The most appropriate response would be:

1. "The medicine ordered by the doctor will make your child well."
2. "Why do you think only prayer will make your child well?"
3. "May I call your minister for you?"
4. "When your child goes home, you can take your child to church."

6 It is important to be aware of a family's religion and culture because:

1. differences in care should not be based on culture or religion.
2. aspects of care might be adapted to meet cultural and religious beliefs.
3. reimbursement is based on cultural and religious beliefs.
4. some cultures and religious groups are more numerous than others.

7 Which of the following statements would indicate that the family is coping well and does not need additional help?

1. "People tell us we need help since the death of our children, but we are fine."
2. "It is nice having my aunt and uncle living so close. We talk with them daily, and they have been so supportive."
3. "If my wife had been home like a good wife should be, the house would not have burned down! It is her fault!"
4. "Look missy, you might be 16, but I'm your dad and if you try sneaking out again, you won't live to be 17. Do you hear me?"

8 If the LPN/LVN suspects that the family is under undue stress, he or she should:

1. set up a meeting with a family counselor.
2. meet with the family as a group to solve the problem.
3. tell the supervising RN.
4. ignore the problem; it is not your concern.

9 A mother and father ask the nurse why she is so interested in how their family functions. The nurse responds:

1. "I'm very interested in the differences between families. I like to compare notes."
2. "I have a responsibility to identify factors that might affect the health of a child."
3. "I have a legal responsibility to search out illegal behavior and alert the police."
4. "I am the only person trained to search out wrongdoing."

10 An LPN/LVN, caring for a child with a progressive terminal illness, is looking for local resources to help a family that needs financial support. Choose the interventions that would be appropriate.

1. Perform a web search.
2. Look in the local yellow pages.
3. Contact social services.
4. Take a quick survey of other patients.
5. Consult with the registered nurse.

Answers for NCLEX-PN® Review and Critical Thinking questions appear in Appendix I.

Thinking Strategically About...

You are an LPN/LVN employed by a home health agency. At 0800, you arrive at the office to receive your assignment. You are expected to visit the clients on your assignment and report to the supervising RN by telephone. You can organize your time as you choose. The clients are all within a 3-mile radius of the home health agency office.

The first client, Jenny, is a 23-year-old married woman who is 35 weeks pregnant with twins. Last week, Jenny experienced preterm labor that was controlled with medication. After 3 days, she was discharged with orders to remain in bed, bathroom privileges only for elimination, and medication every 6 hours. You are to take Jenny's blood pressure, monitor the fetal heart rate, and monitor uterine contractions for 30 minutes. Jenny has many questions about preparing the house for the arrival of the twins.

Your second client is 18-year-old Marie. She delivered her first baby, Jason, 3 days ago. She is not married, has limited financial resources, and has few close friends. She was discharged from the hospital yesterday. She requested a visit from the home health nurse because she has never taken care of a baby and is unsure of herself.

Your third client is Kumiko Hirota, a 17-year-old single woman who delivered a stillborn infant 3 days ago. She is staying with her parents, who practice traditional Japanese customs. Because the infant was delivered at 8 months gestation, a funeral is being planned. The nurse is to complete a postpartum assessment and to assess how the family is coping with the situation.

CRITICAL THINKING

- Using the standard of critical thinking called *depth*, decide what questions should be asked of Kumiko in your assessment of her coping within the Japanese culture?
- Using the standard of critical thinking called *breadth*, what questions should be asked of Jenny in your assessment of her house?
- When visiting Marie, what questions should be asked to determine the risk of her abusing the infant?

COLLABORATIVE CARE

- What agency should Marie be referred to that will provide support and monitoring of this young family?
- What support groups might be helpful for Kumiko?

MANAGEMENT OF CARE AND PRIORITIES IN NURSING CARE

- In what order will you visit these clients?
- What is your rationale for prioritizing care?

DELEGATING

- Is there any care of these three women that could be delegated to a CNA or family members?
- How would you determine that the delegated care has been performed appropriately?

COMMUNICATION AND CLIENT TEACHING

- How would you identify what instruction and supervision needs to be provided to Marie?
- What instruction should be given to Jenny's family about environmental safety?

DOCUMENTING AND REPORTING

- After you have assessed Marie and her baby, if you believe she is at a high risk for neglecting him, what should you do?
- What would you report about Kumiko and her family interaction?

CULTURAL CARE STRATEGIES

- If Marie is of Hispanic origin, what aspects of her culture should be taken into consideration when planning care for her?
- What aspects of Japanese culture, if any, should be taken into consideration when communicating with Kumiko and her family?

Reproductive and Health Issues

UNIT II

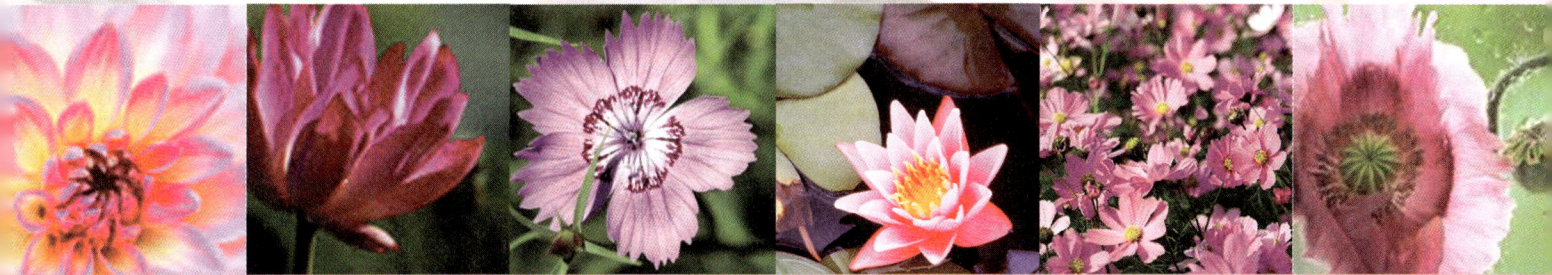

Chapter 5

Reproductive Anatomy and Physiology

BRIEF Outline

Chromosomes and Genes
Male Reproductive System

Female Reproductive System
Nursing Care

LEARNING Outcomes

After completing this chapter, you will be able to:

1. Define key terms.
2. Explain the developmental steps of spermatogenesis and oogenesis.
3. Describe basic information about genes in relation to reproduction.
4. List the essential and accessory organs of the male and female reproductive systems.
5. Describe the general function of each organ of the male and female reproductive systems.
6. Discuss the primary functions of the sex hormones.
7. Discuss the phases of the menstrual cycle, and correlate each with physical changes during a 28-day cycle.
8. Explain the process of lactation.

New human life results from the equal contribution of two parent cells, one from the father and the other from the mother. In both men and women, the reproductive systems have adapted to the specific functions of **gamete** (sex cell) formation and fertilization. (Sex cell formation, or **gametogenesis,** is illustrated in Figure 5-1 ■ .) The female body also has mechanisms for fetal (infant) development and birth.

Male and female infants are not equipped at birth for reproduction. Instead, at about 12 years in females and about 14 years in males, they enter a period of transition and sexual maturation called **puberty.** At puberty, hormonal changes occur that cause the reproductive organs to begin functioning. The external changes of puberty signal

that maturation is occurring. Some of these changes are addressed in the Assessing section of the chapter.

This chapter reviews the normal anatomy and physiology of the male and female reproductive systems.

Chromosomes and Genes

The genetic makeup of each parent plays a critical role in reproduction. The genetic coding carried by gametes from the father and mother creates a unique combination in each fertilized egg. The results can be seen in the variety of individuals who are born from one set of parents. Genetic coding is determined by a person's chromosomes. **Chromosomes** are structures made of DNA and protein that govern

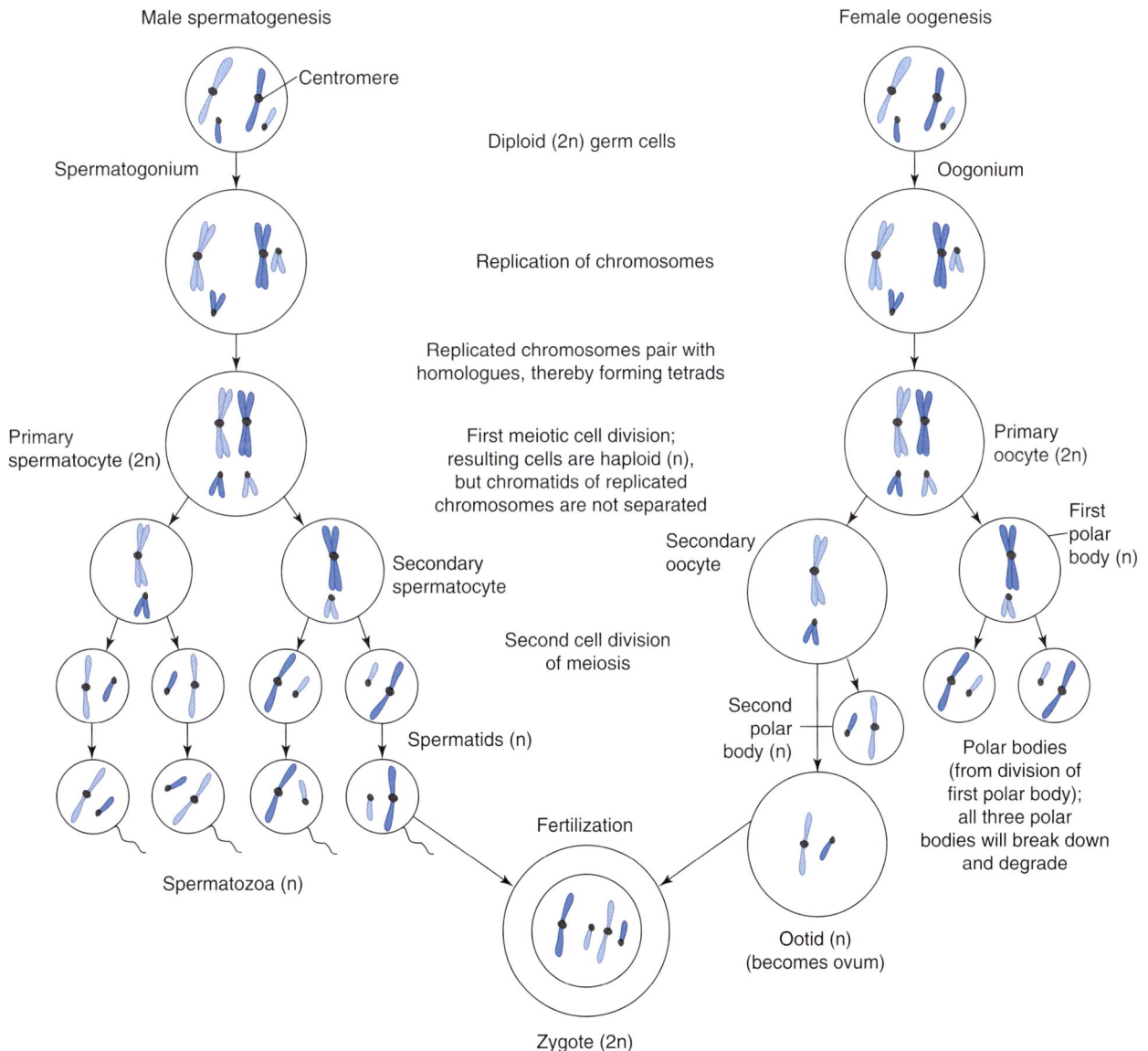

Figure 5-1. ■ Gametogenesis involves meiosis within the ovaries and testicles. (Female) During meiosis, each oogonium produces a single haploid ovum, once cytoplasm moves into the polar bodies. The three polar bodies that remain once the egg is formed are broken down. (Male) Each spermatogonium, in contrast, produces four haploid spermatozoa. When fertilization occurs, they form a zygote. (Pearson Education/PH College.)

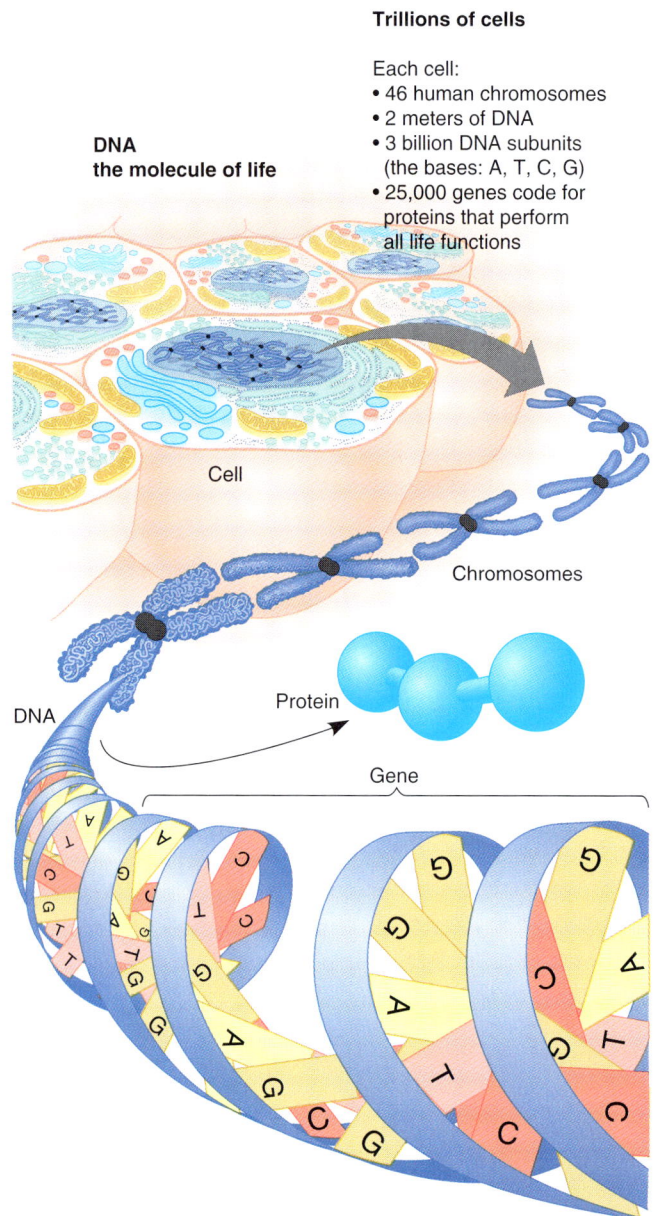

development of an organism. Figure 5-2A ■ and B ■ show a normal set of female and male chromosomes. Abnormalities in the genetic structure of chromosomes can cause lifelong conditions such as Down syndrome (Figure 5-2C ■). In humans, there are 23 sets with 2 chromosomes in each set, for a total of 46 chromosomes.

Genetic information is contained in DNA's pairs of chemical components (bases). These four proteins (adenine and thymine; guanine and cytosine) form pairs creating the "twisted ladder" appearance associated with DNA. Figure 5-3 ■ illustrates structures from chromosomes down to base pairs of protein in DNA.

Trillions of cells

Each cell:
• 46 human chromosomes
• 2 meters of DNA
• 3 billion DNA subunits (the bases: A, T, C, G)
• 25,000 genes code for proteins that perform all life functions

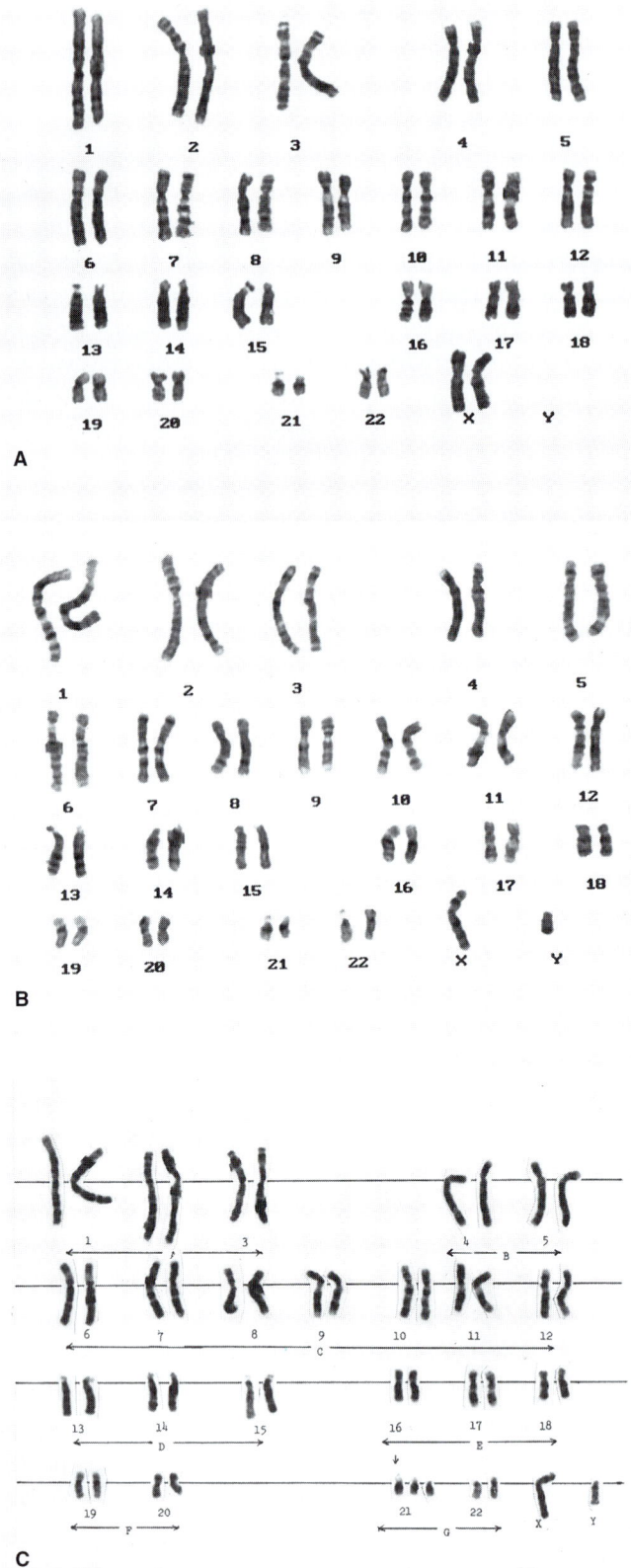

Figure 5-2. ■ (**A**) Normal female sets of genes (karyotype). (**B**) Normal male karyotype. (**C**) Karyotype of a male who has trisomy 21, Down syndrome. Note that position 21 has one extra chromosome. (**A**, **B**: Courtesy of David Peakman, Reproductive Genetic Center, Denver, CO. **C**: Courtesy of Dr. Arthur Robinson, National Jewish Hospital and Research Center, Denver, CO.)

Figure 5-3. ■ Expanding view from DNA strand to chromosome. Each cell nucleus throughout the body contains the genes, DNA, and chromosomes that make up the majority of an individual's genome. The remaining portion of the human genome is in the mitochondria.

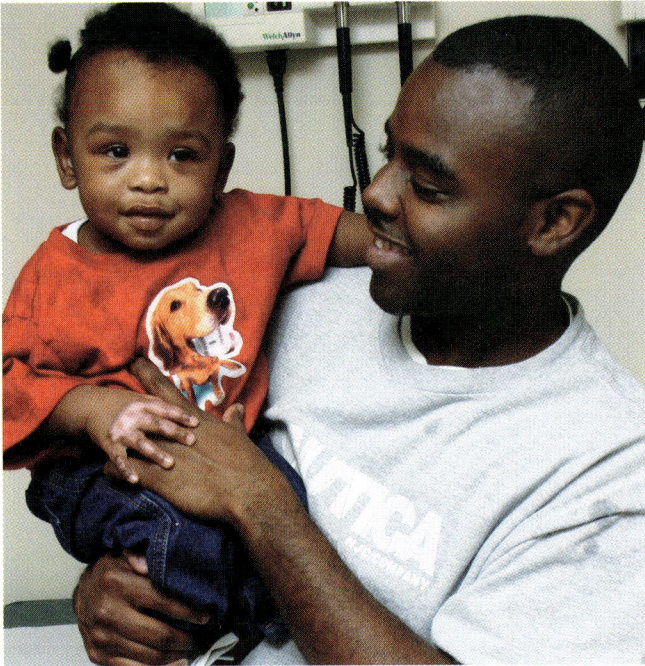

Figure 5-4. ■ Transmission of traits. Children manifest physical characteristics related to their racial or ethnic groups.

The DNA sequence is the unique side-by-side arrangement of bases along the DNA strand. The pattern created by the DNA sequence determines the development of each organism with its own special traits. The DNA sequence determines both the physical traits of a person (Figure 5-4 ■) and the person's basic state of health or disease. Figure 5-5 ■ shows how disease can be passed through a person's genes.

U.S. HUMAN GENOME PROJECT

In 2003, the U.S. Human Genome Project, a long-term project to create the first complete human genetic map, was completed. The human **genome** (our organism's complete set of DNA) contains approximately 3 billion base pairs. (In contrast, the smallest known genome for a free-living organism, the genome for bacteria, contains about 600,000 DNA base pairs.) All organisms are related through similarities in DNA sequences. Therefore, insights gained from nonhuman genomes often lead to new knowledge about human biology.

Some stretches of DNA are unstable and "transposable" (i.e., they can move around, on, and between chromosomes). In fact, nearly half of the human genome is composed of transposable elements (**transposons** or jumping DNA). Scientists now believe that transposons may be linked to some genetic disorders such as hemophilia, leukemia, and breast cancer (U.S. Department of Energy, 2004).

The U.S. Human Genome Project has fueled hope that many inherited diseases may some day be cured. As mentioned in Chapter 3 ⊙⊙, it has also raised some

MediaLink   Human Genome Project

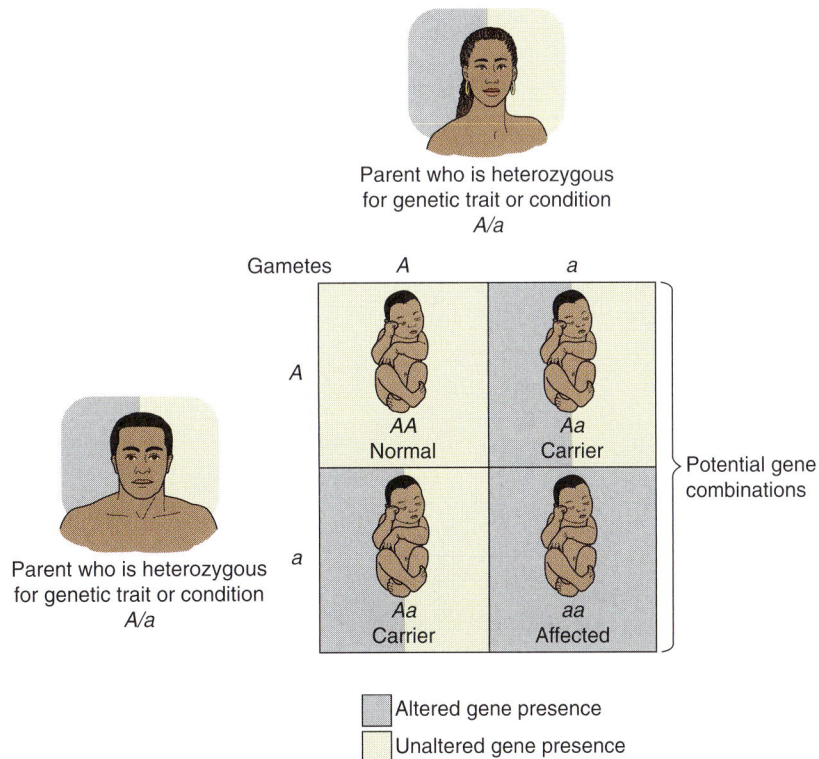

Figure 5-5. ■ Example of transmission of disease. Punnett square shows potential gene combinations (genotypes) and resulting phenotypes of children from parent genotypes with an autosomal recessive altered gene. These are possible genotypes/phenotypes for each pregnancy. Phenotypes are expressed (affected) when a male or female has two copies of the gene alteration.

Superficial inguinal ring (end of inguinal canal)
Spermatic cord
External spermatic fascia
Vas deferens
Autonomic nerve fibers
Testicular artery
Epididymis
Testis

Penis (transection)
Midline septum of scrotum
Cremaster muscle
Superficial fascia containing dartos muscle
Skin

A

ethical questions about the effects of such research. On the one hand, DNA examination may help people who want to identify their heritage and their racial background or ethnicity (U.S. Department of Energy, 2005). However, information may also be used by insurance companies or health care providers to select or to reject customers based on the likelihood of disease (National Institutes of Health, 2005).

Male Reproductive System

ESSENTIAL ORGANS

The essential organs of the male reproductive system are the pair of gonads or **testes.** The testes, formed in the lower abdomen, descend into the scrotum prior to birth. The testes are responsible for production of male hormones and sperm. Figure 5-6 ■ illustrates the structure of the testes.

The environment of the testes is about 3°F (1°C) lower than normal body temperature. This cooler temperature is necessary for normal sperm development. Each testis is egg shaped, approximately 1½ in. long by 1 in. wide (3 cm × 2.5 cm or about the size of a walnut).

clinical ALERT

Testicular cancer is most common in young men. At puberty, adolescent boys should be taught to perform regular self-examination of the testes. Any enlargement or masses should be reported to the care provider. See Procedure 7-2 ⬭, which describes steps in performing a testicular self-examination (TSE).

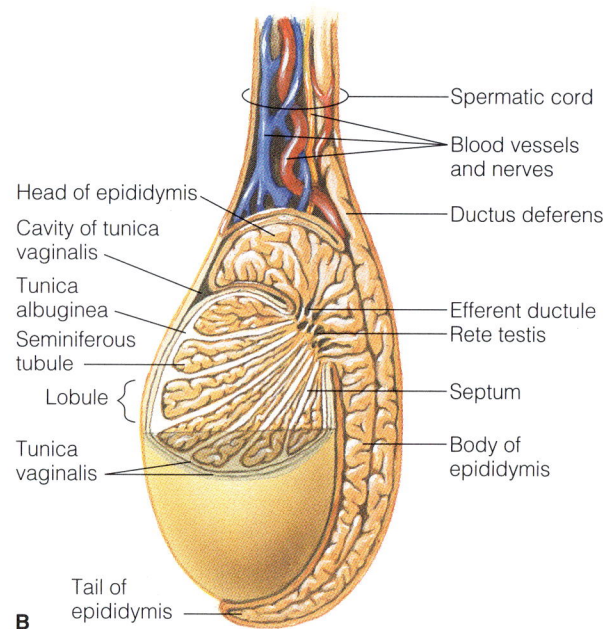

Head of epididymis
Cavity of tunica vaginalis
Tunica albuginea
Seminiferous tubule
Lobule {
Tunica vaginalis

Spermatic cord
Blood vessels and nerves
Ductus deferens
Efferent ductule
Rete testis
Septum
Body of epididymis

Tail of epididymis
B

Figure 5-6. ■ The testes. (**A**) Frontal view. (**B**) Sagittal view showing interior anatomy.

Covering the front and sides of the testes and epididymis is the **tunica vaginalis testis.** This serous membrane is composed of the *parietal* (outer) layer and the *visceral* (inner) layer). Underneath the visceral layer is the tunica albuginea. The **tunica albuginea** covers the outside of the testes and forms the septum between the many sections or lobules. Each lobule consists of long narrow coiled tubes called **seminiferous tubules.** Sperm are produced in the walls of the seminiferous tubules and are released into the lumen to begin their journey to the outside. Specialized interstitial cells located between the septum and seminiferous tubules produce the male hormone testosterone (see Figure 5-6).

Spermatogenesis, sperm production, begins at puberty. Although sperm production slows with age, it continues uninterrupted until death. Shortly before puberty, **spermatogonia** (sperm precursor or stem cells) increase in number by the process of mitosis. As you can see in Figure 5-1, mitosis results in two "daughter cells" identical to the "parent" cell, each containing 46 chromosomes (23 pair).

When the boy enters puberty, the anterior pituitary gland releases **follicle-stimulating hormone** (FSH). Spermatogonia that undergo cell division under the influence of FSH produce two "daughter" cells—each containing 46 chromosomes. One daughter cell remains a spermatogonium; the other develops into a specialized **primary spermatocyte.** The primary spermatocyte divides once by mitosis and then by meiosis. You will recall that in meiosis, the DNA is not replicated; the cells resulting from that division contain 23 chromosomes (one-half of each pair). The result of the meiotic division is four **spermatids** that will develop into sperm.

Of the 46 chromosomes in humans, 22 pair (44 chromosomes) are **autosomes** (alike in males and females), and 1 pair consists of sex chromosomes. Males have an Xy pair, and females have an XX pair. During sperm formation, two spermatids will have the X chromosome, and two will have the y chromosome.

Mature **spermatozoa** (sperm cells) are among the smallest and most highly specialized cells in the body (Figure 5-7). The characteristics the infant will inherit from the father are condensed in the genetic material located in the head of the sperm. The genetic material from both father and mother will fuse if successful fertilization occurs.

For fertilization to occur, sperm deposited in the vagina during ejaculation must move through the female reproductive system and penetrate the outer membrane of the ovum (egg). Note in Figure 5-7 that the head of the sperm is covered by the **acrosome,** a specialized structure containing enzymes that can break down the covering of the ovum. Each sperm also has a midpiece with mitochondria to provide energy for the sperm. A tail moves, propelling the sperm in a "swimming" motion through the female reproductive ducts.

In addition to sperm production, the testes are responsible for the production of testosterone. **Testosterone,** produced in the interstitial cells, is a hormone that causes:

■ Development of male accessory organs.
■ Greater muscle mass and strength.
■ Masculine characteristics such as a deep voice and body hair.

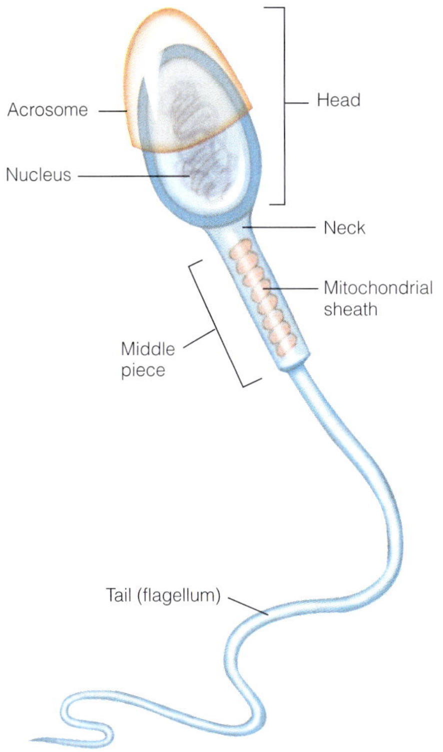

Figure 5-7. ■ Structure of a mature sperm cell.

ACCESSORY ORGANS

The male accessory organs consist of a series of ducts, supportive glands, and external genitalia (Figure 5-8 ■). Each component is discussed separately.

Reproductive Ducts

Located on top of each testis, the **epididymis** consists of a single tightly coiled tube approximately 20 feet long. Here the sperm mature and develop the ability to move. Upon leaving the epididymis, the sperm travel through the **vas deferens** or **ductus deferens.** The **spermatic cord** comprises the vas deferens, blood vessels, and nerves. The spermatic cord passes out of the scrotum, through the inguinal

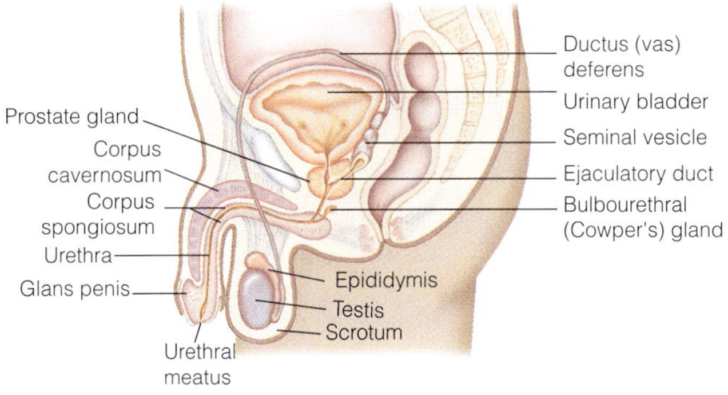

Figure 5-8. ■ Male reproductive organs.

canal, and into the abdominal cavity. It circles the urinary bladder and joins the duct from the seminal vesicle to form the **ejaculatory duct.** The ejaculatory duct passes through the substance of the prostate gland, allowing sperm to empty into the **urethra** and pass through the penis to the exterior at the external urinary meatus.

Infection or inflammation of these structures is described as the gland + -*itis* (e.g., epididymitis or prostatitis).

Accessory Reproductive Glands

Semen or **seminal fluid** is the term used to describe the mixture of sperm and fluid from the reproductive glands. The two **seminal vesicles** are located under and behind the urinary bladder. The seminal vesicles produce a thick, yellowish fluid rich in fructose. This part of the seminal fluid helps provide a source of energy for the highly mobile sperm. The **prostate** gland is a doughnut-shaped gland located just below the urinary bladder (see Figure 5-8). The urethra passes through the center of the prostate gland. The prostate produces a thin milky fluid that helps activate the sperm and maintain their motility.

clinical ALERT

Adult men are encouraged to have regular prostate examinations, including a test for prostate-specific antigen (PSA). They should report any urinary or sexual difficulty to their care provider.

The two **bulbourethral glands** or **Cowper's glands** are located below the prostate. These glands secrete a mucus-like fluid into the penile section of the urethra. This alkaline fluid helps neutralize the acid environment of the urethra and lubricate the end of the penis. Review Figure 5-8 to view the location of these accessory glands.

External Genitalia

The external male genitalia consist of the penis and scrotum. The **penis** is the male organ of copulation or sexual intercourse. The shaft of the penis comprises three separate columns of erectile tissue: one corpus spongiosum, which surrounds the urethra, and two corpora cavernosa, which are along the anterior surface of the penis. During sexual arousal, this tissue engorges with blood, causing the penis to become erect.

The distal end of the penis is the enlarged **glans.** It is encased by loose-fitting, retractable skin called the **foreskin** or **prepuce.** The urethra opens in the center of the glans. Surgical removal of the foreskin is called **circumcision** (see discussion in Chapter 17 🔗).

The **scrotum** is a skin-covered pouch suspended from the groin. Internally, the scrotum is divided by a septum. The scrotum contains the testes, epididymis, and lower end of the vas deferens at the beginning of the spermatic cords.

Female Reproductive System

ESSENTIAL ORGANS

The essential organs of the female reproductive system are the two ovaries (Figure 5-9 ■). Each ovary is the size and shape of a large almond and weighs about 3 grams. Suspended by ligaments in the pelvic cavity on either side of the uterus, the ovaries have a wrinkled appearance. About 1 million **ovarian follicles** are embedded under the surface of each ovary of a newborn girl. Each ovarian follicle contains an **oocyte**, or immature sex cell. By the time the girl reaches

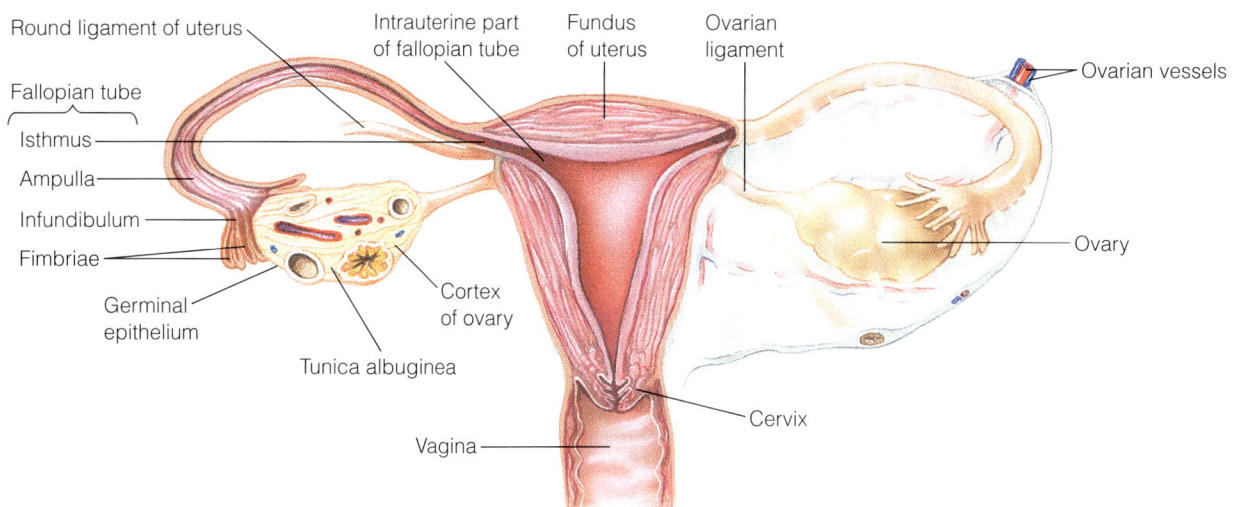

Figure 5-9. ■ Fallopian tubes and ovaries.

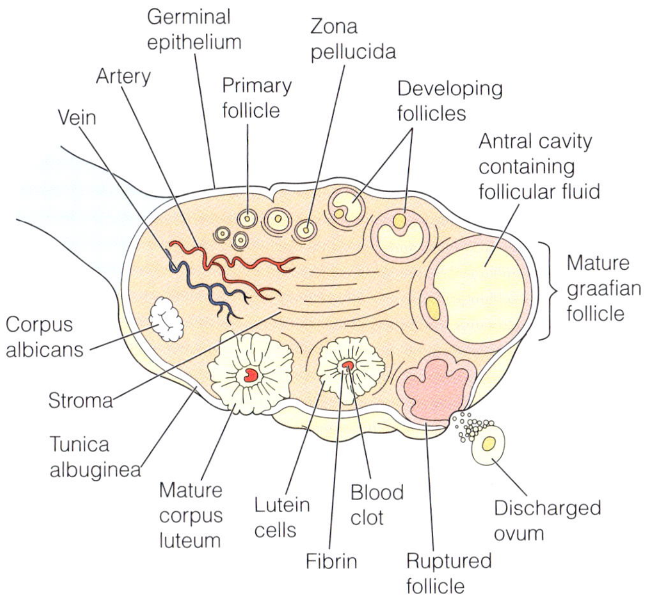

Figure 5-10. ■ Various stages of development of the ovarian follicles.

puberty, the number of follicles has reduced to about 400,000 primary follicles. During her reproductive lifetime, 350 to 500 of the primary follicles develop into **graafian follicles** (mature follicles) and release a ripened **ovum** (egg). The follicles that do not mature degenerate and are absorbed by the ovarian tissue.

The progression of development from a primary follicle to ovulation is illustrated in Figure 5-10 ■. Each primary follicle has a layer of cells surrounding the oocyte (**granulosa cells**). Under the influence of follicle-stimulating hormone (FSH) from the anterior pituitary gland, the layer of granulosa cells thickens, forming a hollow chamber called an **antrum.** The follicle, called a *secondary follicle*, continues to enlarge and move closer to the surface of the ovary until the follicle ruptures and releases the ovum. The ruptured follicle transforms into a glandular structure called the **corpus luteum.** The corpus luteum is also called "yellow body," describing its yellow appearance. The corpus luteum gradually degenerates.

clinical ALERT

At times a sac containing serous fluid or blood forms in the ovary, resulting in an ovarian cyst. The cyst frequently forms in the area of the corpus luteum. The cyst is benign but may cause pain, may rupture into the pelvic cavity, and may need medical or surgical intervention.

Oogenesis, the development of the female gamete or ovum, results from the process of meiosis (see Figure 5-1). Although spermatogenesis begins at puberty, oogenesis occurs during fetal development of the female infant. As a

result of meiosis, the number of chromosomes is reduced equally to 23, one of which will be an X chromosome. However, the cytoplasm does not divide equally in each daughter cell. The result is one large ovum and small **polar bodies** that degenerate. After fertilization, the large supply of cytoplasm will be necessary for nutrition until the developing embryo implants in the uterus.

Besides oogenesis, another function of the ovary is the production and secretion of the two hormones, estrogen and progesterone. Hormone production begins at puberty with the development and maturation of the graafian follicle. The granulosa cells around the ovum produce estrogen. After ovulation, the corpus luteum produces progesterone and some estrogen. **Estrogen** is the hormone responsible for the development and maintenance of the secondary sex characteristics and growth of the **endometrium,** the inner lining of the uterus (Figure 5-11 ■). Progesterone is produced for approximately 11 days after ovulation. **Progesterone** is the hormone that stimulates thickening and vascularization of the endometrium. A decrease in progesterone causes the endometrium to slough off, resulting in **menses.**

ACCESSORY ORGANS

The accessory organs in the female consist of a series of ducts, glands, and external genitalia. Each component is discussed separately. Figure 5-12 ■ illustrates the organization of the female reproductive organs and the ligaments that support them. It also depicts their relationship to surrounding organs and structures.

Reproductive Ducts

The two **fallopian tubes** (also called **uterine tubes** or **oviducts**) serve to transport the ovum from the ovary toward the uterus. However, the structures are not closed

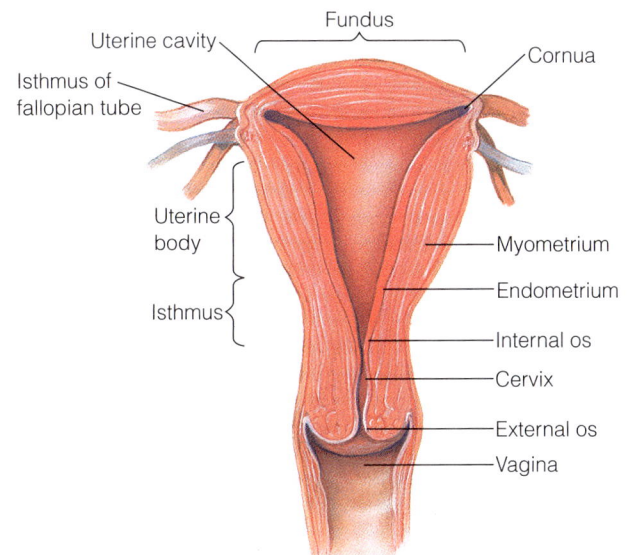

Figure 5-11. ■ Structures of the uterus.

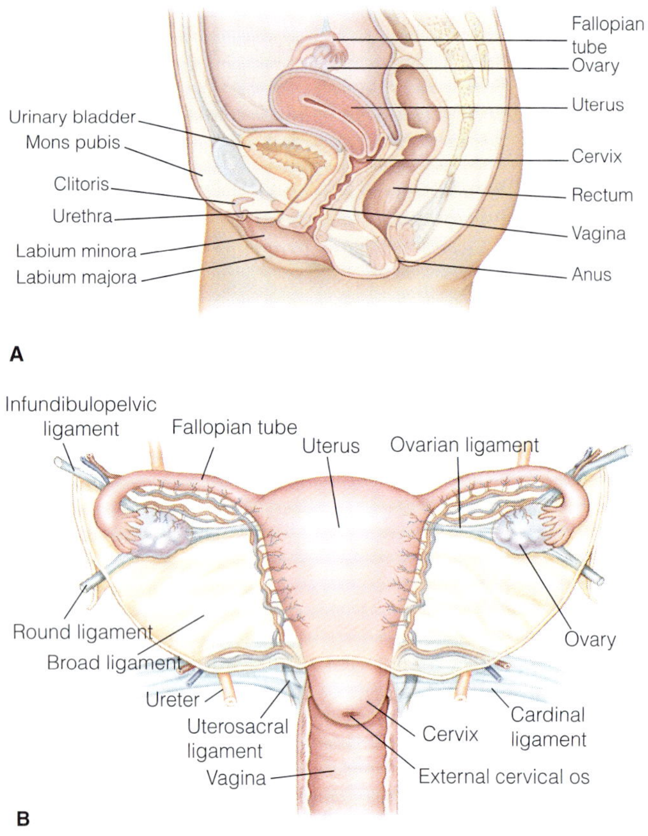

Figure 5-12. ■ (A) Internal female reproductive organs. (B) Uterine ligaments that support reproductive structures.

and connected (e.g., the way the esophagus is connected to the stomach). Because the distal end of the fallopian tube actually opens into the pelvic cavity, the female reproductive system is called an *open system*. The outer end of each fallopian tube is a funnel-shaped structure with finger-like projections called **fimbriae** along the edge (see Figure 5-9). The lumen of the fallopian tube is lined with **cilia**, or minute hairlike structures. Although the fimbriae are not attached to the ovary, the sweeping movements of these finger-like projections, as well as the movement of the cilia, cause the ovum to move into the lumen of the fallopian tube. Fertilization usually occurs in the outer third of the fallopian tube (the third closest to the ovaries).

clinical ALERT

If the fertilized egg implants into the wall of the fallopian tube, the developing embryo enlarges and eventually ruptures the fallopian tube. This results in a surgical emergency (discussed in Chapter 13 ⚭) to stop internal bleeding.

The **uterus** (see Figure 5-11) is a small organ about the size of a pear. The uterus consists almost entirely of muscle (**myometrium**), with a small cavity in the center. The endometrium (inner lining) is a vascular mucous

membrane that responds to hormone influence as described earlier in this chapter. The uterus is suspended in the pelvic cavity between the urinary bladder and the rectum.

The uterus is divided into two parts: the upper portion is the **body,** and the lower region is the **cervix.** Just above the attachment of the fallopian tubes, the uterus forms a round dome called the **fundus.** Except during pregnancy, the normal uterus is tipped forward over the urinary bladder. In some women, atypical uterine positions occur (Figure 5-13 ■). They may make implantation of the embryo more difficult. During pregnancy, the uterus straightens and rises into the abdominal cavity, pressing the intestines backward and the stomach and liver up against the diaphragm.

The **vagina** is a 4-inch-long tube that connects the cervix to the vaginal opening. Composed mainly of smooth muscle, the vagina is lined with mucous membrane. The mucous membrane lies in folds (**rugae**), which allow for stretching of the vagina during delivery. The vagina is the site of deposition of sperm and the passageway for the delivery of the infant. The vaginal orifice is partially covered by a thin membrane called the **hymen.** The hymen usually tears with the first sexual intercourse. It could also tear during insertion of a tampon or from pelvic trauma such as falling on the center bar of a bicycle.

External Genitalia

Figure 5-14 ■ illustrates the external structures of the female reproductive system. The skin-covered fat pad over the symphysis pubis is called the **mons pubis.** This area is covered with coarse hair beginning at puberty and continuing throughout life. Extended downward from the mons pubis are two large folds of skin, the **labia majora.** The **labia minora,** or small folds of tissue, are located inside the labia majora. These folds of tissue join anteriorly at the midline. Located just behind the junction of the labia is erectile tissue called the **clitoris.** The purpose of the clitoris is sexual arousal and pleasure. The area between the labia minora is the **vestibule.** Opening onto the vestibule are the **urinary meatus,** the vagina, and the orifice of several small glands. The **true perineum** is the area between the vaginal opening and the anus.

CULTURAL CONSIDERATIONS. The nurse must be aware of and sensitive to practices by non-Western cultures related to female genitalia. Box 5-1 ■ discusses some of these practices.

ACCESSORY SEX GLANDS

On each side of the vagina are small **Bartholin's glands** or **greater vestibular glands.** The ducts of these glands open onto the vestibule. They secrete a thin, mucus-like substance that provides lubrication during sexual intercourse.

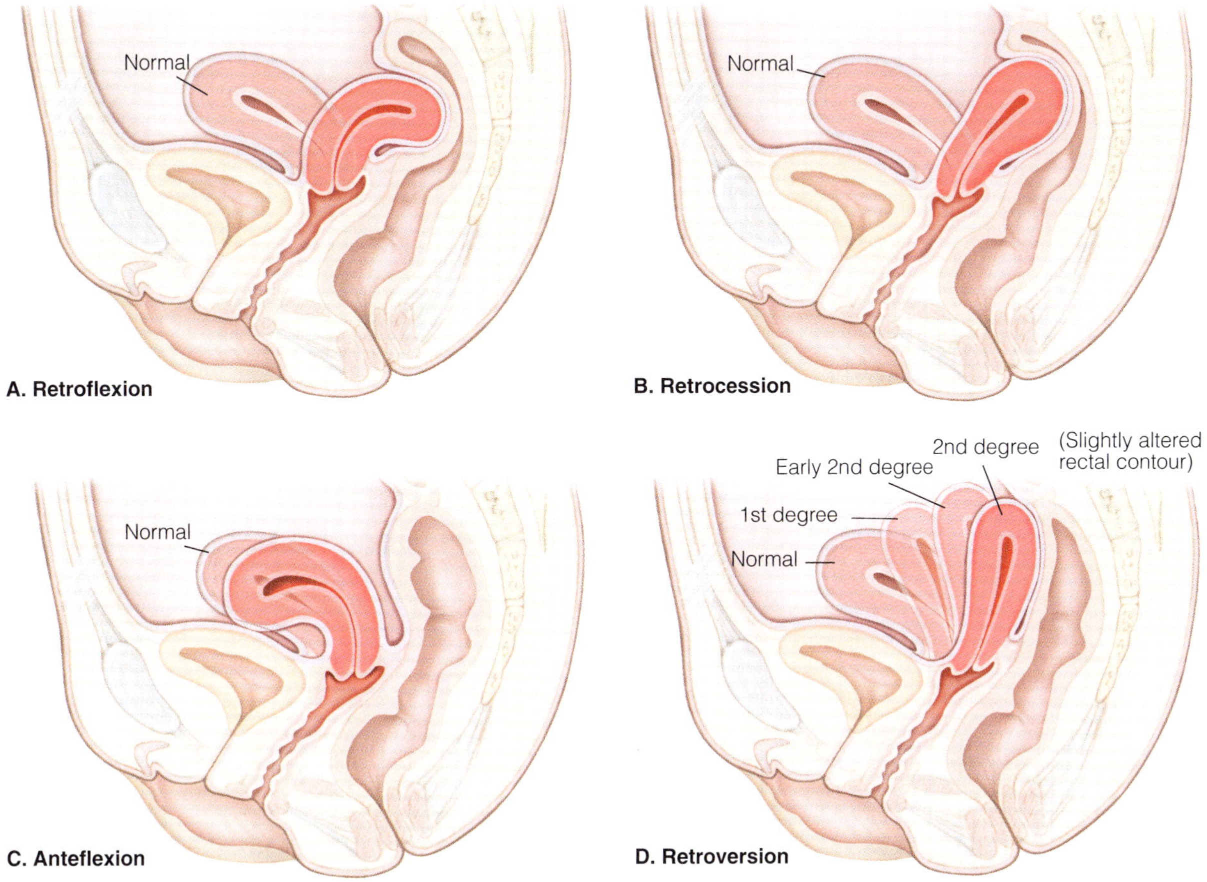

A. Retroflexion

B. Retrocession

C. Anteflexion

D. Retroversion

Figure 5-13. ■ Variations in uterine position. (**A**) Retroflexion. (**B**) Retrocession. (**C**) Anteflexion. (**D**) Retroversion. (Reproduced, with permission, from McGraw-Hill Companies, Inc. DeCherney, A. H., & Pernoll, M. L. [1994]. *Current obstetric and gynecologic diagnosis and treatment* [8th ed.]. Norwalk, CT: Appleton & Lange, p. 16.)

The breasts are located on the anterior chest and are attached to the pectoralis muscles by ligaments. (Figure 5-15 ■ illustrates the structure of the breast.) The mammary glands within the breasts are surrounded by fat tissue. The amount of fat tissue generally determines the size of the breast. The breast consists of 15 to 20 lobes arranged in a circle. Each lobe has several lobules, which contain milk-secreting glandular cells. These glandular

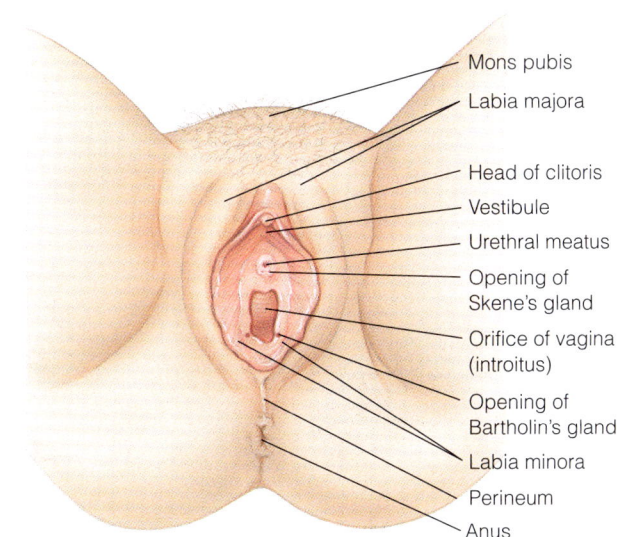

Figure 5-14. ■ External female reproductive organs (adult parous woman).

BOX 5-1   CULTURAL PULSE POINTS

Female Circumcision and Infibulation

Female circumcision and infibulation are practiced in many African countries and by some groups in Malaysia and India. **Female circumcision** is a partial or complete removal of the clitoris, generally performed before puberty. The result is a loss of pleasure during sexual intercourse. **Infibulation** is the removal of the labia majora and labia minora. The excised edges are then sewn together to prevent or limit sexual intercourse. Complications of both procedures include infection, hemorrhage, painful intercourse (**dyspareunia**), difficult childbirth, anxiety, and depression.

Although the international political community has denounced these practices, they are still being performed. The nurse must respect the culture, while creating an environment in which the client is free to discuss the condition, complications, and possible surgical reconstruction.

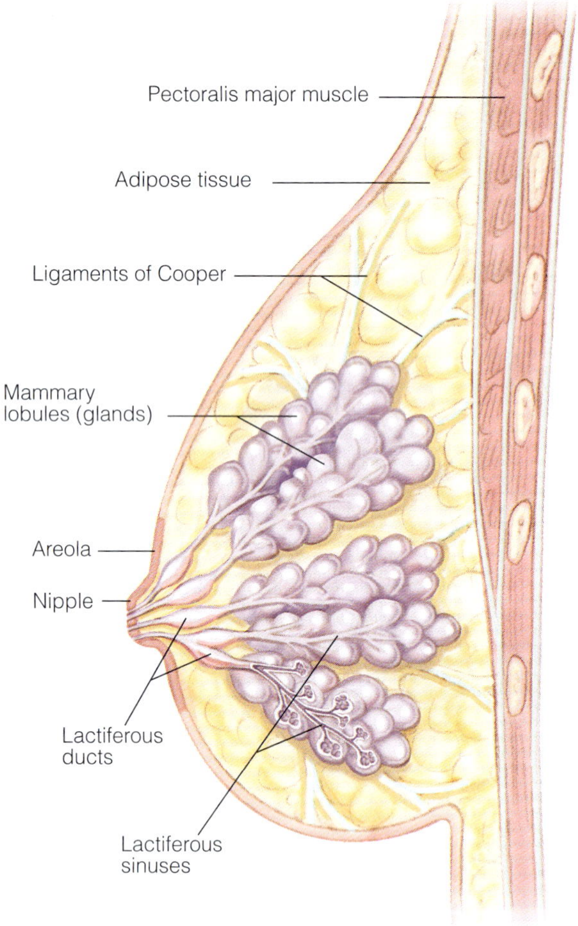

Figure 5-15. ■ Structures of the breast.

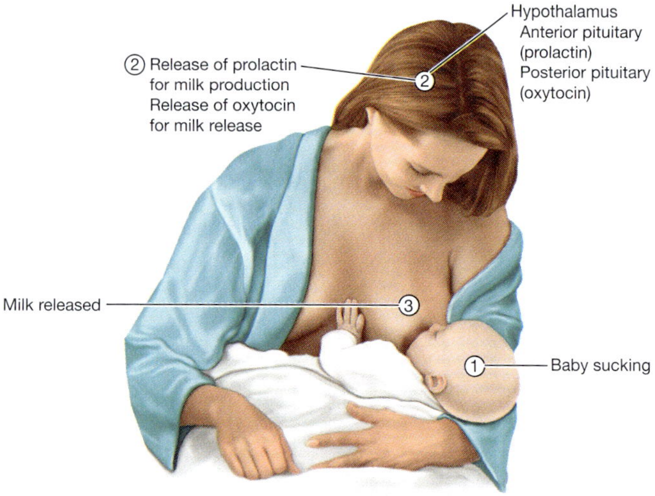

Figure 5-16. ■ Relationship between the pituitary gland and milk production. Sucking of the nipple triggers endocrine release of prolactin (which stimulates new milk production). It also triggers oxytocin (which allows milk to be released from the breast). Oxytocin also stimulates uterine contractions, which help the organ return to its smaller size.

cells are arranged in grapelike clusters called **alveoli.** **Lactiferous ducts** drain each alveoli and converge toward the nipple. Only one lactiferous duct from each lobe drains into the lactiferous sinus located under the colored area around the nipple (the **areola**). The lactiferous sinus drains through a pore on the nipple.

MILK PRODUCTION

Lactogenesis or **lactation** (milk production) begins in pregnancy due to the sustained levels of estrogen and progesterone. The first fluid to be produced by the mammary glands is colostrum. **Colostrum** is a translucent yellow fluid rich in protein, antibodies, and other substances to meet the needs of the newborn. Stimulation of the nipple causes the pituitary gland to secrete pitocin (Figure 5-16 ■). Pitocin causes the milk-ejecting cells in the lactiferous sinus to contract, forcing the colostrum and later the milk from the nipple. (It also stimulates contraction of the uterus, helping it return to its prepregnant size.)

About 1 week after delivery, the level of estrogen and progesterone decreases, causing the mammary glands to change from producing colostrum to producing mature milk. As soon as milk is removed from the breast during feeding, synthesis of more milk begins. If the breast is left full, milk production is limited. (Milk production is discussed further in Chapter 17 ⬭ .)

clinical ALERT

Beginning at puberty, adolescent girls should be taught to perform breast self-examination (BSE) on a monthly basis. See Procedure 7-1 ⬭ , which shows steps in BSE.

FEMALE PELVIC STRUCTURE

Although the pelvis is not part of the female reproductive system, it is important in carrying and delivering an infant. The pelvic structures, their shapes, and their measurements are discussed in Chapter 14 ⬭ . Figure 14-4 ⬭ illustrates the female pelvis and shows typical measurements that can affect the labor and birth process.

MENSTRUAL CYCLE

A review of the female reproductive system would not be complete without discussing the menstrual cycle. Refer often to Figure 5-17 ■ as you review this information.

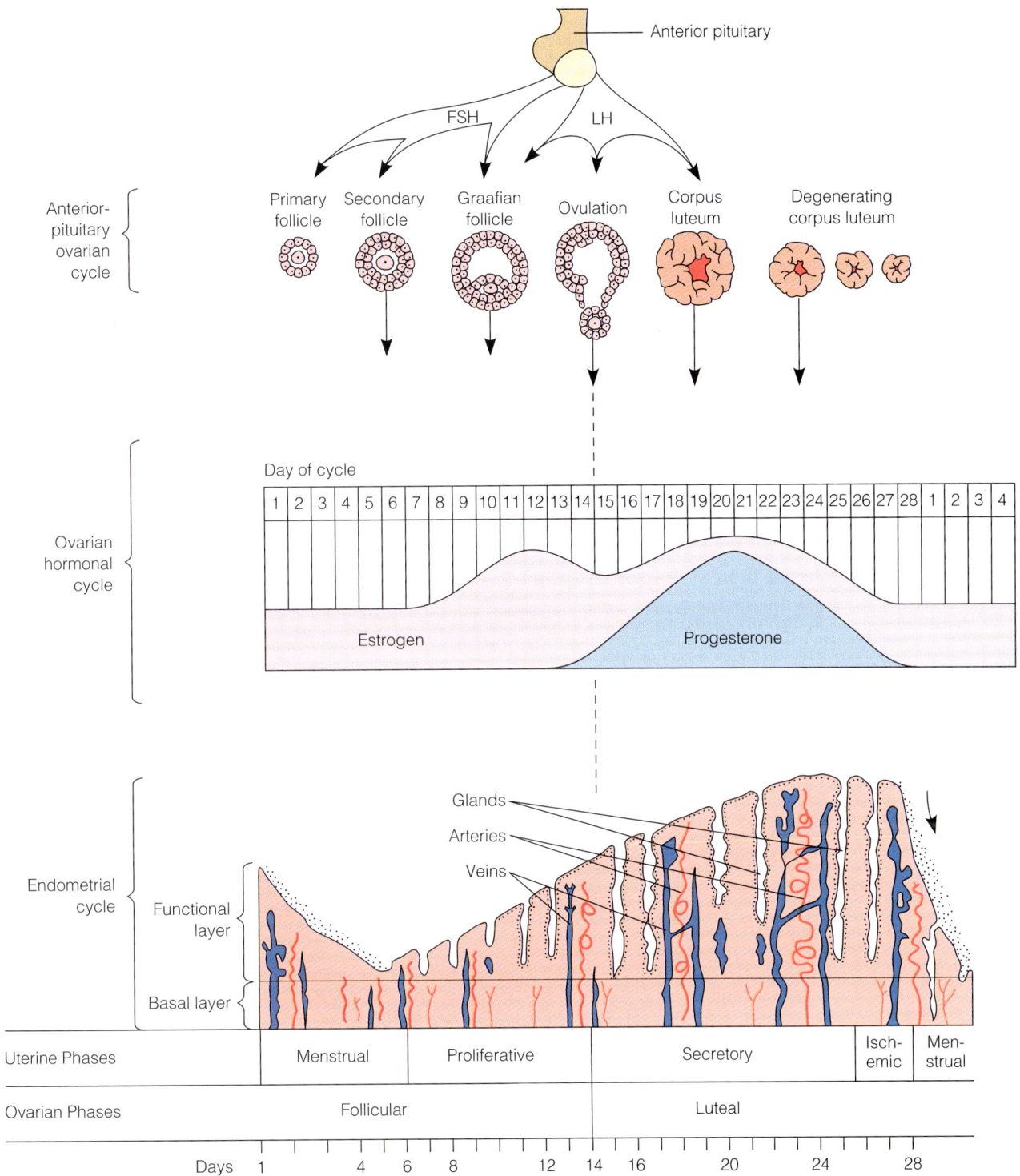

Figure 5-17. ■ Female reproductive cycle showing interrelationships of hormones, phases of the ovarian cycle, and phases of the uterine cycle.

For most women, the events of the menstrual cycle occur with almost precise regularity from their onset (**menarche**) until the cycle ends (**menopause**). Although the length of the cycle varies among women, the average is 28 days. Each cycle can be divided into three phases: menses, proliferative phase, and secretory phase.

The menstrual phase, or menses, begins with menstrual bleeding or flow. The first day of flow is considered the first day of the menstrual cycle; this would be the date listed on the client record as "last menstrual period" (LMP). Menses typically lasts 5 days, with a range of 2 to 10 days.

The **proliferative phase** begins around day 3 when FSH secretion from the anterior pituitary gland begins to increase. You may recall that FHS begins to change the primary follicle into a secondary follicle. The secondary follicle begins to secrete estrogen around day 8. Estrogen helps heal the endometrium and stimulates the production of luteinizing hormone (LH) from the anterior pituitary gland. LH levels increase and cause ripening of one or more graafian follicles by day 11 and ovulation on day 14.

The **secretory phase** begins with ovulation. Following ovulation, FSH and LH levels decrease. The corpus luteum (see Figure 5-10) produces progesterone until day 25 or 26. Progesterone stimulates the endometrium to become more vascular in preparation for a pregnancy. If pregnancy does not occur, the decrease in progesterone causes menses and

stimulates the anterior pituitary gland to again release FSH. If pregnancy does occur, the developing embryo secretes hormones to maintain the endometrium. This process is discussed in more detail in Chapter 8 of this text.

SEXUAL RESPONSE

As anatomic and physiologic development occurs in both genders, sexual responses become more common. When sexual responses become stronger, sexual activity may begin.

In both genders, there is a pattern to sexual response. Masters and Johnson (1966) described phases of sexual response that are still commonly used: excitement, plateau, orgasm, and resolution. Table 5-1 ■ summarizes these changes.

TABLE 5-1			
Physiologic Changes in the Sexual Response Cycle			
PHASE OF THE SEXUAL RESPONSE CYCLE	**SIGNS PRESENT IN BOTH GENDERS**	**SIGNS PRESENT IN MALES ONLY**	**SIGNS PRESENT IN FEMALES ONLY**
Excitement	Increased muscle tension Moderate increase in heart rate, respirations, and blood pressure Sex flush (less prevalent in men than in women; present in 75% of women) Nipple erection (60% of men and most women)	Penile erection Tensing, thickening, and elevation of the scrotum Partial elevation and increase in size of testicles	Enlargement of the clitoral glans Vaginal lubrication Widening and lengthening of vaginal barrel Separation and flattening of the labia majora Reddening of the labia minora and vaginal wall Breast tumescence (enlargement) and enlarged areolae
Plateau	Increased voluntary and involuntary myotonia Abdominal, intercostal, anal, and facial muscle contraction Accelerated heart rate and respiratory rate, and increased blood pressure Sex flush (appearance in some men late in the phase; spread over the entire body in women)	Increase in penile circumference at the coronal ridge (base of the prepuce) and deepening of color 50% increase in testicular size and elevation close to the perineum Appearance of a few drops of mucoid secretions from the bulbourethral glands at tip of penis; may contain sperm	Retraction of the clitoris under the hood Appearance of the orgasmic platform (increase in the size of the outer one-third of the vagina and the labia minora) Slight increase in the width and depth of the inner two-thirds of the vagina Further reddening of the labia minora Appearance of a few drops of mucoid secretion from the Bartholin's glands to lubricate inner labia Further increase in breast size and areolar enlargement

PHASE OF THE SEXUAL RESPONSE CYCLE	SIGNS PRESENT IN BOTH GENDERS	SIGNS PRESENT IN MALES ONLY	SIGNS PRESENT IN FEMALES ONLY
Orgasm	Involuntary spasms of muscle groups throughout the body Diminished sensory awareness Involuntary contractions of the anal sphincter Peak heart rate (110–180 bpm), respiratory rate (40/min or greater), and blood pressure (systolic 30–80 mm Hg and diastolic 20–50 mm Hg above normal)	Rhythmic, expulsive contractions of the penis at 0.8-sec intervals Emission of seminal fluid into the prostatic urethra from contraction of the vas deferens and accessory organs (stage 1 of the expulsive process) Closing of the internal bladder sphincter just before ejaculation to prevent retrograde ejaculation into bladder Orgasm may occur without ejaculation Ejaculation of semen through the penile urethra and expulsion from the urethral meatus; the force of ejaculation varies from man to man and at different times but diminishes after the first two to three contractions (stage 2 of the expulsive process)	Approximately 5–12 contractions in the orgasmic platform at 0.8-sec intervals Contraction of the muscles of the pelvic floor and the uterine muscles Varied pattern of orgasms, including minor surges and contractions, multiple orgasms, or a simple intense orgasm similar to that of the male
Resolution	Reversal of vasocongestion in 10–30 min; disappearance of all signs of myotonia within 5 min Genitals and breasts return to their pre-excitement states Sex flush disappears in reverse order of appearance Heart rate, respiratory rate, and blood pressure return to normal Other reactions include sleepiness, relaxation, and emotional outbursts such as crying or laughing	A refractory period during which the body will not respond to sexual stimulation; varies, depending on age and other factors, from a few moments to hours or days	N/A

NURSING CARE

PRIORITIES IN NURSING CARE

When assessing and caring for clients with reproductive system disorders, keep in mind that many men and women place a high value on their ability to reproduce. Focus your care on being supportive through active listening. Obtaining a comprehensive sexual history is a high priority for the client with pelvic or reproductive system symptoms. A nonjudgmental nurse in a nonthreatening environment is critical in obtaining complete, accurate data. Maintaining confidentiality is also a high priority. Be sensitive to sexual concerns of people from non-Western cultures. Open-ended questions are generally less threatening. Also, spend time promoting sexual health through teaching safe sex practices.

ASSESSING

Reproductive assessment includes recording data of the client's past and present sexual history, and risk factors. Any presenting signs and symptoms are recorded. Observation of the stage of physical maturation is also noted (Figure 5-18A ■ and B ■). The client's understanding of the medical condition is important for the nurse to assess. Because of the close proximity of the urinary system to the reproductive system, the nurse should assess for urinary symptoms.

HEALTH PROMOTION ISSUE

GENETIC TESTING

A young couple, Joe and Amanda, have come to the obstetrician's office to discuss the need for genetic testing before Amanda becomes pregnant. Amanda had a brother with cystic fibrosis (CF). She recalls how difficult it was for her and her parents to watch him die of respiratory complications. She is concerned that she could give this disease to her children. Amanda has been tested and knows she carries the abnormal gene for CF. Because CF is a recessive disorder, both parents must pass on the defective gene in order for the child to have the disease. If Joe is not a carrier of the defective gene, their children may be carriers but will not have CF. It is important to them to understand the risk of conception.

DISCUSSION

Begun in 1990, the U.S. Human Genome Project was a long-term effort coordinated by the U.S. Department of Energy and the National Institutes of Health. The project was completed in 2003. The project goals were to:

- Identify the approximately 20,000 to 25,000 genes in human DNA.
- Determine the sequence of the 3 billion chemical base pairs that constitute human DNA.
- Store this information in a database.
- Improve tools for data analysis.
- Transfer related technologies to the private sector.
- Address the ethical, legal, and social issues (ELSI) that may arise from the project.

The U.S. Human Genome Project was the first large scientific effort to address potential ELSI implications resulting from project data.

Another important aspect of the U.S. Human Genome Project was the federal government's dedication to transferring the technology learned through this study to the private sector. By licensing private companies and awarding grants for continued research, the project could become the catalyst for developing new knowledge.

DNA Structure and Disease

A chromosome is made up of numerous segments called genes. A single gene or genome contains the DNA of the organism. Genes carry the information the organism needs for all life processes. DNA is made of four similar chemicals: adenine (A), thymine (T), guanine (G), and cytosine (C). The order of these chemicals underlies all life's diversity, even determining whether the organism is human or another species, such as

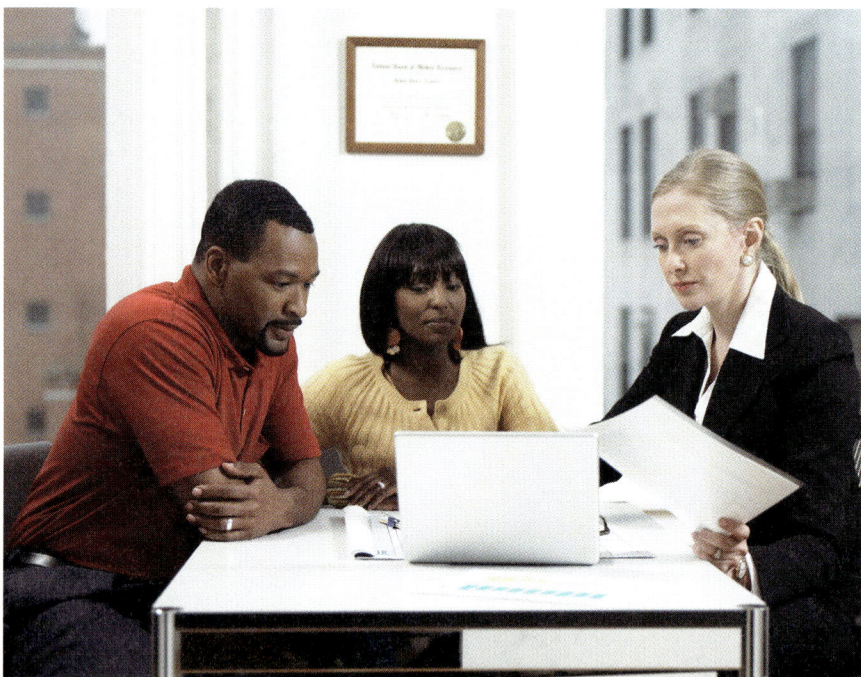

fruit fly or yeast. Identifying and recording the order of these chemicals is the basis of genetic research. Alteration or mutation in the order of A, T, G, and C results in disease. The cause of some disorders has been identified through genetic research.

Prenatal (during pregnancy) genetic testing of the mother and fetus may be recommended if abnormalities are suspected. Although any baby could end up with a genetic disorder caused by a new mutation, babies who have a family history of genetic disorders are at increased risk. In this case, genetic testing before conception is recommended so the parents have an understanding of the risks involved in pregnancy. Once research has identified the exact location of disease-causing genes, it is easier and faster to identify whether parents are carriers of these abnormal genes. If there is a risk that the fetus will inherit a particular genetic disorder, such as cystic fibrosis, genetic counselors can discuss options with the couple.

PLANNING AND IMPLEMENTATION

Although there is never a pregnancy without risk, parents who participate in family planning are requesting information to reduce the risk of abnormalities as much as possible. Genetic testing may be the first in a long line of choices facing the couple. For example, if Joe tests negative for cystic fibrosis, the couple has only a slim chance of having a child with this disorder. However, if Joe tests positive, there is a 50% chance the child will have cystic fibrosis. The couple will need to decide whether to go ahead and have a baby, whether to have artificial insemination with donor sperm, whether to adopt a child, or whether not to have children. If the couple decides to have a baby, they may choose to test the fetus for cystic fibrosis and possibly abort the pregnancy if the disease is present. Before these choices are made, the couple will need accurate, up-to-date information. The best person to help with such decision making is a genetic counselor.

The nurse in the obstetrician's office may need to reinforce information that is presented by the doctor, such as why genetic testing is needed, how specimens are obtained, and what laboratory results mean. The nurse should prepare a list of genetic counselors in the area. When genetic testing is complete, referral to these counselors can be made in a timely manner. If pregnancy does occur, the nurse will need to provide emotional support for the family. Genetic testing is becoming more financially affordable, but finances may prevent many couples from seeking testing before pregnancy. The nurse may be able to suggest financial resources, including research studies, that may be able to perform the tests free of charge.

SELF-REFLECTION

Have you ever had a strong desire to do something, and when you finally had the opportunity, something went wrong and someone was hurt? Do you recall how badly you felt? These are the same feelings parents experience when they have a child with a genetic disorder. They feel guilty. They might blame each other. They tell themselves, "If only I had been tested...." By recalling similar feelings, the nurse can be more empathetic in supporting the parents and helping them work through their feelings.

SUGGESTED RESOURCES

Feigin, R. D. (2005). Prospects for the future of child health through research. *Journal of the American Medical Association, 294,* 1373–1379.

Lea, D. H. (2000). A new world view of genetics service models. *Online Journal of Issues in Nursing, 3* (5).

Nathan, D. G., Fontanarosa, P. B., & Wilson, J. D. (2001). Opportunities for medical research in the 21st century. *Journal of the American Medical Association, 285,* 533–534.

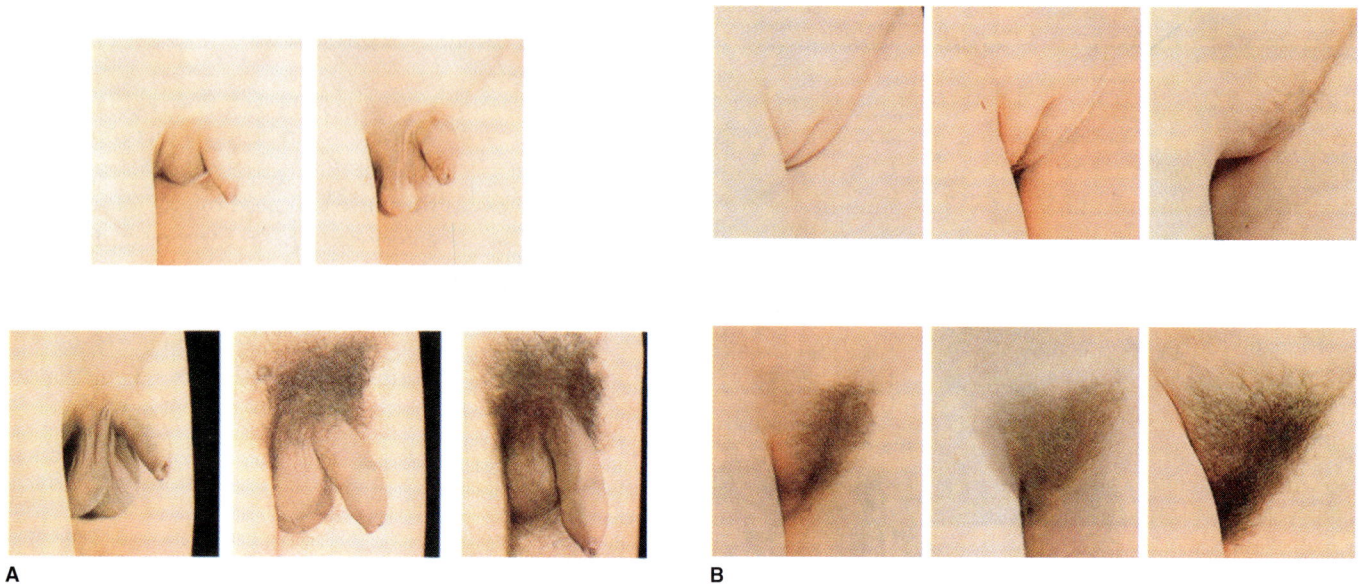

Figure 5-18. ■ **(A)** Stages of male pubic hair and external genital development. **(B)** Stages of female pubic hair development. (From Van Wieringen et al. (1971). *Growth diagrams 1965*. Groningen: Wolters-Noordhoff, the Netherlands.)

DIAGNOSING, PLANNING, AND IMPLEMENTING

Nursing diagnoses are made specifically for the individual client. However, they might include:

- **S**exual Dysfunction reacted to (specific problem)
- **P**ain related to (specific problem)
- Disturbed **B**ody Image related to (specific problem)
- Risk for **I**nfection related to (specific problem)
- **R**ape Trauma Syndrome

Client outcomes might include:

- Expresses understanding of the cause and treatments of sexual dysfunction
- Achieves adequate pain relief
- Expresses acceptance of change in body image
- Maintains infection-free status
- Expresses feelings and initiates positive measures to deal with feelings

To achieve these outcomes, the nurse provides various interventions.

- Assist with screening and diagnostic examinations. *The primary care provider will need to perform a series of diagnostic exams to determine the exact medical diagnosis. The nurse may need to set up equipment, assist with specimen collection, and provide instructions to the client.*

- Teach clients about specific problems. *The primary care provider will provide information to the client about the specific problem. Often, the nurse needs to reinforce teaching and answer questions.*
- Provide pharmacologic and nonpharmacologic pain relief methods. *The care provider will often prescribe medication to relieve pain. The nurse must provide information about the administration, use, and side effects of medication. Other pain relief methods may also be helpful, including heat/cold, positioning, and relaxation techniques.*
- Monitor surgical sites for signs of complications. *Any surgical sites should be observed for signs of bleeding and infection.*
- Refer clients to local support groups as appropriate. *Knowing you are not alone with a medical problem is helpful for emotional support. Many health care facilities have established groups of clients with similar problems. These support groups meet to discuss feelings and solutions for common concerns.*

EVALUATING

The nurse modifies care until expected outcomes are achieved. For example, if vital signs after a complication are altered, the nurse would modify the care plan to take vital signs more frequently.

NURSING PROCESS CARE PLAN
Client with Ovarian Cyst

Janice, 17 years old, was admitted to the postsurgical unit following laparoscopic surgery for a left ovarian cyst. The operative report states that the ovarian cyst was removed with minimal damage to the ovary. The client's mother is at the bedside.

Assessment
VS: T 98.4, P 96, R 24, BP 130/72. Janice states that the nursing assistant just helped her to the bathroom and now she has right upper quadrant pain radiating to right shoulder. She states the pain is a 6 on a 1 to 10 scale. Denies nausea. Abdominal dressings are dry.

Nursing Diagnosis
The following important nursing diagnosis (among others) is established for this client:

- Acute **P**ain (pelvic) related to laparoscopic surgery for left ovarian cyst

Expected Outcome
- Client will verbalize pain as 3 or less on a scale of 1 to 10.

Planning and Implementation
- Teach Janice that she may experience pain in the right upper quadrant and the right shoulder for 24 to 48 hours after laparoscopic surgery. *This teaching will help Janice understand that her pain is normal and should subside in a few days.*

- Teach Janice relaxation techniques to lessen pain and ease breathing. *Diaphragmatic pain can lead to hypoventilation, which could lead to pneumonia. It is important for the client to relax and breathe normally.*
- Teach Janice to lie flat, turning side to side, for most of the day. *Lying flat and turning from side to side will facilitate the absorption of the carbon dioxide gas used in surgery.*
- Teach Janice the use and side effects of prescribed medication. *Taking medication as prescribed can help in the recovery process by allowing Janice to turn, move, and deep breathe. Side effects should be reported and documented.*

Evaluation
Janice's pain level was evaluated 30 minutes after medication and every 2 hours for 24 hours. Her respirations and lung sounds were also evaluated every 2 hours and remained clear. Pain gradually reduced to 3 out of 10 within 12 hours of surgery.

Critical Thinking in the Nursing Process

1. What complications to the ovary might occur because of the ovarian cyst and surgery?
2. Why would diaphragmatic pain be common after laparoscopic abdominal surgery?
3. What are some possible treatments to prevent future ovarian cysts?

Note: Discussion of Critical Thinking questions appears in Appendix I.

Note: The reference and resource listings for this and all chapters have been compiled at the back of the book.

Chapter Review

KEY TERMS by Topic

Use the audio glossary feature of either the CD-ROM or the Companion Website to hear the correct pronunciation of the following key terms.

Introduction
gamete, gametogenesis, puberty

Chromosomes and Genes
chromosomes, genome, transposons

Male Reproductive System
testes, tunica vaginalis testis, tunica albuginea, seminiferous tubules, spermatogenesis, spermatogonia, follicle-stimulating hormone, primary spermatocyte, spermatids, autosomes, spermatozoa, acrosome, testosterone, epididymis, vas deferens, ductus deferens, spermatic cord, ejaculatory duct, urethra, semen, seminal fluid, seminal vesicles, prostate, bulbourethral glands, Cowper's glands, penis, glans, foreskin, prepuce, circumcision, scrotum

Female Reproductive System
ovarian follicles, oocyte, graafian follicles, ovum, granulosa cells, antrum, corpus luteum, oogenesis, polar bodies, estrogen, endometrium, progesterone, menses, fallopian tubes, uterine tubes, oviducts, fimbriae, cilia, uterus, myometrium, body, cervix, fundus, vagina, rugae, hymen, mons pubis, labia majora, labia minora, clitoris, vestibule, urinary meatus, true perineum, Bartholin's gland, greater vestibular gland, female circumcision, infibulation, dyspareunia, alveoli, lactiferous ducts, areola, lactogenesis, lactation, colostrum, menarche, menopause, proliferative phase, secretory phase

KEY Points

- The unique combination of traits a person has results from that person's genetic makeup. Chromosomal abnormalities and genetically inherited illnesses affect a person's physical being and health.

- It is important for the nurse to consider the anatomy and physiology of the male or female reproductive system each time a history or physical is taken.

- The nurse needs to understand the process of sperm and ovum production in order to answer a couple's fertility questions.

- The nurse should understand the function of sex hormones in order to explain the signs of puberty.

- The nurse uses knowledge of the process of lactation when helping the new mother with breastfeeding techniques.

- The nurse must be able to explain the phases of the menstrual cycle and correlate each with physical changes during a 28-day cycle. This information is important when teaching clients about signs of menstrual problems, hormone replacement therapy, and birth control measures.

- The nurse uses knowledge of the sexual response when teaching clients about their own and their partner's sexual responses, and when identifying sexual dysfunction.

EXPLORE Media Link

Additional interactive resources for this chapter can be found on the Companion Website at www.prenhall.com/towle.

Click on Chapter 5 and "Begin" to select the activities for this chapter.

For chapter-related NCLEX®-style questions and an audio glossary, access the accompanying CD-ROM in this book.

Animations

Oogenesis

Spermatogenesis

Ovulation

Conception

Down Syndrome

∞ FOR FURTHER Study

For a complete discussion of ethical questions concerning the U.S. Human Genome Project, see Chapter 3.

For additional information on the surgical treatments for reproductive problems, see Chapter 7.

Procedures 7-1 and 7-2 describe breast and testicular self-examination, respectively.

See Chapter 8 for an in-depth discussion on pregnancy and the developing embryo.

The pelvic structures, their shapes, and their measurements are discussed in Chapter 14 and Figure 14-4.

Circumcision and milk production are discussed further in Chapter 17.

Caring for a Client with Epididymitis
NCLEX-PN® Focus Area: Psychosocial Integrity

Case Study: Juan Martinez, a 24-year-old man, comes to the health clinic with pain and swelling in the scrotum. He admits to burning with urination and a purulent discharge from the penis. He states that he has had unprotected sexual intercourse with several women over the past few weeks. He states, "I hope this will not affect my being able to get an erection."

Nursing Diagnosis: Disturbed Body Image related to infection of the epididymis

COLLECT DATA

Subjective

Objective

Would you report this? Yes/No

If yes, to: _____

Nursing Care

How would you document this? _____

Compare your documentation to the sample provided in Appendix I.

Data Collected
(use only those that apply)

- 24-year-old male
- Pain and swelling in the scrotum
- Burning with urination
- Voice shaky, avoids eye contact
- Purulent discharge from the penis
- States unprotected sexual intercourse with several women over the past few weeks
- "I hope this will not affect my being able to get an erection."

Nursing Interventions
(use only those that apply; list in priority order)

- Teach client about the need for protection from infection during sexual intercourse.
- Obtain a urine specimen for culture and sensitivity.
- Teach client about normal physiology of erection and infection of reproductive system.
- Teach client use and side effects of medication.
- Encourage client to discuss sexuality.
- Obtain a specimen from the penile drainage for culture and sensitivity.

NCLEX-PN® Exam Preparation

1 When teaching clients about the fertilization process, the nurse explains that fertilization usually occurs:
1. in the ovary.
2. in the distal end of the fallopian tube.
3. in the upper uterus.
4. in the vagina.

2 What structure should men check monthly in self-examination? Mark an X over the area in the figure below.

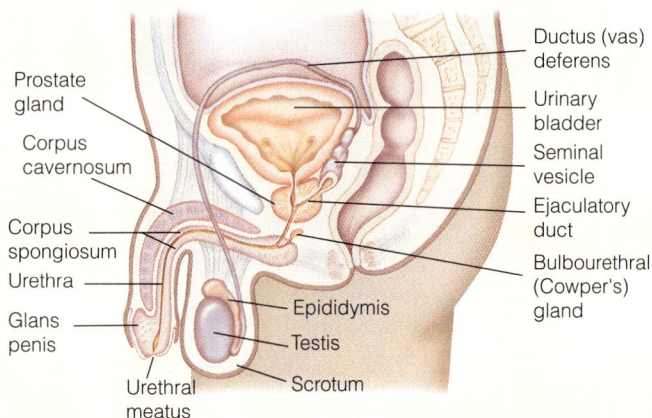

Men's self-exam

3 When teaching parents-to-be about the development of their baby, the nurse includes the fact that:
1. the gender of the baby is determined by the father's sperm.
2. the gender of the baby is determined by the mother's ovum.
3. the gender of the baby is determined by maternal hormones.
4. the gender of the baby is determined by paternal hormones.

4 The female reproductive system is sometimes described as an open system because:
1. the vagina opens to the outside of the body.
2. the cervix opens to allow the baby to leave the uterus.
3. the distal end of the fallopian tubes open into the pelvic cavity.
4. the graafian follicle opens to release the ovum.

5 In the woman with a 30-day menstrual cycle, ovulation would probably occur on:
1. day 1.
2. day 13.
3. day 15.
4. day 30.

6 When teaching a new mother to breastfeed her baby, the nurse stresses that:
1. emptying at least one breast at each feeding stimulates more milk production.
2. the infant will not get enough nutrition if he or she does not drink all of the milk.
3. if milk is allowed to remain in the breast, the breast can get infected.
4. emptying the breast will prevent leaking of milk.

7 When are ova formed in the ovary?
1. continuously after puberty
2. during fetal development
3. just prior to puberty
4. monthly following puberty

8 When assessing a 21-year-old female who comes to the clinic with yellow, odorous vaginal discharge, the nurse should ask which of the following questions? (Select all that apply.)
1. When was your last menstrual period?
2. Are you sexually active?
3. What method of contraception do you use?
4. When was your last bowel movement?
5. Does you sexual partner use condoms?
6. How many children have you had?

9 Following a prostatectomy, the man is generally considered unable to father children. What is the reason for this statement? (Select all that apply.)
1. The urethra is destroyed and sperm cannot leave the body.
2. The vas deferens is cut and the sperm cannot leave the epididymis.
3. The ejaculatory duct is altered.
4. Lack of prostatic fluid makes sperm less mobile.
5. Swelling from the procedure permanently closes the vas deferens.

10 A young client asks the nurse, "Why do I have a period every 26 days and my friend has hers every 29 days?" The nurse's best response would be:
1. "Your menstrual cycle is controlled by hormones from the pituitary gland and uterus."
2. "Your menstrual cycle is controlled by hormones from the ovaries and uterus."
3. "Your menstrual cycle is controlled by hormones from the ovaries and pituitary gland."
4. "Your menstrual cycle is controlled by hormones from the uterus."

Answers for NCLEX-PN® Review and Critical Thinking questions appear in Appendix I.

Chapter 6

Women's Health

BRIEF Outline

Health Promotion and Illness Prevention

Health and Illness

Nurse's Role in Health Promotion for Women

Nutrition

Exercise

Rest and Sleep

Personal Hygiene

Stress and Coping

Tobacco, Alcohol, and Drug Use

Complementary and Alternative Therapies

Nursing Care

LEARNING Outcomes

After completing this chapter, you will be able to:

1. Define key terms.
2. Describe health promotion and illness prevention activities.
3. Describe the nurse's role in health promotion and illness prevention.
4. Describe nutrition, activity, sleep, and rest as they relate to women's health.
5. Describe stress and anxiety as they relate to women's health.
6. Identify alternative therapies that can be used to maintain health and prevent illness.

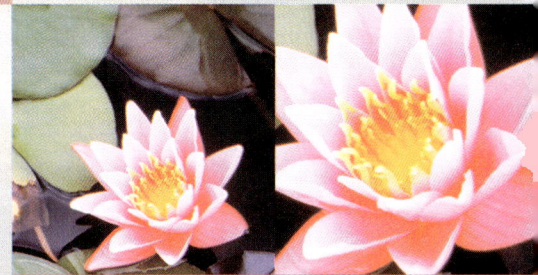

HEALTH PROMOTION ISSUE: Early Sexual Maturation

NURSING CARE PLAN CHART: Planning for Client with Leukorrhea

NURSING PROCESS CARE PLAN: Caring for Woman Who Wants to Stop Smoking

CRITICAL THINKING CARE MAP: Caring for a Woman Seeking Health Information

Health is a state of physical, emotional, and spiritual well-being and not just the absence of disease (WHO, 1948). Many people are becoming aware of the relationship between lifestyle and illness. Usually, changing one's lifestyle to include good nutrition, exercise, and adequate rest and to limit the use of tobacco, alcohol, and other drugs can have a positive impact on the level of health. This chapter will address health promotion and illness prevention in women.

Health Promotion and Illness Prevention

Some people use the terms *health promotion*, *illness prevention*, and *health protection* interchangeably. However, differences appear in the literature regarding these terms. *Prevention* and *protection* mean to avoid something harmful, such as the development of a disease. Leavell and Clark (1965) defined three levels of illness prevention (Table 6-1 ■). Primary prevention includes health promotion activities and protection against specific diseases. An example of primary prevention would be immunization against communicable diseases. Secondary prevention focuses on the early detection and treatment of diseases. An example of secondary prevention would be annual mammograms to detect breast cancer. Tertiary prevention involves the restoration and rehabilitation to return the client to the optimal level of

functioning. An example of tertiary prevention would be early ambulation following a hysterectomy to prevent pneumonia.

Pender, Murdaugh, and Parsons (2002) believe health promotion to be different from illness prevention or health protection. They contend that health promotion is motivated by a desire to increase well-being. Illness prevention and health protection are motivated by a desire to avoid illness, or to detect it early and maintain function within the limitations of the disease. At times, it is difficult to separate health promotion and illness prevention. The goal the client sets becomes the motivation factor and should be clearly communicated. For example, a 50-year-old woman may begin walking 4 miles a day. If the goal is to decrease the risk of cardiovascular disease, the activity would be illness prevention. If the goal of walking is to increase the overall feeling of well-being, the activity is health promotion. Because health promotion and illness prevention activities complement each other, they should be considered together as affecting the quality of health.

Health and Illness

For most people, health is not just the absence of disease or disability. Health is not limited to physical well-being, but includes emotional, social, intellectual, spiritual, occupational, and environmental well-being (Figure 6-1 ■). Each aspect of health is intertwined with the other aspects

---

TABLE 6-1

Levels of Prevention

LEVEL	DESCRIPTION	EXAMPLE
Primary prevention	Applied to healthy individuals, it precedes disease or dysfunction. Generalized health promotion and protection against disease.	■ Health teaching about accident and poisoning at each level of growth and development, prevention, nutrition, exercise, stress reduction, and protection against occupational hazards ■ Immunizations ■ Family planning ■ Safe environment including sanitation, housing, recreation, work conditions
Secondary prevention	Early detection and treatment of disease. Health maintenance and prevention of complications.	■ Screening surveys and procedures ■ Regular medical and dental exams ■ Teaching self-exam (breast and testicular) ■ Nursing assessment and care
Tertiary care	Rehabilitate and restore individuals when illness, defect, or disability is fixed, stabilized, or determined irreversible.	■ Referring to support groups ■ Teaching diabetic to prevent complications ■ Referring to rehabilitation center for life skills retraining

Figure 6-1. ■ Satisfaction with work enhances a sense of well-being and contributes to wellness.

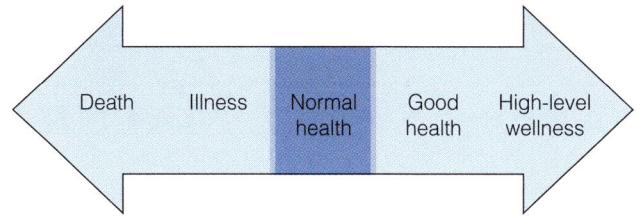

Figure 6-2. ■ Health–illness continuum.

and plays an important role in the individual's sense of well-being. Illness is generally defined as a state in which the individual feels unhealthy. It may or may not be related to a specific disease or infirmity. Many individuals who have physical or mental limitations consider themselves healthy.

High levels of health are on the opposite end of the continuum from extreme illness or premature death. An individual's health can change from day to day. Circumstances outside the individual's control can cause the level of health to decline. The individual can maintain the status quo, or choose to modify their lifestyle and improve their level of health (Figure 6-2 ■). Throughout life, the individual's level of health moves back and forth along the health–illness continuum. For example, a 35-year-old mother of three children may consider herself very healthy. During a breast self-exam she finds a lump that was not present a month ago. Her level of health moves toward the illness side of the continuum. The doctor determines the mass to be a cyst and drains the fluid. The woman's health again moves toward health. If the mass is malignant, the woman's health will remain toward illness during the surgical, pharmacologic, and radiation therapies.

Nurse's Role in Health Promotion for Women

The nurse's role in health promotion for women involves several areas of nursing intervention. The nurse must decide which intervention takes priority in the individual situation. The nurse provides screening for disorders including health assessment, administering standardized screening tests, making referrals to other health care providers or agencies as necessary, and teaching the client activities that promote health or prevent complications.

The nurse has the responsibility to plan and implement care that promotes the normal functioning of all body systems. While the client may present with a specific medical diagnosis, the nurse assesses not only the body system involved but also related body systems. The nurse can then identify problems or potential problems and assist the client to correct or avoid these problems. If the client presents with endometriosis, the nurse must assess pain and vaginal bleeding. Because of the close proximity to the uterus, the nurse should also assess the normal functioning of the gastrointestinal and urinary systems. If the client has developed diarrhea from pelvic inflammation, the nurse must teach the client to prevent dehydration by increasing oral fluids and to prevent skin breakdown by cleaning the perineum following each bowel movement. If the client needs assistance with pericare, the nurse can provide the care or delegate it to the certified nursing assistant.

Health promotion activities for women include teaching and supporting them in the care of their children. Often women have questions such as, "Is my child developing normally?" "What is the correct way to discipline my child?" or "How do I talk with my child about not using drugs?" The nurse should answer questions, provide references, and make referrals as necessary. The Health Promotion Issue on pages 102 and 103 discusses early sexual maturation.

HEALTH PROMOTION ISSUE

EARLY SEXUAL MATURATION

Janice, age 9, and Sue, age 11, share a bedroom in their small house. Their parents are older than their friend's parents and seem to be out of touch with their daughter's needs. When Sue got up one morning, there was blood in her underpants and on the bed sheets. She ran crying to her mother. Janice wakened to her sister's crying. She tried to go into the bathroom with her mother and sister, but was told she had to "stay out." Janice was afraid her sister was dying and no one wanted to tell her. This situation might have been prevented had their mother explained to the girls about their changing bodies.

DISCUSSION

When Should Parents Tell Children About Sexual Maturation?

Parents often are in a quandary as to when and how to tell their children about puberty and sexual relations. Although there are no rules to follow, many authorities believe the topic of sexual maturation is best presented by the parents from a life-span approach.

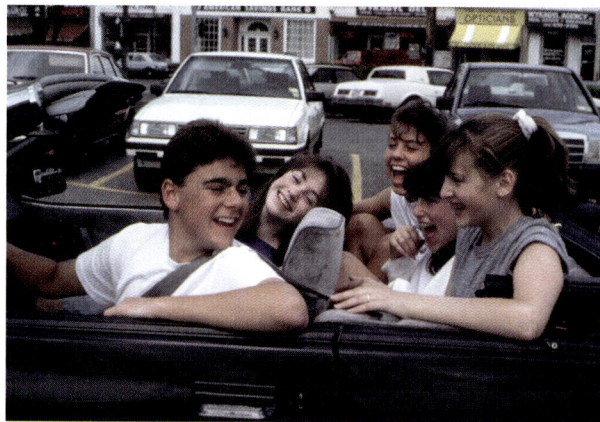

Information about reproduction decreases the child's embarrassment, anxiety, and uncertainty. Middle childhood seems to be the best time to introduce the topic, before early signs of puberty begin.

The time of puberty is slightly different in girls and boys. Girls usually begin puberty with the development of breast buds between 9 and 13. Pubic hair appears approximately 6 months later and menses usually begins 9 months to 2 years after that. For boys, puberty begins with a growth spurt and changing in

body proportions between 9 and 14 years. The lengthening of the penis and enlargement of the scrotum and testes begin about the same time as long, soft, color hair appears at the base of the penis. Over the next 2 years, the penis continues to lengthen, and the pubic hair becomes coarse. As hormone (estrogen and testosterone) levels increase, mood swings often occur. The alert parent will notice the body changes in their children and help them understand what is happening. For more details regarding sexual maturation, see Chapter 5 ⚭ .

Sometimes health promotion activities involve more than one client. The nurse may assist with the set-up and operation of support groups, school health promotion programs, and health clinics such as blood pressure screening, diabetic foot care, and immunization. With each client contact, the nurse provides teaching and referral as necessary.

Nutrition

An essential part of the feeling of well-being is a supply of proper nutrients. To maintain healthy tissue, the body must have a continuous supply of carbohydrates, proteins,

lipids, vitamins, minerals, and water. Table 6-2 ■ shows about how many calories sedentary and active women need at different ages.

Although everyone needs a well-balanced diet, it is essential that during the reproductive years, women pay close attention to eating a balanced diet. For the first few weeks of pregnancy, the woman may be unaware of the presence of the embryo growing inside her. This is a critical time for the developing embryo. Without adequate amounts of protein and vitamins (especially folic acid), the embryo may not develop normally (see Chapter 8). As the woman ages, adequate amounts of calcium are needed to prevent **osteoporosis** (brittle bones).

How Much Should Parents Tell Their Children?

Some parents are reluctant to tell their children about sexual intercourse for fear they will engage in sex. However, research shows that teens whose parents discuss sex with them delay being sexually active longer than teens whose parents do not discuss sex. Once the informed teens become sexually active, they usually do so responsibly. Many children engage in some form of sex play before preadolescence. These activities are a normal aspect of curiosity and not a result of sexual urges. Any adverse emotional consequences of sex play are the result of the parent's reaction. Whether the child views their actions as right or wrong is related to the parent attitude and behavior.

Parents should be encouraged to be informed, honest, and realistic when teaching their children. Because children learn about sex through television, music, and friends, parents should be prepared to answer questions accurately. Children become confused by the concepts of sex, love, and intimacy. It is vital that parents share their values and beliefs with their children. Parents need to give their children the knowledge to make sound choices. They need information about the risks, responsibilities, and realities of being sexually active. Parents need to create an open, ongoing conversation with their children. Items viewed on television, whether in the news or other programs, can be used to open the dialogue about sex, reproduction, and maturation.

What Can the Nurse Do?

The role of the nurse is to provide accurate information to parents, children, and the public. Sex should be treated as a normal part of growth and development. Many times boys and girls should be taught the content separately to prevent embarrassment. The preadolescent needs concrete realistic information so they could answer questions such as: "What if my period starts at school?" "How can I keep people from telling I have an erection?" Children should be told what they want to know and what will happen to them as they mature.

PLANNING AND IMPLEMENTATION

During encounters with parents, the nurse can be open to questions and discussion. By assessing the parents' knowledge and their awareness of their developing child's needs, the nurse can encourage parents to openly discuss sexual maturation with their child. The nurse may need to provide supplemental information to prepare parents for more complex questions as the child grows older.

SELF-REFLECTION

How did your parents explain sexual maturation to you? How did it make you feel? How did you (will you) explain sexual maturation to your child?

SUGGESTED RESOURCE

Hoff, T., Greene, L., & Davis, J. (2003). *National survey of adolescent and young adult sexual health knowledge, attitudes and experiences.* Menlo Park, CA: Henry J. Kaiser Family Foundation.

TABLE 6-2		
Calories Women Need by Age and Activity Level		
AGE	SEDENTARY LIFESTYLE	ACTIVE LIFESTYLE
14–18	1,800	2,400
19–30	2,000	2,400
31–50	1,800	2,200
51+	1,600	2,200
Data from United States Department of Agriculture.		

CARBOHYDRATES

Carbohydrates, needed for energy, are made up of both simple and complex molecules of carbon, hydrogen, and oxygen. Simple sugars are produced by plants including fruits, sugar cane, and sugar beets. Animals also produce simple sugars in the form of milk. Simple carbohydrates can be processed or refined into table sugar, molasses, and corn syrup. Simple sugars are added to many foods such as soft drinks, deserts, candy, and some cereals.

Complex carbohydrates come from starch and fiber. Nearly all starches exist in nature in plants such as grains, legumes, and potatoes. Starch is broken down in the mouth and small intestine into simple sugar. Fiber cannot be digested by humans, but is needed as roughage or bulk in the diet. Bulk satisfies the appetite and helps the digestive system eliminate solid waste by enhancing movement of water into the feces.

PROTEIN

Proteins are made up of amino acids, a combination of carbon, hydrogen, oxygen, and nitrogen. Amino acids are categorized as essential, those that must be supplied in food, and nonessential, those that the body can manufacture. The body takes the ingested protein, breaks apart the amino acids, and uses them to manufacture new protein. *Complete protein* contains all the essential amino acids and some nonessential ones. Animal proteins, including meat, poultry, fish, dairy products, and eggs contain complete protein. *Incomplete protein* lacks one or more essential amino acids. Incomplete proteins come from vegetables. A mixture of vegetable protein must be consumed for all the essential amino acids to be obtained. For example, a combination of corn and dried beans will provide all essential amino acids.

LIPIDS

Lipids are fats, solid at room temperature, and oils, liquid at room temperature. *Glycerides* are the simplest lipids. Lipids are made of fatty acids. *Triglycerides* contain three fatty acids. Saturated triglycerides are found in animal products and are solid at room temperature. The firmer the lipid at room temperature, the more saturated the fat. For example, beef tallow is more saturated than chicken fat or butter. Unsaturated triglycerides are liquid at room temperature. They are found in plant products such as olive oil and corn oil.

Saturated fats (discussed more in Chapter 11 ⊚) contribute to the production of cholesterol in humans. Most of the body's cholesterol is manufactured in the liver, but some is absorbed from the diet. Some cholesterol is needed for the production of bile salts and steroid hormones. Excess cholesterol can build up on the inside of blood vessels leading to hypertension, heart disease, and stroke. Unsaturated fats in the diet lower the blood cholesterol.

Trans fats (hydrogenated fats) are artificial fats made from hydrogen gas and plant oil. Manufacturers started using trans fats in processed foods in 1985 to prolong the shelf life of the foods. However, public health experts have warned that trans fats clog arteries and cause obesity (see Chapter 11 ⊚). The U.S. Food and Drug Administration increased public awareness of the trans fat issue by requiring labeling on products containing trans fats beginning in 2006.

To prevent the effects of trans fats, women can make healthy choices in their own diet and the diet of their children. By avoiding fast foods, preparing food more often than using processed foods, and serving fruits, vegetables, beans, and chicken, trans fats are reduced. Women can become smarter shoppers by:

- Shopping the perimeter of the store (processed foods are usually on the inner isles of supermarkets).
- Avoiding shopping when they are hungry because they are more likely to make poor choices.
- Having a plan for quick meals, such as stir-fry vegetables, rice, chicken, and grilled salmon.
- When eating out, selecting restaurants that do not prepare food with trans fats. Due to research reports linking trans fats and high cholesterol, some fast food restaurants, such as Kentucky Fried Chicken, stopped frying foods in trans fats.

VITAMINS

Vitamins are organic compounds that cannot be manufactured in the body. They are needed in small quantities to facilitate metabolic processes. Vitamins are classified as water soluble and fat soluble. Water-soluble vitamins include C (ascorbic acid), and the B-complex vitamins, including B_1 (thiamine), B_2 (riboflavin), B_3 (niacin or nicotinic acid), B_6 (pyridoxine), B_9 (folic acid), B_{12} (cobalamin), pathothenic acid, and biotin. **Water-soluble vitamins** cannot be stored in the body and therefore must be ingested in the diet daily. **Fat-soluble vitamins** include A, D, E, and K. Fat-soluble vitamins are stored in the body, so a daily intake is not necessary. However, because they are stored in the body, overconsumption can result in toxic levels. All vitamins are found in a variety of fruits and vegetables.

MINERALS

Minerals are necessary for fluid balance, clot formation, strong bones and teeth, and nerve/muscle coordination, among other things. Common minerals include sodium, chloride, potassium, calcium, phosphorus, magnesium, iron, and iodine. Minerals are found in fruits, vegetables, grains, and meat.

WATER

Water is necessary for digestion, transporting nutrients to the cell, removal of waste from the cell and as a cooling agent. The body is able to produce some water, but the majority is obtained orally. To maintain healthy body functions, the average adult needs eight glasses of water daily. Many people think that they can obtain their fluid requirement by drinking any kind of fluid, including coffee, milk, juice, and soda. However, beverages that contain sugar can cause fluid to leave the tissues by osmosis and therefore contribute to dehydration. Flavoring can be added to water, but sugar should be avoided.

HEALTHY DIET

A healthy diet is one that uses these guidelines:

- It emphasizes fruits, vegetables, whole grains, and fat-free or low-fat milk and milk products.
- It includes lean meats, poultry, fish, beans, eggs, and nuts.
- It is low in saturated fats, trans fats, cholesterol, sodium, and added sugars.
- It balances the amount of intake with the energy expended.

Various guides have been developed to assist with planning a healthy diet. One such guide, the new MyPyramid (Figure 6-3 ■), was developed by the U.S. Department of Agriculture to assist individuals of different body types,

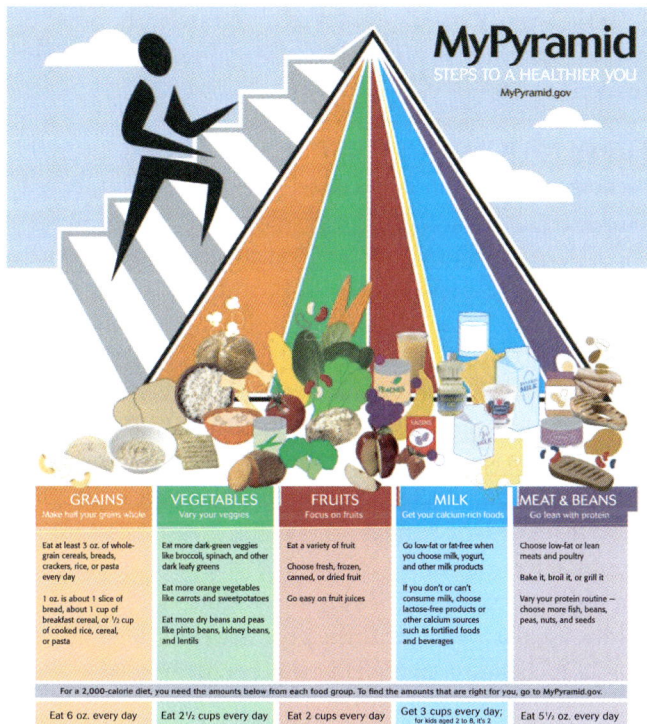

ages, and genders in planning a well-balanced diet. The food guide, found on the U.S. Department of Agriculture website, allows people to personalize a plan for healthy eating. Adjustments can also be made for different ethnic food preferences (Box 6-1 ■). Portion size has been identified as a

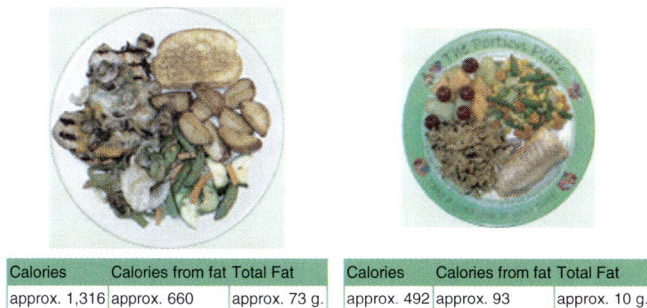

Figure 6-3. ■ (**A**) U.S.D.A. MyPyramid provides information about the different types of food and how much a person needs. (**B**) *Left portion*, typical restaurant amount; *right portion*, a healthful amount of food. (Courtesy of beBetter Networks at www.theportionplate.com.)

BOX 6-1	CULTURAL PULSE POINTS

Alternate Food Guides

Several variations have been made to adapt the food guide pyramid to ethnic diets.

Asian Diet Pyramid

- A wide base of rice, rice products, noodles, breads, and grains; whole grains; and minimally processed foods
- A second level of fruits; vegetables; and legumes, nuts, and seeds
- Daily small amounts of vegetable oils; physical activity; and plant-based beverages (tea, sake, beer, or wine)
- Optional daily fish, shellfish, or dairy
- Weekly eggs or poultry and sweets
- Monthly meats

(Although dairy products are largely absent, the plant-based diet of the Asians results in surprisingly low rates of osteoporosis.)

Mediterranean Diet Pyramid

- An abundance of food from plant sources, including fruits and vegetables, potatoes, breads and grains, beans, nuts, and seeds
- Emphasis on a variety of minimally processed and, wherever possible, seasonally fresh and locally grown foods
- Olive oil as the principal fat, replacing other fats and oils
- Daily consumption of low to moderate amounts of cheese and yogurt
- Weekly consumption of low to moderate amounts of fish and from zero to four eggs per week (including those used in cooking and baking)
- Fresh fruit as the typical daily dessert; sweets with a significant amount of sugar (often as honey) and saturated fat consumed not more than a few times per week
- Red meat a few times per week
- Moderate consumption of wine, normally with meals
- Regular physical activity at a level that promotes a healthy weight, fitness, and well-being

Native American Food Pyramid

- Grain group is divided into bread and cereal group, and rice and pasta group (oats and wild rice); each group allows 6–11 servings per day
- Vegetables: 3–5 servings including corn, squash, and cactus
- Fruits: 2–4 servings including fresh whole fruits
- Dairy: 2–3 servings including cheese, yogurt, and milk
- Meat, poultry, fish, dry beans, eggs, and nuts: 2–3 servings
- Fats and oils sparingly

(continued)

MediaLink Personalized Food Guide

Source: Ramont, R. R., Niedringhaus, D. M., Towle, M. A. (2006). *Comprehensive nursing care*. Upper Saddle River, NJ: Prentice Hall, p. 358, Box 16-1.

BOX 6-1 *(continued)*

Vegetarian Diet
Many ethnic diets are vegetarian based. The following make up a vegetarian food guide pyramid:

- Dairy intake may be 0–3 servings. Individuals who do not use dairy products need to find another source of calcium.
- Protein intake comes from dry beans, soy, and seeds (some do eat eggs).
- Grains and other sources of plant protein need to be varied to provide essential amino acids, which are all only found in animal protein sources.
- The eating patterns of vegetarians vary considerably. The lacto-ovo-vegetarian eating pattern is based on grains, vegetables, fruits, legumes, seeds, nuts, dairy products, and eggs, and excludes meat, fish, and fowl. The vegan (total vegetarian) eating pattern also excludes eggs, dairy, and other animal products. Individual assessment is required to evaluate the nutritional quality of a vegetarian's dietary intake.

major contributor to overweight in the United States. Figure 6-3B contrasts appropriate portion sizes with typical portions provided at American restaurants.

Other food guides have been developed by individuals or companies whose goals are to assist individuals with weight reduction. Examples of weight reduction guides include but are not limited to Weight Watchers, Jenny Craig, the Atkins diet, and the South Beach Diet. These food guides rely on the principles of a balanced diet to guide food choices in an attempt to reduce calorie intake.

Besides varying the kinds of foods, individuals should pay attention to the amount of food consumed. Serving sizes in restaurants have doubled or tripled in the past years. Americans are used to seeing their plate heaped with food, and they eat all of it. Generally serving sizes should be 1/2 to 1 cup of cereals and grains, 1/2 cup of fruits and vegetables, and 3 to 4 ounces of cooked meats. Food labels should be followed regarding serving sizes. Ideally, the food should

TABLE 6-3

Serving Size Estimates

ITEM	APPROXIMATE SIZE
Meat portion	Deck of playing cards
Fruit portion	Tennis ball
Chopped vegetables	Half a baseball or rounded handful
Nuts	Level handful
Ice cream	Tennis ball

be weighed or measured prior to placing it on the plate. If this is not possible, the size can be estimated. Table 6-3 may be helpful in estimating serving sizes.

Exercise

There is no substitution for being physically fit. Exercise is central to almost all other aspects of a healthy lifestyle. The goal is to change from a sedentary lifestyle (couch potato) to doing 30 minutes of activity daily. Daily exercise is necessary for proper utilization of insulin and glucose, weight loss, and increasing muscle strength. Exercise lowers the risk of heart attack and stroke by lowering cholesterol, lowering blood pressure, and improving oxygen consumption. The nurse needs to be prepared to answer women's questions about exercise.

If the woman has a very sedentary lifestyle, the nurse can provide information on adapting intake, such as that shown in Table 6-4.

HOW MUCH EXERCISE?
Generally, the more exercise the better the results. However, some exercise is better than no exercise. To lower the risk of multiple disorders and to improve the general health, people need a total of 30 minutes on most days of the week. Three 10-minute walks are as good as one 30-minute walk, and may be easier to achieve. Increasing the distance the individual needs to walk in a day can provide additional exercise without a lot of extra time spent. For example, parking the car as far away from the grocery store as possible and taking an indirect route to the needed items will increase the walking distance and only require a few additional minutes of shopping. Walking up one flight of stairs and down two flights can increase the cardiovascular workout. If the goal is weight loss, 45 minutes of moderate activity daily is generally needed.

WHAT KIND OF EXERCISE?
Although there are many enjoyable activities, many experts recommend walking 10,000 steps a day. It is simple to do, does not require expensive equipment, and has low risk of injury, and it works. Walking can be done alone, with a friend, or in a group. Using a pedometer to record the number of steps taken will provide instant feedback and may motivate the client to reach the 10,000 step goal. However, self-paced walking is not as effective in lowering the blood pressure and increasing the oxygen utilization as other more aerobic forms of exercise. The client needs to be encouraged to push themselves to a faster paced walk and use arm movements to increase the intensity of the exercise.

Jogging a mile burns the same amount of calories as walking a mile. However, the physically fit person can jog farther in the same amount of time it takes to walk a mile,

TABLE 6-4						
Daily Amounts from Each Food Group by Caloric Level						
CALORIE LEVEL	**1,000**	**1,200**	**1,400**	**1,600**	**1,800**	**2,000**
Fruits	1 cup	1 cup	1.5 cups	1.5 cups	1.5 cups	2 cups
Vegetables	1 cup	1.5 cups	1.5 cups	2 cups	2.5 cups	2.5 cups
Grains	3 oz–eq	4 oz–eq	5 oz–eq	5 oz–eq	6 oz–eq	6 oz–eq
Meat and beans	2 oz–eq	3 oz–eq	4 oz–eq	5 oz–eq	5 oz–eq	5.5 oz–eq
Milk	2 cups	2 cups	2 cups	3 cups	3 cups	3 cups
Oils	3 tsp	4 tsp	4 tsp	5 tsp	5 tsp	6 tsp
Discretionary calorie allowance	165	171	171	132	195	267
CALORIE LEVEL	**2,200**	**2,400**	**2,600**	**2,800**	**3,000**	**3,200**
Fruits	2 cups	2 cups	2 cups	2.5 cups	2.5 cups	2.5 cups
Vegetables	3 cups	3 cups	3.5 cups	3.5 cups	4 cups	4 cups
Grains	7 oz–eq	8 oz–eq	9 oz–eq	10 oz–eq	10 oz–eq	10 oz–eq
Meat and beans	6 oz–eq	6.5 oz–eq	6.5 oz–eq	7 oz–eq	7 oz–eq	7 oz–eq
Milk	3 cups	3 cups	3 cups	3 cups	3 cups	3 cups
Oils	6 tsp	7 tsp	8 tsp	8 tsp	10 tsp	11 tsp
Discretionary calorie allowance	290	362	410	426	512	648

Data from U.S. Department of Agriculture.

and therefore can burn more calories during a 20- to 30-minute workout. Jogging exerts greater force on the bones, muscles, and joints. For the person with bone or joint disorders, this amount of activity may be detrimental. Clients should consult their primary care provider before beginning this or any strenuous activity.

It is important to start slowly and pick up the pace over time. For example, begin walking about 3 miles an hour and increase to a brisk walk of 4 miles an hour. Aerobic walking is around 5 miles an hour. Jogging is faster than this. Other forms of exercise, such as bicycling, roller or ice skating, swimming, and dancing, can be used alone or in combination with walking. Group sports such as basketball, volleyball, or tennis are good forms of exercise but care must be taken to avoid injury. Golf is a good exercise to get the client up and moving, but only the actual time walking (brisk walking preferred) can be counted. Table 6-5 ■ lists the number of calories burned with exercise.

Weight Lifting and Body Building

Aerobic exercise increases the body's use of oxygen and improves cardiovascular health. Lifting weights and body-building increase muscle strength. The straining associated with weigh lifting is dangerous in some cases. The use of resistance training is replacing heavy weight training. Lifting light to moderate weights appears safe for most people. However, the primary care provider should be consulted before beginning any type of weight lifting program.

clinical Alert

Long-term and fairly intense weight training can thicken the heart muscle, increasing the need for blood flow through the coronary arteries and possibly causing a myocardial infarction if the coronary vessels are narrow or blocked. The primary care provider should be consulted prior to beginning any intense activity.

WHEN AND WHERE TO EXERCISE?

The answer to this question is determined, in part, by the environment. If the client lives in a very warm climate, outside exercise should be in the early morning or evening when it is cooler. The client should drink a glass of water before starting exercising and then one glass of water every 30 minutes. In cold climates, the client may be able to exercise more without overheating. However, the cold weather causes vasoconstriction. The heart will have to work harder during exercise to push blood through the

TABLE 6-5

Calories Burned with Exercise* per Hour

Walking 2 mph	240 cals
Walking 3 mph	320 cals
Walking 4.5 mph	440 cals
Bicycling 6 mph	240 cals
Bicycling 12 mph	410 cals
Jogging 5.5 mph	740 cals
Jogging 7 mph	920 cals
Running in place	650 cals
Running 10 mph	1,280 cals
Swimming 25 yards/min	275 cals
Swimming 50 yards/min	500 cals
Jumping rope	750 cals
Tennis (singles)	400 cals
Cross-country skiing	700 cals
Mowing the lawn	500 cals
Shoveling snow	550 cals
Passionate sex	450 cals

*Estimates for a 150-pound person. (Heavier people will burn more, lighter weight people will burn less.)

narrowed vessels. The client should be encouraged to layer clothing and wear a hat, mittens (not gloves), and a scarf. An outer wind- and water-resistant covering may be needed. In both cases the client could choose to exercise inside at home, a gym, or the mall.

Exercise can be done at any time. Some feel more refreshed if they exercise in the morning, shower, and then go to work. Others prefer to exercise after work as a way of relieving work stress. A strenuous physical workout on a full stomach may result in nausea, but walking after a meal may increase peristalsis and improve digestion. Generally, exercise just before bedtime may not be ideal. Exercise increases the release of epinephrine, speeds up the heart, and may prevent the client from relaxing enough to sleep. Allowing 1 hour between exercise and bedtime may be needed.

Rest and Sleep

Rest is a state of calmness and relaxation without emotional stress or anxiety. Rest does not necessarily mean inactivity. A person may find light activity such as slow walking or hobbies restful. Rest restores a person's energy. When a

person is unable to rest, they become irritable, depressed, and emotional. **Sleep** is a state of altered consciousness, in which the person's perception and reaction to the environment are decreased. Sleep is characterized by decreased activity, variable levels of consciousness, changes in the body's physiological state, and a decreased response to stimuli. The individual responds to meaningful stimuli and disregards unmeaningful stimuli. For example, a woman may awaken to the crying of her infant or the alarm of a smoke detector, but continues to sleep when the furnace fan turns on or a truck drives past the house.

Plants, animals, and humans respond to rhythmic biological clocks (biorhythms). In humans these biorhythms are controlled from within the brain as responses to light, dark, gravity, and electromagnetic energy. The most familiar biorhythm is the circadian rhythm (circadian comes from the Latin term *circa dies*, meaning about a day). Ideally, the individual's circadian rhythm coincides with their daily activities. For example, if the person is awake when the rhythms are most active and asleep when the rhythms are most inactive, the individual is in synchronization. This synchronization allows the individual to become renewed. If the circadian rhythm is not synchronized with life activities, as seen when mothers are awakened by their children or a nurse works all night and is unable to sleep during the day, the individual will not be rested and health will decline.

STAGES OF SLEEP

There are two types of sleep characterized by eye movement or lack of it. Rapid eye movement (REM) sleep occurs about every 90 minutes and lasts 5 to 30 minutes. The individual does not rest during REM sleep as the brain increases its activity by 20%. Most dreams occur during REM sleep and are stored in the memory. During this stage of sleep, the pulse and respirations become irregular, the gastric secretions increase, muscle tone is decreased, and the individual may awaken spontaneously or be difficult to awaken.

Non-REM (NREM) makes up most of the sleep throughout the night. It is a deep, restful sleep resulting in a decrease in all metabolic functions. NREM sleep is recorded in four stages. Stage I, lasting only a few minutes, is very light sleep where the individual feels drowsy and relaxed. The sleeper can be easily awakened. Stage II lasts only 10 to 15 minutes but makes up approximately 45% of the total sleep time. The sleeper's temperature, pulse, and respirations decrease. In Stage III, the body functions continue to decrease. The sleeper becomes more difficult to awaken as they stop responding to stimuli. Muscles become very relaxed and snoring may occur. Stage IV, the deepest level of sleep, is called delta sleep. The individual's vital signs drop 20% to 30 % below the

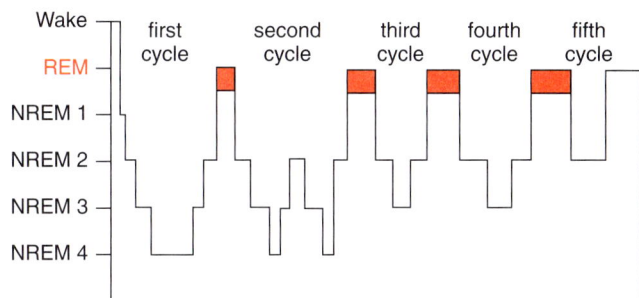

Figure 6-4. ■ Time spent in REM (red portion) and non-REM parts of the sleep cycle.

awake values. The sleeper is very relaxed and rarely moves. The body is restored physically during Stage IV sleep. The individual cycles through the stages of sleep, experiencing four to six cycles during an 8-hour period (Figure 6-4 ■).

WOMEN AND SLEEP

Many women who work outside the home are also responsible for household chores and the care of the children. Being able to have 8 hours of uninterrupted sleep is a rare occurrence for these women. Sleep deprivation results in fatigue, depression, decreased mental alertness, and emotional instability. The nurse must assist the woman to find alternative solutions for her responsibilities that will allow her to obtain adequate sleep and rest. The nurse may need to facilitate communication with her significant others in the problem-solving process. The woman may need to use relaxation techniques, such as those addressed later in this chapter. She may find herbal tea, warm bath, and lavender or other fragrances relaxing. If other methods of relaxation are not effective, she may need to discuss the use of sleeping medication with her primary health care provider.

Personal Hygiene

Cleanliness is both a health promotion and illness prevention activity. When body secretions are allowed to build up, microorganisms grow resulting in potential infection. Personal hygiene (skin, hair, mouth, nails, perineal area) promotes a feeling of well-being. Although the procedures of personal hygiene are not included in this text, a review of key concepts as they apply to women's health follows.

ORAL HYGIENE

Mouth care, including brushing the teeth and tongue and flossing, is necessary to prevent cavities and gum disease. The teeth should be professionally cleaned every 6 months. Estrogen affects the gums resulting in bleeding. Low blood calcium levels seen in women after menopause can

result in dental cavities if good dental practices have not been maintained.

GENERAL HYGIENE

Hygiene is affected by many factors (Table 6-6 ■). Although some general guidelines are accepted by most social groups, variations may occur. It is important for the nurse to avoid being judgmental about people's choices in maintaining hygiene.

Women need to pay close attention to keeping the skin clean and dry, especially in body folds, under the arms, under the breast, and in the groin. A shower is preferred to a tub bath to prevent water from flowing into the vagina and urethra. However, this is generally not a problem unless the woman reclines for long periods of time in a bubble bath solution. An antiperspirant should be used in the axilla and may be used under pendulous breasts if moisture is a problem. Powder mixes with sweat and may cake in body folds, resulting in skin irritation.

The breasts should be cleaned daily. If the woman is pregnant or breastfeeding, care must be taken to prevent infection of the mammary glands. Breast care in these circumstances is addressed in Chapter 16 ◯◯. A well-supportive bra should be worn to prevent the breast tissue from sliding away from the chest wall.

TABLE 6-6	
Factors Influencing Personal Hygiene Practices	
FACTOR	**HYGIENE PRACTICE**
Culture	■ Body odor is offensive in some cultures and accepted as normal in others.
	■ In North American culture, most people bathe or shower daily. In some cultures, people bathe once a week.
	■ In North America, privacy during bathing is essential. In other cultures, communal bathing is the norm.
Religion	■ Some religions practice ceremonial washings.
Finances	■ Finances affect the individual's ability to bathe. The homeless person may not have warm water, soap, shampoo, etc. Those with limited resources may be unable to purchase hygiene products.
Role models	■ Children learn hygiene practices from their parents.
Health status	■ Ill people may be physically unable to bathe. Some may lack the motivation or energy to provide self-hygiene.

The perineal area should be washed and dried daily. Smegma accumulates between the labia folds and should be removed to prevent infection. After elimination, the perineum should be wiped with toilet tissue from front to back to prevent contaminating the urethra and vagina with stool. Following sexual intercourse, some women feel a **douche** (vaginal irrigation) is needed to remove secretions and odor. Frequent douching can remove normal vaginal mucosa, resulting in infection. Therefore, douching is not necessary unless recommended by the primary care provider. Urinating after sexual intercourse will wash secretions from the vaginal opening. Sitting on the toilet for several minutes will allow secretions to drain out of the vagina. The perineum should then be washed with warm water, or the woman could shower to clean the area.

At one time, women were taught that they should not bathe during the monthly period. This is not true. Cleaning the perineum prevents odor and infection. Douching should not be done during menses because the upward flow of water could force endometrial tissue back through the cervix and increase the chance of developing endometriosis (see Chapter 7).

In early times, women made pads and tampons from strips of cloth, washing and reusing them monthly. Today, adhesive strip minipads, maxipads, and flushable tampons are readily available. Although an increased absorbency of pads provides reassurance that leaks will not occur, increased absorbency in tampons may be harmful. Regular absorbent tampons are safe to use during heavy flow days, if they are changed every 3 to 4 hours. If used in the absence of heavy flow, the tampon causes drying of the mucous membrane, which could lead to ulcer formation. If the tampon is hard to pull out or if the vagina becomes dry, the tampon is too absorbent. Regular tampons that expand in width offer protection from leaks without being too absorbent.

The use of super-absorbent tampons has been linked to toxic shock syndrome (TSS). TSS is caused by *Staphylococcus aureus*, a common organism found on the hands of many women. Women should be instructed to wash the hands before inserting the tampon, and then to avoid touching the tip and sides of the applicator during insertion.

A woman may choose to use a tampon during the day and then switch to a pad at night. She should avoid using a tampon on the last "spotty" days, and never use one for mid-cycle spotting, **leukorrhea** (a white mucus discharge from the vagina that may or may not be pathological). If irritation, itching, soreness, or dryness occurs, she should stop using the tampon, change brands, or switch to pads. If itching or soreness continues or a foul odor is present, she should consult her primary care provider. (The Nursing Care Plan Chart that starts on this page discusses nursing interventions for leukorrhea.)

NURSING CARE PLAN CHART

Planning for Client with Leukorrhea

GOAL	INTERVENTION	RATIONALE	EXPECTED OUTCOME
1. Deficient Knowledge related to physiologic patterns of vaginal discharge			
The client or couple will obtain information about variation in vaginal discharge as the result of the normal biological patterns versus the signs of disease.	Provide written information regarding anticipated normal changes in the quantity and thickness of cervical mucous produced in response to ovulation and/or pregnancy.	*Written information allows clients to review information at home.*	Client or couple will understand the self-limiting nature of normal increases in production of vaginal discharge.
	Explain that changes in a female's own established pattern of vaginal discharge is expected as the result of normal hormonal changes, including after menarche and during ovulation, pregnancy, and perimenopause. (Observation of these changes is the basis for *Natural Family Planning*.)	*Verbal instructions meet the needs of auditory learners.* *Not all increases in the quantity or thickness of vaginal discharge indicate disease. Providing factual information can reduce the patient or couple's anxiety.*	Client or couple will demonstrate understanding the difference between normal and infectious discharge by listing three main distinguishing factors: Color, odor, and discomfort (including pain or itch).

GOAL	INTERVENTION	RATIONALE	EXPECTED OUTCOME
2. Risk for Infection			
The client or couple will understand causes and treatment of vaginal infection.	Provide written information on the three most common vaginal infections that produce abnormal discharge: *Monilia* (*Candida* or "yeast"), *Gardnerella* (bacterial vaginosis), and *Trichomonas*.	*Written information allows clients to review information at home.*	Client or couple will list at least two comfort measures for coping with increased vaginal discharge.
An existing infection will be successfully treated.	Provide written information on medical treatment (including antibiotic therapy) for vaginal infection. Explain that hormonal changes of pregnancy and immune disorders (including diabetes mellitus) increase a woman's risk of developing a vaginal infection, especially candidiasis (yeast infection). Explain distinguishing factors between normal discharge and infectious vaginal exudates.	*Verbal instructions meet the needs of auditory learners.* *Increased physical comfort promotes increased emotional comfort and enhanced self-esteem.* *Sexually acquired vaginal infections (such as* Trichomonas vaginalis*) require treatment for the couple. Couples may need to alter their style of sexual expression to avoid reinfection or transmission to a partner.*	Client or couple will list chief components of the medical treatment plan. The client or couple will explain the rationale behind the requests to enhance personal hygiene and limit sexual encounters.
3. Disturbed Body Image			
Client or couple will understand hygienic measures to manage symptoms associated with vaginal discharge.	Provide a written list of recommended comfort measures for perineal care. Discuss comfort measures for managing changes in vaginal discharge (such as wearing loose-fitting garments and natural cotton underwear). Address client's concerns regarding personal hygiene and sexual activity through gentle inquiry, through active listening, and by providing emotional support and culturally sensitive care.	*Written information allows clients to review information at home. Verbal instructions meet the needs of auditory learners.* *Increased physical comfort promotes increased emotional comfort and enhanced self-esteem.* *Alteration in sexual functioning and changing perceptions of the client's own level of personal cleanliness can cause a negative change in body image.* *In some cultures, loss of genital secretions can cause extreme anxiety due to perceived loss of spiritual vitality and/or sexual vigor.*	Client or couple will share any concerns they may have regarding the client's normal vaginal discharge or vaginal infection.

Stress and Coping

Stress is a response to internal or external changes in the client's state of balance (**homeostasis**). A **stressor** is any event that results in stress. The response to a stressor is referred to as **coping response (coping mechanisms).**

Stressors can result in positive coping responses or negative coping responses. For example, the birth of a child is generally a happy experience. With the change in lifestyle that accompanies the new addition, the parents learn to adjust to the stress and within a short time have stabilized their family environment. The changing body image associated with aging and menopause is viewed as a normal change by many women. Both of these life events could become a negative experience. If the new mother becomes overwhelmed with the responsibilities of parenting, she may become depressed. If the new father is unable to adjust to a crying baby, he might lose control and shake the infant, causing brain damage. The aging woman could become upset by her changing body and could request numerous plastic surgeries in an attempt to stay young.

SOURCES OF STRESSORS

There are many sources of stressors. Internal stressors originate from within the person such as diabetes, cancer, or depression. External stressors originate from the external environment such as moving, marriage, or death in the family. Some stressors are anticipated or are predictable. For example, parents anticipate the time when their children will be raised and leave home. Even though the change in the family is anticipated, the child leaving the home results in some stress for each family member. Stressors can also be

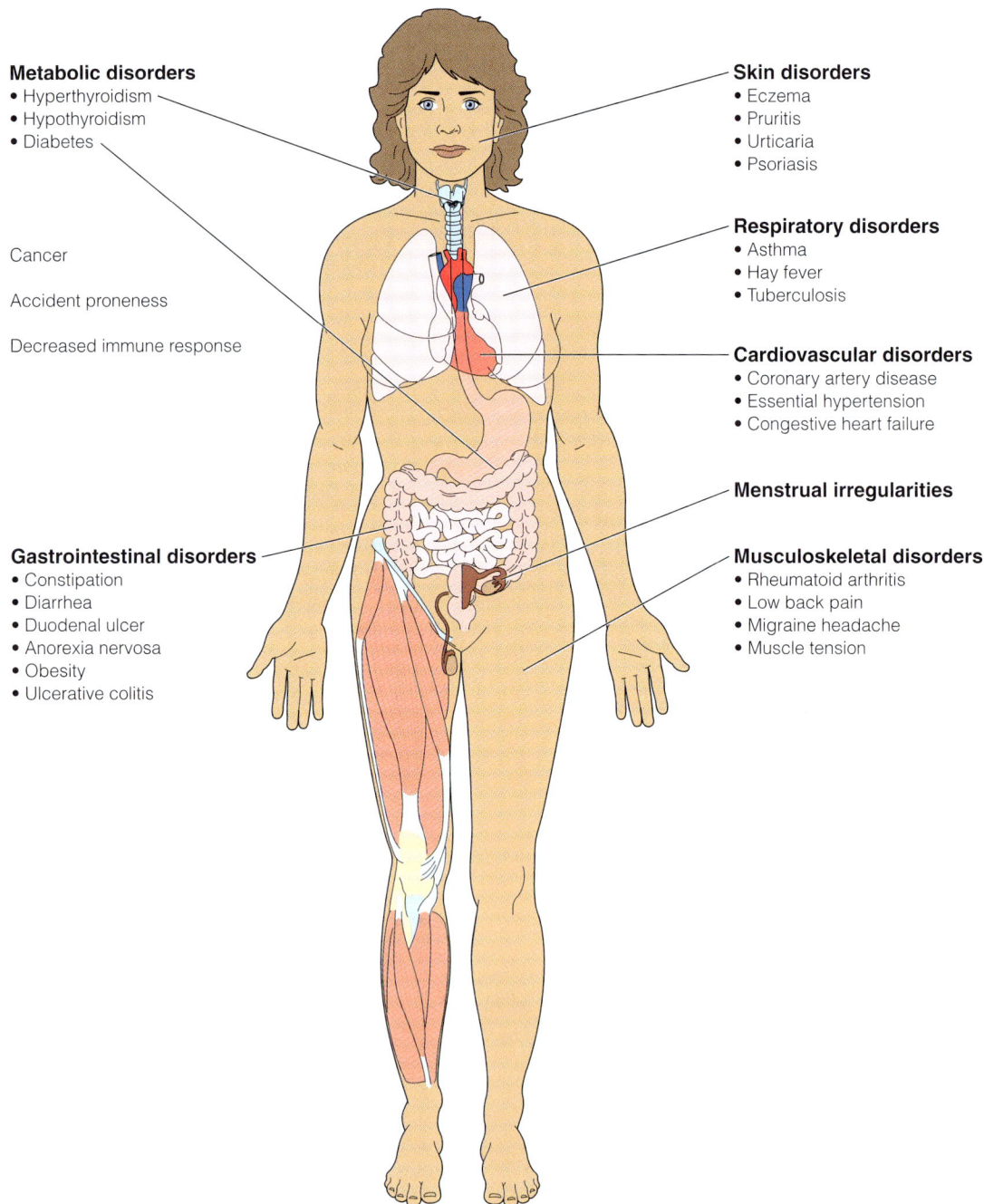

Metabolic disorders
• Hyperthyroidism
• Hypothyroidism
• Diabetes

Cancer

Accident proneness

Decreased immune response

Gastrointestinal disorders
• Constipation
• Diarrhea
• Duodenal ulcer
• Anorexia nervosa
• Obesity
• Ulcerative colitis

Skin disorders
• Eczema
• Pruritis
• Urticaria
• Psoriasis

Respiratory disorders
• Asthma
• Hay fever
• Tuberculosis

Cardiovascular disorders
• Coronary artery disease
• Essential hypertension
• Congestive heart failure

Menstrual irregularities

Musculoskeletal disorders
• Rheumatoid arthritis
• Low back pain
• Migraine headache
• Muscle tension

Figure 6-5. ■ Multisystem effects of stress.

unpredictable. For example, an automobile accident resulting in a physical deformity is not anticipated or predictable.

EFFECTS OF STRESS

Stress affects the whole person and can result in physical, psychological, emotional, social, and spiritual consequences. Stress threatens the person's physiologic homeostasis and can aggravate or cause pathology in the individual (Figure 6-5 ■). Stress can cause individuals to have negative or unconstructive feelings about themselves. Stress can alter a person's perception and problem-solving ability. Stress interferes with relationships and can cause people to question their values and beliefs.

Stress can be seen as changes in the body structure and chemical balance. Stress increases the secretion in the gastrointestinal tract and can result in hyperacidity in the stomach. Stress causes an increase in adrenal hormones, and prolonged stress can result in an enlargement of the adrenal gland. Lymphatic structures—the thymus, spleen, and lymph nodes—atrophy (shrink), and the individual is less resistant to infection. Box 6-2 ■ identifies physiologic indicators of stress.

Anxiety, a common reaction to stress, is a state of mental uneasiness, apprehension, or dread or a feeling of helplessness related to actual or unidentified threat to self or significant relationships. Anxiety results from psychological or emotional conflict, the source of which may not be identifiable. Anxiety can be identified on four levels.

- Mild anxiety produces a mental awakening that enhances learning, perception, and productivity. Most people find mild anxiety a motivating force to seek more information.
- Moderate anxiety produces tension, nervousness, or concern. Perception is narrowed and the individual focuses on particular aspects of the situation rather than the surrounding activities. Learning may be impaired. The vital signs will be slightly elevated and the individual may describe "butterflies in the stomach."
- Severe anxiety takes all the individual's energy and requires intervention. The individual is only able to focus on one thing, usually only one detail of the situation. Communication is difficult to understand, as the individual may repeat or mix up details. The individual experiences tachycardia, hyperventilation, headache, dizziness, and nausea. They will have a fearful facial expression.
- Panic is an overpowering, fearful level of anxiety resulting in loss of control. The individual has increased motor activity, is agitated, and is unpredictable. Perception is often distorted. The person may express a feeling of impending doom and may experience dyspnea, palpitations, and chest pain.

Typically, women are nurturing, caring individuals. They have a strong desire to take care of their loved ones by trying to "fix" the situation. Many women internalize stress and anxiety. Instead of acting out their feelings, their self-talk may be directed toward putting themselves down for being unable the change their situation.

COPING MECHANISMS

To deal with life stressors, individuals develop conscious and unconscious skills or behavior to make themselves feel comfortable. Table 6-7 ■ identifies some commonly used defense mechanisms. Generally when the stressor is relieved or removed, the individual no longer needs to use the defense mechanism. Effective coping results in adaptation to the situation. At times the individual continues to use the defense mechanism beyond the stressful situation, resulting in ineffective coping and maladaptive behavior.

Tobacco, Alcohol, and Drug Use

Due to peer pressure, parental role modeling, or personal stress, many individuals begin using tobacco, alcohol, or other drugs to cope with life issues. Some begin using these chemicals during their adolescent years to "look cool" or fit in with the crowd. Others begin using drugs, alcohol, and

---

BOX 6-2

Physiologic Indicators of Stress

Pupils dilate to increase visual perception when serious threats to the body arise.

Sweat production (diaphoresis) increases to control elevated body heat due to increased metabolism.

The heart rate and cardiac output increase to transport nutrients and by-products of metabolism more effectively.

Skin is pallid because of constriction of peripheral blood vessels, an effect of norepinephrine.

Sodium and water retention increase due to release of mineralocorticoids, which results in increased blood volume.

The rate and depth of respirations increase because of dilatation of the bronchioles, promoting hyperventilation.

Urinary output decreases.

The mouth will be dry.

Peristalsis of the intestines decreases, resulting in possible constipation and flatus.

For serious threats, mental alertness improves.

Muscle tension increases to prepare for rapid motor activity or defense.

Blood sugar increases because of release of glucocorticoids and gluconeogenesis.

Source: Kozier, B., Erb, G., Berman, A., & Snyder, S. (2004). Fundamentals of nursing: Concepts, process, and practice (7th ed.). Upper Saddle River, NJ: Prentice Hall, Box 40-1, p. 1016.

TABLE 6-7

Selected Defense Mechanisms

DEFENSE MECHANISM	EXAMPLE	USE/PURPOSE
Compensation: covering up a weakness by emphasizing a more desirable trait	A high school student too small to play football becomes the star piano player.	Allows individual to overcome weakness and achieve success
Denial: screening or ignoring hurtful or unwanted realities by refusing to acknowledge them	Woman diagnosed with terminal cancer continues to plan a family reunion for 18 months in the future.	Temporarily isolates individual from full impact of traumatic event
Displacement: the discharging of emotion from one object or person to another object or person	Following an argument with the boss, a woman comes home and kicks the dog.	Allows feeling to be released through less threatening means
Projection: blaming others, the environment for unacceptable thoughts, shortcomings, mistakes	Student who is failing college blames the instructor for poor teaching.	Allows person to deny mistakes or shortcomings
Rationalization: justification of behavior by faulty logic	Woman thinks it is all right to shoplift because "everyone" does it.	Helps person cope with inability to meet goals

tobacco later in life to relax and cope with personal, work, or school stress. Although the U.S. government and private agencies spend millions of dollars annually to educate the public on the hazards of chemical use, women's health is still being impacted daily.

Individuals who use tobacco in the form of cigarettes, cigars, pipe tobacco, or chewing tobacco have an increased risk for cancer of the mouth, throat, lung, esophagus, pancreas, and prostate. The risk for hypertension, heart disease, stroke, and peripheral vascular disease is increased by tobacco use as well. Many individuals who smoke also use alcohol and other drugs.

Alcohol is the most commonly abused substance. Alcohol is a central nervous system (CNS) depressant that is readily absorbed into the blood. Within minutes of consumption, the effects of alcohol, including relaxation and euphoria, can be felt. Overconsumption can result in slurred speech, **ataxia** (staggering gait), aggressive behavior, respiratory depression, and death. Because alcohol impairs judgment, an intoxicated individual may make choices, such as speeding or having unprotected sex, that they would not normally make. Some individuals mix alcohol with other CNS depressants such as narcotics resulting in respiratory depression and death.

Other drugs, including narcotics, cocaine, methamphetamine, and marijuana, alter women's health. These drugs are addicting, making it difficult to stop taking them. To have the money to purchase drugs, many women become prostitutes or get involved in the production and sale of drugs. When a woman is high on drugs, she may not eat well or maintain hygiene. All of these result in a lower level of health and lead to disease, including heart, liver, and kidney failure.

Women who become pregnant while using drugs endanger the fetus as well as themselves. Table 6-8 ■ identifies some specific effects of drug use on the embryo, fetus, or neonate.

Complementary and Alternative Therapies

The term **complementary and alternative medicine (CAM)** is defined as those practices that do not form part of the dominant system of health management in the area. Many complementary and alternative therapies have been used for centuries, and their effectiveness has been documented in local custom. Since 1991, the National Institute of Health has been investigating and evaluating promising unconventional medical practices. Today, many insurance plans cover CAM including chiropractic care, acupuncture, and massage therapy.

Holistic nursing theories proposed by Parse (1981), Newman (1986), Watson (1988), and others imply that all living organisms are interacting parts of the whole. Any disturbance in one part affects the whole being. Therefore, the nurse must keep the whole individual in mind when assessing any part, and consider how that part interacts with other parts. The nurse must also consider how the individual interacts with and relates to the environment and other individuals in society. The goal of holistic nursing is to enhance the healing of the whole person from birth to death.

Some CAM techniques can be used by any nurse with a holistic orientation to nursing practice. Other CAM techniques require advanced training, certification, or licensure. The nurse must be familiar with the legal scope of nursing

TABLE 6-8

Selected Drugs and Possible Effects on Embryo/Fetus/Neonate

DRUG	EFFECT
Alcohol	Mental retardation, microcephaly, midfacial hypoplasia, cardiac anomalies, intrauterine growth restriction, potential teratogenic effects, fetal alcohol syndrome, fetal alcohol effects
Heroin	Intrauterine growth retardation, withdrawal symptoms, respiratory depression, convulsions, tremors, sneezing, irritability, vomiting, fever, diarrhea, neonatal death
Methadone	Fetal distress, preterm labor, rapid labor, placenta abruption, meconium aspiration, neonatal drug withdrawal
Valium	Possible cleft lip and palate, respiratory depression, hypotonia, hypothermia, low Apgar score, poor sucking reflex
Amphetamines	Learning disabilities, poor motor coordination, generalized arthritis, possible cleft lip and palate, transposition of the great vessels
Marijuana	Fetal growth retardation
Cocaine	Spontaneous abortion, fetal death, low birth weight, cerebral infarctions, microcephaly, learning disabilities, CNS anomalies, cardiac anomalies, genitourinary anomalies, sudden infant death syndrome (SIDS)
Hallucinogens (phencyclidine [PCP], LSD)	Withdrawal symptoms, newborn behavioral and developmental abnormalities, chromosomal breakage
Nicotine (1/2 to 1 pack of cigarettes/day)	Increased rate of spontaneous abortion, abruptio placentae, small for gestational age, small head circumference, decreased length, SIDS, attention deficit/hyperactivity disorder

under which they practice. Many state boards of nursing include aspects of CAM in their nurse practice acts. Several therapies will be mentioned here, but are not intended to provide complete instruction in CAM.

TOUCH THERAPIES

Touch therapies, including massage, foot reflexology, acupressure, and Reiki, date back to early civilization. Many religions believe that the "laying on of hands" has a healing effect. Touch can stimulate the immune system, cause relaxation, and promote a sense of comfort and well-being. Some techniques involve hand-to-body contact between the nurse or therapist and the client, whereas other techniques involve the invisible energy field that surrounds the client. The energy field can be visualized by use of thermography, but this is unusual. With instruction and practice, the nurse can feel the energy field. The energy field is congested over areas of pain, injury, or other physical dysfunction and feels farther away from the client or warmer than other areas.

Massage

Massage, the rubbing of the skin and underlying muscles, improves circulation and promotes relaxation. It releases lactic acid that accumulates during exercise and causes muscle fatigue and pain. Massage can relieve anxiety and

provide a sense of balance and harmony. A variety of massage strokes can be used, including effleurage (stroking), pétrissage (kneading or large quick pinches of skin and muscle), light touch, and pressure (Figure 6-6 ■).

Foot Reflexology

Foot **reflexology** is based on work by William H. Fitzgerald in the early 1900s. He believed that the hands and feet are a mirror of the body, and reflex points on the hands and feet

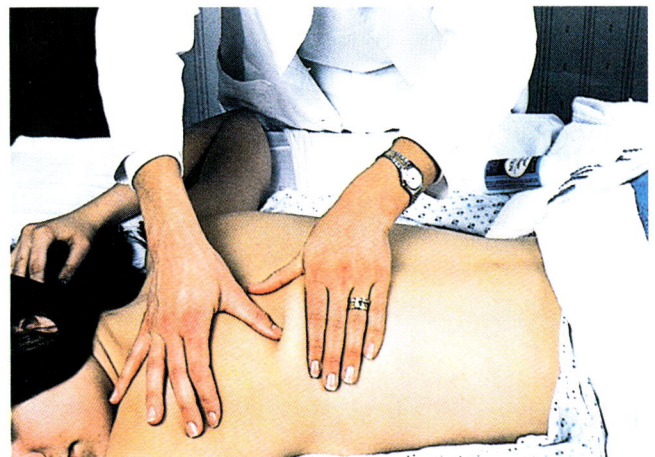

Figure 6-6. ■ Back rubs are one way of reducing stress.

correspond to the body's glands, structures, and organs (Figure 6-7 ■). According to this theory, when the flow of energy in the body is blocked or congested, massaging the corresponding reflex points in the feet can relieve the congestion. At this time, no research validates the theory. However, massaging the feet can stimulate relaxation and affects the autonomic response including the endocrine and immune systems. Although foot reflexology is a relatively safe procedure, an experienced reflexologist should be consulted if the client has a circulatory disorder of the extremities.

Acupressure

Acupressure is a form of healing in which the therapist uses finger or thumb pressure over specific pressure points. These points are run along body meridians that connect each side of the body. According to theory, pressure on these points can free up the flow of energy between the body parts, thus allowing the body to heal itself. These pressure points are similar to those used in acupuncture. The nurse can use acupressure, but is not licensed to perform acupuncture.

Reiki

Reiki (pronounced RAY-key) and therapeutic touch are similar therapies in which the therapist interacts with and redistributes the client's energy fields. In Reiki, the therapist places his or her hands on the client and there is an exchange of energy. With therapeutic touch, the therapist touches the client's energy field. By moving the hands, the energy is redistributed to areas of less congestion. In both cases, the changing of the energy field stimulates the body to heal itself.

MIND–BODY THERAPIES

Mind–body therapies are techniques that utilize mental processes to bring about healing. The focus of mind–body therapies is to bring balance between the thoughts and emotions in order to bring a sense of physical and spiritual well-being. Mind–body therapies include relaxation, imagery, prayer, music therapy, and aromatherapy. Many times it is beneficial to utilize these mind–body therapies in combination to achieve maximum effect.

Relaxation

Relaxation has been used extensively in women's health to reduce stress and decrease chronic pain. Relaxation encourages the client to take control over the body's response to tension and anxiety. In many instances, relaxation can decrease discomfort to a tolerable level and decrease the need for pain medication. For many years, nurses have used relaxation techniques and rhythmic breathing patterns to assist the laboring client. Although the mother could still feel the delivery, she was able to work with the natural body process for a positive outcome.

For relaxation techniques to be beneficial, the client must be in correct posture, have a restful mind, and be in a quiet environment. The body position must be in proper alignment, with joints slightly flexed, and no strain on

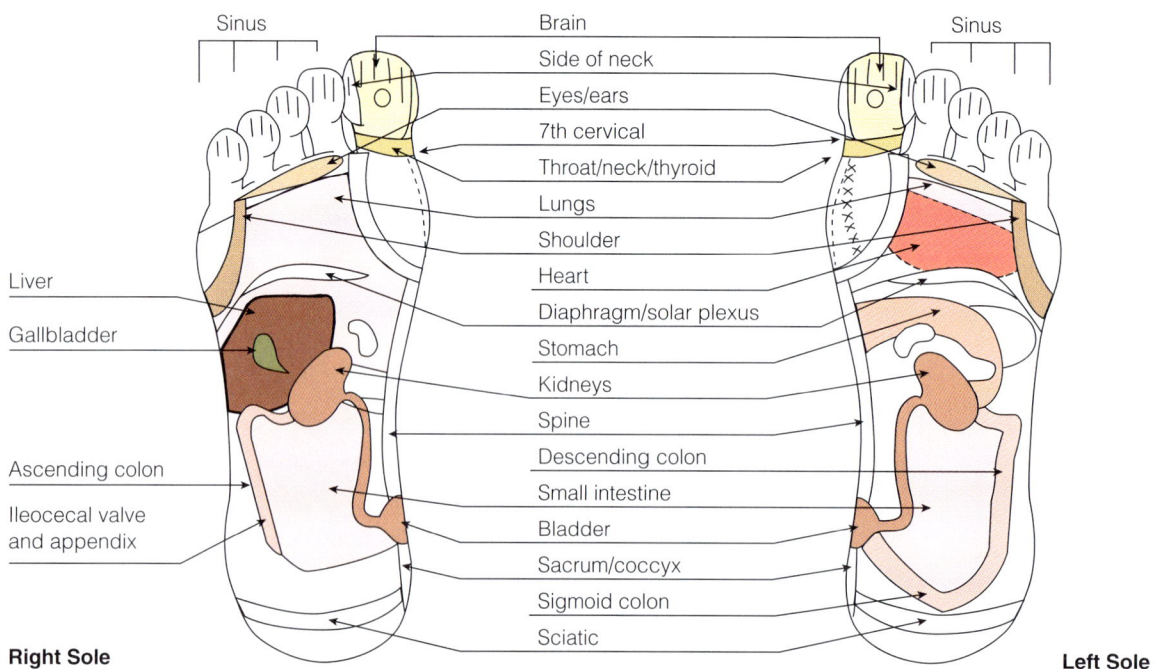

Right Sole

Left Sole

Figure 6-7. ■ Foot reflex areas for massage or pressure points.

muscles. Pillows can be used to support the limbs. To relax the mind, ask the client to slowly gaze around the room and focus on some object such as the pattern on the curtain before moving the gaze to another area of the room. The activity creates a center of concentration. The environment must be free of distractions, with dim light.

The client is asked to contract a muscle group for 3 to 5 seconds, focusing the mind on the feeling of the tight muscle. The muscle group is then relaxed and the sensation of relaxation becomes the focus. Progressively tighten and relax each muscle group in the body. Many clients begin at the feet and work up toward the head. Clients should be encouraged to enjoy the feeling of the muscles relaxing.

Imagery

Imagery is the use of the imagination with the intent of stimulating mind, body, and spiritual healing. Different kinds of images can be used. All body senses should be incorporated into the image. Images are reinforced by asking the client to describe the image including sounds, smells, tastes, etc. If the client is becoming tired and depressed by the situation, imagining a beautiful place such as a beach can stimulate relaxation and a mental escape for a time. Asking the client to listen to the surf and smell the salt air increases the effect of the image. Playing music or using fragrances can enhance the image and subsequent relaxation.

Prayer

Prayer and the reading of the Bible, Koran, or other religious literature of the client's choosing provide healing for the spirit. The nurse may be asked to participate in these religious events or to contact the client's clergy, rabbi, or priest. The nurse supports client's beliefs without imposing other beliefs upon the client.

NURSING CARE

PRIORITIES IN NURSING CARE

To focus on the overall health of a women, a holistic assessment is done. The physical, emotional, and spiritual aspects of the client are reviewed. Attention is paid to clarifying the client's current status, identifying potential health risks, and providing information so that the client can achieve a greater degree of wellness. Box 6-3 ■ provides a brief listing of aspects of an overall health assessment.

ASSESSING

When assessing a client, the nurse collects data related to not only the functioning of each body system, but also nutritional status, quality of the diet, the amount and

---

BOX 6-3	ASSESSMENT

Data Collection About Health Risks
- Demographic information (age, gender, height, weight)
- Type and amount of exercise
- Occupation
- Smoking
- Twenty-four-hour dietary history
- Family history of heart disease, diabetes, cancer
- History of screening tests
- Oral hygiene and dental care history
- Immunization history
- Personal history of illness
- Safety measures (seatbelt, sunscreen, condom)
- Sexual activity and reproductive history
- Use of alcohol, illicit drugs, prescription drugs
- Emotional state or mood

Source: D'Amico, D., & Barbarito, C. (2007). *Health & physical assessment in nursing.* Upper Saddle River, NJ: Prentice Hall, Box 2-1, p. 44.

---

quality of sleep and rest the client receives daily, and the client's ability to cope with daily stressors. Obtaining a sexual history is an important part of assessment, even though it may cause the client and the nurse some degree of anxiety. Most people do not discuss the details of their sexual experiences, especially if they believe their behavior would offend or upset the listener. The nurse must ask questions related to sexual relations, the number of sexual partners, and the use of contraceptives and barriers to prevent sexually transmitted infections. The nurse must listen with an open mind and display a nonjudgmental attitude.

Some indicators of health problems are determined through a nursing history, whereas others are obtained by direct observations. The nurse must look for subtle indicators and compare them to the subjective data the client relates. For example, if the client denies stress in her life, but talks rapidly, bites her nails, avoids eye contact, and has increased weight gain over the past 3 months, the nurse might suspect that the client's denial of stress is inaccurate. More detailed questioning is warranted.

DIAGNOSING, PLANNING, AND IMPLEMENTING

Nursing diagnoses related to women's health could include but are not limited to:

- Health-Seeking **B**ehaviors (specify)
- Readiness for Enhanced **K**nowledge (specify)
- Readiness for Enhanced **N**utrition
- Disturbed **S**leep Pattern

Expected outcomes might include:

- Agrees to stop smoking
- Verbalizes understanding of teaching (specify)
- Follows diet guideline as evidenced by weight loss (or maintenance)
- Sleeps 8 hours each night

The nurse might provide some of the following interventions:

- Work with the client to identify the specific problem, desired outcome, and next steps to be taken. *Assisting the client to verbalize the area that needs change is the first step. It is crucial to reframe the problem in terms of what the client desires to accomplish, so that incremental steps can be made toward the client's goal. If steps are not identified, the client may become overwhelmed and discouraged.*
- Provide client teaching and resources, including support groups, written material, Internet websites, or agency referrals. *The client will need support to make changes in lifestyle. Resources and support groups can help the client to maintain focus and to start again when lapses occur.*
- Make a follow-up appointment. *Follow-up appointments are an important part of the ongoing plan. They provide opportunities to discuss successes and failures and to maintain a positive direction.*

EVALUATING

Many health promotion and illness prevention activities take time before changes are seen in the client's health. The nurse would evaluate the client's health status at each clinic visit. By pointing out positive changes, the nurse encourages the client to continue to improve her health. If positive changes are not identified, the nurse would need to explore with the client the reason for the lack of change. The plan of action would then be updated.

NURSING PROCESS CARE PLAN
Caring for Woman Who Wants to Stop Smoking

Barbara, a 24-year-old woman, is hoping to become pregnant in the next few months. She has read that smoking increases the risk of having a low birth weight or premature baby. Barbara has been smoking since she was 16. She currently smokes 3/4 of a pack of cigarettes per day. She states she really wants to quit smoking, but is not sure where to begin.

Assessment

- BP 132/88, P 82, R 24
- Lung sounds of fine crackles
- Clothing smells of tobacco smoke

Nursing Diagnosis
The following important nursing diagnosis (among others) is established for this client:

- Deficient **K**nowledge related to stop smoking programs

Expected Outcomes

- The client will verbalize stop smoking programs available to her, how to access support groups and the need for follow-up health care.

Planning and Implementation

- Assist client to set realistic plan to stop smoking with dates for compliance. *Making expectations reachable will encourage compliance and promote success.*
- Discuss available stop smoking programs that are offered at local hospitals, treatment centers, and some private businesses. *Programs can provide motivation and support.*
- Discuss the need for a combination of medication and nicotine replacement therapy (NRT), aversion therapy, alternative therapies such as hypnosis, acupuncture or herbs, and counseling. *This approach validates the fact that eliminating an addiction is not just a matter of "having willpower."*
- Provide a list of local stop smoking support groups. *Reinforcement and encouragement are especially useful when people can empathize with one another.*
- Schedule a return visit to the clinic in 1 month. *The return visit sets a goal and provides an opportunity to help the person further if the first attempts have not been successful.*

Evaluation
Barbara stopped smoking by the date established. If she became noncompliant with her plan, she reestablished a target date and began the program again.

Critical Thinking in the Nursing Process

1. What are some other topics that should be discussed with Barbara while she is trying to stop smoking?
2. What should the nurse say if Barbara has not been able to stop smoking in one month?
3. Have you ever tried to quit smoking or complete any similar life-altering activity? What did you do to keep from getting discouraged?

Note: Discussion of Critical Thinking questions appears in Appendix I.

Note: The reference and resource listings for this and all chapters have been compiled at the back of the book.

Chapter Review

KEY TERMS by Topic

Use the audio glossary feature of either the CD-ROM or the Companion Website to hear the correct pronunciation of the following key terms.

Nutrition
osteoporosis, carbohydrates, proteins, lipids, trans fats , vitamins, water-soluble vitamins, fat-soluble vitamins, minerals

Rest and Sleep
rest, sleep

Personal Hygiene
douche, leukorrhea

Stress and Coping
stress, homeostasis, stressor, coping response, coping mechanisms, anxiety

Tobacco, Alcohol, and Drug Use
ataxia

Complementary and Alternative Therapies
complementary and alternative medicine, massage, reflexology, acupressure, Reiki, mind–body therapies, imagery

KEY Points

- Health promotion and illness prevention must become a part of each client interaction.
- The nurse has the responsibility to plan and implement care that permits normal functioning of all body systems.
- The LPN has the responsibility to assist the RN in health promotion activities.
- Health promotion activities include client teaching regarding nutrition and fluids, exercise, sleep and rest, and cleanliness.
- Many alternative treatments such as relaxation, massage, and imagery aid in stress reduction.
- The nurse may work with other health care professionals in planning and implementing health promotion and illness prevention activities for individuals and groups.
- The nurse can apply the principles of health promotion and illness prevention in helping to improve the health of the entire community.
- Stop smoking and substance abuse programs are examples of health promotion and illness prevention activities.

EXPLORE MediaLink

Additional interactive resources for this chapter can be found on the Companion Website at www.prenhall.com/towle. Click on Chapter 6 and "Begin" to select the activities for this chapter.

For chapter-related NCLEX®-style questions and an audio glossary, access the accompanying CD-ROM in this book.

FOR FURTHER Study

For endometriosis and other reproductive disorders, see Chapter 7.

For normal fetal development, see Chapter 8.

Saturated fats and trans fats are discussed in Chapter 11.

For information about breast care when breastfeeding, see Chapter 16.

Critical Thinking Care Map

Caring for a Woman Seeking Health Information
NCLEX-PN® Focus Area: Psychological Adaptation

Case Study: Wendy, 23 years old, has recently moved across the country due to work commitments. She comes to the Woman's Clinic for a health examination and to establish a relationship for future health maintenance or treatment. She has no family in the area. Wendy has no specific health complaints, but is anxious and tearful. She said that it has been hard to move away from her family. She is concerned she will not be able to meet her work commitments. She states she has been staying in her apartment and eating too much because it makes her feel safe, but she is upset because she has gained 15 pounds in 3 months.

Nursing Diagnosis: Health-Seeking Behaviors related to recent move

COLLECT DATA

Subjective	Objective
_____	_____
_____	_____
_____	_____
_____	_____
_____	_____
_____	_____

Would you report this? Yes/No

If yes, to: _____

Nursing Care

_____
_____
_____
_____
_____
_____
_____
_____
_____
_____

How would you document this? _____
_____
_____
_____

Compare your documentation to the sample provided in Appendix I.

Data Collected
(use only those that apply)

- Tearful
- Afraid
- Overeating
- Anxious
- States she eats too much
- Little exercise
- No family or friends in local area
- Staying home
- No specific physical complaints
- Stressed by work commitments
- BP 114/72, T 98.4° F, P 76, R 18
- Establish relationship for health maintenance

Nursing Interventions
(use only those that apply; list in priority order)

- Provide list of health clubs in the area.
- Draw blood for CBC.
- Identify nutrition needs.
- Obtain a baseline weight.
- Set up equipment for a complete physical examination.
- Identify learning needs.
- Provide information on balanced diet.
- Provide relaxation techniques.
- Obtain a health history.

NCLEX-PN® Exam Preparation

1 The nurse is teaching a group of young women about birth control methods. This activity is an example of:

1. primary prevention.
2. secondary prevention.
3. health promotion.
4. tertiary prevention.

2 The LPN/LVN documents that a client with a broken leg is experiencing moderate anxiety based on the assessment of which of the following symptoms?

1. Client asks for more information about crutching walking.
2. Client is easily agitated.
3. Client's learning is impaired.
4. Client is experiencing palpitations.

3 A client complains she has a hard time sleeping even though she exercises right before bedtime. Which of the following suggestions should the LPN/LVN recommend?

1. Exercise earlier in the evening.
2. Lift weights before bedtime.
3. Take a short walk before going to sleep.
4. Exercise only on the weekend.

4 A client expresses concern about feeling fatigued and unable to relax in the evenings. Which of the following recommendations would the LPN/LVN suggest to help improve sleep? Select all that apply.

1. Drink herbal tea in the evening.
2. Exercise right before bedtime.
3. Avoid working on hobbies in the evening.
4. Take a warm bath before bedtime.
5. Practice imagery techniques.
6. Increase fluids containing carbohydrates.

5 The nurse is conducting a class on nutrition for women. Which of the following statements made by a client requires further teaching about healthy nutrition?

1. "I will shop for food after I have eaten lunch."
2. "I will select foods that are low in trans fat."
3. "Vitamin A is good for you, so I can eat as much as I want."
4. "I will try to drink at least 8 glasses of water a day."

6 The LPN/LVN is caring for a client who has frequent vaginal infections and reviews the client's hygiene practices. Which of the following would increase the client's risk for vaginal infections?

1. frequent douching
2. avoiding douching during menstruation
3. cleansing the perineum with water
4. changing tampon every 3 hours

7 The nurse is preparing to teach a class to young adolescents on the use of tampons. Which of the following instructions should be included in the class? Select all that apply.

1. To insert the tampon, hold the side of the applicator.
2. Douche on the second day of menses.
3. Avoid super-absorbent tampons.
4. Tampons may be used for heavy mucus discharge.
5. Wash hands prior to inserting the tampon.
6. Change regular absorbent tampons every 3 to 4 hours.

8 The LPN/LVN is assisting a client to relax using imagery. Which of the following nursing strategies will increase the effects of imagery?

1. performing acupuncture
2. administering sleep medication
3. increasing fluid intake
4. playing music

9 Which of the following nursing actions by the LPN/LVN provides an example of secondary prevention?

1. screening for osteoporosis
2. administering a hepatitis B vaccine
3. providing a list of foods to increase calcium intake
4. teaching proper foot care to a diabetic client

10 The nurse is explaining how physical activity promotes health in older women. Which of the following activities would the LPN/LVN suggest to help women increase muscle strength?

1. aerobic activity
2. group sports
3. lifting weights
4. walking 10,000 steps per day

Answers for NCLEX-PN® Review and Critical Thinking questions appear in Appendix I.

Chapter 7

Reproductive Issues

LEARNING Outcomes

After completing this chapter, you will be able to:

1. Define key terms.
2. Describe possible causes of reproductive issues.
3. Discuss the medical and surgical interventions used to treat the client with reproductive issues.
4. Identify nursing diagnoses and nursing interventions to assist the couple with reproductive issues.
5. Provide appropriate care for the couple with reproductive issues.

Since the mid-1960s, more emphasis and support have been placed on reproductive issues than at any other time in recent history. Many of these issues carry with them emotional, moral, and ethical concerns. This chapter presents common reproductive issues and currently accepted interventions. For a more in-depth study of specific disorders, pathology, and medical treatment, the reader should refer to a medical-surgical textbook.

WOMEN'S REPRODUCTIVE HEALTH ISSUES

Throughout her life, a woman faces many reproductive system issues. Some are minor, easily treatable conditions. Others are major life-threatening disorders. Some disorders affect the woman's ability to conceive, carry a pregnancy to term, or breastfeed the infant. Some disorders may occur early in life but have an impact on the woman's ability to reproduce years later.

Breast Disorders

Breast disorders may be detected by the woman during a monthly breast self-examination (BSE), during a physical examination by the primary care provider, or by **mammog-**raphy (diagnostic x-ray of the breast). Because early detection is critical to the treatment of malignancy, women should be taught the BSE technique and encouraged to seek annual physical examination and mammogram. Procedure 7-1 ■ describes steps in performing a BSE.

NONMALIGNANT BREAST DISORDERS

Fibrosis is the replacement of inflamed or damaged tissue with connective or scar tissue. In the breast, the result is a painless encapsulated tumor or fibroid. Frequently, the fibroid degenerates, accumulating fluid in the process. This fluid-filled mass or **fibrocyst** puts pressure on surrounding tissue and becomes painful. Commonly, more than one

| PROCEDURE 7-1 | **Breast Self-Examination** |

Purpose

- To provide instruction in monthly self-examination of the breasts
- To identify abnormalities in the breast tissue

Equipment

- Mirror
- Small pillow or folded towel

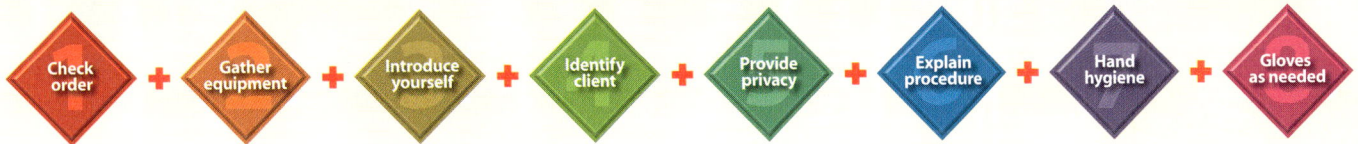

Check order + Gather equipment + Introduce yourself + Identify client + Provide privacy + Explain procedure + Hand hygiene + Gloves as needed

Interventions and Rationales

1. Perform preparatory steps (see icon bar above).

2. Instruction is provided by demonstration, return demonstration, and written material. *Showing the client what to do and then watching her return the demonstration ensures proper technique. Written material is a useful reference when at home.*

3. Stand in front of a mirror in good light with both breasts exposed. *Standing in front of a mirror with good light provides the opportunity to visually inspect all areas of the breast.*

4. Observe the breasts individually for lumps, dimpling, deviation, recent nipple retraction, irregular shape,

edema, or discharge. Compare the right and left breast for symmetry. *Tissue should be consistent throughout the breast. Inconsistent tissue could indicate abnormalities.*

5. Observe the breasts in these positions (Figure 7-1 ■). *Changing position allows for adequate inspection.*
   - With her arms relaxed at her sides
   - With her arms lifted over her head
   - With her hands pressed against her hips while leaning forward

6. While sitting or standing in the shower, place one hand behind the head. Use the finger pads of the other hand to palpate the breast, moving in small, dime-sized circles. *Soap and water make the skin slick and decrease discomfort.*

MediaLink

Breast Cancer

Figure 7-1. ■ Positions for inspection of the breast. (**A**) Both arms relaxed at sides. (**B**) Both arms above the head. (**C**) Both arms on hips while leaning forward. (Data from the American Cancer Society; National Breast Cancer Foundation, Inc®; *Breast Health Access for Women with Disabilities,* produced by The Susan G. Komen Breast Cancer Foundation of San Francisco.)

7. Palpate the area from the collarbone to below the breasts, and from the middle of the armpit to the breastbone. Gently press the breast tissue against the chest wall, feeling for lumps or thickening of the tissue. *This pattern ensures all areas of the breast are examined.*

8. Repeat on the other side.

9. Position supine with a small pillow or folded towel under one shoulder. Place the arm on that side under the head (Figure 7-2 ■). *In this position, gravity pulls the breast into a different position, allowing for more complete examination.*

10. Using the pads of the fingers, palpate the breast again as in step 6. Move down and up across the breast, starting at the axilla (see Figure 7-2A).

11. Repeat on the other side.

12. Palpate the areola and the nipple. Compress the nipple between the thumb and finger to check for discharge (Figure 7-3 ■). *Gently compressing the nipple forces any drainage from the lactiferous duct.*

13. Use a calendar to record when BSE was performed. BSE should be performed once a month, usually on the fifth day after onset of menses. *Recording when BSE was performed is a useful reminder of when to do the next BSE as well as providing documentation should abnormalities occur. On the fifth day after menses begins, the breast tissue has the least hormonal influence.*

14. Report any lumps, dimpling, asymmetry, or discharge to the primary health care provider.

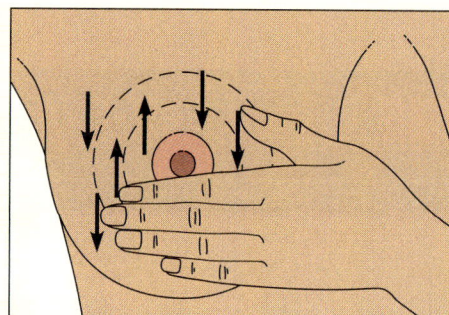

Move the hand vertically down and up across the breasts, starting at the axilla and working toward the center of the body. Press with the finger-pads in small, dime-sized circles to feel the chest wall.

A

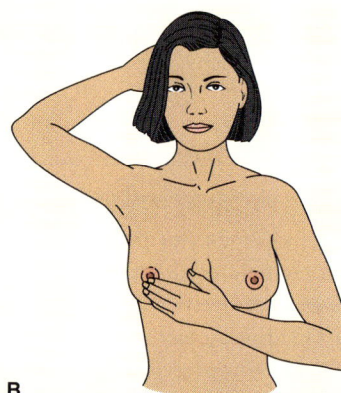

Repeat the same procedure sitting up with your hand still behind your head.

B

Figure 7-2. ■ (**A**) Check each breast in a circular manner, feeling all parts of the breast. (**B**) While holding one hand behind your head, palpate your breast. (Data from the American Cancer Society; National Breast Cancer Foundation, Inc®; *Breast Health Access for Women with Disabilities,* produced by The Susan G. Komen Breast Cancer Foundation of San Francisco.)

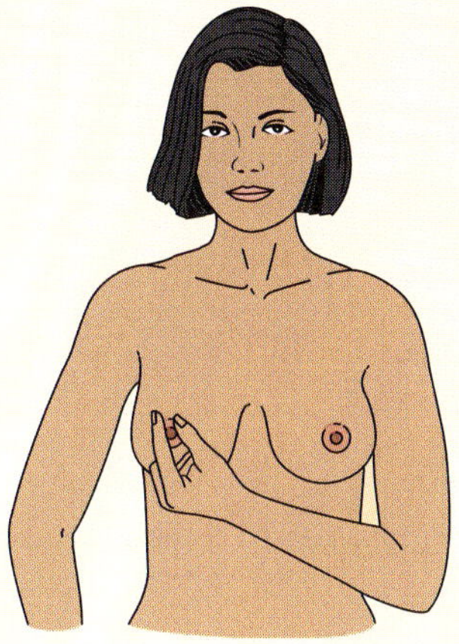

Squeeze your nipple between your thumb and forefinger; look for any clear or bloody discharge.

Figure 7-3. ■ Squeeze the nipple and look for any drainage. (Data from the American Cancer Society; National Breast Cancer Foundation, Inc®; *Breast Health Access for Women with Disabilities,* produced by The Susan G. Komen Breast Cancer Foundation of San Francisco.)

SAMPLE DOCUMENTATION

(date/time)   Instruction in BSE provided. Return demonstration indicates appropriate technique. Written material provided. _____
C. Downey, LPN

fibrocyst forms in each breast, resulting in breast irregularities or "lumpiness." Occasionally, the cyst will drain into the nipple. Table 7-1 ■ describes symptoms and treatment of fibrocystic and other breast disorders.

Fibrocystic breast disease is most common in women between 30 and 50 years of age. Fibrocystic changes in the breast are an excessive response to cyclic hormonal changes. After menopause, these breast changes usually decrease.

TABLE 7-1

Breast Disorders: Symptoms and Treatment

DISORDER	SYMPTOMS	DIAGNOSIS/TREATMENT	NURSING INTERVENTIONS
Fibrocystic breast disease	Fluid-filled movable mass Drainage from nipple Localized pain No skin retraction	Diagnosed by history, mammography, aspiration Medication to suppress estrogen and stimulate progesterone Mild analgesic	Teach BSE. Encourage to limit caffeine in diet. Provide emotional support.
Fibroadenoma	Freely movable mass with well-defined edges Rubbery in texture Nontender mass Most common in teens and early twenties	Fine-needle biopsy Excision with caution to prevent structural damage	Teach postoperative wound care. Provide emotional support.
Intraductal papillomas	Small ball-like nonpalpable mass May have nipple drainage of serosanguineous or brownish-green fluid	Found on mammogram Potential for malignancy Surgical removal	Reinforce teaching by health care provider. Provide emotional support. Provide referral to support group as appropriate.
Breast cancer	Small, hard painless lump, change in the size or shape of the breast, nipple Discharge, dimpling, pulling, or retraction of the skin of the breast resembling an orange peel	BSE, mammography, biopsy Surgical removal, chemotherapy, radiation Long-term therapy with tamoxifen	Reinforce teaching by health care provider. Teach postoperative care. Teach medication use and side effects. Provide emotional support. Provide referral to support group as appropriate.

If cell growth occurs in conjunction with cyst formation, the woman is at a greater risk for breast cancer. Oral intake of caffeine found in coffee, tea, cola, and chocolate may contribute to fibrocystic breast disease. Medical management of fibrocystic breast disease focuses on diagnosis, screening for malignancy, and suppressing estrogen while stimulating progesterone. Aspirated fluid from the cysts is used for diagnosis as well as for relieving pressure and discomfort. There is no evidence that fibrocystic breast disease prevents breastfeeding.

Fibroadenoma is a freely movable, rounded mass with well-defined borders and a solid rubbery texture. These nontender masses are most common in women in their teens and early twenties. Diagnosis is by history and fine-needle biopsy. Excision may be indicated, but caution is exercised to prevent damage to the developing breast structure. Fibroadenomas are not associated with breast cancer.

Intraductal papillomas are tumors growing in a mammary duct. They most commonly occur during menopause. Although they are not malignant, they have the potential of becoming cancerous. These small ball-like tumors are often not palpable but are found on mammography. If they occur near the nipple, a serosanguineous or brownish-green discharge may be present. Because of the risk for malignancy, papillomas are usually removed surgically.

BREAST CANCER

Breast cancer is the second leading cause of cancer-related deaths among women. The most significant risk factor is the woman's age, with most breast cancer occurring after 50. Box 7-1 ■ describes breast cancer risk factors.

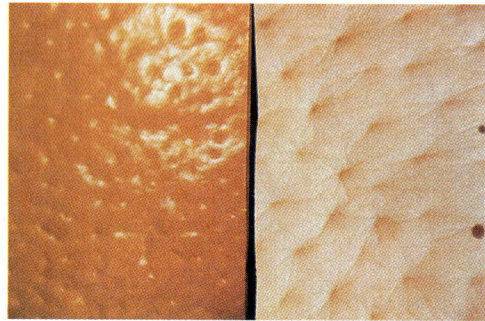

Figure 7-4. ■ *Left*, orange peel; *right*, peau d'orange cancerous changes in a breast.

Breast cancer is an uncontrolled growth of abnormal cells in the breast. Women who have never had functioning ovaries and who have never had estrogen replacement do not develop breast cancer. Most cancerous tumors occur in the ductal areas of the breast.

Noninvasive (also called *in situ*) malignancies develop within the ducts or lobes of the breast without invading the surrounding tissue. Diagnosis of these tumors, which often lie under the areola and nipple, is usually made by mammography rather than palpation.

Invasive tumors grow from the intermediate ducts of the breast. Tumors are classified by cell type. However, prognosis and treatment depend on the progression of the disease (stage of development). Symptoms of breast cancer include a small, hard painless lump; change in the size or shape of the breast; nipple discharge; dimpling; or pulling or retraction of the skin of the breast resembling an orange peel (Figure 7-4 ■).

BOX 7-1   ASSESSMENT

Breast Cancer Risk Factors

- *Personal Data*: Female, over 50
- *Race*: White
- *Family History*: Mother or sister with breast cancer
- *Genetic History*: Defective genes BRCA1 and BRCA2
- *Medical History*: Cancer of breast, endometrial cancer, proliferative fibrocystic breast changes
- *Menstrual/Reproductive History*: Early menarche (before age 12), late menopause (after age 50), first birth after age 30, use of estrogen replacement therapy more than 5 years
- *Radiation Exposure*: Multiple chest x-rays or fluoroscopic exams, particularly before age 30
- *Lifestyle*: More than two alcoholic drinks daily, obesity, smoking, high economic status, breast trauma

---

clinical ALERT

The type of breast cancer that causes *peau d'orange* is called *inflammatory breast cancer*. Physicians may mistakenly diagnose this condition as an insect bite or a breast infection, but the lesion does not resolve within a week or two. Client teaching about this type of breast cancer is important to prevent potentially fatal delays in treatment.

Breast cancer can metastasize to the ribs, sternum, or lungs. In this case, the woman may also exhibit pain, spontaneous bone fractures, and respiratory symptoms such as labored breathing, cough, and **hemoptysis** (bloody sputum).

Treatment of breast cancer depends on the stage of cancer progression. Surgical intervention may include a **lumpectomy** (removal of the lump), breast-conserving surgery (removal of the tumor, a disease-free margin

MediaLink Inflammatory Breast Cancer

TABLE 7-2				
Pharmacology: Common Drug for Clients with Breast Cancer				
DRUG (GENERIC AND COMMON BRAND NAME)	USUAL ROUTE/DOSE	CLASSIFICATION	SELECTED SIDE EFFECTS	DON'T GIVE IF (CALL HEALTH CARE PROVIDER IF)
Tamoxifen (Tamofen, Tamone, Nolvadex)	10–20 mg once or twice a day for 5 years	Antiestrogen, antineoplastic	Bone pain, blood clot formation, alteration in CBC, GI upset	Suspected blood clots, signs of thrombophlebitis, or pulmonary embolism

surrounding the tumor, and adjacent lymph nodes), simple **mastectomy** (removal of the breast), or radical mastectomy (removal of the breast, surrounding lymph nodes, and underlying muscle structure). Radiation and chemotherapy may also be used to shrink and destroy the cancer cells. Long-term treatment with tamoxifen (Nolvadex) is usually recommended (Table 7-2 ■). Due to the change in the body image, women who have had mastectomies may need additional emotional support and referral to a mastectomy support group.

Many women who must undergo a mastectomy assume they are unable to afford reconstructive surgery. Some think that reconstructive breast surgery is cosmetic surgery, which typically is not covered by health insurance policies. Women need to be informed of their rights under the Federal Women's Health and Cancer Rights Act of 1998 (WHCRA). WHCRA requires insurance companies to provide benefits for:

- Reconstruction of a surgically removed breast
- Surgery and reconstruction of the other breast to produce a symmetrical appearance
- Prostheses and treatment for physical complications from all stages of mastectomy, including lymphedema

Under WHCRA, if insurance provides benefits for mastectomy for any reason, it must also provide benefits for reconstruction to ensure a symmetrical appearance. Benefits are subject to terms and conditions of the health insurance plan, including deductibles, copayments, coinsurance, and medical insurance limitations and exclusions. It is important for the woman to become informed about her health insurance policy and applicable federal and state regulations. Information on WHCRA can be obtained through the U.S. Department of Labor and Health and Human Services.

BREAST SURGERY

Surgery on the breast can be done for several reasons. As mentioned, surgery can be performed to remove a tumor or the entire breast and surrounding tissue due to a malignancy. Breast reconstruction **(mammoplasty)** may be performed at the time of the mastectomy or at a later date if extensive therapy is required. (This information is covered in depth in medical-surgical courses.)

Some women have breasts that are large and heavy, putting strain on the shoulders and upper back. These women sometimes request that a **reduction mammoplasty** be performed. In women of childbearing age, the size of the breast will be reduced by removing fat tissue with an attempt to leave the mammary glands intact. This would allow the woman to breastfeed if she desires. In older women, the breast may be reduced by removing mammary glands and fat tissue.

Some women have smaller breasts. The ability to breastfeed is not related to the size of the breast. However, breast augmentation or implants may help these women improve their self-image. Implants contain either saline or silicone. In recent years, there has been controversy over the safety of silicone implants. Continued research should resolve this controversy.

Postoperatively, the woman may have drains leading away from the surgical site. The dressings are usually large and may be cumbersome. It will take 1 week or more for the swelling and bruising to subside. Before discharge, the woman should be taught to care for the incision, apply dressings, and empty the drainage container. During this time, she should be encouraged to look at the breast with a mirror and to begin to adjust to her new image. If a mastectomy has been performed, the woman will need to perform arm exercises on the affected side in order to facilitate lymphatic drainage and achieve full range of motion (Figure 7-5 ■). Due to the change in body image, she may need additional emotional support and referral to a mastectomy support group.

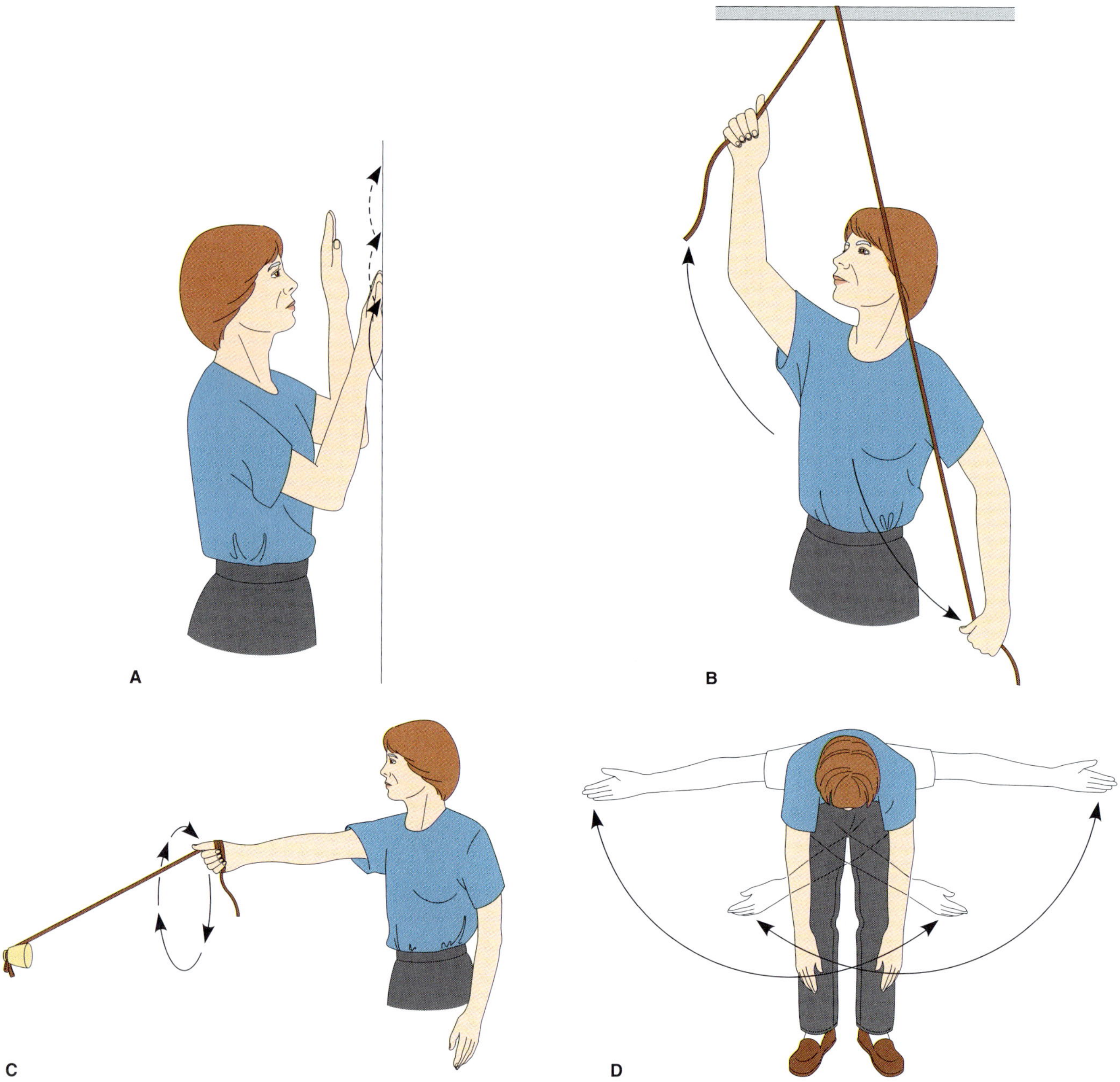

Figure 7-5. ■ Postmastectomy exercises. (**A**) Wall climbing: Stand facing wall with toes 6 to 12 inches from wall. Bend elbow and place palms against wall at shoulder level. Gradually move both hands up the wall parallel to each other until incisional pulling or pain occurs. (Mark that spot on wall to measure progress.) Work down to shoulder level. Move closer to wall as height of reach improves. (**B**) Overhead pulley: Using operated arm, toss 6-foot rope over shower curtain rod (or over top of a door that has a nail in the top to hold the rope in place for exercise). Grasp one end of rope in each hand. Slowly raise operated arm as far as comfortable by pulling down on the rope on opposite side. Keep raised arm close to your head. Reverse to raise unoperated arm by lowering the operated arm. Repeat. (**C**) Rope turning: Tie rope to door handle. Hold rope in hand of operated side. Back away from door until arm is extended away from body, parallel to floor. Swing rope in as wide a circle as possible. Increase size of circle as mobility returns. (**D**) Arm swings: Stand with feet 8 inches apart. Bend forward from waist, allowing arms to hang toward floor. Swing both arms up to sides to reach shoulder level. Swing back to center, then cross arms at center. Do not bend elbows. If possible, do this and other exercises in front of a mirror to ensure even posture and correct motion.

Neurologic
- Syncope
- Dizziness
- Paresthesias
- Headache
- Inability to concentrate
- Depression
- Irritability
- Anxiety
- Mood swings
- Anger
- Aggressive behavior

Sensory
- Conjunctivitis
- Visual disturbances

Cardiovascular
- Bruising
- Palpitations

Urinary
- Cystitis
- Oliguria

Gastrointestinal
- Constipation
- Nausea
- Vomiting

Musculoskeletal
- Backache
- Pelvic stiffness

Integumentary
- Acne
- Herpes recurrence
- Urticaria

Immune System
- ↑ Susceptibility to infection
- Asthma
- ↑ Allergic reactions

Metabolic Processes
- Breast tenderness
- Edema
- Transient weight gain
- Food cravings

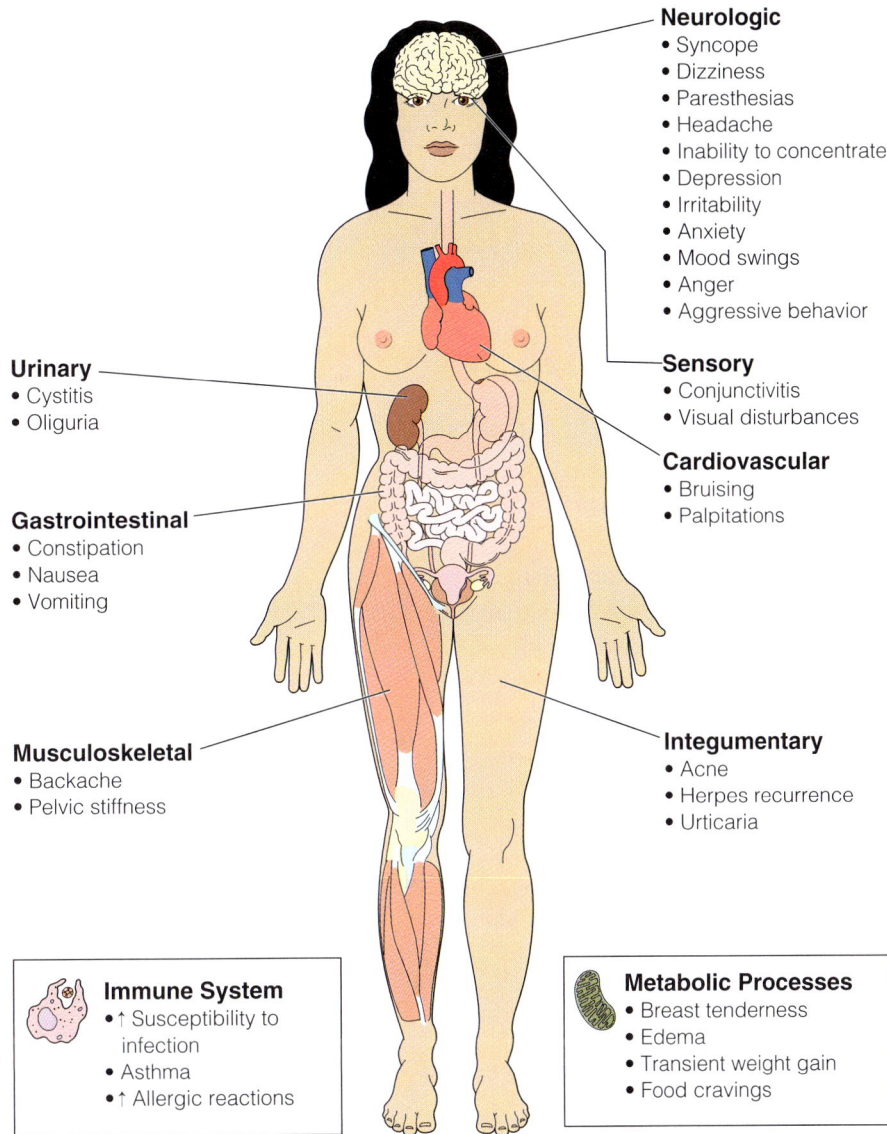

Figure 7-6. ■ The multisystem effects of premenstrual syndrome.

Uterine Disorders

MENSTRUAL DISORDERS

Most women experience minor discomforts just prior to and during menstruation. These include bloating, breast tenderness, cramping, and backache. Other effects can be symptoms of more serious disorders.

Premenstrual syndrome (PMS) is a group of symptoms resulting from an imbalance of estrogen and progesterone, as well as increased prolactin and aldosterone levels. Rising aldosterone causes sodium and water retention. The neurotransmitters monoamine oxidase (MAO) and serotonin may also play a role in PMS. Symptoms, including irritability, depression, edema, and breast tenderness, begin 7 to 10 days before menses and stop with the beginning of the

menstrual flow. The manifestations of multisystem effects of PMS (shown in Figure 7-6 ■) vary for each client and each month.

Management of PMS focuses on diet, exercise, and relaxation techniques to reduce stress. A diet high in complex carbohydrates with limited simple sugars and alcohol is recommended. Restricting caffeine may reduce irritability. Limiting salt intake is useful in reducing fluid retention. An increased intake of calcium, magnesium, and vitamin B$_6$ may be helpful. A balance between exercise and rest can also help reduce irritability. Relaxation techniques and stress management include muscle relaxation, deep abdominal breathing, guided imagery, and meditation.

Other common conditions associated with menses include **menorrhalgia** (painful menses, also known as

Herbal Therapy

Black cohosh (*Cimicifuga racemosa*) is popular in the treatment of PMS and menopausal symptoms. No interaction with other drugs has been reported. Recommended doses may cause gastrointestinal upset. Black cohosh is contraindicated in pregnancy and lactation.

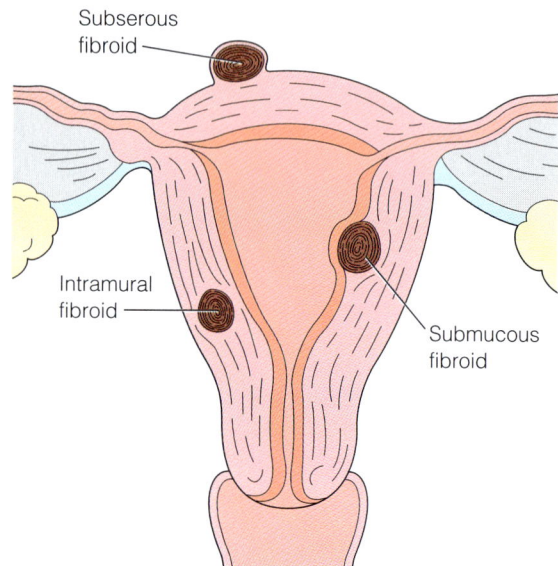

Figure 7-7. ■ Sites of uterine fibroid tumors.

dysmenorrhea), **menorrhagia** (excessive menstruation in volume or number of days), **metrorrhagia** (bleeding between periods), and **amenorrhea** (absence of periods). These conditions are signs of underlying pathology and should be investigated by a health care provider.

Menopause (**climacteric**), the permanent cessation of menstruation, occurs between 35 and 58 years of age. Menses may stop suddenly or may decrease in volume until cessation occurs, or the time between periods becomes longer. Women who have short menstrual cycles or who smoke usually experience menopause 1 to 2 years sooner than women with longer menstrual cycles or women who do not smoke.

Symptoms of menopause begin shortly after the ovaries stop functioning whether menopause occurs naturally or due to surgical removal of the ovaries (**oophorectomy**). Symptoms include hot flashes, irritability, fatigue, apathy, depression, crying episodes, palpitations, vertigo, and vaginal dryness. Decalcification of bones occurs more commonly after menopause. Hormone replacement therapy (HRT) is recommended for many women to ease the menopausal symptoms and promote bone health. Some women choose herbal or food-based supplements instead of HRT (Box 7-2 ■). The Nursing Care Plan Chart on page 131 discusses a client with surgically induced menopause (hysterectomy).

UTERINE TUMORS

Common uterine tumors include nonmalignant fibroids, endometrial cancer, and cervical cancer. Fibroid tumors of the uterus, common among women of all ages, are classified by their location within the uterus (Figure 7-7 ■). Although the exact cause of fibroid uterine tumor is unclear, they are probably related to estrogen secretion. Small tumors may go unnoticed for some time. Large tumors can enlarge the uterus, cause menorrhagia, put pressure on surrounding tissues, and cause lower abdominal and pelvic pain. In asymptomatic women who want to bear children, the fibroid tumors are monitored. In some cases, a laparoscopic **myomectomy** (removal of tumor and surrounding myometrium) may be performed. If tumors are large, a **hysterectomy** (removal of the uterus) may be necessary.

Endometrial cancer is common, affecting women between 50 and 70 years of age. Risk factors include an early menarche,

late menopause, use of estrogen preparations without progestin for prolonged periods, obesity, and diabetes. These slow-growing tumors begin with endometrial **hyperplasia** (excessive proliferation of normal cells). The tumor usually begins in the fundus, spreads to the myometrium, and invades the entire female reproductive system. Metastasis occurs through the lymphatic system, with common sites being lungs, liver, and bone. Treatment includes a hysterectomy with bilateral **salpingo-oophorectomy** (removal of the uterus and both ovaries). Radiation may be used to shrink the tumor prior to surgery and postoperatively to eliminate cancer cells in lymphatic tissue.

Most cervical cancers result from an infection by the human papillomavirus (HPV). Other risk factors include early sexual intercourse, unprotected sex, multiple sex partners, HIV infection, smoking, and poor diet. Early detection and intervention have reduced the incidence of invasive cervical carcinoma.

Most cervical cancers begin as **cervical dysplasia** (abnormal changes in the tissue of the cervix) or cervical intraepithelial neoplasia (CIN), including changes in the squamous cells of the cervix. Over time these cellular changes develop into carcinoma *in situ*, a localized cancer that becomes invasive if not treated. Cervical cancer invades the surrounding tissue, including the vagina, urethra, bladder, and rectum.

In the early stages, cervical cancer is asymptomatic. Once invasion occurs, bleeding, back and thigh pain, hematuria, bloody stools, and anemia are common. Diagnosis is made by a "thin prep" or a Papanicolaou (Pap) smear. In these tests, cells and secretions from the cervix are collected and sent to the laboratory for examination.

NURSING CARE PLAN CHART

Planning for Client with Surgically Induced Menopause

GOAL	INTERVENTION	RATIONALE	EXPECTED OUTCOME
1. Deficient Knowledge related to physiological impact of oophorectomy/ovariectomy			
The client or couple will obtain information about biological changes and the start of menopause as the result of the loss of the ovaries.	Provide written information regarding surgical removal of the ovaries, and on menopause. Explain that only removal of *both* ovaries will cause menopause; the symptoms experienced may be more intense than with ordinary menopause, especially in regard to a decline in sexual desire.	*Written information allows clients to review information at home.* *Verbal instructions meet the needs of auditory learners.* *In the natural female climacteric, ovaries gradually lose their ability to produce hormones at levels necessary to maintain a normal menstrual cycle. However, minimal levels of the hormones estrogen and testosterone continue to be produced even after menses have stopped.* *The activity of one ovary is generally sufficient to produce minimal levels of hormones.* *The severity of menopausal symptoms is closely linked to the level of circulating hormones. Testosterone is the hormone responsible for sexual desire in humans.*	Client or couple will understand the difference between postsurgical and natural menopause. Client or couple will demonstrate understanding by explaining the underlying rationale for menopause after removal of both ovaries, and why this occurs *only* when both ovaries are removed.
2. Readiness for Enhanced Decision Making related to effects of upcoming surgery			
The client or couple will make informed decision treatment options.	Provide written information on health risks associated with surgically induced menopause. Provide written information on the risks and controversial nature of hormone replacement therapy (HRT) to treat menopause. Provide written information on methods to preserve fertility for young women of child-bearing age, such as ovarian tissue cryopreservation.	*Written information allows clients to review information at home.* *Verbal instructions meet the needs of auditory learners.* *HRT has been associated with a significant increase (3 x normal) in the risks of breast cancer, cardiovascular events, including stroke, and Alzheimer's disease.* *Freezing can preserve ovarian tissue containing human eggs. Eggs may be harvested and later fertilized "in-vitro" (IVF).* *Parameters exist regarding the efficacy of different treatment options. The choice for ovarian tissue cryopreservation depends on the underlying disease (e.g., type of cancer), chemotherapy, the client's age and partner status. The physician's knowledge of the client's unique clinical profile is essential in evaluating the risks and benefits of fertility options.*	The client or couple will state understanding of the risks and benefits of pre- and postsurgical treatment options, and will share plans and/or preferences for treatment.

GOAL	INTERVENTION	RATIONALE	EXPECTED OUTCOME
	Explain that the hormonal decline of menopause increases the risk of diseases such as heart disease and osteoporosis.		
	Explain that bilateral oophorectomy/ovariectomy is associated with an increased risk of developing Parkinson's disease.		
	Explain the risks and benefits of HRT.		
	Explain to young women that options to preserve fertility exist; these options should be explored with guidance of the gynecologist and/or oncologist.		
3. Risk for Imbalanced Nutrition: Less than Body Requirements			
Client will maintain balance in body nutrients, especially calcium.	Provide written information on the relationship between dietary calcium and bone health after menopause.	*Written information allows clients to review information at home.*	Client will receive the RDA of calcium each day through diet and/or by calcium supplement intake (dose level as determined by the physician).
	Provide written information on the recommended daily allowance (RDA) for calcium, and a list of high-calcium foods. Recommend consultation with a registered dietitian.	*Verbal instructions meet the needs of auditory learners.* *Change in the rate of bone remodeling occurs as the result of estrogen loss.*	
	Provide information on dietary calcium supplements (e.g., calcium carbonate tablets) and prescription medications to facilitate calcium balance. Administer supplements as per physician order.	*Insufficient dietary calcium intake can worsen demineralization of the bones, the cause of osteoporosis.* *Dietary supplements serve as safeguards for individuals whose diets are lacking in necessary nutrients.*	
	Explain the relationship among diet, calcium balance, menopause, and bone health. Explain the mechanisms of action of prescription medications to reduce bone loss. Administer medications per physician order.	*Professional nutritional counseling facilitates good dietary management.* *HRT reduces bone loss by providing estrogen. Other drug categories include bisphosphonates that inhibit bone resorption, selective estrogen receptor modulators that cause estrogen-like activity in the body, and parathyroid hormone that helps to build new bone.*	

If cancerous cells are identified, magnetic resonance imaging (MRI) or a computed tomography (CT) scan of the pelvis, abdomen, and bones may be ordered to determine the extent of invasion.

When the tumor is localized within the cervix, it may be removed by laser, heated or cooled probes, or cauterization.

A **conization** (removal of a cone-shaped wedge of cervical tissue) may be done if lesions extend into the endocervical canal (Figure 7-8 ■). If the client becomes pregnant, it is important for her to discuss the cervical conization with her health care provider. As the pregnancy progresses, the cervix may dilate under pressure, and premature delivery

Figure 7-8. ■ Conization: removal of a cone-shaped section of the cervix.

may result. If the cancer has spread to surrounding organs, radical surgery, radiation, and chemotherapy may be needed.

Endometriosis occurs when endometrial tissue grows outside the uterine cavity (Figure 7-9 ■). Although the exact cause is unknown, it is theorized that endometrial cells migrate to deeper uterine tissue (myometrium) during fetal development or are washed through the fallopian tubes during menstruation. Endometrial cells can also be picked up in the lymph vessels and transported throughout the body. Endometrial cells that are **ectopic** (outside the uterus) respond to cyclic hormone influence just as uterine endometrium does. The cyclic bleeding results in inflammation, scar tissue formation, adhesions, and occlusions. Endometriosis may lead to infertility.

No single symptom is diagnostic of endometriosis. Often the client will complain of dysmenorrhea with pelvic pain or premenstrual **dyspareunia** (painful intercourse). Dysuria may indicate involvement of the urinary bladder. Premenstrual **tenesmus** (painful straining to defecate) and diarrhea may indicate colon involvement. Diagnosis is made by laparoscopic examination and biopsy of suspected tissue.

The goal of treatment is to preserve fertility for as long as possible. The woman who wants to have children is encouraged to become pregnant as soon as she can. Hormones may be prescribed to cause endometrial atrophy. Table 7-3 ■ identifies common medications used to treat endometriosis.

Surgical treatment may include endometrial obliteration with a laser or electrocautery via a laparoscope. If adequate symptom relief is not achieved, a hysterectomy with bilateral salpingo-oophorectomy may be required.

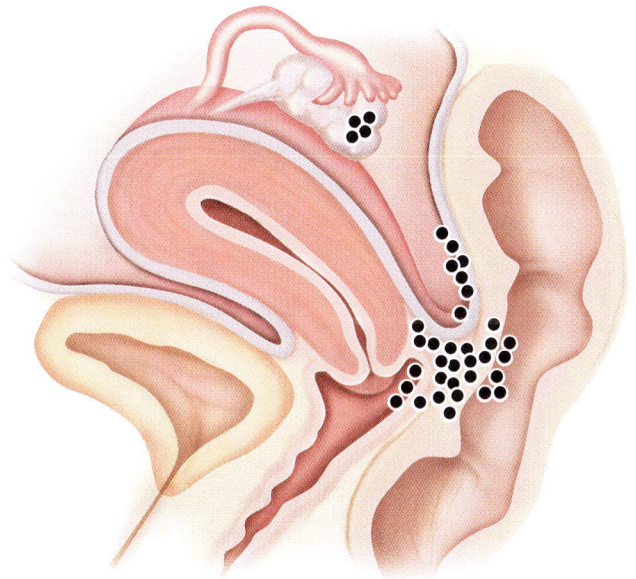

Figure 7-9. ■ Common sites for endometriosis. (Reproduced, with permission, from McGraw-Hill Companies, Inc. Way, L. W. [Ed.]. [1994]. *Current surgical diagnosis and treatment* [10th ed.]. Norwalk, CT: Appleton & Lange, p. 985.)

Ovarian Disorders

Cysts (fluid-filled sacs) commonly form in the ovary, whether from the graafian follicle or from the corpus luteum. Most cysts regress spontaneously in two to three menstrual cycles. Some cysts become so large that they rupture and drain into the pelvis. Bleeding and a surgical emergency could occur.

TABLE 7-3

Pharmacology: Drugs Used to Treat Endometriosis

DRUG (GENERIC AND COMMON BRAND NAME)	USUAL ROUTE/DOSE	CLASSIFICATION	SELECTED SIDE EFFECTS	DON'T GIVE IF (CALL HEALTH CARE PROVIDER IF)
Oral contraceptives	mg/tab depends on specific drug, one tablet daily	Contraceptive hormone	GI upset, depression, increased blood clotting, weight change	History of blood clotting disorders Pregnancy
Progesterone	Individual	Hormone	GI upset, depression, increased blood clotting, weight change	History of blood clotting disorders Pregnancy
Androgen hormone (Danozol)	100–400 mg twice daily	Androgen hormone	Decreased breast size, decreased libido, emotional lability	Pregnancy

Polycystic ovary syndrome (PCOS) results from numerous follicular cysts. This endocrine disorder is characterized by higher than normal LH, estrogen, and androgen levels, and low FSH levels. This hormone imbalance results in irregular menstrual cycles, **hirsutism** (excessive hair growth), acne, obesity, and infertility. The woman may develop type 2 diabetes mellitus and has an increased risk for endometrial cancer, hypertension, and high cholesterol.

Diagnosis of ovarian cysts is made by pelvic ultrasound. Hormone levels are evaluated to diagnose PCOS. Laparoscopic surgery may be necessary to drain large cysts or control bleeding. Hormone therapy may be useful to prevent cyst formation.

Ovarian cancer is the most lethal of female reproductive cancers. Ovarian cancer is asymptomatic until the cancer has spread to surrounding tissue or has been transported by the lymphatic system to other parts of the body. Risk factors for ovarian cancer include older age, early menarche, late menopause, history of infertility, treatment of infertility with Clomid (clomiphene), and a history of breast or ovarian cancer.

Diagnosis of ovarian cancer is made by pelvic ultrasound and laparoscopic biopsy. The treatment of choice is abdominal hysterectomy with bilateral salpingo-oophorectomy. The pelvic organs are examined for metastasis. Radiation and chemotherapy are used to destroy remaining malignant cells.

Pelvic Floor Disorders

Relaxation or damage of the pelvic muscles may result in prolapse or displacement of pelvic organs, including the urinary bladder, uterus, and rectum. A **cystocele** is prolapse of the urinary bladder into the vagina. It develops when the ligaments supporting the bladder are stretched,

thinned with aging, or damaged during delivery. The client may experience stress incontinence, urgency, and difficulty emptying the bladder. Frequent bladder infections may develop.

A **rectocele** develops when the anterior rectal wall protrudes into the vagina. This condition may be caused by childbirth trauma or chronic constipation with straining to defecate. Symptoms include pelvic pressure and difficulty defecating. The woman may need to push up on the perineum or press against the back wall of the vagina to assist proper bowel alignment for defecation.

Uterine prolapse develops when the ligaments supporting the uterus in the pelvic cavity are stretched or damaged. The result is a slipping of the uterus into the vagina. The woman may notice a heavy or dragging sensation in the pelvis. She may also experience stress incontinence, constipation, and dyspareunia. She may be able to feel or see the cervix or entire uterus protrude from the vagina, especially after bearing down or heavy lifting.

Kegel exercises may be ordered to strengthen the pelvic muscles (see Figure 10-8). Pelvic organ prolapse is often treated with surgery to shorten the muscle and supportive ligaments, and resuspend the pelvic organs in their natural position. In postmenopausal women, a hysterectomy is the preferred treatment for significant uterine prolapse. When surgery is contraindicated, the uterus and bladder may be supported with a vaginal pessary. The pessary must be removed, cleaned, and reinserted at regular intervals.

Violence Against Women

Violence against women is a major health concern, causing physical injury, psychological trauma, and sometimes death. Violence affects women and children of all socioeconomic levels, races, ethnic backgrounds, ages, and educational levels. Two of the most common forms of violence against women are domestic violence and rape. Often the blame for the violence is placed on the woman by asking questions such as: "What did she do to make him mad?" "Why doesn't she just leave?" or "Why does she dress so provocatively?"

DOMESTIC VIOLENCE

Domestic violence is defined as methods used to exert power and control over another person in an adult or intimate relationship. It may also be termed **intimate partner violence.** Domestic violence is not limited to married, heterosexual adults. Gay and lesbian individuals and single teens also experience domestic violence. This section focuses on violence against women who are married to their abusers, or who are living with, dating, or divorced from them.

Many people think of domestic violence as physical injury, but it also includes insults, intimidation, ridicule, verbal attacks, threats, emotional abuse, social isolation, economical deprivation, and stalking. Physical attacks may include slapping, kicking, shoving, punching, torture, attacks with weapons, and sexual assault. Women who are physically abused are often psychologically and emotionally abused as well.

CYCLE OF VIOLENCE

Walker (1984) explained that battering takes place in a cycle of three phases:

1. During the tension-building phase, the batterer takes control and demonstrates power. The baterer is angry, argues, and blames the woman for external problems. Minor battering may occur. The woman feels she can prevent escalation of the batterer's anger.
2. During the acute battering incident, which is triggered by some external event, the batterer loses control and violently strikes out at the woman. The batterer is unpredictable and often breaks or damages property as well as injuring the woman.
3. During the tranquil, loving phase (also called the honeymoon period), the batterer tries to make up for the abuse by a show of kind, loving behavior. Without intervention, this phase will end and the cycle of violence will continue. Over time, the violence increases in severity and frequency.

CHARACTERISTICS OF BATTERERS

Batterers come from all backgrounds and socioeconomic levels. Often they have witnessed their mother being abused, or they themselves were abused as children. Male batterers accept traditional values of male dominance. When they are not angry, they appear dependent, seductive, manipulative, and in need of nurturing. They often experience conflict between the image of the "macho man" that they must live up to and feelings of inadequacy in their marriage and intimate relationships. They have a low frustration level and poor impulse control.

CHARACTERISTICS OF BATTERED WOMEN

Many battered women were raised to be passive, submissive, and dependent upon their partners. Some were exposed to violence between their parents, while others first experience battering from their partner. Most battered women do not work outside the home. Over time, the batterer manipulates the woman and isolates her from family and friends. The woman becomes totally dependent on the batterer for financial and emotional needs.

The woman is told the family problems are all her fault. When women are isolated, they find it harder to judge who is right. Eventually they believe they are inadequate and deserve to be beaten. They have deep feelings of guilt, fear, and depression. Their low self-esteem and feelings of hopelessness and helplessness decrease their problem-solving ability.

NURSING RESPONSIBILITIES

Nurses often fail to recognize the abused woman, especially if bruises are not obvious. The woman may be seeking health care for another reason, such as pregnancy, drug use, or alcohol abuse. She may be bringing her child to the doctor for illness or injury. Therefore, the nurse must always be alert for expressions of helplessness or powerlessness. The woman's low self-esteem may be exhibited by her dress, appearance, fatigue, depression, aches, pains, or insomnia. She may have a history of missed or frequently changed appointments.

Because of the incidence of domestic abuse, many primary care providers are recommending screening of all female clients at every health visit. Screening should be done in a quiet, private environment. Possible screening questions include: (ACOG, 1999)

- In the past year, has your partner threatened to harm you?
- In the past year, has anyone hit, kicked, choked, or hurt you physically?
- Has anyone ever forced you to have sex?

During the screening, it is important to be nonjudgmental and to assure the woman that her privacy will be respected. When caring for a woman's injuries, be alert for cues that the injury was the result of abuse. The signs might include:

- Hesitation in discussing the cause of the injury
- Inappropriate emotional response to the situation
- Explanation of injuries that does not match with physical findings
- Lack of eye contact
- Pattern of injury consistent with abuse, such as bruising and abrasion of the head, face, back of neck, throat, chest, abdomen, and genitals
- Battering partner does most of the talking; the woman shows increased anxiety in presence of the partner

The nurse must provide a safe environment for the client. If the partner is with her, ask him or her to remain in the waiting room during the examination. Allow the woman to discuss the situation at her own pace. Provide reassurance that her feelings are normal and expected in the situation. Anticipate that the woman may blame herself for the situation. She may believe that the batterer loves her and will not hurt her again. The woman may need help in identifying the problem and developing realistic solutions. It is important for the nurse to stress that no one should be abused and that the abuse is not the woman's fault. The LPN/LVN in this situation should inform the supervising RN and primary care provider of the abuse. Facility security and local police may need to be notified to offer protection to the woman and health care providers.

Rape Trauma Syndrome

Rape is forced sexual intercourse that involves vaginal, anal, or oral penetration. The rape can be forced by physical or psychological coercion, and drug or alcohol ingestion may be used to decrease the woman's awareness of the situation. The rapist can be a stranger, friend, or relative. Rape may occur by a sudden attack, or it may occur in a social situation (date rape). Date rape is on the increase, but in most situations, it is preventable. Box 7-3 ■ provides some guidelines for preventing date rape.

Incest is sexual intercourse between close blood relatives and may or may not be consensual.

Sexual abuse affects the woman physically and mentally. Rape can cause trauma to the reproductive organs and lead to infection and scarring. Scarring may result in painful intercourse and may prevent future pregnancy. Following a rape, many women have a strong urge to shower and "wash away" all traces of the experience. Showering can actually destroy vital evidence the police will need to apprehend and prosecute the offender. It is, therefore, important for the

woman to seek help from police and medical personnel prior to cleaning herself.

The psychological trauma is as great as or greater than the physical trauma. (Refer to a medical-surgical or psychiatric nursing text for more information.) The woman may feel guilty that she allowed the sexual abuse to occur, that she might have done something to encourage the assailant, or that she could not defend herself. She may be afraid that sexual abuse will recur with the same person or another person.

| BOX 7-3 | CLIENT TEACHING |

Preventing Date Rape

- Meet dates in public places or stay around others, especially when with a new acquaintance.
- Let someone know when you are leaving, where you are going, and when you expect to return. If possible, take a cell phone along and leave your number with a trusted friend.
- Attend parties with a friend and plan ahead how you will get home.
- Pour your own beverages and keep them with you and within sight at all times. Some drugs that cause loss of muscle control or loss of consciousness can be undetectable in drinks.
- Avoid drugs and alcohol. Substance abuse makes it harder to think clearly and harder to resist aggressive behavior.
- Date rape drugs may have no color, taste, or smell and may be easily added to flavored drinks without being detectable. Common date rape drugs include:
  - GHB (gamma hydroxybutyric acid)
  - Rohypnol (flunitrazepam)
  - Ketamine (ketamine hydrochloride)
- Don't drink from punch bowls or other people's drinks.
- Don't drink anything that smells, looks, or tastes strange. (GHB sometimes tastes salty.)
- Know your own limits and values. Communicate them clearly. Respect the limits and values of your date.
- Trust your intuition. If you feel that someone is pressuring you for sex or not respecting your limits, you are probably right. Verbalize your feeling assertively (loudly, if necessary). Don't be afraid to make a scene to keep yourself safe.
- Remember that it is never too late to say "no." Both boys and girls have a right to say "no."
- Be clear that forced sex is rape when you say "no," even if you previously agreed to intercourse with that person. You always have the right to say "no."
- Remember that even if you drank alcohol or used some substance before a rape, you are NOT at fault for being assaulted. Go to a police station or hospital right away. Do not urinate or douche before going. Crisis centers and hotlines are available to talk about the feelings you may experience after a rape.
- Be aware that both males and females can be victims of sexual assault.

The woman may be asked to testify in court regarding the sexual abuse, which could open her past sexual relationships to public scrutiny. Following this emotional trauma, it may be difficult for her to develop trusting relationships and enjoy future sexual encounters.

A woman might present in the emergency department or clinic stating that she has been raped, or she might present with physical trauma suspicious of a violent sexual encounter. The nurse's responsibilities are to provide emotional support and assist in data collection. Most facilities have a "rape kit" containing specimen containers, comb, slides, and other supplies necessary to collect evidence. It is important that all evidence be collected and secured according to legal standards. Guidelines and procedures for collecting this evidence should be outlined in a facility's policy and procedure manual. Respect for confidentiality is essential.

Before collecting data, the woman needs to sign an informed consent form (see Chapter 3 for legal responsibilities of the nurse). A detailed history is obtained using the woman's own words to describe the events. The caregiver should use a nonjudgmental approach and must avoid coaching or leading the woman. The collecting of physical evidence serves the purpose of:

- Confirming recent sexual contact.
- Showing that force or coercion was used.
- Identifying the assailant.
- Collaborating the woman's story.

The woman will be asked to remove all her clothing, and each item will be placed in a separate paper bag and labeled. Samples of stains and body fluids will be obtained for sperm analysis. The absence of sperm does not indicate that a rape did not occur because the assailant could have used a condom or might not have ejaculated. Hair samples will be pulled from the woman's head and pubic area to compare with other hair found on her body. The pubic hair will be combed to check for loose hairs that may have been transferred from the assailant. Debris will be collected from under her fingernails to check for blood or tissue from the assailant. Photographs should be taken of any injuries. A colposcope with photographic capability can be used to photograph intravaginal injury. All evidence must be labeled, be placed in a paper bag, and remain in the possession of a professional until it is turned over to the police.

Because the psychological trauma during a rape is so great, the woman should receive counseling immediately. Many areas have rape crisis centers and personnel trained to provide the psychological support and counseling required in this situation. The psychological response to rape can be described in a series of overlapping phases. The acute phase begins during the rape and can last for a few days or longer. The woman feels fear, shock, disbelief, powerlessness, or helplessness. She may feel angry, humiliated, and unclean. She may suppress her feelings or exhibit an outward response in the form of crying or being tense and restless. She may experience alterations in sleep patterns such as insomnia or nightmares.

Within a few weeks, the woman may appear calm and composed as though she has adjusted to the situation. Frequently, however, these are outward signs of denial. She may go about her daily activities and return to work or school. This resumption of routine is important for her to regain a sense of control over her life. She may seek some forms of self-protection such as installing extra locks on her doors, taking a self-defense course, or buying a weapon. These activities do not resolve the emotional trauma. Instead, they give the impression to her support system that she is "over it." The support system may then withdraw.

However, denial does not last long. She may become depressed and anxious. She may want to talk about the rape (Figure 7-10 ■). She may develop phobias, especially to situations similar to those in which the rape occurred. For example, if she was attacked at night, she may fear leaving her home after dark. If the rape occurred in her home, she may fear returning to an empty house. If her attacker was a stranger, she may fear crowds. She may continue to have nightmares in which she relives the rape. She may replay the incident repeatedly until she finally resolves that the attack was out of her control. It is important for the nurse to be a good, nonjudgmental listener and to make appropriate referrals to the registered nurse, physician, or counselor.

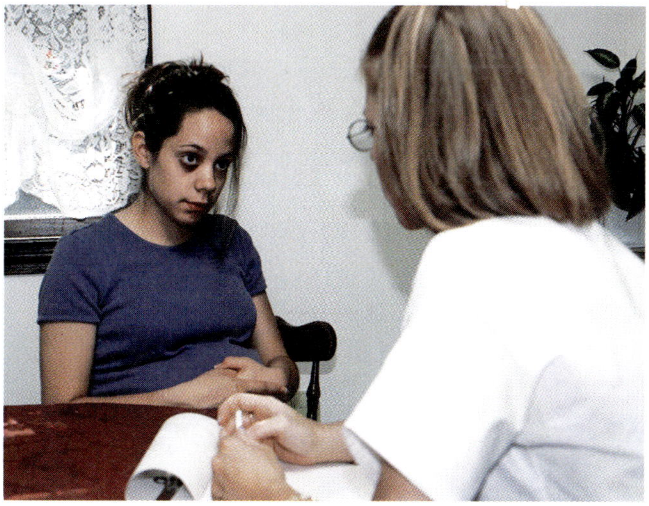

Figure 7-10. ■ Privacy is always a client right, but it is especially important when asking a client questions about abuse or rape.

MEN'S REPRODUCTIVE HEALTH ISSUES

A discussion of reproductive issues would not be complete without reviewing male reproductive conditions. Only common conditions are discussed here. For more detailed information, pathology, medical treatment, and nursing interventions, refer to a medical-surgical textbook.

Testicular and Epididymal Disorders

Testicular cancer is the most common cancer of men between 15 and 35 years of age. Fortunately, testicular cancer has a greater than 90% cure rate. Most men with testicular cancer have no risk factors. Therefore, beginning at 15 years of age, all men should perform testicular self-exam. Procedure 7-2 ■ describes steps in performing a testicular self-examination (TSE).

Testicular cancer grows within the testicle, eventually replacing all normal tissue. Normal tissue will feel soft, while the tumor will be a hard painless mass. Most commonly, only one testicle is affected. Testicular cancer spreads rapidly through the lymph vessels into the retroperitoneal lymph nodes (located behind the peritoneum but outside the abdominal/pelvic cavity). Enlarged lymph nodes may be palpated in the groin. If the cancer cells reach the vascular system, they commonly metastasize to the lungs, liver, and bone.

Treatment usually involves a radical **orchiectomy** (removal of one testis and spermatic cord) with removal of the retroperitoneal lymph nodes. The surgery is accomplished through an inguinal incision, taking care not to damage the nerves needed for ejaculation. Following surgery, radiation and chemotherapy are used to destroy any remaining cancer cells. If only one testicle is removed, reproduction may still be possible. However, the banking of sperm prior to surgery, radiation, and chemotherapy should be discussed with the client and his partner. If the client is a minor, teaching and support must also be provided to the parents.

An infection of the male reproductive system may result in **epididymitis** (inflammation of the epididymis) and

---

| PROCEDURE 7-2 | **Testicular Self-Examination** |

Purpose

■ To provide instruction in monthly self-examination of the testes
■ To identify abnormalities in the testicular tissue

Equipment

■ Hand mirror

Check order + Gather equipment + Introduce yourself + Identify client + Provide privacy + Explain procedure + Hand hygiene + Gloves as needed

Interventions and Rationales

1. Perform preparatory steps (see icon bar above).

2. Instruction is provided by demonstration, return demonstration, and written material. *Showing the client what to do and then watching him return the demonstration ensures proper technique. Written material is a useful reference when at home.*

3. Stand in front of a mirror in good light with genitals exposed. *Using a hand mirror with good light provides the opportunity to inspect all areas of the genitals.*

4. Observe the scrotum and penis for lumps, edema, sores, or discharge. *The scrotum and penis should be free of lumps, swelling, sores, and discharge.*

5. While standing in the shower, support the scrotum with one hand. Place the fingers of the other hand under one testicle and the thumb on top. *Soap and water make the skin slick and decrease discomfort.*

6. Gently roll each testicle between the thumb and fingers feeling for lumps, thickening, or hardening of the tissue (Figure 7-11 ■). *The testes should feel smooth.*

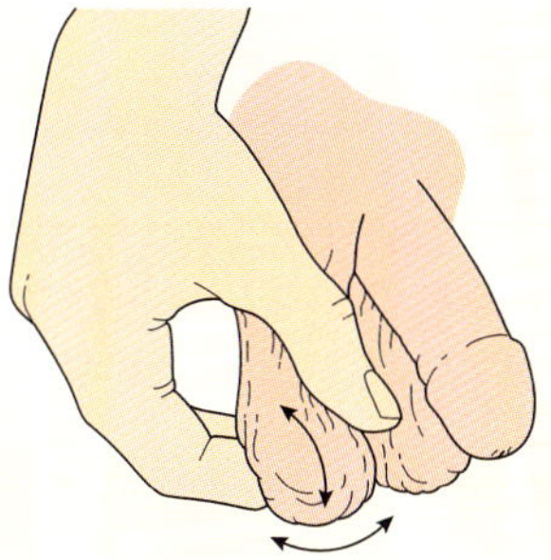

Figure 7-11. ■ Self-examination of the testes should be done monthly to check for the possibility of testicular cancer. Young men are at higher risk for this than other groups.

7. Palpate the epididymis, a cordlike structure on top and back of the testicle. The epididymis feels soft but not as smooth as the testicle. *Feel for firm masses in the epididymis.*

8. Palpate the vas deferens (spermatic cord), which extends upward toward the base of the penis. The vas deferens should feel firm and smooth. *Feel for hard masses in the vas deferens.*

9. Use a calendar to record when TSE was performed. TSE should be performed on the same day of each month. *Recording when TSE was performed is a useful reminder of when to do the next TSE as well as providing documentation should abnormalities occur.*

10. Report any lumps, dimpling, asymmetry, or discharge to the primary health care provider.

SAMPLE DOCUMENTATION

(date/time)   Instruction in TSE provided. Return demonstration indicates appropriate technique. Written material provided. W. Clark, LPN

---

orchitis (inflammation of the testes). In young men, the infection is most commonly caused by sexually transmitted infections (STIs) such as chlamydia or gonorrhea. (Sexually transmitted infections will be discussed later in this chapter.) In older men, epididymitis is associated with urinary tract infection or **prostatitis** (inflammation of the prostate).

Manifestations of epididymitis include pain and swelling of the scrotum, at times interfering with ambulation. Medical treatment includes antibiotics and analgesics. Nursing care focuses on relieving symptoms with ice packs and scrotal support. Epididymitis can cause infertility and should be evaluated after the infection is resolved.

Orchitis may be caused by the same organisms as epididymitis, as well as by a mumps virus that is excreted in the urine, or by trauma. Manifestations include severe testicular pain and swelling. Complications include **hydrocele** (fluid in the scrotal sac) and abscess. These complications can result in infertility and erectile dysfunction.

Erectile Dysfunction

Erectile dysfunction (ED, or impotence) is the inability to achieve or maintain an erection that allows for satisfactory sexual intercourse. Most commonly, this disorder affects men over 65 years of age. Any disorder that impairs circulation (e.g., atherosclerosis) or interrupts nerve or hormone intervention (e.g., diabetes and multiple sclerosis), or trauma that results in scar tissue (e.g., chronic infection or prostate surgery), may cause ED. Drugs that also alter circulation (e.g., antihypertensives) depress the central and peripheral nervous system (e.g., antidepressants), and some hormones may also have side effects of ED.

Diagnostic exams include:

■ Blood tests for chemistry, testosterone, prolactin, thyroxine, and prostate-specific antigen (PSA).
■ Nocturnal penile tumescence and rigidity monitoring. This test monitors the number and firmness of erections during sleep. It is useful in determining if ED is physical or psychological.

Medical or surgical treatment may influence the degree of erection but have little effect on fertility. ED can be treated with drugs such as Viagra (sildenafil), which enhances natural response to sexual stimuli. Testosterone replacement may be used if blood levels are low. Alprostadil (prostaglandin E$_1$) pellets may be inserted into the urethra or injected into the penis. This drug stimulates an erection but may be an unacceptable option for many men (Table 7-4 ■).

When ED does not respond to less invasive treatment, penile implants may be surgically inserted into the penis. Two types of penile implants are available (Figure 7-12 ■). The semirigid implant maintains a constant state of partial erection. The inflatable penile implant has a fluid-filled reservoir that is inserted in the lower abdominal cavity, cylinders are inserted in the penis, and a pump is inserted in the scrotum. Erection is obtained when the pump is

MediaLink Erectile Dysfunction

TABLE 7-4

Pharmacology: Drugs Used to Treat Erectile Dysfunction

DRUG (GENERIC AND COMMON BRAND NAME)	USUAL ROUTE/DOSE	CLASSIFICATION	SELECTED SIDE EFFECTS	DON'T GIVE IF (CALL HEALTH CARE PROVIDER IF)
Sildenafil (Viagra)	50 mg taken 1 hr before sexual activity; not more than once daily	Anti-impotence agent	GI upset, headache, cardiovascular collapse	There are numerous drug–drug interactions that could result in death. Teach client to contact health care provider if erection lasts longer than 4 hours.
Protaglandin E$_1$ (Alprostadil)	5–20 mcg injected into penis or urethral pellets; not more than one dose three times a week with 24 hr between doses	Tissue hormone	Dizziness, low blood pressure, drug allergy including redness at site, and respiratory distress	Teach client to contact health care provider if erection lasts longer than 4 hours.

A Semirigid

Reservoir
Cylinders

Pump

B Inflatable

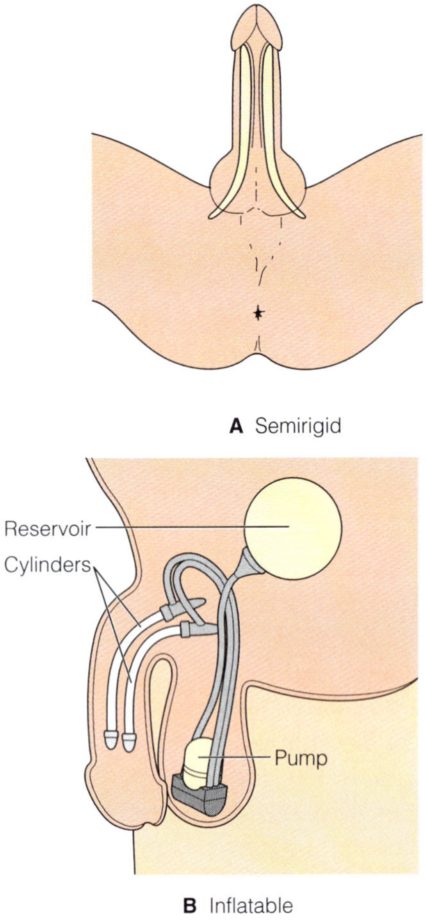

Figure 7-12. ■ Types of penile implants. **(A)** Semirigid rods implanted in the corpora cavernosa keep the penis in a constant state of semierection. **(B)** With an inflatable penile implant, the client compresses a pump in the scrotum to fill cylinders in the corpora cavernosa and achieve an erection. Pressing a release valve returns the fluids to a reservoir.

compressed, filling the cylinders with fluid. A release valve returns the fluid to the reservoir.

Prostate Disorders

Benign prostatic hyperplasia (BPH) most commonly affects men over the age of 50. Normally testosterone is converted to dihydrotestosterone (DHT) in the prostate. DHT, along with estrogen (normally found in small amounts in men), may contribute to the growth of the prostate gland. The prostate gland enlarges in the center, compressing surrounding tissue and narrowing the urethra.

The primary symptoms include **nocturia** (the need to void frequently at night), difficulty getting the stream of urine started, a narrow stream of urine, dribbling after voiding, incomplete emptying of the bladder, frequency, and urgency. Diagnostic exams include:

- Digital rectal exam (DRE) to assess the size and consistency of the prostate.
- PSA—this chemical produced by the prostate gland indicates prostate cancer when elevated. Note that incidence of prostate cancer is affected by race (Box 7-4 ■).
- Routine urinalysis and urine culture to determine if a urinary tract infection is present.
- Uroflowmeter to determine the degree of urinary obstruction.

Treatment includes medication to shrink the prostate or relax the smooth muscles of the prostate, urethra, and bladder neck. Some of these drugs can cause a decrease in **libido** (the sexual drive). The herbal remedy saw palmetto reduces the

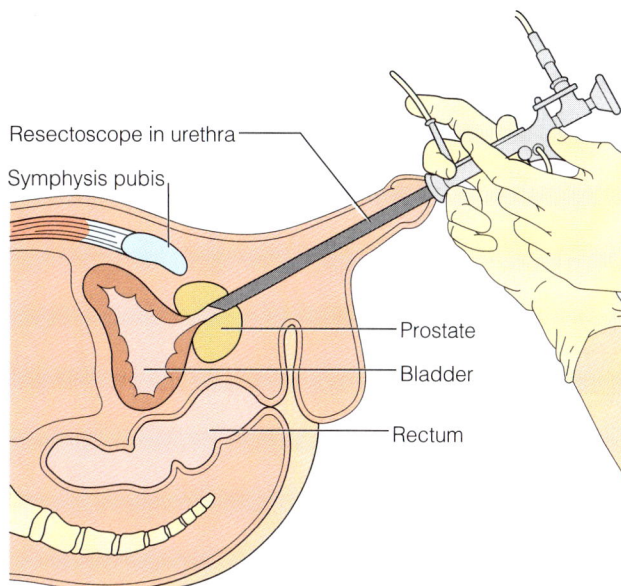

Figure 7-13. ■ TURP. A resectoscope inserted through the urethra is used to remove excess prostate tissue.

symptoms of BPH and has few side effects. Often, surgery to remove the prostate will be required. The most common surgical approach is through the urethra or transurethral resection of the prostate (TURP; Figure 7-13 ■). Following surgery, a large three-lumen catheter is left in the urethra, and a continuous bladder infusion is instituted to prevent blood clots from obstructing the flow of urine. Following surgery, retrograde ejaculation (discharge of seminal fluid into the bladder instead of the urethra) may occur, resulting in a low sperm count. However, it should not be assumed that the man is sterile.

Prostate cancer is a leading type of cancer in men. Prostate cancer rarely occurs before the age of 40. When diagnosed early and confined to the prostate, the 5-year cure rate is 100%. The cancerous tumor usually begins in the posterior region of the prostate and may spread into the seminiferous tubules or bladder. If metastasis occurs in the lymph nodes, tumors may also involve the lung, liver, and bone, especially the pelvis and spine. Besides a DRE and PSA, other diagnostic tests include transurethral ultrasound to help differentiate BPH from prostate cancer. Tissue biopsy is done to confirm diagnosis. A bone scan, MRI, or CT is done to identify possible metastasis.

Treatment includes drugs to block the effects of testosterone, radiation, and surgery. If the tumor is isolated in the prostate, a TURP may be performed. If metastasis has occurred, a radical prostatectomy is done through a different approach.

FAMILY PLANNING ISSUES

Infections

SEXUALLY TRANSMITTED INFECTIONS

STIs result from sexual contact with an infected person. Many people believe that only sexual intercourse can result in STIs. The reality is that infection can occur not only through sexual intercourse, but also through genital-genital, oral-genital, or rectal-genital contact. The most common STIs are chlamydia, genital herpes, gonorrhea, genital warts, trichomoniasis, and syphilis. Table 7-5 ■ lists these common infections, their manifestations, and their medical treatment.

Reportable STIs are those sexually transmitted infections that must be reported to the public health department and Centers for Disease Control. The reportable STIs are chlamydia, gonorrhea, and syphilis. The public health department will notify all identified sexual partners of their possible exposure to an STI and assist them with diagnosis and treatment.

COMMON SEXUALLY TRANSMITTED INFECTIONS

Chlamydia

Chlamydia is caused by *Chlamydia trachomatis*. In males, chlamydia is the major cause of nongonorrhea urethritis. In females, it infects the vagina, cervix, uterus, fallopian tubes, and urethra. The infection can be passed to the newborn during the birth process, resulting in eye infection

MediaLink CDC Presentation of STIs

TABLE 7-5

Summary of Sexually Transmitted Infections

DISEASE	ORGANISM	MANIFESTATIONS	MEDICAL TREATMENT
Chlamydia	*Chlamydia trachomatis*	Males: urethritis Females: permanent scarring	Erythromycin Amoxicillin
Genital herpes	Herpes simplex virus (HSV-2)	Burning, itching sensation prior to blister formation; blisters break, resulting in painful open lesions	Acyclovir
Gonorrhea	*Neisseria gonorrhoeae*	Females: asymptomatic, permanent scarring Males: urethritis, purulent urethral drainage, burning on urination	Ceftriaxone Cefixime with erythromycin or amoxicillin
Genital warts (condylomata acuminata)	Human papillomavirus (HPV)	Grayish-pink cauliflower-like lesions appear on the vulva or penis approximately 3 weeks after exposure	Cryotherapy Trichloroacetic acid
Trichomoniasis	*Trichomonas vaginalis*	Inflammation of the vagina and cervix, yellow-green, frothy, odorous discharge	*Note:* Metronidazole (Flagyl) is *contraindicated* in the first trimester of pregnancy due to its effects on the fetus (can cause birth defects).
Syphilis	*Treponema pallidum*	Stage 1: painless open sore, chancre, slight fever, and malaise Stage 2: fine red rash over the body, palms, and soles Stage 3: damage to heart, nervous system, bone, and skin Aneurysm, gait disturbances, blindness, dementia	Benzathine Penicillin G

and pneumonia. Complications include pelvic inflammatory disease, scarring of the fallopian tubes, and ectopic pregnancy. The newborn of an infected, untreated woman is at risk for developing ophthalmia neonatorum (an infection of the eye that can result in blindness; see Chapter 17 ⬮⬮). In men, chlamydia can cause scarring of the urethral mucosa.

Gonorrhea

Gonorrhea is caused by *Neisseria gonorrhoeae*. In males, gonorrhea is associated with urethritis, purulent urethral drainage, and burning on urination. Females are usually asymptomatic. Prior to pregnancy, gonorrhea can ascend through the cervix and infect the uterus, fallopian tubes, and pelvis. After the third month of pregnancy, the cervical mucous plug prevents gonorrhea from ascending into these organs. When the fetal membranes rupture during the birth process, gonorrhea can infect the infant's eyes and respiratory tract.

Like chlamydia, gonorrheal infection of the reproductive organs can lead to permanent scarring of the fallopian tubes and seminiferous tubules. The scarring may result in infertility.

Chlamydia and gonorrhea are commonly found together. Adequate treatment of both partners is essential to cure the infections. Abstinence or condom use is needed to prevent reinfection until cure is achieved. Further cultures must be taken to verify that treatment was successful.

Syphilis

Syphilis is an infection by the bacteria *Treponema pallidum*. Syphilis is divided into three stages with different symptoms at each stage.

- Primary syphilis: Initially, a **chancre** (painless open sore) forms at the entry site (Figure 7-14A ▪). General signs of infection, including slight fever and malaise, may occur. If left untreated, the chancre disappears in 3 to 4 weeks.

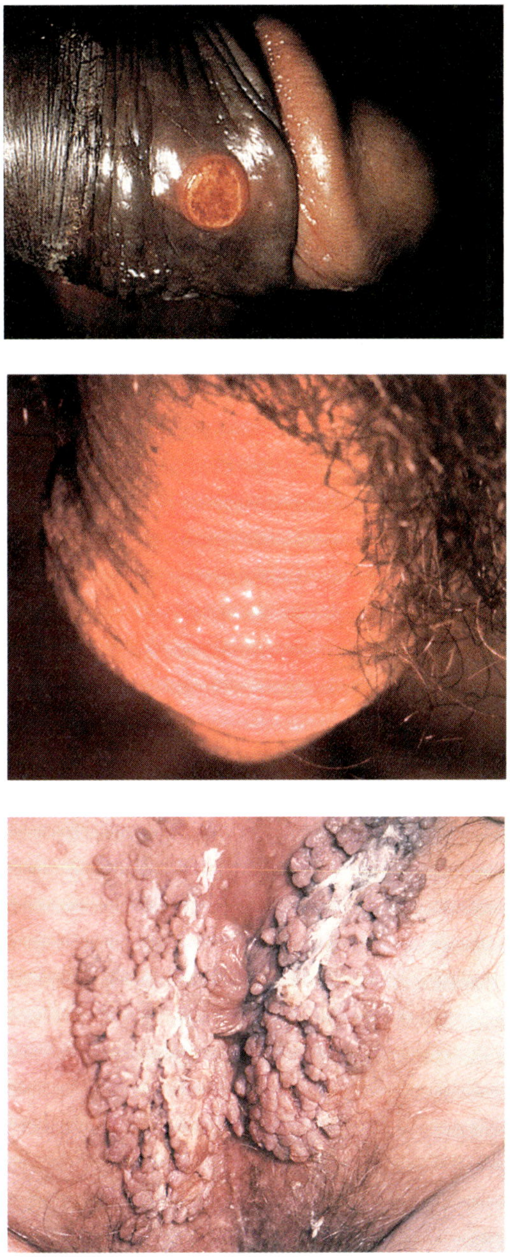

Figure 7-14. ■ Some sexually transmitted infections. (**A**) Primary syphilis. The entry point of syphilis develops a chancre. (**B**) Genital herpes blisters on the penile shaft signal the infectious phase. (**C**) Condylomata acuminata (genital warts) on the labia. (**A**: Custom Medical Stock Photo. **B**: Camera MD Studios, Carroll Weiss, Director, 8290 NW 26th Place, Sunrise, FL 33322. **C**: Ken Greer Visuals Unlimited.)

- Secondary syphilis: Several months later, the symptoms of secondary syphilis appear. These include a fine red rash over the body, palms, and soles of the feet. Highly infectious moist papules may appear on the perineum. If untreated, these symptoms will also disappear in a few weeks. Symptoms of infection may not recur for many years.
- Tertiary syphilis: In the tertiary stage, damage to the heart, nervous system, bone, and skin become apparent.

Aneurysm, gait disturbances, blindness, and dementia are a few disorders that can result from untreated syphilis.

Genital Herpes

Herpes is caused by one of two types of herpes simplex virus (HSV). HSV-1 causes cold sores and typically occurs above the waist. HSV-1 is not sexually transmitted. HSV-2 is associated with sexual contact. The symptoms include a burning, itching sensation prior to blister formation (Figure 7-14B ■). The blisters break and result in painful open lesions. Many viruses are shed at this time, and an infection is highly contagious. Lesions heal spontaneously in several weeks.

Genital herpes also results in lifelong health problems that will affect infected people and their partners. Therefore, during an acute outbreak, the couple should abstain from sexual intercourse. If a pregnant woman has an acute outbreak and goes into labor, a cesarean section delivery should be performed to prevent infection of the infant.

Genital Warts

Genital warts (or condylomata acuminata) are caused by HPV. The grayish-pink cauliflower-like lesions appear on the vulva (Figure 7-14C ■) or penis approximately 3 weeks after exposure. Because genital warts resemble other lesions and can undergo malignant transformation, they should be biopsied and treated. Some strains of HPV, for which a vaccine is available, are associated with cancer of the cervix.

Trichomoniasis

Trichomoniasis, caused by the protozoa *Trichomonas vaginalis*, is most commonly transmitted through sexual contact. It can also be transmitted through shared bath facilities, wet towels, and wet swimwear. Symptoms in women include inflammation of the vagina and cervix as well as a yellow-green, frothy, odorous discharge. In men, trichomoniasis causes burning on urination due to urethral irritation. The treatment consists of administration of metronidazole (Flagyl) to all partners. Flagyl is contraindicated in the first trimester of pregnancy because it acts as a **teratogen** (a chemical that can cause abnormal fetal development). Clotrimazole vaginal suppositories are used to provide symptomatic relief during the first 12 weeks of pregnancy, and then Flagyl can be given.

HIV and AIDS

Human immunodeficiency virus (HIV) is a retrovirus that attacks and destroys the body's immune system. The method of transmission is by direct contact with body fluids. **Acquired immunodeficiency syndrome (AIDS)** is a life-threatening, end-stage infection with HIV. Although HIV is being treated with increased success, HIV infection is still considered fatal. Refer to an adult medical-surgical textbook for further information.

Candidiasis

Candidiasis (monilia or **yeast infection)** is a common organism causing vaginitis. Characteristics of a yeast infection are thick white patches resembling cottage cheese adhering to the cervix, vaginal wall, and labia. There is intense itching of the vulva and vagina. The mucous membrane is red and inflamed. When a specimen is viewed under the microscope, *hyphae* (threadlike filaments) and spores may be seen.

Treatment includes medicated creams, vaginal tablets, or suppositories. The sexual partner should also be treated because *Candida* can grow on the foreskin, glans, and outer skin of the penis.

Contraception

Contraception is the prevention of pregnancy. Although several methods are addressed here, it is important to encourage teens and others to discuss methods of contraception with their health care provider (Figure 7-15 ■). Some methods may not be recommended with certain physical disorders. Table 7-6 ■ lists facts about conception and contraception.

FERTILITY AWARENESS

Fertility awareness is based on the assumption that ovulation occurs at the same time each month. By collecting data regarding physical changes that take place throughout the menstrual cycle, the time of ovulation can be identified. The couple then abstains from intercourse or uses other methods of contraception during ovulation. Objective data to identify ovulation include a **basal body temperature** taken every morning before activity and assessment of cervical mucus (*spinnbarkeit*) (Figure 7-16 ■). Subjective data include increased libido, bloating, and breast changes. Some women may also experience *mittelschmerz* (abdominal pain with ovulation). Once the data are collected for several months, patterns can be identified. Abstinence is generally recommended for several days prior to ovulation and until 3 days after ovulation. The calendar method is the least effective method of contraception.

SPERMICIDES

Spermicides are chemicals in the form of creams, foams, jellies, or suppositories that are inserted into the vagina prior to sexual intercourse. They destroy the sperm or prevent sperm mobility. The chemical must be inserted deep in the vagina and come in contact with the cervix. Suppositories

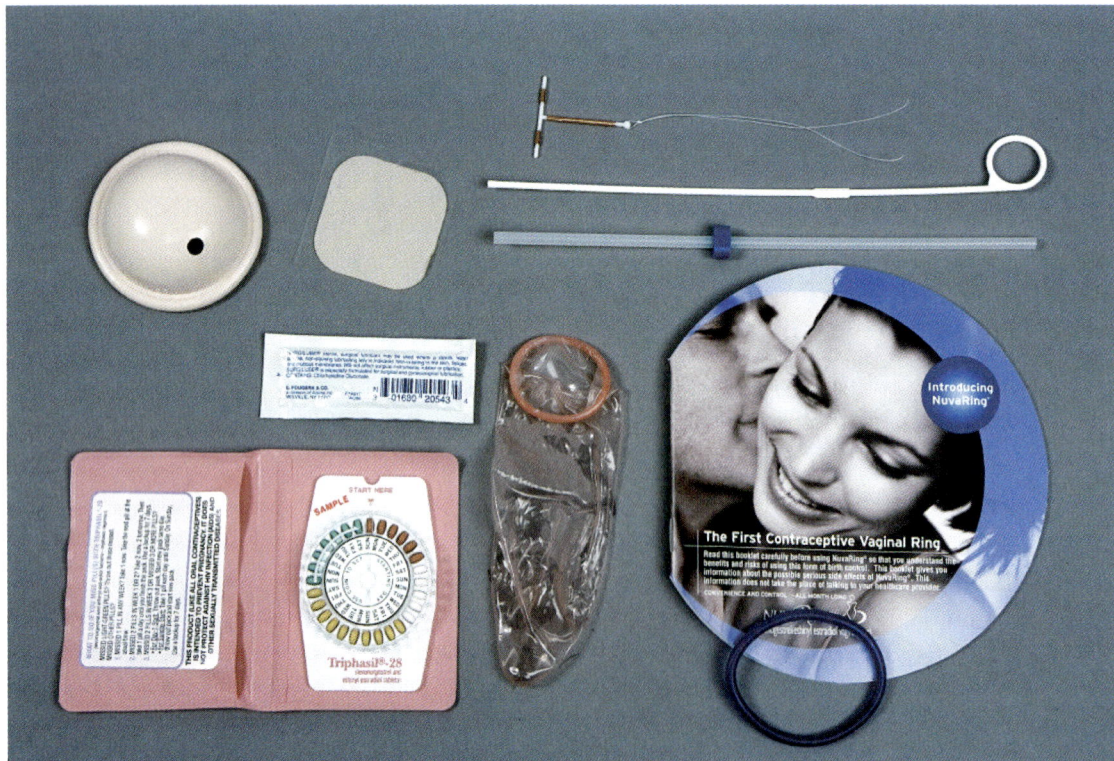

MediaLink Contraception Online

Figure 7-15. ■ Methods of contraception (from top right): Mirena intrauterine device (IUD), applicator for female condom, delivery catheter, Norplant subcutaneous contraceptive, vaginal ring, male condom, "the pill," diaphragm, and contraceptive patch.

TABLE 7-6

Facts About Conception and Contraception

1500 BC	First record of vaginal contraception	One of the earliest mentions of contraceptive vaginal suppositories appears in the Ebers Medical Papyrus. The guide suggests that a fiber tampon moistened with an herbal mixture of acacia, dates, colocynth, and honey would prevent pregnancy. The fermentation of this mixture can result in the production of lactic acid, which today is recognized as a spermicide.
16th century	Male condom	The condom was first created out of sheep intestines by a physician in the court of King Charles II of England. The condom became widely used as a birth control device after the vulcanization of rubber in 1844.
1838	Barrier methods of contraception—female; diaphragm and cervical cap	The modern diaphragm was invented by a German physician. The cervical cap was invented in 1860, but it did not receive the approval of the U.S. Food and Drug Administration for use in the United States until the late 1980s, despite its widespread use in Europe.
1921	Margaret Sanger	An advocate for birth control in the United States, she founded the American Birth Control League, which became the Planned Parenthood Federation of America in 1942.
1960	Gregory Pincus	Developed an oral contraceptive.
1965	Birth control pills or oral contraceptives	First approved for use in the United States. These early pills, known as combination pills, contained both estrogen and progestin (a synthetic form of progesterone). In 1973, progestin-only pills also became available.
1980s	Artificial insemination	Initiated as a means of fertilization. Many couples now resort to various methods of *in vitro* fertilization ("test tube" babies) or transplantation of fertilized ova from one womb to another.

may take up to 30 minutes to dissolve, and they will not offer protection until then. The spermicide must be inserted before each ejaculation.

clinical ALERT

It is important to teach clients that spermicides do not prevent STIs.

BARRIERS

Barriers, including male and female condoms, vaginal diaphragms, and cervical caps, are devices placed in the vagina or over the penis to prevent sperm from entering the cervix. To be effective, these devices must be correctly applied. The use of spermicide increases their effectiveness.

The male condom is applied to the erect penis before contact with the vulva or vagina. A small space must be available at the end of the condom to contain the ejaculate. After ejaculation, the man should withdraw the penis from the vagina while it is still erect and hold the rim of the condom to prevent spillage. Figure 7-17 ■ illustrates correct male condom use.

The female condom contains a ring at the closed end. It is inserted into the vagina so the ring rests around the cervix. The open end extends from the vagina and partially covers the vulva. The female condom can be inserted up to 8 hours prior to intercourse. A fresh condom must be used with each sexual episode. Figure 7-18 ■ illustrates application of a female condom.

The vaginal diaphragm consists of a metal ring covered with rubber. When inserted high in the vagina, the rubber covers the cervix (Figure 7-19 ■). The cervical cap is a similar device: a small ring covered with rubber that fits over the cervix. Both the vaginal diaphragm and cervical cap are most effective when spermicide is applied to the inner surface and rim before being placed next to the cervix. The devices should be left in place for 6 hours after intercourse to ensure that sperm do not enter the cervix. If intercourse is desired again within 6 hours, the diaphragm or cervical cap should remain in place and another method of contraception should also be used.

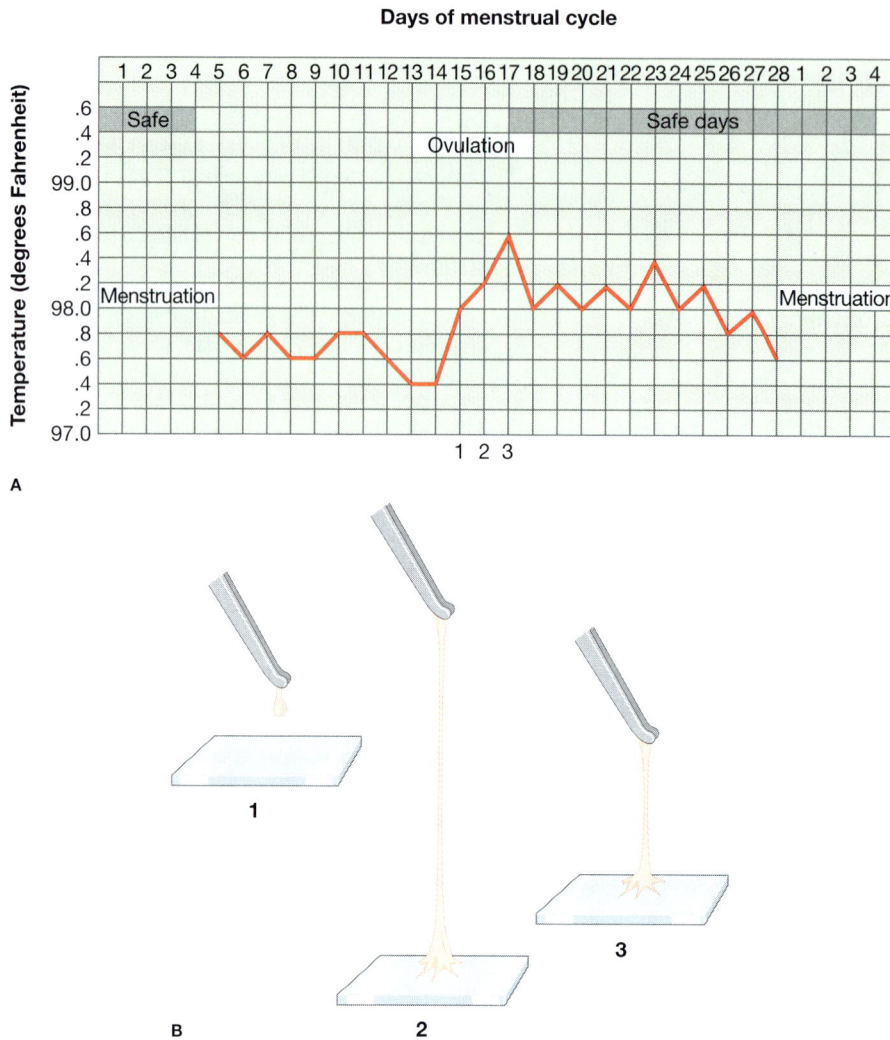

Figure 7-16. ■ (**A**) Basal body temperature chart with ovulation indicated. If this method is used for contraception, some sources recommend abstaining from intercourse for an additional day prior to ovulation and an additional day after ovulation (end of the fourth day). (**B**) Determining elasticity of cervical mucus (*spinnbarkeit*) to predict day of ovulation: 1. Three days before ovulation. 2. Day of ovulation. 3. Day after ovulation.

INTRAUTERINE DEVICE

The **intrauterine device** (IUD) is a small T-shaped piece of metal covered with copper or levonorgestrel (see Figure 7-15). The exact mechanism of action of an IUD is unclear. It is believed that the copper or levonorgestrel either kills the sperm or alters its motility to prevent conception. The IUD also disrupts the normal turbulence inside the uterus and may prevent implantation of the fertilized egg. The IUD is inserted into the uterus by a qualified health professional so that a string attached to the lower end of the "T" protrudes from the cervix. The woman is instructed to feel the string once a week for the first month and then after each menses to be sure it is in the proper position. If she develops signs of infection or pregnancy, she should consult her health care provider immediately. In case of pregnancy, the IUD is generally removed, but its removal could cause a spontaneous abortion.

HORMONAL CONTRACEPTIVES

Hormonal contraceptives are usually a combination of estrogen and progestin. They may be supplied in oral pill form taken once a day for 21 days (followed by 7 days "off"), a dermal patch applied weekly (see Figure 7-15), an intramuscular injection given every 3 months, or a ring that encircles the cervix for 21 days each menstrual cycle (Figure 7-20 ■). Women who smoke or who have a history of clotting disorders, liver disease, hyperlipidemia, hypertension, or diabetes should not take oral contraceptives. For further information, please refer to a pharmacology text.

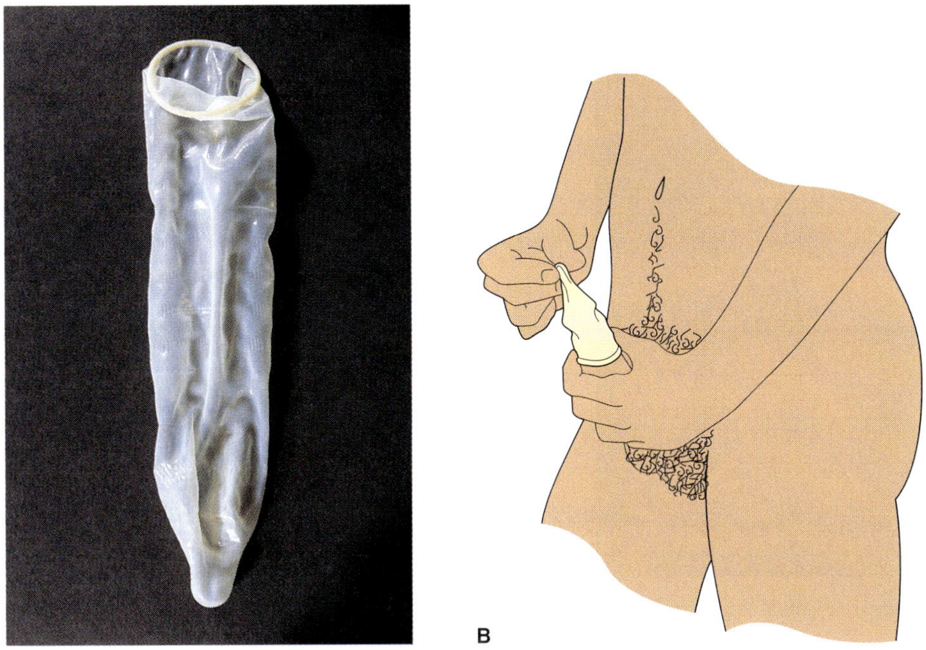

Figure 7-17. ■ The male condom. (**A**) Unrolled condom with reservoir tip. (**B**) Correct application of a condom. After use, it is crucial for the man to keep the condom in place until it is fully removed from the vagina.

In August 2006, the Food and Drug Administration approved "Plan B," an *emergency contraceptive* formulation of progestin (levonorgestrel). Available over the counter to 18-year-olds and by prescription to girls 17 and younger, the drug acts by delaying ovulation and perhaps preventing fertilization and implantation. (It is not effective if an embryo is already implanted; the pregnancy would continue.) One dose of 0.75 mg is taken as soon as possible after unprotected vaginal intercourse, with a second dose of 0.75 mg taken 12 hours later (FDA, 2006). Although it was dubbed the "morning-after" pill, it is effective up to 72 hours after intercourse. As with all hormonal contraceptives, Plan B does not provide protection against STIs.

SURGICAL STERILIZATION

Surgical sterilization—vasectomy or tubal ligation—is the tying and cutting of the vas deferens or fallopian tubes (Figure 7-21 ■). In rare instances, the procedure can be reversed. However, the couple should understand that the procedure is usually permanent. Following a vasectomy, it might take six or more ejaculations to clear the vas deferens of sperm. The couple must use other methods of birth control until negative sperm counts are obtained.

A tubal ligation might be performed at the time of a cesarean section delivery, through a laparoscopy following delivery, or at another time. The woman is encouraged to abstain from sexual intercourse until her healing is complete. She can then engage in unprotected intercourse.

SEXUALITY AND FERTILITY ISSUES

Infertility Issues

INFERTILITY

Infertility is the inability to achieve pregnancy after 1 year or more of unprotected intercourse. There are several causes of infertility. The simplest and least invasive diagnostic exam is to obtain a semen sample and analyze the number and quality of sperm. If the sperm count is low, the testes may not be producing enough sperm or there may be occlusion of the seminiferous tubules or vas deferens, preventing the transport of sperm. Some occlusions of the vas deferens may be correctable with surgery. Spermatogenesis may be stimulated by hormone therapy with varying degrees of success. If the quality of sperm is poor, little can be done to correct the problem.

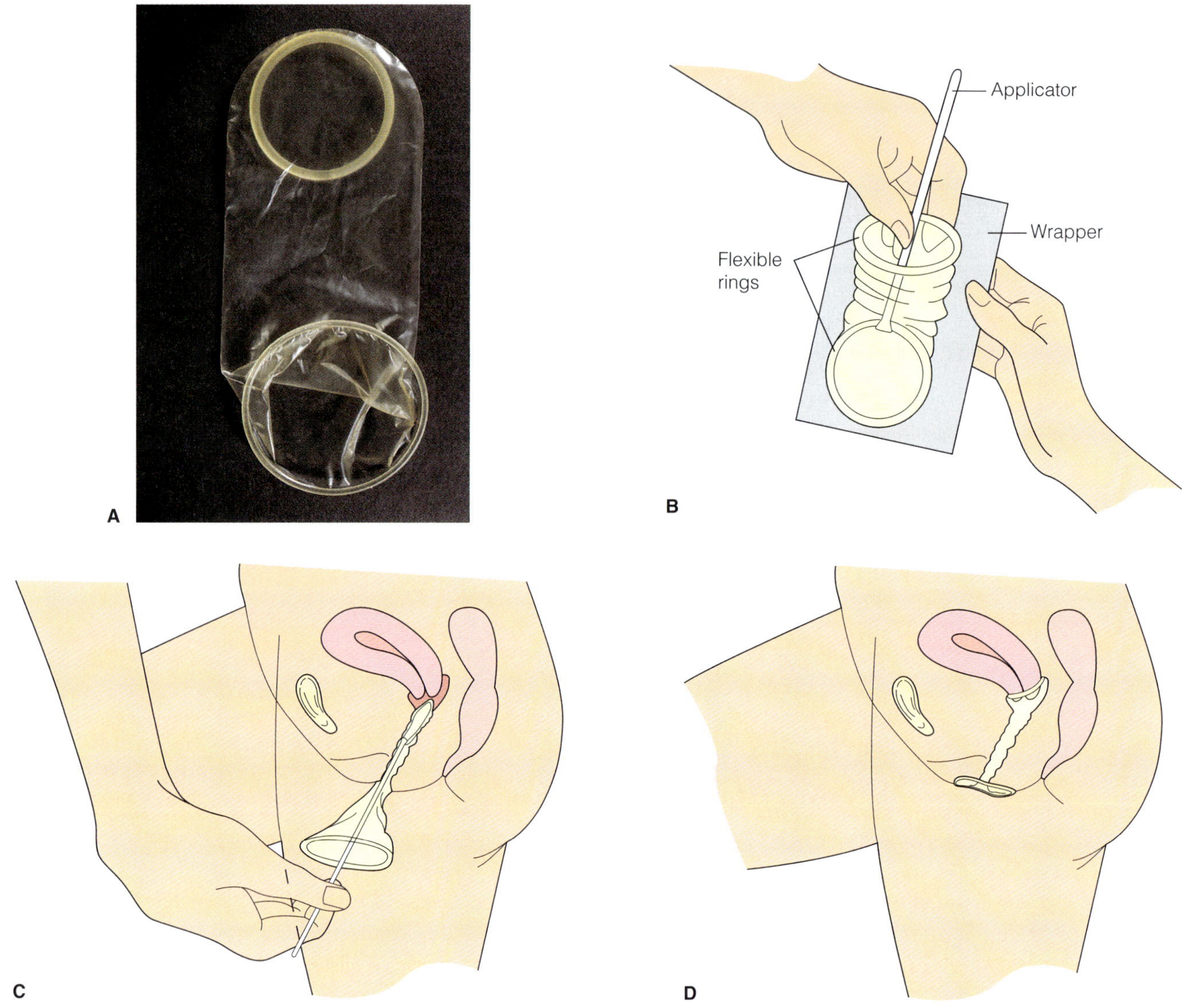

Figure 7-18. ■ (**A**) The female condom. To insert the condom: (**B**) Remove condom and application from wrapper by pulling up on the ring. (**C**) Insert condom slowly by gently pushing the applicator toward the small of the back. (**D**) When properly inserted, the outer ring should rest on the folds of skin around the vaginal opening, and the inner ring (closed end) should fit loosely against the cervix.

Infertility in women is generally easier to treat. Diagnostic tests, including hormone levels and ultrasound of the reproductive organs, are used to determine the exact cause. Hormone therapy may be used to stimulate ovulation. Narrow fallopian tubes can sometimes be enlarged, and pregnancy may then be obtained by natural means.

If the couple remains infertile, other methods may be used to become pregnant. The man's sperm can be obtained, stored, and concentrated to obtain a high sperm count. The semen can then be instilled by **artificial insemination.** The eggs can be obtained through a laparoscopic procedure (see Figure 7-21C), fertilized in the laboratory, and then implanted into the uterus. This process is known as *in vitro* **fertilization.** When pregnancy takes place by

in vitro fertilization, several fertilized eggs are instilled in an attempt to have at least one embryo implant in the uterus. Hormone therapy, used to stimulate ovulation, frequently results in more than one egg being released from the ovary. Therefore, there is an increased risk of a multifetal pregnancy.

Nursing Considerations

The nursing responsibilities include emotional support and teaching. When the couple desiring a child learns that one partner is infertile, feelings of sadness, guilt, and blame put strain on the relationship. Counseling may be needed to help the couple explore these feelings and keep lines of communication open. The nurse, working with the

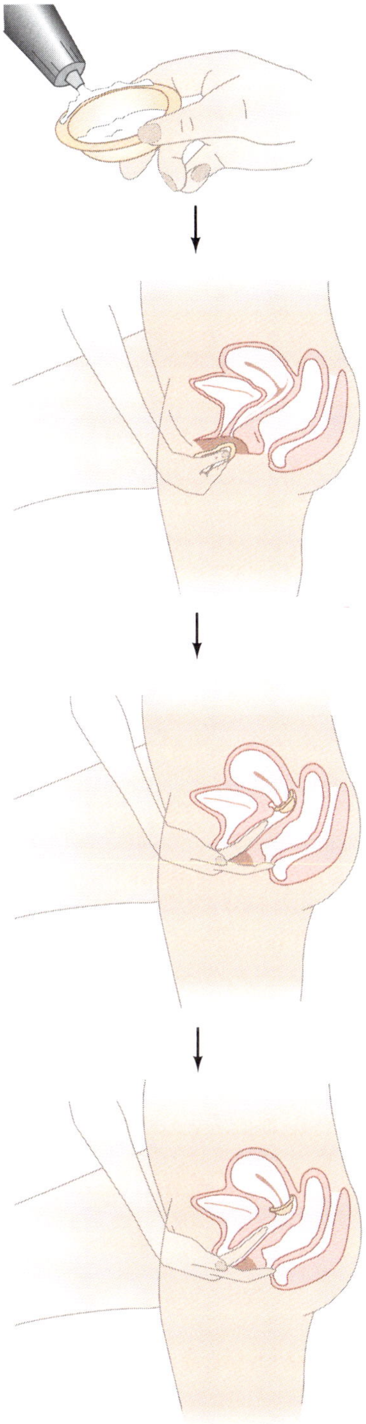

Figure 7-19. ■ Application of spermicide and placement of vaginal diaphragm. Apply gel to the rim and center of the diaphragm. Fold and insert the diaphragm. Check placement; the cervix should be felt through the diaphragm. Push the rim of the diaphragm up under the symphysis pubis.

obstetrician, can be helpful in clarifying medical and surgical options. The treatment of infertility can be quite costly, and the couple may need assistance in exploring financial resources.

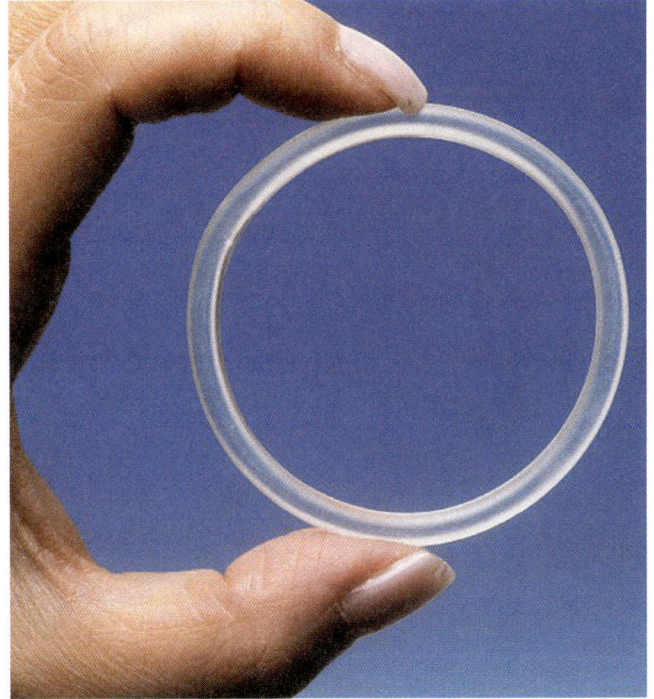

Figure 7-20. ■ The NuvaRing, a flexible hormonal contraceptive ring, encircles the cervix for 21 days and is removed. A new ring is placed 1 week later. The woman is advised to use a backup contraceptive if she removes the ring for more than 3 hours during the 21-day period. A woman with marked vaginal prolapse should check the ring often early in use to be sure it has not been expelled.

MULTIPLE PREGNANCY

Multifetal pregnancy, also known as multiple pregnancy, is the carrying of more than one fetus at a time. Twins, the most common naturally occurring multifetal pregnancy, occur in approximately 1 of 250 births. Triplets occur in about 1 of 7,600 pregnancies. Naturally occurring quadruplets, quintuplets, and sextuplets are extremely rare. Multifetal pregnancies, other than twins, occur most commonly from the use of fertility drugs or *in-vitro* fertilization (see Chapters 8 and 13 ⬭ for additional information).

ADOLESCENT SEXUALITY AND TEENAGE PREGNANCY

Over 50% of adolescent girls and 75% of adolescent boys report engaging in sexual intercourse before the age of 18. This high-risk behavior not only increases the incidence of teenage pregnancy, but also exposes the teens to STIs. Decreasing the incidence of adolescent pregnancy and STIs is an objective of the U.S. Department of Health and Human Services and many school systems (Figure 7-22 ■). Due to the complex nature of adolescent sexuality and

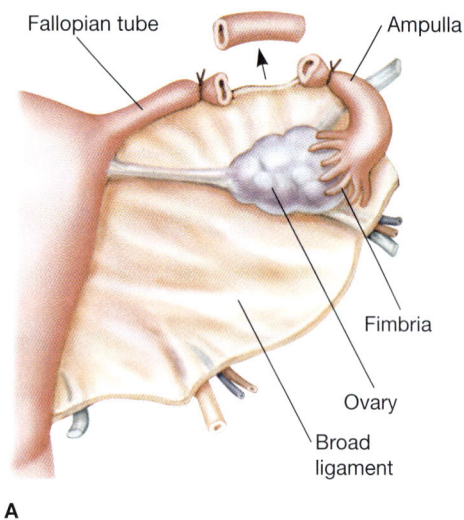

A

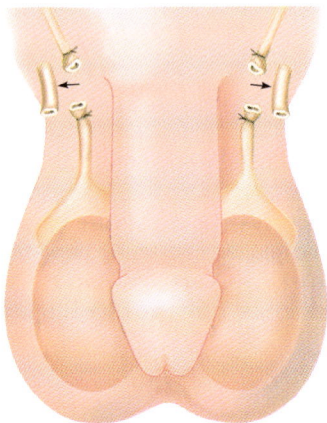

B

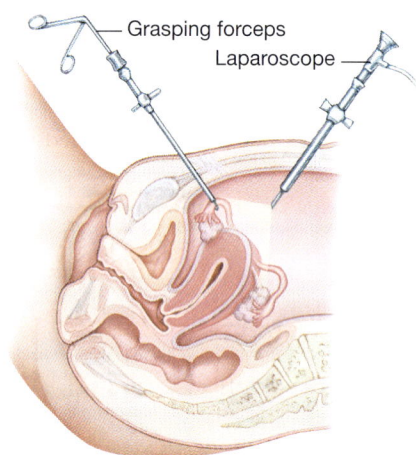

C

Figure 7-21. ■ Permanent sterilization. (**A**) Tubal ligation. (**B**) Vasectomy. (**C**) Laparoscopy. The laparoscope is used to visualize tubal sterilization accomplished through minilaparotomy incision at level of pubic hair line. (C: Redrawn, with permission, from Hatcher, R. A. et al. [1994]. *Contraceptive technology* [16th rev. ed.]. New York: Irvington.)

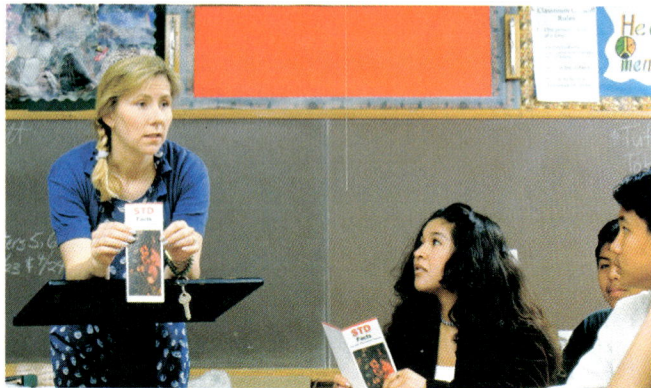

Figure 7-22. ■ Adolescents require age-appropriate teaching about sexuality and sexually transmitted infections.

teenage pregnancy, an entire chapter (Chapter 12 ⦿) is devoted to this issue.

UNINTENDED PREGNANCY

Unintended pregnancy can occur any time a couple has unprotected sexual intercourse. If the couple is married or in a long-standing relationship, a pregnancy may be inconvenient. However, the couple can generally make adjustments without undue strain on the relationship. If the couple consists of two adolescents who are unmarried or in a casual relationship, an unintended pregnancy may be overwhelming. This couple will need more support.

Once pregnant, the mother and father have some difficult decisions to make. How should they tell their family? Should they get married? Should the pregnancy be continued or terminated? Will the child be raised in the family? Will the child be adopted by another family? Some family members may provide emotional and financial support when there is an unintended pregnancy. Other family members may refuse any form of support because they believe the teen has committed a "terrible sin."

If there were several sexual partners, the mother may not know the identity of the father. Even if she knows the father, he may or may not accept responsibility and offer support. The young teen mother may not have the cognitive or emotional resources to make objective decisions for her own well-being or the well-being of her child.

Nursing Considerations

The nurse must encourage early and continued prenatal care. Prenatal care is outlined in Chapter 10 ⦿. The nurse must make appropriate referrals to social services. Professional staff must assist the mother, father, and family members in the decision-making process. With early and appropriate care, the health of both the mother and infant can be protected. This increases the likelihood of a positive outcome for the pregnancy and the family unit.

ABORTION

Abortion is the termination of a pregnancy before the fetus is able to live outside the mother. Abortion can be a spontaneous event, commonly called a miscarriage (see Figure 13-2 🔗). If the pregnancy is terminated for medical reasons such as saving the mother's life, it is termed a **therapeutic abortion.** If the abortion is performed at the request of the mother, the term **elective abortion** is used. The condition of the mother and the gestational age and size of the fetus determine the method used in performing an abortion. In 1973, the U.S. Supreme Court ruled that first-trimester abortions were permissible. Second-trimester abortions were left to the discretion of the individual states. The nurse must know the laws of the state regarding abortion prior to offering abortion counseling or teaching.

The physical care of the mother before and after an abortion is similar to the physical care of other pregnant women before and after delivery (see Chapters 10 and 13 🔗). The emotional care is different. The mother, father, and entire family need support and grief counseling similar to the family that has experienced a stillbirth or other death of a child. Prior to and following a therapeutic or elective abortion, the mother and father will need assistance to make the best-informed decision. The values and moral convictions of the mother and father, their families, and the nurse are involved in the planning and implementing of care. Conflicts and doubts can be communicated.

Health care professionals need assistance in identifying and accepting their own feelings prior to helping the mother and her family. The nurse who objects to abortion for ethical or religious reasons may refuse to care for a woman having an abortion as long as the woman's life is not in danger.

ADOPTION

Adoption is the legal transfer of the responsibility for raising a child from the birth mother to the adoptive parent(s). State laws determine the procedure of adoption. The birth mother may choose an adoption agency or a private attorney to handle the arrangements. In a *closed adoption*, the birth mother does not share identifying information with the adoptive parents and there is no future contact. In an *open adoption*, the birth mother shares information, holds the baby, and may have frequent contact with the adoptive parents and the child.

The nurse has a responsibility to assist the birth mother in decision making, make appropriate referrals, and provide emotional support during the separation process. Even in an open adoption, the birth mother will experience grief over the loss of her child. She needs to be encouraged to share her feelings in order to make positive adjustments. A referral to a professional counselor may be needed.

PREGNANCY AFTER 35

Two groups of women are becoming pregnant after 35. One group consists of women who have other children and now find themselves pregnant again. The older multiparous woman may be one who has never used birth control methods due to personal choice or lack of knowledge or one who chooses to have another baby at this time in her life. The second group consists of women who have postponed pregnancy until their late thirties or early forties. The older nulliparous woman may have delayed pregnancy in order to complete her education or establish a career. She may believe that "time is running out," and that if she does not have a child now, she never will.

Some of the possible negative consequences of having children later in life include:

- Higher risk of fetal anomalies.
- Difficulty in changing from a child-free lifestyle to a child-rearing lifestyle.
- Feelings of anger and resentment toward the parents or infant about having a "second" family later in life.
- Feelings of isolation if parents feel "tied down" and adult friends withdraw.

Due to these consequences, older parents have special needs that should be addressed (before pregnancy occurs if possible). Because the risk for fetal anomalies is greater, an amniocentesis will generally be performed at approximately 16 weeks' gestation. If anomalies are found, decisions about continuing or terminating the pregnancy must be made. In either case, the parents will need emotional support and teaching. The Care Plan Chart in Chapter 4 🔗 discussed issues related to pregnancy at advanced maternal age.

The couple may need assistance in discussing the lifestyle changes required by the raising of an infant. Some couples, excited to have a child later in life, may believe that the ability to bear children indicates that they are still young. Others may be upset by the pregnancy, feeling they will be tied down for the next 18 years. They should be encouraged to express their feelings and develop positive coping skills. Referral to social services may be needed.

HEALTH PROMOTION ISSUE

TEACHING ABOUT SEX

The LPN/LVN works at a family practice clinic. During the weekly staff meeting, client cases were reviewed and two issues were noted. The teenage pregnancy rate for their practice had increased slightly over last year's rates, and several mothers of prepubescent girls had asked for help in discussing issues of puberty with their daughters. The staff, consisting of an RN, two LPNs/LVNs, a family nurse practitioner, and a family practice physician, discussed how they might address these issues. It was decided that young girls and mothers needed more information, as well as tools to manage the changes that occur before, during, and after puberty. One nurse noted that the challenges of puberty also impact young boys. However, it was decided to develop a plan to address the female issues first. The first task was to look more specifically at the issues.

DISCUSSION

According to the 2004 annual survey of adults and teens conducted by the National Campaign to Prevent Teen Pregnancy, teens state that parents greatly influence their decisions about sexual behavior. Yet, in 2002, the National Survey of Family Growth reports that 14.5% of females and 17.4% of males ages 15 to 19 had no formal education on methods of avoiding sexual behavior. Parents also reported difficulty in communicating with their teens about sex, love, and relationships. They also report being unsure of when to approach these topics with their teens.

Teens report that their personal morals and values influence decisions

about delaying sexual behavior and preventing teen pregnancy. Both teenagers and parents state that more help from their religious institutions would be appreciated. In 2002, the National Survey of Family Growth reported that 13% of females and 10.7% of males had taken a vow or pledge to remain a virgin until they married. Teaching surrounding these vows or pledges is usually provided by religious or faith institutions.

IMPLEMENTATION

After reviewing growth and development tasks for the school-age child and the adolescent, the staff decided that they would need to develop two community-based education programs. The first class would be for prepubescent girls, ages 8 to 11, and their moms.

School-age children are interested in how things work; therefore, the class should contain a detailed description of the physical changes occurring during the puberty process. They enjoy books, games, and interactive learning. The staff decided to plan fun activities to learn more about how to care for yourself during puberty. They would

purchase age-appropriate books for the girls to read. Posters and graphics would need to be colorful and cartoon-like, and contain correct terms.

Mothers attending the class would be seated with their daughters. Tables that would seat several families would be used. This would encourage friends to attend together. Nutritious snacks would be served to assist in teaching nutritional concepts. Because young girls enjoy thinking about growing older, the staff would provide a gift bag containing items they would need as puberty approaches. These items would include different types of feminine protection with a decorative zippered pouch, deodorant, a safety razor, shampoo, soap, and a pocket calendar.

The tone of the class needed to be fun, energetic, celebratory, and encouraging. Attention would also need to be given to protecting the privacy of the girls so they would feel free to discuss the issues. The agenda needed to be light enough to allow for variation and discussion. The staff agreed that girls this age were sure to giggle during these discussions. Giggling would be allowed, if not encouraged, to release

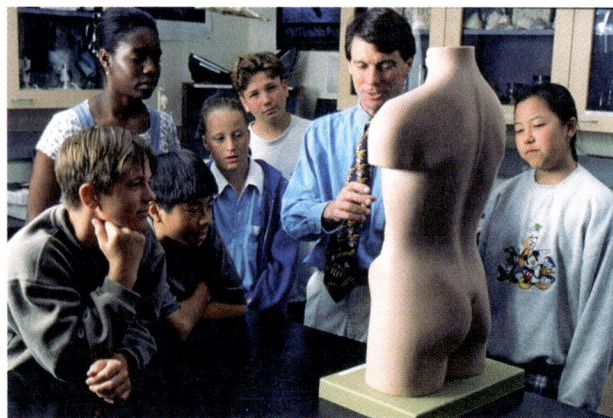

feelings of embarrassment. The young LPN/LVN was chosen as the instructor for this course because she relates well to school-age children.

The proposed agenda for this class is as follows:

- *Opening question:* Name the one thing that excites you most about growing up.
- *What is puberty?*
- *Physical changes during puberty:* What is it, and what do I do about it?
  - Growth spurts
  - Body shape changes
  - Fatigue
  - Growing pains
  - Perspiration and body odor
  - Pimples and acne
  - Body hair
  - Breast changes
  - Vulva changes
  - Changes to internal organs: vagina, ovaries, fallopian tubes, uterus, and cervix
  - Menstruation
- *Emotional changes during puberty:* What is it, and what do I do about it?
  - Emotions come and go.
  - Feelings can be unreliable.
  - Desire for independence increases.

The next class that the staff decided to offer to the community was a class for 12- to 15-year-olds discussing age-appropriate topics related to puberty and sexuality.

Adolescents are more comfortable with their peers, so the staff decided that mothers would not attend this class. Adolescent thinking is concrete, and abstract thinking is beginning to develop. So, a mix of frank discussions with true-to-life visual aids would be mixed with scenarios for the class to consider.

The instructor for this class should be credible, knowledgeable, and between the ages of 25 and 35 so she is not quite as old as their mothers. It was also suggested that they attempt to find a young teen who had experienced a teenage pregnancy to give her testimony. This teen should describe the experience in her own words. She should be encouraged to be frank and honest about the positive and negative aspects of her situation. The staff decided that it would be too distracting for the infant to attend the class with this teenage mom, although assistance with child care would be offered.

The proposed agenda for this class is as follows:

- *Opening:* "You have the right to say 'I pass' to anything tonight. You can be bored by any topic or grossed out by anything I say. You may ask any and all questions that come to mind, and I promise to answer honestly. Please realize that what is said in this room is confidential and private."

- *Maturity*
  - Definition
  - Physical maturity
  - Emotional maturity
- Self-esteem
- Peer pressure
- Dating and sex
  - Emotional differences of males and females
  - Emotional consequences of early sex
  - Creative dating
  - Setting standards
  - Physical consequences of early sex
    - Conception control
    - Pregnancy
    - Sexually transmitted infections
    - Abortion
- Other issues
  - Smoking
  - Alcohol
  - Drugs
  - Eating disorders

SELF-REFLECTION

Were you raised in a family that discussed reproductive issues openly or where such topics were not directly discussed? What aspect of reproduction or sexuality would be most awkward for you to discuss? How could you respond nonjudgmentally to a teenager who is worried that he might be homosexual?

SUGGESTED RESOURCES

For the Nurse

Butts, J., & Hartman, S. (2002). Project BART: Effectiveness of a behavioral intervention to reduce HIV risk in adolescents. *The American Journal of Maternal/Child Nursing, 27*, 163–170.

Hershberger, P. (1998). Smoking and pregnant teens: What nurses can do to help. *Lifelines, 2*, 26–31.

For the Client

Gravelle, K., & Gravelle, J. *The period book.* (2006). New York: Walker & Company.

Kitzinger, S., & Nillsson, L. *Being born.* (1986). New York: Grosset and Dunlap.

Madaras, L., Madaras, A., Sullivan, S., & Aher, J. (2001). *What's happening to my body? Book for girls* (3rd ed.). New York: Newmarket Press.

McDowell, J., & Hostetler, B. *Don't check your brains at the door. How to help your child say "no" to sexual pressure.* (1992). Word Publishing. Available on the Internet.

Future Issues

Although common reproductive issues are discussed here, stem cell research is also worth mentioning. Many believe that stem cells, harvested from embryos, may be useful in treating and curing a variety of disorders. Others believe that harvesting of stem cells from embryos for research purposes is unethical. Questions about stem cell research and government funding of such research will undoubtedly continue to be debated on many levels in the future. It is important for the public to receive accurate information about the procurement of embryos, the harvesting process, and the use of the harvested stem cells. The nurse can be a key player in obtaining and disseminating accurate and useful information.

NURSING CARE

PRIORITIES IN NURSING CARE

The priority of nursing care for a client with a reproductive system disorder is to identify the nature of the disorder, provide emotional support, and teach clients to care for themselves and prevent complications.

ASSESSING

When assessing men and women for reproductive issues, the nurse must use a nonjudgmental attitude and open communication. Many clients are uncomfortable discussing their sexuality and sexual activity. The nurse must approach the topic in a matter-of-fact manner, with reassurance of confidentiality within the law. Some questions are the same for both genders.

- Ask about history of sexual activity, including the age at first sexual intercourse.
- Ask about the number of sexual partners, currently and in the past.
- Ask about the use of contraceptives.
- Ask about the use of barriers to prevent STIs.
- Ask about a history of sexual trauma, including abuse, rape, or incest.

Women
- Ask about risk factors for breast cancer, including family history.
- Ask about breast self-exam, how often they do it, and any abnormal findings.

- Perform a breast examination, palpating the breast for masses, irregularities in contour, and drainage, if warranted.
- Ask about menstrual history, including onset of menstruation, the date of the last menses, and any irregularities.

Men
- Ask about testicular self-examination, how often they do it, and any abnormal findings.
- Perform a testicular examination, palpating for masses and inspecting the genitals for lesions and drainage, if warranted.
- Ask about difficulty voiding, including difficulty starting or stopping and the size of the stream. Include symptoms of burning, frequency, urgency, or nocturia.
- Ask about sexual functioning, including premature ejaculation, impotence, or other sexual problems.

DIAGNOSING, PLANNING, AND IMPLEMENTING

Possible nursing diagnoses include the following:

Risk for Disturbed Body Image
- Encourage verbalization of feelings. *Alterations in sexual functioning from surgery or disease can change body image. Verbalizing helps the client cope with feelings of loss and change.*
- Provide resources (pamphlets, books, tapes, referrals to support groups and counselors) as appropriate. *Referrals and resources assist with coping and adaptation.*
- Encourage client (and significant other if appropriate) to look at physical changes in body. *Often, the imagined alteration of physical characteristics is worse than the real changes.*

Sexual Dysfunction
- Encourage discussion of sexual function among client, partner, and health care provider. *Open discussion assists with decision making about diagnosis and treatment.*
- Reinforce information given by the health care provider regarding treatment options. *The health care provider is responsible for discussing treatment options with the client. The nurse must reinforce teaching and answer questions. The client can then make an informed decision about treatment.*
- Encourage the client to discuss concerns of sexuality with a therapist or counselor. *The therapist or counselor may be able to offer alternatives for expressing sexuality.*

Deficient Knowledge Related to Risk Factors, Disease Prevention, and Treatment, Including Medications

- Teach clients about risk factors for reproductive dysfunction. For example, STIs increase the risk of infertility. *By understanding risk factors for reproductive dysfunction, clients can make better choices.*
- Teach clients about disease prevention. For example, teach about use of contraceptives and application of condoms. *By understanding disease prevention, clients can take measures to protect themselves.*
- Teach clients (and significant others if appropriate) about their specific disease and prescribed treatment. *When clients and significant others understand the specific condition, prescribed treatment, and possible complications, they are more compliant and make healthier choices.*

EVALUATING

To evaluate the effectiveness of nursing interventions, collect data such as the following:

- Makes informed decisions about treatment based on the extent of the disorder and individual choice
- Verbalizes understanding of information presented
- Expresses feelings openly

NURSING PROCESS CARE PLAN
Care of the Client with Rape Trauma Syndrome

Ms. Kelly is an 18-year-old college student living in a coed dorm. She is an average student, a member of the marching band, and a participant in a weekly campus religious organization. While walking home alone after band practice, she was attacked and raped. At the urging of her roommate and resident assistant, she contacted the campus health organization.

Assessment. VS: T 98.3, P 110, R 22 and labored, BP 122/78. Ms. Kelly reports intense perineal and back pain. Weight 110 pounds. Height 5′ 6″. Skin is moist and pink with bruising noted on the upper arms, buttocks, and back. She also has a small 2-cm gash on her forehead. She is alert, yet easily distracted. She is crying frequently. She asks the nurse to call her parents for her. A cervical specimen is obtained for sperm analysis. Hair specimens are obtained. Debris is removed from under Ms. Kelly's fingernails and from her back. A blood sample is obtained for screening of

other STIs, including HIV and pregnancy testing. X-rays are taken to determine fractures.

Nursing Diagnosis. The following important nursing diagnoses (among others) have been established for this client:

- Acute **P**ain related to injuries received during the rape
- **A**nxiety related to status of physical health and the act of violence experienced
- **F**ear related to future violence and concern for personal safety

Expected Outcomes. The expected outcomes for the plan of care are that Ms. Kelly will:

- Demonstrate a decrease in pain within 48 hours of initiating treatment as evidenced by lower rating on pain scale and less facial grimacing.
- Demonstrate decreased symptoms of anxiety in 2 weeks as evidenced by pulse and respirations within normal limits (WNL) and statement of supportive social interactions with family members.
- Demonstrate decreased fear in 2 weeks as evidenced by a report of safety measures implemented to provide personal protection.

Planning and Implementation. The following nursing interventions are implemented for Ms. Kelly:

- Reassess perineal and back pain by telephone follow-up call within 48 hours of initiating treatment.
- Have Ms. Kelly apply moist heat to the perineum and back. *Moist heat provides comfort and aids healing.*
- Encourage Ms. Kelly to self-administer analgesics prior to pain levels of 5 or above.
- Reassess anxiety levels at follow-up clinic visit. *Feelings of anxiety may emerge slowly or be long lasting.*
- Encourage Ms. Kelly to express her feelings, anxieties, and fears related to her diagnosis. *Verbalization allows appropriate follow-up.*
- Encourage and support effective coping behaviors.
- Refer Ms. Kelly to a rape counselor. *Psychological effects of the rape may surface over time and are sometimes difficult to overcome.*
- Include Ms. Kelly's parents in counseling if Ms. Kelly agrees.

Evaluation. At the follow-up visit, Ms. Kelly's vital signs are T 98.6, BP 120/80, P 66, R 16. She has seen the rape counselor daily and is dealing with her fears and anxiety. She has decided to take a leave of absence from her coursework and return to her hometown. Her back and perineal pain have subsided, and STI and pregnancy tests remain negative. The criminal investigation into the rape continues.

Critical Thinking in the Nursing Process

1. List conditions and procedures for collecting data regarding the specific events of the rape.
2. What types of personal protection should be recommended to Ms. Kelly and why?

3. Describe the psychological support necessary for Ms. Kelly.

Note: Discussion of Critical Thinking questions appears in Appendix I.

Note: The reference and resource listings for this and all chapters have been compiled at the back of the book.

Chapter Review

KEY Points

- Reproductive issues involve physical disorders that can have an impact on psychological health.
- Physical disorders, including infection, hormonal imbalance, and structural defects, may be treated medically or, at times, surgically.
- Some disorders cannot be treated and result in infertility.
- Couples wanting to postpone pregnancy need information about contraception.
- The couple experiencing psychological and emotional problems about reproductive issues may require long-term support and professional counseling.
- Discussing the personal subject of sexual relations can be uncomfortable for the client, the partner, and the nurse. It is important for the nurse to express compassion and understanding, and to be open-minded and nonjudgmental.

🔗 FOR FURTHER Study

For information about informed consent, see Chapter 3.

The Nursing Care Plan Chart in Chapter 4 discusses pregnancy at advanced maternal age.

For initial development of secondary sex characteristics, see Figure 5-18.

See placental layers in Figure 8-3. See more about pregnancy in Chapter 10; see muscles strengthened by Kegel exercises in Figure 10-8.

For a full discussion on the complex nature of adolescent sexuality and teenage pregnancy, see Chapter 12.

See discussion of high-risk pregnancies in Chapter 13.

For a discussion of ophthalmia neonatorum, see Chapter 17.

Critical Thinking Care Map

Caring for a Client with Genital Warts
NCLEX-PN® Focus Area: Physiologic Integrity

Case Study: Claire presents to the family planning clinic for her Pap smear with complaints of vaginal spotting and a slight headache. Upon cervical examination, gray-pink lesions are identified. The tissue culture of the lesion reveals condylomata acuminata.

Nursing Diagnosis: Impaired Tissue Integrity related to infection with HPV

COLLECT DATA

Subjective	Objective
_____	_____
_____	_____
_____	_____
_____	_____
_____	_____
_____	_____
_____	_____

Would you report this? Yes/No

If yes, to: _____

Nursing Care

_____
_____
_____
_____
_____
_____
_____
_____
_____
_____

How would you document this? _____
_____
_____
_____

Compare your documentation to the sample provided in Appendix I.

Data Collected
(use only those that apply)

- Diet high in fat and calories
- States vaginal spotting has occurred for 4 days
- LMP (month/day/year)
- Exercises two times a week
- Small amount of dark red vaginal discharge noted
- Multiple cervical lesions measuring 1/2 to 1 cm in diameter
- Headache pain level 4
- Labia with diffuse redness
- Breasts without tenderness
- States has had three sexual partners in 3 months

Nursing Interventions
(use only those that apply; list in priority order)

- Teach the importance of regular Pap smears.
- Teach the client about cryotherapy treatment.
- Teach the importance of informing all sexual partners.
- Assess characteristics of the lesion.
- Discuss importance of low-fat, high-fiber diet.
- Assess fears and anxieties related to sexual activity.

1 The nurse is reviewing the charts of four clients. Which of the following assessment findings is consistent with a client who has been diagnosed with a cystocele?

1. difficulty defecating
2. difficulty emptying the bladder
3. dyspareunia
4. pelvic pressure

2 When collecting data related to the client's sexual history, which of the following sexual practices would put the client at risk for contracting HIV? Choose all that apply.

1. heterosexual intercourse
2. homosexual activity
3. oral sex
4. French kissing
5. rectal sex
6. a monogamous relationship

3 The nurse is teaching a client the proper use of an IUD. Which of the following teaching points would the nurse include in her teaching? Choose all that apply.

1. Feel for the string weekly for the first month.
2. Feel for the string monthly after menses.
3. Report fever and chills to the physician immediately.
4. Report symptoms of pregnancy immediately.
5. Use a spermicide with each act of intercourse.
6. This is a permanent form of contraception.

4 The nurse is assisting with the prenatal care of a 36-year-old client. Which of the following statements would the nurse need to explore first?

1. "I would like to have an amniocentesis."
2. "The child might have a fetal anomaly."
3. "I blame my husband for this pregnancy."
4. "I hope to spend time with my neighbor who is pregnant."

5 The LPN/LVN is taking a menstrual history on a 26-year-old client. The client states that menses usually last for more than 10 days a month with a heavy flow. The nurse anticipates the client will be evaluated for which of the following disorders?

1. premenstrual syndrome
2. endometriosis
3. human papillomavirus
4. fibroid tumors

6 A client is 10 weeks pregnant and has a repeat infection of trichomoniasis. The client states she has taken Metronidazole (Flagyl) in the past and now questions why the physician has prescribed Clotrimazole vaginal suppositories. The nurse's best response is:

1. "Flagyl is contraindicated during the first trimester of pregnancy."
2. "Flagyl is not prescribed to treat trichomoniasis."
3. "Flagyl is not prescribed for repeat infections."
4. "Flagyl is contraindicated during the entire pregnancy."

7 The LPN/LVN is evaluating a return demonstration on a client performing a breast self-examination. Which of the following techniques require further teaching from the LPN/LVN?

1. Client compresses the nipple with the thumb and finger.
2. Client uses palm of hand to palpate breast tissue.
3. Client palpates tissue from the axilla to the sternum.
4. Client inspects breast by lifting arms over her head.

8 Which of the following nursing interventions is appropriate for the client giving her child up for adoption?

1. caring for the mother and infant in the same postpartum room
2. separating the mother and infant and not allowing visitation
3. withholding information about the baby's physical characteristics from the client
4. providing opportunities for the client to express her true feelings

9 The nurse works in the emergency department. She is caring for a woman admitted following a rape. Which option is the most appropriate for providing hygiene for this client?

1. Help the woman immediately with a shower.
2. Wash only her face and hands.
3. Avoid washing the perineum.
4. Avoid showering and bathing at this time.

10 Which of the following places the client at greater risk for developing cervical cancer?

1. history of endometriosis
2. repeat gonorrheal infections
3. history of human papillomavirus infection
4. history of fibroid tumors

Answers for NCLEX-PN® Review and Critical Thinking questions appear in Appendix I.

Thinking Strategically About...

You are an LPN/LVN employed by a small acute care hospital. You are to provide routine care for the following three stable postoperative clients from 7:00 A.M. until 7:00 P.M.

- Curt is a 66-year-old man who had TURP 4 days ago. He can be discharged as soon as he can empty his bladder. His catheter was removed at 6:00 A.M.
- Roma, 56 years old, had an abdominal hysterectomy with bilateral salpingo-oophorectomy 1 day ago. She has IV fluids, patient-controlled analgesia (PCA) for pain, a Foley catheter, and an abdominal dressing.
- Anita, 32 years old, had a 3-cm cancerous lump removed from her left breast 1 day ago. She has a Jackson-Pratt (JP) drain and IV fluids.

CRITICAL THINKING

- What questions should you ask Roma to add the intellectual standard of *clarity* to your assessment of her feelings about having a hysterectomy?
- What questions should you ask Curt to add the intellectual standard of *accuracy* to your assessment of his postoperative pain?

COLLABORATIVE CARE

- To what agency should Anita be referred that will provide support for breast cancer clients?

MANAGEMENT OF CARE AND PRIORITIES IN NURSING CARE

- In what order will you visit these clients?
- What is your rationale for prioritizing care?

DELEGATING

- When visiting Roma, how would you determine what care can be delegated to the CNA?

COMMUNICATION AND CLIENT TEACHING

- What health promotion activities can Roma do to help her heal?
- What instruction should be given to Curt regarding discharge?

DOCUMENTING AND REPORTING

- Since the catheter was removed at 6:00 A.M., when should Curt void? What data should be documented and reported?

CULTURAL CARE STRATEGIES

- Anita is of Filipino origin. How will you determine if there are cultural aspects of her care you should plan for?

Nursing Care During the Prenatal Period

Chapter 8

Fetal Development

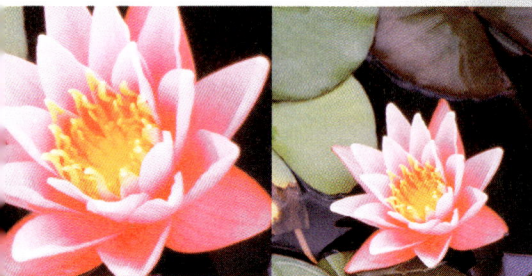

LEARNING Outcomes

After completing this chapter, you will be able to:
1. Define key terms.
2. Describe fetal development.
3. Describe factors that influence fetal development.
4. Discuss nursing measures that can help to ensure healthy fetal development.

Fetal development is a complex process of cell division, tissue formation, and a series of openings and closings that form organs. The entire process must progress in an organized sequence of events in order for the developing baby to be formed normally. This chapter discusses the process of fetal development and some causes of fetal malformation, as well as preconception planning as it relates to fetal development.

FETAL DEVELOPMENT

Fertilization

Fertilization is the process of uniting two sex cells (Figure 8-1 ■). **Pregnancy** is the carrying of the resulting offspring in the uterus. Pregnancy can be described by the events that occur throughout the 40 weeks of development.

For pregnancy to occur, sperm from the male must be deposited near the cervix of the female. Although this most commonly occurs with coitus or copulation, sperm can also be deposited by artificial means. Once deposited, sperm must "swim" through the mucus inside the cervix, through the uterus, and through the fallopian tube. The ovum and sperm usually unite in the outer one third of the fallopian tube (Figure 8-2 ■). The timing of sperm deposition has an effect on the success of the sperm in reaching the ovum. Sperm can survive in the female reproductive tract for up to 72 hours, but they are believed to be healthy and highly fertile for only about the first 24 hours (DeJonge, 2000). The ovum is fertile for only about 12 to 24 hours after ovulation. Therefore, fertilization or **conception** (the uniting of ovum and sperm) is only possible for a short time.

The fertilized egg is called a **zygote.** As it travels through the fallopian tube, the zygote divides rapidly to form a many-celled, mulberry-shaped mass called a **morula.** By the time the morula reaches the uterus in 4 to 5 days, the cells have become a two-layer ball called a **blastocyst.** The outer layer or **trophoblast** will become the placenta and fetal membranes (or bag of waters, discussed below). The inner layer or **embryonic disc** will become the embryo. Figure 8-3 ■ illustrates the first days of development after fertilization and beginning embryonic development.

Implantation

Implantation is the embedding of the blastocyst into the endometrium (see Figure 8-3). One area of the trophoblast develops finger-like projections, called **chorionic villi** (singular, *villus*) that secure the blastocyst to the uterus. The chorionic villi begin producing the chemical **human chorionic gonadotropin** (hCG) 8 to 10 days after

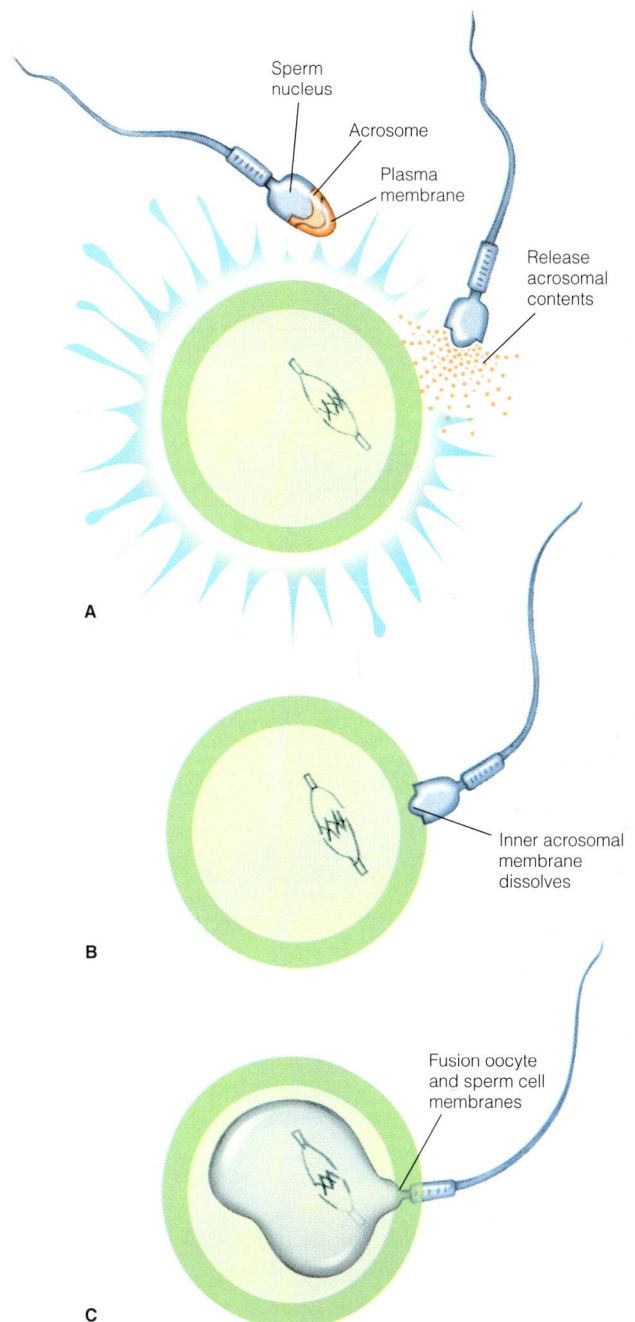

Figure 8-1. ■ At fertilization, the following sequence (called an *acrosome reaction*) occurs: (**A**) Perforations in the acrosome release chemicals onto the cell membrane of the ovum. (**B**) The acrosomal membrane continues to dissolve as the sperm penetrates the ovum. (**C**) The membranes of the sperm and oocyte cell fuse.

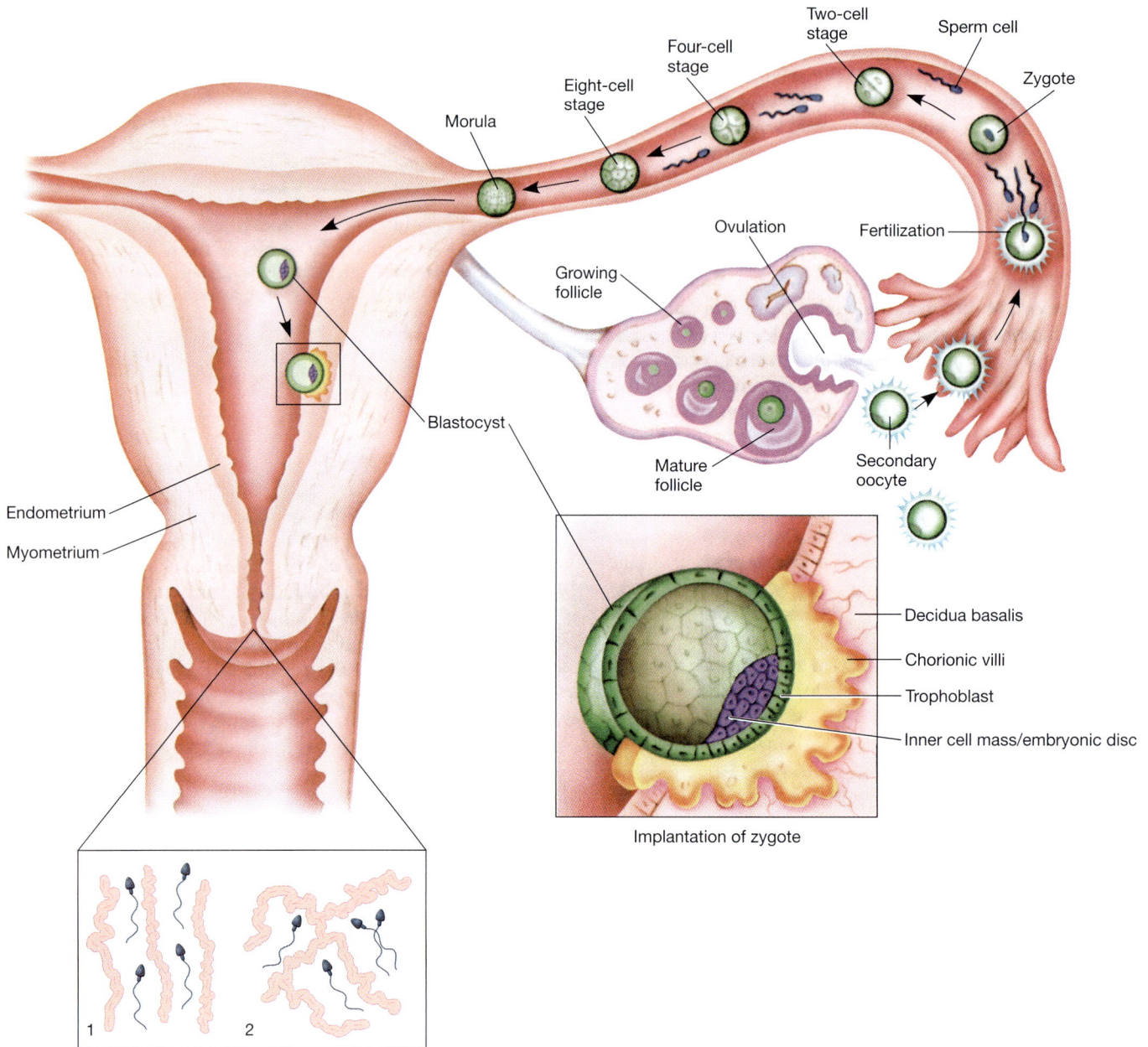

Figure 8-2. ■ Ovulation, fertilization, and implantation. During ovulation, the ovum leaves the ovary and enters the fallopian tube. Fertilization generally occurs in the outer third of the fallopian tube. Subsequent changes in the fertilized ovum from conception to implantation are shown. (*Left inset*) Sperm passage through cervical mucus. (1) During ovulation the mucoid strands become more parallel, allowing sperm to pass through easily. (Corson, S. [1990]. *Conquering infertility: A guide for couples* [4th ed.]. Vancouver, BC, Canada: EMIS-Canada, p.16.) (2) When the client is not ovulating, tangled mucus strands prevent many sperm from passing. (*Right inset*) Implanted zygote.

fertilization. The hCG is the chemical that pregnancy kits identify in order to determine pregnancy. The hCG maintains the *corpus luteum* (the fully developed ovum discharged from the ovary). It stimulates the corpus luteum to continue producing estrogen and progesterone until 11 to 12 weeks. By that time, the placenta is developed enough to produce estrogen and progesterone and maintain the pregnancy.

Development of Support Structures

FETAL MEMBRANES

The chorionic villi develop into the placenta. The remainder of the trophoblast becomes the outer layer of the membranes called the **chorion** (see Figure 8-3). The inner layer

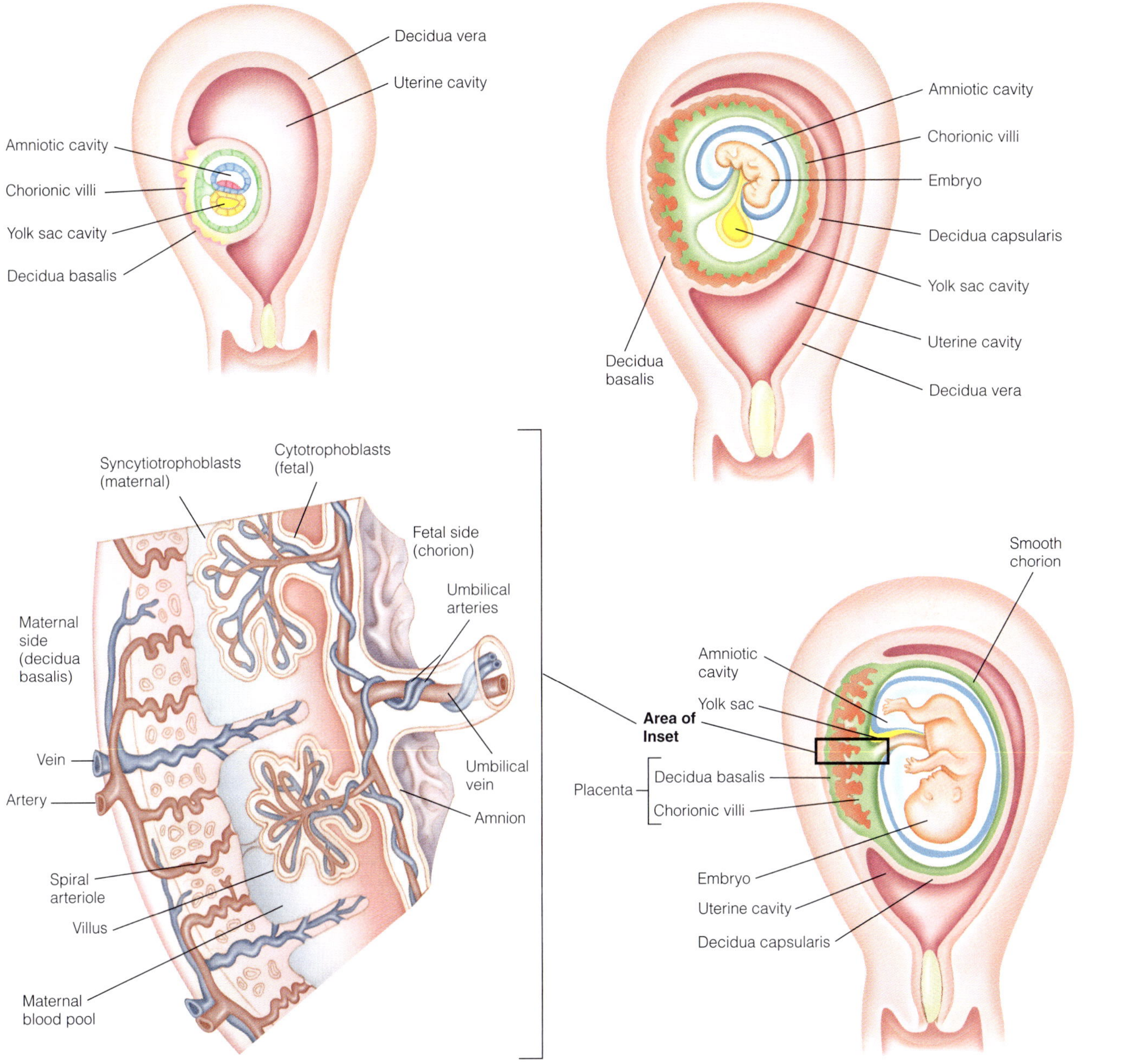

Figure 8-3. ■ Sequence of development of the embryo from primary germ layers. The stages show the implanted blastocyst and development of the embryo, fetal membranes, and yolk sac during the preplacental phase. The *inset* illustrates vascularization of the placenta.

of the placenta, the **amnion,** originates from the inside of the blastocyst. The amnion grows as the fetus grows until it comes into contact with the chorion. Together the two layers form the **fetal membranes,** also called the **"bag of waters."**

AMNIOTIC FLUID

The **amniotic fluid** is formed by the amnion (see Figure 8-3). Amniotic fluid consists of about 98% water. It also contains glucose, proteins, urea, **lanugo** (fine fetal hair), and **vernix caseosa** (white, cheesy covering of the fetus's skin).

The fetus drinks the amniotic fluid and urinates into it. Amniotic fluid is absorbed and replaced every 3 hours. The amniotic fluid has the following important functions for the developing fetus.

- Maintains constant temperature
- Equalizes the pressure around the fetus to allow for growth
- Cushions the fetus from injury and the umbilical cord from compression
- Prevents the fetal membranes from adhering to the fetus
- Allows the fetus to move freely
- Provides the fetus with fluid to swallow

PLACENTA

By the 3rd week post fertilization, the placenta has formed, but it is not fully functional until the 12th week. The **placenta** is a highly vascular organ connecting the mother and the fetus. The maternal side of the placenta is divided into irregular sections called **cotyledons.** Both the color and the texture are like liver. The fetal side of the placenta is white and shiny with the large blood vessels leading to the umbilical cord visible. Figure 8-4 ■ illustrates the inner and outer surfaces of the placenta. At the time of delivery, the placenta is about 8 inches in diameter and weighs approximately 1 pound.

The placenta has three main functions.

1. The placenta's first function is transport. Oxygen, glucose, amino acids, electrolytes, and vitamins are transported from the mother's blood to the infant's blood. At the same time, carbon dioxide, urea, creatinine, and other fetal waste are transported from the infant's blood to the mother's blood.

   Drugs that are in the maternal blood may be transported to the infant's blood. Though chemicals are transported between mother and infant, the blood cells themselves do not cross the placenta.

2. The second function of the placenta is to produce hormones.
   * hCG, the basis for pregnancy tests, has already been discussed.
   * **Human placental lactogen** (hPL) stimulates changes in the maternal metabolism. These changes make protein, glucose, and minerals more readily available to the fetus. The hPL is an *insulin antagonist* (it decreases the woman's metabolism of glucose). The mother's body prepares for lactation because of an increase in hPL. The placenta also produces estrogen and progesterone to maintain the endometrium, stimulate breast development, and prevent uterine contractions.
   * **Relaxin** is a hormone produced by the corpus luteum and placenta that decreases uterine activity, decreases the strength of uterine contractions, softens the cervix, and causes softening of the collagen connective tissue of the symphysis pubis and sacroiliac joints. In late pregnancy, these joints become moveable, making a larger passageway for the delivery.

3. The third function of the placenta is production of fatty acids, glycogen, and cholesterol for fetal use. Enzymes that are necessary for the transport of nutrients to the fetus are also produced by the placenta.

UMBILICAL CORD

The **umbilical cord** connects the fetus to the placenta. The umbilical cord consists of a white gelatinous tissue called **Wharton's jelly.** Wharton's jelly protects and supports the two umbilical arteries and one umbilical vein. At term, the umbilical cord is 23 to 24 inches long. When the Wharton's jelly comes in contact with air following delivery, it contracts, clamping the blood vessels to prevent bleeding.

Stages of Fetal Development

Fetal development or **gestation** is marked in weeks following conception. (Figure 8-5 ■ illustrates stages of fetal development through week 30.) The term **embryo** is used to describe the developing baby from weeks 3 through 8. From week 9 until delivery, the developing baby is called a **fetus.** Fetal development is described in terms of three stages.

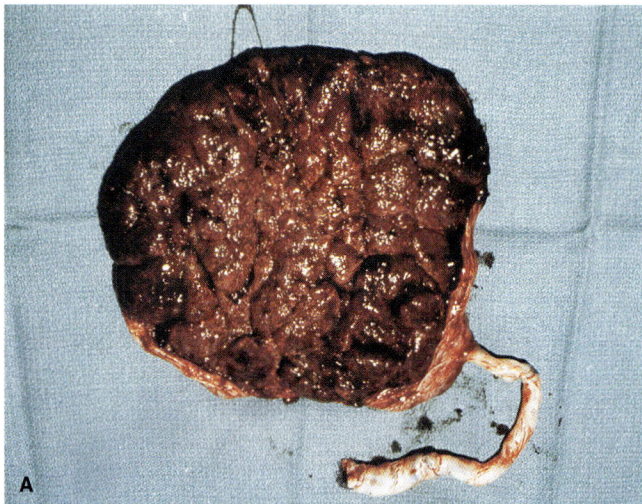

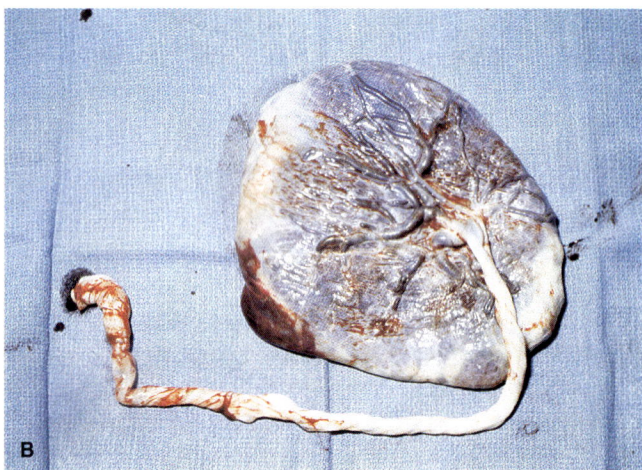

Figure 8-4. ■ Placenta. (**A**) Maternal side or Duncan mechanism ("Dirty Duncan"). (**B**) Fetal side or Schultze mechanism ("Shiny Schultze"). (Courtesy of Marcia London, RNC, MSN, NNP.)

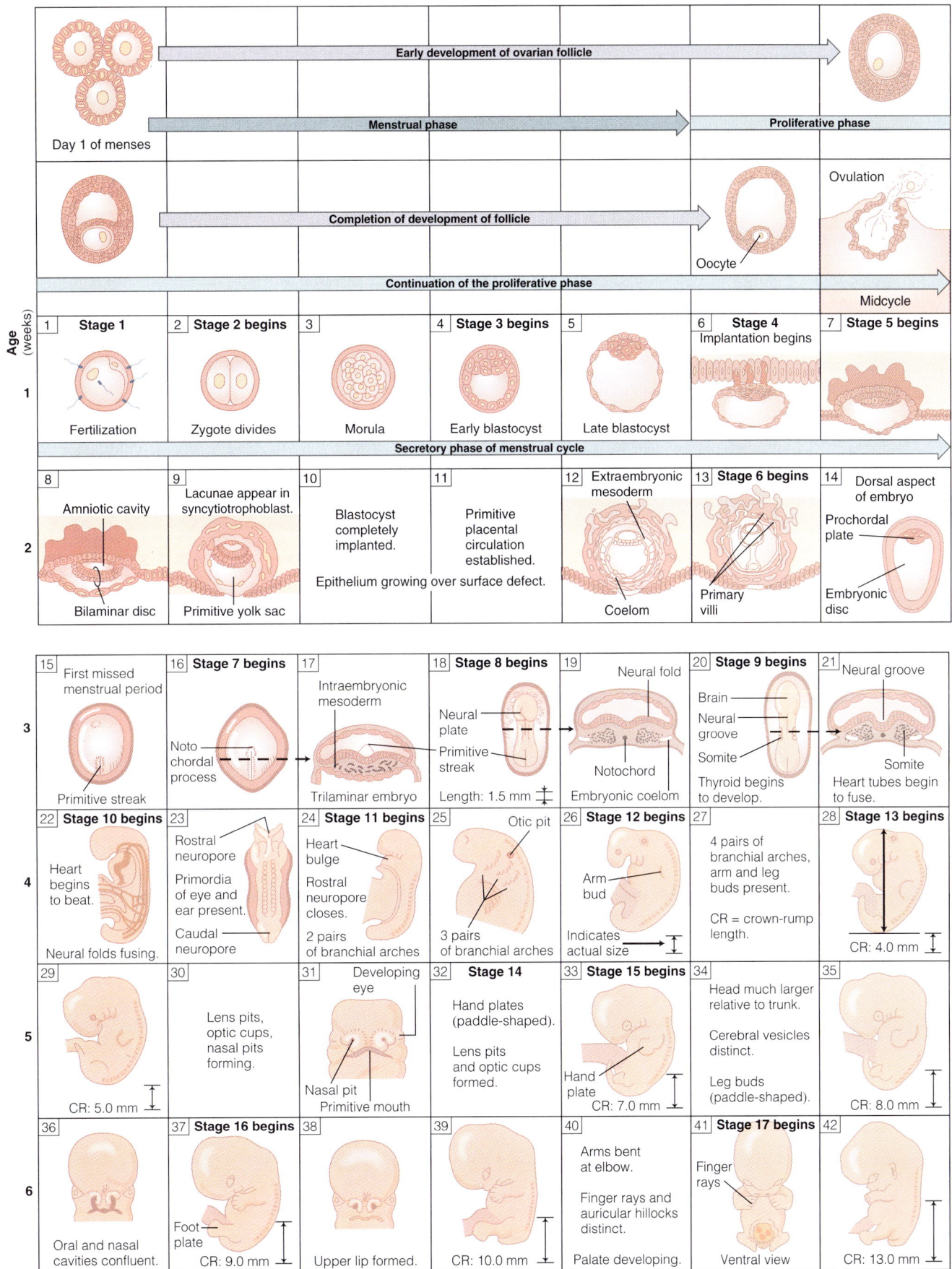

Figure 8-5. ■ (**A**) Human prenatal development from conception to 10 weeks. (**B**) Human fetal development: 12 weeks, 20 weeks, 24 weeks, and 30 weeks. (**A**: Reprinted from Moore, K. L. [1989]. *The developing human: Clinically oriented embryology* [3rd ed.]. Philadelphia: W. B. Saunders, pp. 2–4, with permission from Elsevier, Inc.)

A (continued)

Age (weeks)						
7	43 CR: 16.0 mm.	44 **Stage 18 begins** Eyelids beginning	45 Tip of nose distinct. Toe rays appear. Ossification may begin. CR: 17.0 mm	46 Loss of villi Smooth chorion forms.	47 Genital tubercle Urogenital membrane Anal membrane ♀ or ♂	48 **Stage 19 begins** Trunk elongating and straightening. / 49 CR: 18 mm
8	50 Upper limbs longer and bent at elbows. Fingers distinct.	51 Anal membrane perforated. Urogenital membrane degenerating. Testes and ovaries distinguishable.	52 **Stage 21 begins**	53 **Stage 21** External genitalia still in sexless state but have begun to differentiate.	54 **Stage 22 begins** Genital tubercle Urethral groove Anus ♀ or ♂	55 Beginnings of all essential external and internal structures are present. / 56 **Stage 23** CR: 30 mm
9	57 Beginning of fetal period	58	59 Genitalia show some ♀ characteristics but still easily confused with ♂.	60 Phallus Urogenital fold Labioscrotal fold Perineum ♀	61 Genitalia show fusion of urethral folds. Urethral groove extends into phallus.	62 Phallus Urogenital fold Labioscrotal fold Perineum ♂ / 63 CR: 50 mm
10	64 Face has human profile. Note growth of chin compared to day 44.	65	66 Face has human appearance.	67 Clitoris Labium minus Urogenital groove Labium majus ♀	68 Genitalia have ♀ or ♂ characteristics but still not fully formed.	69 Glans penis Urethral groove Scrotum ♂ / 70 CR: 61 mm

B

12 weeks   20 weeks   24 weeks   30 weeks

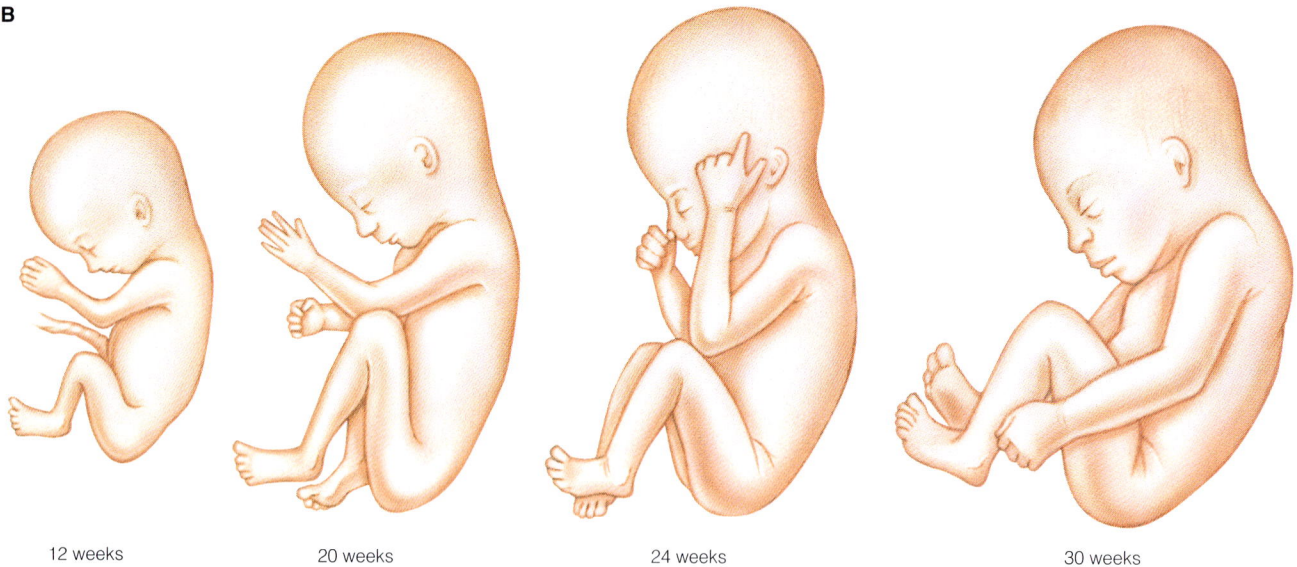

Figure 8-5. ■ *Continued.*

- Stage I, the **preembryonic stage**, is from fertilization through 14 days or 2 weeks. This is the time when the fertilized ovum travels through the fallopian tube, differentiates into trophoblast and *embryonic disc* (the cells that become the embryo), and attaches to the endometrium.

- Stage II, the **embryonic stage**, is from weeks 3 through 8. During this stage, all body systems are formed. Developing cells are at greatest risk to environmental teratogens, infections, and drugs at this time.

- Stage III, the **fetal stage**, is from weeks 9 through 38 to 40. During this stage all body systems are refined and begin to function. Some body systems will take several years to reach their maximum functioning.

Development of Fetal Body Systems

The embryonic disc forms three germ layers from which all body systems develop. Table 8-1 ■ identifies the three germ layers and the body systems derived from each. Development is very systematic, occurring from head to toe **(cephalocaudal),** from proximal to distal, and from general to specific.

CARDIOVASCULAR SYSTEM

The cardiovascular system begins with the development of a series of tubes, carrying a primitive blood. On day 21, one area of vessels begins to beat. This area will develop into the heart through a series of foldings, openings, and closings. Most heart anomalies occur between weeks 6 to 8.

Fetal Circulation

Because fetal circulation must carry blood to and from the placenta, and because the fetal respiratory system does not oxygenate blood, several structures in the fetus are unique. Blood flows from the internal iliac arteries in the fetus to the placenta through two **umbilical arteries** (Figure 8-6 ■). In the placenta, blood gases are exchanged, waste is removed, and nutrients are received. The fetal blood then flows back to the fetus through one **umbilical vein.** After entering the fetal abdomen, the umbilical vein divides into two branches. The umbilical vein carries blood to the fetal liver. The other branch, the **ductus venosus,** carries blood to the inferior vena cava.

Two structures limit the amount of blood going to the fetal lungs. Inside the fetal heart, the **foramen ovale** is an opening in the septum between the right atrium and left atrium. The higher pressure in the right atrium pushes some blood through the foramen ovale into the left atrium. Outside the fetal heart, the **ductus arteriosus,** connects the main pulmonary artery to the aorta. Some blood flows from the pulmonary artery to the aorta, thus bypassing the lungs. The small amount of blood actually reaching the lungs is necessary for the development of the respiratory system (see Figure 8-6). Usually, shortly after birth, these fetal structures close, and the cardiovascular system adjusts to normal functioning.

Fetal blood is initially formed on day 14 in the **yolk sac,** a structure inside the ovum. The liver will not be able to make blood cells until the 5th week, and the bone marrow will not function until the 10th week. Fetal hemoglobin (HgbF) has a greater attraction for oxygen than maternal hemoglobin does. This helps ensure that the fetus receives an adequate supply of oxygen. The actual blood type is determined at the time of conception.

RESPIRATORY SYSTEM

The respiratory system begins as lung buds during the 6th week of development and is well formed by the 23rd week, but still there are not enough alveoli to maintain gas exchange outside of the uterus. By week 20 to 23 the primitive lungs begin to produce surfactant. **Surfactant,** composed of phospholipids, is a substance that decreases the surface tension of fluid inside the alveoli, allowing the lungs to expand. It takes a great deal of pressure for a newborn to take its first breath and expand the lungs. Surfactant lowers the surface tension within the alveoli, allowing some air to remain in the alveoli after exhalation. Lung function is stabilized by the presence of surfactant. By the 24th week, the lungs are developed enough to oxygenate the blood with ventilatory support. Therefore, the age of **viability** (the ability to live outside the uterus) is 24 weeks. An infant born at this time would require intensive nursing care, including ventilation support. Surfactant production matures by the 35th week, making the prognosis more favorable. The lungs continue to add alveoli until adulthood.

NERVOUS SYSTEM

The head and brain develop rapidly in the fetus. By the 4th week, the brain has differentiated into lobes. A week later the cranial nerves are present and functioning. By the 6th week, the entire central nervous system is present. The peripheral nervous system, however, will not be functioning completely for another 7 to 10 years.

TABLE 8-1	
Germ Layers and Body System Development	
EMBRYONIC (GERM) LAYER	**BODY SYSTEM INTO WHICH GERM LAYER DEVELOPS**
Endoderm (inner layer)	Respiratory system Gastrointestinal system, liver, pancreas Bladder and urethra
Mesoderm (middle layer)	Muscular system Skeletal system Heart, blood, and blood vessels Spleen Urinary Reproductive
Ectoderm (outer layer)	Skin Nervous system Sense organs Mouth and anus

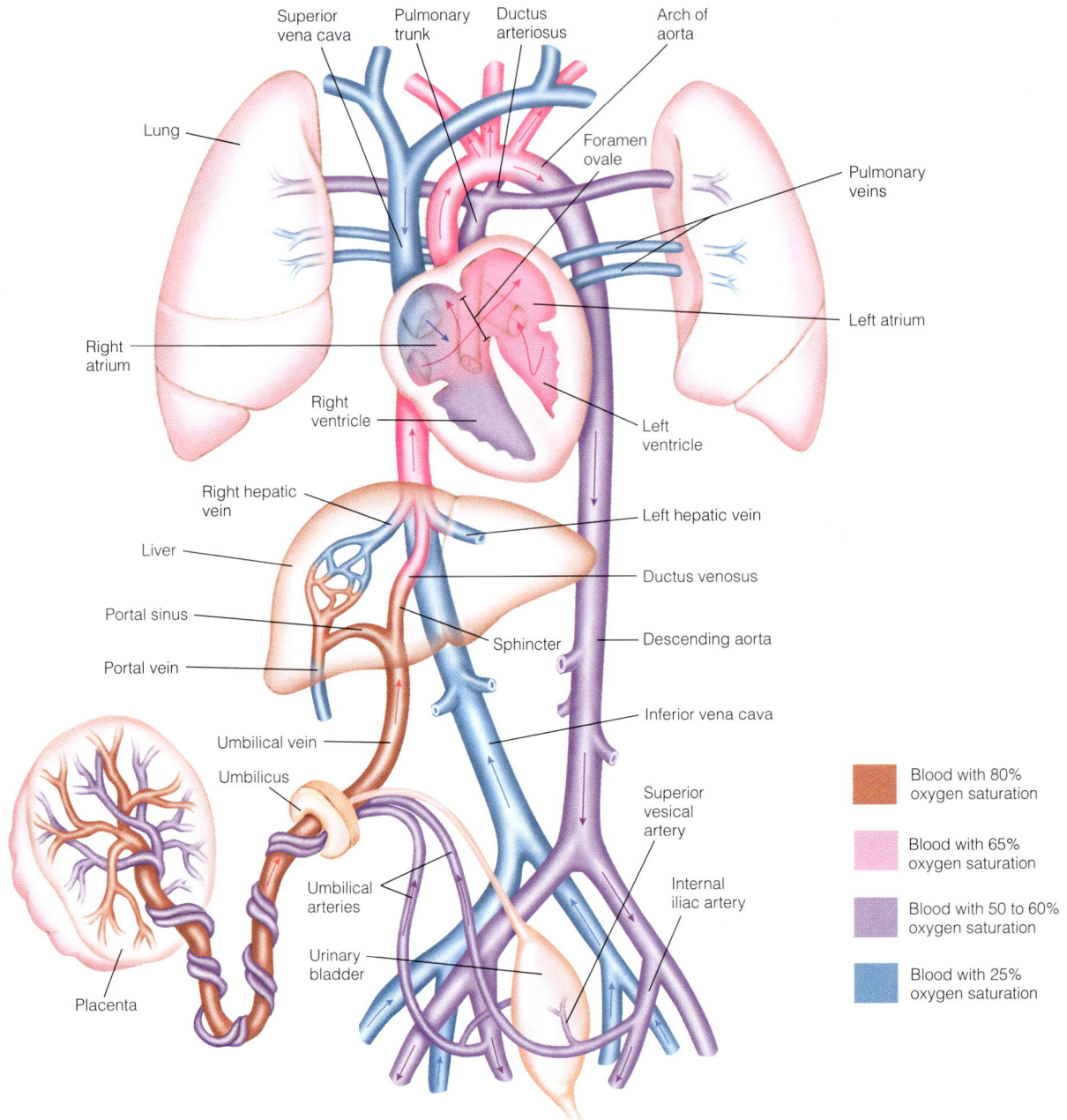

Figure 8-6. ■ Fetal circulation. Note that there are two umbilical arteries and one umbilical vein. Differences in these structures are an indicator of possible urinary abnormalities.

Special Senses

The ears begin to appear in the 3rd week, low on the head, in the region of the lower jaw. They gradually move upward to their designated place on the head by the 8th week. The infant can hear and respond to sound by the 12th week.

In the 3rd week, the eyes can be seen as large dark discs on the side of the developing head. By the 7th week, eyelids form and seal to protect the developing retina (Figure 8-7 ■). A week later the eyes have moved to the front of the face. The eyelids will remain closed until the 28th week of development.

GASTROINTESTINAL SYSTEM

The gastrointestinal system begins formation in the 4th week. The esophagus, stomach, small intestines, liver, pancreas, and most of the colon are developed from the same germ layer, the endoderm. (Refer to Table 8-1.) The oral cavity, pharynx, and anus are formed from the ectoderm. Occasionally there is incomplete development in the area where the germ layers meet, resulting in congenital anomalies.

By the 12th week, the fetus swallows amniotic fluid, and the liver is making bile. In the 16th week, **meconium** (the

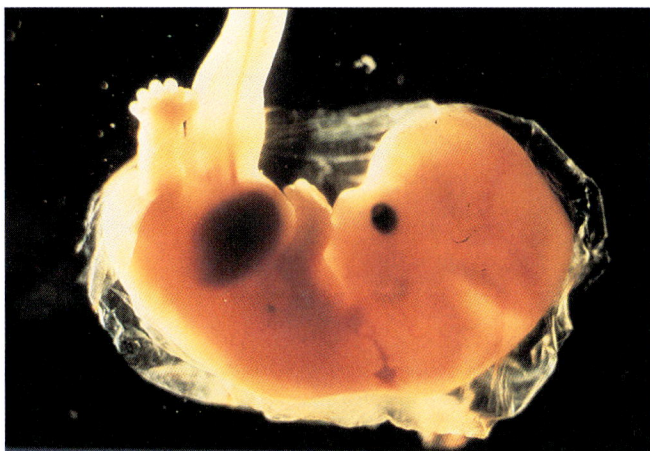

Figure 8-7. ■ The embryo at 7 weeks. The head is round and nearly erect. The eyelids begin to form. The eyes will shift forward and move closer together. (Used with permission from Petit Format/Nestle/Science Source/Photo Researchers, Inc.)

first fetal stool) is made from amniotic fluid, bile, and epithelial cells. Meconium should remain in the colon until after delivery.

clinical ALERT

The passage of meconium prior to delivery signals some type of fetal distress.

RENAL SYSTEM

The urinary system is another body system that develops from more than one germ layer. (Refer to Table 8-1.) The kidneys, ureters, and *trigone*, or lower section of the bladder, come from the mesoderm. The remainder of the bladder, female urethra, and proximal male urethra come from the endoderm. The distal male urethra develops from the ectoderm. Any disruption in development results in complex anomalies.

The kidneys develop in several stages in the pelvis and ascend to their normal location. The kidneys begin producing urine in the 10th week, and the fetus urinates into the amniotic fluid by the 11th week of development.

REPRODUCTIVE SYSTEM

The sex of the fetus is determined at conception. The fetus develops undifferentiated gonads until the 7th week. In the presence of the Y chromosome, testosterone stimulates the gonads to differentiate into testes. Sperm will not be produced until puberty. Testosterone will also stimulate the development of male genitalia. Without testosterone, the gonads develop into ovaries, and female genitalia form internally (Figure 8-8 ■). Ova will be produced and will

remain in the ovary until puberty. External male and female genitalia can be identified in the 12th week of development. (Refer to Table 8-1.) Rarely, malformation of the genitalia occurs and the genitalia are not clearly male or female. This condition, called *ambiguous genitalia*, is discussed in more detail in Chapter 18 ⬯.

MUSCULOSKELETAL SYSTEM

Limb buds appear in the 4th week. Cartilage forms a primitive skeleton covered by muscles by the 6th week. A week later fetal movement can be seen on ultrasound. However, **quickening** (the first fetal movements felt by the mother) will not occur until the 16th to 20th week. By the end of the 8th week, **ossification** (formation of bone) begins, marking the transition from embryo to fetus (Figure 8-9 ■).

INTEGUMENTARY SYSTEM

The skin of the fetus is thin and pink. Because the skin lacks fat until 34 to 36 weeks of gestation, the blood vessels can readily be seen. Fingernails and toenails reach the end of the digit by the 36th week. Lanugo (a fine, downy hair that covers the body) begins to disappear in the 28th week, leaving only hair on the scalp and at times the shoulders and upper back at birth. Vernix caseosa covers the skin to protect it from the amniotic fluid. The white cheesy substance is gradually absorbed by the skin, leaving a small amount in the body folds and the lower back. Skin color is determined at conception.

Multifetal Pregnancy

Multifetal pregnancy (multiple gestation) is a pregnancy with more than one fetus such as twins, triplets, or quadruplets. Twins occur naturally in approximately 31 in 1,000 pregnancies and triplets occur in 1.87 in 1,000 pregnancies (National Center for Health Statistics, 2005). Twins are more common in Black women than in White women or women of Asian origin. The use of fertility drugs and ***in-vitro* fertilization** (uniting ova and sperm in a laboratory setting) has resulted in a higher incidence of multiple gestation (Moore & Persaud, 2003). The Health Promotion Issue on pages 174 and 175 provides more information about *in-vitro* fertilization.

Fraternal twins or dizygotic twins occur when two ova are fertilized by two sperm. Each fertilized ova develops into a fetus in the same manner a single fetus would develop (Figure 8-10 ■). The embryos could implant close together in the uterus resulting in overlapping placentas. In this case it may be necessary to examine the fetal membranes to determine whether the twins are fraternal or identical. Fraternal twins have two separate chorion and amnion layers.

Identical twins or monozygotic twins develop from one fertilized ovum. They have the same genetic makeup and therefore are the same sex. Identical twins can originate at

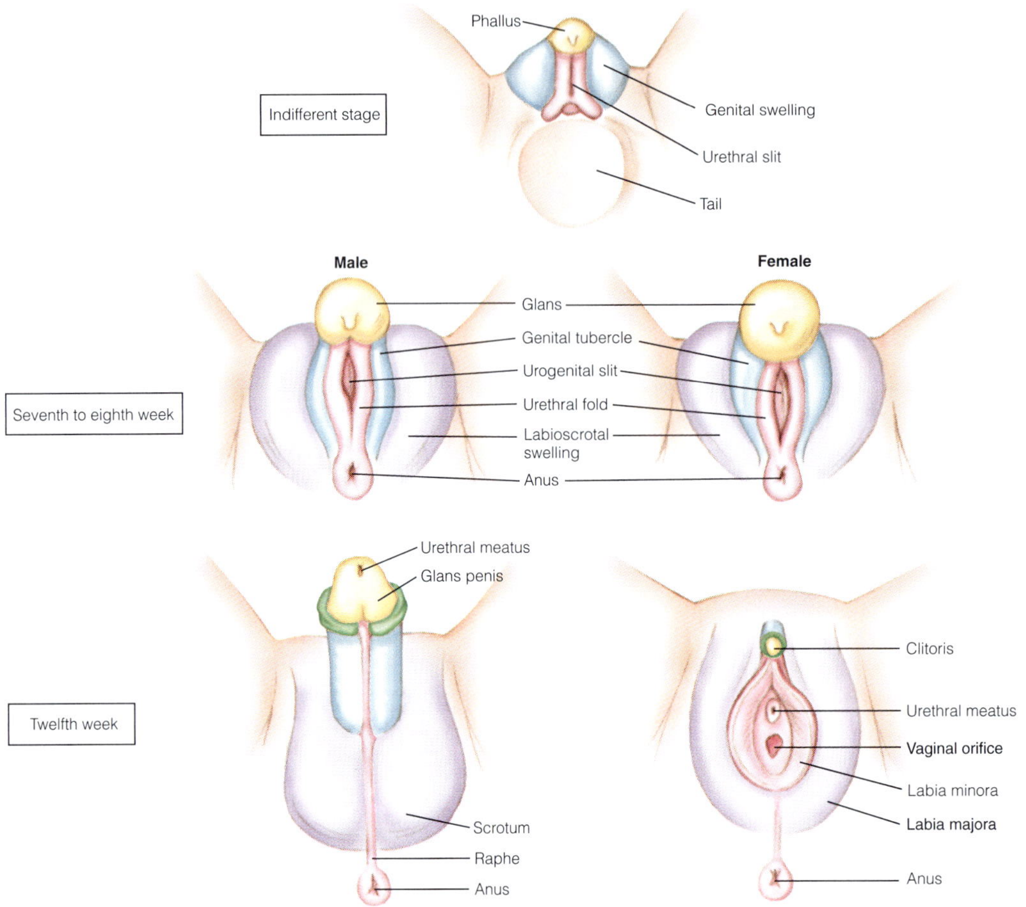

Figure 8-8. ■ Development of the external reproductive structures. (Reproduced with permission from McGraw-Hill Companies, Inc. Ganong, W. F. [1995]. *Review of medical physiology* [17th ed.]. Norwalk, CT: Appleton & Lange, p. 384.)

different stages of early development after the zygote has reached thousands of cells. Complete separation of the cell mass into two parts is necessary for normal formation of the embryos. If complete separation does not occur, conjoined

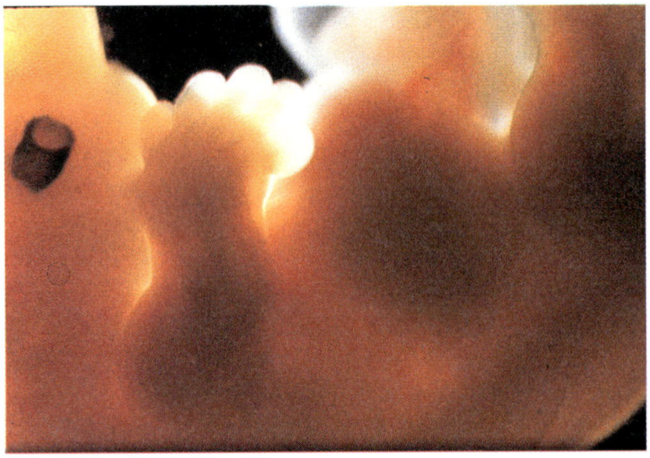

Figure 8-9. ■ The embryo at 8 weeks. Although only 3 centimeters in crown-to-rump (C-R) length, the embryo clearly resembles a human. Facial features continue to develop.

twins could result. If the cell mass separates within the first 3 days before the inner cell mass and chorion are formed, two embryos, two amnions, and two chorions will develop. If the cell mass separates about day 5 after the chorion has developed, two embryos will form with separate amnion sacs. If the cell mass separates approximately day 7 to 13 after the amnion has developed, there will be one amnion and one chorion surrounding the two embryos.

Other multiple gestations can be fraternal, identical, or a combination of these. For example, three ova fertilized by three sperm would result in fraternal triplets. Two ova fertilized by two sperm and then one zygote separating would result in two identical siblings and a fraternal sibling.

RISKS OF MULTIPLE PREGNANCY

The risks of a multiple pregnancy include preterm labor, pregnancy-induced hypertension, and gestational diabetes. These disorders are discussed in Chapter 13 ⚭ . As the uterus enlarges to accommodate the fetuses, there is an increased risk of rupturing. Cesarean birth may be indicated because of prematurity or malpresentation of one or more of the infants.

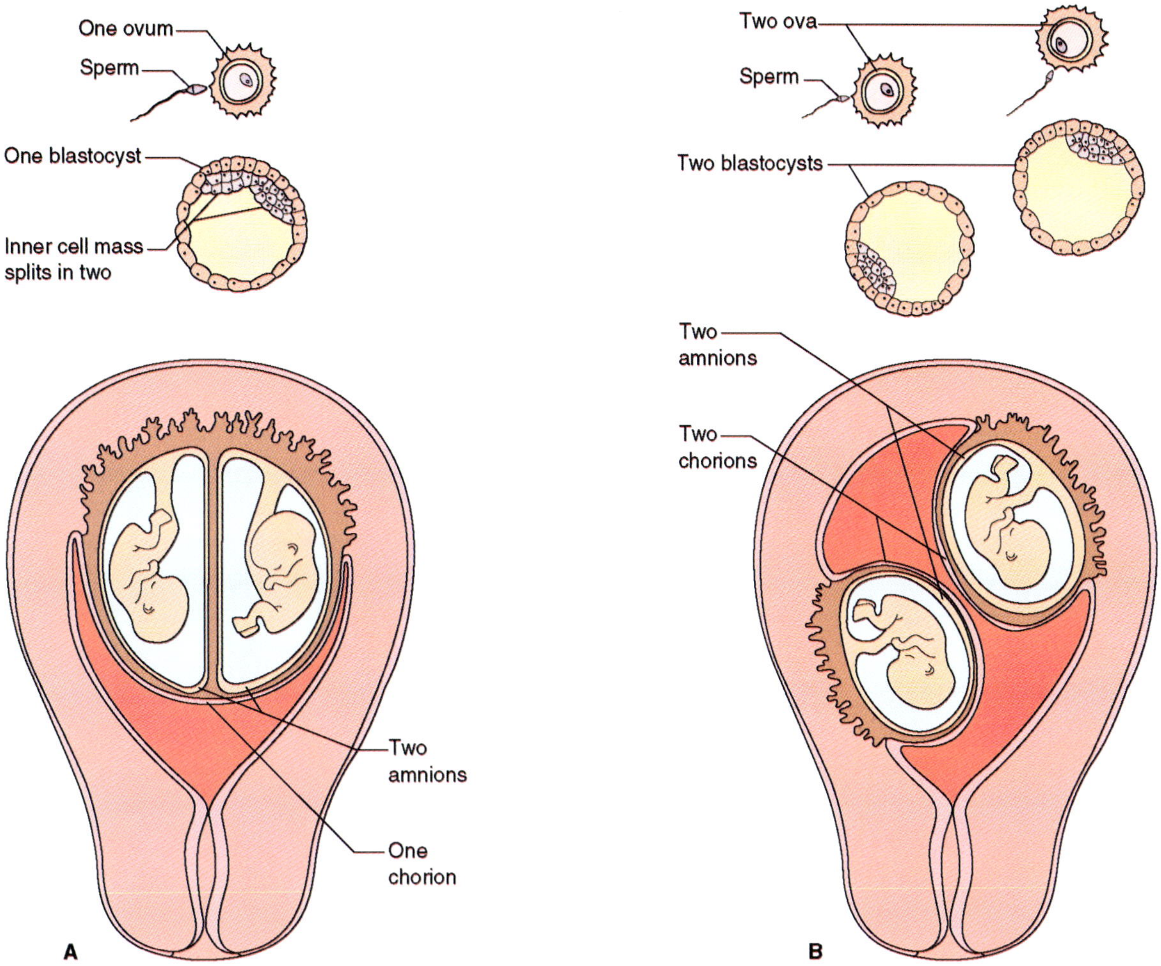

Figure 8-10. ■ (**A**) Formation of identical (*monozygotic*) twins. (**B**) Formation of fraternal (*dizygotic*) twins.

Chromosomal Abnormalities

Young teenage girls, women over 30, and couples who have a family history of genetic anomalies are at a higher risk for conceiving a fetus with chromosomal abnormalities than other parents. The **karyotype,** a picture analysis of the chromosomes, is usually obtained from stained cells (see Figure 5-2 ⬤⬤). Samples of placental tissue can also be used to determine the karyotype of the fetus. The chromosome pairs are numbered 1 through 22 and designated XX or XY. Abnormalities can be **autosomal** (found on chromosomes 1 through 22) or **sex-linked** (found on the X or Y chromosome). Abnormalities are also either **dominant** (exerting a controlling influence) or **recessive** (incapable of expressing control). A person who has one dominant gene and one recessive gene is said to be a **carrier** of the disorder. A child will have the genetic disorder if he or she receives a recessive gene from both parents.

Couples with a family history of genetic disorders may choose to have genetic testing done before they become pregnant. An informed decision regarding parenting can then be made. Pregnant women at risk may have placental tissue sampling completed to determine the presence of genetic disorders. Informed decisions can then be made regarding termination or continuation of the pregnancy.

Chromosomal defects result from an altered number of chromosomes (one chromosome—called *monosomatic,* or three chromosomes—called **trisomy**) or abnormalities of structure (deletion of one part of the chromosome). Common chromosomal (genetic) anomalies include Down syndrome (trisomy 21), trisomy 18, trisomy 13, and Klinefelter syndrome (extra A chromosome in male XXY).

Chromosomal defects can result in a variety of physical anomalies, including malformations and underdeveloped structures or body systems. Other chromosomal defects result in mental delays, retardation, or behavioral problems. When testing is completed before delivery and diagnosis of genetic anomalies are made, the parents can be better prepared to care for the infant. The Nursing Care Plan Chart on page 176 provides some information about nursing care for clients with genetic traits for disease.

HEALTH PROMOTION ISSUE

IN-VITRO FERTILIZATION

Julie and Daniel Dawson have been trying to have a baby for a year and a half without success. Julie has been tested for ovulation patterns and structural abnormalities including open fallopian tubes and uterine or cervical anomalies. Daniel has been tested for sperm count and quality. The couple comes to the fertility clinic to discuss options for assisted fertility.

DISCUSSION

Approximately 10% of men and women of reproductive age are unable to become pregnant after 1 year of unprotected sexual intercourse. (Infertility issues are discussed in Chapter 7 ⟲⟳.) Since 1981, trained obstetricians have had the ability to assist reproduction using a variety of techniques. Each attempt at assisted reproduction, called a cycle, may cost the couple $12,000 or more. Although often several embryos develop, there is no guarantee that a pregnancy will occur. Couples are encouraged to explore the risks and benefits of assisted reproduction.

In-vitro fertilization (IVF) is used in cases when infertility results from narrow, blocked, or absent fallopian tubes or vas deferens, male and female immunologic infertility, decreased sperm count, or poor sperm quality. IVF is the combining of egg and sperm in a laboratory dish and then implanting the embryo into the uterus. The success of IVF is improved when three to four embryos (rather than one) are placed in the uterus. To obtain multiple ova, the woman may be asked to take fertility drugs to induce ovulation. Ultrasound is then used to monitor follicular development. When follicles appear mature, hCG is given to stimulate final egg maturation and control ovulation. Using ultrasound as a guide, the obstetrician surgically aspirates ova through a needle instated through the vagina. The ova are placed in a sterile laboratory dish. (See illustration inset.)

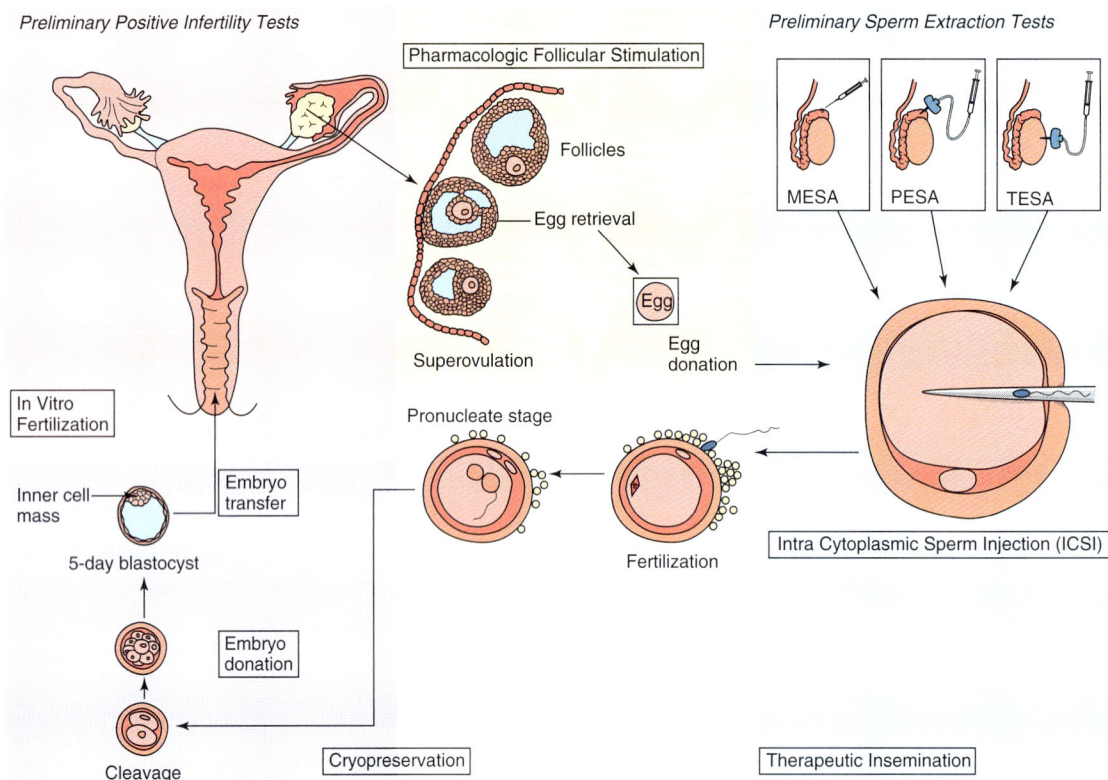

Assisted reproductive techniques.

The man is asked to abstain from ejaculation for 2 to 3 days prior to obtaining a semen sample. The semen sample is usually obtained by masturbation and ejaculation into a specimen cup. If there is blockage of vas deferens, a needle may be inserted into the epididymis or testes, and sperm aspirated. These procedures are termed microsurgical epididymal sperm aspiration (MESA), percutaneous epididymal sperm aspiration (PESA), and testicular sperm aspiration (TESA). (See the inset figure.) The semen is placed in the laboratory dish along with the ova. The laboratory dish is placed in a controlled warm environment.

After several days, the ova are examined to determine whether fertilization has taken place. If so, the obstetrician inserts a catheter through the woman's cervix, and three to four embryos are transferred to the uterus. The woman is asked to remain in a supine position for approximately an hour to decrease the possibility of the embryos being expelled through the cervix. If the embryo implants into the endometrium, pregnancy should progress as with natural fertilization.

At times, other assisted reproduction techniques are used. Once the ova are obtained, they may be immediately placed in a catheter with motile sperm and inserted into the fimbriated end of the fallopian tube. Fertilization occurs in the fallopian tube rather than in the laboratory. This procedure is called **gamete intrafallopian transfer (GIFT).** Similar procedures include **zygote intrafallopian transfer (ZIFT)** and **tubal embryo transfer,** in which the fertilized ova are placed into the fallopian tube at an earlier stage of development.

Intracytoplasmic sperm injection may be used if there is a very low sperm count or the sperm have poor mobility. In this technique, the mature ovum is held in a pipette (small glass tube). A delicate, sharp needle containing a single sperm is gently inserted into the cytoplasm of the ovum. The sperm is slowly pushed into the ovum. The fertilized ovum is allowed to incubate for several days and then is placed into the uterus.

Sometimes many ova are obtained and fertilized. They are then frozen by a process called **cryopreservation,** and stored for future use. The couple must decide whether to use these embryos themselves, give them to another woman, or destroy them. Controversy remains regarding use of these embryos for stem cell research.

PLANNING AND IMPLEMENTATION

The nurse working in a fertility clinic should realize that couples seeking help to reproduce are under great pressure. They have a strong desire to have a baby, and in most cases have been unsuccessful for a year or more. They need accurate, up-to-date information in a format they can understand. They will need to be seen in the clinic frequently, which may take time away from their work schedules. Assisted reproduction is expensive, and there is no guarantee that pregnancy will occur. Many insurance companies will not cover assisted reproduction procedures. The couple may need help locating financial resources.

The nurse must be prepared to explain all procedures to the couple, answer questions, and provide resource information. The nurse assists in obtaining ovum and sperm, ensures proper handling of specimens, and assists with insertion of embryos into the uterus. It is critical that specimens are properly labeled and the correct embryos are inserted into the uterus. There are legal ramifications if the improper handling results in death of embryos or embryos are implanted into the wrong woman.

Many times, support groups can provide couples with encouragement, information, and resources. The nurse should have a list of support groups in the area.

SELF-REFLECTION

Assess your own desire to parent. How would you feel if you or your partner were unable to become pregnant? How would you feel if you and your partner wanted to have children, but were unable to because of your health problem? How would you feel if you were unable to conceive because of your partner's health problem?

SUGGESTED RESOURCES

Armour, K., & Clark Callister, L. (2005). Prevention of triplets & higher order multiples: Trends in reproductive medicine. *Journal of Perinatal & Neonatal Nursing, 19*(2), 103–111.

Squires, J., & Kaplan, P. (2007). Developmental outcomes of children born after assisted reproduction technologies. *Infants and Children 20*(1), 2–10.

NURSING CARE PLAN CHART

Planning for Couple with Sickle Cell Trait

John and Trina Lewis, an African American couple, recently married. They are planning a family in the near future. They are concerned about giving sickle cell anemia to their children. John's cousin has suffered from sickle cell anemia since birth. Trina was adopted as a baby and does not have information regarding her family history. They have come to the clinic to obtain information and testing prior to becoming pregnant. (*Note:* sickle cell anemia is used here as an example of a genetic disorder. For complete discussion of sickle cell anemia, consult a pediatric textbook.)

GOAL	INTERVENTION	RATIONALE	EXPECTED OUTCOME
1. Deficient Knowledge related to sickle cell anemia			
The couple will obtain information about testing for sickle cell disease.	Provide written information regarding sickle cell anemia.	*Written information allows clients to review information at home.*	Couple will make decision about genetic testing for sickle cell anemia.
	Explain what "recessive autosomal disorders" are.	*Parents need an understanding of the cause of the disorder in order to understand how it may affect offspring.*	
	Explain the difference between having the disorder and being a carrier of the trait.	*Client can be a carrier of trait without having disorder. Both parents must at least be carriers for child to have the disorder.*	
	Explain procedure of obtaining a blood sample.	*This prepares the clients for the procedure. Genetic markers in the blood identify the disorder.*	
	Explain need for follow-up appointment to obtain results of testing.	*Several days are needed to obtain test results.*	
2. Readiness for Enhanced Family Coping			
Couple will make informed decision about childbearing.	When test results are obtained, provide explanations and reinforce understanding. Provide written materials for the couple to read at home.	*This is a stressful experience for the couple. They may be unable to absorb all the information at once and may need some information repeated.*	Couple will state understanding of the result of testing and will begin to shape their plans around it.
3. Anticipatory Grieving			
Couple will develop a plan for their life and family that includes new data.	Provide therapeutic listening to allow each person to express feelings openly.	*The news that they cannot proceed without concern can be devastating initially. The couple needs time to express and process their feelings in order to be able to move ahead.*	Couple will recognize the grief they feel at the loss of "the perfect child." They will come to some resolution about how to go forward to have a family.
	Provide a nonjudgmental response to strategizing.	*To come to clear decisions, the couple must weigh all possibilities against their beliefs and values. They should not be swayed by the nurse's beliefs.*	
	Provide referrals to local groups; provide information for researching more information online.	*No one is better able to assist this couple in their grief than people who have dealt with the same disease. Support groups can be of help no matter what the couple decides.*	

PRECONCEPTION PLANNING

For many years, health professionals have recognized that a healthy pregnancy begins before conception with good health habits. The focus of preconception care is to help the couple identify their pregnancy risk and prepare for conception. When possible, the nurse should help the couple establish a healthy lifestyle prior to conception. It must be acknowledged, however, that many pregnancies are not planned. Unhealthy habits can affect the embryo before the mother knows she is pregnant. If the client presents pregnant, reviewing the preconception lifestyle of the couple can provide important data on which to plan care during pregnancy.

At times couples have difficulty becoming pregnant.

Assessment

The LPN/LVN can assist in data collection regarding risk factors for both partners. Some questions specifically address smoking, drinking alcohol, using illicit drugs, and being exposed to environmental hazards, because of their possible effects on the fetus (see Table 6-8 ⬭). Individuals may be unaware of exposure to chemicals, but when a work history is explored chemical exposure may become apparent. For example, a cashier in an automobile parts store may feel relatively safe from chemical exposure. However, if the store is in the same building as a mechanic shop, the cashier may be exposed to fumes from the gas and oil used in repair of cars.

Data about family history of genetic anomalies is also collected. (Family history is also discussed in Chapter 4 ⬭.) Research has determined that various ethnic groups are at risk for genetic disorders (Box 8-1 ■).

MALE CONTRIBUTION
The health of the fetus is not just related to the mother. Smoking decreases sperm production and motility. Men who have been exposed to industrial chemicals are the fathers of more stillborn and small-for-gestational-age infants. They are the fathers in more pregnancies that end in preterm labor or spontaneous abortion. Because production of sperm (*spermatogenesis*) is a continuous process, men can decrease these risks by avoiding smoking and industrial chemicals for 3 to 4 months prior to conception. It is important to ask the male partner about smoking and exposure to chemicals.

FEMALE CONTRIBUTION
To carry a pregnancy with minimal risk, the mother should develop a healthy lifestyle well before conception. A healthy lifestyle includes eating a low-fat, high-fiber

BOX 8-1	CULTURAL PULSE POINTS

Suggested Genetic Testing by Ethnic Group

Because subpopulations of women have an increased tendency toward carrying children with certain genetic abnormalities (Ladewig et al., 2006), screening tests are recommended. The following list provides a sampling of these groups:

- Africans, Arabs, Asian Indians, Egyptians, Hispanics from Central or South America or Caribbean—sickle cell anemia
- All women (especially from British Isles or Ireland)—neural tube defects
- Ashkenazi Jews—cystic fibrosis, Gaucher disease, Tay-Sachs disease
- Cajuns and French Canadians—Tay-Sachs disease
- Caucasian (especially Northern Europeans and Celtic)—cystic fibrosis
- Mediterranean (Greeks, Italians, Sicilians, etc.)—thalassemia
- Southeast Asian (Cambodian, Filipino, Laotian, Vietnamese) and Filipino—alpha-thalassemia
- Women over 35—chromosomal trisomies

diet with an adequate amount of folic acid; exercising at least three times per week; and being within 15 pounds of one's ideal weight. Because pregnancies are not always planned, women of childbearing age should be advised that avoiding unhealthy or risk-taking behavior will help ensure a healthy infant. The nurse should ask about smoking, drinking alcohol, and using illicit drugs, and about exposure to chemicals.

NUTRITIONAL DEFICITS
Because fetal development occurs on a strict timeline, the lack of certain nutrients at specific times can have a profound effect on the developing organism. Maternal nutrition can affect brain and neural tube (spinal column) development. Amino acids, glucose, fatty acids, and folic acid are needed for normal development. Subtle damage associated with the brain's capacity, possibly leading to learning delays or disabilities, may be caused by nutritional deficiency. Supplements containing folic acid can reduce the incidence of neural tube defects, including **spina bifida** (a defect in the spinal column), **meningomyelocele** (protrusion of the meninges and spinal cord through a defect in the spinal column), and **anencephaly** (absence of neural tissue in the cranium). (See Chapter 18 ⬭ for more discussion on neural tube defects.)

Iron is needed for red blood cell formation in the mother and fetus. Iron deficiency could cause inadequate oxygenation of fetal tissue, resulting in delayed development or

Food Sources of Iron, Vitamin B₁₂, and Folic Acid

Iron-Rich Foods
Beef, chicken, pork loin, turkey, veal, egg yolk
Bran flakes, oatmeal, brown rice, whole-grain breads
Clams, oysters
Dried beans
Dried fruits
Greens

Folic Acid Food Sources
Asparagus, broccoli, green leafy vegetables
Eggs, liver, milk, organ meats
Kidney beans
Wheat germ
Yeast

Vitamin B₁₂ Food Sources
Eggs, cheese, milk
Fresh shrimp and oysters
Meats, organ meats (liver, kidney)

fetal death. In the woman, a decrease in vitamin B_{12} results in pernicious anemia, causing infertility. (See Chapters 10 and 11 ⬭ for more discussion on nutrition during pregnancy.) Box 8-2 ▪ provides a list of foods that are high in iron, vitamin B_{12}, and folic acid. Because many of these problems occur before the woman knows she is pregnant, it is important for women of childbearing age to eat a well-balanced diet daily. The nurse should collect and record data regarding dietary practices.

HARMFUL CHEMICALS
The woman may be exposed to **teratogens** (agents that cause defects in the developing embryo). Cigarettes, alcohol, and illicit drugs can have negative effects on pregnancy. Exposure to or lack of a chemical can have a huge effect, especially during certain crucial weeks of fetal development (Figure 8-11 ▪). Smoking during pregnancy can cause low birth weight and spontaneous abortion. Alcohol, even in moderate amounts, may cause fetal alcohol syndrome (discussed in Chapter 18 ⬭), including **craniofacial** (head and face) malformation and central nervous system dysfunction. Illicit drugs can cause a variety of **anomalies** (developments of abnormal organs or structures). Clients should be encouraged to stop using these substances prior to and during pregnancy.

Medications, both prescription and over the counter, may interfere with normal pregnancy and should be discussed with the health care provider. It is important to keep the health care provider informed if pregnancy is suspected. If prescribed medication is necessary, the primary care provider should be consulted regarding present or future

pregnancies. Some medication is so potentially harmful to the fetus that unplanned pregnancy must be prevented. For example, in the 20th century, women were sometimes prescribed the tranquillizer *thalidomide* until it was realized that the drug interfered with normal limb development. Children born to these mothers had only partially developed limbs. Today, pregnancy would be prevented in a woman taking thalidomide.

To prevent teratogenic effects, the FDA has established five categories of potential risk for the development of birth defects. Box 8-3 ▪ identifies these categories. It is important to recall that herbal medicines are categorized as dietary supplements rather than drugs. Therefore, the testing, regulation, and standardization of herbs may not be as strict as other prescription or over-the-counter medication. See Chapter 10 ⬭ for more discussion regarding herbal supplements during pregnancy.

The nurse should collect and record data about exposure to any harmful chemicals. Women of childbearing age should be aware of harmful chemicals and avoid them when possible. For example, the woman of childbearing age can avoid skin contact with cleaning supplies by wearing rubber gloves while using these agents, and she can work in a well-ventilated room to prevent inhaling fumes.

Infectious Disease Complications

Infectious diseases and other disorders can have a negative impact on pregnancy. Routine testing should be done for such infections as syphilis, gonorrhea, HIV, chlamydia, human papilloma virus, herpes simplex, and group B streptococcus. (See Chapter 7 ⬭ for a full discussion.) If the client tests positive, treatment should begin as soon as possible. Infection of the fallopian tubes, **salpingitis,** can cause scarring and narrowing of the lumen. A narrow fallopian tube can lead to infertility or tubal pregnancy. Some infections such as rubella (measles) and syphilis can cause malformation in the developing fetus. (See Chapter 13 ⬭ for full discussion.) The nurse should collect and record data regarding previous infections.

NURSING CARE

PRIORITIES IN NURSING CARE

In fostering optimal fetal development, the nurse's priorities are to gather data for ongoing assessment of fetal and maternal well-being and to encourage consistent prenatal care. The nurse also reinforces client learning about nutrition, exercise, rest, and hygiene.

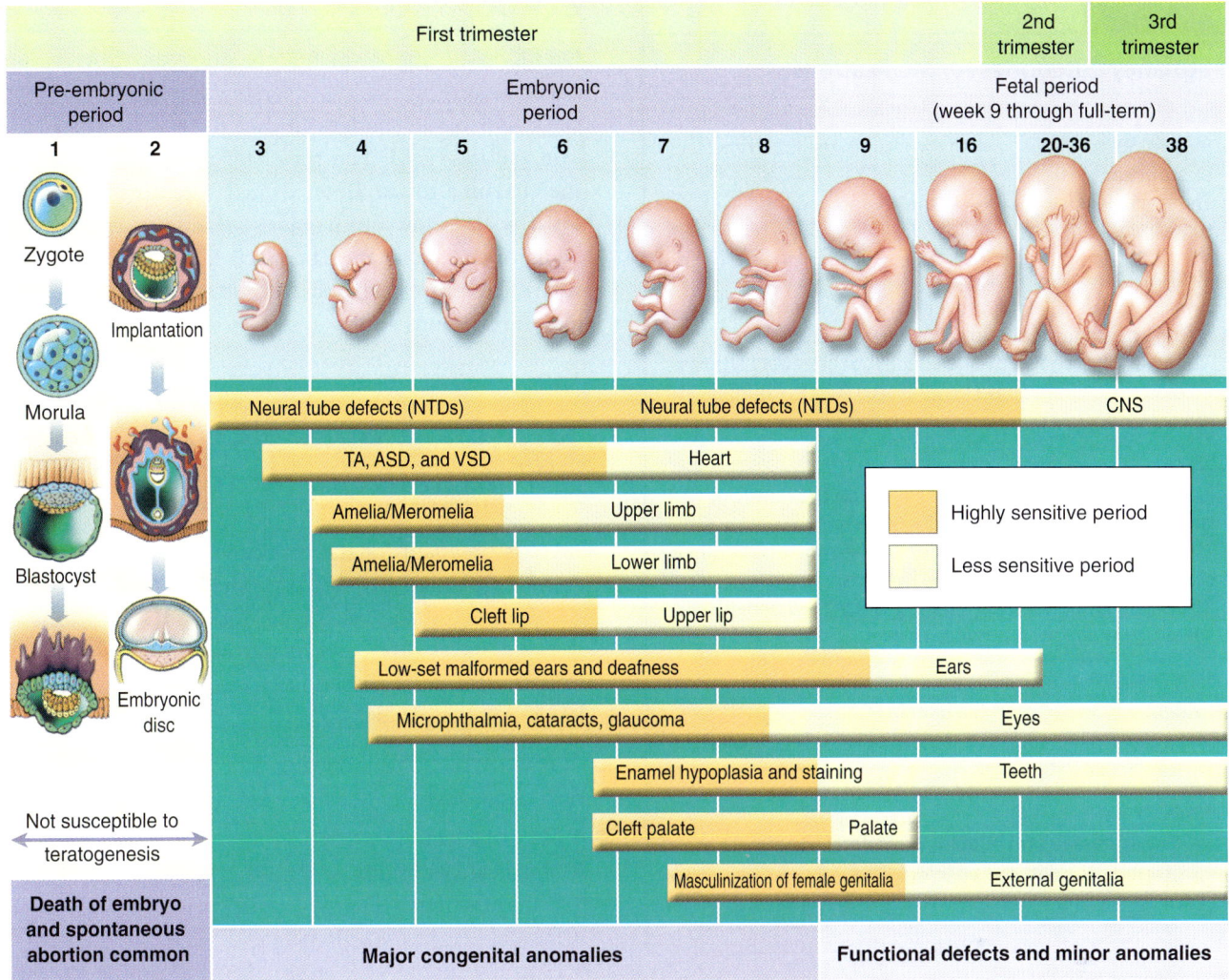

	First trimester		2nd trimester	3rd trimester

Figure 8-11. ■ Highly sensitive periods during the embryonic stage. For the first 2 weeks after conception, exposure to a teratogen has an all-or-nothing effect. It either disrupts implantation and causes spontaneous abortion or leaves the embryo unharmed. From about the 3rd through the 8th week of pregnancy (when organs form), exposure to a hazardous agent may cause serious anomalies. After organ formation and for the remainder of the pregnancy, exposure to fetal toxins will not cause malformation but can interfere with maturation of the central nervous system and retard intrauterine growth. It may also cause cognitive or behavioral abnormalities.

ASSESSING

The nurse uses the data collected to help determine the risk of genetic or developmental anomalies in the fetus. The nurse should review aspects of the client's lifestyle and help her understand where changes are needed for the benefit of the fetus.

DIAGNOSING, PLANNING, AND IMPLEMENTING

Nursing diagnoses related to fetal development might include the following:

■ Deficient **K**nowledge related to risk for alterations in fetal development

■ Readiness for Enhanced **K**nowledge related to *in-vitro* fertilization

Expected outcomes might include:

■ Verbalizes understanding of risks for alterations in fetal development.
■ Verbalizes understanding of the *in-vitro* fertilization process.

In relation to fetal development, the nurse has the following responsibilities:

■ Identify families at risk for genetic or reproductive problems. *The first step in helping the family is to identify problems or potential problems.*

BOX 8-3

Pregnancy Categories for Medications

Category A
- Studies do not show a risk to the fetus in the first trimester of pregnancy.
- There is no evidence of risk in the second and third trimesters.

Category B
- Animal studies have not proven a risk to the fetus, but there are no adequate studies in pregnant women.
- Animal studies show adverse effects, but adequate studies on pregnant women have not shown risk to the human fetus.

Category C
- Animal studies show an adverse effect on the fetus, but there are no adequate studies in humans.
- There are no animal reproduction studies, and no adequate studies have been performed in humans.
- The drug may be used during pregnancy if the benefits of the drug outweigh its possible risks.

Category D
- Evidence shows a risk to the human fetus.
- The potential benefits from the use of the drug may outweigh the risk to the fetus.

Category X
- Studies in animals and humans prove fetal abnormalities, or reports indicate evidence of fetal risk.
- The risks of using these drugs clearly outweigh any possible benefits.

- Determine how the genetic or reproductive problem for which a family is at risk is perceived, and what further information is needed. *The nurse must assess what information the family has in order to determine what further information is needed.*
- Assist families in acquiring accurate information about the specific problem. *When the family has accurate information, they can make the best decision for themselves.*
- Assist the family in understanding and dealing with information received. *Information about genetic or reproductive problems is complex and can stimulate an emotional response. Families may need to have the information explained in simple terms. Family members may need emotional support.*
- Provide information about support groups. *Support groups not only provide emotional support but can be instrumental in helping family members.*
- Aid families in coping with the crisis they are experiencing. *Reproductive and genetic problems can place a lot of strain on marital relationships. The family under stress may not hear or understand instructions. The nurse can facilitate communication and coping.*

EVALUATING

On follow-up appointments, the nurse should question the client regarding lifestyle changes. For example: How has the client made changes in diet to increase the intake of iron and folic acid? Has the client stopped smoking? Does she continue to use illicit drugs? The nurse may need to assist with follow-up diagnostic exams to assess the well-being of the fetus. (See Chapter 9 ⬭ for further discussion.) The nurse may assist in setting up an appointment for genetic counseling.

NURSING PROCESS CARE PLAN
Woman Pregnant for First Time

Joyce is pregnant for the first time. Her husband, George, attends each monthly checkup. They are very excited about the pregnancy and ask many questions. The fetus is 20 weeks gestation and appears normal. Joyce asks the nurse, "When will our baby be fully developed? When will we know if it is a girl or boy?"

Assessment. The following data should be collected with each clinic visit:
- Maternal weight
- Maternal vital signs
- Fetal heart rate
- Fundal height measurement
- Learning needs

Nursing Diagnosis. The following important nursing diagnosis (among others) is established for the client:
- Deficient **K**nowledge related to fetal development

Expected Outcome
- The couple will explain major milestones in fetal development.

Planning and Implementation
- Provide written information illustrating fetal development on a weekly basis. *Pictures of developing fetus aids in understanding of fetal development process. Couple can refer to pictures to see how their baby is growing and developing.*
- Explain written information and answer questions. *Visual aids may need to be explained and questions answered for complete understanding.*
- Ask primary care provider to identify fetal body parts if an ultrasound is performed. *If an ultrasound is performed, the primary care provider may help couple compare their fetus to the pictures provided. This would reinforce the normal development of their baby.*

Evaluation.   The couple will explain how the fetus is growing at each scheduled clinic visit.

Critical Thinking in the Nursing Process

1. What else should the nurse teach the couple at this routine clinic visit?
2. What would be some signs the nurse can observe that the fetus is not developing normally?

3. What signs would make the nurse suspect a multifetal pregnancy?

Note: Discussion of Critical Thinking questions appears in Appendix I.

Note: The reference and resource listings for this and all chapters have been compiled at the back of the book.

Chapter Review

KEY TERMS by Topic

Use the audio glossary feature of either the CD-ROM or the Companion Website to hear the correct pronunciation of the following key terms.

Fertilization
fertilization, pregnancy, conception, zygote, morula, blastocyst, trophoblast, embryonic disc

Implantation
implantation, chorionic villi, human chorionic gonadotropin

Development of Support Structures
chorion, amnion, fetal membranes, bag of waters, amniotic fluid, lanugo, vernix

caseosa, placenta, cotyledons, human placental lactogen, relaxin, umbilical cord, Wharton's jelly

Stages of Fetal Development
gestation, embryo, fetus, preembryonic stage, embryonic stage, fetal stage

Development of Fetal Body Systems
cephalocaudal, umbilical arteries, umbilical vein, ductus venosus, foramen ovale, ductus arteriosus, yolk sac, surfactant, viability, meconium, quickening, ossification

Multifetal Pregnancy
multifetal pregnancy, multiple gestation, in-vitro fertilization, fraternal twins, identical

twins, gamete intrafallopian transfer (GIFT), zygote intrafallopian transfer (ZIFT), tubal embryo transfer, intracytoplasmic sperm injection, cryopreservation

Chromosomal Abnormalities
karyotype, autosomal, sex-linked, dominant, recessive, carrier, trisomy

Assessment
spina bifida, meningomyelocele, anencephaly, teratogens, craniofacial, anomalies

Infectious Disease Complications
salpingitis

KEY Points

- Fetal development progresses in an orderly, predictable sequence over the normal 40 weeks of gestation.
- All body systems are established in the embryo within the first 8 weeks after conception.
- From the 9th week of gestation until delivery the baby is called an embryo.
- Nutrients from the mother enter the fetal blood in the placenta.
- Waste from the fetus enters the maternal blood in the placenta.
- Maternal and fetal blood does not mix.
- The umbilical cord has 2 umbilical arteries and 1 umbilical vein.
- The fetus is viable with life support after the 24th week of gestation, but viability is greatly improved after the 35th week of gestation.
- Couples having difficulty conceiving may seek additional assistance from a fertility specialist.
- Couples with a family history of genetic abnormalities may seek additional information prior to or after conception.
- The LPN/LVN assists the RN in providing instruction to families about fetal development.

EXPLORE MediaLink

Additional interactive resources for this chapter can be found on the Companion Website at www.prenhall.com/towle. Click on Chapter 8 and "Begin" to select the activities for this chapter.

For chapter-related NCLEX®-style questions and an audio glossary, access the accompanying CD-ROM in this book.

Animations
Conception
Cell division

FOR FURTHER Study

Family history is discussed in Chapter 4.

The karyotype, a picture analysis of the chromosomes, is usually obtained from stained cells; see Figure 5-2.

The effects on fetal development of smoking, alcohol, and illicit drugs are discussed in Table 6-8.

For a discussion about routine testing for sexually transmitted infections, see Chapter 7.

See Chapters 10 and 11 for more on nutrition, including herbal supplements.

See Chapter 13 for risks of multiple pregnancy and for discussion of infections such as rubella (measles) and syphilis that can cause malformations in the developing fetus.

For more discussion on neural tube defects and fetal alcohol syndrome, see Chapter 18.

Caring for a Pregnant Woman Whose Fetus Has a Genetic Abnormality

NCLEX-PN® Focus Area: Physiologic Integrity

Case Study: Juanita, a 22-year-old, married woman, comes to the clinic for a follow-up appointment following genetic testing on the fetus. She is 5 months pregnant. Her husband is in the military and out of the country. The obstetrician has told her the diagnostic tests indicate the fetus has spina bifida.

Nursing Diagnosis: Deficient <u>K</u>nowledge related to the effects of spina bifida

COLLECT DATA

Subjective	Objective
_____	_____
_____	_____
_____	_____
_____	_____
_____	_____
_____	_____

Would you report this? Yes/No

If yes, to: _____

Nursing Care

_____
_____
_____
_____
_____
_____
_____
_____
_____
_____
_____

How would you document this? _____
_____
_____

Compare your documentation to the sample provided in Appendix I.

Data Collected
(use only those that apply)

- Weight: 137 pounds
- States she does not know what she did wrong
- Vital signs within normal limits
- Crying
- Urine negative
- States she does not know how to tell her husband

Nursing Interventions
(use only those that apply; list in priority order)

- Refer to WIC program.
- Teach about spina bifida.
- Provide written information about spina bifida.
- Schedule an appointment for 2 weeks.
- Provide information about support groups.
- Place a hand on her shoulder.
- Provide facial tissue.
- Teach about folic acid.

NCLEX-PN® Exam Preparation

1 After fertilization of the ova, when does the production of hCG begin?

1. 8–12 hours
2. 18–36 hours
3. 4–6 days
4. 8–10 days

2 Which of the following substances produced by the placenta prevents uterine contractions?

1. human placental lactogen
2. human chorionic gonadotropin
3. progesterone
4. relaxin

3 Which of the following statements about fetal circulation are true? Choose all that apply.

1. The fetal respiratory system oxygenates blood.
2. The ductus arteriosus is located inside the fetal heart.
3. Osmosis is the means of blood exchange between placenta and fetus.
4. The umbilical cord contains two arteries and one vein.
5. The fetal blood and maternal blood do not mix.

4 A client's history reveals a previous infection of the fallopian tubes. The client asks the nurse if the previous infection will affect the possibility of becoming pregnant. The nurse explains that becoming pregnant after an infection in the fallopian tube may be difficult because:

1. fertilization occurs in the outer third of the fallopian tube.
2. production of hCG may be decreased.
3. ovulation may be delayed.
4. the ovum is only fertile for 72 hours.

5 A client at 24 weeks gestation is about to give birth. The nurse is preparing to assist the physician. It is most appropriate for the nurse to be prepared to offer:

1. assistance with breastfeeding.
2. ventilation support to the newborn.
3. guidance with holding the newborn.
4. information regarding cord care.

6 A nurse is reviewing prenatal records in the clinic. Which of the pregnant clients are most at risk for conceiving a newborn with a chromosomal abnormality? Select all that apply.

1. A 36-year-old woman pregnant for the first time.
2. A client expecting twins.
3. A woman who smokes during pregnancy.
4. A 15-year-old girl.
5. A woman who has a child with Down syndrome.
6. A woman lacking folic acid in her diet.

7 A client who is 12 weeks pregnant says she hasn't felt the baby move yet. Which of the following statements by the nurse is correct about fetal movement?

1. "Fetal movement can be felt between 16 and 20 weeks."
2. "You should be able to feel the baby kick by now."
3. "Keeping a full bladder will help you feel the baby."
4. "It is too early for the limbs to move freely."

8 A 12-week pregnant client asked how to reduce the risk of spina bifida during pregnancy. The nurse instructs the client to increase which of the following foods during pregnancy?

1. dried fruits
2. fresh seafood
3. brown rice
4. green leafy vegetables

9 The nurse is teaching a class to pregnant women about healthy lifestyles. Which statement made by one of the pregnant women requires further teaching?

1. "The placenta will not prevent all medications from entering the fetal blood circulation."
2. "Over-the-counter medications are better to take during pregnancy than prescription medications."
3. "It is important to increase the amount of folic acid in the diet."
4. "It is a good idea to exercise 3 times a week."

10 A nurse is teaching a class about genetic disorders. Which statement by the nurse best explains how a child can be a carrier of a genetic disorder?

1. The child receives one dominant gene and one recessive gene.
2. The child receives an extra chromosome.
3. The child receives recessive genes from both parents.
4. The child is missing part of a chromosome.

Answers for NCLEX-PN® Review and Critical Thinking questions appear in Appendix I.

Chapter 9

Prenatal Fetal Assessment

BRIEF Outline

General Assessment
Diagnostic Tests of Fetal Status
Signs of Fetal Distress

Medical Care
Nursing Care

LEARNING Outcomes

After completing this chapter, you will be able to:
1. Define key terms.
2. Discuss common techniques used to assess fetal well-being.
3. Provide teaching and support of the pregnant woman undergoing tests to assess fetal well-being.
4. Discuss signs of fetal distress.
5. Discuss nursing care of the mother when the fetus is distressed.

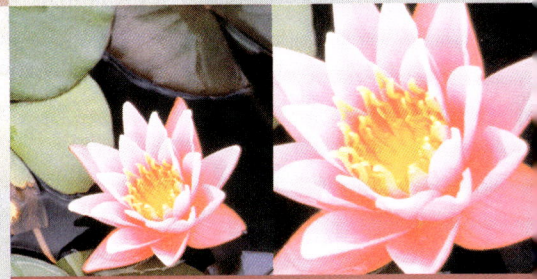

NURSING CARE PLAN CHART:
Planning for Client with Hydatidiform Mole

HEALTH PROMOTION ISSUE:
Fetal Surgery

NURSING PROCESS CARE PLAN:
Woman Undergoing Chorionic Villus Sampling

CRITICAL THINKING CARE MAP:
Caring for a Pregnant Woman Undergoing NST

During pregnancy, health care providers are responsible for the care of two clients, the mother and the developing fetus. Collecting subjective and objective data from the mother is a relatively simple process. However, assessing the well-being of the fetus is more complex because the examiner is unable to see the fetus. This chapter will discuss fetal assessment techniques, common tests, and the role of the LPN/LVN in data collection.

General Assessment

Fetal assessment begins by questioning the mother regarding her health. If the mother is feeling well, there is a greater possibility the fetus is well. For example, if the mother experiences vomiting and becomes dehydrated, the fetus may become dehydrated, too. Assessment of maternal well-being is discussed in Chapter 10 ⬭.

The mother should be able to feel fetal movements (quickening) at 18 to 20 weeks gestation (see Chapter 10 ⬭). After that point, the mother should be questioned about fetal activity. A healthy fetus may sleep for 20 to 30 minutes and then become active for some time. As the fetus grows, muscle strength increases and fetal movements become stronger. Several methods of keeping track of fetal movement have been developed. They all focus on having the mother count the number of fetal movements over a short time period and recording the data. The woman should count for 20 to 30 minutes, at the same time every day, usually 1 hour after a meal. Lying on her side, she should record every fetal movement during the desired time period. If there are fewer than 3 movements in 30 minutes she should continue to count for 1 hour or more until 10 fetal movements are recorded. She should contact the primary care provider if:

- there are fewer than 10 movements in 3 hours.
- it takes longer each day to record 10 movements.
- fetal movements are absent.

She should bring the fetal movement record with her to each clinic visit so the primary care provider can review the data.

MANUAL READING OF THE FETAL HEART RATE

The fetal heart rate (FHR) can be heard by a Doppler (an instrument that uses ultrasound to magnify sound) at 10 to 12 weeks gestation. A **fetoscope** (an older assessment tool similar to a stethoscope) can be used to obtain the FHR by 14 to 16 weeks. The nurse may perform manual FHR monitoring at most prenatal visits. The normal fetal heart rate is 120 to 150 beats per minute. If complications develop, continuous electronic monitoring of the FHR may be required.

clinical ALERT

If the FHR is less than 100 or greater than 160 the charge nurse and primary care provider should be notified immediately.

Procedure 9-1 ■ provides steps in obtaining a manual FHR.

PROCEDURE 9-1

Assessing the Fetal Heart Rate with Doppler

Purpose

- To provide information about the status of the fetus
- To monitor the status of the fetus

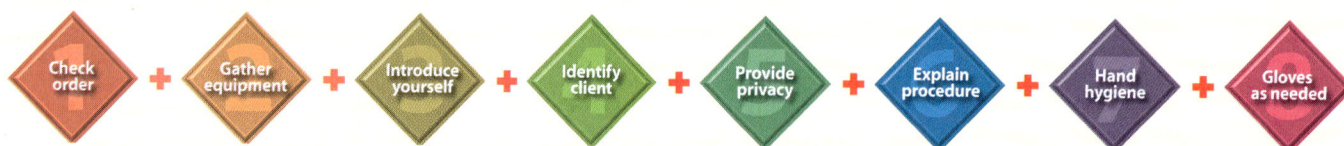

Equipment

- Doppler device
- Ultrasonic gel

Check order + Gather equipment + Introduce yourself + Identify client + Provide privacy + Explain procedure + Hand hygiene + Gloves as needed

Interventions and Rationales

1. Perform preparatory steps (see icon bar above).

2. Apply gel to the diaphragm of the Doppler. *Gel aids sound transmission and helps maintain contact between the Doppler diaphragm and the abdomen.*

3. Uncover the woman's abdomen. Position the diaphragm in the midline of the woman's abdomen halfway between the umbilicus and the symphysis pubis (Figure 9-1 ■). *This is the most likely position in which to hear the fetal heartbeat.*

4. When pulse is heard, check it against the woman's pulse. If they are the same, reposition the Doppler diaphragm. If the pulse is not heard, move the diaphragm laterally. *If the rates are the same, they are probably both the mother's pulse.*

5. If the rates are not the same, count the beats for 1 minute. Count each double rhythm as one beat. *The fetal heart sound has a double rhythm. The beats per minute are the FHR.*

6. Auscultate the FHR at each office visit during pregnancy. FHR is also assessed before, during, and for

Figure 9-1. ■ Ultrasound scanning permits visualization of the fetus *in-utero.* The woman may experience some discomfort as the probe moves over a full bladder.

30 seconds after a uterine contraction during labor. *This can provide information about fetal health or distress.*

7. Follow recommendations for frequency of auscultation and documentation. *The health and risk status of the woman will determine the usual frequency of auscultation.*
   a. FHR should be assessed at each office visit.
   b. FHR should be assessed anytime the mother accesses health care for any reason during the pregnancy.
   c. FHR should be assessed if the woman believes she is in labor. Fetal assessment during labor is discussed in Chapter 14 🔗.

SAMPLE DOCUMENTATION

(date) 0800 FHR 144. Mother reports increase in fetal activity over the past 2 weeks, especially after periods of maternal activity. Reassured that this is usual during the 6th month of pregnancy. K. Doss, LPN

Diagnostic Tests of Fetal Status

At times the mother develops symptoms of complications during the pregnancy. The primary care provider may order a variety of diagnostic tests to assess fetal well-being. The LPN/LVN may be required to assist with these diagnostic tests.

BLOOD TESTS

A blood sample is obtained from the mother between 15 and 22 weeks gestation to test for maternal serum alpha-fetoprotein (MSAFP), unconjugated estriol (UE), human chorionic gonadotropin (hCG), and inhibin-A. Sometimes only MSAFP is done, but more commonly the four tests can be done together (*quad marker screen*). The quad marker screen is gradually replacing the triple-marker screen, which omits inhibin-A.

Maternal serum alpha-fetoprotein or MSAFP is a blood marker that is elevated when the fetus has an open neural tube defect, anencephaly, omphalocele, or *gastroschisis* (a defect in the abdominal wall). It is also elevated in multiple gestations. Low MSAFP is associated with Down syndrome (Jenkins & Wapner, 2004). **Unconjugated estriol** (UE), **human chorionic gonadotropin** (hCG), and **inhibin-A** are blood markers that are used to determine the likelihood of Down syndrome. With Down syndrome, high levels of hCG and inhibin-A, and a low level of UE, are seen. Because the most common cause of abnormal results is inaccurate data, it is important that further testing be done. The mother will need encouragement and emotional support.

ULTRASOUND

Ultrasound is used to outline the shape and determine the consistency of various organs. High-frequency sound waves are transmitted through a transducer that is applied to the woman's abdomen or through a probe inserted into the vagina. The sound waves bounce off tissues within the woman's abdomen, showing structures of varying densities. Not only is ultrasound used to diagnose pregnancy, but it can also be used to determine the exact position (Figure 9-2 ■), size, and gender of the fetus and to identify some developmental anomalies. At times several ultrasound tests are done over time to assess the continual development of the fetus. Ultrasound can be used in conjunction with other diagnostic

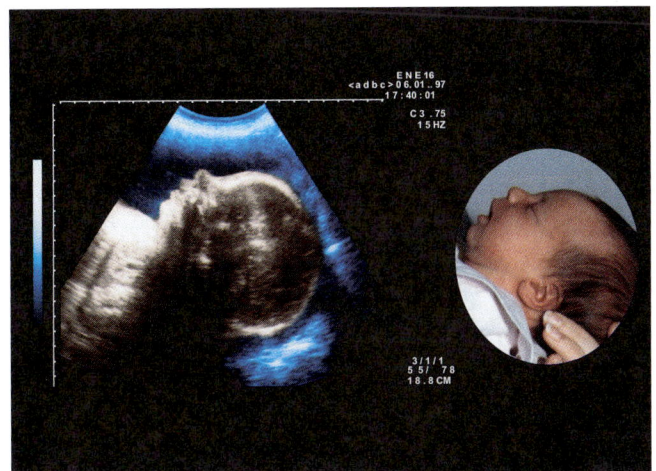

Figure 9-2. ■ This ultrasound study shows a fetal image at 20 weeks.

tests. The technology produces photolike pictures allowing the health care provider to visualize fetal structures and provide guidance during invasive procedures like amniocentesis and chorionic villus sampling.

Transabdominal Ultrasound

When the ultrasound is obtained through the abdomen **(transabdominal ultrasound)**, the woman is generally requested to have a full bladder. When the bladder is full, the lower uterine segment is supported in the upper pelvis and the cervix can be visualized. This is extremely important when the position of the placenta is questioned. The woman may be asked to drink 1 to 1.5 quarts of water 2 hours before the test and refrain from emptying the bladder until after the test is completed.

A generous amount of mineral oil or transducer gel is spread over the abdomen. The transducer is slowly rolled across the abdomen and the contents of the uterus are recorded. The woman may experience slight discomfort when the transducer is rolled across a full bladder. She may be uncomfortable lying on her back. The head of the bed can be elevated slightly. A small pillow or towel should be placed under the right hip to prevent the heavy uterus pressing on the vena cava. (See Chapter 10 ⚭.)

Transvaginal Ultrasound

When ultrasound is obtained through the vagina **(transvaginal ultrasound)**, a small probe is inserted into the vagina. The client is asked to assume the lithotomy or dorsal recumbent position with appropriate drapes. The small probe is covered with a condom, sterile sheath, or finger of a glove, and ultrasound gel is applied to the end and sides of the probe. The examiner inserts the probe into the upper area of the vagina. If the examiner is male, a female attendant should be in the room. At times, the client is asked to insert the probe and then the examiner moves the probe to obtain the required pictures.

When the transvaginal ultrasound is used, a full bladder is generally not required. Because the probe is inserted next to the cervix, the lower uterine segment does not need to be supported in the upper pelvis for adequate visualization of the cervix. There might be slight discomfort when the probe is moved in various directions to obtain the necessary images.

The LPN/LVN may be requested to prepare the woman for ultrasound by explaining the procedure. With additional training, the LPN/LVN may perform ultrasound testing, making the images available for the primary care provider. A description of nursing care for clients undergoing fetal assessment is given in the Nursing Care Plan Chart on this page.

NURSING CARE PLAN CHART

Planning for Client with Hydatidiform Mole

GOAL	INTERVENTION	RATIONALE	EXPECTED OUTCOME
1. Deficient Knowledge related to hydatidiform mole			
The client or couple will obtain information about hydatidiform mole and treatment options.	Provide written information on hydatidiform mole.	*Written information allows clients to review information at home. Verbal instruction meets the needs of auditory learners.*	Client or couple will state understanding of hydatidiform mole and explain their understanding of treatment options.
	Explain what a hydatidiform mole is, and the difference between complete and partial mole.	*Hydatidiform moles are tumorlike masses that occur due to abnormal overgrowth of placental tissue. Partial moles may develop when there are twins at conception and one placenta is abnormal. In general, partial moles may contain fetal tissue or be attached to a fetus. Complete moles do not contain fetal tissue.*	
	Explain signs and symptoms of a mole: Primary signs and symptoms include vaginal bleeding and absence of fetal heart tones. Dark vaginal discharge and hyperemesis, are associated with complete mole. Other signs include uterine enlargement, ovarian cysts, hyperthyroidism, and preeclampsia.	*Bleeding occurs as the result of the separation of tissues in the uterus (similar to abruption).*	
	Explain diagnostic test results indicating presence of a mole.	*Ultrasonography can often detect the presence of a mole before the onset of symptoms. Elevated serum human chorionic gonadotropin (hCG) may be indicative. Serum inhibin-A and activin-A levels are seven times higher in molar pregnancies.*	

GOAL	INTERVENTION	RATIONALE	EXPECTED OUTCOME
2. Readiness for Enhanced Family Coping			
The client or couple will make informed decision about mole treatment and future childbearing.	When test results are obtained, provide explanations and reinforce understanding. Provide written materials for the couple to read at home. Discuss age as a significant risk factor for developing hydatidiform mole. Explain that following a molar pregnancy, a woman is at increased risk for developing uterine cancer. When there is no live fetus attached to the mole, the mole may be removed via curettage or a hysterectomy may be performed. Reinforce teaching that it is extremely important for the woman to avoid pregnancy and keep follow-up appointments for a year following a procedure to remove hydatidiform mole.	*This is a stressful experience for the couple. They may be unable to absorb all the information at once and may need some information repeated.* *Teenagers and perimenopausal women are at increased risk, especially women over 40 years old. Nutritional deficiencies (such as carotene) are risk factors, too.* *Symptoms of hydatidiform mole are similar to a missed abortion.* *Emergency hysterectomy may be necessary to treat hemorrhage.* *Prophylactic hysterectomy may be preferred by women approaching menopause.* *Lab beta-hCG values, x-rays, and physical examination must be done to monitor for the possibility of cancer (choriocarcinoma) and/or metastases. If hCG values are within normal limits for a year after molar pregnancy, the women is likely to have a normal pregnancy with a low risk of recurrent hydatidiform mole.*	Client or couple will state understanding of the test results and will explain their understanding of the potential outcome of the current pregnancy and the impact it will have on future childbearing potential.
3. Anticipatory Grieving			
Couple will develop a plan for their life and family that includes new data.	Engage in therapeutic listening to allow each person to express feelings openly. Recommend that the client or couple include their primary spiritual care provider (rabbi, priest, minister, etc.) during decision making. Provide spiritual care. Offer emotional support to client or couple dealing with anticipated termination of pregnancy. Provide hope instillation to the client or couple with a partial mole attached to a live fetus. Provide referrals to local groups; provide information for researching more information online.	*The news that there is no fetus or that an existing pregnancy cannot proceed without danger can be devastating. The client or couple needs time to express and process feelings in order to be able to move ahead.* *To make rational decisions, the client or couple must have the opportunity to evaluate treatment options in light of their personal beliefs and values.* *Some religions prohibit the voluntary termination of a viable pregnancy as well as elective surgeries that result in infertility. Pastoral care following diagnosis and during the decision-making process is essential to treat spiritual distress and/or to prevent spiritual crisis.* *Clergy are equipped to assist the client or couple in reaching a treatment decision that is in the best interests of the family and in keeping with their own faith tradition. Clients who choose to continue a difficult pregnancy need hope and emotional support.* *Support groups can be of help no matter what the couple decides. Pro-active fact-seeking is an activity than can reduce anxiety and feelings of powerlessness.*	Client or couple will recognize the grief they feel at the loss of "the ideal child." They will reach a decision regarding the outcome of the current pregnancy and regarding future childbearing.

Figure 9-3. ■ Amniocentesis is an invasive test often performed between weeks 15 and 18. It is used as a test for genetic abnormalities, maternal–fetal incompatibilities, and maturity of fetal lungs.

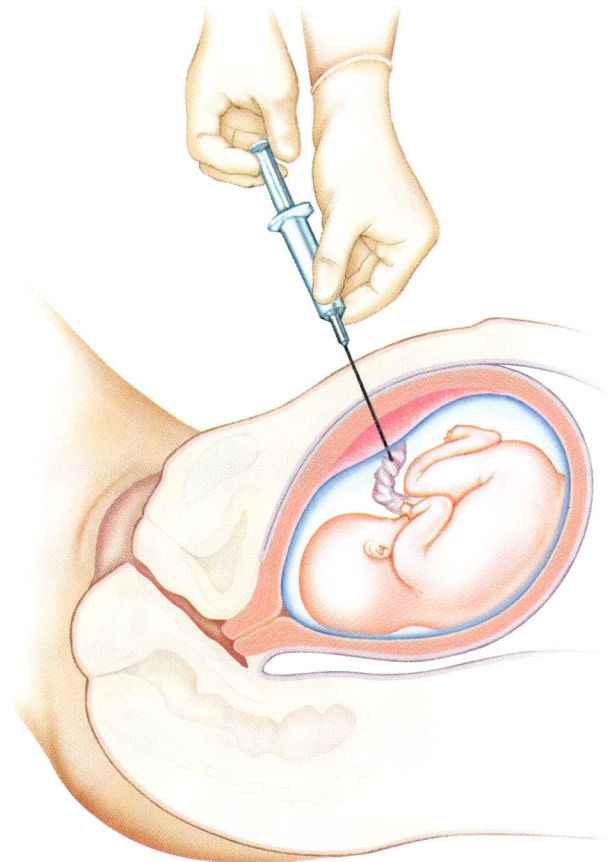

Figure 9-4. ■ Umbilical cord blood sampling is performed in the second or third trimester to diagnose inherited blood disorders or fetal infection, and to determine acid–base balance.

AMNIOTIC FLUID ANALYSIS

Amniotic fluid may be obtained for chemical analysis and chromosome analysis of fetal cells. Amniotic fluid is obtained by **amniocentesis** (Figure 9-3 ■), the withdrawal of amniotic fluid through a needle inserted into the abdomen and the uterus. The amniotic fluid and fetal cells contained in the fluid are studied to determine genetic abnormalities, maternal–fetal blood incompatibilities, and the maturity of the fetal lungs. Amniocentesis is usually performed between 15 to 18 weeks gestation to determine normal fetal development, but it may be done later in the pregnancy to determine lung maturity. It is common for amniocentesis to be repeated several times in a high-risk pregnancy.

Procedure 9-2 ■ describes the nurse's role in assisting with amniocentesis and similar tests.

PERCUTANEOUS UMBILICAL CORD SAMPLING

Similar to amniocentesis, **percutaneous umbilical cord sampling** (Figure 9-4 ■) is the removal of umbilical cord blood through a needle inserted into the uterus. It is done in the second and third trimesters when the umbilical cord is large enough to accommodate a needle. The physician locates the fetal parts, and identifies the placenta and umbilical cord by ultrasound. A needle is then inserted through the maternal abdomen into an umbilical vessel in the umbilical cord, approximately 1 to 2 inches (2.5–5 cm) from the placenta. Fetal blood is aspirated and analyzed for chemical content. The test is useful in diagnosing inherited blood disorders, detecting fetal infection, and determining acid–base balance. It is used for diagnosing **erythroblastosis fetalis** (a serious anemia, usually resulting from maternal antibodies to Rh-positive fetal blood), as well as *thrombocytopenia* (a lack of platelets in circulating blood). If necessary, a blood transfusion can be completed. (Rh incompatibility is discussed in Chapter 13 ⬭.)

CHORIONIC VILLUS SAMPLING

Chorionic villus sampling, obtaining a small piece of the chorionic villus from the placenta, can be done by

Assisting with Amniocentesis, Umbilical Cord Sampling, or Chorionic Villus Sampling

Purpose

- To provide information about the genetic makeup of the fetus
- To provide information about the status of the fetus

Equipment

- Ultrasound equipment
- Ultrasonic gel

- Amniocentesis kit containing skin prep (Betadine), sterile drapes, 22-gauge spinal needle with stylet, and amber-colored test tubes. If a kit is not available, the nurse must assemble the supplies from stock. *Amniotic fluid must be protected from light. If amber-colored test tubes are not available, place tape over the test tube to protect the specimen.*
- Sterile gloves
- Local anesthetic (1% lidocaine)

Check order + Gather equipment + Introduce yourself + Identify client + Provide privacy + Explain procedure + Hand hygiene + Gloves as needed

Interventions and Rationales

1. Perform preparatory steps (see icon bar above).

2. Ensure that a signed informed consent form is in the chart. If not, inform the care provider. *This procedure requires an informed consent signature.*

3. Obtain the mother's vital signs and the FHR. Monitor maternal vital signs and FHR every 15 minutes during the procedure, and for a minimum of 30 minutes after the procedure. *The first vital signs and FHR readings provide a baseline. Later readings give information about the status of the mother and the fetus. Changes can signal complications.*

4. Position the woman on her back, with a wedge placed under her right hip to displace the weight to the left side. External fetal monitor may be used during the exam to monitor the fetus. *This position will promote better blood flow and prevent supine hypotension.*

5. The physician uses ultrasound to locate the placenta and fetus. Provide ultrasound gel and assist as needed. *Gel creates a seal between the monitor and the woman's skin and improves the quality of the ultrasound reading.*

6. The physician dons sterile gloves and cleanses the woman's abdomen. *Cleansing the abdomen prior to needle insertion helps prevent infection.*

7. The physician applies sterile drapes, then inserts the needle into the uterus and withdraws a sample of amniotic fluid, umbilical cord blood, or chorionic villi. *Note: If a sample of the placenta is obtained*

for chorionic villus sampling or blood is obtained from an umbilical vessel, other specimen containers may be needed. The nurse may be required to assist with continuous ultrasound monitoring. *Sterile technique is essential to prevent infection of the mother and fetus.*

8. Obtain specimen containers from physician, attach proper labels, and send to lab with appropriate lab slips. *It is the nurse's responsibility to be sure materials are labeled properly. Prompt delivery to the lab helps ensure accurate results.*

9. Assist physician to apply a small dressing over puncture site.

10. Monitor the woman and fetus for 30 minutes, paying close attention to the mother's vital signs, FHR, and any contractions she may be having. *Changes from normal may indicate complications that would need to be reported.*

11. Assess the woman's blood type and determine if Rh immune globulin (RhoGAM) is needed and administer if necessary (see Chapter 10 🔗). *To prevent Rh sensitization of an Rh-negative woman during the procedure, Rh immune globulin is administered.*

12. Instruct the woman to report any of the following changes immediately to her primary care provider:
    a. Unusual increase in fetal activity or lack of fetal movement

b. Vaginal discharge, either clear fluid or bloody drainage
c. Uterine contractions or abdominal cramping
d. Fever or chills

These are signs of complications that will require further medical investigation and treatment.

13. Encourage the woman to engage in only light activity for 24 hours and to increase her fluid intake. *Light activity will decrease uterine irritability. Fluid is needed to replace the amniotic fluid.*

14. Complete the client record. *Full documentation includes date and time, vital signs, type of procedure, name of provider who performed the procedure, number of specimens obtained and disposition of specimens, repeat VS and client status, record of discharge teaching, and follow-up care.*

SAMPLE DOCUMENTATION

(date) 0800 T 98.2, P 82, R 24, BP 136/72, FHR 150. No uterine contractions noted at this time. Dr. Lopez here. Amniocentesis completed without incident. 3 specimens sent to lab.
0830. Vital signs have remained stable since amniocentesis. P. 78, R. 22, BP 130/70, FHR 144-150. No contractions noted on monitor. Written instructions provided and reviewed regarding home care, activity, and warning signs to report to the physician. Instructed to return to clinic in 1 week for follow-up. J. Sole, LPN

amniocentesis or through the vagina and cervix (Figure 9-5 ■). Using ultrasound to locate the baby, a needle is inserted through the mother's abdomen into the uterus and the placenta. If the placenta is located on the posterior surface of the uterus, a transvaginal approach may be used. A sample of placental tissue is aspirated through the needle. The tissue, formed from the zygote, reflects the genetic makeup of the fetus. The procedure, done between the 10th and 12th weeks of gestation, identifies chromosomal anomalies early in the pregnancy. The parents can then make an informed decision regarding the welfare of the baby or possible termination of the pregnancy.

RISKS OF INVASIVE TESTING
Amniocentesis, chorionic villus sampling, and percutaneous umbilical blood sampling carry some risk to the mother and infant. Complications could include premature rupture of the fetal membranes, placental detachment, hemorrhage (for both mother and infant), and infection. The mother and fetus are monitored closely for an hour or more after the procedure. Follow-up ultrasound may be used to ensure that bleeding or hematoma formation has not occurred. If complications do arise, all efforts will be made to protect both mother and infant. However, in the case of fetal hemorrhage, death may not be preventable.

Nursing Considerations
Parents need emotional support when an amniocentesis or other invasive tests are performed. They will be concerned not only about the welfare of the infant during the test, but also about the possibility of a life-altering diagnosis such as Down syndrome. Test results may not be obtained

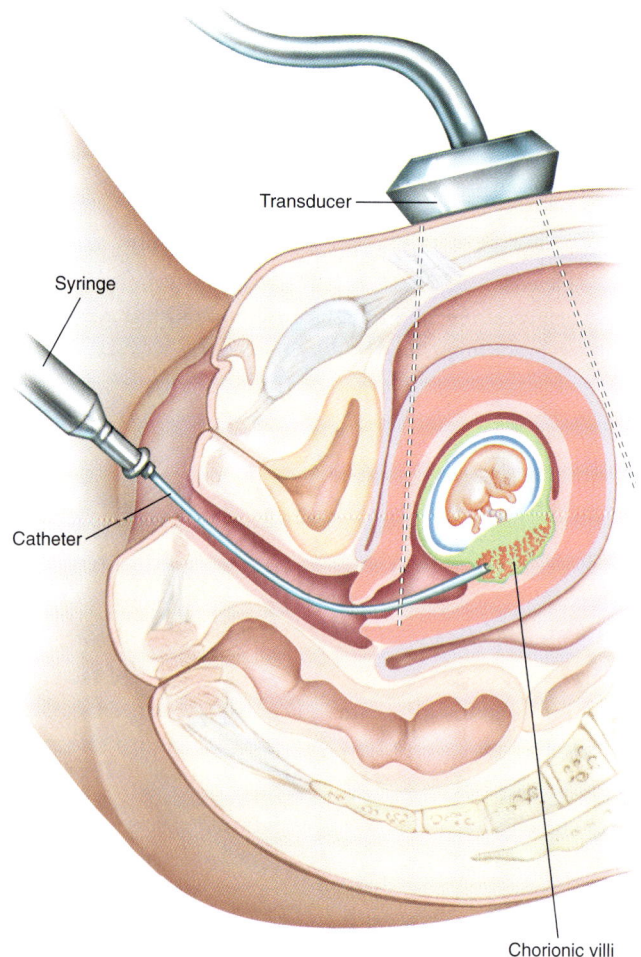

Figure 9-5. ■ Chorionic villus sampling, done between weeks 10 and 12 of gestation, uses a piece of placental tissue for early identification of chromosomal anomalies.

for several days or weeks, and the period of waiting may seem unbearable. If a life-altering diagnosis is made, the parents may decide to keep the pregnancy and accept responsibility for a sick infant, or they may decide to terminate the pregnancy. Either decision brings tremendous emotional strain requiring support, understanding, and nonjudgmental care.

NONSTRESS TEST

A **nonstress test** (NST) is used to assess fetal movement and fetal heart rate.

When the fetus has adequate oxygen and an intact central nervous system, the fetal heart rate increases with activity. The NST is quick, inexpensive, and easy to perform in the office or clinic. In a high-risk pregnancy, NST is generally performed at 30 to 32 weeks and repeated

frequently until delivery. The LPN/LVN may perform the NST but is generally not able to interpret the findings.

The woman is positioned in a recliner or bed in semi-Fowler's position or side-lying position. External fetal monitoring equipment (see Procedure 9-3 ■) is used to provide written documentation of the FHR and fetal movement. Two belts are applied to the client's abdomen, one to hold the device for monitoring uterine and fetal movement and the other to hold the device to monitor the FHR. The client identifies episodes of fetal movement. If the fetus is not active, fetal movement can be stimulated with a low-frequency vibrator (Figure 9-6 ■). Each episode consists of a FHR increase of 15 bpm, lasting 15 seconds. The test is reactive or normal if two episodes occur in a 20-minute period. If decelerations are noted, the primary care provider should be contacted.

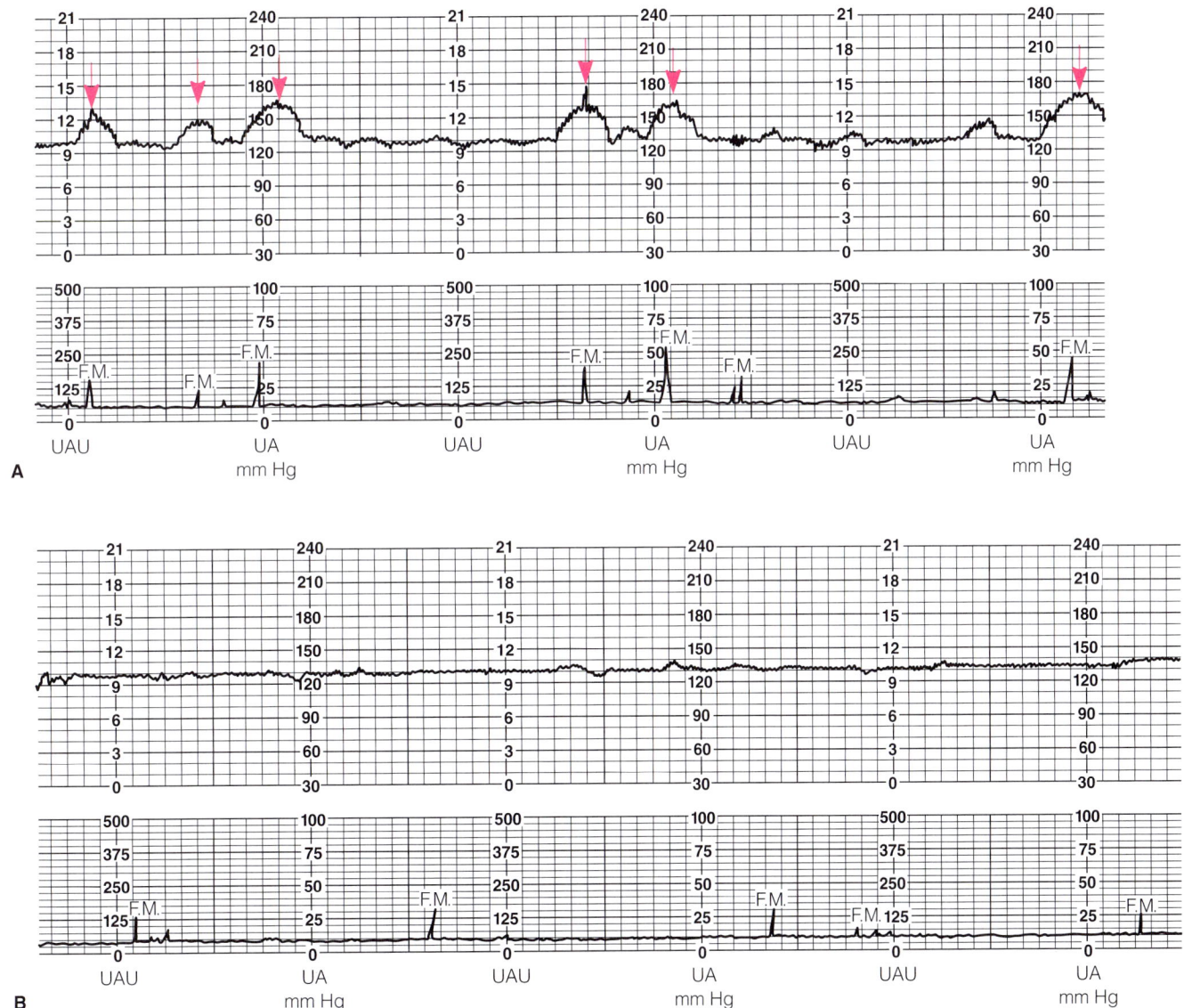

Figure 9-6. ■ (A) Normal findings of a reactive nonstress test (NST). (B) Examples of a nonreactive NST.

External Electronic Fetal Heart Rate Monitoring

Purpose

■ To obtain a continuous reading on the status of the fetus prior to delivery

Equipment

■ Electronic fetal monitor
■ Elastic monitor belts (2)
■ Tocodynamometer, also called a "toco"
■ Ultrasound transducer
■ Ultrasound gel

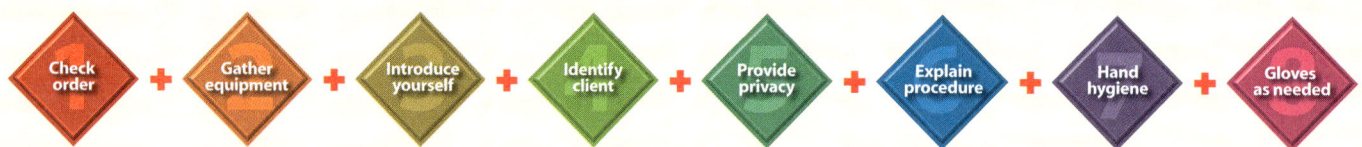

Interventions and Rationales

1. Perform preparatory steps (see icon bar above).

2. With the monitor turned on, place the two monitor belts around the woman's abdomen (Figure 9-7 ■).

3. Palpate the area off midline and over the uterine fundus that is most firm during contractions. Place the "toco" in this area, and secure it with one elastic belt. *Because the fundus is the area where contractions are greatest, this placement will provide the best graph of uterine contractions.*

4. Adjust the tracing so it shows 10 or 15 mm Hg between contractions. *Adjustment to this level prevents background static.*

5. Apply gel to the diaphragm of the transducer, and place the diaphragm on the mother's abdomen halfway between the symphysis pubis and the umbilicus. *The gel seals contact between the diaphragm and the maternal abdomen to produce the best quality sound. The midline of the mother's abdomen is most often closest to the fetal heart. When the uterus contracts, pressure is exerted against the "toco" and information is relayed to the electronic fetal monitor and recorded on graph paper.*

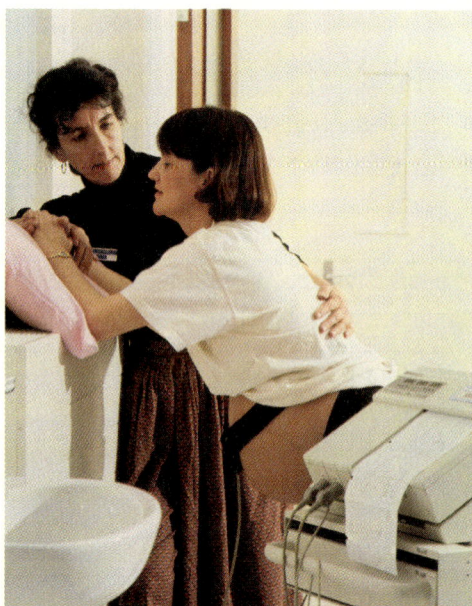

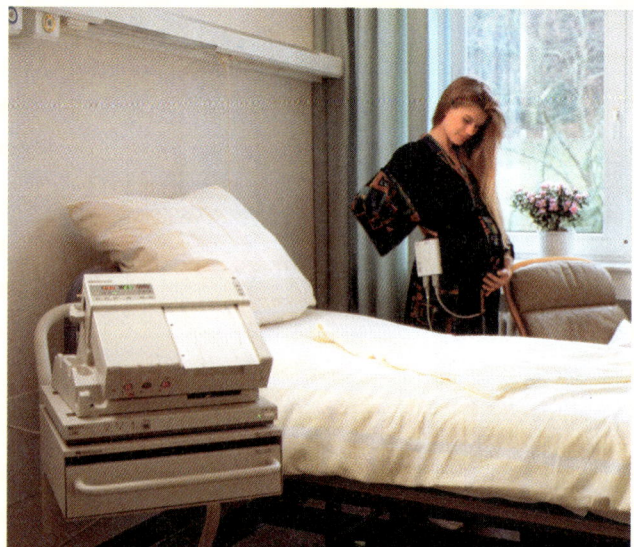

A   **B**

Figure 9-7. ■ **(A)** External electronic fetal monitoring device showing graph readout. **(B)** Beltless tocodynamometer system features remote telemetry that allows the laboring woman more mobility.

6. Move the diaphragm laterally or vertically until the strongest heart sound is heard. (If the fetus is breech, the heart sound will be above the umbilicus.) Attach the second elastic belt snugly to the transducer at this point. *Note*: If a beltless monitor is available (Figure 9-7B), follow specific directions for attaching it. *When the diaphragm directs the ultrasonic beam toward the fetal heart, the whiplike sound of the heartbeat will be heard. Moving the transducer laterally helps determine the position that is most directly over the fetal heart. The belt keeps the transducer in position. A beltless FHR monitor allows the mother to move around the room.*

7. At the beginning of the fetal monitor tape, record the following information: date, time, woman's name, gravida, para, membrane status, and name of the care provider (physician or certified nurse midwife). Follow facility guidelines. *Documentation is a continuous part of quality care. Individual facilities may require additional information to be recorded on the tape.*

8. Follow facility policy about ongoing documentation of information gathered by electronic FHR monitoring, as well as documentation of procedures performed, changes in position, any therapy that might be initiated, etc. The LPN/LVN is not responsible for interpretation of findings but must report unusual findings as directed. *The baseline rate in bpm, plus acceleration and decelerations of FHR in response to maternal contractions, are some of the data that will be recorded. Data either can be reassuring or can provide an early warning of possible complications. Prompt reporting of designated information allows therapeutic intervention. Documentation according to facility policy provides for safe practice and quality care.*

SAMPLE DOCUMENTATION

(date/time)   External fetal monitor applied, FHR 140 bpm, "C" q4m, lasting 45 sec, mod intensity. _____
Margaret Messenger, LPN

BIOPHYSICAL PROFILE

Biophysical profile is a test that assesses five variables:

- Fetal breathing
- Fetal movement
- Fetal tone
- Amniotic fluid volume
- Fetal reaction

To complete a biophysical profile, a combination of ultrasound and NST are used. The LPN/LVN is sometimes taught to collect the data; the trained registered nurse, certified nurse midwife, or physician interprets the data. A score of 8 or more indicates positive fetal well-being.

LEOPOLD'S MANEUVERS

Leopold's maneuvers are performed to determine the position and presentation of the fetus. Procedure 9-4 ■ describes Leopold's maneuvers.

Signs of Fetal Distress

Because the fetus cannot be seen or monitored all the time, signs of fetal distress during the pregnancy often go unnoticed. This is especially true if the fetus is distressed for a short period of time. At times, the mother will feel that "something is wrong" even though she may not be able identify what specifically is different. The mother may notice a decrease or absence of fetal movement. In either case, the mother should be encouraged to be evaluated by the primary health care provider.

When the mother is being monitored inside a health care facility, nonreassuring fetal status may be identified. Nonreassuring fetal status results from lack of oxygen to the fetus that may be temporary or chronic. The most common causes are umbilical cord compression or placental complications. Signs of fetal distress include decreased fetal movement and decreased fetal heart rate. It is critical that the LPN/LVN report decreased fetal heart rate to the supervising RN or primary health care provider immediately. The woman should be positioned on her left side and oxygen applied. If medication is being administered, the rate may need to be adjusted.

Medical Care

Once the primary care provider has evaluated the conditions of mother and fetus, diagnoses of any complications can be made. Medical treatment might include medication, bed rest with frequent monitoring, induction of labor, or cesarean birth. If fetal malformation has occurred, decisions must be made to keep or terminate the pregnancy. In recent years, a few surgeons across the country have been performing corrective surgery on the fetus while it is still in the uterus. Although surgery in the womb is still in beginning stages, early results appear promising. The Health Promotion Issue on page 198 provides more information about fetal surgery.

PROCEDURE 9-4	**Performing Leopold's Maneuvers**

Purpose

■ To determine fetal position and presentation for fetal monitoring or other reasons

Equipment

■ Gloves (optional)

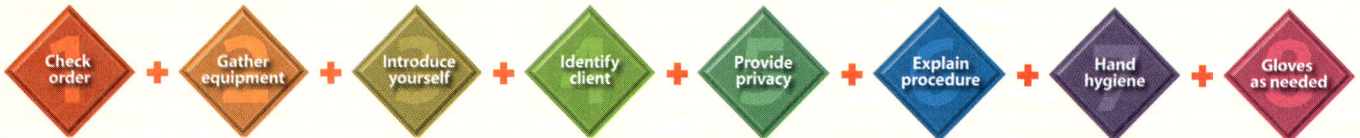

Check order + Gather equipment + Introduce yourself + Identify client + Provide privacy + Explain procedure + Hand hygiene + Gloves as needed

Interventions and Rationales

1. Perform preparatory steps (see icon bar above).

2. The first maneuver (Figure 9-8A ■) is to palpate the fundus with two hands, feeling for the fetus's body parts. *The fetal head is firm and round, and it moves independently of the body. The buttocks are softer and round with small bony prominences; they move with the trunk.*

3. The second maneuver (Figure 9-8B) is to find the fetal back and determine if it is to the right or left side of the mother's abdomen. Using the palms, the nurse uses firm but gentle pressure to explore one side of the abdomen and then the other. Supporting the uterus with one hand, the other hand feels for the fetal limbs and back. *The back should feel firm and smooth and connected to the part found in the fundus. The limbs will feel hard and have bony projections.*

4. The third maneuver (Figure 9-8C) is to determine the fetal part lying in the pelvic inlet by grasping the abdomen just above the symphysis pubis with the thumb and forefingers. *Findings should be opposite those found in the fundus. If the presenting part is the head and it is not yet engaged, it will be able to be moved back and forth.*

5. The fourth maneuver (Figure 9-8D) is to locate a prominence on the fetal head (usually the brow). Using the fingers, the nurse gently palpates down the sides of the uterus toward the pubis. *The brow should be located on the opposite side from the fetal back. If the fetal head is*

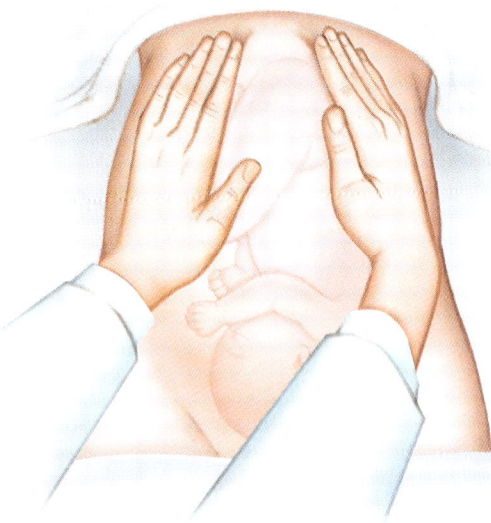

A

B

Figure 9-8. ■ Performing Leopold's maneuvers to determine fetal lie. (**A**) First maneuver. (**B**) Second maneuver. (**C**) Third maneuver. (**D**) Fourth maneuver. (Reproduced, with permission, from McGraw-Hill Companies, Inc. Cunningham, F. G., et al. [eds.]. [1997]. *Williams obstetrics* [20th ed.]. Stamford, CT: Appleton & Lange, p. 258.)

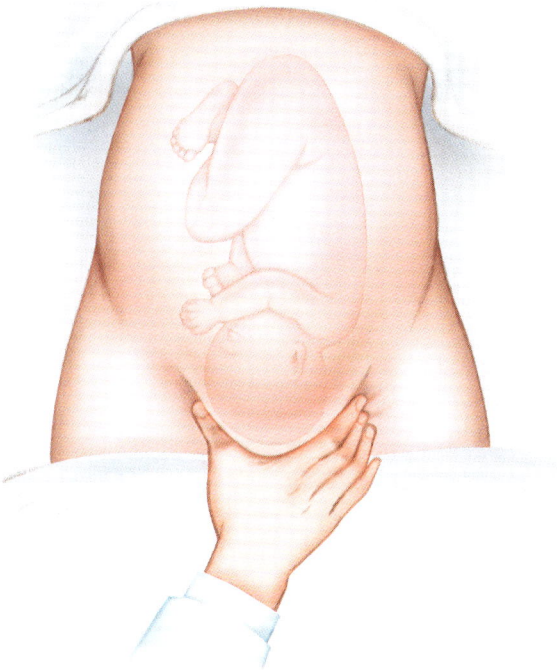

C

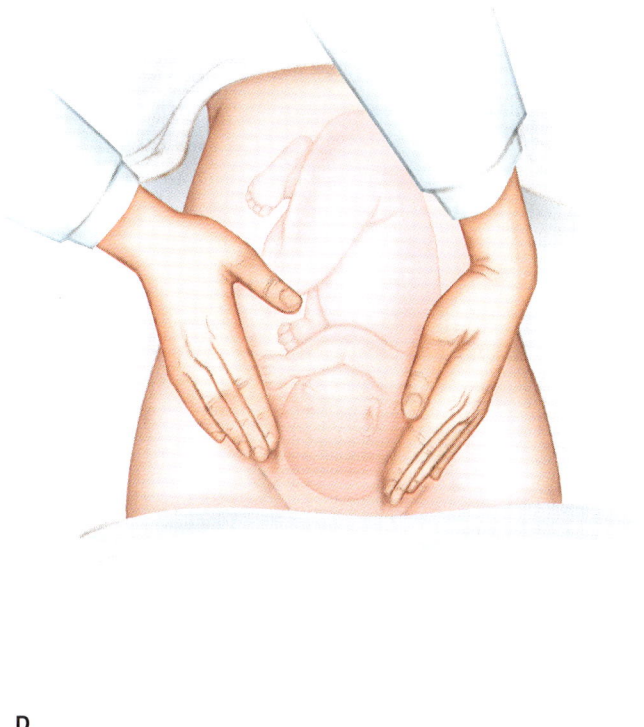

D

Figure 9-8. ■ *Continued.*

extended, the fetal occiput will be felt on the same side as the back (see Figure 14-11 ⦾).

clinical ALERT

Some nurses perform the fourth maneuver first. They begin the maneuvers by identifying the fetal part located in the pelvic outlet.

SAMPLE DOCUMENTATION

(date, time)   Leopold's maneuvers.
Presentation LOA. Client "eager
to hear heartbeat." _____
J. Roe, LVN

NURSING CARE

PRIORITIES IN NURSING CARE

The priorities for caring for women undergoing fetal assessment are to provide information as needed and to ensure that equipment and supplies are available and in good order for procedures. It is important to maintain a calm and professional manner because tests, especially invasive ones, may cause anxiety in the client.

ASSESSING

The role of the LPN/LVN in fetal assessment is mostly supportive. LPNs/LVNs take vital signs of the mother and compare them to baseline. They check fetal heart rate by external monitoring. They ask about the client's subjective status and document these findings. They report any measurement or subjective symptoms described by the client that are outside the normal range.

DIAGNOSING, PLANNING, AND IMPLEMENTING

Possible nursing diagnoses that might apply to clients who are undergoing fetal assessment would include the following:

- **A**nxiety related to lack of knowledge or concern about status of fetus
- Readiness for Enhanced **K**nowledge
- Risk for **I**njury related to invasive fetal testing
- Risk for **I**nfection related to invasive fetal testing

(Text continues on p. 199.)

FETAL SURGERY

A young married couple comes to the obstetrician's office for a follow-up visit after receiving information that blood tests indicate a neural tube defect in their 21-week fetus. The diagnosis of spina bifida is confirmed by ultrasound. The obstetrician explains that spina bifida is a defect in the protective bone and skin that covers the spinal cord. In severe forms, spina bifida results in leg paralysis and chronic hydrocephaly, a persistent buildup of cerebrospinal fluid that can cause mental delays and death. The shocked couple wants to know what can be done for their baby before it is born.

DISCUSSION

Once a diagnosis of spina bifida meant life-long disability. Besides leg paralysis, the children often had no control of their bowel or bladder, were wheelchair bound and prone to skin breakdown. Surgical repair of the spinal defect resulted in an accumulation of spinal fluid in their brain. As cranial pressure increased, the brain tissue was damaged resulting in mental delays.

Doctors in three U.S. hospitals (Children's Hospital of Philadelphia, Vanderbilt University Medical Center in Nashville, and the University of California at San Francisco) believed that surgical repair of spina bifida during early pregnancy might allow fetal limb and neurologic function to develop normally. Since the late 1990s these doctors have been operating before birth on such fetuses.

Fetal surgery is still in an experimental stage. At first, fetal surgery was undertaken only to correct defects that otherwise would kill the infant. Today, fetal surgeons are attempting to correct defects and enhance life. With the use of modern technology, surgery is being performed through laparoscopes, as well as open procedures. Although not all procedures are successful, many children are reaching developmental milestones on time or only slightly behind normal children.

These miracle cures are not without risk. A team of medical specialists opens the mother's uterus, repairs the defect on the fetus's back with a patch made from human skin, and closes the uterus. For women who receive the surgery, there is a risk of bleeding, infection, and fatal side effects from drugs used to control preterm labor. All infants who have had this surgery were born prematurely, which increased their risk of complications.

Fetal surgery may increase quality of life, but there are also ethical issues that need to be addressed. Is this the best use of resources? Each operation costs more than $35,000. Providing high-quality prenatal care and nutrition to all women in the United States may prevent many neural tube defects and be a better use of financial resources.

PLANNING AND IMPLEMENTATION

The nurse should provide emotional support for the couple. With the approval of the primary care provider, the nurse can provide written information about surgical options. Due to the limited facilities and surgical personnel who are performing fetal operations, the couple may need to travel great distances to obtain care. Travel and room and board add to the expenses.

At times, decisions need to be made rapidly with little time for the couple to adjust to the diagnosis. By helping the couple to write down the pros and cons of the proposed treatments, the couple may be able to make an informed, objective decision.

SELF-REFLECTION

What are your feelings about fetal surgery? If you were in a situation of having a baby with spina bifida, would you risk your life in an attempt to give the baby a higher quality of life? How would you feel if a couple decides not to have the surgery?

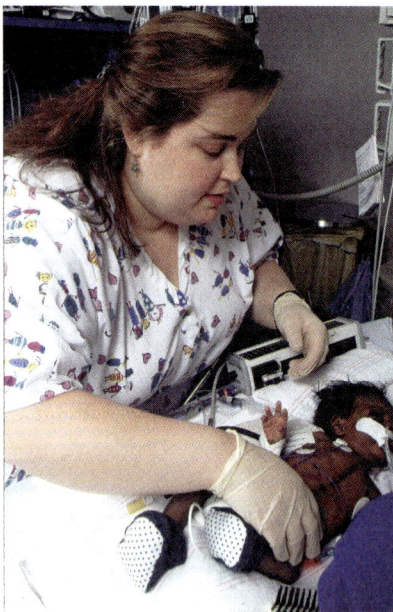

SUGGESTED RESOURCE

Chervenak, F., & McCullough, L. B. (2002). Comprehensive ethical framework for fetal research & its application to fetal surgery for spina bifida. *American Journal of Obstetrics and Gynecology, 187* (1), 10–14.

Possible outcomes for this client would be:

- Client will express reduced feelings of anxiety.
- Client will verbalize understanding of test.
- Client will maintain stable vital signs and fetus will maintain stable heart rate.

The following interventions would be part of nursing care for the client undergoing fetal assessment. The nurse working with pregnant women should anticipate the need to assist with fetal assessment. The LPN/LVN would:

- Keep equipment clean and ready to use. *Keeping the equipment clean and ready to use prevents spread of infection and facilitates efficiency in the office environment.*
- Ask if woman understands the reason for the test and the procedure that is about to occur. *By providing an opportunity for the client to ask questions, the nurse sets up a situation in which the client is the center of care, and any confusion or misunderstanding can be corrected. If the LPN/LVN does not know the answer to a specific question, he or she should say so and refer the question on or provide the answer at a later time.*
- For the normal pregnancy, obtain fetal heart rate with external monitor, document findings, and report any findings outside normal range. *The LPN/LVN may perform external fetal heart monitoring.*
- If ordered, the LPN/LVN may set up and attach the electronic fetal monitor. Before attaching the monitoring equipment, the nurse will need to assess for fetal position. *Correct placement of the monitor will provide a strong, clear recording of the FHR.*
- When amniocentesis, NST, and ultrasound are ordered, provide reassurance and emotional support. Frequently, the father or other family members are present during testing. *Anxiety is a normal response to testing. Both the woman and the support person may need support.*
- Monitor client's physical status during and after the testing and report any sudden changes to the health care provider. *Changes in client status or report by the mother of sudden fetal changes could signal a complication.*
- Monitor client's emotional status during the test. Encourage the client to practice some form of relaxation. *A sudden attack of anxiety may cause the mother to tense and may interfere with testing. It could also signal some physical change in the client or fetus.*
- Reinforce teaching about procedures (before and after care) and possible complications. *Clients may need reminders prior to fetal assessment tests. For example, if an ultrasound is planned for the next routine appointment, the client should be instructed to drink 1 to 1.5 quarts of water prior to coming to the office. Clients also need reinforcement of*

information for follow-up to the testing. For example, a client who has had an amniocentesis needs to be told to watch for signs of infection, and to call the office if she notices leaking vaginal fluid or a change in fetal activity.

- Provide follow-up care as directed. *Depending on the facility, the nurse may set follow-up appointments or provide information about test results.*

EVALUATING

The evaluation of the mother and fetus following assessment procedures must occur prior to the mother leaving the clinic or examination area. Maternal vital signs and fetal heart rate must return to normal baseline readings. The mother should verbalize understanding of any teaching, when to notify the primary care provider of signs of complications, and when to return for follow-up care.

NURSING PROCESS CARE PLAN
Woman Undergoing Chorionic Villus Sampling

Jackie, a 38-year-old mother of three sons, is 8 weeks pregnant. She is at the clinic for her first prenatal visit. Jackie states she is worried about possible genetic abnormalities in the fetus because of her age. There were no complications in her other pregnancies. A chorionic villus sampling is planned in 2 weeks. An ultrasound will be performed during the chorionic villus sampling to locate the placenta.

Assessment.   The following data were collected about this client:

- Age 38 years
- Eight weeks pregnant
- Gravida 4 Para 3
- No complications with previous pregnancies
- Worried about possible genetic abnormalities

Nursing Diagnosis.   The following important nursing diagnosis (among others) is established for this client:
- **A**nxiety related to possible genetic abnormalities in fetus and diagnostic test

Expected Outcomes
- Client verbalizes decreased anxiety, appears relaxed.

Planning and Implementation
- Provide written information regarding upcoming diagnostic test. *Written information allows clients to know what to expect during testing.*
- Encourage client to discuss fears and concerns. *Verbalization decreases anxiety.*

■ Encourage client to bring husband, family, or friend to be with her during testing. *Support from family and friends can help to decrease anxiety.*

Evaluation. Client verbalizes understanding of testing procedure and a decrease in anxiety. States she may be a bit anxious until the diagnosis is made, but states she feels more in control of her emotions.

Critical Thinking in the Nursing Process

1. What are some other topics that should be discussed with this client as she plans for a new baby at this time of her life?

2. What is the role of the LPN/LVN in providing emotional support?

3. If diagnostic testing reveals a genetic abnormality, how can the LPN/LVN locate resources for the client?

Note: Discussion of Critical Thinking questions appears in Appendix I.

Note: The reference and resource listings for this and all chapters have been compiled at the back of the book.

Chapter Review

🔊 KEY TERMS by Topic

Use the audio glossary feature of either the CD-ROM or the Companion Website to hear the correct pronunciation of the following key terms.

General Assessment
fetoscope

Diagnostic Tests of Fetal Status
maternal serum alpha-fetoprotein, unconjugated estriol, human chorionic gonadotropin, inhibin-A, ultrasound, transabdominal ultrasound, transvaginal ultrasound, amniocentesis, percutaneous umbilical cord sampling, erythroblastosis fetalis, chorionic villus sampling, nonstress test, biophysical profile

KEY Points

- The nurse must assess the fetus with each maternal contact.
- General fetal assessment, done at each clinic visit, includes fetal movement and fetal heart rate.
- The primary health care professional may request additional fetal testing and monitoring throughout the pregnancy.
- The role of the LPN/LVN is to assist with fetal testing.
- The nurse must teach the mother about fetal testing and how to assist as needed.
- The nurse should provide emotional support to the couple before, during, and after fetal testing.
- The nurse must accurately document all assessment data.

∞ FOR FURTHER Study

See Chapter 10 for information about the discomforts of and blood work in normal pregnancy.

Rh incompatibility and pregnancy-induced hypertension are discussed in Chapter 13.

See Chapter 14 for assessment during labor; Table 14-6 provides a timeline for collecting fetal and maternal data during labor.

Chapter 15 discusses use of fetal tests during labor.

🌐💿 EXPLORE MediaLink

Additional interactive resources for this chapter can be found on the Companion Website at www.prenhall.com/towle. Click on Chapter 9 and "Begin" to select the activities for this chapter.

For chapter-related NCLEX®-style questions and an audio glossary, access the accompanying CD-ROM in this book.

Animation
Leopold's Maneuvers

Critical Thinking Care Map

Caring for a Pregnant Woman Undergoing NST
NCLEX-PN® Focus Area: Physiologic Integrity

Case Study: Marsha is 35 weeks pregnant with her first baby. She has been experiencing an elevation of her blood pressure. She is retaining fluid and has positive protein in her urine. Her doctor has diagnosed pregnancy-induced hypertension and has ordered an NST to evaluate the fetus. (Pregnancy-induced hypertension is discussed in Chapter 13.) Marsha states, "I don't know anything about all this electronic equipment. Is it safe for the baby?" The LPN is to perform the NST in the office.

Nursing Diagnosis: Deficient Knowledge related to NST procedure

COLLECT DATA

Subjective	Objective
_____	_____
_____	_____
_____	_____
_____	_____
_____	_____
_____	_____

Would you report this? Yes/No

If yes, to: _____

Nursing Care

_____
_____
_____
_____
_____
_____
_____
_____
_____
_____

How would you document this? _____
_____
_____
_____

Compare your documentation to the sample provided in Appendix I.

Data Collected
(use only those that apply)

- Weight: 137 pounds (up 4 pounds since last month)
- BG 120
- States "I don't know anything about all this electronic equipment. Is it safe for the baby?"
- Blood pressure: 162/94
- Crying
- Urine positive for protein
- Edema in feet and hands
- Urine cloudy

Nursing Interventions
(use only those that apply; list in priority order)

- Instruct to record fetal movements during NST.
- Refer to WIC program.
- Teach about safety of electronic monitoring equipment.
- Provide written information about pregnancy-induced hypertension.
- Place in semi-Fowler's position.
- Schedule an appointment for 2 weeks.
- Provide information about support group.
- Apply belts and monitoring equipment.
- Teach about nutrition.
- Teach about FHR increasing with fetal movement.

1 The earliest the nurse will be able to hear the fetal heart tones by using a Doppler is by week number:

1. 2.
2. 6.
3. 10.
4. 20.

2 When assessing the fetal heart rate using the Doppler, the nurse finds it to be the same as the maternal heart rate. The nurse will:

1. count the rate again for 30 seconds.
2. reposition the Doppler.
3. call the physician.
4. document the rate in the client's chart.

3 The nurse has requested the client to return tomorrow for an ultrasound. Which of the following instructions is most appropriate prior to the ultrasound?

1. Do not eat prior to the ultrasound.
2. Empty your bladder right before the ultrasound.
3. Drink 1 quart of water 2 hours before the ultrasound.
4. Do not drink fluids prior to the ultrasound.

4 The LPN/LVN is preparing a client for an ultrasound. Which of the following nursing interventions are appropriate? Select all those that apply.

1. Raise the head of the bed slightly.
2. Begin intravenous infusion.
3. Place a towel under the right hip.
4. Position the client on her right side.
5. Insert a Foley catheter.
6. Position the client in the supine position.

5 Which of the following nursing interventions would the LPN/LVN be expected to implement following a chorionic villus sampling procedure?

1. Having the client remain on bed rest for 12 hours.
2. Monitoring the fetal heart rate for 30 minutes.
3. Decreasing the client's fluid intake for 4 hours.
4. Encouraging the client to resume normal activity.

6 A client expresses concern about having an amniocentesis. Which of the following statements by the nurse is most helpful?

1. "You should have read the information we gave you at your last visit."
2. "You may want to ask your husband to come with you."
3. "It is not healthy for you to worry."
4. "The amniocentesis is a very quick procedure."

7 The LPN/LVN is assisting with a nonstress test and asks the client if she understands the procedure. She knows that the client has a proper understanding of the procedure when the client says she will:

1. take slow deep breaths during the test.
2. remain flat on her back during the test.
3. avoid emptying her bladder.
4. identify any fetal movement.

8 A client is 6 weeks pregnant and has been scheduled for chorionic villus sampling. For this procedure, the LPN/LVN will schedule the client to return in:

1. 4 weeks.
2. 10 weeks.
3. 12 weeks.
4. 30 weeks.

9 Which of the following lab reports should be reported immediately to the nurse prior to obtaining a chorionic villus sampling?

1. Rh factor: Rh negative
2. Urine protein: negative
3. Blood glucose: 90 mg/dL
4. Hemoglobin: 14

10 The LPN/LVN will be assisting with a biophysical profile. Which of the following equipment should the LPN/LVN gather prior to the procedure? Select all those that apply.

1. amber-colored lab tubes
2. electronic fetal monitor
3. low-frequency vibrator
4. 1% lidocaine
5. ultrasonic gel
6. 2 × 2 gauze dressing and tape

Answers for NCLEX-PN® Review and Critical Thinking questions appear in Appendix I.

Chapter 10

Care During Normal Pregnancy

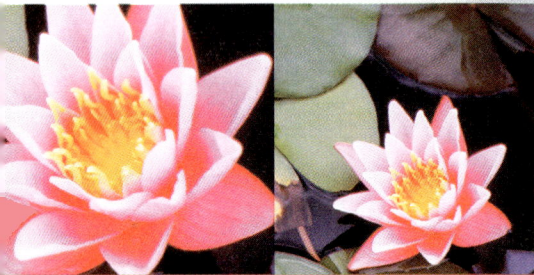

LEARNING Outcomes

After completing this chapter, you will be able to:

1. Define key terms.
2. Identify signs of pregnancy and maternal changes throughout pregnancy.
3. Discuss common maternal discomforts during pregnancy and their treatment.
4. Discuss prenatal care and client teaching related to prenatal care.

Pregnancy is a powerful and a complex time in a woman's life. She may be happily looking forward to the birth of a long-awaited first child. She may be wondering how to make adjustments for another of many children. She may be waiting fearfully through the period of pregnancy to give the baby up for adoption. In any case, she will face physical changes and processes that are unique and life-altering. The role of the nurse in caring for pregnant women involves a great deal of emotional support and client education.

PREGNANCY

Signs of Pregnancy

During pregnancy, many physiological changes will be reported by the mother or observed by the health care provider. These changes can be categorized as presumptive, probable, and positive signs of pregnancy.

PRESUMPTIVE SIGNS

The subjective signs the mother experiences during pregnancy are **presumptive signs.** They may be indicators of other conditions besides pregnancy, so are not diagnostic in nature. Presumptive signs include amenorrhea, nausea and vomiting, breast changes, urinary frequency, fatigue, abdominal enlargement, and quickening.

Amenorrhea

Amenorrhea, or the absence of menses, is usually the first sign a woman notices that may cause her to think she is pregnant. Although pregnancy is the most common cause of amenorrhea, other causes could be hormone imbalance, stress, menopause, or tumors.

Nausea and Vomiting

Nausea and vomiting usually occur in the morning, but could occur at any time. Sometimes called morning sickness, these symptoms are commonly experienced during early pregnancy. However, nausea and vomiting are also associated with many other conditions.

Breast Changes

Breast changes, such as tenderness, tingling, and enlargement of the breast, occur in early pregnancy. Many women also experience these changes with the monthly period.

Urinary Frequency

Urinary frequency occurs because the enlarging uterus presses on the bladder, giving the woman the feeling of needing to urinate often. Other disorders, including urinary infection and abdominal tumor, could also elicit this sensation.

Fatigue

Fatigue is most often noted in the first few months of pregnancy, but many other conditions result in fatigue as well.

Abdominal Enlargement

Abdominal enlargement is noted by the 12th week, but may be earlier in the very thin woman or later in the large woman. Abdominal enlargement may be noted when tumors are present.

Quickening

Quickening is a fluttering sensation felt as the fetus moves. The sensation begins between 16 and 20 weeks and gradually becomes stronger and more frequent. Other causes, such as muscle twitch or intestinal gas, can mimic this sensation. Because the mother is experiencing this subjective sensation, quickening is a presumptive sign.

Pregnancy is usually diagnosed before the woman experiences all of the presumptive signs. Denial of pregnancy could keep the woman from noticing the presumptive signs. False pregnancy, also known as **pseudopregnancy,** occurs when the nonpregnant woman so strongly wants to be pregnant that she experiences the presumptive signs. Treatment of pseudopregnancy is by psychiatric means.

PROBABLE SIGNS

The health care provider can identify objective signs that could indicate pregnancy. Because these signs could also indicate other conditions, they are not diagnostic. Probable signs include positive pregnancy tests, ballottement, and uterine changes.

Positive Pregnancy Test

Pregnancy tests screen for the presence of hCG in the urine or blood. Most home tests are based on the amount of hCG in the urine. A test may be positive 8 to 14 days after conception. Some medication, the timing and accuracy of specimen collection, and the presence of hormone-producing tumors can affect the accuracy of the test.

Ballottement

Ballottement is a test for pregnancy in which the examiner puts two fingers into the vagina and pushes upward on the uterus. If the woman is pregnant, the fetus will rebound against the fingers.

Uterine Changes

There are physical signs that can be checked to assess the probability of pregnancy (Figure 10-1 ■). **Hegar's sign** (a softening of the lower uterine segment), **Goodell's sign** (a softening of the cervix), and **Chadwick's sign** (a bluish purple discoloration of the cervix and vagina) can be observed in the first few weeks of pregnancy. The fundus of the uterus can be palpated just above the pubis at 12 weeks. Tumors can also cause uterine enlargement.

When probable signs are combined with presumptive signs, there is a strong indication of pregnancy.

POSITIVE SIGNS

Positive signs are diagnostic of pregnancy. No other condition can cause these signs. Positive signs of pregnancy include hearing fetal heart tones, visualization of the fetus, and fetal movement felt by an examiner.

Hearing Fetal Heart Tones

Fetal heart tones (FHT) or the fetal heartbeat, can be heard with a Doppler by 10 to 12 weeks. The normal fetal heart rate is 120 to 150 bpm. It is important to distinguish the FHR from the maternal heart rate. When auscultating the abdomen, a soft blowing sound can be heard. The sound occurring at the same rate as the maternal pulse is called **uterine soufflé** and is caused by increased maternal blood flow to the uterus. The sound occurring at the FHR is called **funic soufflé** and is caused by fetal blood flowing through the umbilical cord.

Visualization of the Fetus

An abdominal ultrasound can detect a pregnancy by the 6th week. A transvaginal ultrasound can detect a trophoblast by the 10th day after conception. X-ray examination of the pelvis is rarely done due to the risk of radiation exposure to the fetus and maternal reproductive organs.

Fetal Movement Felt by Examiner

The fetus usually does not kick strongly enough for the examiner to feel the movement until the 20th week.

Diagnostic tests to determine fetal status are discussed in Chapter 9 ⬤⬤.

Maternal Changes During Pregnancy

Typically, the progression of the pregnancy is described in 3-month blocks of time called **trimesters.** This might seem confusing when fetal development is described by weeks. A normal pregnancy takes three trimesters equaling 9 calendar months, or 40 weeks equaling 10 lunar months.

Pregnancy causes many changes in a woman's body and additional work in each body system that increases the need for oxygen (Figure 10-2 ■). A healthy woman's body can tolerate the additional work. However, if disease is present, the additional stress may be harmful or life threatening to the mother.

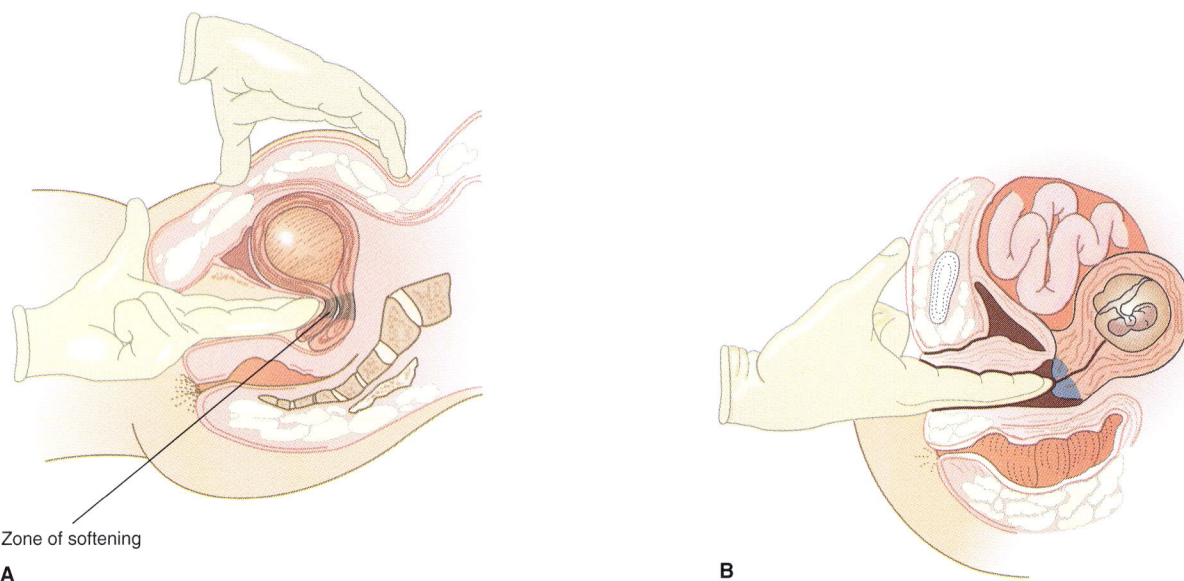

Zone of softening

A

B

Figure 10-1. ■ (**A**) Hegar's sign. (**B**) Goodell's sign and Chadwick's sign. (Reproduced, with permission, from McGraw Hill Companies, Inc. DeCherney, A.H., & Pernoll, M.L. [1994]. *Current obstetric and gynecologic diagnosis and treatment* [8th ed.]. Norwalk, CT: Appleton & Lange, p. 187.)

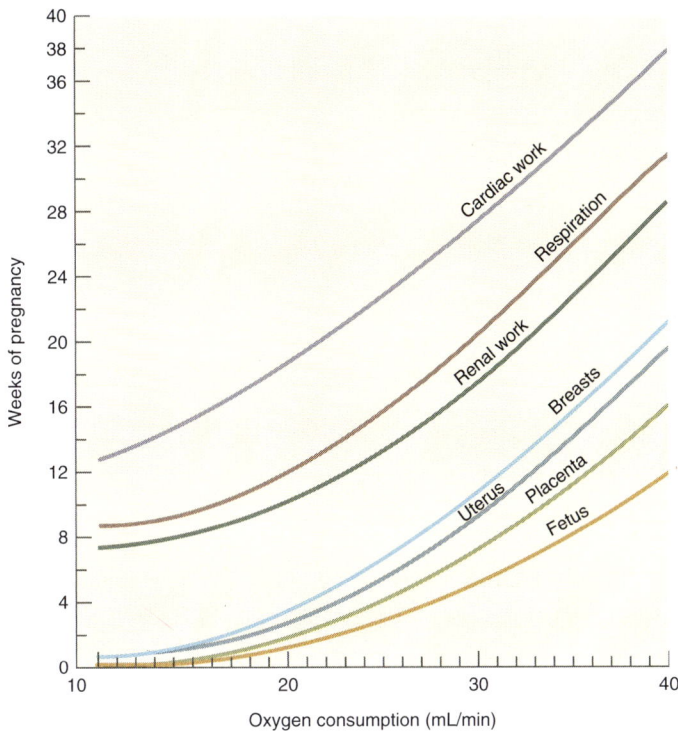

Figure 10-2. ■ Increase in oxygen consumption among body organs during pregnancy.

REPRODUCTIVE SYSTEM

The most obvious changes occur in the reproductive system. Prior to pregnancy, the uterus (see Figure 5-11 🔗) is a small, pear-shaped, thick-walled organ weighing 60 g (2 oz) with a capacity of 10 mL. By the end of pregnancy, the uterus is a large, thin-walled organ weighing 2 pounds and having a capacity of 5 L. The structure of the three muscle layers of the uterus allows the uterus to expand evenly in all directions. Painless contractions called **Braxton-Hicks contractions** occur throughout the pregnancy, but become more noticeable after the 20th week and during periods of rapid fetal growth.

The fundus should enlarge 1 cm/wk. If the fundus is not enlarging at this rate, the fetus is not growing at a normal rate. Enlargement of more than 1 centimeter each week would indicate the fetus is growing too rapidly or that a multiple pregnancy may exist.

clinical ALERT

From 20 to 36 weeks, the fundal measurement is normally 2 centimeters plus or minus the number of weeks' gestation. So, for example, at 24 weeks' gestation, fundal measurement is typically 22 to 26 centimeters.

The cervix secretes thick, sticky mucus that plugs the os to prevent micro-organisms from entering the uterus. When the cervix dilates, the mucus plug is expelled. Certain changes that occur in the presence of estrogen are present by the 8th week.

These signs (Goodell's sign, Chadwick's sign, and Hegar's sign) were described previously under Signs of Pregnancy.

The ovaries do not release ova during pregnancy. The corpus luteum produces estrogen and progesterone for approximately 12 weeks until the placenta takes over this function. Ovulation usually returns within 3 months following delivery.

The breasts enlarge due to hormonal influence. The areolae darken, and the nipple becomes more erect. **Colostrum,** a yellowish fluid rich in antibodies, is secreted in the last trimester and the first few days following delivery. The colostrum is then replaced with milk.

CARDIOVASCULAR SYSTEM

The female's pulse rate increases by 10 to 15 bpm by the end of pregnancy. Cardiac output also increases, and there is an increased blood flow to the uterus and kidneys. The blood pressure decreases slightly in the second trimester due to the influence of progesterone on the smooth muscles of blood vessels, but returns to normal during the third trimester.

clinical ALERT

Any increase in blood pressure above the normal range should be monitored and reported to the health care provider.

Supine Hypotensive Syndrome

The enlarging uterus puts pressure on the deep veins of the pelvis, resulting in venous stasis in the lower extremities. Venous stasis leads to dependent edema and varicose veins of the legs, vulva, and rectum. **Supine hypotensive syndrome** occurs after the 20th week when the mother lies supine (Figure 10-3 ■). The heavy uterus presses on the inferior vena cava, resulting in reduced blood flow back to the right atrium. The mother will experience low blood pressure, dizziness, and pale skin. The mother should be encouraged to sleep on her side to prevent hypotension. Positioning on the left side allows greater blood return than the right.

Physiologic Anemia of Pregnancy

There is an increase in blood volume during pregnancy. The red blood cell count is only slightly elevated, but there is a considerable increase in plasma volume. **Physiologic anemia of pregnancy** occurs between 26 and 32 weeks' gestation. It results from this hemodilution, as evidenced by a hematocrit of 34% to 40%. The number of white blood cells increases beginning in the second trimester. An increase in platelets, fibrin, fibrinogen, and other coagulation factors coupled with venous stasis increases the risk of thrombus formation.

RESPIRATORY SYSTEM

The enlarging uterus presses upward on the diaphragm. The ribs move outward and the diameter of the chest increases. Progesterone relaxes smooth muscles, decreasing airway

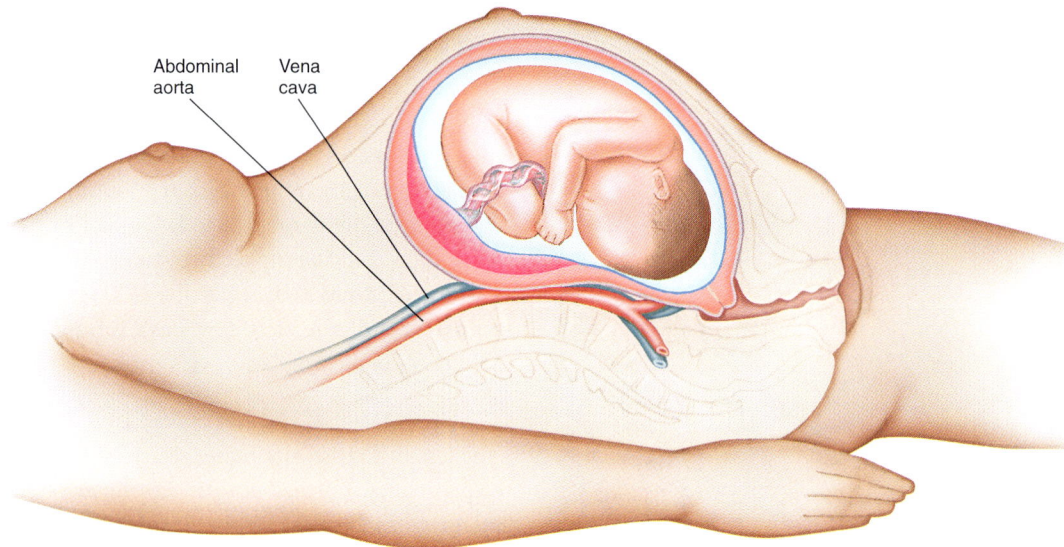

Figure 10-3. ■ Supine hypotensive syndrome. When the woman lies on her back, the large, heavy uterus compresses the vena cava and abdominal aorta against the spinal column, interfering with circulation.

resistance and allowing more oxygen into the lungs. Estrogen may cause swelling of the nasal mucosa, so the pregnant woman may experience nasal stuffiness or nosebleeds (epistaxis). As shown in Figure 10-2, oxygen demand is greatly increased during pregnancy.

RENAL SYSTEM

In the first trimester, urinary frequency is caused by the enlarging uterus that presses on the bladder. During the second trimester, the uterus has elevated out of the pelvis and the pressure is relieved. In the third trimester, the infant descends into the pelvis, again pressing on the bladder.

Glomerular infiltration and tubular reabsorption increase to remove the added waste products from the fetus. If the kidneys are unable to reabsorb all of the glucose, glucosuria will result.

clinical ALERT

Any amount of glucose over a trace should be reported to the health care provider.

GASTROINTESTINAL SYSTEM

"Morning sickness," usually beginning in the 6th week and ending in the 12th week, results from an increase in progesterone. Although not always experienced in the morning, nausea and vomiting can range from mild to severe. Prolonged vomiting or **hyperemesis gravidarum** leads to dehydration and electrolyte imbalance. It should be reported to the health care provider. Relaxation of the cardiac sphincter can cause gastric reflux. Medication may be prescribed for these discomforts.

The enlarging uterus puts pressure on the stomach and intestines. Progesterone relaxes the smooth muscle of the intestine, resulting in a decrease in peristalsis. Together these two factors increase the likelihood of constipation.

MUSCULOSKELETAL SYSTEM

The increased size and weight of the uterus cause an alteration in the mother's center of gravity. To compensate, the mother increases the lumbar curve (*lordosis*) and widens her stance. The pelvic joints become more relaxed in preparation for childbirth. These factors result in low backache and waddling gait.

Muscle cramps, especially in the lower legs, result from venous stasis and possible electrolyte imbalance. Low calcium and phosphorus levels are the most common cause. The mother should be encouraged to consume adequate amounts of milk products to prevent muscle cramps.

INTEGUMENTARY SYSTEM

Changes in skin color result from an increase in maternal hormones. The areolae, nipples, and vulva darken. **Linea nigra** (Figure 10-4 ■) is a dark line on the abdomen from the umbilicus to the pubis. **Chloasma,** or "mask of pregnancy," is a darkening of the forehead, cheeks, and area around the eyes. Both are more obvious in later pregnancy.

Striae gravidarum, or "stretch marks," occur when the underlying connective tissue separates during periods of rapid growth. Following pregnancy, these dark red streaks gradually lighten and become white, but they never disappear.

ENDOCRINE SYSTEM

Prolactin, from the anterior pituitary gland, stimulates the production of milk by the mammary glands (see Figure 5-16 ⬤). **Oxytocin,** a hormone produced by the posterior

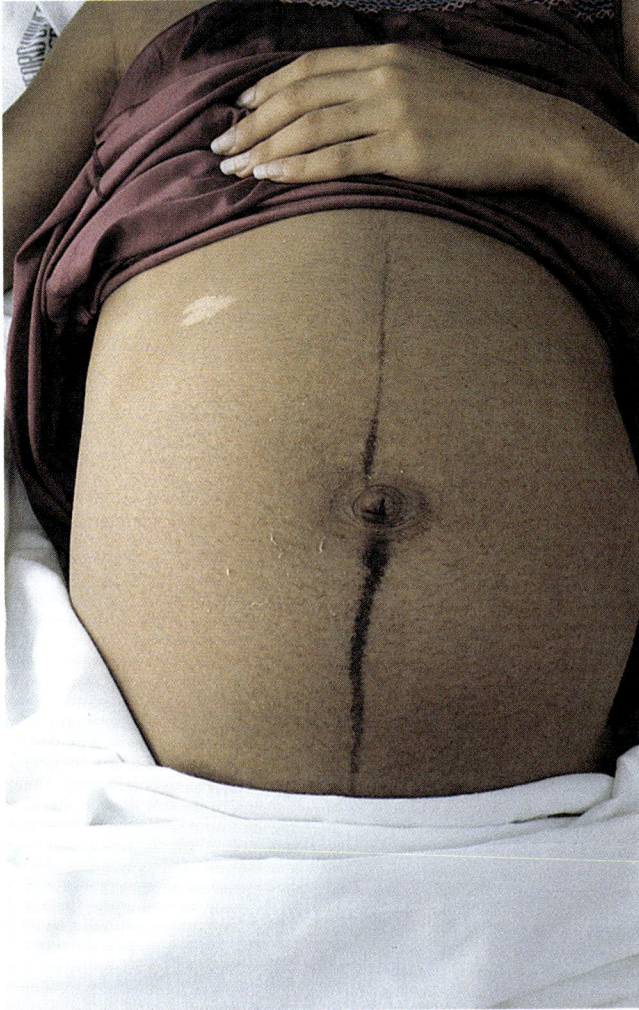

Figure 10-4. ■ Linea nigra.

pituitary gland, stimulates uterine contractions, and the **"let-down reflex,"** or release of milk after delivery.

The placenta hormones are insulin antagonists, which means they counteract insulin. As a result, the pancreas needs to produce more insulin to meet the mother's requirements. If the mother is marginal in meeting the need for more insulin, gestational diabetes results. Gestational diabetes is discussed in detail in Chapter 13 ◎◎.

Hormonal increases affecting the reproductive system are discussed under that system.

PSYCHOLOGICAL CHANGES

A diagnosis of pregnancy brings many emotions. The woman may be very happy and excited if she desires to be pregnant. She may be sad and angry if the pregnancy is unwanted. She may be ambivalent about the pregnancy. Some women become depressed and apathetic. Even when pregnancy is planned, marked anxiety and apprehension are common. As the pregnancy progresses, emotions usually change, resulting in a change of behavior that significant others may have difficulty understanding.

Early in the pregnancy, the woman often feels a little overwhelmed by the rush of emotions she has been experiencing. Even when the pregnancy is planned, it is common for the woman to feel insecure in her ability to be a mother. She may be anxious about the health of her baby, about the physical changes that are ahead of her, and about the financial drain as she adjusts her wardrobe and purchases supplies for the baby. She usually looks for signs, such as enlarging abdomen, to verify she is pregnant.

In the second trimester, the woman's feelings change. As her abdomen enlarges and the fetus moves, the pregnancy becomes real. She turns her feeling inward and becomes more introspective. Her thoughts and speech are centered on her baby, the pregnancy, and how she is feeling.

During the third trimester, she begins to think of the baby as a separate person, often beginning to select a name for the baby. She remains self-centered, frequently talking about herself and the baby. As the time of labor approaches, she begins to feel restless. She may say that labor will never begin, and that she cannot stand another day of being pregnant. She may become so emotionally drained that she cries frequently. It is important for the nurse to help her and her significant others understand these emotional outbursts.

PRENATAL CARE

Research has shown that prenatal care, beginning as soon as possible, has a dramatic effect on the outcome of the pregnancy. The goals of prenatal care include:

- A healthy, prepared mother who has minimal discomforts during the pregnancy.
- The safe delivery of a healthy fetus.
- A prepared family, including father or partner, siblings, grandparents, and any significant others.

Access to and Use of Prenatal Care

Although prenatal care is the best way to ensure a healthy child, it does not universally occur. *Healthy People 2010* (U.S. Department of Health and Human Services, 2000) has identified a real shortfall of prenatal care in certain populations. For example, Black Americans are generally less likely to obtain early and regular prenatal care. Certain

Views on Prenatal Care

A frequent complaint of labor and delivery nurses is the lack of prenatal care by many mothers-to-be from other cultures. Western medicine places high value on prenatal care. Many Americans view pregnancy and childbirth as a medical condition and begin to be followed by a physician almost from the day they discover they are pregnant. Women from other cultures, such as many Hispanic women, view pregnancy as a normal condition. They do not feel that consultation with a physician is necessary. Instead, they depend on older women to supply them with the information and support they need. If the woman does seek prenatal care, it is important to stress the need to continue to see the physician, especially if the mother is considered to be a high-risk client.

Source: Data from Centers for Disease Control and Prevention, Division of Reproductive Health, National Center for Chronic Disease Prevention and Health Promotion; and Division of Vital Statistics, National Center for Health Statistics. Washington, DC: U.S. Government Printing Office.

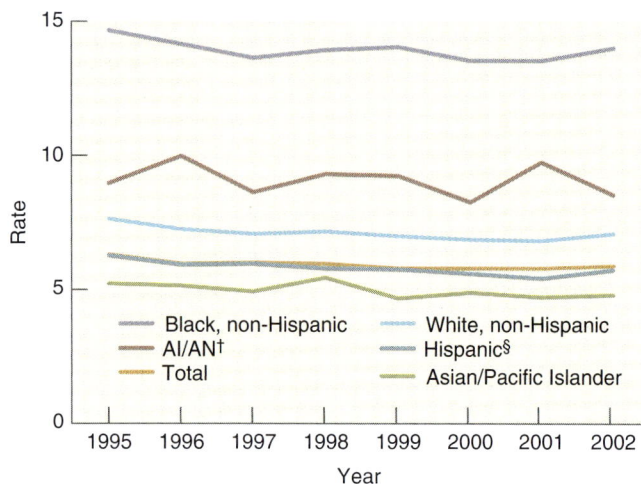

Figure 10-5. ■ U.S. infant mortality rate* by race and ethnicity from 1995 to 2002. (Courtesy of Centers for Disease Control and Prevention, Rockville, MD.)

*Per 1,000 live birth.

†American Indian/Alaska Native.

§Hispanic mothers might be of any race.

other cultures may look to sources outside the Western health care establishment for prenatal information and care. Box 10-1 ■ provides more information on this topic.

Figure 10-5 ■ illustrates the U.S. infant mortality rate by race and ethnicity from 1995 to 2002. It is clear from this illustration that there is more work to be done in finding and eliminating the cause of infant mortality. (See also Tables 1-2 and 1-3 🔗 for more data on infant and maternal mortality.)

Initial Visit

The initial visit to a health care provider can be happy or sad, depending on the women's feelings about being pregnant.

A comfortable environment, open communication, and the nurse's attitude are important in putting the woman at ease. At times, the father or partner attends the initial visit, and the nurse assesses the degree of support the woman receives from this person. The initial visit is generally longer than subsequent visits.

HEALTH HISTORY

Unless a health history has been obtained prior to pregnancy, it must be done at this time. The health history includes identifying all past medical issues that could have an impact on the pregnancy. A menstrual history will be obtained, including any past pregnancies. (Table 10-1 ■ identifies descriptive terms used to refer to pregnancy.) The woman's **gravida** (G—number of pregnancies), **para** (P—number of deliveries after 24 weeks' gestation), and the outcome of past pregnancies will be recorded. Possible outcomes include **abortion** (A—the loss of pregnancy before the 20th week), **preterm delivery** (P—delivery after the 24th week but before the 38th week), **term delivery** (T—delivery between

TABLE 10-1	
Common Terms Describing Pregnancy	
TERM	**DEFINITION**
Abortion	Loss of pregnancy prior to viable age (usually 24 weeks)
GP/TPAL	Gravida, Para/Term, preterm, abortion, live birth
Gravida	Number of pregnancies, including present pregnancy
Multigravida	Pregnant two or more times
Multipara	Delivered two or more times after 24 weeks' gestation
Nulligravida	Never been pregnant
Nullipara	Never delivered an infant after 24 weeks' gestation
Para	Number of deliveries after a viable age, including infants born alive and dead
Postterm	A delivery after 42 weeks' gestation
Preterm	A delivery after 24 weeks but before 38 weeks' gestation
Primigravida	First pregnancy
Primipara	First delivery after 24 weeks' gestation
Term	A pregnancy between 38 and 42 weeks' gestation

38 and 42 weeks), **postterm delivery** (delivery after 42 weeks' gestation), and whether the infant lived (L—live birth). It is important to remember that the word *abortion* is used medically to describe the loss of a pregnancy, whether that is a planned, elective event or a spontaneous occurrence **(miscarriage).** A woman who has been pregnant three times, had one abortion at 8 weeks, and had two live births at term would be designated G3P2/T2A1.

PHYSICAL ASSESSMENT

A physical assessment, done by the health care provider, will include a detailed assessment of the reproductive organs. An ultrasound may be performed to diagnose pregnancy. Blood may be drawn to determine a baseline for future reference.

NAEGELE'S RULE

If pregnancy is diagnosed, the duration of pregnancy will be determined. Terms used to refer to the expected delivery date are:

- estimated date of delivery (EDD)
- estimated date of birth (EDB)
- estimated date of confinement (EDC)

The EDB can be determined by several methods. **Naegele's rule** is the most common method for determining the due date. To apply the rule, take the first day of the LMP, subtract 3 months, and add 7 days. For example, if the LMP was on January 18, the EDB would be October 25. Adjustments to the rule have to be made if the LMP falls at the end of a month, for example, on July 29. Subtracting 3 months would be April, and adding 7 days would be April 36. April has only 30 days, so the EDB would be advanced to May 6. A gestational wheel or chart can be used for quick reference. Figure 10-6 ■ illustrates a gestational wheel that provides expected dates for the EDB and other pregnancy landmarks.

Follow-up Visits

The pregnant woman should return to the clinic for follow-up care on the following schedule:

- Every 4 weeks for the first 28 weeks
- Every 2 weeks during weeks 29 to 36
- Every week after 36 weeks until delivery

LABORATORY TESTS RELATED TO PREGNANCY

Laboratory blood values often change while a woman is pregnant. Laboratory tests (Table 10-2 ■) can provide valuable data for assessing a woman's health. Nurses should be familiar with values that are normal for women during pregnancy.

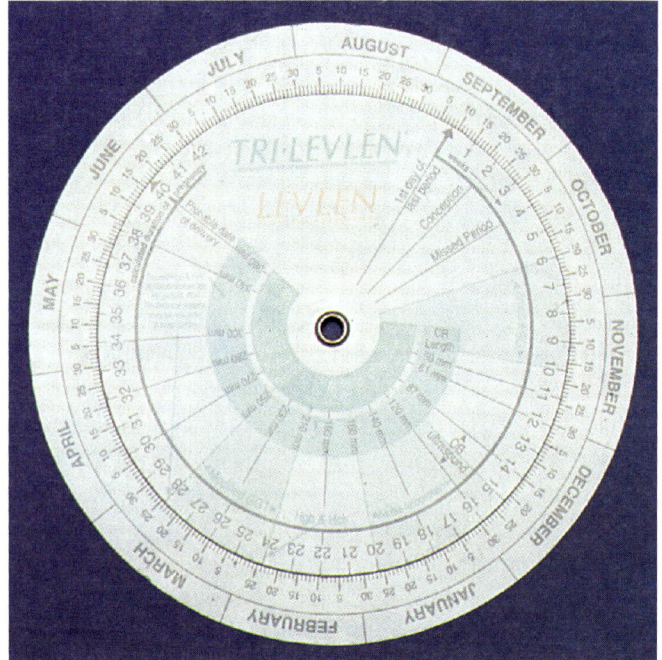

Figure 10-6. ■ The gestational wheel can be used to calculate the EDB (estimated date of birth). To use, place the "last menses began" arrow on the date of the woman's last menstrual period (LMP). Then read the "EDB date" at the arrow labeled 40. In this case, the LMP is September 8 and the EDB is June 17.

TABLE 10-2		
Pregnant and Nonpregnant Laboratory Values		
TEST	**PREGNANT VALUES**	**NONPREGNANT VALUES**
Hematocrit (%)	32–42	37–47
Hemoglobin (g/dL)	10–14	12–16
Platelets (mm³)	Significant increase 3–5 days after birth	150,000–350,000
White blood cells (mm³)	5,000–15,000	4,500–10,000
Fibrinogen (mg/dL)	Up to 600	175–400
Serum glucose (mg/dL)	65 (fasting) Less than 140 (2hr PP)	70–80
Sodium (mEq/L)	135–145	135–145
Potassium (mEq/L)	3.5–5.1	3.5–5.1
Chloride (mEq/L)	100–108	100–108
Bicarbonate (mEq/L)	22–26	22–26
Calcium (mg/dL)	Falls 10% by term	8.5–10.5

MEDICATIONS DURING PREGNANCY

The use of any medication—prescription, nonprescription, or herbal—during pregnancy carries a risk to the fetus. A *teratogen* is any chemical that can cause abnormal development in the fetus. Drugs are one form of teratogen. To prevent teratogenic effects, the FDA has established five categories of potential risk for the development of birth defects. See Box 8-3 ⚭ for identification of these categories. It is important to recall that herbal medicines are categorized as dietary supplements rather than drugs. Therefore, the testing, regulation, and standardization of herbs may not be as strict.

Although the first trimester is the most critical for teratogenic effects of drugs, some drugs can be harmful in the second and third trimesters as well. If medications must be taken during pregnancy, it is wisest to use the lowest dose for the shortest period of time. It is usually safer to select well-known medications than to choose newer medications whose teratogenic effect may be unknown. Pregnant women should be advised to avoid all herbs during the first trimester. During the second and third trimesters, whole plant extracts are safer than concentrated extracts. Certain categories of herbs should be avoided throughout the pregnancy, including **abortifacients** (abortion-inducing herbs that induce menstruation), nervous system stimulants, stimulant laxatives, and others. Box 10-2 ■ lists common herbs to avoid during pregnancy because they are considered abortifacients.

BOX 10-2	NUTRITION THERAPY

Common Herbs to Avoid in Pregnancy*

Aloe spp.	Kava kava
Black cohosh	Licorice
Buckthorn	Ma huang
Cascara sagrada	Pennyroyal
Chamomile, Roman	Rue
Chaste tree berry	Sage
Dong quai	Senna
Feverfew	St John's wort
Goldenseal	Stinging nettle
Gotu kola	Tansy
Guggul	Wormwood
Horehound	Yarrow
Horseradish (fresh)	

Use with caution
Garlic
Ginger
Turmeric

*Avoid excessive consumption relative to usual and customary food use.
Source: Hardy, M. (2000). Herbs of special interest to women. *Journal of the American Pharmaceutical Association, 40*(2) 234–242; American Pregnancy Association. (2002–2006). Natural herbs & vitamins in pregnancy; Krieger/Elchai, L. (1996–1997). *Herbs of special interest to women.* Herbs for a Health Balance. Creative Minds Unlimited.

Most care providers prescribe a prenatal multivitamin with iron to be taken once a day. This nutritional supplement will help ensure that adequate amounts of vitamins and iron are ingested for the developing fetus. Some women may want to omit the vitamin due to nausea in the early weeks of pregnancy. However, at this time, the woman may not be consuming adequate amounts of nutritious foods. She should be encouraged to adjust the time of day the medication is taken instead of omitting a dose.

Pregnant women may develop headaches, respiratory infections, allergies, or flu as often as the nonpregnant woman. Commonly, over-the-counter medications are used to treat these conditions. Many physicians, nurse midwives, and nurse practitioners provide their clients with a list of over-the-counter medications that are acceptable to use during pregnancy. If the client wishes to use another medication or herbal supplement, she should contact her health care provider. It is important for the client to communicate to any health care provider that she is pregnant (or suspects pregnancy) before she takes any prescribed medication. For example, a woman who is 6 months pregnant could be taken to an emergency room for treatment following an automobile accident. Because the pregnancy may not be obvious, it is important for her to communicate to the nurses, doctor, and x-ray technician that she is pregnant. When getting a new prescription medication filled at the drug store, the pregnant woman should inform the pharmacist that she is pregnant and question the safety of the drug at this time.

DISCOMFORTS OF PREGNANCY

Numerous changes occur in a woman's body during pregnancy. Initially, there may be feelings of "fullness" or morning sickness, heavier breasts, and a slight sensation of bloating. Later changes affect the woman's center of gravity and her circulation. They alter how a woman stands, walks, and rests, and many of these changes involve some level of discomfort. It is helpful for women to be prepared for these changes ahead of time. Table 10-3 ■ identifies the common discomforts and possible interventions to alleviate or decrease the discomforts of pregnancy. Some alternate therapies for relief of pregnancy-related muscle pain are summarized in Box 10-3 ■.

Nutrition

Nutrition is a vital part of prenatal care. Good nutrition provides crucial ingredients to supply the developing fetus. It also provides energy for the extra demands being made on the mother's body. For a complete discussion of nutrition during pregnancy, see Chapter 11 ⚭. The Health Promotion Issue on pages 216 and 217 describes nutritional needs of pregnant women who are vegetarians.

MediaLink Safe and Unsafe Herbs

TABLE 10-3

Common Discomforts of Pregnancy and Treatment

DISCOMFORT	CAUSE	INTERVENTION
Nausea and/or vomiting	Increased hormones Enlarged uterus pushing on stomach	Limit fluids upon waking. Eat dry toast or crackers. Eat small amounts frequently. Avoid fried or spicy foods.
Heartburn	Gastric reflux due to relaxed cardiac sphincter from effects of progesterone and pressure from enlarged uterus	Avoid fried or spicy foods. Eat small amounts and avoid overeating. Sit up for 30 minutes after eating. Take antacids ONLY with care provider's approval.
Flatulence	Slowing of GI motility due to progesterone and pressure from enlarged uterus	Omit gas-forming foods. Increase bulk in diet. Have regular bowel movements.
Constipation	Slowing of GI motility due to progesterone and pressure from enlarged uterus Decreased activity Inadequate fiber and fluids in diet Iron supplements	Increase fiber from fruits and vegetables (raisins, prunes, apples). Engage in daily activity (walking). Increase fluids.
Hemorrhoids	Straining to have bowel movement Pressure from enlarged uterus on rectal veins	Prevent constipation. Use cool compresses. Take a warm sitz bath. Apply topical analgesic ointment.
Varicose veins	Pressure from enlarged uterus on deep pelvic veins Relaxation of vessel walls due to progesterone Inactivity, long periods of sitting or standing	Rest with feet elevated. Avoid restrictive clothing, crossing legs. Wear support hose. Engage in daily activity (walking).
Ankle edema	Inactivity, long periods of sitting or standing Sodium retention	Engage in daily activity (walking). Rest with feet elevated. Avoid salty foods. If edema increases or is routinely present upon arising, contact health care provider.
Leg cramps	Calcium/phosphorus imbalance Muscle fatigue/strain Restricted circulation	Increase calcium in diet. Have frequent rest periods with legs elevated.
Backache	Relaxation of pelvic joints Exaggerated lordosis due to change in center of gravity Fatigue Poor body mechanics	Rest lying on side. Wear low-heeled shoes. Use proper body mechanics.
Urinary frequency	Pressure of enlarging uterus on bladder Urinary tract infection	Empty bladder frequently. Do NOT limit fluids. Contact health care provider if other signs of urinary infection are present.
Dyspnea	Decreased lung capacity due to pressure of enlarged uterus on diaphragm	Lie on side or semi-Fowler's position.

(continued)

TABLE 10-3

Common Discomforts of Pregnancy and Treatment (continued)

DISCOMFORT	CAUSE	INTERVENTION
Vaginal discharge	Increased vaginal secretions due to estrogen Vaginal infection	Maintain good hygiene. If other signs of vaginal infection are present, contact health care provider.
Itchy skin	Dehydration Stretching skin	Increase fluids. Avoid drying soaps. Apply lotion.
Mood swings	Hormonal change Fatigue Inadequate diet	Express fears and concerns. Eat adequate diet and drink fluids. Take adequate rest periods.

BOX 10-3   COMPLEMENTARY THERAPIES

Physical Modalities for Relief of Pregnancy-Related Muscle Pain

Massage Therapy for Low Back Pain

Massage often helps relieve the low back pain associated with pregnancy. During the first 4 months of pregnancy, the body should be massaged with a gentle, soft touch. The best position for lumbar massage is with the women sitting on a stool, resting her arms on a table and leaning her forehead against her arms. The person doing the massage kneels on the floor behind her, which enhances the ability to apply an effective amount of pressure to the back muscles.

Yoga

Yoga builds and tones muscles, increases flexibility, improves endurance, and promotes a state of relaxation. Many of the techniques taught in childbirth classes, such as focus, relaxation, and systematic breathing, have their roots in yoga. The gentle stretching of the poses helps ease the muscle aches of pregnancy and strengthens the muscles that will be used during childbirth. The breathing techniques may lessen the shortness of breath that often accompanies advanced pregnancy.

Some yoga poses are contraindicated while pregnant. These poses are the extreme stretching positions and any position that puts pressure on the uterus. Full forward bends will probably be uncomfortable for both woman and baby. A woman's center of balance has shifted completely, and thus she must be careful with balance poses. Pregnant women should never lie on the stomach for any pose. If any pose feels uncomfortable, the woman should stop at once. If she experiences dizziness, sudden swelling, extreme shortness of breath, or vaginal bleeding, she should see her midwife or doctor immediately.

Reflexology for Sciatica

Reflexology uses specific touch techniques to stimulate "reflex points and areas" on the feet, hands, and ears. Reflexologists believe that each of these points corresponds to a specific part of the body. The growing baby can put pressure on the large sciatic nerve. The pressure inflames the nerve, causing severe lower back pain that radiates into the legs. The reflex points for the sciatic nerve are on the heel. A woman in her second or third trimester can press gently and release with her thumbs to stimulate first one whole heel, then the other. Each heel can be worked for 1 to 2 minutes twice a day until the pain is gone.

Women who are in the first trimester of pregnancy should not have reflexology that stimulates the uterine points on the hands, feet, or ears. In general, pregnant women should receive reflexology that uses light, gentle pressure (Gottlieb, 2000).

Source: Olds, S. B., London, M. L., Ladewig, P. A. W., & Davidson, M. R. (2004). *Maternal-newborn nursing & women's health care* (7th ed.). Upper Saddle River, NJ: Prentice Hall, p. 367.

Adequate fluid intake is important for the pregnant woman. Drinking 1.5 to 2 L of water, milk, or juice every 24 hours is recommended. It is best to limit caffeine-containing beverages. Women in low socioeconomic levels may have difficulty buying adequate amounts of milk and high-protein foods. These women should be referred for aid. Programs such as Women, Infants, and Children (WIC) may provide assistance (see Chapter 3).

Exercise

Exercise is increasingly recognized as an important part of a health maintenance program. Healthy, active women are more likely to have healthy infants. Women who are overweight and sedentary are more likely to encounter problems in themselves such as gestational diabetes, and in their children (see Chapter 13). It is important to maintain activity throughout pregnancy. However, modifications should be made to adapt exercise to the physical changes pregnancy causes and the demands it makes on the body. Figure 10-7 ■ illustrates some simple exercises that help relax muscles and also help prepare the body for childbirth.

KEGEL EXERCISES

Kegel exercises are promoted during the prenatal period. These exercises help women identify muscle groups that are affected by delivery and that need conditioning after birth.

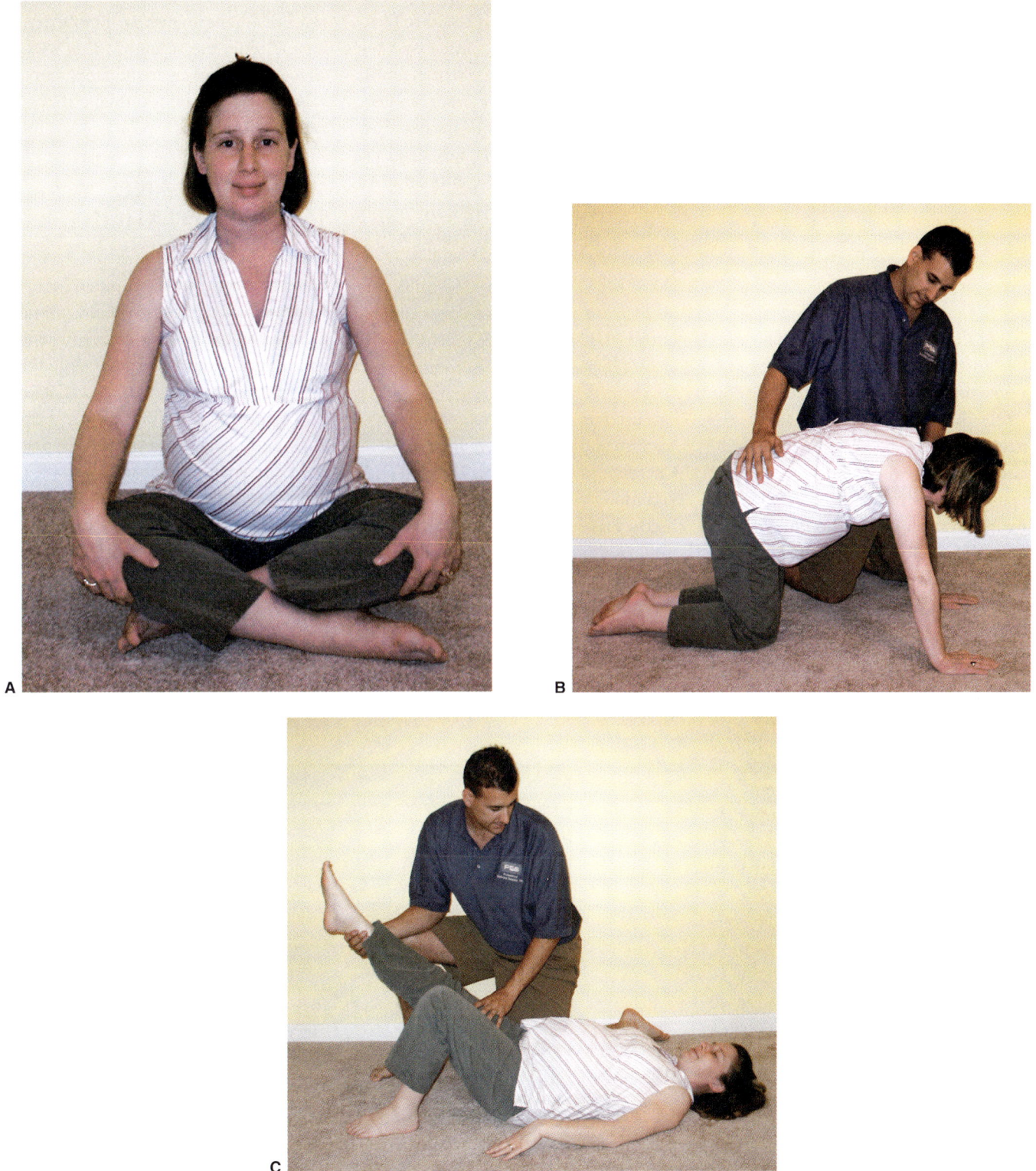

Figure 10-7. ■ Prenatal exercises. (**A**) Tailor sitting. (**B**) Pelvic tilt on hands and knees: The woman arches her lower back and then relaxes it to a flat position. (**C**) Leg raises: To strengthen abdominal muscles, a pregnant woman may be taught to alternately raise one leg, then the other, from a bent position straight up off the floor as shown here.

HEALTH PROMOTION ISSUE

PREGNANCY AND VEGETARIANISM

The nurse is taking an initial history of a G2 P1, 29-year-old, married client who is 12 weeks pregnant. Her weight today is 135 pounds and her height is 5'8". The client works full-time as an accountant. She is concerned about her diet and reports being faithful to take her prenatal vitamins. She states she doesn't have time to eat right, eats out frequently because her 3-year-old son loves fast food and claims that she really can't cook too well. She also states that she is a vegetarian, although her husband and her son are not. The nurse understands that there are several issues that need to be addressed with this client. She needs help with food choices and food preparation. She needs to be advised of the hazards of poor nutrition during pregnancy and its effect on her children's health. It would also be helpful if she had some sample menus after which to model her diet.

DISCUSSION

Increasing the protein content to 60 to 80 g/day can be especially challenging for the vegetarian pregnant client. Added protein is essential to support the increased metabolic needs of pregnancy and to aid the growth of maternal and fetal tissues. Protein also aids increased energy levels, muscular contractions, and immunity. Lack of protein in the diet of a pregnant woman has been linked to increased incidence of low birth weight infants, pregnancy-induced hypertension, and poor fetal brain development.

Nonanimal proteins are said to be incomplete proteins. Incomplete proteins do not contain all of the essential amino acids. However, the vegetarian can get these essential amino acids in their diet by combining complementary plant proteins. Examples of these combinations are beans and grains or dairy and grains. Many nonanimal foods provide good sources of protein such as chick peas, baked beans, tofu, cow or soy milk, cereals such as muesli, peanuts or peanut butter, and breads. Some vegetarians are not opposed to eggs in their diet.

The pregnant vegetarian woman also needs to be careful to get enough calcium and vitamin D in her diet. Choosing soy milk that is fortified with vitamin D will aid in meeting these needs. Prenatal vitamins should contain iron, vitamin B_{12}, zinc, and vitamin D.

Proper parental food choices and dietary restraint have been found to have a direct effect on childhood obesity. Fast-food meals are typically high in calories and contain a high fat content. Parents who are intent on preventing obesity should avoid prepackaged foods, as well as foods high in sugar and fat. A child's diet should contain less than 30% of calories from fat.

PLANNING AND IMPLEMENTATION

The nurse should help the client understand that proper planning and advanced preparation will aid in making proper food choices and in the long run save time and energy. Encouraging her to create a detailed weekly menu and resulting shopping list will prevent making unhealthy purchases. Explain to the pregnant client that her weekly food preparation will be aided if upon returning from the grocery store she prepares the food by slicing meats and cheeses, washing and cutting fruits and vegetables, and boiling eggs.

Mornings are typically difficult for working mothers of young children. Time demands rarely allow for meal

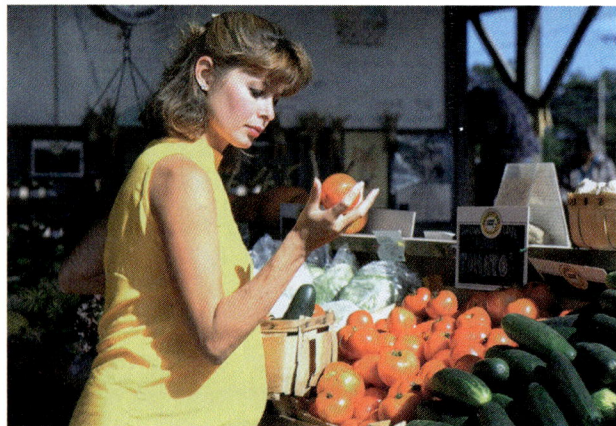

	MENU 1	MENU 2	MENU 3
Breakfast	One orange, whole wheat toast with peanut butter, 1 cup low-fat yogurt, 20 oz water	Scrambled egg, cream of wheat with raisins, 1 cup soy milk	Whole wheat waffles with pureed fruit spread, low-fat cream cheese and peanut butter, 1 cup soy milk
Snack	Trail mix of raisins and almonds, 20 oz water	Frozen low-fat yogurt with fresh blueberries and granola with walnuts, 20 oz water	Whole wheat English muffin toasted with Swiss cheese and tomato, handful pecans, 20 oz water
Lunch	Spinach salad with tomatoes, feta cheese, sunflower seeds; 5 whole wheat crackers; 1 cup of herbal tea	Steamed broccoli and asparagus with cheese, baked beans, 2 slices whole wheat bread, 1 cup herbal tea	Lettuce wraps with black bean spread, onions, and shredded cheddar cheese; baked tortilla chips with salsa; 20 oz water
Snack	Carrots and celery with cottage cheese	Apple slices with peanut butter, crackers, 20 oz water	Whole wheat cereal such as Cheerios, cheese cubes, flax seeds, 20 oz water
Dinner	Veggie burger on whole wheat bun with cheese, lettuce, and tomato; serving of brown rice; 1 cup soy milk	Stir fry of squash, zucchini, slivered almonds, and tofu; serving of brown rice; 1 plum; 1 cup soy milk	Mushrooms, green pepper, and onions, sautéed, and served over whole wheat pasta with cream sauce made with soy milk and mozzarella cheese, 1 cup herbal tea
Snack	Banana, bran muffin, 1 cup herbal tea	Mixed fruit cup, 10 oz water	Pure fruit sorbet with graham crackers

planning and preparation. The nurse could encourage the client to fix lunches and begin the next night's dinner preparation before bedtime. Above are several choices of easy-to-prepare vegetarian meals.

Because it would be virtually impossible to avoid eating out, living in a fast-paced American society, the nurse should assist the client in making healthy choices when dining out. Fortunately, the majority of fast-food restaurants offer healthy, low-fat menu choices. Many restaurants offer a wide range of salads containing fresh vegetables, cheeses, and nuts. Combined with a low-fat salad dressing, this option makes a smart choice for the vegetarian. Some fast-food restaurants offer fruit cups, coleslaw, and yogurt parfaits. For the nonvegetarian, there are grilled chicken sandwiches and deli sandwiches on whole wheat breads.

SELF-REFLECTION

Carefully assess your own nutritional habits. Record your intake for a 24-hour period. Determine excesses and deficiencies in your dietary and fluid intake. What is your weight? Is it appropriate for your height? What poor nutritional habits are you role modeling to your clients? Actions often speak louder than words.

SUGGESTED RESOURCES

For the Nurse

Fowles, E. (2004). Prenatal nutrition and birth outcomes. *Journal of Obstetric, Gynecologic, and Neonatal Nursing, 33*(6), 809–822.

Hood, M.Y., Moore, L.L., Sundarajan-Ramamurti, A., Singer, M., Cupples, L.A., & Ellison, R.C. (2000). Parental eating attitudes and the development of obesity in children. The Framingham Children's Study. *International Journal of Obesity Related Metabolic Disorders, 24*(10), 1319–1325.

Moran, R. (1999). Evaluation and treatment of childhood obesity. *American Family Physician, 59*(4), 861–877.

For the Client

Eisenberg, A., Murkoff, H., & Hathaway, S. (1986). *What to eat when you're expecting.* New York: Workman Publishing.

Mangels, R. (1996). Vegetarian diets during pregnancy. *Vegetarian Nutrition.* American Dietetic Association.

Somer, E. (2002). *Nutrition for a healthy pregnancy: The complete guide to eating before, during, and after your pregnancy.* New York: Owl Books.

Figure 10-8 ■ shows the effect of Kegel exercise on the pubococcygeus muscle; it also shows the muscles of the pelvic floor. To identify the muscles of the pelvic floor, some nurses suggest stopping urination in midstream. However, it is not recommended to perform the exercise while urinating.

The woman is asked to visualize the pelvic floor muscles as an elevator. In relaxed position, the muscles are on the "ground floor." Then the woman draws the muscles in and up raising the "elevator" to the first, second, third, and fourth "floor." She holds the muscles in that position, then gradually allows them to return to starting position.

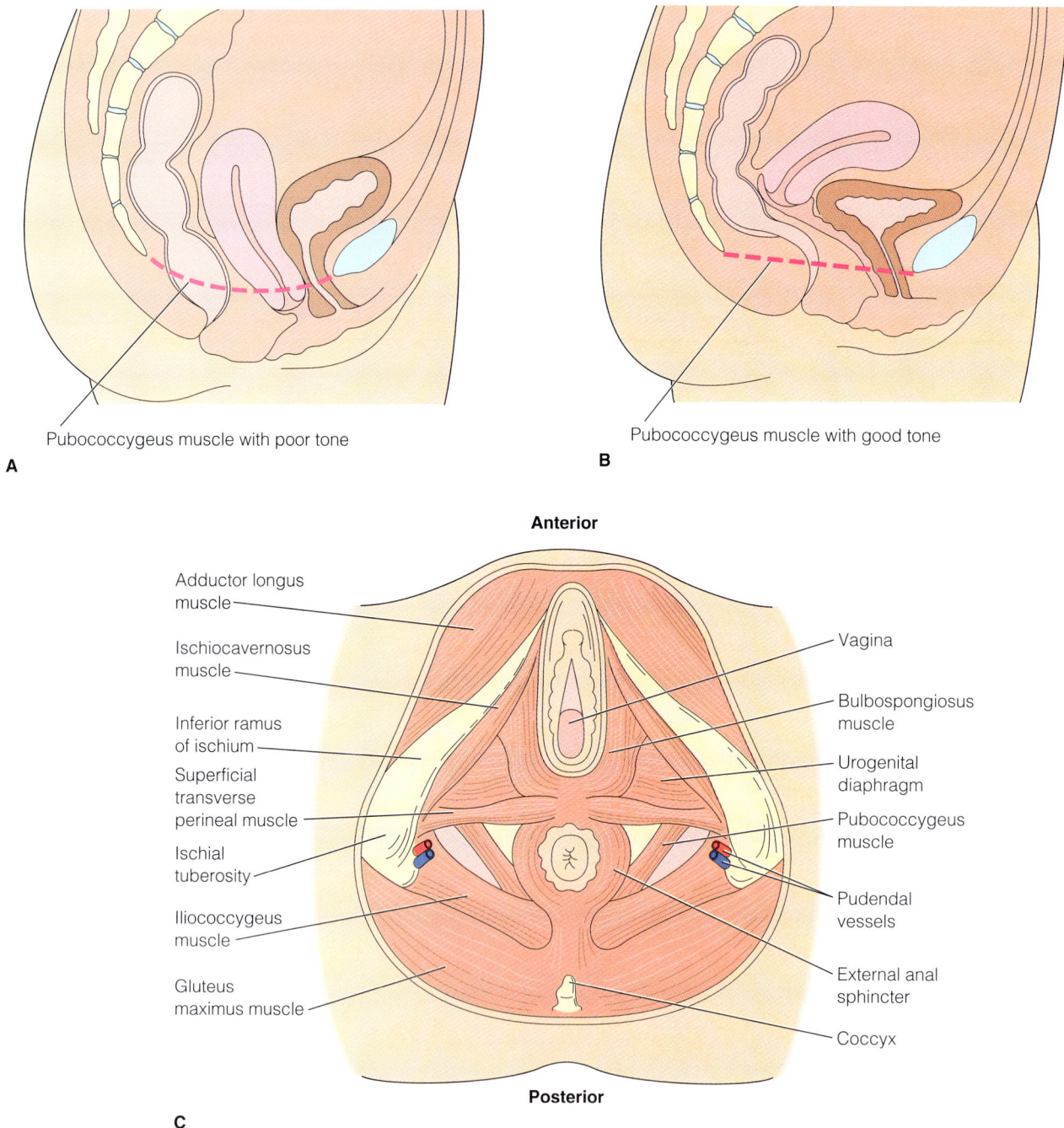

Pubococcygeus muscle with poor tone

A

Pubococcygeus muscle with good tone

B

Anterior

Adductor longus muscle

Ischiocavernosus muscle

Inferior ramus of ischium

Superficial transverse perineal muscle

Ischial tuberosity

Iliococcygeus muscle

Gluteus maximus muscle

Vagina

Bulbospongiosus muscle

Urogenital diaphragm

Pubococcygeus muscle

Pudendal vessels

External anal sphincter

Coccyx

Posterior

C

Figure 10-8. ■ Kegel exercises are often taught during pregnancy. They help the woman become familiar with muscles that support the pelvic floor. After birth, these exercises will be useful in regaining muscle tone. (**A**) The pubococcygeal muscle with poor tone. (**B**) The pubococcygeal muscle with good tone. (**C**) The muscles of the pelvic floor (the puborectalis, pubovaginalis, and coccygeal muscles cannot be seen from this view).

Kegel exercises can be done while standing, sitting, or lying down. Some women use visual cues (e.g., standing in a grocery line, stopping for a red light) to remind them to do Kegel exercises. If properly done, the exercise does not engage the muscles of the thigh or buttocks. It is important to emphasize taking full, smooth breaths during the exercise.

AVOIDING HYPERTHERMIA

The pregnant woman, in part due to increased blood volume, has an increased tendency toward hyperthermia. Although women generally may continue the types of exercise they did before pregnancy, they will need to make adjustments in the intensity and duration of exercise. Many women are advised to avoid sports such as jogging and tennis that can put excessive strain on joints. Walking and swimming are often recommended to promote circulation and muscle tone. Swimming is especially good, because water provides support while the aerobic workout occurs.

SAFETY CONCERNS

The home and work environment must be safe for the pregnant client. In late pregnancy, the woman is at risk for falls because her center of gravity has shifted. The home should be inspected for hazards and corrections should be made. Chemicals (including cleaning supplies, insecticides, and weed control agents) can harm the fetus. These chemicals should be avoided if possible. If the woman must use these chemicals, she should avoid skin contact and inhalation of fumes. Excessive heat from hot tubs, saunas, or hot humid weather should be avoided, because water 106° F can cause maternal hyperthermia (Rogers & Davis, 1995).

Prenatal Teaching

Every clinical visit is an opportunity for the nurse to provide prenatal teaching. The nurse can answer questions, offer new information, and reassure parents-to-be of things they are doing right. Office visits are an opportunity to review the importance of good nutrition, regular exercise, and adequate rest. Most women are open to learning in this period of their lives. This gives the nurse the opportunity to promote steps toward a healthier lifestyle that can have long-term effects. Some important areas of client teaching during pregnancy are listed in Box 10-4 ■.

PRENATAL CLASSES

Prenatal classes are advisable for all mothers, not just those in their first pregnancies. Topics that are generally covered in these classes are:

- Health considerations during pregnancy, including:
  - Nutrition, diet, and exercise

- Pets (especially cats because of the potential for being infected with toxoplasmosis when handling cat feces)
- Signs that labor is beginning
- Contraction patterns and timing
- Breathing techniques to assist the woman through contractions (e.g., Lamaze method)
- Chemical and nonchemical methods of providing pain relief during labor (large birthing tub, etc.)
- Possible complications in the mother and warning signs
- Possible complications of labor, including emergency cesarean birth and fetal anomaly or death
- Infant feeding (breast or bottle, positions, burping; see Chapter 11)
- Infant care (diapering, dressing, bathing)
- Infant safety (see Chapters 14 and 17)
- Siblings

BOX 10-4   CLIENT TEACHING

Health Promotion Topics During Pregnancy

Nutrition, Diet, and Exercise (affecting both mother and fetus)
- Prenatal vitamins and/or foods to supply pregnancy needs
- Importance of fluids
- Hygiene, clothing adaptations, dental care
- Pattern of weight gain, desired weight gain (individualized teaching)
- Referral, if needed, to WIC program or other community assistance
- Alcohol's effects on the fetus
- Limiting or eliminating caffeine

Safety
- Adapting to body changes and changes in balance
- Techniques for relieving physical stresses of pregnancy
- Checking all medications (even OTC) with physician before use
- Smoking cessation
- Pets (especially cats because of the potential for being infected with toxoplasmosis when handling cat feces)
- Toxins and exposure to dangerous chemicals in the home and environment (wearing gloves when gardening)

Work
- Learning to balance work and rest
- Adaptations to jobs requiring long periods of standing

Travel Considerations
- Car travel—seatbelt adjustment
- Air travel—restrictions

Prenatal Classes
- Physical and mental preparation for childbirth and parenting
- Effects of pregnancy on sexuality
- Awareness of possible complications requiring medical aid
- Value of prenatal health care visits
- Planning for effects of pregnancy on home life

ADOLESCENT PARENTS

It can be beneficial to provide prenatal classes specifically for pregnant teens. An all-teens class can offer a safe environment in which to discuss impending parenthood. Issues such as altered self-image can be much more difficult for adolescents to handle than for adults. There may be resentment about having life plans interrupted by the pregnancy. There may be issues about parental criticism that need to be aired, or disagreement over who will raise the child after birth. In a peer environment, teens can express their views

NURSING CARE PLAN CHART

Planning for a Client with an Abnormal Pap Smear During Pregnancy

GOAL	INTERVENTION	RATIONALE	EXPECTED OUTCOME
1. Deficient Knowledge related to treatment options for possible cervical cancer			
The client or couple will obtain information about further testing, including repeat PAP smear, culposcopy, biopsy, and/or diagnostic conization procedure.	Provide written information regarding PAP interpretation, cervical cancer stages, and treatment options.	*Written information allows clients to review information at home.*	Client or couple will make decision regarding woman's treatment.
	Explain the difference between having an "abnormal PAP smear" and having cancer.	*Verbal instructions meet the needs of auditory learners.*	
	Explain that conization during the first trimester of pregnancy is likely to precipitate a spontaneous abortion (miscarriage). It should only be performed during the second trimester, and when there is convincing evidence of *invasive* cancer.	*Not all abnormal PAP smears indicate cancer. Providing factual information can reduce the client's or couple's anxiety. Explanation prepares the client or couple for potential diagnostic testing and enables them to choose an appropriate method of treatment to protect the fetus.*	
2. Readiness for Enhanced Decision Making			
Client or couple will make an informed decision about childbearing.	When test results are shared, provide a detailed explanation to facilitate understanding. Provide written materials for the client or couple to read later.	*Diagnosis of cancer (or the anticipation of such news) is a fear-evoking event. Stress triggered by the event is likely to impair the client's or couple's ability to process new information immediately after such news.*	Client or couple will state understanding of test report and resulting impact on future decision making.
3. Death Anxiety			
Client or couple will voice their fears regarding an unfavorable diagnosis.	Engage in therapeutic listening to allow each person to express feelings openly and with confidentiality.	*The client or couple needs to be able to share feelings in order to move forward with decision making.*	Client or couple will recognize signs and symptoms of anxiety and when it becomes necessary to receive further help for such symptoms.
	Demonstrate unconditional positive regard for the client (mother) or couple and provide emotional support.	*To make a rational decision, the couple must be free of excessive anxiety, so they may evaluate the facts according to their personal beliefs and values.*	Client or couple will explain to the nurse the extent of their ability to recognize such signs and symptoms.
	Explore with client or couple the extent of their emotional support network.	*Demonstrated acts of caring by others close to the client or couple can help to alleviate stress.*	
	Provide referrals as needed for mental health services and spiritual care.	*Spiritual and mental health care are effective means of treating anxiety.*	

TABLE 10-4

Warning Signs During Pregnancy

WARNING SIGN (NEED MEDICAL EVALUATION RIGHT AWAY)	POSSIBLE CAUSE
Vaginal bleeding (any)	Spontaneous abortion, placenta previa, abruptio placentae
Fluid gushing or leaking from vagina	Rupture of membranes (leaking urine may appear similar)
Persistent vomiting	Hyperemesis gravidarum
Swelling of hands, face, legs, feet	Gestational hypertension (also called pregnancy-induced hypertension or PIH), preeclampsia
Visual disturbance: blurred vision, double vision, seeing spots or flashes of light	Gestational hypertension, preeclampsia
Dizziness, fainting, persistent headache	Gestational hypertension, preeclampsia
Fever over 100° F (37.8° C) and chills	Infection
Abdominal pain, cramping	Ectopic pregnancy, spontaneous abortion, abruptio placentae, labor
Thick, white/yellow, irritating vaginal discharge	Vaginal infection
Dysuria	Urinary infection
Oliguria	Dehydration, PIH
Notable decrease or absence of fetal movement	Fetal distress, fetal death

more openly and can receive support from others who share their situation. (See Chapter 12 .)

MONITORING FOR COMPLICATIONS

The client should be taught warning signs of possible complications. Usually, the sooner interventions are begun, the better the outcome. Signs of impending labor should be discussed with the client in the third trimester of pregnancy. Table 10-4 identifies warning signs.

Complications and high-risk pregnancy are discussed in Chapter 13 . The Nursing Care Plan Chart on page 220 discusses nursing care for one potential complication during pregnancy.

Birthing Facilities and Staff

The settings in which women give birth are varied. Women may go to a local hospital and deliver the baby in a delivery room. They may choose a maternity center where labor and birth occur in a homelike atmosphere. A few elect to deliver their babies at home.

As care providers, women may have a physician, a nurse midwife, or a **doula** (a supportive companion who accompanies the woman through birth, providing physical and emotional support and information, and advocating for the woman and the family). The obstetrician, although no

longer the sole person assisting births, is on call to other caregivers in case of emergency.

NURSING CARE

PRIORITIES IN NURSING CARE

The highest priority in providing prenatal care is monitoring the mother and fetus for signs of complications. Signs of complications must be reported immediately. Teaching the mother, father, and significant others is important in health maintenance and preparation for childbirth. The nurse must be prepared to provide instruction at every client contact.

ASSESSING

The assessment of the pregnant family includes collecting physical data, determining the psychological response to pregnancy, and evaluating family functioning. An important piece of data to collect is information about the woman's culture and cultural expectations related to pregnancy.

Cultural Considerations

Families are influenced by their cultures, perhaps especially during times of great change, such as marriage, death, and birth. The nurse must be open to and respectful of their beliefs. Language barriers may pose a challenge in providing client and family teaching. It is important to have an interpreter available when possible. Printed material should be available in the woman's language. Table 10-5 ■ presents activities encouraged or prevented by some cultures.

Initial Visit

■ Provide a pleasant environment and therapeutic listening skills. Use open-ended questions when inquiring about the effect of the pregnancy on the woman's life. *The pregnant woman will have positive or negative feelings about the pregnancy. For her to feel safe about expressing them,* *the nurse's feeling about pregnancy must not affect the interview. The client and her needs are the focus. There may be a difference of opinion between the woman and her partner. The nurse assists by providing a place in which issues can be raised. In the case of difficult family issues, the nurse would bring in a qualified social worker or counselor.*

■ A health history will be obtained (in depth, if necessary), including menstrual history and history of past pregnancies. The LPN/LVN will assist the RN in collecting data. *A complete health history is needed to identify any past medical issues that might affect the pregnancy. A history of past pregnancies is important, because labor time is usually*

TABLE 10-5		
Activities Encouraged or Avoided by Some Cultures During Pregnancy		
TOPIC	**BELIEF**	**NURSING CONSIDERATIONS**
Nutrition	**Italian descent:** Desire for certain foods must be satisfied to prevent congenital anomalies. Also they must smell the food to prevent miscarriage. (Spector, 2000) **African descent:** Eat clay, dirt, or starch to benefit mother and fetus. (Spector, 2000) **Korean descent:** Practice Tae Kyo, rules for safe childbirth, which lists food taboos. (Choi, 1995)	Obtain a diet history. Discuss need for well-balanced diet during pregnancy. If the dietary practice is not harmful, there is no reason to ask the client to discontinue the practice.
Exercise	**Italian descent:** Fear that moving in certain ways can cause fetal anomalies. (Spector, 2000) **Southeast Asian descent:** Inactivity during pregnancy results in difficult labor. (Mattson, 1995) **European, African, Mexican descent:** Reaching over head during pregnancy can harm the baby.	Obtain exercise history. Ask client if there are activities she is afraid to do because of the pregnancy. Assure her that reaching over her head will not harm the baby. Help her to identify safe forms of activity. Teach need for activity related to general health and weight control.
Home remedies	**Native-American descent:** May use herbal remedies (milky juice from dandelion to increase breast milk). (Spector, 2000) **Chinese descent:** Drink ginseng tea for faintness. Adding bamboo leaves will have sedative effect. **African descent:** Self-medicate for common discomforts of pregnancy (take laxatives to prevent/treat constipation).	Many clients fail to report use of home remedies for fear of being judged unfavorably. When obtaining a health history, ask about home remedies. Teach that some herbs can be harmful when taken with prescribed medication.
Spirituality	**Native-American descent:** May use the "medicine man" to ensure safe birth and healthy baby. Tribal spiritual leaders may be invited by family to attend birth, pray, and perform "ceremonies." Many cultures pay attention to spirituality to lessen fear.	Encourage the use of support systems. Be sensitive to "tribal ceremonies" as long as they do not disrupt others.
Alternate health care providers	Women of many cultures may choose to use alternate health care providers. **Mexican descendants:** May seek care from a partera (midwife). The partera can speak their language, understands the culture, and may deliver the infant in the home or possibly at a birthing center. (Spector, 2000)	Discuss a variety of health care provider choices. Help the client explore the risks and benefits of different prenatal care and delivery settings. Provide reassurance that the goal is a healthy mother and the delivery of a healthy baby with respect for the client's beliefs. *Note:* Some midwives are RNs with advanced education and certification. Others are lay midwives with little or no formal education. During a home delivery, equipment may not be available during an emergency.

significantly reduced after the first delivery (see Chapter 14 ⦿). History of abortion, whether elective or spontaneous, is recorded at this time. Important precautions would be instituted for a woman wanting children who has had a spontaneous abortion in the past (see Chapter 13 ⦿). Review Table 10-1 for the proper terms to use in describing a woman's parous state.

■ Assist with an in-depth physical assessment. *The health care provider will perform a detailed assessment of the reproductive organs. An ultrasound may be done to diagnose pregnancy. Blood may be drawn to determine a baseline for future reference.*

Follow-up Visits

■ Collect data on the woman's vital signs and changes related to pregnancy. Ask about any current concerns or discomforts. Inquire about how the woman and the family are coping with the pregnancy. Provide client teaching related to gestational changes and ways of monitoring the fetus between visits. *Data must be monitored throughout the woman's pregnancy. Client teaching is a regular part of each prenatal visit. Open-ended questions about how the woman and family are responding to the pregnancy allow the woman to bring issues forward for discussion.*

■ Assist or collect data on the fetal heart rate. (See Chapter 9 ⦿.) *Once audible, the FHR is a useful indicator of fetal health.*

■ Inquire about any medications, over-the-counter drugs, herbal remedies, or recreational drugs the woman may be using. Encourage the woman to take prenatal vitamins as prescribed. *The nurse should collect information about all types of drugs and preparations and should report any unusual or potentially harmful drugs to the care provider. Client teaching should include information about safe and unsafe chemicals. (See Box 8-3 ⦿.) Prenatal vitamins help ensure a healthy fetus.*

■ Report a blood pressure increase of 30 mmHg systolic and 20 mmHg diastolic over previous measurement to the health care provider. If a previous blood pressure measurement is not available, report a recording of 140/90. *A rise in BP could indicate pregnancy-induced hypertension.*

■ Track the woman's weight from visit to visit. A total weight gain should be 25 to 35 pounds, with the most rapid weight gain occurring in the last half of the pregnancy. From weeks 1 to 12, the client should gain 3 to 4 pounds. From weeks 13 to 40, she should gain 1 pound per week. *Weight gain less than this could indicate poor nutrition and low fetal growth. A weight gain of more than this could indicate improper nutrition or fluid retention (Figure 10-9 ■).*

■ Measure the height of the fundus in centimeters above the pubis (Figure 10-10 ■). Compare this measurement

to previous measurements and the weeks of gestation. *The fundus should enlarge 1 cm/wk. The fundus not enlarging at this rate would indicate the fetus is not growing at a normal rate. The fundus enlarging more than this rate would indicate the fetus is growing too rapidly or a multiple pregnancy is suspected (see Chapter 13 ⦿).*

■ Monitor for edema. *A small amount of dependent edema is often present in the last few weeks of pregnancy. A large amount of edema in the feet, or edema of the calves, thighs, hands, and face should be reported to the health care provider.*

■ Collect a urine sample at each visit and perform a dipstick test for glucose, protein, and ketone bodies. *A glucose tolerance test might be ordered in the 20th week to determine the presence of gestational diabetes. (Review Table 10-2 for normal lab values during pregnancy.)*

DIAGNOSING, PLANNING, AND IMPLEMENTING

In planning nursing interventions for the prenatal client, the nurse should consider the woman's knowledge, past experiences, behaviors that increase risk, family support system, and socioeconomic status. Most nursing interventions involve teaching or anticipatory guidance. Specific topics and time frame depend on when prenatal care is begun and complications. Nursing diagnoses might include:

■ **A**nxiety
■ Disturbed **B**ody Image
■ **C**onstipation
■ **F**atigue
■ Readiness for Enhanced Family **C**oping
■ **F**ear
■ Deficient **F**luid Volume
■ Imbalanced **F**luid Volume
■ Risk for **I**njury
■ Deficient **K**nowledge (specify)
■ Imbalanced **N**utrition: Less Than Body Requirements
■ Impaired Physical **M**obility
■ **S**exual Dysfunction
■ Disturbed **S**leep Pattern

Some suggested outcomes for clients might include:

■ Client exhibits no signs of fluid excess or fluid deficit.
■ Client verbalizes understanding of teaching.
■ Client verbalizes consuming a balanced diet.
■ Client verbalizes she sleeps for 6 to 8 hours every night.

One of the main functions of the nurse is educating the client and family about the pregnancy process and prenatal care. Topics for client and family teaching are included here.

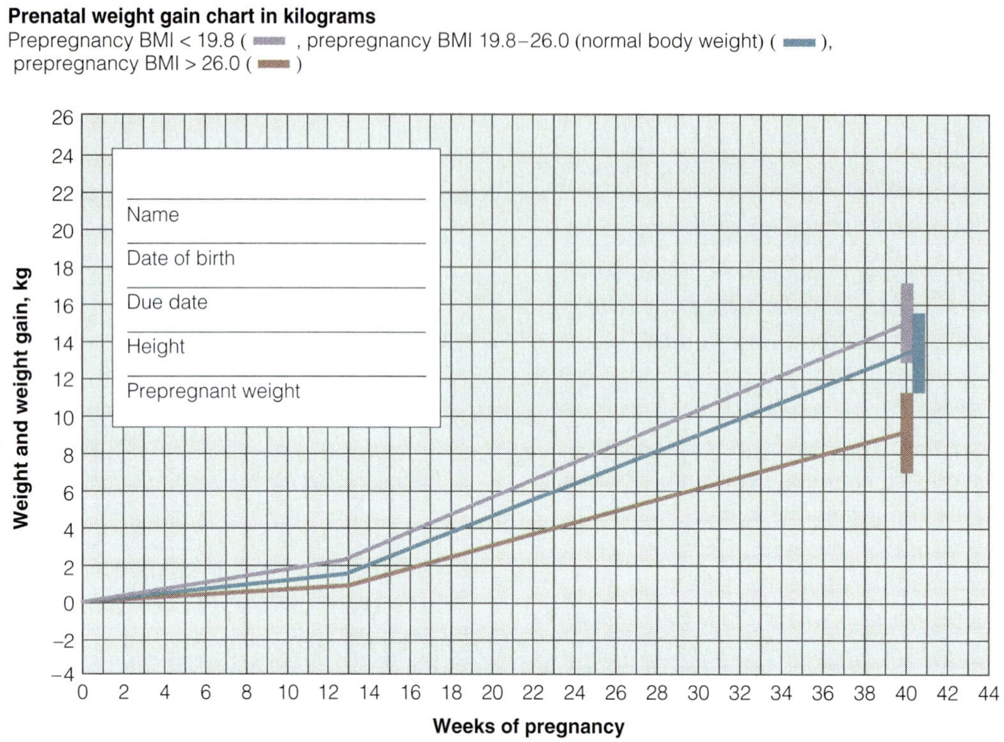

Prenatal weight gain chart in kilograms
Prepregnancy BMI < 19.8 (▬▬▬), prepregnancy BMI 19.8–26.0 (normal body weight) (▬▬▬),
prepregnancy BMI > 26.0 (▬▬▬)

Name
Date of birth
Due date
Height
Prepregnant weight

Weight record

Date	Weeks of gestation	Weight	Notes

Please bring this chart with you to each prenatal visit.

Figure 10-9. ■ Weight gain form shows the typical pattern of weight gain in pregnancy. (From the National Academy of Sciences Institute of Medicine, Subcommittee of Nutritional Status and Weight Gain During Pregnancy. [1992]. *Supplemental materials on nutrition during pregnancy and lactation: An implementation guide.* Washington, DC: National Academy Press.)

- Encourage good nutrition and moderate, regular exercise. Remind the woman to drink plenty of fluids. Provide suggestions for discomforts associated with pregnancy. *Good nutrition and regular exercise can help the woman overcome some of the discomforts of pregnancy (see Box 10-3 and Table 10-3). It is recommended that pregnant women drink 1.5 to 2 liters of fluid per day and that caffeine intake be limited.*

- If necessary, refer the woman to programs that can supply milk and protein. *Some women may not be able to afford the extra high-calcium and high-protein foods that are useful when pregnant. Assistance programs are available to help provide these nutrients.*

- Remind the woman to consult a physician before taking cold, headache, allergy, flu, or other medications or supplements. *Many physicians, nurse midwives, and nurse*

interventions are begun, the better. Giving the woman informa-tion allows her to relax when there are no warning signs and to report them promptly if they should occur. Prompt attention may prevent complications.

Client Self-Care

Self-care generally involves a minimal adjustment of normal habits.

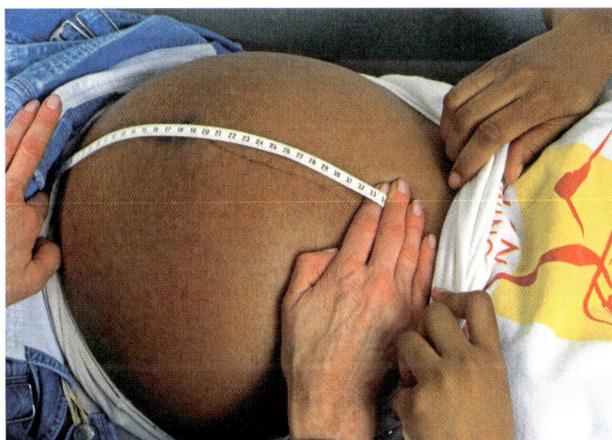

Figure 10-10. ■ (**A**) Height of the fundus during the second trimester at 16, 20, and 24 weeks. (**B**) The height of the fundus is measured at prenatal visits during the third trimester.

practitioners provide their clients with a list of over-the-counter medications that are acceptable to use during pregnancy.

- Review safety hazards for pregnant women and encourage them to take them seriously. Women in late pregnancy are at risk for falls. Exposure to chemicals may harm the fetus. Excessive heat can cause maternal hyperthermia.
- Encourage the client to make and keep regularly scheduled appointments throughout the prenatal period. The pregnant woman should return every 4 weeks for the first 28 weeks, every 2 weeks during weeks 29 to 36, and every week thereafter until delivery.
- Teach the client warning signs of possible complications (see Table 10-4). Discuss signs of impending labor with the client in the third trimester. Usually, the sooner

- Teach the client the importance of personal hygiene during pregnancy. Bathing daily is important due to an increase in perspiration and vaginal secretions. Either a tub bath or shower may be used with warm water. In late pregnancy, the woman may have difficulty rising from a sitting position in the bathtub. Care should be taken to prevent falls in the tub or shower. Douching should be avoided.
- Teach the client to clean the breasts with water, rubbing the nipple with a washcloth, and air-drying the breast. Leakage of fluid from the nipple is common. This fluid should be rubbed into the nipple to lubricate the skin and promote breast health. Clients may benefit from wearing a maternity bra. Prenatal washing and air-drying will toughen breast tissue prior to breastfeeding. A properly fitting maternity bra promotes comfort, supports the enlarged heavy breast, and prevents back strain.
- Encourage continued activity and periods of rest. The pregnant woman should have regular activity. Activities routinely practiced before pregnancy can generally be continued as long as there are no complications and the woman can safely participate. Walking and swimming are best (Figure 10-11 ■), and very strenuous activity should be avoided. Fatigue should be avoided. Periods of rest, with the legs elevated to promote venous return, should be scheduled throughout the day.
- Discuss the importance of clothing for the self-image and comfort during pregnancy. Clothing that is attractive, loose fitting, and easy to care for should be selected. Teach client to avoid using stockings that constrict at knees or thighs and to choose low-heeled shoes for everyday wear. Because maternity clothing is only worn for a short time, clothing may be shared among friends, or secondhand clothing may be purchased at reasonable prices. Knee-high or thigh-high stockings can interfere with circulation. Low-heeled shoes are generally recommended due to the difficulty of maintaining balance in high-heeled shoes.
- Advise women to continue dental care on a regular schedule, but not to have x-rays during pregnancy. The woman should inform her dentist that she is pregnant. Dental care is necessary for ongoing good health. X-ray examinations are postponed until after the pregnancy because of the risk of radiation to the fetus.

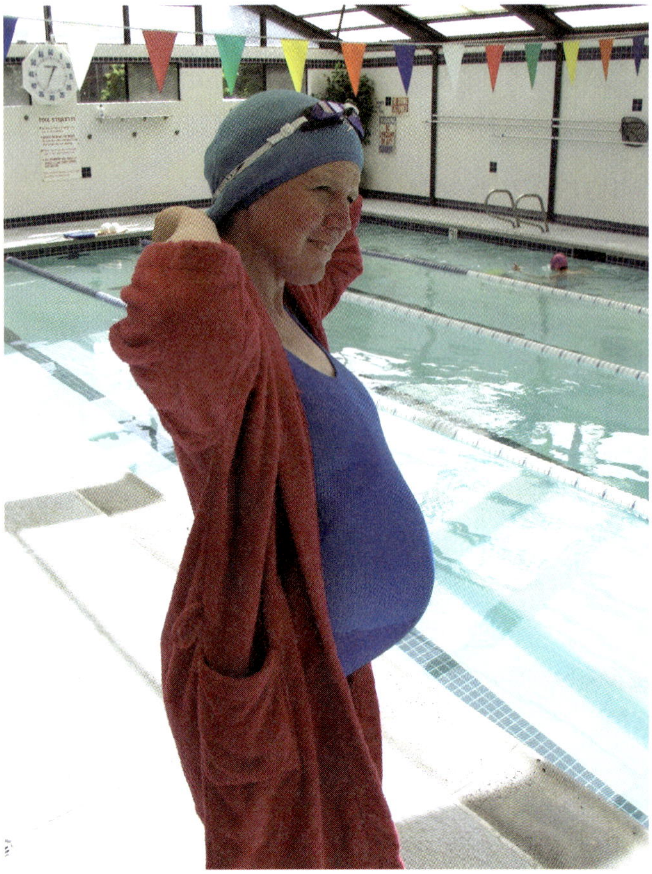

Figure 10-11. ■ Swimming is one of the best exercises during pregnancy. Walking is also recommended as a low-impact, aerobic activity.

- Teach that sexual activities may continue throughout the pregnancy unless there are complications. *There may be a decreased desire for sexual activity during pregnancy. After the 4th month, the woman should not lie flat on her back due to hypotensive syndrome. A pillow can be placed under her right hip or an alternative position can be used.*
- Advise the woman to review the employment environment in terms of her needs while pregnant and to discuss areas of concern with the health care provider. *The decision to continue employment should be based on several factors. Are there hazards in the workplace that would place additional risk on the pregnancy? Would the woman be under undue physical strain? Would periods of rest be available?*
- Discuss effect of pregnancy on travel. *Travel need not be restricted unless complications develop. Generally, the best time to travel is in the second trimester, when the risks of complications are less. Some airlines may not accept passengers past a certain week of pregnancy. When traveling, the woman should walk for about 10 minutes every 2 hours to prevent venous stasis. The seat belt should be worn snuggly, below the abdomen.*

- Encourage the woman to attend childbirth education classes. *Preparation for childbirth usually begins in the third trimester. Many hospitals and birthing centers present childbirth classes. Women should be encouraged to attend these classes so that they will be well prepared mentally as well as physically. Printed resources are also available to assist in childbirth preparation.*

EVALUATING

Clients should be able to verbalize an understanding of the instructions. A change, or lack of change, in client's behavior is also used to evaluate the instruction provided.

Although the majority of pregnancies are completed with a minimum of discomfort, complications can happen at any time. It is the role of the LPN/LVN to assist in data collection and to report any signs of complications. Chapter 13 ∞ describes the most common complications of pregnancy and the related nursing care.

NURSING PROCESS CARE PLAN
Caring for a Pregnant Woman Who Wants to Travel

Mrs. Taylor, expecting her first baby, comes to the clinic for a routine visit. She is 22 weeks pregnant and states she is feeling well, and the baby is becoming very active. She states she would like to go on a trip with her husband in a few weeks. She also states she is getting excited about labor, but is a little scared.

Assessment
- BP 134/72
- Negative protein in urine
- No edema in ankles
- Weight increase by 1 1/2 pounds in last month

Nursing Diagnosis
The following important nursing diagnosis (among others) is established for this client:
- Deficient **K**nowledge related to travel during pregnancy and childbirth

Expected Outcomes
- The mother will verbalize an understanding of travel guidelines, symptoms of complications, and how to access health care.

Planning and Implementation
- Discuss travel at this point of the pregnancy, including need for exercise and fluids. Provide information regarding signs of complications and how to access health care

if needed. *Having information ahead of time will enable the client to travel without undue anxiety.*

■ Provide information regarding childbirth education classes in the area. *The woman may want to continue childbirth education classes if she will be away from home for an extended period of time.*

■ Schedule a return visit to the clinic in 1 month. *The return visit will be an opportunity to determine whether any significant changes have occurred.*

Evaluation

Pregnancy progressing in a normal pattern. Mrs. Taylor should verbalize signs of complications and when to contact health care provider. She should be able to begin childbirth education classes.

Critical Thinking in the Nursing Process

1. What are some other topics that should be discussed with Mrs. Taylor at this point of the pregnancy? (Hint: Think about changing body shape and safety.)
2. What topics should the nurse plan to discuss at the next appointment in 1 month?
3. What is the role of the LPN/LVN in providing care to the pregnant client in a physician's office?

Note: Discussion of Critical Thinking questions appears in Appendix I.

Note: The reference and resource listings for this and all chapters have been compiled at the back of the book.

Chapter Review

KEY TERMS by Topic

Use the audio glossary feature of either the CD-ROM or the Companion Website to hear the correct pronunciation of the following key terms.

Signs of Pregnancy
presumptive signs, amenorrhea, quickening, pseudopregnancy, ballottement, Hegar's sign, Goodell's sign, Chadwick's sign, fetal heart tones, uterine soufflé, funic soufflé

Maternal Changes During Pregnancy
trimester, Braxton-Hicks contractions, colostrum, supine hypotensive syndrome, physiologic anemia of pregnancy, hyperemesis gravidarum, linea nigra, chloasma, striae gravidarum, oxytocin, "let-down reflex"

Initial Visit
gravida, para, abortion, preterm delivery, term delivery, postterm delivery, miscarriage, GP/TPAL, multigravida, multipara, nulligravida, nullipara, para, primigravida, primipara, Naegele's rule

Follow-up Visits
abortifacients

Birthing Facilities and Staff
doula

KEY Points

- Most pregnancies progress as planned. The LPN/LVN is responsible for collecting data and reporting symptoms of complications.

- The key to a healthy pregnancy is regular prenatal care, including client teaching and early detection of complications.

- Nurses have a responsibility to teach good health practices, including nutrition, exercise, and eliminating risky behaviors.

- The nurse must know the signs of pregnancy to anticipate data needing to be collected, client teaching needs, and what equipment the primary care provider will need for diagnostic exams.

- The nurse must teach the client about physical and psychological changes that occur during pregnancy.

- The nurse must teach the client common discomforts of pregnancy and methods of lessening them.

- The nurse must provide client instruction in verbal and written format to ensure client understanding.

FOR FURTHER Study

For additional information on infant and maternal mortality, and for programs that may provide assistance to pregnant women, see Chapter 1.

See Chapter 3 for information on federal assistance programs for women and infants.

For information on the reproductive system, including the let-down reflex, see Chapter 5.

For additional information on potential risks to the developing fetus, see Chapter 8.

Fetal assessment and diagnostic tests are discussed in Chapter 9.

For a complete discussion of nutrition (for the mother and for the neonate), see Chapter 11.

See Chapter 12 for a full discussion of adolescent pregnancy.

For all high-risk pregnancy issues and related nursing care, see Chapter 13.

For a full discussion of normal labor and delivery, see Chapter 14.

For information on infant safety, see Chapters 14 and 17.

EXPLORE MediaLink

Additional interactive resources for this chapter can be found on the Companion Website at www.prenhall.com/towle. Click on Chapter 10 and "Begin" to select the activities for this chapter.

For chapter-related NCLEX®-style questions and an audio glossary, access the accompanying CD-ROM in this book.

Animation
Preeclampsia

Caring for a Woman with an Uncomplicated Pregnancy

NCLEX-PN® Focus Area: Physiologic Integrity

Case Study: Jessica is a 21-year-old, married woman who is 36 weeks pregnant. She has a healthy 2-year-old son at home. Jessica is an elementary school teacher. Classes will end next week for summer break. During a routine prenatal check, Jessica's blood pressure is mildly elevated, she has 1+ ankle edema, and she states she is very tired because she is unable to sleep all night. She gets up every 2 hours to void.

Nursing Diagnosis: Activity Intolerance related to third trimester pregnancy

COLLECT DATA

Subjective	Objective
_____	_____
_____	_____
_____	_____
_____	_____
_____	_____
_____	_____

Would you report this? Yes/No

If yes, to: _____

Nursing Care

_____
_____
_____
_____
_____
_____
_____
_____
_____

How would you document this? _____
_____
_____

Compare your documentation to the sample provided in Appendix I.

Data Collected
(use only those that apply)

- Urine trace for glucose
- Resp 24
- Respiration shallow, slightly labored
- States tired
- 2-year-old son
- Working
- BP 138/76
- Lungs sounds clear
- Not sleeping all night
- Voiding every 2 hours
- FHR 142
- Urine negative for protein

Nursing Interventions
(use only those that apply; list in priority order)

- Teach use and side effects of tocolytic medication.
- Discuss need to get more child care.
- Drink cranberry juice.
- Teach need for additional rest in third trimester.
- Enforce bed rest with bathroom privileges.
- Recommend afternoon naps.
- Discuss the need to quit work.
- Recommend frequent rest periods with feet elevated.

NCLEX-PN® Exam Preparation

1 The nurse, working with a pregnant woman in the last trimester, will advise the woman to sleep on her side mainly to:

1. relieve pressure on the bladder.
2. relieve pressure on the fetus.
3. facilitate sleep.
4. prevent hypotension.

2 You are trying to determine the estimated date of delivery for a client whose last menstrual period began on May 6 and ended on May 11. The estimated date of delivery using Naegele's rule is which of the following dates in February?

1. 6
2. 11
3. 13
4. 18

3 A 17-year-old single woman is 12 weeks pregnant. She says to the nurse, "I don't want to be pregnant. How can I take care of a baby and still do all the things I want?" The nurse should reply:

1. "I can make you an appointment for an abortion."
2. "You should have thought about that before you had unprotected sex."
3. "How can I help you problem solve what will be best for you to do?"
4. "You should contact a lawyer who handles adoption."

4 A woman 32 weeks pregnant comes to the office stating that the baby has not been moving as much as usual. All of the following must be assessed. Place them in priority order.

1. Report findings to the doctor.
2. Take her vital signs.
3. Measure her weight.
4. Listen to the FHT.
5. Check her urine for glucose and protein.

5 During a physical examination, a client states that she is pregnant. Which of the following data collected during the exam would be considered probable signs of pregnancy? Select all that apply.

1. uterine soufflé
2. Chadwick's sign
3. abdominal enlargement
4. ballottement
5. positive pregnancy test
6. amenorrhea

6 The nurse is measuring the fundus of a client who is 14 weeks' gestation and documents fundal height to be 14 cm. At the next appointment, the nurse would expect her fundus to measure:

1. 16 cm.
2. 18 cm.
3. 20 cm.
4. 22 cm.

7 Prepregnant vital signs for a client includes: temp: 98.8 F, pulse: 115, respirations: 12, and BP: 116/78. Which of the following current set of vital signs assessed during the second trimester should the LPN/LVN report to the charge nurse?

1. Temp: 98.0 F
2. Pulse: 130 bpm
3. Respirations: 14 per minute
4. BP: 136/88

8 A pregnant client states she had a boy at 40 weeks' gestation and a girl at 38 weeks' gestation. The nurse documents this as:

1. G3P2/T2A0.
2. G2P2/T2A0.
3. G2P1/T1A0.
4. G3P1/T1A0.

9 The nurse is discussing interventions with a client complaining of varicose veins. Which of the following statements made by the client requires further teaching?

1. "I will decrease intake of foods high in sodium."
2. "When I am sitting, I will not cross my legs."
3. "I will start wearing support hose."
4. "After work, I will elevate my feet and rest."

10 A pregnant client states that maternity clothing is not necessary. Which of the following recommendations should the nurse advise the client to include when selecting clothing?

1. Select comfortable shoes with heels.
2. Wear a loose-fitting bra.
3. Avoid knee high stockings.
4. Wear firm fitting pants.

Answers for NCLEX-PN® Review and Critical Thinking questions appear in Appendix I.

Chapter 11

Prenatal, Postpartum, and Neonatal Nutrition

BRIEF Outline

Nutrients
Nutrition Before Pregnancy
Nutrition During Pregnancy
Nutrition During the Postpartum Period

Nutrition During the Newborn Period
Nursing Care

LEARNING Outcomes

After completing this chapter, you will be able to:

1. Define key terms.
2. Describe each nutrient and its normal function within the body.
3. Describe the need for adequate nutrition before pregnancy occurs.
4. Describe the changes in nutritional requirements during pregnancy and lactation.
5. Describe nutritional requirements of the newborn.
6. Provide instruction to the mother on breastfeeding or bottle-feeding techniques.

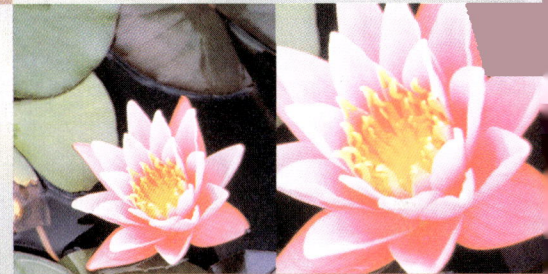

NURSING CARE PLAN CHART: Planning for a Client with Hyperemesis Gravidarum

HEALTH PROMOTION ISSUE: Folic Acid Intake and Pregnancy

NURSING PROCESS CARE PLAN: Client Wanting to Breastfeed

CRITICAL THINKING CARE MAP: Caring for an Undernourished Pregnant Woman

Nutrition is a vital part of a healthy life before pregnancy. During pregnancy adequate nutrients are needed to supply the needs of the mother and growing fetus. Good nutrition provides crucial ingredients to supply the needs of the growing newborn. Good nutrition is also important for the mother in order for her to lose weight, replenish nutrient stores, and provide breast milk. To provide nutrition teaching to the woman during pregnancy and following delivery, the nurse needs to understand the importance of each nutrient and the common food sources. This chapter will begin with a review of the nutrients, and then will address nutrition for the pregnant or lactating mother and for the newborn.

Nutrients

CARBOHYDRATES

Carbohydrates include simple carbohydrates (sugars) and complex carbohydrates (starches and fiber). Simple sugars are described as **monosaccharides,** a single sugar, or **disaccharides,** sugar composed of pairs of monosaccharides. Complex carbohydrates are described as **polysaccharides** or large compounds composed of chains of monosaccharides.

Three monosaccharides important in nutrition are glucose, fructose, and galactose. Commonly known as blood sugar, **glucose** serves as the major source of energy for all body activities. Glucose is the basis of the common disaccharides and the polysaccharides. Through digestion and metabolism, the chemical bonds in disaccharides and polysaccharides are broken and glucose is released. **Fructose,** found naturally in fruits and honey, is the sweetest of the simple sugars. Because it stimulates the taste buds to produce the sweet taste, fructose is commonly used in soft drinks, cereals, and desserts that have been sweetened with corn syrup. **Galactose,** seldom occurring free in nature, combines with glucose in milk.

Disaccharides are pairs of the three monosaccharides. When two units of glucose combine, the result is **maltose.** Maltose, found in a few plants, is the result of the fermentation process that yields alcohol. **Sucrose** is a combination of glucose and fructose. Because of the natural sweetness, the juices of sugarcane and sugar beets are refined into table sugar. The principal sugar in milk, **lactose,** is made from glucose and galactose.

Three polysaccharides are important in nutrition: glycogen, starches, and fiber. In animals, energy is stored as glycogen. To release the glucose, a hormone message must be received at the storage sites and enzymes must break the complex chemical bonds. Glycogen stored in meat is not a significant source of rapid energy.

Plants store glucose as starch, long chains of glucose molecules. These long chains are packaged side-by-side in grains such as wheat, corn, and rice; in tubers such as yams and potatoes; and in legumes such as peas and beans. Through digestion, the long strands of starch are broken and glucose is released for energy.

Nonstarch polysaccharides are found in food in the form of plant fiber. Fiber makes up the structure of plants such as stems, roots, leaves, and skins of fruit. Nonstarch polysaccharides also include cellulose, pectins, gums, and mucilages that make up the pulp of fruit.

Carbohydrate digestion begins in the mouth through the action of the salivary enzyme amylase. Because gastric acid inactivates salivary amylase, further digestion does not take place until the food enters the small intestine. The pancreatic amylase continues to break down complex carbohydrates. Maltase, sucrase, and lactase (found in intestinal enzymes) complete the process. Simple sugars are absorbed into the blood. Fiber in the large intestine attracts water to soften the stool for easy passage.

PROTEINS

Proteins are substances made up of about 20 amino acids. Proteins are required for cell growth and repair. Over half of the amino acids can be made by the human body. They are considered **nonessential amino acids;** that is, they do not need to be included in the diet because the body can create them. There are nine amino acids that the body cannot make or cannot make in sufficient quantities. These amino acids must be included in the diet and are therefore considered to be **essential amino acids.** In some circumstances, nonessential amino acids become **conditionally essential amino acids.** For example, the body uses the essential amino acid phenylalanine to make the nonessential amino acid tyrosine. If the diet does not supply enough phenylalanine or if the body cannot make tyrosine (as happens in the inherited disease *phenylketonuria*), then tyrosine becomes, conditionally essential. Within cells, amino acids are linked together to form proteins. The distinctive sequence of the amino acids in each protein determines its function.

Large clumps of proteins (such as meat) are mechanically broken into smaller pieces by chewing. However, the chemical digestion of protein begins in the stomach. Hydrochloric acid and the enzyme *pepsin* break down pieces of protein into smaller pieces called *polypeptides*, releasing some amino acids from the large clumps of protein. The food mass (chyme) moves into the small intestine where the pancreatic enzyme *protease* and the intestinal enzyme *peptidase* complete the digestive process. The amino acids are absorbed into the blood.

LIPIDS

Lipids (often called fats) are made up of triglycerides (fats and oils), phospholipids, and sterols. Of these lipids, triglycerides predominate in foods and in the body.

Triglycerides contain one molecule of glycerol and three fatty acids. Fatty acids can carry a varying amount of hydrogen. If the fatty acid is carrying the maximum amount of hydrogen, it is **saturated.** An **unsaturated** fatty acid is one that does not carry the maximum amount of hydrogen, resulting in a double bond between two carbon atoms. There are varying degrees of unsaturation. If the fatty acid has only one double carbon bond, it is a **monounsaturated** fatty acid. A **polyunsaturated** fatty acid has two or more double carbon bonds. Chemists, identifying polyunsaturated fatty acids by the location of the double carbon bonds, describe the fatty acid by an omega number. An *omega-3 fatty acid*, for example, has its first double bond three carbon atoms away from the end of the acid chain.

The degree of unsaturation determines the firmness of fats at room temperature. Generally, polyunsaturated vegetable oils are more liquid than the more saturated animal fats. Some margarines are less saturated (less firm) than the more saturated (firmer) butter. Some vegetable oils, such as cocoa butter, palm oil, and coconut oil, are saturated. Because they have shorter carbon chains, they are softer than most animal fats.

Saturation also affects the shelf life or stability of the fat. When exposed to oxygen, all fats become rancid. Saturated fats cannot bond easily to oxygen, so they are less likely to become rancid. Manufacturers can protect unsaturated fats from becoming rancid in three ways. First, products can be sealed air-tight and refrigerated, which is expensive and inconvenient. Second, manufacturers can add antioxidants to compete with oxygen and protect the oil. Examples of antioxidants are vitamins C and E. Third, manufacturers can add hydrogen (hydrogenation) to saturate the double bond points. Hydrogenation prolongs shelf life and alters the texture of foods. Because hydrogenation results in saturation, the health benefit of polyunsaturated fats is lost. Another disadvantage of hydrogenation is the hydrogen changes the configuration of the fatty acid resulting in **trans fats** (*trans-fatty acids*). The relationship between trans-fatty acids and heart disease has been the subject of recent research.

The effects of trans fats on health are worse than natural fat, including saturated fats. Natural fats found in butter, cheese, and beef raise total cholesterol. Trans fats however, not only contribute to the total cholesterol levels but also cause a drop in the healthy HDL cholesterol. Over time, trans fats clog the arteries of the heart and brain. Trans fats double the risk of heart disease in women. Children who begin eating trans fats in fast food, toaster pastries, microwave popcorn, cookies, and prepared fish sticks can be expected to get heart disease at an earlier age than children who eat foods without trans fats.

Like triglycerides, phospholipids contain fatty acids, but they also contain a phosphate group of molecules. In the body, phospholipids are constituents of cell membranes. They serve an important function by helping lipids and fat-soluble substances (vitamins and hormones) move into and out of the cell. Phospholipids also act as emulsifiers, helping fats stay suspended in blood and body fluids.

Lipids contain sterols, a compound with a multi-ring structure. The most famous sterol is cholesterol. Dietary sterols come from both plants and animals, but cholesterol only comes from animal fats, such as meat, milk, poultry, and eggs. The body makes many valuable substances from sterols, including bile acids, sex hormones, adrenal hormones, vitamin D, and cell membranes. Over 90% of cholesterol is found inside cells.

Not all of the body's cholesterol comes from dietary sources. The liver manufactures more cholesterol from carbohydrates, proteins, and fats than is eaten in a day. Some dietary cholesterol becomes bound to fiber and is eliminated in the feces.

Lipid digestion begins in the mouth as some firm triglycerides begin to melt at body temperature. Lingual lipase, found in saliva, plays a role in beginning digestion of milk fat, especially in infants. Only a little fat digestion takes place in the stomach. The churning action of the stomach muscles prevents the fat from floating to the top of the chyme. When fat enters the small intestine, bile is released from the gall bladder. Bile emulsifies fats, breaking large fat molecules into smaller fat molecules. Lipase from the pancreas and the small intestine complete the process of fat digestion. Fatty acids, phospholipids, and sterol are absorbed into the blood through the lymphatic system.

VITAMINS

Vitamins are organic compounds that are essential in small amounts to perform specific functions within the body. Deficiency in any of the vitamins can have devastating consequences. For example, blindness can result from vitamin A deficiency, retarded bone growth can be caused by vitamin D deficiency, and birth defects can result from lack of the B vitamin folic acid. Much of the credit given to low-fat diets in preventing disease belongs to the vitamins found in diets rich in vegetables, fruits, and whole grains. Vitamins also promote normal body functions, such as supporting a strong immune system. Table 11-1 ■ provides a summary of vitamins and minerals and their food sources.

TABLE 11-1

Vitamins and Minerals: Functions and Food Sources

VITAMIN/MINERAL	FUNCTION	FOOD SOURCES
Vitamin A	Antioxidant: protects brain and body from toxins	Animal foods (as retinal): dairy, meat, fish, eggs Plant foods (as beta-carotene): fruits and vegetables
Vitamin C	Antioxidant: protects brain and body from toxins—helps with iron absorption	Fruits: citrus, kiwi, berries Vegetables: green vegetables, tomatoes, bell peppers
Vitamin E	Antioxidant: protects brain and body from toxins	Nuts, seeds, and various oils
B vitamins	Essential for brain function, healthy nervous system, and energy metabolism	Whole grains, brown rice, green vegetables, eggs, meat, fish, legumes, nuts, seeds
Calcium	Relax nerve and muscle cells	Dairy products, almonds, green leafy vegetables, apricots, sardines
Magnesium	Relax nerve and muscle cells	Whole grains, nuts, soybeans, green leafy vegetables, meat
Choline (vitamin-like compound)	Helps in the process of conducting electrical impulses to brain and nervous system	Sardines, egg yolk, nuts, legumes, grains
Zinc	Memory and brain function, helps produce serotonin	Shellfish, whole grains, beans, turkey meat (dark)
Iron	Carries oxygen in blood	Red meat, eggs, parsley, cocoa
Chromium	Helps control blood glucose levels	Cheese, red meat, seafood, whole grains, eggs

Vitamins are divided into two categories based on their solubility: water-soluble or fat-soluble vitamins. (Fat-soluble vitamins are discussed below.)

Water-Soluble Vitamins

As the name implies, **water-soluble vitamins** dissolve in and are transported in water. Water-soluble vitamins can be found in all water-filled compartments within the body. When the blood level of water-soluble vitamins rises, small excesses are readily excreted in the urine. Large excesses may overwhelm the kidneys, resulting in adverse effects. Because they are excreted to some extent daily, water-soluble vitamins must be replenished in the diet. The water-soluble vitamins are vitamin C and the B vitamin complex, which is made up of eight separate vitamins.

VITAMIN C. Vitamin C, or *ascorbic acid*, becomes a cofactor in helping enzymes in some settings and as an antioxidant in other settings. As a cofactor, vitamin C helps to form the connective tissue, collagen. Collagen forms a matrix on which bones and teeth are formed, "glues" separated tissue together forming scars, and holds cells together preventing tissue breakdown. This action is especially important in blood vessels because they expand and contract with each pulse and must withstand the pressure of the blood without giving way.

To understand the function of vitamin C as an antioxidant, a brief review of oxidation is necessary. The body uses oxygen in metabolic reactions, sometimes producing highly unstable molecules known as **free radicals.** These free radicals lack an atomic particle called an electron. Free radicals steal an electron from a neighboring molecule. The molecule that loses the electron becomes a free radical, beginning a chain reaction of damage to molecules. Occasionally, free radicals are helpful. For example, cells of the immune system use free radicals to destroy disease-causing viruses and bacteria. Most often, however, free radicals damage polyunsaturated fatty acids and lipoproteins in cell membranes and disrupt the free movement of substances into and out of the cell. The body's defenses try to repair the damage of free radicals, but these defense systems become less effective with age, resulting in **oxidative stress.** Dietary antioxidants defend the body against oxidative stress. Vitamin C sacrifices its electrons to neutralize free radicals. In the intestine, vitamin C enhances the absorption of iron by protecting iron from oxidation.

Fruits and vegetables provide generous amounts of vitamin C. Citrus fruits are famous for having vitamin C, but other fruits and vegetables such as broccoli, bell peppers, strawberries, and potatoes are also good sources. Because vitamin C can be damaged by heat, raw fruits and vegetables are higher in nutrient value.

B VITAMINS. The eight B vitamins play a critical role in the functioning of the body. Because of the interdependent nature of the B vitamins, it is difficult to tell which vitamin is responsible for an effect. Contrary to advertising claims, the B vitamins do not provide the body with energy. Energy comes from carbohydrates, proteins, and fats. The B vitamins help the body make use of the energy. For example, thiamin, riboflavin, niacin, pantothenic acid, and biotin form part of coenzymes that assist in the release of energy from carbohydrates, fats, and protein. This section will discuss each of the B vitamins separately, but with an understanding that they all work in concert.

Thiamin.   Thiamin plays two important roles in the body. First, thiamin is part of thiamin pyrophosphate (TPP), a coenzyme that is pivotal in the energy metabolism in all cells. Second, thiamin is found on the cell membrane of nerve cells. Inadequate thiamin intake occurs most commonly in malnourished people, including the homeless and those who have a high intake of empty calories like alcohol. Thiamin deficiency results in **beriberi**, a disease that damages the nervous system, heart, and other muscles. Thiamin is found in a variety of food groups, including whole grains, green vegetables, legumes, and meat. Pork is especially rich in thiamin.

Riboflavin.   **Riboflavin** serves as a coenzyme in many chemical reactions, especially the release of energy from nutrients inside cells. In the United States, riboflavin deficiency is rare. Although riboflavin is found in all food groups, several servings of milk and milk products would meet daily requirements.

Niacin.   **Niacin** is found in coenzymes that are needed to metabolize glucose, fat, and alcohol. The body can make niacin from the amino acid tryptophan. Niacin deficiency is called **pellagra,** which causes diarrhea, dermatitis, dementia, and death. Foods from the meat group are the richest in niacin. Because the body can make niacin from tryptophan, an essential amino acid found in animal and fish protein, diets high in animal protein are not lacking in niacin.

Biotin.   **Biotin,** a coenzyme in metabolism, is crucial in the synthesis of glucose from noncarbohydrate sources (such as amino acids and glycerol), in the synthesis of fatty acids, and in the breakdown of some amino acids. Biotin is needed in very small amounts and is found in a wide variety of foods. Therefore, deficiency rarely occurs.

Pantothenic Acid.   Pantothenic acid is involved in numerous steps in the synthesis of lipids, neurotransmitters, steroids, and hemoglobin. Pantothenic acid is found in a wide variety of foods, but it is easily destroyed by freezing, canning, and refining processes.

Vitamin B_6.   Vitamin B_6 occurs in three forms: pyridoxal, pyridoxine, and pyridoxamine. All three are converted to a coenzyme that is active in amino acid metabolism. Vitamin B_6 influences thought processes, immune function, and steroid hormone activity. Unlike other water-soluble vitamins, vitamin B_6 is stored in muscle tissue. Some drugs, including alcohol and INH (used to treat tuberculosis), destroy vitamin B_6. Without adequate vitamin B_6, the production of key neurotransmitters decreases, and abnormal compounds accumulate in the brain. Initially, vitamin B_6 deficiency causes depression and confusion, but eventually it can lead to seizures. A variety of foods including yellow and green vegetables, yellow and red fruits, and red meat are rich in vitamin B_6.

clinical ALERT

Some women take high doses of vitamin B_6 in an attempt to treat premenstrual syndrome (PMS). Other people take vitamin B_6 to cure carpal tunnel syndrome or sleep disorders. No evidence suggests that these treatments are effective. Neurologic damage can result from high doses of vitamin B_6. It is important that the upper levels of RDA not be exceeded without approval from the primary care provider.

Folic Acid.   **Folic acid,** also know as *folate* and *folacin,* helps synthesize DNA required for all rapidly growing cells. For folic acid to function properly, an adequate amount of vitamin B_{12} must be present. The liver excretes any excess folic acid into the bile. Folic acid can then be reabsorbed in the gastrointestinal system. Folic acid deficiency prevents cell division and protein synthesis, which is critical to growing tissue. Many foods contain folic acid. Dark green vegetables, dried beans, and fortified cereals are especially rich in folic acid.

Vitamin B_{12}.   Vitamin B_{12} and folic acid are closely related because they depend on each other for activation. Vitamin B_{12} is released from food by the action of hydrochloric acid and pepsin in the stomach. Intrinsic factor, produced in the stomach lining, binds with vitamin B_{12} for transport to the small intestine, where absorption takes place. If the stomach is unable to produce adequate amounts of intrinsic factor, vitamin B_{12} will not be absorbed.

Because folic acid and vitamin B_{12} are required for normal cell division in rapidly growing cells, a deficiency of one or both vitamins generally results in anemia. There may be a connection between deficiency of folic acid and vitamin B_{12} and chronic diseases. For example, maternal anemia during the critical period of placenta formation alters the pattern of blood vessel growth that may affect the cardiovascular formation in the fetus. Vascular malformation in the brain may not become apparent until the blood vessel ruptures, resulting in a cerebral hemorrhage and stroke.

Fat-Soluble Vitamins

The **fat-soluble vitamins** differ from water-soluble vitamins in several ways. Fat-soluble vitamins require bile for their absorption from the small intestine. Fat-soluble vitamins are transported through the lymphatic system before entering the bloodstream. Excess fat-soluble vitamins are stored in the liver and adipose tissue. Because the body can retrieve fat-soluble vitamins from storage, individuals can eat less than their daily requirement. The fat-soluble vitamins are A, D, E, and K.

VITAMIN A. Vitamin A and its precursor, **beta-carotene,** have diverse roles in the body. A precursor is a chemical that can be converted into an active vitamin. Three forms of vitamin A are active in the body: retinol, retinal, and retinoic acid. Foods from animals are easily changed to retinol in the intestine. Foods from plants provide carotenoids, which can be changed to retinol in the intestine and liver. Beta-carotene, the orange pigment in plants, is the carotenoid with the greatest vitamin A activity.

Vitamin A has three major roles in the body. Retinal is needed for vision and in the conversion of retinol to retinoic acid. In the eye, vitamin A helps maintain a clear cornea. Vitamin A participates in the conversion of light energy to nerve impulses in the retina. Retinol is needed for sperm production and cell growth, both in fetal development and in growing children. Most of the vitamin A is in the form of retinoic acid, which acts as a hormone, regulating cell differentiation, cell growth, and protein synthesis. Not all of the beta-carotene that is consumed in foods is converted to vitamin A. Some beta-carotene is used as an antioxidant.

Vitamin A is found in large quantities in organ meat (such as liver), fish, eggs, and milk products. Because vitamin A is fat soluble, some is lost when skim milk is used. Dark green leafy vegetables, such as spinach and broccoli, and deep yellow and orange fruits and vegetables, such as winter squash, cantaloupe, carrots, and sweet potatoes, also have a high content of beta-carotene. Although liver is an excellent source of many nutrients, symptoms of toxic levels of vitamin A have been reported when too much liver is eaten. One ounce of beef liver contains more than three times the RDA for vitamin A.

VITAMIN D (CALCIFEROL). Vitamin D (calciferol) is different from other nutrients, in that the body can make vitamin D with the help of sunshine. When ultraviolet light from the sun strikes precursor chemicals in the skin, previtamin D_3 is made. Over the next 36 to 38 hours, vitamin D_3 becomes activated by body heat. Whether vitamin D_3 is made in the body or obtained in the diet, the liver and kidneys add important oxygen and hydrogen elements (OH group) for the vitamin D to be fully activated.

Vitamin D plays a role in bone growth and health by maintaining blood concentration of calcium and phosphorus. Vitamin D does not work alone but in cooperation with parathyroid hormone and calcitonin. Vitamin D enhances the absorption of calcium and phosphorus from the intestine, the reabsorption of these minerals from the kidney, and their movement from the bone to the blood.

Vitamin D deficiency can result in three major bone disorders. Without adequate amounts of vitamin D in childhood, the bones fail to calcify properly, leading to soft, easily bendable bones. This disease is called **rickets. Osteomalacia** is softening of the bones in adults, most often in young women who had low intake of vitamin D and calcium and who had repeated pregnancies and lactation. Figure 11-1 ■ illustrates rickets and osteomalacia. At times, women have healthy bones until after menopause when calcium is lost from the bones because of a decrease in estrogen. **Osteoporosis** can develop, resulting in brittle bones that break easily.

Scientists are discovering other vitamin D target tissues, including the brain, nervous system, skin, muscles, and many cancer cells. Continued research may discover other health disorders that can be treated with vitamin D.

VITAMIN E. Vitamin E is a fat-soluble antioxidant. Its main action is to stop the chain reaction of free radicals. Vitamin E, therefore, protects cell membranes from destruction. Vitamin E may reduce the risk of heart disease by protecting low density lipoproteins (LDL) from oxidation. Research has proved that vitamin E does not improve physical performance, prevent sexual dysfunction in men, slow the aging process, or slow Parkinson's disease.

Vitamin E deficiency from poor oral intake is rare. Without vitamin E, red blood cells break. Known as **erythrocyte hemolysis,** this condition is seen in premature infants because the transfer of vitamin E from the mother takes place in the last few weeks of pregnancy. Erythrocyte hemolysis corrects with vitamin E treatment. Two other disorders—nonmalignant breast disease and intermittent claudication (cramping in the legs due to decreased circulation)—seem to respond to vitamin E treatment, but with inconsistent results.

Vitamin E is found in a variety of foods, predominantly in vegetable oils, seeds, and nuts. Vitamin E is easily destroyed by heating, so cooking with vegetable oil is not an effective food source.

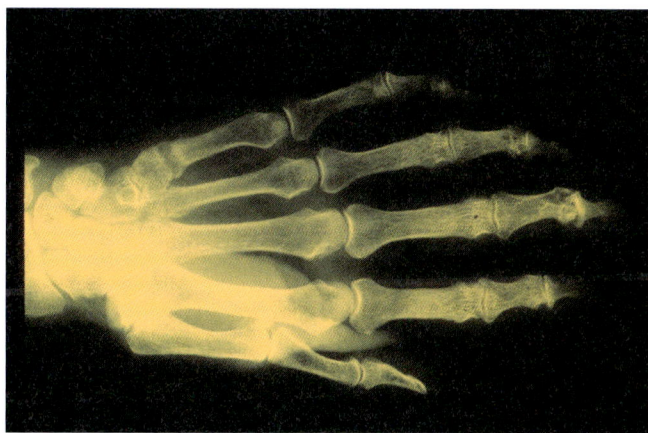

A

B

Figure 11-1. ■ Effects of specific vitamin deficiencies. (**A**) Rickets in an infant. The legs bow out at the knees. (**B**) Osteomalacia.

VITAMIN K.   Vitamin K, like vitamin D, is produced in the body. Vitamin K, made by bacteria in the intestinal tract, is essential in the blood clotting process. Without vitamin K, even a small pinprick would cause life-threatening hemorrhage. The body produces only half of the amount required. The other half must be provided from foods rich in vitamin K, such as liver and dark green, leafy vegetables. Other meats, eggs, cereals, fruits, and vegetables provide smaller, but significant, amounts of vitamin K.

Primary vitamin K deficiency is rare, but it can occur secondarily to other conditions. When bile secretion decreases, vitamin K absorption declines. Some antibiotics can kill the bacteria required for vitamin K synthesis.

Anticoagulant therapy interferes with vitamin K metabolism and activity. Newborn infants are unable to make vitamin K, because they are born with a sterile intestinal tract. Vitamin K–producing bacteria take several weeks to establish themselves. Vitamin K is routinely administered to the newborn infant shortly after birth.

MAJOR MINERALS

Minerals play an important role in fluid balance, nerve/muscle conduction, and strong bones and teeth. The major minerals, those that are required in large amounts, will be discussed here.

Sodium

Sodium, found primarily in the extracellular fluid, is the primary regulator of fluid balance. Sodium is also an important factor in acid–base balance by the kidney. Sodium is essential in nerve transmission and muscle contractions. The body loses sodium through perspiration, vomiting, and diarrhea, and replacement may be required. However, because foods contain more sodium than the body requires, more often individuals need to decrease their sodium intake. Too much sodium can lead to hypertension, renal failure, and heart disease.

Potassium

Potassium is primarily an intracellular element. Potassium plays a major role in fluid and electrolyte balance. During nerve transmission and muscle contraction, sodium and potassium briefly trade places. If normal levels of potassium and sodium are not maintained, the heart cannot contract normally and death could occur. Like sodium, potassium loss occurs through prolonged vomiting and diarrhea. Fresh fruits and vegetables provide an abundance of potassium.

Chloride

Chloride is found in conjunction with both sodium and potassium. It assists with fluid and electrolyte and acid–base balance. Chloride is abundant in foods, and diets rarely lack this essential mineral.

Calcium

Calcium is not only essential for strong bones and teeth, but also necessary for the regulation of muscle contraction, the transmission of nerve impulses, the clotting of blood, and the secretion of hormones. Calcium balance is regulated by both the thyroid and parathyroid glands. Recall that vitamin D is required for the absorption of calcium from the gastrointestinal tract. Although milk products are the richest source of calcium, green leafy vegetables, fruits, and legumes are also important sources of calcium.

Phosphorus

Phosphorus is most often bound to calcium in bones and teeth. Phosphorus is part of the DNA and RNA molecules and therefore is vital to normal cell function and growth. Diets that are adequate in protein also supply adequate amounts of phosphorus.

Magnesium

Magnesium is found in bones, muscles, and soft tissue. Magnesium is necessary for energy metabolism. Magnesium, together with calcium, is needed for muscle contraction and blood clotting. It is estimated that most adults fall below the daily recommendations, but they rarely exhibit symptoms of deficiency. In areas where the drinking water is "hard," individuals may get a significant amount of magnesium and calcium from water.

Iron

Iron is not considered a major mineral because of the daily requirement, but it is an essential nutrient. Iron is found in the proteins hemoglobin in red blood cells and myoglobin in muscle cells. Iron is primarily responsible for carrying and releasing oxygen. Iron is also used by the enzymes involved in making amino acids, collagen, hormones, and neurotransmitters. Red blood cells live approximately 4 months and then are destroyed by the liver and spleen. The iron is salvaged, transported to the bone marrow, and reused in making new red blood cells. A small amount of iron is lost daily through the GI tract and if bleeding occurs.

Iron deficiency is the most common nutrient deficiency. Without an adequate supply of iron, red blood cells lack hemoglobin, the oxygen-carrying molecule. The result is iron-deficiency anemia. Without oxygen, all cells are unable to metabolize glucose.

Some stages of life demand more iron. For example, during the reproductive years, women require additional iron because of blood loss with menstruation. The pregnant woman requires additional iron to meet her needs of increased red blood cells to support the growth of the fetus and in preparation for blood loss during delivery. Infants and young children require iron to support their rapid growth, but their high-milk diets are generally poor in iron.

During the childbearing years, women need 18 milligrams of iron a day. Their diet supplies 6 to 7 milligrams per 1,000 kcalories, or 12 to 13 milligrams of iron. Meat, fish, and poultry supply the most iron. Legumes, dark green, leafy vegetables such as spinach, and eggs are also good sources of iron. Adding fruit and vegetables rich in vitamin C is essential in the absorption of iron from the diet.

WATER

Water is needed to transport nutrients in the blood, to transfer nutrients through the interstitial space into cells, and to eliminate waste products. Water participates in most metabolic reactions, acts as a lubricant, and regulates body temperature. Water is the most essential nutrient in that humans can only survive a few days without water. They can survive weeks without food.

Although water is lost in small amounts through skin, respirations, and feces, water is lost mainly through the kidneys. Water volume is regulated in part by two hormones: antidiuretic hormone from the pituitary gland and aldosterone from the adrenal glands. Because the minerals sodium, potassium, and chloride are readily dissolved in water, fluid imbalance also affects these important minerals. Although the body can conserve water by decreasing urinary output, a daily intake of water is essential.

Nutrition Before Pregnancy

Nutrition before pregnancy plays an important role in a healthy lifestyle. Table 11-2 ■ shows amounts of healthful

TABLE 11-2

Daily Food Recommendations vs. Foods Consumed

| FOOD GROUP | DAILY FOOD RECOMMENDATIONS | | AVERAGE AMOUNT CONSUMED | |
	FEMALES 31–50	MALES 31–50	FEMALES 31–50	MALES 31–50
Fruits	1.5 cups	2 cups	0.8 cups	0.8 cups
Vegetables	2.5 cups	3 cups	1.6 cups	2.1 cups
Grains	6 oz eq	7 oz eq	5.9 oz eq	8.0 oz eq
Meat and beans	5 oz eq	6 oz eq	4.6 oz eq	7.4 oz eq
Milk	3 cups	3 cups	1.4 cups	1.8 cups

Consumption data is based on National Health and Nutrition Examination Survey 01–02 data.

foods that should be consumed versus what is commonly consumed per day. The young woman must consume adequate amounts of all nutrients in order for her tissues and body systems to function normally. She also needs to store adequate amounts of nutrients to support a developing fetus should pregnancy occur. (Review Box 8-2 ⚭ for specific nutritional information related to fetal development and Chapter 6 ⚭ for nutrition and overall health.) Although all nutrients are important, inadequate amounts of folic acid and iron can have a devastating impact on the developing fetus even before the woman knows she is pregnant. (See Health Promotion Issue on pages 242 and 243 for a discussion of the importance of folic acid.)

Nutrition During Pregnancy

If the woman is already eating a well-balanced diet, she will not need to make major changes during pregnancy. During pregnancy, the woman should add 300 kcalories a day to her diet. The addition of two milk servings and one serving of meat will meet the need for increased calories as well as calcium and protein. Steady weight gain through the second and third trimester is expected (Figure 11-2 ■).

Many women, however, do not eat a well-balanced diet prior to or during pregnancy. Malnutrition during pregnancy can result in devastating, life-long complications in the baby. For example, malnutrition during a critical period of pancreatic cell growth may result in the development of diabetes in adulthood. Pancreatic cells increase over a hundred fold between the 12th week of gestation and 5 months after birth. Infants who have suffered malnutrition during this time have significantly fewer pancreatic beta cells. There may not be enough beta cells to produce adequate insulin during times of overnutrition later in life.

If the mother does not have enough iron, her red blood cells and the red blood cells of the fetus will be unable to carry adequate amounts of oxygen to perfuse all tissues. Menstruation stops during pregnancy, and absorption in the intestinal tract increases. However, the mother's blood volume and the number of red blood cells increase during pregnancy in preparation for blood loss during delivery. The developing fetus requires iron for red blood cell formation and to store for use during the first 6 months of life when the diet of milk may be low in iron.

Some women are vegetarians and need to seek other alternatives for protein. The nurse must provide these women with more in-depth information or refer them to a dietitian. Many health care providers prescribe a daily

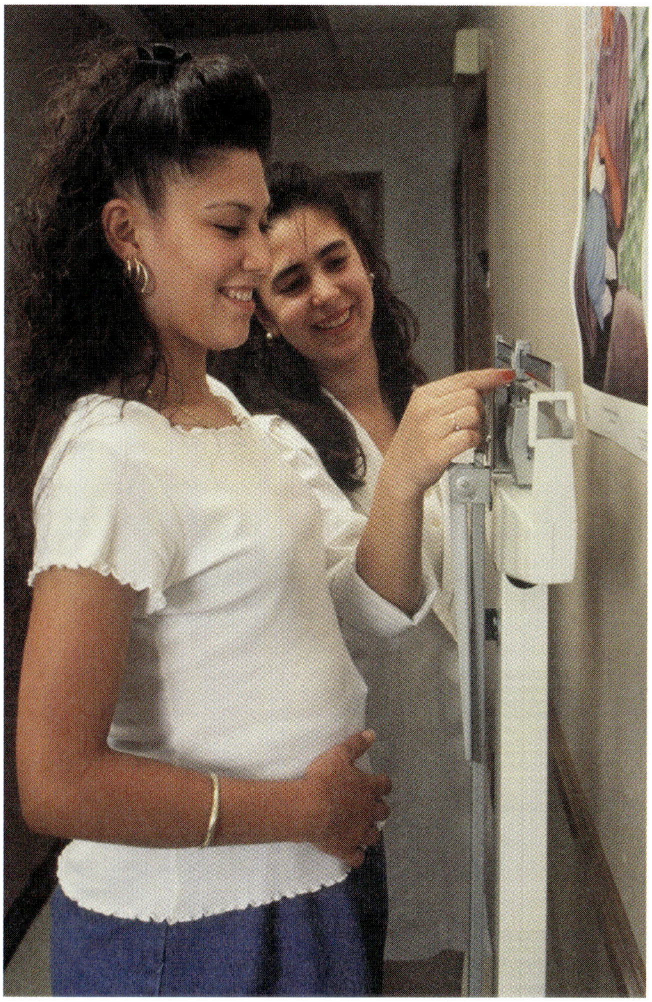

Figure 11-2. ■ Monitoring the weight of a pregnant woman is important. Sudden increases in weight could signal complications.

multiple vitamin with calcium and iron. Table 11-3 ■ identifies a food guide to meet nutritional needs during pregnancy and breastfeeding.

Many women get adequate daily calories but are still at risk for improper nutrition because of food choices. Choosing to eat high-carbohydrate, high-fat foods adds many calories to the diet. These foods, however, are usually lacking in vitamins and minerals. Many women are overweight when they become pregnant. These women may lack knowledge to make good food choices. Other women choose to diet during pregnancy in order to limit body changes or to keep the baby small for easier delivery. The consequence of improper nutrition during pregnancy is a malnourished fetus.

Adequate fluid intake is important for the pregnant woman. Drinking 1.5 to 2 L of water, milk, or juice every 24 hours is recommended. It is best to limit caffeine-containing beverages. Women in low socioeconomic

MediaLink   Nutrition Before and During Pregnancy

TABLE 11-3

Food Guide During Pregnancy and Lactation

FOOD GROUP	SERVING SIZE	SUGGESTED SERVINGS PER DAY	
		DURING PREGNANCY	DURING LACTATION
Grain products (whole grain breads, cereals, pasta, rice)	1 slice bread ½ bun, bagel ½ cup cereal	6–11	6–11
Vegetables (dark green leafy, deep yellow, dry beans/peas)	1 cup leafy greens ½ cup all others	3–5 eat dry beans & peas often	3–5
Fruits (citrus fruits and others)	1 medium apple, banana, orange, etc. ½ cup canned ¾ cup juice	2–4	2–4
Meat/poultry/fish Beans/nuts/eggs Limit peanut butter and nuts due to fat content Trim fat, remove skin from poultry	½ cup cooked dry beans 1 egg, 1½ tbsp peanut butter = 1 oz meat	Up to 6 oz total	Up to 6 oz total
Milk and milk products	1 cup milk or yogurt 1½ oz cheese	3 or more	4 or more

NURSING CARE PLAN CHART

Planning for a Client with Hyperemesis Gravidarum

GOAL	INTERVENTION	RATIONALE	EXPECTED OUTCOME
1. Deficient Fluid Volume related to severe vomiting			
The client will achieve and maintain adequate hydration and physiological balance of fluid and electrolytes.	Intravenous fluid replacement therapy Specimen collection for laboratory testing and interpretation of results Vital signs and fluid monitoring Urinary elimination management	*Delivery of fluids and electrolytes via intravenous catheter bypasses the gastrointestinal system, permitting absorption.* *Altered vital signs, decreased urine output, and abnormal laboratory values (e.g., BUN and serum K+) are indicators of disease severity and progression.*	Client will avoid physiological complications of severe dehydration and will continue to excrete bodily fluids (urine, sweat, tears) at a normal rate.
2. Imbalanced Nutrition: Less than Body Requirements			
Client will maintain current body weight and will achieve normally anticipated gains appropriate to the stage of the pregnancy.	Total Parenteral Nutrition (TPN) Administration of enteral feedings Intravenous pulsed steroid therapy Nutritional counseling, monitoring and management Weight monitoring	*Dietary nutrients are necessary for optimal fetal growth and development. Nutrient deficiency (e.g., folic acid) is associated with birth defects.* *Feeding routes that bypass taste and swallowing decrease sensory stimuli that worsen nausea and vomiting.* *Nausea and vomiting associated with pregnancy may result from adrenocortical hormone deficiency. Benefits of steroid therapy include increased appetite, weight gain and enhanced sense of emotional well-being.*	Client's daily caloric expenditure (energy output) will not exceed daily caloric intake.

GOAL	INTERVENTION	RATIONALE	EXPECTED OUTCOME
3. Impaired Skin Integrity related to infusions:			
Client will maintain skin integrity of body areas unaffected by therapeutic devices. Client will experience restoration of the integrity of the skin currently impaired by the presence of therapeutic devices.	Wound care of intravenous insertion site(s) or operative site (PEG tube insertion) Skin care: topical treatments Bathing and oral care Urinary catheter care Positioning and pressure ulcer prevention Circulatory precautions	*Wound and skin care measures (dressing changes, topical treatments, etc.) as well as acts of personal hygiene guard against infection and facilitate skin comfort.* *Severe, prolonged emesis can cause chemical injury to the oral mucosa and the teeth.* *Nutritional deficits increase the client's risk of developing pressure ulcers. Furthermore, severe fluid and electrolyte imbalance may cause profound fatigue, necessitating increased bed rest. Prolonged bed rest increases the risk of pressure ulcers and blood clots (thrombi or emboli).*	Wound sites will remain free of redness, swelling, purulent drainage and other signs of infection. Oral mucosa will remain pink and moist, and free of ulceration. Color and integrity of the teeth will be maintained (i.e. no loosening or darkening of the enamel as a result of vomiting). Throat will remain free of exudates or other signs of infection. Client's skin will remain intact, and free of chronic redness over bony prominences or other signs of impending pressure ulcer development.

levels may have difficulty buying adequate amounts of milk and high-protein foods. These women should be referred for assistance from programs such as WIC (see Table 3-1 🔗).

Women may experience extreme nausea and vomiting, especially in the early stages of pregnancy. The Nursing Care Plan Chart on pages 240 and 241 discusses this complaint.

Nutrition During the Postpartum Period

The new mother needs a balanced diet in order to regain her strength. Client teaching is a priority at this time. Most facilities provide written information about proper nutrition after delivery. The hospital dietitian is also a valuable resource.

- Teach the client that her diet should be high in fiber and fluids. *This diet will prevent constipation.*
- If the woman has a good understanding of basic nutrition, it may be sufficient to advise her to decrease her daily caloric intake by 300 kcalories and resume her prepregnancy level of other nutrients. *The 300 kcalories a day that provided for the needs of the fetus are no longer necessary. The woman will return to her prepregnancy weight more quickly if she reduces the daily intake of calories.*

- Teach the breastfeeding mother to consume an additional 500 kcalories per day, to drink an additional 8 glasses of fluid a day (1,000 mL), and to consume 65 g of protein and 1,000 mg of calcium. Most physicians request that the new mother continue to take prenatal vitamins with iron for 3 months. *These will balance the nutrients used up by milk production and breastfeeding. The prenatal vitamins help ensure that the woman's system is balanced.*

Nutrition During the Newborn Period

A full-term infant needs 50 to 55 kcal/lb (110–120 kcal/kg), which equals 20 ounces (600 mL) of breast milk or formula per day. At birth, the newborn's stomach will hold 20 mL or slightly less than 1 ounce. Because the newborn is initially unable to consume enough nutrition to meet its needs, the infant will lose weight during the first few days. By the end of the first week of life, the newborn can retain 2 to 3 ounces (60–90 mL) with each feeding. The infant will need to be fed every 2 to 4 hours in order to meet nutritional needs.

It is important for parents to receive information about the benefits of both breastfeeding and bottle-feeding. Table 11-4 ■ illustrates benefits for each method of feeding. Some women may choose to breastfeed in the privacy of their homes and bottle-feed when they are in public or with

HEALTH PROMOTION ISSUE

FOLIC ACID INTAKE AND PREGNANCY

Kathy, a 16-year-old high school cheerleader, comes to the health clinic after missing one period. She reports that an over-the-counter pregnancy test is positive. Her weight today is 112 pounds. Kathy tells the nurse that to be a cheerleader she must keep her weight low. To do this, Kathy skips breakfast, eats yogurt for lunch, and has fast food or pizza for dinner. She has 3 to 4 cans of soda pop during the day. The nurse understands that while there are several issues that need to be addressed with this client, her nutritional status is a high priority. She needs to be advised of the hazards of poor nutrition during pregnancy. She needs to be advised on better food choices for her health and that of the fetus. It would be helpful if she had some sample menus after which to model her diet.

DISCUSSION

A lack of adequate nutrients in the diet during pregnancy has been linked to an increased incidence of low birth weight infants, gestational hypertension, and poor fetal brain development. Although major congenital anomalies occur in 2% to 3% of live births, neural tube defects (NTDs) are among the most common (Toriello, 2005). The brain, spinal cord, and protective bone structures of the skull and vertebra are formed within the first 28 days after conception. Research has shown that without adequate amounts of folic acid, the brain fails to develop normally, resulting in **anencephaly**, and the vertebrae fail to close, resulting in **spina bifida** with meningomyelocele. Because many pregnancies are unplanned, and NTDs occur within the first month after conception (which is before the recognition of pregnancy), NTDs are best prevented by adequate folic acid intake throughout the reproductive years.

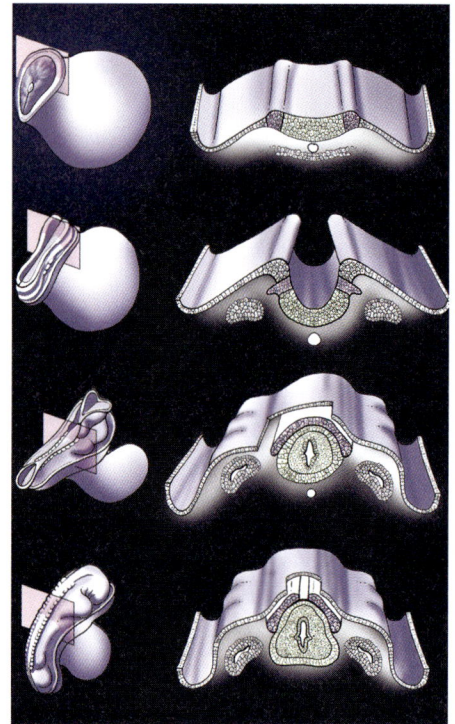

visitors. Once the parents have decided how to feed their baby, the nurse should support the decision. It is not appropriate to make the parents feel guilty about their decision.

BREASTFEEDING

The American Academy of Pediatrics recommends breast milk for the first year of life. Commercially prepared formula closely approximates breast milk.

Breast milk is produced to meet the newborn's needs and changes as the infant grows. Breast milk contains easily digested nutrients and antibodies. *Colostrum*, the first fluid produced by the breast, is a thin yellow fluid, rich in protein, calories, and immune globulins. Colostrum protects the newborn from intestinal infections. Colostrum also contains a laxative that assists the passage of *meconium*, the first feces of the newborn.

Breast stimulation and emptying of the mammary glands stimulate the secretion of prolactin by the mother's anterior pituitary gland (see Figure 5-16 ⬤⬤). Prolactin increases milk production. As the newborn nurses more frequently and for longer periods of time, more milk is produced.

The breastfeeding mother needs a balanced diet in order to provide nutritious breast milk and maintain her own nutritional needs. An extra 500 calories and 1,000 milliliters of fluid are needed per day to support breastfeeding. Most health care providers recommend the woman continue taking prenatal vitamins throughout lactation.

The mother and newborn do not automatically know how to breastfeed. Teaching and support will be needed during the learning process. Several positions (Figure 11-3 ■) can be used for breastfeeding. The *cradle hold*, with the infant's head in the bend of the mother's elbow and the infant's body resting against the mother's abdomen, is the most common. Another position is a *football hold* with the infant's body tucked beneath the mother's axilla and the

Research is still being conducted on folic acid deficiency and other anomalies such as heart defects, cleft lip, and cleft palate. Because folic acid is needed for all rapidly growing cells, insufficient folic acid can result in anemia. Iron deficiency during pregnancy also contributes to anemia in both the mother and fetus. Anemia during pregnancy can lead to premature delivery. Delivery requires endurance, physical effort, and a physically fit woman. The anemic woman has more complications during delivery, including hemorrhage, cardiovascular collapse, and maternal death.

In 1998, the Food and Drug Administration mandated that enriched cereals be fortified with 140 micrograms of synthetic folic acid per 100 grams of grain. This fortification of staple foods is effective, inexpensive, and increased the overall folic acid intake without the need for behavior change. Since that time, the incidence of NTDs have decreased but have not been eliminated. The Center for Disease Control and the American College of Medical Genetics recommend supplementation of 400 micrograms (0.4 mg) of folic acid daily beginning at least 1 month prior to conception.

PLANNING AND IMPLEMENTATION

The nurse should help the client understand that planning and food preparation will aid in making proper food choices and improve nutrition. The nurse should encourage the client to make a detailed weekly menu and to follow it. The nurse can encourage the client to prepare lunches before bedtime and store them in the refrigerator. If fast food is necessary, the nurse can help the client make healthy choices.

SELF-REFLECTION

Carefully assess your own nutritional habits. Record your intake for a 24-hour period. Determine excesses and deficiencies in your diet. If you were to become pregnant, is your diet adequate in iron and folic acid? What changes should you make to ensure adequate nutrition?

SUGGESTED RESOURCES

For the Nurse

Toriello, H. V. (2005). Folic acid and neural tube defects. *Genetics in Medicine, 7*(4), 283–284.

For the Client

Brown, J. E., & Carlson, M. (2000). Nutrition and multifetal pregnancy. *Journal of the American Dietetic Association, 100*(3), 343–348.

infant's head positioned against the mother's breast. A *sidelying position* is frequently used in bed. The mother lies on her side with pillows supporting her head and back. The newborn is positioned next to her with the infant's head against the breast and the body parallel to the mother's body. It is important to use a pillow under the mother's forearm to support the weight of the infant.

Latching On

Once the newborn is positioned against the breast, the infant must open the mouth wide enough to take the nipple and areola into the mouth. To help the newborn to latch onto the breast (Figure 11-4 ■), the mother holds the breast in her hand with the thumb and forefinger in the shape of a "C" around the breast and well behind the areola. She tickles the infant's lips with the nipple. The infant will open the mouth (part of the sucking reflex). When the mouth is wide open, and the tongue is down, the infant is brought rapidly to the breast. When latched on properly, the nipple and areola will be in the mouth, with the tongue under the nipple and the lips flared outward. The suction will be strong, but there will be no discomfort. If the mother experiences discomfort, the infant should be removed from the breast, repositioned, and allowed to latch on again.

Protecting the Nipple

When removing the newborn from the breast, the mother should gently insert a finger into the corner of the infant's mouth to break the suction. If the nipple becomes sore, cracked, or bleeds, or if blisters form, the nipple needs treatment. Leaving a small amount of milk on the nipple after feeding can help to heal sore nipples. Also the tannic acid obtained by gently rubbing the nipple with a cool wet tea bag can help with healing. A light film of an approved emollient (such as Eucerin) may be applied after feedings.

TABLE 11-4

Reasons for Breastfeeding and Bottle-Feeding

FEEDING METHOD	BENEFIT TO MOTHER	BENEFIT TO INFANT
Breastfeeding	Decreases incidence of ovarian, uterine, and breast cancer	Breast milk enhances maturation of the GI tract; it is *species specific* (human milk for human babies) so it supplies the exact nutrients needed by the infant; it assists in passage of meconium and stools
	Promotes involution	Breast milk contains antibodies that can protect against some infections
	Return to prepregnant weight sooner	Lower incidence of allergies among breastfed infants
	Unique bonding experience	Breastfed infants have lower incidence of SIDS
	Convenient, no formula and bottles to carry	
	Saves money	
Bottle-feeding	Personal preference	Bonding still can occur
	Provides a good option if mother has breast scarring or HIV infection or if maternal medication precludes breastfeeding	Others besides mother can feed infant
	Is good choice if mother's place of employment (such as hair salon) contains chemicals that could contaminate expressed milk	Provides adequate nutrition
		Commercial formula comes in three forms for convenience
	Provides solution if mother's workplace is intolerant of breastfeeding	Commercial formula comes in cow's milk and soy milk
	Allows several people to share bonding experience while feeding infant	WIC program provides iron-fortified formula
	May allow mother to get more rest if others take night feedings	

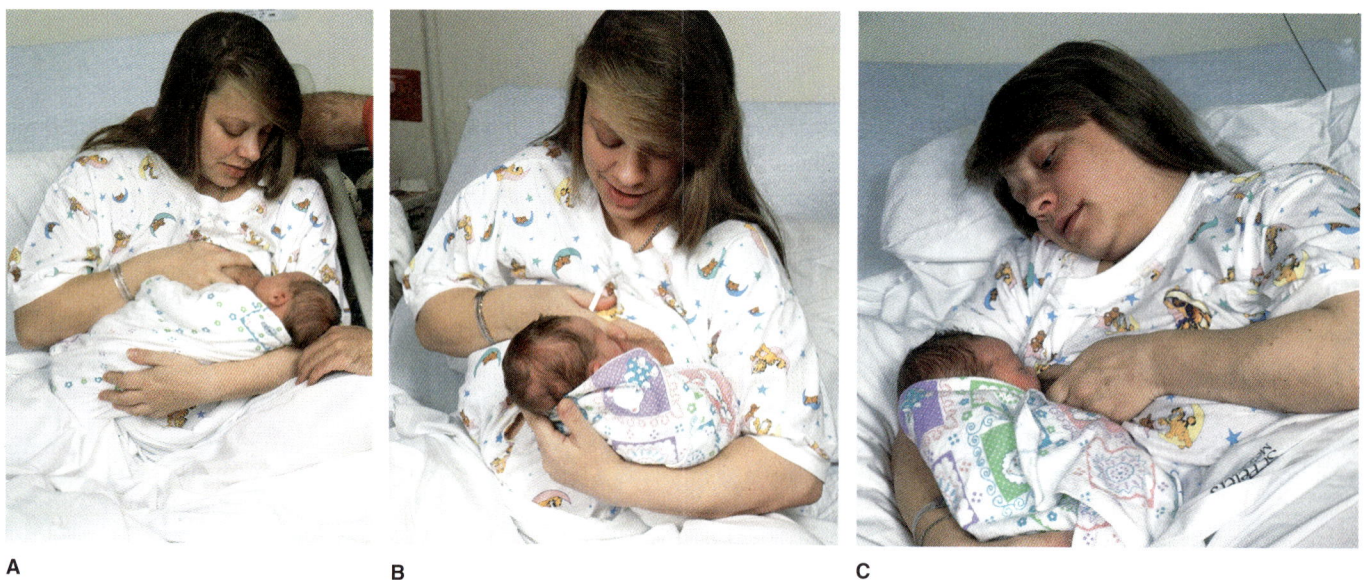

Figure 11-3. ■ Three positions that are often used for breastfeeding. (**A**) Cradle hold. (**B**) Football hold. (**C**) Side-lying position.

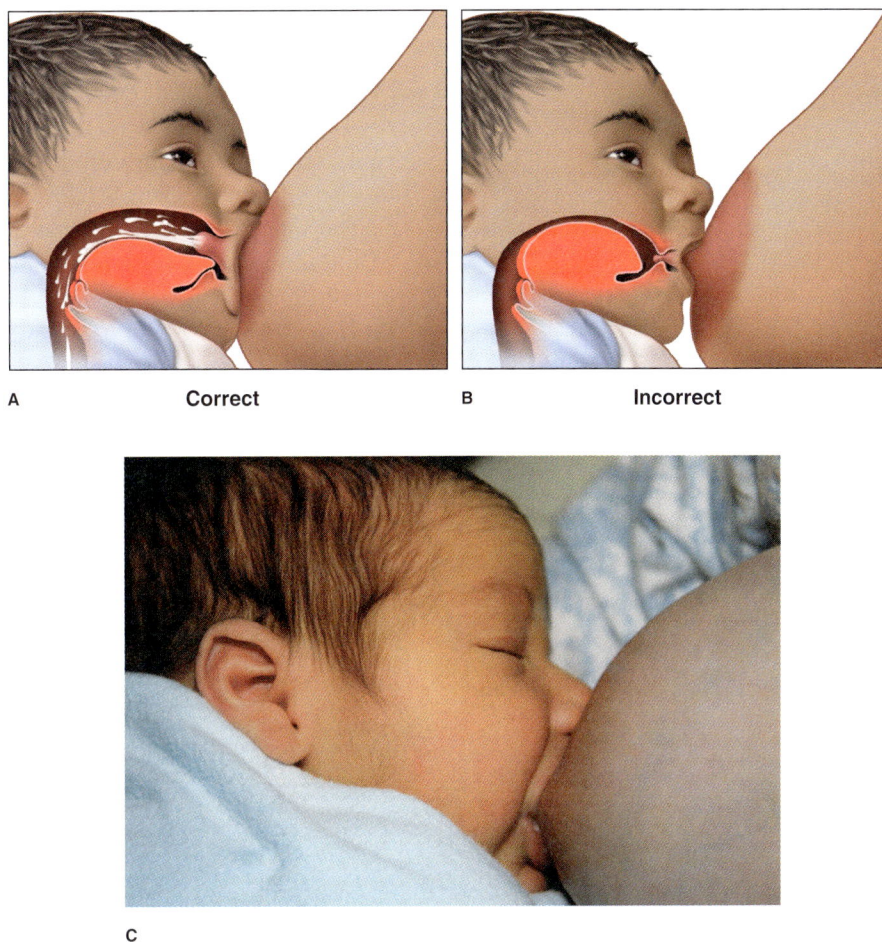

Figure 11-4. ■ Latching on. (**A**) Correct position with tongue over gum ridge. Nipple is down far into mouth and milk flows. (**B**) Incorrect position with tongue behind the lower gum ridge. Only the tip of the nipple is in the mouth. The nipple is pinched and milk cannot flow. (**C**) Newborn properly latched onto mother's breast.

Feeding at Both Breasts

Breastfeeding may range from 10 to 30 minutes a side, depending on the size and health of the infant. Frequency is at least 8 to 12 times a day. However, it is more important to know when the infant is full than to follow the clock. Infants will nurse vigorously at first, then slow when they become full. The breast will become soft when empty. Infants should be allowed to empty one breast and then be moved to the other breast until they are full. At the next feeding, the infant is started on the breast used last at the previous feeding. This technique allows each breast to be emptied completely every other feeding. As infants grow, both breasts may be emptied with each feeding. Breastfed infants generally do not swallow as much air as bottle-fed infants, but they still should be burped halfway through and again at the end of the feeding.

Engorgement

Engorgement is swelling of the breast tissue caused by an increase in blood and lymph preceding true lactation. Over the first 3 to 5 days after giving birth, the mammary glands release colostrum and then begin to produce true milk. The breasts gradually fill until they become hard, warm to the touch, and uncomfortable. This engorgement may last until the breast is emptied during breastfeeding or for approximately 48 to 72 hours.

The following tips will help to relieve the pressure and discomfort:

■ Apply a warm, wet compress to your breasts for 3 to 5 minutes before feeding.
■ Using the tips of your fingers, gently massage your breasts from your chest down toward your nipple in a circular motion.

Cabbage Leaves for Treatment of Breast Engorgement

If the client does not feel relief from the suggestions provided in the text, suggest that the woman try using a few cabbage leaves. An enzyme found in green cabbage leaves has been effective in decreasing the swelling and increasing milk flow in breastfeeding mothers. Instructions for use of cabbage leaves follow:

- Wash and dry crisp, cold green cabbage leaves.
- Gently bend the leaves to release some of the natural juice.
- Apply a cabbage leaf directly to the skin for approximately 1 hour; then try feeding the baby or expressing milk.
- Reapply cabbage leaves 3 to 4 times a day. (Additional times may lead to a decrease of the woman's milk supply.)
- Discontinue use immediately if skin rash occurs. (This reaction is very rare.)

- Hand express or pump a little milk to soften breasts and reduce fullness so infant can latch on.
- Apply an ice pack for a few minutes after feeding if breasts remain uncomfortable.
- Pump only for comfort. Avoid pumping to empty the breasts completely.
- Avoid pacifiers and bottles during these days.
- Nurse frequently, even if this means waking the baby during the day.
- Nurse on the most engorged breast first.
- Call your lactation consultant for additional tips if engorgement does not subside.

Box 11-1 ■ provides some complementary therapy for engorged breasts.

BOTTLE-FEEDING

Bottle-feeding will take some forethought and preparation. Bottles and nipples should be cleaned with a brush and soapy water and thoroughly rinsed. If there is question about the safety of the water supply, bottles and nipples should be boiled.

A variety of nipples are available. Generally, babies will feed well from any bottle and nipple, but may eventually prefer one style. Formulas are available in ready-to-feed, concentrated liquid, and powder forms. There is a great range of prices for formula, and finances should be a factor in choosing what type of formula to use. Accurate mixing is essential to provide the necessary nutrients, the proper number of calories, and an easily digested concentration.

The physician orders the brand of formula. It is important to note that, if the woman is participating in the WIC program, some brands of formula may not be funded.

Adjustments can usually be made between the physician and the WIC program.

Most newborns will take 15 mL (1/2 ounce) the first few days but gradually increase the amount of each feeding over time. To avoid wasting formula, only a few ounces should be made until the infant is taking higher volumes.

The infant should be positioned with the head higher than the stomach. The infant should be burped when about half of the feeding is consumed and again at the end of the feeding. To facilitate burping, the infant can be held upright against the feeder's shoulder (Figure 11-5 ■),

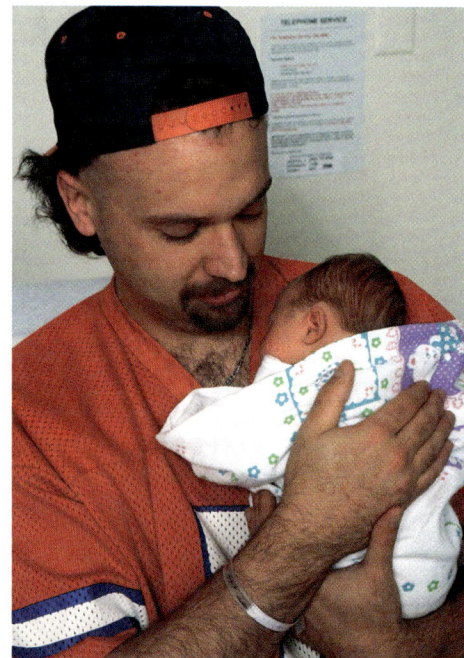

A

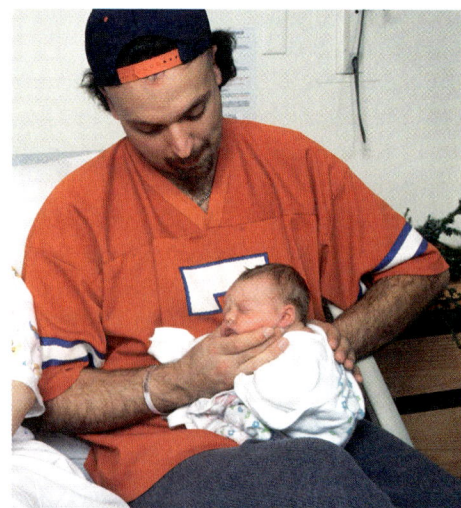

B

Figure 11-5. ■ Positions in which a neonate may be burped. (**A**) Upright. (**B**) Sitting leaning forward. The infant may also be laid across the lap.

leaned forward in a sitting position with the head and chest supported, or laid prone across the feeder's lap. Gently rubbing or patting the infant's back can also facilitate burping.

NURSING CARE

PRIORITIES IN NURSING CARE

The highest priority in care of the pregnant woman related to her nutrition is to provide instruction regarding the essential nutrients, their use within the body, and their food source. All adults providing care of the newborn should have instruction regarding feeding, but the priority in care is to provide nutrition teaching to the parents.

ASSESSING

The assessment of the woman, either before or during pregnancy, should include subjective and objective data related to nutrition. Obtain a diet history. By asking the woman to identify the foods she consumes on a regular basis, the nurse can identify the adequacy of the diet or any culturally based ideas of food (Box 11-2 ■). Because poor nutrition results in skin lesions, dull hair, and thin flexible nails, objective observations of the skin, hair, and nails alert the nurse to possible nutrition problems. Check the laboratory results for hematocrit, hemoglobin, and iron levels. Notify the primary care provider of abnormal values that require medical attention.

In collecting information about the nutritional status of the newborn, the nurse should question the parents about the frequency and amount of feeding, monitor the baby's weight, palpate the fontanels, and discuss stool changes with the parents. (See Chapter 17 🔗 for techniques in assessing the newborn.)

BOX 11-2	CULTURAL PULSE POINTS

Culturally Based Ideas About Nutrition

Some beliefs about food and pregnancy are culturally determined. The following are a few examples of culturally based ideas about nutrition.

- Italian descent: Desire for certain foods must be satisfied to prevent congenital anomalies. Also, pregnant women must smell the food to prevent miscarriage (Spector, 2000).
- African descent: Eat clay, dirt, or starch to benefit mother and fetus (Spector, 2000).
- Korean descent: Practice *Tae Kyo* (set of rules for safe childbirth, which lists food taboos) (Choi, 1995).

Note: If the dietary practice is not harmful, there is no reason to ask the client to discontinue it.

DIAGNOSING, PLANNING, AND IMPLEMENTING

Common nursing diagnoses for both the mother and newborn might include the following:

- Imbalanced **N**utrition: Less Than Body Requirements
- Deficient **K**nowledge related to basic nutrition
- Deficient **K**nowledge related to breastfeeding

Expected outcomes for these diagnoses include, but are not limited to, the following:

- Neonate will maintain normal weight pattern during the first week of life.
- Mother will state how often baby should be fed in a 24-hour-period.
- Mother will state that she will empty one breast completely at each feeding before moving the baby to the second breast.

Nursing care for a woman in pregnancy or the postpartum period includes the following interventions:

- Reinforce information about prenatal nutrition early in the pregnancy. *Proper nutrition early in pregnancy can prevent congenital disorders and malformations.*
- Provide written information as well as verbal discussion for prenatal or postpartum teaching. *Written materials help the client consolidate new learning. They are more useful than verbal teaching for visual learners.*
- Provide referral to a dietitian as indicated. *Clients who need careful review of their nutritional practices would benefit by visiting a dietitian.*
- Provide written information about proper nutrition for the postpartum client. *A tired new mother may not remember how important her own self-care is to herself and the infant. Written materials can be helpful to the mother and the family.*
- Reinforce teaching about breastfeeding and bottle-feeding to both parents. *Parents may have questions in the prenatal period that will help them decide whether to breastfeed, bottle-feed, or both. Breastfeeding techniques generally are addressed in the late prenatal or early postpartum period. Both parents should be taught to prepare formula for the bottle-fed infant.*

EVALUATING

The most common method of evaluating the nutritional status of the client during and after pregnancy is to monitor the weight gain and loss. The client should verbalize the dietary allowances and restrictions. The breastfeeding mother should be observed helping the baby to latch onto the breast, removing the baby from the breast, and burping the baby. Both parents should be able to verbalize how to prepare the formula and demonstrate feeding the baby.

NURSING PROCESS CARE PLAN
Client Wanting to Breastfeed

Maria, a 17-year-old primigravida, had a 7-lb 6-oz baby girl by spontaneous vaginal delivery 1 hour ago. She wants to breastfeed her baby. She has no experience handling a newborn.

Assessment
- 17-year-old primigravida
- Delivered 7-lb 6-oz baby 1 hour ago
- Wants to breastfeed baby
- Has no experience handling a newborn

Nursing Diagnosis.
The following important nursing diagnosis (among others) is established for this client:
- Deficient **K**nowledge related to breastfeeding

Expected Outcomes
- Maria will learn to breastfeed the baby with minimal assistance.
- Maria will verbalize and demonstrate use of different positions for breastfeeding.
- Maria will verbalize signs of possible complications of breastfeeding.

Planning and Implementing
- Assist Maria to a comfortable position. *Relaxation is necessary to let-down reflex.*
- Provide detailed instructions on breastfeeding. *Maria is young and inexperienced, so detailed instruction is needed for understanding and confidence.*
- Observe Maria burp the baby. *Burping is needed to expel air from stomach.*
- Observe Maria feeding the baby on opposite breast. *Observation of breastfeeding is needed to ensure proper technique and limit complications.*

Evaluation.
Maria begins to breastfeed her newborn. The baby feeds for 8 minutes each side. Maria initially has trouble getting the baby to latch on, but was eventually successful.

Critical Thinking in the Nursing Process

1. What other topics regarding nutrition should be discussed with this client?
2. If the client has difficulty breastfeeding, what would the LPN do next?
3. What follow-up should be done with this young mother regarding her nutritional status and that of the baby?

Note: Discussion of Critical Thinking questions appears in Appendix I.

Note: The reference and resource listings for this and all chapters have been compiled at the back of the book.

Chapter Review

KEY TERMS by Topic

Use the audio glossary feature of either the CD-ROM or the Companion Website to hear the correct pronunciation of the following key terms.

Nutrients
monosaccharides, disaccharides, polysaccharides, glucose, fructose, galactose, maltose, sucrose, lactose, proteins, nonessential amino acids, essential amino acids, conditionally essential amino acids, lipids, saturated, unsaturated, monounsaturated, polyunsaturated, trans fats, water-soluble vitamins, free radicals, oxidative stress, beriberi, riboflavin, niacin, pellagra, biotin, folic acid, fat-soluble vitamins, beta-carotene, rickets, osteomalacia, osteoporosis, erythrocyte hemolysis, anencephaly, spina bifida

Nutrition During the Newborn Period
engorgement

KEY Points

- Adequate nutrients are essential to maintain healthy tissues.
- It is important to build up nutritional reserves prior to pregnancy.
- Deficiency of folic acid can result in life-altering anomalies in the newborn.
- Deficiency in nutrients during fetal development can result in health issues later in life.
- The nurse has a responsibility to teach parents health nutrition practices for themselves and their children.
- Women should not be made to feel guilty if they choose to bottle-feed instead of breastfeed their baby.
- Women choosing to bottle-feed need instruction in formula preparation, feeding techniques, and how to burp the baby.
- Women choosing to breastfeed need instruction in positioning the baby, helping the baby latch on to the nipple, and removing the baby from the nipple.

EXPLORE MediaLink

Additional interactive resources for this chapter can be found on the Companion Website at www.prenhall.com/towle. Click on Chapter 11 and "Begin" to select the activities for this chapter.

For chapter-related NCLEX®-style questions and an audio glossary, access the accompanying CD-ROM in this book.

Animation
Breastfeeding and first foods

FOR FURTHER Study

See Table 3-1 for federal programs to assist women and newborns.

Figure 5-16 illustrates the processes involved in lactation.

See Chapter 6 for general women's health topics.

See Box 8-2 for specific nutritional information related to fetal development.

See Chapter 17 for techniques in assessing the newborn.

Critical Thinking Care Map

Caring for an Undernourished Pregnant Woman
NCLEX-PN® Focus Area: Physiologic Integrity

Case Study: Jean, a 17-year-old, comes to the clinic for her first visit. She appears pale and thin. Her weight is 135 lbs. Her vital signs are within normal limits. Her urine is negative for protein. It is determined she is 10 weeks pregnant. She states she is living with her boyfriend in a one-bedroom basement apartment. Both Jean and her boyfriend have had to drop out of high school to get jobs. They are barely able to pay the rent and buy food. Jean begins to cry, stating she does not know what to do.

Nursing Diagnosis: Imbalanced Nutrition: Less than Body Requirements related to pregnancy

COLLECT DATA

Subjective	Objective
_____	_____
_____	_____
_____	_____
_____	_____
_____	_____
_____	_____
_____	_____

Would you report this? Yes/No

If yes, to: _____

Nursing Care

_____
_____
_____
_____
_____
_____
_____
_____
_____
_____
_____
_____

How would you document this? _____
_____
_____
_____

Compare your documentation to the sample provided in Appendix I.

Data Collected
(use only those that apply)

- Crying
- States she does not know what to do
- Wt. 135 lbs
- Vital signs
- Urine negative for protein
- Pale
- Thin
- Money only for rent and food

Nursing Interventions
(use only those that apply; list in priority order)

- Teach need for milk products.
- Refer to WIC program.
- Teach need for increased protein and lower carbohydrates in diet.
- Arrange follow-up appointment with the boyfriend.
- Teach need for prenatal vitamins.
- Refer to therapist for depression.

NCLEX-PN® Exam Preparation

TEST-TAKING TIP   Eat a nutritious snack before beginning the test.

1 The mother of 1-month-old Jason tells the nurse that she props the baby's bottle on pillows because he wiggles so much. The best response from the nurse would be:
1. "It is probably a good idea to prop the bottle until you feel more comfortable holding him."
2. "It is not a good idea because he could choke on the formula."
3. "You need to hold the baby when you are feeding him."
4. "Are you afraid of dropping him?"

2 Kathy, a new mother, is learning to breastfeed before she leaves the hospital. Kathy demonstrates correct breastfeeding technique when she:
1. has the baby take only the nipple in his mouth.
2. nurses on one side at each feeding.
3. has the baby take as much of the areola as possible into his mouth.
4. nurses for 20 minutes on each side.

3 The LPN/LVN is conducting preconception classes. While discussing nutrition, it is important for the LPN/LVN to explain that which of the following nutrients should be consumed prior to pregnancy to prevent neural tube defects?
1. folic acid
2. vitamin A
3. protein
4. potassium

4 The LPN/LVN is discussing prenatal nutrition for a client who is anemic. Which of the following foods should the LPN/LVN recommend to increase the client's red blood cell count? Select all that apply.
1. oranges
2. milk
3. broccoli
4. strawberries
5. white bread
6. hamburger
7. eggs

5 Which of the following assessment findings would alert the LPN/LVN to poor nutritional intake during pregnancy?
1. moist mucous membranes
2. hematocrit level of 34%
3. hemoglobin level of 12 g/dL
4. dull hair

6 A pregnant client states that she consumes 2,200 calories every day and asks the LPN/LVN how many calories should she consume while breastfeeding. The LPN/LVN suggests she increase her caloric intake by _____ calories per day.

7 A pregnant client needs to increase calcium in her daily diet. The LPN/LVN suggests she increase her intake of which of the following vitamins?
1. vitamin A
2. vitamin B
3. vitamin C
4. vitamin D

8 A breastfeeding client states that she will wait and breastfeed when her milk comes in. The LPN/LVN explains that colostrum is good for the newborn because it:
1. helps the newborn sleep.
2. aids in the passage of meconium.
3. assists with bonding.
4. slows digestion.

9 A breastfeeding mother states her nipples are sore because it is difficult to remove the newborn from the breast after feeding. Which of the following instructions by the LPN/LVN is most helpful in removing the newborn from the breast?
1. Slide one finger into the corner of the newborn's mouth to break the suction.
2. Allow the newborn to fall asleep at the breast then remove.
3. Slide the breast out of the newborn's mouth with two hands.
4. Support the newborn's head and pull the newborn away from the breast.

10 An LPN/LVN is teaching a class on bottle-feeding. Which statement made by one of the class participants indicates understanding of caring for the bottles and nipples?
1. "I will not boil the bottles and nipples."
2. "All bottles and nipples will be placed in the dishwasher."
3. "I will clean the bottles and nipples with a brush in soapy water."
4. "I will add a teaspoon of vinegar to the water when cleaning bottles and nipples."

Answers for NCLEX-PN® Review and Critical Thinking questions appear in Appendix I.

Chapter 12

Care of the Pregnant Adolescent

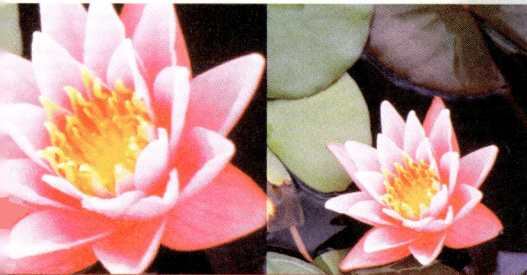

BRIEF Outline

LEARNING Outcomes

After completing this chapter, you will be able to:

1. Define key terms.
2. Describe factors contributing to adolescent pregnancy.
3. Describe risk factors for the child of an adolescent mother.
4. Describe characteristics of fathers who have children with adolescent mothers.
5. Discuss the reactions of the adolescent's family.
6. Assist in formulating a plan of care to meet the needs of a pregnant adolescent.
7. Describe approaches to prevent adolescent pregnancy.

Pregnancy is a time of great adjustment for a woman. She must adjust to the physical demands of carrying a growing fetus as well as the psychological demands of preparing to become a parent. These challenges are even greater when the pregnant mother is an adolescent. The adolescent has not completed all of the developmental tasks associated with maturation. Many describe this reality as children having children. This chapter explores the issues surrounding adolescent pregnancy, the impact on the father, the reaction of family members, and efforts to prevent adolescent pregnancy.

Review of Adolescent Growth and Development

Before discussing adolescent pregnancy, it is important to review the normal growth and development process. Adolescence spans a period of 6 years from age 13 to 19. The work of the adolescent period is to mature physically into the "adult" body and to develop a strong identity.

Physical maturation begins with the increase of hormones from the pituitary gland. A combination of follicle-stimulating hormone, luteinizing hormone, estrogen and progesterone in the female, and testosterone in the male results in body changes. In the female, these changes include the development of axillary and pubic hair, a widening of the hips, breast development, and menstruation. In the male, these changes include the appearance of body hair, deepening of the voice, muscle and skeletal development, lengthening of the penis, and sperm production. (See Chapter 5 ⚭ for a complete discussion of reproductive anatomy and physiology.) Although these physical changes usually occur without incident, emotional development is generally more difficult for the adolescent.

Prior to adulthood and emotional maturity, the limbic system in the brain has primary control of behavior. Found deep inside the brain, the limbic system is activated by behavior and arousal, and is responsible for primitive drives, including the sex drive. The adolescent can think in abstract, plan for the "what if," and make logical choices in many situations. The limbic system, however, gives the adolescent a feeling that "nothing bad will happen to me" when faced with situations that stimulate the primitive drives. Until the frontal lobe of the cerebrum is able to control the primitive drives, the adolescent often engages in risk-taking behaviors.

A changing body, increasing hormones, and primitive drives bring about confusion and doubt. The adolescent wants to feel attractive, but the skin changes, awkwardness of a rapidly changing body, and mood changes can make them feel ugly. Wanting to "fit in," the adolescent may purchase numerous skin products, lie in the sun for hours to "get the perfect tan," and wear revealing clothing. They may decorate their bodies with unusual hairstyles, colors, and body piercing and tattoos in order to express their individuality.

Striving for identity and reassurance, adolescents turn to their peers who can "understand what they are going through." Peers can have a positive or negative influence on behavior. If the peer group is active in sports, religious activities, or other organized activities, the adolescent can develop a strong identity and positive self-image. On the other hand, if the peer group indulges in drinking, uses illicit drugs, and engages in violent behavior, the adolescent can develop conflict between the values of the parent and those of the peer group. This conflict can lead to a poor self-image.

Adolescence is the time of identity versus role confusion. The teenager is developing a sexual identity, is becoming more independent, and is beginning the process of separation from the parents. The teenager has a strong desire to make his or her own decisions and "live my own life" but at the same time has a real need to know boundaries or rules. The teenager is examining the world and trying to decide where he or she fits, what his or her life's work will be, and how to accomplish goals. He or she is beginning to use peers for support instead of relying on parents for help in making decisions.

With positive reinforcement of their progress, teens can develop a strong identity. With continual negative feedback coupled with feelings of inferiority and guilt, teens are more likely to become confused, ambivalent, and withdrawn. If parents do not allow them to separate from parental influence, to develop peer relationships, and to make their own decisions, teens will either remain dependent or rebel. In either case, they will miss the opportunity to learn important life skills.

Contributing Factors of Adolescent Pregnancy

Each year about 750,000 teens become pregnant (Figure 12-1 ■). Of these pregnancies, about 33% are terminated by therapeutic abortion and about 14% end in miscarriage. More than half of the pregnant teens keep their babies (National Campaign to Prevent Teen Pregnancy, 2006). Very few adolescent mothers choose adoption. Although the rate of adolescent pregnancy in the United States has decreased dramatically (30%) since 1991, it remains the highest in the world (Martin et al., 2003). This section explores some of the factors contributing to adolescent pregnancy.

Pregnancy, birth, and abortion rates for teenagers 15–17 years

Rate per 1,000 women aged 15–17

NOTE: Rates are plotted on a log scale.
SOURCE: CDC/NCHS, Division of Vital Statistics, Published reports.

Pregnancy, birth, abortion, and fetal loss rates for teenagers 15–17 and 18–19 years: 1990, 1995, 2000, and 2002

Rates per 1,000 women in specified group

- Fetal loss
- Abortion
- Birth

15–17 years: 77.1, 67.4, 50.8, 44.4 (1990, 1995, 2000, 2002)
18–19 years: 167.7, 153.4, 134.5, 125.0 (1990, 1995, 2000, 2002)

SOURCE: CDC/NCHS, Division of Vital Statistics, Published reports.

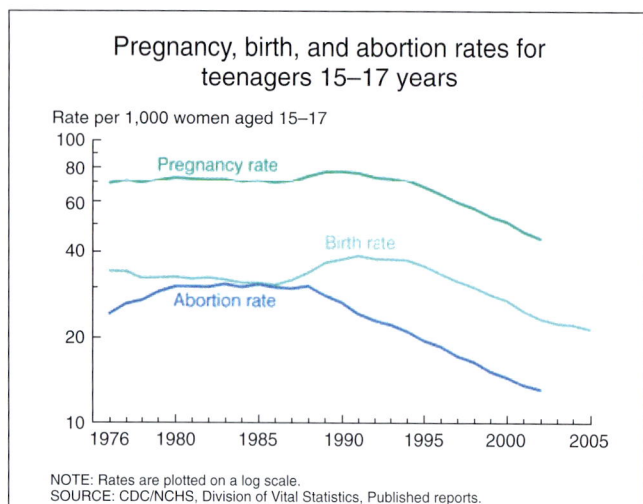

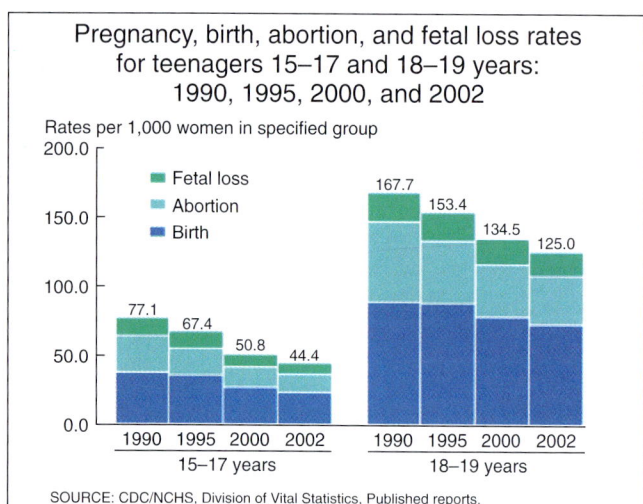

Figure 12-1. ■ Statistics showing teenage pregnancy birth, abortion, and fetal loss in the United States. (Source: Ventura, S.J., Abma, J.C., Mosher, W.D., & Henshaw, S.K. *Recent trends in teenage pregnancy in the United States, 1990–2002.* Centers for Disease Control and Prevention. Hyattsville, MD: National Center for Health Statistics.)

SOCIOECONOMIC FACTORS

A major risk factor for adolescent pregnancy is poverty. Approximately 85% of pregnancies in unmarried teens occur to those from poor or low-income families (Alan Guttmacher Institute, 2002). These adolescents tend to maintain the pregnancy and keep the baby. Teens from low-income families generally do not participate in adult-supervised extracurricular activities. Research indicates that adolescents who have limited time in adult supervision have a greater level of sexual activity. These girls may see pregnancy as a way to gain attention or adult status. Also, they may have had to carry adult responsibilities from a young age while the parent or parents were out at work. Duties may have included caring for younger siblings,

preparing meals, and so on. If young girls perceive these tasks as the role they are meant to play (and do not see other options), they may be more inclined to become sexually active and keep a child if they become pregnant.

CULTURAL FACTORS

Since 1991, the pregnancy rates in African American and Hispanic teens have declined. Pregnancy rates remain higher in Black and Hispanic teens than in White teens (Martin et al., 2003). However, as noted in the section on Socioeconomic Factors, a disproportionately higher number of African American and Hispanic teens live in poverty. Internationally, in countries where Islam is the predominant religion, where larger families are desired, where most childbearing occurs within marriage, and where social change is slow in coming, women are more likely to become married and pregnant during the adolescent years.

Family values and experiences affect adolescent pregnancy rates. If the mother or sisters of an adolescent had a baby in their early teens, the adolescent is more likely to indulge in sexual intercourse and is therefore at risk for adolescent pregnancy (Short & Rosenthal, 2003). The younger the teen when she first gets pregnant, the more likely she is to have a second adolescent pregnancy (Key, Barbosa, & Owens, 2001).

EDUCATIONAL FACTORS

Teens with low educational achievement are at greater risk of pregnancy. Teens with high future goals (college, career) are more consistent in using birth control. If they do become pregnant, they are more likely to have an abortion. There is an increased likelihood of adolescent pregnancy when the teen drops out of school (Cohen et al., 2002).

PSYCHOLOGICAL FACTORS

Poor self-esteem is a contributing factor to adolescent pregnancy. Some teens plan to get pregnant for conscious or subconscious reasons. They may want to punish their parent(s), to escape their home situation, or to have someone to love and who will love them. Intentional pregnancy may also be a form of acting out to gain attention.

Family dysfunction is a contributing factor to adolescent pregnancy. Compared to nonpregnant teens, more teens who become pregnant have been physically, emotionally, or sexually abused (Montgomery, 2003). When the very young adolescent becomes pregnant, incest or sexual abuse should be suspected.

HIGH-RISK BEHAVIOR

Sexual activity among American teens is more commonplace today than it was in the past. The peer pressure to become sexually active during the teen years is tremendous.

The Allen Guttmacher Institute reports that three-fourths of teens are sexually active by late adolescence and more than two-thirds have had more than one partner (Allen Guttmacher Institute, 2002).

High-risk behaviors include multiple partners, lack of protection from sexually transmitted diseases, and lack of contraceptive use. Recent statistics show an increased use of condoms among adolescents, but the use of contraception is inconsistent (National Campaign to Prevent Teen Pregnancy, 2000). When teens discuss contraception before engaging in sex and when they have waited to have sex until the relationship has been established for a longer time, contraceptive use is more consistent (Manlove, Ryan, & Franzetta, 2003).

The use of contraception is a common topic in sex education classes. However, many teens lack accurate or adequate knowledge. Debate continues about the appropriateness of sex education in public schools (Figure 12-2 ■). Opponents claim that discussion about sex increases sexual activity among teens. They contend that sex education is the responsibility of parents and should be provided in the home. Research reveals, however, that sex education in public schools does not cause an increase in sexual activity or sexual activity at an earlier age (Doniger, Adams, Utter, & Riley, 2001).

Other factors affecting the use of contraception and protection against infection include availability and cost of supplies. Teens may have difficulty purchasing condoms at local stores for fear of embarrassment and concern about confidentiality. Oral contraception requires a prescription, and teens may have difficulty obtaining one. If they are able to obtain protection from infection and pregnancy, they may need to hide contraceptives from their parents. The fear of discovery increases their psychological stress.

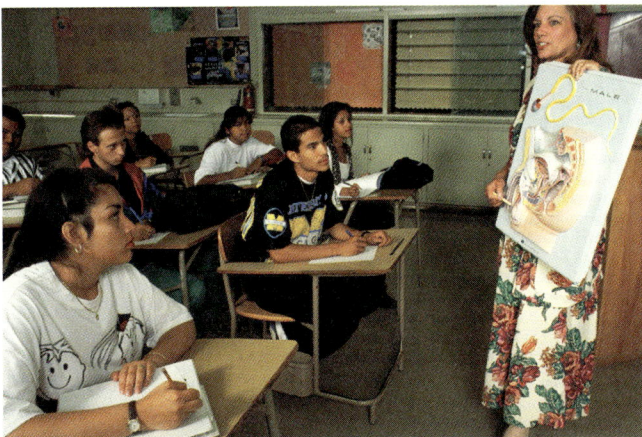

Figure 12-2. ■ Sex education in schools is one means of challenging myths about sex and sexuality.

Nurse's Role with Pregnant Adolescents

The nurse's role is to be supportive and nonjudgmental. The pregnant teen is often frightened, overwhelmed, and alone. The nurse can provide needed support and adult guidance. The nurse may need to assist in informing parents of the pregnancy. The nurse may become a mediator should conflict arise.

If the pregnancy has resulted from abuse, the nurse has a responsibility to inform the authorities (see Chapter 3 ⏺⏺). If the abuse occurred in the home, the adolescent may be placed in foster care or a home for pregnant adolescents. The adolescent will need support from the nurse to deal with the abuse, the pregnancy, and pending legal actions.

Risks of Pregnancy to the Adolescent Mother
PHYSICAL RISKS

The adolescent over age 15 who receives early prenatal care is at no greater risk of negative consequences from pregnancy than the 20-year-old. The adolescent under age 15 is at greatest risk during pregnancy. The young adolescent is still growing and developing physically. The pregnant adolescent already has an increased need for adequate nutrients to maintain her own growth. The needs of the fetus can actually compete with demands of the young teenager's own body. Also, because the bone structure of young teens is still developing, the dimensions of the pelvis may not be adequate to deliver a baby at term.

clinical ALERT

The pregnant teen under age 15 should gain 35 pounds during the pregnancy. To obtain adequate nutrients, the teen should eat 9 to10 servings of grains, 5 servings of vegetables, 4 servings of fruit, 5 servings of milk, and 3 servings of meat daily.

Adolescents typically do not seek prenatal care until later in the pregnancy. The risks for the pregnant adolescent include preterm birth, iron deficiency anemia, pregnancy-induced hypertension, and its **sequelae** (conditions that occur because of another condition). Adolescents have a high incidence of sexually transmitted infections. Some vaginal infections are curable with antibiotics; others are not. Vaginal infections during pregnancy greatly increase the risk to the fetus. (For further discussion of sexually transmitted infections, see Chapter 7 ⏺⏺.)

Substance abuse is high in many adolescents. Adolescents who smoke cigarettes and use drugs (including alcohol) are at increased risk of developing complications of pregnancy, including abnormalities in the fetus. Because of irregular menstrual periods, the young adolescent may not be aware of the pregnancy for some time. By the time the pregnancy is confirmed, the fetus may already have been harmed.

PSYCHOLOGICAL RISKS

The major psychological risk to the pregnant adolescent is the added pressure on her developmental tasks. Delaying these developmental tasks may have lifelong implications. The adolescent should be gaining autonomy, independence, and a sense of achievement. However, pregnancy often causes the adolescent to remain dependent on her parents, or public assistance, for financial support for many years. Often the pregnant adolescent's school performance decreases, outside-of-school activities stop, and she no longer takes pride in her accomplishments. Low school performance limits access to higher education and employment opportunities.

The adolescent may be fearful of telling peers and parents that she is pregnant. She may be overwhelmed and confused about keeping or terminating the pregnancy. She may be frightened about the delivery process. Table 12-1 ■ identifies some initial reactions when pregnancy begins in

early, middle, and late adolescence. The nurse should realize other factors may also affect the psychological response of the adolescent.

Risks to the Child of an Adolescent Mother
PHYSICAL RISKS

The adolescent mother requires additional nutrition to support her growth as well as the growth of the fetus. The adolescent lacks knowledge of nutritional requirements and has limited financial resources to purchase nutritious foods. Limited nutrition can result in intrauterine growth retardation, premature birth, and increased death rate in the fetus.

PSYCHOLOGICAL RISKS

Because teens are not developmentally or economically prepared to be parents, the children of adolescent mothers are at risk for becoming developmentally disadvantaged. Many teen mothers face adverse social and economic conditions. Children of adolescent mothers have a high rate of abuse and neglect (Koniak-Griffin, Anderson, Verzemnieks, & Brecht, 2000). These children do not do well in school and are less likely to complete high school. The Nursing Care Plan Chart on pages 257 and 258 discusses some aspects of nursing care for a single adolescent mother.

TABLE 12-1
Adolescent Reactions to Pregnancy

AGE	REACTION	NURSING IMPLICATIONS
Early adolescent (under 15)	Self-conscious about changing body with adolescents coupled with changes due to pregnancy Lack of knowledge about signs of early pregnancy Denial Fear of confiding in anyone Dependent on parents Fear of pregnancy, labor, delivery, motherhood Unable to develop maternal role at this time	Use a nonjudgmental approach Focus on needs of adolescent Encourage expression of feelings of pregnancy and options Include parents in discussion Explain physical changes in simple terms Refer to counseling as appropriate
Middle adolescent (15–17 years)	Fear of rejection by peers, parents May seek confirmation of pregnancy on own through pregnancy kits, Planned Parenthood, etc. Possible conflict with parent's and personal values	Use a nonjudgmental approach Assure confidentiality Be aware of state laws regarding abortion and parental consent Encourage communication with parents Refer to counseling as appropriate
Late adolescent (18–19 years)	May confirm pregnancy on own Understands consequences of actions Personal values, relationship with father, and future plans help in decision about pregnancy	Use a nonjudgmental approach Refer to counseling as appropriate Encourage to be realistic about pregnancy

NURSING CARE PLAN CHART

Planning for Adolescent Single Parent

GOAL	INTERVENTION	RATIONALE	EXPECTED OUTCOME
1. Risk for Impaired Parenting related to developmental stage			
Client will effectively bond with her newborn and will provide attentive, loving direct care to the baby to meet the neonate's physical, developmental, psychosocial, and spiritual needs.	Provide anticipatory guidance and parent education.	*Adolescent mothers (especially the youngest) generally lack the developmental maturity necessary to put aside self-centeredness and to focus on the many needs of a newborn.* *Adolescent mothers may put more emphasis on their personal relationships with members of the opposite sex than on their own offspring.*	Client will demonstrate personal interest in her newborn, shown by active participation in the neonate's daily care routine (feeding, bathing, diapering, etc.). Client will anticipate and respond appropriately to the newborn's cues (e.g., she will attempt to comfort the crying baby, to check for a soiled diaper, etc.).
	Provide emotional support. Help the mother learn ways to be responsible for herself and the baby.	*Guidance, support, and facilitation are ways to meet the adolescent's own developmental needs, enabling the client to focus on her child.* *Adolescent mothers generally know less about newborns' needs and the basics of child care than mature women do. They tend to be less sensitive to, and less accepting of, the newborn's behavior.*	
	Promote attachment. Encourage the mother to hold, look at, and talk to her child.	*Impaired bonding has been linked to the development of mental illness in the child.*	
2. Situational Low Self-Esteem related to unexpected pregnancy			
Client will demonstrate improved self-esteem and a positive self-concept. Client will avoid development of mental disorders associated with poor self-esteem, such as major depression.	Provide emotional support and active listening. Help the mother become more self-aware. Help her clarify what her values are.	*In highly developed nations, adolescent pregnancy is generally discouraged. In many cultures, pregnancy outside of marriage is considered taboo. Single adolescent parents may feel guilt and shame regarding their sexual behavior. Social stigma contributes to poor self-concept.* *Adolescent parents may experience social isolation, as the demands of parenting consume time and energy, taking them away from normal peer interaction and social events. Such social marginalization contributes to negative alterations in self-concept and to poor self-esteem.*	Client will verbalize a self-affirming, yet realistic self-perception. Client will demonstrate continued interest in her environment and activity in her social network. Client will avoid negative self-talk indicative of a poor self-image. Client will engage in personal goal setting and will list three key goals she wants to meet in the next 3 months (e.g., "I will return to high school").

(Continued)

GOAL	INTERVENTION	RATIONALE	EXPECTED OUTCOME
		Emotional support in the form of unconditional positive regard for the client serves to build the client's self-esteem, as does active listening. Self-awareness enhancement and values clarification, in the context of active listening, assist the client in developing an affirming, yet realistic, self-perception.	
	Instill hope.	*Hope is a necessary human capacity for mental and spiritual well-being.*	
3. Risk for Other-Directed Violence related to inexperience and stresses of motherhood			
Client will be able to manage personal emotions effectively without resorting to violence.	Provide parent education about the risk factors for domestic violence and/or child abuse. Support the young mother to recognize the need to protect the infant from anger and abuse.	*Adolescent mothers with few social supports tend to demonstrate more anger and more punitive parenting methods than older mothers. Such adolescents are likely to discipline harshly and to reject the child. Rejection and harsh discipline can be emotionally and physically damaging to the child. Extreme types are forms of child abuse.*	Client will identify signs and symptoms of escalating anger that may result in violence. Client will identify current personal and environmental stressors likely to trigger anger. Client will share a personal behavioral plan for avoiding or lessening the impact of situations likely to provoke intense anger.
	Encourage self-awareness. Ask the mother to verbalize her own anger triggers.	*Self-awareness enables the client to recognize situations and events that contribute to the escalation of personal anger and to acts of violence.*	Client will list key components of her personal support network and available community support resources.
	Help the mother identify family and caregiver support.	*Social support, especially practical assistance with direct child care, reduces the burden of care giving, and therefore, reduces the client's emotional stress.*	Client will identify behaviors requiring professional crisis intervention and the steps to be taken to obtain such services.
	Provide information about crisis intervention. Give anticipatory referrals.	*Anticipatory referral for crisis intervention is a prevention strategy designed to protect the child.*	Client will enter a behavioral contract: she will agree to seek immediate professional mental health care when in crisis. She will seek routine pastoral and/or mental health care for regular assistance with managing emotions, especially anger.
	Offer to contact a resource for spiritual care of the mother.	*Spiritual care facilitates mental and emotional well-being.*	

Partners of Adolescent Mothers

Adolescent males tend to have sexual relations at an earlier age than adolescent girls, and they tend to have more partners. Half of the fathers of infants of adolescent mothers are also teens. Like the adolescent mother, the adolescent father has not completed developmental tasks and is no better prepared financially or psychologically to become a parent. Adolescent fathers tend to seek less prestigious careers and have less formal education. They often marry at a younger age and have more children.

Half of fathers of infants of adolescent mothers are 20 years of age or older. However, many times the older partner of a pregnant adolescent is at the same emotional, educational, and financial level as adolescent fathers. They are no more likely than adolescent fathers to support the adolescent mother. In the case of the early or middle adolescent who is pregnant by an older father, authorities may need to be notified.

LEGAL RIGHTS AND RESPONSIBILITIES RELATED TO PATERNITY

The father has the right to participate in the life of the child. He also has the responsibility to provide financial support. It is the responsibility of the mother to complete the information for the birth certificate. Including the father's name on the birth certificate helps ensure his rights and encourages him to meet his responsibilities. Legal paternity gives children access to the father's medical information, military benefits (if they exist), and social security benefits. At times, such as in rape, incest, or casual sex, the adolescent mother may not want to identify or contact the father of her child. If paternity is questioned, genetic testing may be required to establish legal rights and responsibilities.

INVOLVING THE PARTNER IN PREGNANCY AND BIRTH

Many adolescent couples have meaningful relationships. The male partner may wish to be involved in the pregnancy. Health care providers need to be supportive of the father's needs, rights, and responsibilities. He may lack knowledge of the physical and psychological changes associated with pregnancy, childbirth, and parenting.

Although the father may have been included in the pregnancy, many pregnant adolescents want their mother as their primary support during labor and delivery. It is important to support the adolescent mother's wishes. The father will need support as appropriate in the situation. Unfortunately, even when the father is involved with the mother during the pregnancy and birth, if the couple does not marry, there is decreasing contact between the father, mother, and infant over time (Taylor et al., 1999). Box 12-1 ■ provides some considerations specific to teenage mothers in labor (Nichols & Humenick, 2000).

Family's Response to Adolescent Pregnancy

The reaction of both maternal and paternal family members to an adolescent pregnancy is varied. In families that foster education and career goals, an adolescent pregnancy may cause shock and disbelief. Anger, shame, and sorrow are also common reactions for these families. The majority of the adolescents from these families choose abortion, except when culture or religious beliefs prevent such decisions. There may be conflict between the adolescent parents and family members about how to deal with the pregnancy.

In families with a history of adolescent pregnancy, substance abuse, poverty, or low education goals, an adolescent pregnancy may cause anger or sorrow. On the other hand,

---

| BOX 12-1 | LIFESPAN CONSIDERATIONS |

Teen in Labor

- Teens often have greater need for emotional support. Emotional needs are often more complex than those of an adult woman.
- Adequate pain control must be provided. Teens need teaching prior to labor about the progression of pain in labor.
- Age, preparation, and family support will all affect the quality of the labor experience.
- Teen may want to have a friend come for labor support. (Friend may compete with teen's partner or parent for position; this problem occurs at a time that the young mother is most vulnerable; this needs to be discussed in prenatal class.)
- Peer support programs are effective in prenatal education programs.
- Teens' attitude of immortality and narcissism may make it difficult to address potential complications. ("Of course my body can give birth! Why shouldn't it?" This is part of the "it can't happen to me" way of thinking that is typical of this age group.)
- Any procedure (vaginal exam, epidural, IV lines, cesarean) may be terrifying to a teen. Be honest but gentle in providing an explanation prior to the procedure.
- Teens may be skeptical about relaxation and breathing techniques. They may want to prepare a tape or CD of their own music to use for relaxation during labor. (The nurse educator may prepare a tape or CD of music with phrases about deep breathing interspersed and provide it to the prenatal class.)

---

these families may be more accepting, because adolescent pregnancy is more common and part of their life experience. Most commonly, these pregnancies are maintained, and the adolescent mother chooses to raise the baby.

The mother of the pregnant adolescent is usually the first to be told about the pregnancy. She typically becomes involved in the decision making about issues such as maintaining the pregnancy, abortion, or adoption. She often accompanies the pregnant adolescent on the first prenatal visit. She may be instrumental in supporting the adolescent couple through the pregnancy, childbirth, and parenting.

Social Considerations

Adolescent pregnancy affects all of society. Typically the adolescent mother accesses public services such as the WIC program, Aid to Dependent Children, welfare, and food stamp programs. If employed, the adolescent generally holds a low-paying job. The adolescent couple has little advanced education and, therefore, has little chance for career advancement. See the Health Promotion Issue on pages 260 to 261 for further discussion of the social impact of adolescent pregnancy.

HEALTH PROMOTION ISSUE

IMPACT OF ADOLESCENT PREGNANCY ON SOCIETY

Sonya Adams is the mother of three teenagers and has recently been elected to public office. Sonya has a good relationship with her children and their friends. Her oldest daughter's girlfriend has just discovered she is pregnant. Sonya wants to be able to help her children, their friends, and also her community. She needs more information regarding the impact of adolescent pregnancy on society.

DISCUSSION

Adolescent pregnancy has a widespread effect on society. For example, in 2002, only 10% of teen mothers aged 15 to 17 had completed high school. It is estimated that only 33% of teen mothers will eventually graduate from high school and only 1.5% will receive a college degree by the time they reach 30 years of age (Annie E. Casey Foundation, 2004). When teens are undereducated, their employment opportunities are limited. Nearly 80% of teen mothers eventually go on welfare.

Although less severe than for teen mothers, the effects of early parenting are also negative for adolescent fathers. Teen fathers are more likely to have behaviors such as alcohol abuse or drug dealing, and they complete less formal education than their childless peers. Fathers of children born to teenage mothers earn an estimated $3,400 less per year than fathers of children born to older mothers. Only 30% of teenage mothers receive child support payments from the child's father.

Children born to teen mothers are at greater risk of lower intelligence, lower academic achievement, and social behavioral problems. Children born to teen mothers face inadequate nutrition, poor health care, and less cognitive and social stimulation. Children of teen mothers are more likely to become teen parents. Children of teenage mothers are more likely to be incarcerated during their adolescence or early twenties.

Experts estimate the annual costs of births to teens is about $7 billion in tax revenues, public assistance, child health care, foster care, and involvement in the criminal justice system. During her first 13 years of parenthood, the average teen mother receives approximately $1,400 per year in support from Aid to Families with Dependent Children (AFDC) and federal food stamps (Annie E. Casey Foundation, 1998).

Besides keeping and rearing the child, there are other options to consider. Many teens are choosing to terminate the pregnancy. In 1999, nearly 40% of teen pregnancies ended in abortion. In recent years, teen abortion rates have declined, but statistics regarding teen abortion are slow in being published. Teens who choose to terminate the pregnancy identify several reasons: being too young, not having enough money, and wanting to finish their education are among the most common.

Although terminating a pregnancy may be beneficial to the future of the individual, there are also costs. In 2001, the average charge for abortion was $468. Most women (74%) paid for the abortion themselves. Medicaid and private insurance paid for the remainder. Congress has barred the use of federal Medicaid funds to pay for abortions, except when the woman's life is endangered by the pregnancy, or in case of rape or incest. Some states use their own money to subsidize abortion for poor women (Allen Guttmacher Institute, 2002).

Some women may initially believe that abortion is their best option. However, the long-term effects of abortion have not been extensively explored. Physical complications, including infection, hemorrhage, future miscarriages, and infertility, have an impact on the woman, her future partners, and society as a whole.

Psychological complications associated with abortion are identified as post-abortion syndrome (PAS). Often years after the abortion, some women begin to have psychological difficulties dealing with grief and guilt over their choice. PAS may present with physical and psychological symptoms that may appear to be associated with other diagnoses. Upon further exploration, these symptoms are associated with unresolved feelings about the abortion. These women need professional help.

Another option for the pregnant adolescent is adoption. Adoption is a way for the birth parents to place their baby in a loving family when they are unable to care for the child themselves. Only 1% of teen pregnancies result in adoption. In many cases, the birth mother can identify criteria the adoptive family must meet and thereby have a voice in her child's future. Some adoptions are **open adoptions,** meaning that the birth mother and adoptive parents can meet and communicate about the child. Other adoptions are **closed adoptions,** and the birth parents and adoptive parent do not communicate. Many times, once adoptive children become 18 years of age, they can locate their birth parents.

Adoption impacts society. The adoptive child becomes a member of a family. The adoptive parents are legally responsible for providing food, clothing, shelter, and education for the child. In many instances, the adoptive family is better prepared, emotionally and financially, to raise the child than the adolescent birth parents. Therefore, the child has an increased opportunity for becoming a productive citizen.

PLANNING AND IMPLEMENTATION

The nurse has a responsibility to society. The nurse assists the adolescent parents in making informed decisions and accessing resources. The nurse also participates in research, publishing findings and keeping elected officials informed of the issues. The elected officials can therefore make informed decisions and provide needed resources.

SELF-REFLECTION

What are your thoughts about the impact of teen pregnancy on society? How has teen pregnancy affected you personally? How can you help teen parents to make the best decisions possible for the child and for themselves?

SUGGESTED RESOURCES

For the Nurse

Abma, J.C., Martinez, G.M., Mosner, W.D., & Dawson, B.S. (2004). Teenagers in United States: Sexual activity, contraceptive use and childbearing, 2002. *Vital Health Statistics, 23*(24).

Doniger, A., Adams, E., Utter, C., & Riley, J. (2001). Impact evaluation of the "not me, not now" abstinence-oriented adolescent pregnancy prevention communication program, Monroe County, New York. *Journal of Health Communication,* 6(1), 45–60.

The Guttmacher Institute. (2006). *U.S. Teenage pregnancy statistics national and state trends and trends by race and ethnicity.* New York: The Guttmacher Institute.

For the Client

Cohen, D.A., Farley, T.A., Taylor, S.N., Martin, D.H., & Schuster, M.A. (2002). When and where do youths have sex? The potential role of adult supervision. *Pediatrics, 110*(6), 66–69.

National Campaign to Prevent Teen Pregnancy. (2003). *With one voice: American adults and teens sound off about teen pregnancy.* Washington, DC: Author.

NURSING CARE

PRIORITIES IN NURSING CARE

The first priority in working with the pregnant adolescent is to establish a trusting relationship. The adolescent will need help to make a plan of how to proceed with the pregnancy, including but not limited to telling the father and their parents and seeking additional medical assistance. Although each situation is different, the nurse can provide support and objectivity.

ASSESSING

The nurse needs to establish data from which to plan interventions for the mother-to-be and family. Because the amount of data that needs to be collected is extensive, the initial interview may take some time. If time is not available, or if the adolescent mother becomes upset or uncooperative, a second interview should be planned in a few weeks. The following areas should be assessed:

- Family and personal health history, including support systems and socioeconomic situation
- Medical history
- Menstrual history
- Obstetric and gynecologic history, including sexually transmitted infections
- Substance abuse history
- Maturational level of pregnant teen and her partner
- The pregnant teen's self-concept, including body image
- The pregnant teen's attitude toward and anticipated ability to care for the coming baby

clinical ALERT

The pregnant teen may be so distraught by the pregnancy that she sees suicide as her only option. Be alert for signs of impending suicide, including giving away possessions, not keeping appointments, and verbalizing a desire to die. If such signs occur, the adolescent should not be left alone, and the parent or nurse should summon assistance.

DIAGNOSING, PLANNING, AND IMPLEMENTING

Nursing diagnoses for a pregnant adolescent would include those for any pregnant woman. Additional nursing diagnoses might include:

- Imbalanced **N**utrition: Less than Body Requirements related to poor eating habits
- Health Seeking **B**ehaviors related to expressed desire to parent effectively
- Risk for Situational Low **S**elf-Esteem related to unanticipated pregnancy

Expected outcomes might include:

- Gains weight within normal limits for stage of pregnancy
- Fetal growth within normal limits for gestational age
- Verbalizes information regarding pregnancy and child care practices
- Develops positive attitude about her body and physical changes

To achieve these outcomes, the nurse provides various interventions.

- Make the teenager feel more comfortable by assuming a nonjudgmental attitude, by explaining procedures, and by showing compassion through tone of voice and touch. *The first step in planning and implementing care of the pregnant adolescent is to establish a trusting relationship. The adolescent may feel nervous and vulnerable at her first clinic visit, which may include her first vaginal examination.*
- Assist the adolescent in her decision-making and problem-solving skills. *Providing support will help the teen proceed with her developmental tasks and begin to assume responsibility for her life and that of her infant. With an open, nonjudgmental manner, without imposing personal values, the nurse can educate the adolescent about her options of maintaining or terminating the pregnancy, and keeping or relinquishing the infant for adoption.*
- Encourage the adolescent to express her feelings regarding each option. *Helping the teen to express her feelings will help her make the decisions that are best for her.*
- Provide information regarding community resources to assist with each option. *Providing community resources will give the adolescent additional information and support needed throughout the pregnancy.*
- Help the pregnant teen to discuss options with her partner, her family, and his family in a timely manner. *The decision to terminate the pregnancy may need to be made rapidly to remain within the time frame of a legal abortion. Other options may not require rapid decisions.*
- Refer the families to the RN, primary care provider, or counseling to resolve conflicts. *The families may not agree with the decision of the pregnant teen. The LPN/LVN needs help to resolve complex family conflict.*
- If the pregnancy is terminated, the adolescent, her partner, and family members may need counseling to accept the loss. *It is common for the mother to experience grief and guilt, even when she believes abortion is her best option. If she does not deal with these feelings early, they can become life-long mental health issues.*
- Help the adolescent enroll in education programs especially designed for pregnant adolescents. Some programs provide resident, 24-hour services where the pregnant teen can live and attend classes. Day classes are available for teens who do not need a place to live. *Classes help the*

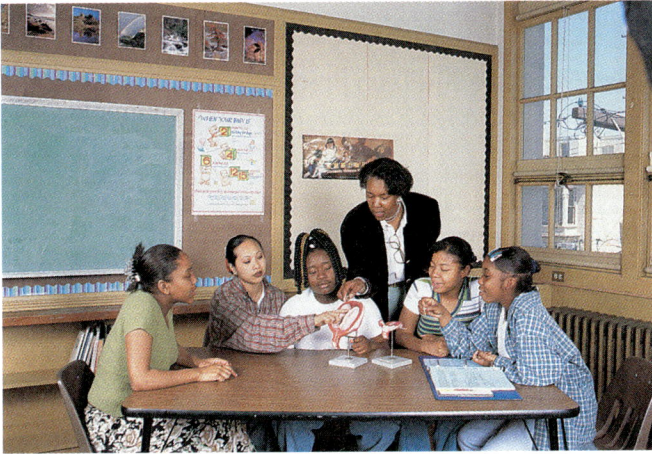

Figure 12-3. ■ Providing prenatal classes specifically for teens can improve the learning environment for young mothers.

adolescent to understand pregnancy and the changes happening within their body (Figure 12-3 ■). Classes can be designed to teach life skills, complete her high school education, and help her learn to care for her infant.

- Adapt teaching materials to meet the needs of the cognitively challenged pregnant adolescent. Box 12-2 ■ lists some methods of reaching the low-level learner (Nichols & Humenick, 2000). *The nurse must provide instruction in a format the client can understand.*
- Provide printed information regarding specific foods to eat to obtain the needed nutrients. *Printed information should include recommendations for meeting the*

| BOX 12-2 | CLIENT TEACHING |

Reaching the Low-Level Learner

Teens become pregnant across the spectrum from high to low socioeconomic and academic backgrounds. When a teen presents at a very young age or at a low reading level, additional client teaching is needed. The following recommendations can be of use with the low-level learner:

- Ensure that written materials are at a fifth-grade level.
- Include various types of media to help with different learning styles.
- Use posters that address only one topic at a time.
- Use games (flashcards, "bingo") as a means of reinforcing information.
- After teaching, ask students to create a poster and present it to the class to see where learning has occurred and whether any misconceptions need to be addressed.
- Role-play phone calling the physician or midwife when the teen thinks labor is beginning.
- If the father is also involved in prenatal education, use sports analogies. For example, crowning may be compared to being one yard from the end zone in football (one last big push).

adolescent's nutritional needs as well as the needs of the fetus (see Chapter 11 ⬭).

- Provide information on the WIC program in her area. *The WIC program provides assistance with the purchase of nutritious foods.*

EVALUATING

As the pregnancy progresses, the adolescent will become more involved in her care. She will verbalize acceptance of her changing body. She will understand that following delivery, some effects of pregnancy (such as linea nigra will fade) and she will be able to regain abdominal muscle tone. Other effects of pregnancy, such as striae, will be permanent.

She will comply with her nutritional plan and any prescribed treatments.

She will be able to set goals for herself and her infant. She will establish a plan of action and show evidence of working toward her goals.

NURSING PROCESS CARE PLAN
Caring for a Client with Situational Low Self-Esteem

Janet, 16 years old, comes to the clinic for the first time. She is 10 weeks pregnant. She states that her parents "kicked her out of the house" when they discovered she was sexually active with her 17-year-old boyfriend, Joe. Janet and Joe live together in a one-bedroom basement apartment. Neither attends school. Joe works at a grocery store during the day and at a fast-food restaurant in the evening. They can barely pay the rent and utilities and buy food. Joe has been angry recently over their lack of money to "have fun." Janet is fearful he will leave her when he discovers she is pregnant.

Assessment

- 16 years old
- 10 weeks pregnant
- Low income
- Unemployed
- Not attending school
- "Kicked out" of parents home
- Conflict with boyfriend

Nursing Diagnosis.   The following important nursing diagnosis (among others) is established for this condition:

- Situational Low Self-Esteem related to pregnancy, being "kicked out of parents' house," and fear of Joe leaving her

Expected Outcome

- Client will verbalize goals and plan for changing present living situation.

Planning and Implementation

- Assist in identifying personal strengths. *During periods of stress, individuals lose sight of personal strengths. Identifying personal strengths gives individuals some power and control over their situation.*
- Assist in identifying resources. *The pregnant adolescent needs to identify resources (individuals, groups, or agencies) that will be able to assist with planning and problem solving.*
- Assist in identifying alternatives to present living situation. *Identifying alternatives to present situation provides emotional strength.*

Evaluation.   Client states that she will talk with her friends about ways to change her situation. She will feel safe and be prepared to begin decision making regarding pregnancy.

Critical Thinking in the Nursing Process

1. What are two other nursing diagnoses for Janet?
2. To what agencies should Janet be referred for assistance?
3. How often should the nurse follow up with Janet's care?

Note: Discussion of Critical Thinking questions appears in Appendix I.

Prevention of Adolescent Pregnancy

Preventing adolescent pregnancies is a monumental task. Over the past decade, the rate of adolescent pregnancy has declined. The reasons for this decline may be due to improved contraception. However, teen pregnancy rates in the United States are the highest among developed countries.

Teens who have a set of values, pride in themselves, respect for their bodies and their health, and constructive plans for their future are most likely to resist peer pressure to engage in sex. Box 12-3 ■ discusses some aspects of the teen culture that need to be addressed in preventing teen pregnancy.

Parents, teachers, and other significant adults need to give teenagers the knowledge to make sound choices and take responsibility for their actions. Teens who discuss sex with their parents delay being sexually active. Teens want to discuss sex with their parents, but some parents have difficulty discussing sex with their teens. An important part of communicating with teens is to actively listen to them. Parents can use the "I hear" checklist as a tool that creates open lines of communication (Figure 12-4 ■).

BOX 12-3	CULTURAL PULSE POINTS

Teen Culture and Teen Pregnancy

Teen culture and media promote casual sex among teens and adults and rarely show negative consequences of early sexual behavior. In television shows, films, songs, and advertising, sex has little meaning, partners are often unmarried, and unplanned pregnancies seldom occur.

To combat this barrage of misinformation, parents need to take an active role in discussing the facts about sexual involvement. They need to share the importance of values in life and the possible consequences to health and livelihood of early sexual intercourse. They also need to equip their teens with tools to use to combat peer pressure.

Parents must make sure the information they give their children about risks, responsibilities, and realities of being sexually active is accurate. The nurse can be a valuable resource for the parents who need assistance talking with their teens. Parents should tell their teens about the risk of sexually transmitted infections and pregnancy. Teens need to be taught about contraception, including how to apply a condom. (See Chapter 7 ⊙⊙ for information about contraception.) Parents can teach their teens to say "no" by learning the lines used by peers to encourage them to engage in sexual activities. For example: "If you really loved me, you would have sex with me," or, "Everyone is having sex." In reality, if he (or she) really loved her (him), the person would want to wait until they were older and ready to handle the responsibility of sex and parenthood. Also, it is not true that everyone is having sex. There has been an increase in abstinence in teens over the past few years. Some teens are making a written contract to abstain from sexual activity.

Although there is no rule on when to talk with children about sex, most authorities believe open discussion about body parts, functions, and sexual behavior should take place as the child asks questions. With the widespread exposure to sexual content in the media, children have more information and at a younger age than their parents did. Parents have a responsibility to relay their family values to their

---

"I HEAR"	
I	Be **i**nformed.
H	Be **h**onest.
E	Initiate conversations **e**arly.
A	Be **a**vailable and **a**skable.
R	Be **r**ealistic.

Figure 12-4. ■ The mnemonic "I hear" can be used to recall approaches that help the nurse connect well with teenagers.

children. By discussing situations with children and helping them think through solutions, parents can give children the skills necessary to say "no" to peer pressure until they are mature enough to be responsible for their actions.

Parents need to make time to interact with their children. By being available and approachable, parents establish an atmosphere in which children will feel comfortable to ask questions. Children learn about sexuality by watching how warmly, respectfully, and affectionately their parents treat one another. Children learn that having sexual feelings does not make them a bad person. However, children need to learn that the consequences of acting on their sexual feelings may prevent them from reaching their goals.

Note: The reference and resource listings for this and all chapters have been compiled at the back of the book.

Chapter Review

KEY TERMS by Topic

Use the audio glossary feature of either the CD-ROM or the Companion Website to hear the correct pronunciation of the following key terms.

Risks of Pregnancy to the Adolescent Mother
sequelae

Social Considerations
open adoption, closed adoption

KEY Points

- Adolescent pregnancy is an individual, family, and societal problem.
- Lack of education, poverty, and high-risk behavior contribute to adolescent pregnancy.
- Because the adolescent is still growing and developing, pregnancy puts additional stress on her physically and psychologically.
- The child of an adolescent mother is at risk for abuse, neglect, and becoming an adolescent parent.
- The adolescent has difficult decisions to make regarding the pregnancy and will need information and support in making these decisions.
- The pregnant adolescent has a need for additional nutrition to meet her growth needs and the needs of the fetus.
- The nurse must provide support to the pregnant teen, her partner, and parents.
- The pregnant teen needs assistance with problem solving in order to make an informed decision regarding the pregnancy.
- The teen needs referral to education and financial assistance programs.

EXPLORE MediaLink

Additional interactive resources for this chapter can be found on the Companion Website at www.prenhall.com/towle. Click on Chapter 12 and "Begin" to select the activities for this chapter.

For chapter-related NCLEX®-style questions and an audio glossary, access the accompanying CD-ROM in this book.

Animation
Teens: Mental & Spiritual Health

FOR FURTHER Study

See Chapter 5 for a complete discussion of reproductive anatomy and physiology.

For further discussion about contraception and sexually transmitted infections, see Chapter 7.

For information on adolescent's nutritional needs as well as the needs of the fetus, see Chapter 11.

Critical Thinking Care Map

Pregnant Adolescent Exploring Options
NCLEX-PN® Focus Area: Psychosocial Integrity

Case Study: Maria, age 14, comes to the clinic with her mother. Maria has been having nausea and vomiting every morning for a week. She began her menses at age 12 and has been having regular periods for the past year. She missed her period the last 2 months. Maria's mother states she is afraid Maria is pregnant. Maria at first denies being sexually active, but then begins to cry and states she had sex one time with her 14-year-old boyfriend. She states she does not know what to do. Maria's mother wants to know their options at this point. A pregnancy test performed in the clinic is positive.

Nursing Diagnosis: Health Seeking Behavior related to adolescent pregnancy

COLLECT DATA

Subjective

_____
_____
_____
_____
_____
_____
_____

Objective

_____
_____
_____
_____
_____
_____
_____

Would you report this? Yes/No

If yes, to: _____

Nursing Care

_____
_____
_____
_____
_____
_____
_____
_____
_____
_____

How would you document this?_____
_____
_____
_____

Data Collected
(use only those that apply)

- Positive pregnancy test
- Crying
- Menarche at age 12
- Nausea and vomiting
- Requests information regarding options
- Missed period for 2 months
- Denies sexual activity
- States does not know what to do

Nursing Interventions
(use only those that apply; list in priority order)

- Give Maria prenatal vitamins.
- Instruct Maria in birth control methods.
- Tell Maria what to expect during a pelvic examination.
- Provide Maria and her mother with information on nutrition.
- Encourage Maria to discuss her sexual experience.
- Provide Maria and her mother with information about abortion and adoption.
- Tell Maria what to expect with an ultrasound examination.
- Provide information for Maria and her mother about sexually transmitted infections.

Compare your documentation to the sample provided in Appendix I.

NCLEX-PN® Exam Preparation

1 The LPN/LVN gathers the following information from a 16-year-old pregnant female during an initial visit in the prenatal clinic. Which of the following information would be considered contributing factors to adolescent pregnancy? (Select all that apply.)

1. Is active in after-school activities.
2. Mother had first pregnancy at age 16.
3. Spends weekends at home alone while parents work.
4. Plans to attend college and study music.
5. Prepares evening meal for two younger siblings.

2 The LPN/LVN has completed a physical assessment on a 15-year-old pregnant client. Which of the following data indicates a risk for the client?

1. hemoglobin level of 10
2. mild contractions at 38 weeks' gestation
3. menarche at age 13
4. blood pressure of 120/84

3 The nurse is reviewing a list of nutritious foods with a pregnant 15-year-old. The nurse encourages the adolescent to select foods that are high in:

1. fat.
2. sugars.
3. protein.
4. starch.

4 The nurse is preparing to visit a 16-year-old client who recently had an abortion. The nurse understands that the client may project feelings of (select all that apply):

1. guilt.
2. disbelief.
3. grief.
4. joy.
5. doubt.

5 The nurse is counseling a group of pregnant teenagers. Which of the following teenagers are more likely to terminate the pregnancy?

1. Teenagers who are high achievers in school.
2. Teenagers whose family struggle financially.
3. Teenager whose mother became pregnant at an early age.
4. Teenagers with a family history of substance abuse.

6 Which of the following statements indicates that the pregnant adolescent understands how to protect the father's rights relating to paternity?

1. "The father will come to the hospital to see his baby."
2. "I will include his name on the birth certificate."
3. "The father will attend the birth of his baby."
4. "I will wait until he states he wants to see his baby."

7 A nurse is teaching a class on adolescent pregnancy to a group of high school parents. Which of the following are true about adolescent males? (Select all that apply.)

1. Adolescents males engage in sexual relations earlier than females.
2. Adolescent males tend to have more sexual partners.
3. Adolescent males are more mature than their partners.
4. Adolescent males tend to have fewer sexual partners.
5. Adolescent males often do not complete their education.

8 The nurse is discussing nutritional requirements with the parents of a pregnant 14-year-old. The nurse explains that young adolescents who have a poor nutritional intake are at risk for:

1. prolonged labor.
2. post mature birth.
3. intrauterine growth retardation.
4. dystocia.

9 A nurse is discussing teen pregnancy with a group of high school parents. Which of the following recommendations by the nurse would help parents reduce the risk of teen pregnancy?

1. Encourage parents to send their teen to a sex education class.
2. During the early teen years, provide accurate information about the responsibilities of sexual activity.
3. Delay discussing sexually activity until the teen is older.
4. Provide reading material and avoid open discussions about sex.

10 A 16-year-old pregnant client has arrived for her first prenatal visit. During the initial visit, it is most important for the nurse to:

1. assess the 16-year-old's attitude toward pregnancy.
2. evaluate the client's socioeconomic situation.
3. identify educational plans during the pregnancy.
4. establish a trusting relationship.

Answers for NCLEX-PN® Review and Critical Thinking questions appear in Appendix I.

Care During High-Risk Pregnancy

BRIEF Outline

Risk Factors

Tests Used to Assess Maternal Well-Being

COMPLICATIONS OF PREGNANCY

Complications with Bleeding

Hypertensive Disorders

Gestational Diabetes Mellitus

Hemolytic Disorders of Pregnancy

Hyperemesis Gravidarum

Multiple Pregnancy

MEDICAL CONDITIONS COMPLICATED BY PREGNANCY

Respiratory Disorders

Cardiac Disorders

Urinary Disorders

Neurologic Disorders

Hematologic Disorders

Infections

Trauma

Homelessness

Psychosocial Effects of Medical Conditions During Pregnancy

ANTEPARTAL LOSS

Fetal Demise

Maternal Death

Grief Process

Family Response to Fetal Loss

Nursing Care

High-Risk Postpartum Care

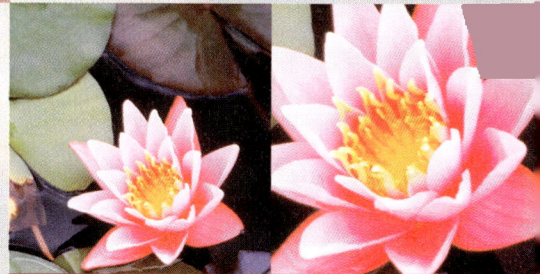

HEALTH PROMOTION ISSUE: Smoking and Pregnancy

NURSING CARE PLAN CHART: Planning for Mother at Risk for Premature Labor

NURSING PROCESS CARE PLAN: Woman with Gestational Diabetes

CRITICAL THINKING CARE MAP: Woman Presenting with Gestational (Pregnancy-Induced) Hypertension

LEARNING Outcomes

After completing this chapter, you will be able to:

1. Define key terms.
2. Describe factors that put a woman at risk for complications of pregnancy.
3. Describe tests used to monitor the pregnant woman's status.
4. Describe common complications of pregnancy including symptoms, medical treatment, and nursing care.
5. Describe medical conditions that are complicated by pregnancy.
6. Describe loss and grief in association with high-risk pregnancy.
7. Describe the role of the LPN/LVN in caring for the high-risk woman with a pregnancy at risk.

The role of the LPN/LVN is generally one of caring for stable clients, including identifying and reporting signs of complications and teaching clients to prevent them. At times, the RN needs assistance in providing care to clients who are seriously ill. In these cases, the LPN/LVN needs to have a deeper understanding of pathophysiology and treatment. This chapter contains information about care of the woman at risk for life-threatening complications during pregnancy.

Risk Factors

Factors associated with high-risk childbearing are grouped according to the threat to health and the outcome of the pregnancy. Box 13-1 ■ identifies these risk factors. Figure 13-1 ■ shows various high-risk issues for which referrals are likely. Risk factors are interrelated and cumulative. Therefore, a pregnant woman who has multiple risk factors is considered to have a high-risk pregnancy even if each risk factor is not major by itself. Risk factors may also be identified by verbal interview or written survey. The LPN/LVN may help collect data about risk factors.

The Health Promotion Issue on pages 272 and 273 discusses the topic of smoking during pregnancy.

Ideally, women prepare for pregnancy by maintaining healthy behaviors, including proper nutrition and the avoidance of risky behavior prior to conception. As stated in Chapter 10 ⚭ , the woman should obtain prenatal care as soon as she suspects she is pregnant or within the first 6 to 8 weeks. However, many women do not plan for pregnancy. Some engage in a variety of risk-taking behaviors (large intake of alcohol or other substances, unguarded sexual intercourse with multiple partners, smoking, poor nutritional habits, or fad diets). These behaviors may be part of a woman's lifestyle, and they increase the woman's risk of complications. Once the pregnant woman obtains health care and risk factors are identified, teaching can begin and a plan of care can be implemented to decrease the number and severity of complications.

Even with the best prenatal care, complications can occur. With frequent monitoring and evaluation, though, the severity of complications may be kept to a minimum. See Table 10-4 ⚭ for signs of complications. If signs of complications are detected, further testing is warranted to evaluate fetal well-being. Common tests used to evaluate fetal well-being include ultrasound, amniocentesis, nonstress test, and biophysical profile. These tests are described in detail in Chapter 9 ⚭ .

Tests Used to Assess Maternal Well-Being

Besides evaluating fetal well-being, prenatal care must include an assessment of maternal well-being. Recall that routine prenatal maternal assessment includes vital signs,

---

| BOX 13-1 | ASSESSMENT |

Risk Factors for High-Risk Pregnancy

Biophysical Factors

  Genetic makeup: Abnormalities may interfere with normal fetal development.

  Nutritional status: Normal fetal growth and development cannot progress without adequate nutrients.

  Medical and/or obstetric history: Mother's health can lead to complications. Examples include history of preterm labor, diabetes, and kidney disease.

Psychosocial Factors

  Smoking: Maternal smoking leads to low birth weight infants.

  Caffeine: Heavy consumption may lead to slight decrease in birth weight.

  Alcohol: Consumption of alcohol can lead to fetal disabilities, including fetal alcohol syndrome, learning disabilities, and hyperactivity.

  Drugs: Many drugs can affect the fetus, including prescription, over-the-counter, and illicit drugs.

  Psychological status: Pregnancy triggers complex psychological responses that affect maternal well-being.

Sociodemographic Factors

  Low income: Inadequate financial resources lead to no prenatal care, poor diet, and poor general health.

  Lack of prenatal care: Early diagnosis and treatment of complications affect the outcome of the pregnancy.

  Age: Adolescents have a higher incidence of complications, including anemia, gestational hypertension, and difficult labor. The mature woman is at higher risk for low birth weight, macrosomia, chromosomal abnormalities, congenital malformation, and neonatal mortality.

  Parity: First pregnancies and multigravida (especially when pregnancies are close together) carry higher risk.

  Marital status: Mortality and morbidity rates are higher for the fetus of nonmarried women.

  Residence: Residence alone is not a risk factor, but health care in some areas is not available or of poor quality.

  Ethnicity: Ethnicity alone is not a risk factor, but it may be impacted by other sociodemographic factors.

Environmental Factors

Many environmental substances can impact the pregnancy, including air quality, chemicals such as pesticides, radiation, and stress. These are found in the workplace, the home, and the community.

---

weight, and urine analysis for glucose and protein. Baseline blood tests are usually done during the initial prenatal visit and then repeated as indicated. Refer to Table 10-2 ⚭ for normal values during pregnancy.

Early pregnancy risk identification

Medical history/conditions	Recommended consultation *
Asthma	
Symptomatic on medication	■
Severe (multiple hospitalizations)	△
Cardiac disease	
Cyanotic, prior MI, prosthetic valve, AHA Class ≥ II	△
Other	■
Diabetes mellitus	
Class A–C	■
Class ≥ D	△
Drug/alcohol use	■
Epilepsy (on medication)	■
Family history of genetic problems (Down Syndrome, Tay Sachs)	△
Hemoglobinopathy (SS, SC, S-thal)	△
Hypertension	
Chronic, with renal or heart disease	△
Chronic, on medication or diastolic ≥ 90	■
Prior pulmonary embolus/deep vein thrombosis	■
Psychiatric disease	■
Pulmonary disease	
Severe obstructive or restrictive	△
Moderate	■
Renal disease	
Chronic, creatinine ≥ 3 with/without hypertension	△
Chronic, other	■
Requirement for prolonged anticoagulation	△
Severe systemic disease (examples: SLE, hyperthyroidism)	△

Obstetric history/conditions	
Age > 35 at delivery	■
Cesarean delivery, prior classical or vertical	■
Incompetent cervix	■
Prior fetal structural or chromosomal abnormality	△
Prior neonatal death	■
Prior stillbirth	■
Prior preterm delivery or preterm PROM	■
Prior low birthweight (< 2500 g)	■
Second trimester pregnancy loss	■
Uterine leiomyomata or malformation	■

*At the time of consultation, continued patient care should be determined to be by collaboration with the referring care provider or by transfer of care

Initial laboratory	
HIV	
Symptomatic or low CD4 count	△
Other	■
Rh/other blood group isoimmunizations (excl. ABO, Lewis)	△

Initial examination	
Condylomata (extensive, covering vulva/vaginal opening)	■

Key
■ Specialty
△ Subspecialty

Figure 13-1. ■ Early pregnancy risk identification, showing the likely referral for each condition. Depending on the condition, the client may stay with the original health care provider, who would collaborate with the specialist, or the client might be transferred to the specialist for the duration of the pregnancy. (Reproduced, with permission, from Committee on Perinatal Health, 1995.)

SMOKING AND PREGNANCY

Juanita, pregnant for the second time, comes to the clinic for her second prenatal checkup. She comments to the LPN that she hopes this baby is as small as her son, Don, who is now 2 years old. She explains that if the baby is small she will have fewer stretch marks and labor will be easier. When questioned about Don, she states that he weighed 5 pounds, 10 ounces at term. He is still small but is growing steadily. Juanita states she smokes one pack of cigarettes a day. She smokes outside because Don has difficulty breathing in a smoky house. She intends to continue smoking throughout the pregnancy.

DISCUSSION

Smoking cigarettes is a widespread health problem that affects nearly every American. For years, research and education has been directed at campaigns designed to help smokers quit and to prevent teens from starting smoking. Most people have general knowledge of the effects of smoking on the individual's lungs. Smoking leads to chronic obstructive pulmonary disease (COPD), hypertension, cardiovascular disease, and stroke. However, because symptoms of these disorders do not appear right away, the individual may deny the effects of smoking on health. The pregnant woman who smokes may not acknowledge that these disorders will impact their ability to care for and raise their children.

Cigarette smoking during pregnancy does not just affect the woman. Cigarette smoking causes low birth weight in the infant. Like Juanita, some women, fearful of a difficult labor, are thinking of themselves instead of their unborn baby. Low birth weight can lead to life-threatening complications such as hypothermia, hypoglycemia, and neonatal death. Besides low birth weight, cigarette smoking during pregnancy is related to other health problems.

Cigarette smoke contains over 1,000 different chemical compounds. Two main compounds, carbon monoxide and nicotine, are suspected of causing the most damage to the developing fetus. Carbon monoxide, having a high affinity for hemoglobin, prevents the blood from carrying adequate amounts of oxygen to the tissues. The result is hypoxia in the fetus. Nicotine has both cardiovascular and central nervous system effects. Nicotine is able to cross the placenta in levels in the fetus that exceed those in the mother. Nicotine is measurable in the breast milk of smoking mothers and to some extent in nonsmoking mothers who have been exposed to secondhand smoke.

Nicotine causes vasoconstriction, reducing blood flow to the uterus and

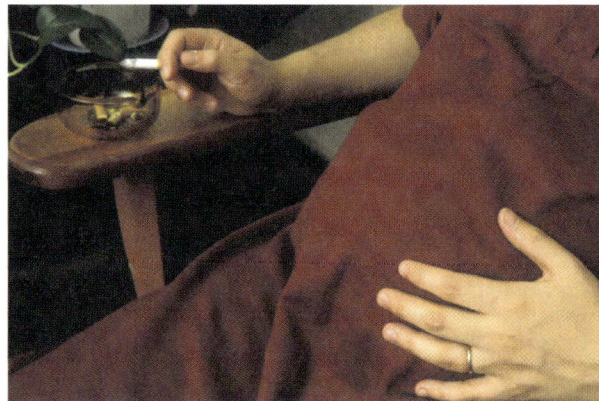

MATERNAL HEMOGLOBIN TEST

A **maternal hemoglobin test** is repeated at 7 months to assess for anemia. Recall that hemoglobin, found inside the red blood cell, is the chemical made from iron that carries oxygen. If the hemoglobin level is less than 11 g/dL, an increased intake of iron or iron supplements may be necessary. There is a tendency for anemia to occur in certain cultural groups, as discussed in Box 13-2 ■.

INDIRECT COOMBS' TEST

An **indirect Coombs' test** is done at 28 weeks on Rh-negative woman. If the indirect Coombs' changes from a normal value of negative to a positive value, it indicates that the woman's blood has been sensitized by fetal Rh-positive blood. RhIgG prophylaxis must be given to prevent the mother's Rh-negative blood from destroying the fetal blood. This condition, one of the hemolytic disorders of pregnancy, is discussed later in this chapter.

BOX 13-2	CULTURAL PULSE POINTS

Erythroblastic Anemia

Women of Mediterranean descent are prone to developing thalassemia, a type of erythroblastic anemia. These women may have a chromosomal defect that results in fragile red blood cells. The stress of pregnancy could cause these fragile cells to be destroyed, resulting in anemia.

placenta. This may account for the increased rate of spontaneous abortion in smoking women. Vasoconstriction also accounts for an increase in abruptio placentae. The placenta in smoking women is generally larger than in non-smoking women, which is believed to be a compensatory mechanism for decreased oxygen. A large placenta increases the chance of developing placenta previa. There is an increase in perinatal (after 20 weeks' gestation) and neonatal (in the first 28 days) deaths in smoking women. This increase does not include the increase mortality for low birth weight infants. Of the risk factors for sudden infant death syndrome (SIDS), maternal smoking is the most predictable.

Nicotine damages brain cell quality. Numerous studies over the past 25 to 30 years indicate that children of smoking mothers are more likely to have attention deficit hyperactive disorder (ADHD), learning disabilities, and behavior problems. Many of these problems continue as the child moves into adulthood.

It has been known for many years that individuals who smoke have a much higher risk of developing cancer. Components of cigarette smoke have been shown to be transplacental carcinogens in animals. Researchers confirm an increased risk of all cancers, including acute lymphocytic leukemia and lymphoma, in children of smoking mothers.

It is important to keep the baby in a smoke-free environment. Babies who are exposed to cigarette smoke have a higher incidence of SIDS, asthma, ear infections, and tonsillitis. Babies who live in a smoke environment are more likely to be hospitalized for pneumonia in the first year of life.

PLANNING AND IMPLEMENTATION

It is important for the nurse to question the pregnant woman regarding cigarette smoking, including the smoking behavior of others in the household. When cigarette smoking is identified, the nurse should inform the parents of the risks to themselves and to the fetus and other children in the household. The nurse must be able to answer questions about the impact of cigarette smoking on the fetus and young children. Many times, after she is informed of the risks to the fetus, the pregnant woman is more motivated to stop smoking. The nurse may need to seek help from the primary care provider to obtain supervised medical treatment and prescriptions for a stop smoking program. The nurse may refer the pregnant woman to support groups.

SELF-REFLECTION

If you were a smoking mother, how might you feel if you were told of the risk you were placing on your baby? How might you feel if you had a baby with respiratory distress, low birth weight, or SIDS? Knowing the high risk of smoking on the fetus and newborn, should smoking during pregnancy be illegal? In your opinion, what should be the consequences for knowing the risks and continuing to expose the baby to cigarette smoke?

SUGGESTED RESOURCES

Pressinger, R. W. (1998). Cigarette smoking during pregnancy: Links to learning disabilities, attention deficit disorder—A.D.D.—hyperactivity, and behavior disorders. Tampa, Florida: University of South Florida, Special Education Department.

Van Meurs, K. (1999). Cigarette smoking, pregnancy and the developing fetus. Stanford, CA: Stanford University Schools of Medicine, *Stanford Medical Review*, 1(1): 14–16.

MULTIPLE MARKER SCREEN TEST

A **multiple marker screen** (also called *triple screen*) test, done at 15 to 20 weeks, evaluates maternal serum alpha-fetoprotein (MSAFP), estriol, and hCG levels. If abnormal values are obtained, further diagnostic evaluation of amniotic fluid is warranted.

1-HOUR GLUCOSE SCREEN TEST

A **1-hour glucose screen** is a test done at 24 to 28 weeks' gestation. To do a 1-hour glucose tolerance test (GTT), the woman drinks 50 grams of oral glucose, and a blood sample is obtained in 1 hour. If the glucose level is above 140 mg/dL, a 3-hour GTT may be ordered. To do a 3-hour GTT, the woman eats at least 150 grams of carbohydrate daily for 3 days. She fasts for at least 8 hours before a blood sample is obtained. She then drinks a 100-gram carbohydrate solution. Blood samples are obtained at 1, 2, and 3 hours. Gestational diabetes is diagnosed if the following values are exceeded.

Fasting	95 mg/dL
1 hour	180 mg/dL
2 hour	155 mg/dL
3 hour	140 mg/dL

A glucose level below 65 mg/dL would indicate hypoglycemia. Blood values above or below accepted levels must be reported to the primary care provider.

VAGINAL CULTURE

Vaginal culture for group B streptococcal infection is a test obtained at 35 to 37 weeks. Beta streptococcus, commonly found in the vagina, is easily treated with antibiotics. If the infection is not diagnosed and treated, it is possible for the fetus to become exposed during vaginal delivery. Treatment involves the administration of penicillin G or ampicillin IV at the onset of labor and every 4 hours until delivery. For women who are allergic to penicillin, clindamycin or erythromycin can be used.

COMPLICATIONS OF PREGNANCY

Complications are grouped here by those that only occur during a pregnancy, and those that are associated with other medical disorders. At times, the pregnant woman may develop more than one complication, placing her health and that of the fetus at greater risk.

Complications with Bleeding

Bleeding during pregnancy is always a potential life-threatening condition for both the mother and the fetus. Bleeding should be evaluated by the health care provider. Although bleeding could happen at any time, it more commonly occurs in the first and third trimesters.

MENSTRUATION

Menstruation could occur after conception. If the blastocyst implants a few days late, there may not be enough hCG produced to prevent the breakdown of the corpus luteum. A decrease or a lack of increase in progesterone would lead to menstrual bleeding. If this occurs, the blastocyst may become detached and the pregnancy could end before the client knew she was pregnant. However, the blastocyst may remain attached to the endometrium and the pregnancy could continue.

SPONTANEOUS ABORTION

Abortion is the term used to identify any pregnancy that terminates before the 20th week of gestation. Although in medicine abortion is used to describe any pregnancy that ends before the fetus is viable, the public often uses the term to describe a planned termination, either a therapeutic or a criminal action. The public uses the term **miscarriage** to describe the spontaneous event. Some cultures use abortion to describe either occurrence. It is important for the nurse to question the client in a nonjudgmental manner to determine the cause of the abortion.

Spontaneous abortion (Figure 13-2 ■) occurs more commonly in the first trimester and can be classified as follows:

- *Threatened*. Bleeding and cramping with the cervix closed and membranes intact.
- *Inevitable*. Bleeding and cramping with the cervix beginning to dilate. The membranes may or may not rupture.
- *Complete*. All products of conception are expelled.
- *Incomplete*. Some of the products of conception are expelled, but some remain attached. Heavy bleeding and severe cramping continue until the placenta or other matter is removed.
- *Missed*. The embryo or fetus dies but is not expelled. If the fetus is not expelled within 6 weeks, other complications, including infection and disseminated intravascular coagulation (DIC), can occur.
- *Septic*. An infection of the uterus is present. The infection can be caused by premature rupture of the membranes, an intrauterine device, or an abortion attempted in unsterile conditions.
- *Habitual*. The occurrence of any of the above in three consecutive pregnancies. Most commonly, a weak cervix dilates in the second trimester, expelling the fetus. This condition is called **incompetent cervix.**

The treatment of abortion depends on the cause. For a threatened abortion, the client would be placed on bed rest for several days. If the bleeding stops, she should be advised

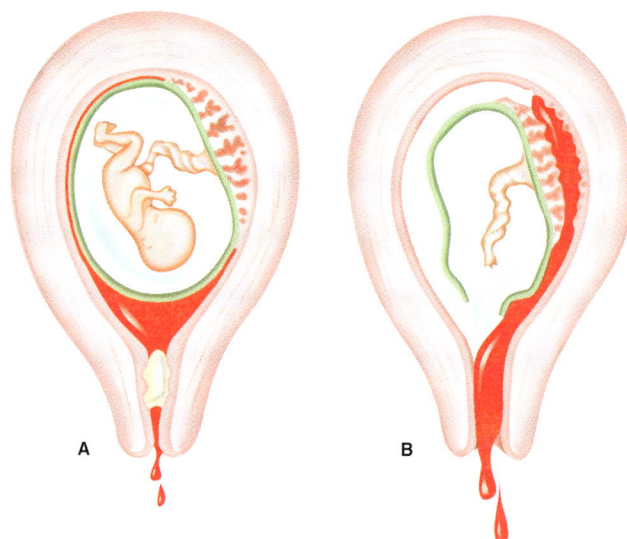

Figure 13-2. ■ Spontaneous abortion (or miscarriage). **(A)** Threatened abortion. **(B)** Incomplete abortion.

Figure 13-4. ■ Implantation sites of ectopic pregnancy in order of frequency. (1) Ampulla of fallopian tube. (2) Remainder of tube. (3) Interstitial portion of tube. (4) Ovary. (5) Broad ligament (*intraligamentary*). (6) Surface of peritoneum (abdominal). (7) Rudimentary horn. (8) Cervix. (9) Tubouterine junction (angular).

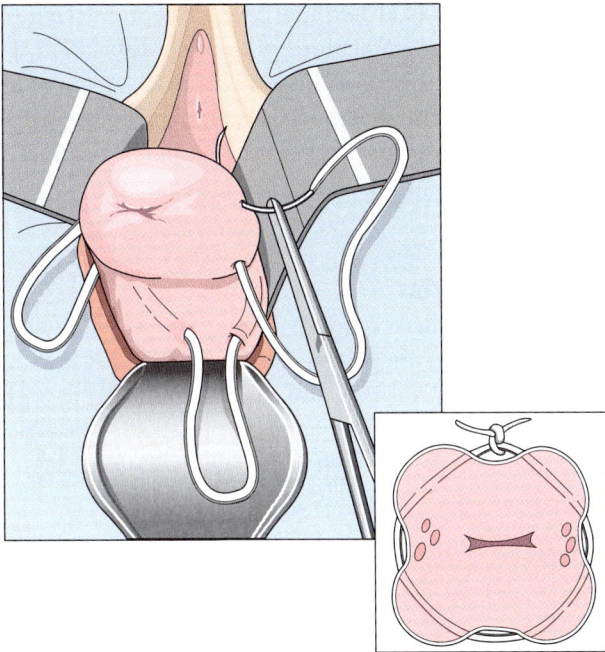

Figure 13-3. ■ A cerclage or purse-string suture is inserted into the cervix to prevent cervical dilation and pregnancy loss. After placement, the string is tightened and secured anteriorly.

to avoid strenuous activity, fatigue, and sexual intercourse until the pregnancy seems to be progressing normally. If the bleeding does not stop, the pregnancy may be lost and surgical intervention may be necessary. For an inevitable or incomplete abortion, a **D & C (dilatation and curettage)** is usually performed under anesthesia. In this procedure, the cervix is dilated, a curette is inserted into the uterus, and the endometrium is scraped, removing all products of conception. For a missed abortion, a D & C may be preformed or labor may be induced, depending on the gestational age of the fetus. For habitual abortion caused by an incompetent cervix, a **cerclage (Shirodkar procedure)** is used (Figure 13-3 ■). This procedure, done at 16 weeks' gestation, involves surgically placing a suture in the cervix in a purse-string design to hold the cervix closed. The suture can be removed at term, and the fetus can be delivered vaginally. Alternatively, the suture can remain in place for future pregnancies, and then the fetus will be delivered by cesarean section.

ECTOPIC PREGNANCY

Ectopic pregnancy occurs when the blastocyst implants outside the uterine cavity (Figure 13-4 ■). The most common site of an ectopic pregnancy is the fallopian tube **(tubal pregnancy).** Because the fallopian tubes are not attached to the ovaries, the blastocyst could attach to the ovary or any intra-abdominal structure. The blastocyst could also travel through the uterus and implant in the cervix. As the embryo grows, it damages the organ.

Manifestations

The symptoms of ectopic pregnancy may mimic normal symptoms of early pregnancy. There may be slight uterine enlargement, but because implantation is outside the uterine cavity, uterine enlargement is not expected. The ectopic implantation causes abnormal fluctuation of hormones, which may result in vaginal bleeding. Usually there is *adnexal tenderness* (sensitivity of areas surrounding the site), and a mass may be palpable. Symptoms may be vague, such as nausea, vomiting, diarrhea, and abdominal fullness. If internal hemorrhage has occurred, the woman may have unilateral or diffuse lower abdominal pain, fainting, or dizziness. Referred shoulder pain may occur if blood pools under the diaphragm. A rigid abdomen will develop, and vaginal examination will be very painful. With extensive bleeding, the woman will experience symptoms of hypovolemic shock, including low blood pressure, and pale, cold, clammy skin.

Diagnosis

Diagnosis includes menstrual history and laboratory tests for low hCG, hemoglobin, and hematocrit levels and rising leukocyte count. Careful examination for pelvic masses and pain is performed. Ultrasound is used to identify an intrauterine pregnancy (which virtually eliminates the possibility of an ectopic pregnancy). Laparoscopy may be necessary if other measures fail to identify ectopic pregnancy.

Treatment

In the event of tubal pregnancy, the fallopian tube may rupture, causing bleeding into the abdominal cavity, some vaginal bleeding, and shock. Surgery must be performed immediately to stop the bleeding and save the client's life. In most cases, the embryo will not survive an ectopic pregnancy.

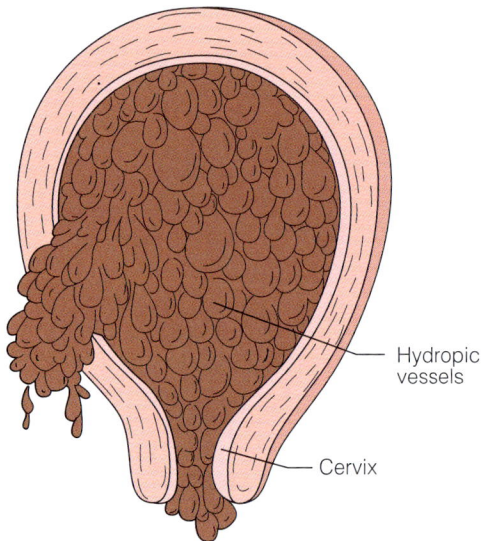

Figure 13-5. ■ Hydatidiform mole. A common sign is vaginal bleeding, often brownish (the characteristic "prune juice" appearance) but sometimes bright red. In this figure, some of the hydropic vesicles are being passed. This confirms the diagnosis of hydatidiform mole.

At times, an ectopic pregnancy is diagnosed before the growing embryo ruptures the fallopian tube or other structures. When this is the case, methotrexate may be given. Methotrexate interferes with DNA synthesis and metabolism, so the growth of the embryo would stop. Generally, the embryo would spontaneously detach from maternal tissue and be expelled. In some instances, surgical removal of the embryo tissue is necessary.

HYDATIDIFORM MOLE

Hydatidiform mole (also called *gestational trophoblastic disease* or *molar pregnancy*) is a rare condition in which the chorionic tissue increases abnormally and forms sacs (*vesicles*) that resemble drops of water (Figure 13-5 ■). It is most likely to

occur in women at either end of their reproductive life. Especially in older women, it has a strong association with cancer (choriocarcinoma) when left untreated.

In hydatidiform mole, tissue proliferates within the uterus. The tissue may proliferate with no fetus at all (*complete mole*) or a fetus with chromosomal abnormalities (*partial mole*).

Manifestations

The woman may have vaginal bleeding (brownish or bright red). Vesicles may be passed. The uterus often grows at a greater rate than normal, and hCG levels will be higher than normal. The woman may experience hyperemesis gravidarum (discussed later in this chapter). Preeclampsia may occur prior to 24 weeks' gestation.

Diagnosis and Treatment

Ultrasound confirms the diagnosis. Treatment is by vacuum evacuation and curettage of the uterus. Hysterectomy is recommended if the woman has completed her childbearing. Follow-up for 1 year is crucial to monitor for choriocarcinoma or metastases. If a woman has hCG within normal limits for 1 year, she can be reassured of the expectation of a normal pregnancy.

Nursing care for a woman with hydatidiform mole was discussed in the Nursing Care Plan Chart in Chapter 9 .

PLACENTA PREVIA

Placenta previa results from the blastocyst implanting low in the uterus, allowing the placenta to grow partially or totally across the cervical opening. There are three classifications of placenta previa (Figure 13-6 ■).

■ *Marginal or low lying*. The placenta is near the internal cervical opening, but does not cover it.

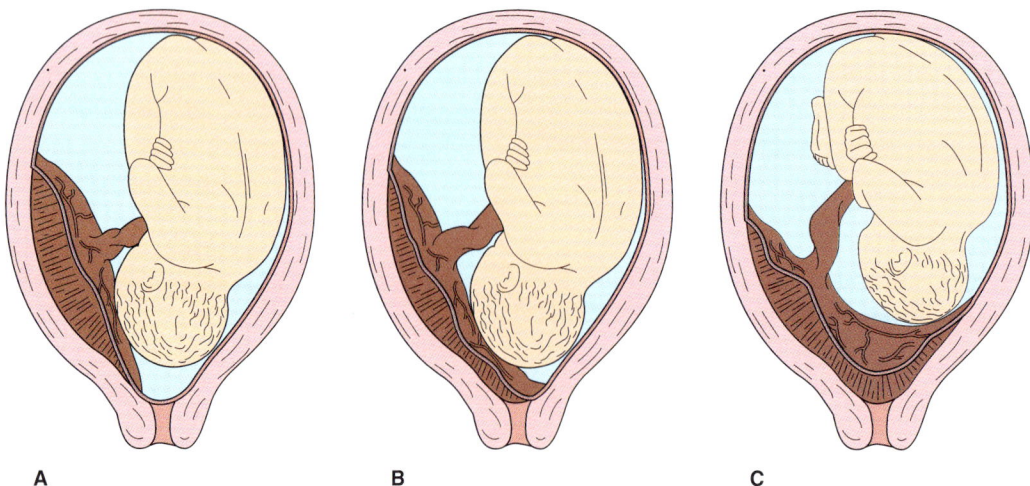

Figure 13-6. ■ Placenta previa. (**A**) Lower placental implantation. (**B**) Partial placenta previa. (**C**) Total placenta previa.

- *Partial.* The placenta covers part of the cervical opening.
- *Total or complete.* The placenta totally covers the cervical opening.

Manifestations

During the later part of pregnancy, the cervix begins to efface and dilate, resulting in the placenta being torn away from the endometrium. This causes the classic symptoms of painless bleeding in the third trimester. The uterus will be relaxed and nontender. Bleeding could be spotting or more profuse, but is usually intermittent.

Diagnosis

Vaginal exams are contraindicated until diagnosis can be made by ultrasound. In placenta previa, a vaginal examination could dislodge the placenta resulting in hemorrhage and fetal death. If ultrasound is unavailable, the health care provider may perform a vaginal exam once preparations for an emergency cesarean section delivery are made.

clinical ALERT

If ultrasound is not available and bleeding is present, preparations for emergency cesarean delivery are made prior to any vaginal examination by the health care provider.

Treatment

The goal of treatment for placenta previa is to stop the bleeding, allowing the fetus time to mature. This may be accomplished by placing the client on bed rest. At times, drugs such as betamethasone (Celestone) may be given to accelerate fetal lung maturity (Table 13-1 ■). If the placenta is marginal or low lying, it may be possible for the cervix to dilate without the placenta becoming detached. In this case, a vaginal birth may be attempted. Careful monitoring of the fetus and mother would be required during the labor and birth process. If bleeding continues, delivery by cesarean section is begun immediately. The infant and mother should be assessed for anemia.

ABRUPTIO PLACENTAE

Abruptio placentae, or premature separation of the placenta, may occur in late pregnancy or during labor (Figure 13-7 ■). The cause is unknown, but contributing factors include maternal hypertension, multiple pregnancy, smoking, use of alcohol and other illicit drugs, uterine trauma, and pregnancy continuing past the due date.

Manifestations

There are three classifications of abruptio placentae, and they have different manifestations:

- *Marginal.* Edge of the placenta separates and bright red vaginal bleeding occurs.
- *Central.* The center of the placenta separates, trapping blood between the placenta and the uterus. There is no vaginal bleeding, but the uterus becomes painful.
- *Complete.* The entire placenta separates, resulting in profuse bleeding.

If the fetal head is tight against the cervix and maternal pelvis, some blood can be trapped inside the uterus. Bleeding into the myometrium causes a rigid, painful abdomen.

Diagnosis

Because the amount of vaginal bleeding is not a guide to the degree of placental separation, it is important to assess for changes in the size of the uterus as a sign of concealed bleeding. The size of the uterus is determined by measuring the abdominal girth at the umbilicus and by measuring the distance from the top of the fundus to the symphysis pubis. These measurements are obtained hourly. An increase in size must be reported immediately to the RN and primary care provider.

Treatment

The goal of treatment for abruptio placentae is delivery as soon as possible. If the separation is small and there are no signs of fetal distress, labor may be induced and allowed to progress. If the separation is moderate or severe, or if the fetus is in distress, an immediate cesarean section is performed. The

TABLE 13-1				
Pharmacology: Drug to Encourage Fetal Lung Maturity				
DRUG (GENERIC AND COMMON BRAND NAME)	**USUAL ROUTE/DOSE**	**CLASSIFICATION**	**SELECTED SIDE EFFECTS**	**DON'T GIVE IF**
Betamethasone (Celestone)	12 mg IM daily for 2 to 3 days before delivery	Systemic corticosteroid	Low-dose, short-term use has few side effects, fluid retention	Client has active untreated infections (unlabeled use in pregnancy)

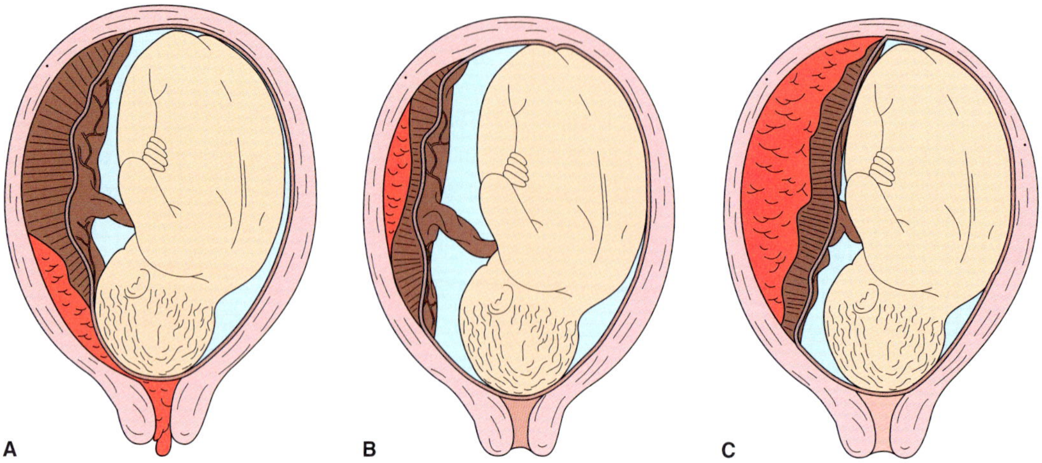

Figure 13-7. ■ Abruptio placentae. (**A**) The marginal abruption with external hemorrhage. (**B**) The central abruption with concealed hemorrhage. (**C**) Complete separation.

LPN/LVN would follow the direction of the primary care provider or RN when providing care in these situations.

Possible Complications

Following delivery, the fetus should be evaluated for anemia and hypoxia. After delivery, the uterus may contract poorly. Therefore, the mother should be evaluated for continued vaginal bleeding and hypovolemia.

DISSEMINATED INTRAVASCULAR COAGULATION

Disseminated intravascular coagulation (DIC) is a life-threatening pathologic process of the blood clotting mechanism. The overactivation of the blood clotting mechanism results in a depletion of clotting factors and platelets. Clots form in small blood vessels, blocking circulation to body tissues. Because blood clotting factors are tied up within these small clots, hemorrhage occurs in areas of trauma, such as intravenous puncture sites, the uterus following delivery, and lacerations.

Manifestations

There are many causes of disseminated intravascular coagulation, and it is not limited to the events surrounding pregnancy. DIC is seen as a complication of systemic disorders, such as preeclampsia or septicemia, lengthy surgery, and pulmonary embolism. Other causes may include fetal demise and abruptio placentae. In addition to bleeding from wounds, manifestations include bleeding gums, nosebleeds, bruising, and petechiae on the chest and under the blood pressure cuff.

Diagnosis

Diagnosis is based on laboratory findings and clinical symptoms. Laboratory tests show a decrease in platelets and blood clotting factors, coagulation time shows no clot, and partial thromboplastin time (PTT) is increased.

Treatment

Medical treatment involves removing the cause if possible. Intravenous fluids and blood transfusions are used to replace lost fluids. Oxygen is administered to improve tissue perfusion. Anticoagulants such as intravenous heparin may be given to release the blood clotting factors that are tied up in the small vessels.

The nurse must carefully and continuously assess the functioning of all body systems by monitoring vital signs every 15 minutes. It is crucial to measure intake and output, paying close attention to urinary output and the amount of blood loss.

Because DIC could begin prior to delivery, the condition of the fetus must be evaluated frequently. Nursing care focuses on stopping bleeding by pressure and elevation where possible, administering prescribed medical treatment, and providing support to the client and family. Because of the seriousness of this life-threatening condition, the client and family members experience fear, anxiety, and anticipatory or actual grieving. The nurse provides support but may need to contact other resources such as social workers or clergy to assist.

Hypertensive Disorders

Several hypertensive disorders can occur during pregnancy. The National High Blood Pressure Education Program (2000) recommends the following classification:

- Chronic hypertension
- Gestational hypertension (formerly called pregnancy-induced hypertension or PIH)
- Preeclampsia
- Eclampsia
- Preeclampsia superimposed on chronic hypertension

CHRONIC HYPERTENSION

Chronic hypertension occurs when the blood pressure is 140/90 or higher before pregnancy and continues for more than 12 weeks after delivery. It is important for the woman with chronic hypertension to be monitored closely for signs of preeclampsia.

GESTATIONAL HYPERTENSION

Gestational hypertension is a transient disorder characterized by an increased blood pressure of 140/90 or higher. The hypertensive event occurs for the first time during pregnancy. It is not accompanied by proteinuria. The blood pressure returns to normal by 12 weeks after the pregnancy.

Clients may be advised about herbs and supplements that affect hypertension (Box 13-3 ■).

PREECLAMPSIA AND ECLAMPSIA

Preeclampsia and **eclampsia**, once called *toxemia*, is a common, complex condition that develops after 20 weeks' gestation. It is most often seen in primigravidas younger than 20 or older than 35 years of age who have a poor nutritional status. Chronic hypertension, diabetes, and multiple pregnancy (more than one fetus) increase the risk of preeclampsia. The only cure is delivery of the baby. This complication of pregnancy ranges from mild preeclampsia to severe preeclampsia and eclampsia, depending on the severity of the symptoms.

Although the cause is unknown, preeclampsia begins in the placenta. Two prostaglandins—prostacyclin (a potent vasodilator) and thromboxane (a potent vasoconstrictor)—are

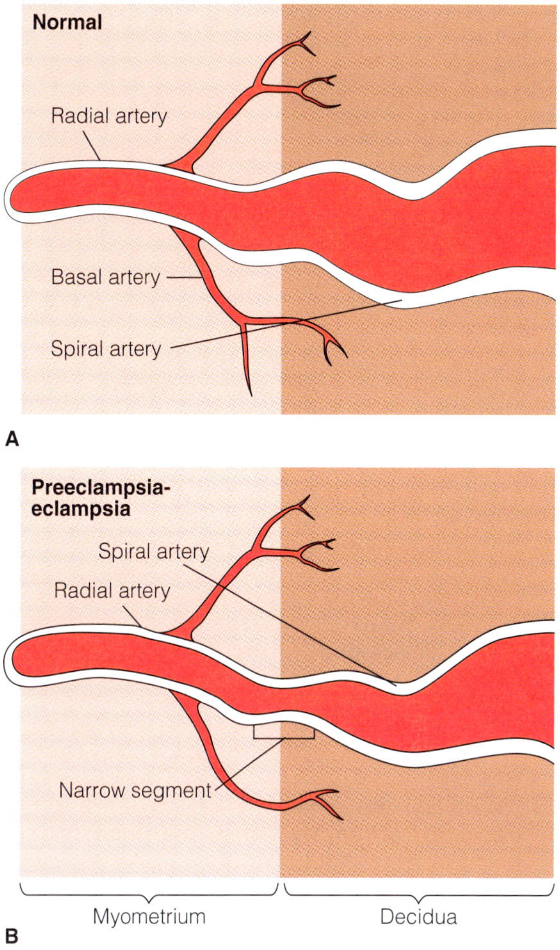

Figure 13-8. ■ (**A**) In a normal pregnancy, the passive quality of the spiral arteries permits increased blood flow to the placenta. (**B**) In preeclampsia, vasoconstriction of the myometrial segment of the spiral arteries occurs. This restricts blood flow to the placenta.

| BOX 13-3 | COMPLEMENTARY THERAPIES |

Herbs, Supplements, and Hypertension

Certain herbs and supplements can affect blood pressure (heighten or reduce it). Advise the client to check with a qualified health care provider before using any of the following.

Compounds That Reduce Hypertension

Burdock seeds can be found as an extract, tincture, or tea. They help reduce hypertension. DO NOT USE the root of the plant, because it may be a uterine stimulant.

Dandelion root is found as an extract, tincture, capsule, or tea. It has an antihypertensive effect and also is a diuretic.

Hawthorn leaf and flower can be administered in extract, tincture, capsule, or tea form for an antihypertensive effect. DO NOT USE hawthorn berries, which can be a uterine stimulant.

Coenzyme Q10 is a vitamin-like compound used at times for hypertension.

Compound That Heightens Hypertension

DO NOT USE licorice during pregnancy, because it has a hypertensive effect.

produced by the placenta. In preeclampsia, prostacyclin is reduced, allowing the vasoconstrictor and platelet-aggregating effects of thromboxane to dominate.

Effects on the Fetus

Vasoconstriction of uterine arteries decreases circulation to the uterus and to the placenta (Figure 13-8 ■). The effects on the fetus may be growth restriction, decreased fetal movement, chronic hypoxia, fetal distress, and death. Often the fetus is delivered prematurely in order to reverse the effects of preeclampsia. In this case, the fetus is at risk for respiratory distress and other complications of the preterm infant. See Chapter 18 ⚭ for care of the high-risk newborn.

Manifestations

PREECLAMPSIA.   The classic symptoms include sustained hypertension and proteinuria. Edema, once included as one of the classic signs, is such a common finding during

Preeclampsia and Eclampsia (Toxemia)

INDICATIONS
Progressive hypertension
Proteinuria

RESULTS

| Vasoconstriction decreases circulation to uterus and placenta. | Blood flow to kidneys slows; glomerular filtration decreases; protein in urine increases; marked edema occurs. | Fluid overload with:
• Cerebral edema
• Headaches
• Visual disturbances
• Hyperactivity
• Deep tendon reflexes | Liver enlarges; epigastric pain and liver damage occur. |

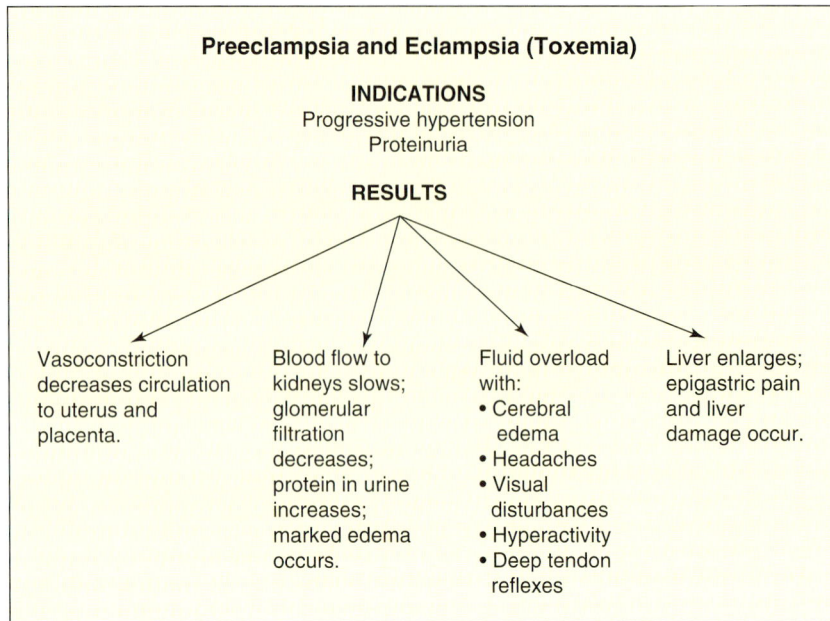

Figure 13-9. ■ Preeclampsia edema.

pregnancy it is no longer listed as a symptom of preeclampsia or eclampsia. To be considered sustained hypertension, the blood pressure elevation must be obtained on two occasions 6 hours apart.

Blood flow to the mother's kidneys slows, which decreases filtration through the glomerulus, resulting in protein in the urine and edema. Fluid overload leads to cerebral edema, headache, visual disturbances, and hyperactive deep tendon reflexes (Procedure 13-1 ■). The liver enlarges, resulting in epigastric pain and liver damage.

Mild preeclampsia is exhibited by a blood pressure of 30 mmHg systolic or 15 mmHg diastolic above the client's normal blood pressure reading or a blood pressure reading of 140/90. Edema may be seen in the hands and face, and the client will have a weight gain of more than 1 pound per week (Figure 13-9 ■). The urine may show 1+

PROCEDURE 13-1 **Assessing Deep Tendon Reflexes and Clonus**

Purpose

- To detect hyperreflexia, which may be a sign of preeclampsia
- To determine the presence of clonus, which indicates CNS irritability
- To establish a baseline when beginning medication for preeclampsia
- To determine the effectiveness of magnesium sulfate therapy

Equipment

- Percussion hammer (bell of a stethoscope or the radial side of hand may be used if hammer is not available)

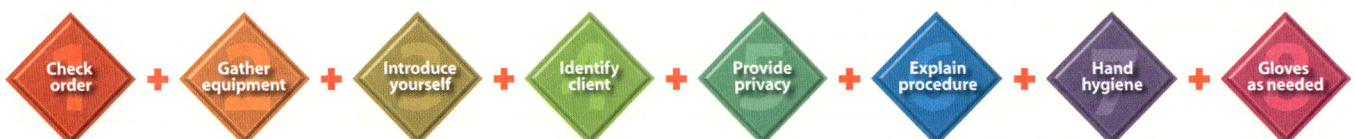

Check order + Gather equipment + Introduce yourself + Identify client + Provide privacy + Explain procedure + Hand hygiene + Gloves as needed

Interventions and Rationales

1. Perform preparatory steps (see icon bar).

2. Elicit reflexes. Usually the patellar reflex and one other reflex are elicited. *Test of more than one reflex helps to ensure that assessment of response is accurate.*

   a. *Patellar reflex:* Woman in position with legs hanging over the bed or table and not touching the floor. Strike the patellar tendon quickly (just below the patella or "kneecap"). In a normal response the foot thrusts ("jerks") forward in extension.

   b. *Biceps reflex:* Support woman's relaxed arm flexed at 45 degrees at the elbow. Place your thumb on the biceps tendon in the antecubital space and your fingers on the posterior elbow. Strike your thumb in a downward motion. In a normal response, the arm flexes.

   c. *Triceps reflex:* Abduct the woman's upper arm up to 90 degrees and have her allow the hand to drop down loosely from the elbow. Strike the triceps tendon (just above the elbow). In a normal response the muscle contracts and the arm extends (straightens).

   d. *Brachioradialis reflex:* Flex the woman's arm and lay it on your own forearm, with the hand slightly pronated. Strike the brachioradialis tendon, about 1 to 2 inches (2.5 to 5 cm) above the wrist. In a normal response the elbow will flex and the forearm will pronate.

3. Grade reflexes on a scale of 0 to 4+. *Normal reflexes are 1+ or 2+. With CNS irritation (associated with preeclampsia), reflexes may be abnormally high (hyperreflexia). If magnesium levels become too high, reflexes may be abnormally low or absent.*

   a. 4+ = Hyperreactive; very brisk, jerky, or clonic response

   b. 3+ = Brisker than normal, but may not be abnormal

   c. 2+ = Average or normal response

   d. 1+ = Diminished or less than normal response

   e. 0 = No response

4. Assess for clonus. With woman's knee flexed, support the leg and vigorously dorsiflex the foot (Figure 13-10 ■). Hold the foot in dorsiflexion briefly and then release. Note and document normal or abnormal response as 1 to 4 beats or sustained. *Normal response is a return to normal*

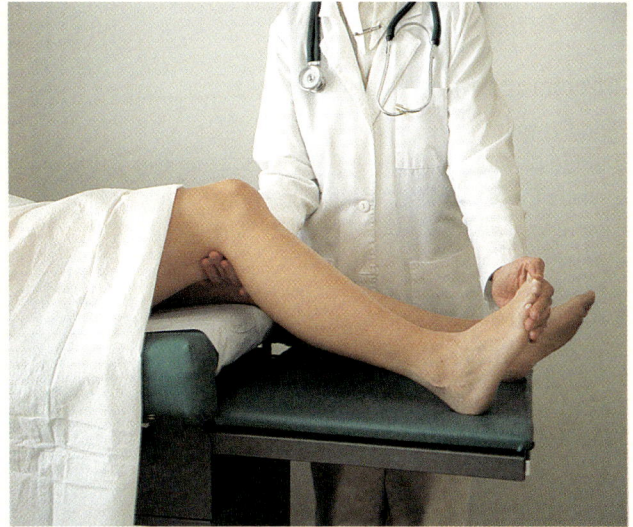

Figure 13-10. ■ To elicit clonus, the nurse sharply dorsiflexes the foot. In an abnormal reaction, the foot performs one or a series of "taps" against the examiner's hand. The nurse records the reaction and the number of taps.

position. Abnormal response is a "jerk" or tap of the foot against the examiner's hand before the foot returns to rest in normal plantar flexion. The number of taps or beats must be recorded. This abnormal reaction indicates CNS irritability and a more pronounced hyperreflexia.

SAMPLE DOCUMENTATION

(date) 1530   T 98.6F, R 20, P 75, BP 176/100. Assessed reflexes. Patellar 4+, Brachioradialis 4+, clonus sustained; reported reflexes and clonus to care provider. _____
S. Kimini, LVN

protein on a dipstick. Box 13-4 ■ highlights manifestations of mild versus severe preeclampsia and eclampsia.

In severe preeclampsia, the blood pressure increases to 160/110 or higher. Generalized edema is noted in the hands, face, sacrum, lower extremities, and abdomen. Weight gain may be 2 or more pounds in a few days to a week. Protein will be 2+ or more on a dipstick. Urine output may drop to less than 500 mL in 24 hours. The client may exhibit other symptoms, including headache, blurred vision, scotoma (spots before eyes), irritability, hyperreactive

reflexes, and epigastric pain. Procedure 13-1 reviews the procedure for testing deep tendon reflexes for hyperreactive reflexes.

ECLAMPSIA.   If left untreated, the condition may progress to eclampsia, as evidenced by grand mal seizures. The client may slip into a coma. The seizures may recur, and the client, the fetus, or both may die. The seizure activity may induce uterine contraction, but the comatose client may be unable to let anyone know.

BOX 13-4 ASSESSMENT

Preeclampsia and Eclampsia

Mild Preeclampsia

- Blood pressure of 30 mmHg systolic or 15 mmHg diastolic above the client's normal blood pressure reading *or* BP reading of 140/90
- Possible edema in hands and face
- Weight gain of more than 1 pound per week
- Possible urine output reduction
- Urine may show 1+ protein on a dipstick
- Hyper reflexes
- Complaints of headache, blurred vision, scotoma (spots before eyes), irritability, epigastric pain

Severe Preeclampsia

- Blood pressure increases to 160/110 or higher
- Generalized edema in hands, face, sacrum, lower extremities, and abdomen
- Possible weight gain of 2 or more pounds in a few days to a week
- Urine protein 2+ or more on a dipstick
- Urine output reduced, possibly less than 500 mL in 24 hours

Eclampsia

- Grand mal seizures
- Possible coma
- Initiation of contractions (The seizure activity may induce uterine contractions, but the comatose client may be unable to let anyone know.)
- Death

---

clinical ALERT

The client with chronic hypertension who develops preeclampsia often progresses quickly to eclampsia. The woman with chronic hypertension must be taught to notify the health care provider immediately if any symptoms of preeclampsia appear. The nurse must also be alert to and report any manifestations of a seizure. These include:

- **Parietal seizures.** Brief change in consciousness with blank stare, blinking of the eyes, fluttering eyelids, or lip smacking.
- **Generalized seizures.** Loud cry (called an epileptic cry), loss of consciousness, tonic (back arching) contractions, any cyanosis, followed by clonic (jerking, contracting, and relaxing) contractions, possible frothing, tongue biting, and incontinence.

Anticonvulsants (magnesium sulfate or Dilantin) should be available at the bedside for immediate administration.

Complications

Preeclampsia with liver damage is characterized by hemolysis, elevated liver enzymes, and low platelet count or **HELLP syndrome.** *Hemolysis* (breakdown of RBCs) occurs when vasospasms cause platelets to aggregate and a fibrin

network to form. As RBCs are forced through the fibrin network, they break, resulting in a large decrease in hematocrit. It is believed that the elevation of liver enzymes (AST and ALT) is due to microemboli in vessels in the liver that cause ischemia. A low platelet count of less than $100,000/mm^3$ occurs when platelets aggregate in the arteries. HELLP syndrome results in ischemia and tissue damage. The low platelet count may increase postdelivery bleeding.

Preeclampsia may cause a placental infarction. Placental infarction may in turn cause intrauterine growth retardation (IUGR) and acute hypoxia in the fetus, leading to intrauterine death. Abruptio placentae is more common with preeclampsia. The fetus may be born preterm due to spontaneous labor or obstetric induction to save the lives of the mother and the infant.

Treatment

The goals of treatment of preeclampsia are to lower the blood pressure, prevent convulsions, and deliver a healthy infant. The client with mild preeclampsia may remain at home but is advised to rest in bed. The client is taught not to lie on her back because in this position the uterus compresses the vena cava and abdominal aorta against the spinal column (see illustration of supine hypotensive syndrome, Figure 10-3). Blood flow will be best with the woman positioned on her left side, but she will need to shift position for comfort by lying on either side. A well-balanced diet, high in protein and moderate in sodium, should be provided for the client. Excessively salty foods should be avoided, but salt is not restricted. Antihypertensive drugs, diuretics, and sedatives may be prescribed.

If severe preeclampsia develops, the client is hospitalized and CNS depressants such as magnesium sulfate ($MgSO_4$) are given for 24 to 48 hours after delivery to ensure that seizures do not develop (Table 13-2).

---

clinical ALERT

A syringe containing calcium carbonate, the antidote for magnesium sulfate, must be at the bedside in case magnesium toxicity develops.

Nursing Considerations

Nursing assessment involves monitoring blood pressure, urine output, proteinuria, and deep tendon reflexes (see Procedure 13-1). In mild preeclampsia, the client feels healthy and must be encouraged to follow the plan of care. Teaching about diet, activity, and medication must be provided.

In severe preeclampsia, the client is hospitalized, and fetal and maternal monitoring is more frequent. The nurse

TABLE 13-2

Pharmacology: Drug to Reduce CNS Activity and Risk of Seizures

DRUG (GENERIC AND COMMON BRAND NAME)	USUAL ROUTE/DOSE	CLASSIFICATION	SELECTED SIDE EFFECTS	DON'T GIVE IF
Magnesium sulfate (MgSO$_4$)	4 g/IV infusion then 1–2 g/hr continuous	Mineral/electrolyte	Arrhythmias, bradycardia, hypotension	Vital signs are not within normal limits (unlabeled use in pregnancy, but it is routinely given)

should be prepared to assist in induction of labor or cesarean section delivery if the client does not improve. Preeclampsia slowly decreases following delivery, but the client remains at risk of seizure for several days. For this reason, clients usually remain hospitalized. Blood pressure, urine protein, and deep tendon reflexes are monitored frequently.

Gestational Diabetes Mellitus

Appearing only during pregnancy, **gestational diabetes mellitus** (GDM) is an abnormal glucose metabolism caused by the additional requirement for insulin. Many women who develop GDM will develop diabetes mellitus later in life. The client who develops diabetes prior to pregnancy has the same risks to the pregnancy as does the client who develops gestational diabetes, but the blood glucose is more difficult to control. Testing for gestational diabetes mellitus was described at the beginning of this chapter.

In early pregnancy, the mother's pancreas increases insulin production due to an increase in hormones. The tissue's response to the high insulin level is also increased. After the 20th week of pregnancy, an increased resistance to insulin develops as a result of increased placental hormones. Fat is more readily metabolized, resulting in ketonuria.

Because the maternal glucose provides energy for the developing fetus, balancing blood glucose levels is more difficult.

After delivery of the placenta, there is a rapid decrease in the amount of insulin required. The diabetic client is at greater risk for preeclampsia and ketoacidosis than the nondiabetic client. Refer to a medical-surgical text for information on ketoacidosis.

Nursing Considerations

The client who develops diabetes during pregnancy will need to be taught to monitor her blood sugar (Figure 13-11 ■) and possibly to administer insulin. She will also need instruction in diet and activity. Many areas have diabetes centers where nurses and dietitians who are trained in diabetes management provide this instruction. If a diabetic center is not available, the clinic nurse will need to provide demonstration, written material, and follow-up evaluation.

Complications

Maternal hyperglycemia can result in **macrosomia** (excessive growth in the fetus) (Figure 13-11B). Hyperglycemia stimulates fetal insulin production. After birth, the source of glucose is removed, and the infant can develop hypoglycemia within 2 to 4 hours or actually be born in a hypoglycemic

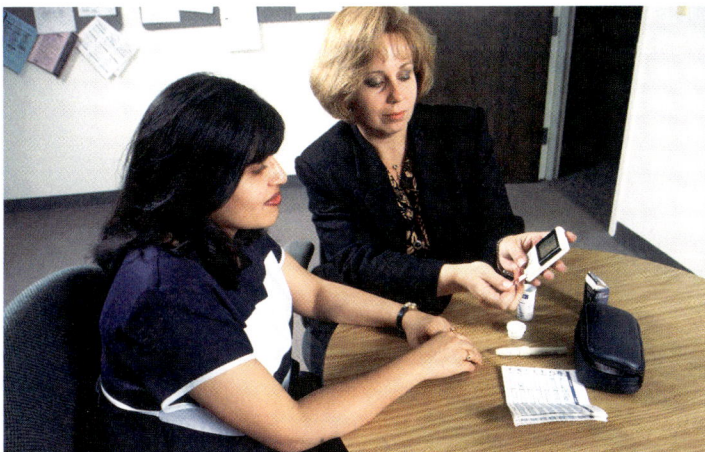

MediaLink   Diabetes

A

B

Figure 13-11. ■ (**A**) Pregnant woman learning to do serum glucose monitoring. (**B**) Macrosomia. This infant's mother had diabetes during the pregnancy.

state. Gradually, the fetus will produce only the amount of insulin needed. Chapter 18 🔗 also discusses hypoglycemia in the newborn.

Hemolytic Disorders of Pregnancy

Hemolytic disorders are those conditions that cause fetal red blood cells to break during pregnancy, during labor, or immediately following delivery. There are two types of hemolytic disorders: Rh incompatibility and ABO incompatibility.

RH INCOMPATIBILITY

Rh incompatibility can only occur when the mother is Rh negative and the fetus is Rh positive. It is a condition in which antibodies in the mother's blood react to fetal blood as a foreign substance. The placenta normally keeps the maternal and fetal blood from mixing. However, there could be times when tears occur in the placenta. Examples include abruptio placentae, placental infection, abortion, and birth. At that time, fetal blood can enter the maternal circulation (Figure 13-12 ■).

The maternal Rh-negative blood produces antibodies against the Rh-positive fetal blood. This fetus is not harmed because this mixing of blood usually occurs at delivery. However, the mother has been sensitized to the Rh factor. If a future pregnancy is an Rh-positive fetus, the maternal antibodies will attack the fetus, resulting in hemolysis (*erythroblastosis fetalis*). The infant will develop severe anemia, congestive heart failure, and jaundice. The fetus may need blood transfusion upon delivery. In some cases, intrauterine blood transfusion may be indicated.

Diagnosis

Blood screening tests done at the first prenatal visit determine the mother's Rh factor. An indirect Coombs' test (discussed previously) detects Rh antibodies. The indirect Coombs' test may be repeated throughout the pregnancy as necessary.

Treatment

Every Rh-negative mother, following delivery of every Rh-positive fetus, should receive Rh immune globulin (RhoGAM or HypoRho-D) within 72 hours of delivery. (Some facilities say within 48 hours.) It is also recommended that RhoGAM be given at 28 weeks' gestation to protect the fetus from hemolysis. RhoGAM is administered by IM injection (Table 13-3 ■).

ABO INCOMPATIBILITY

The second hemolytic disorder affecting the fetus is ABO incompatibility. The most common type of **ABO incompatibility** is a clash between the mother's type O and the fetus's type A, B, or AB blood. The mother's blood contains anti-A and anti-B antibodies. If the mother's blood enters the fetal circulation, these antibodies attack the fetal blood. Because only a small amount of maternal blood enters the

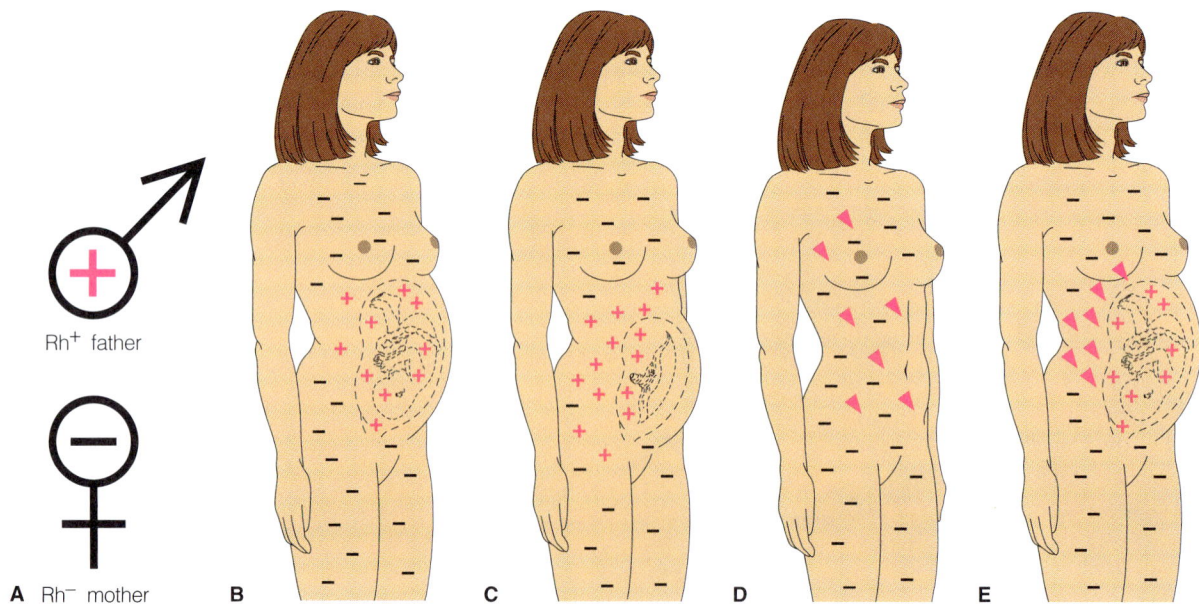

Figure 13-12. ■ Rh isoimmunization sequence. (**A**) Rh-positive father and Rh-negative mother. (**B**) Pregnancy with Rh-positive fetus. Some Rh-positive blood enters the mother's bloodstream. (**C**) As the placenta separates, the mother is further exposed to the Rh-positive blood. (**D**) The mother is sensitized to the Rh-positive blood; anti-Rh-positive antibodies (see *triangles*) are formed. (**E**) In subsequent pregnancies with an Rh-positive fetus, Rh-positive red blood cells are attacked by the anti-Rh-positive maternal antibodies, causing hemolysis of red blood cells in the fetus.

TABLE 13-3				
Pharmacology: Drug for Prevention of Hemolysis				
DRUG (GENERIC AND COMMON BRAND NAME)	**USUAL ROUTE/DOSE**	**CLASSIFICATION**	**SELECTED SIDE EFFECTS**	**DON'T GIVE IF**
Rh immune globulin (RhoGAM, HypoRho-D)	300 mcg at 28 weeks' gestation; 300 mcg within 72 hours after delivery	Immune globulin	Injection site irritation, fever, myalgia	Mother is Rh positive. Infant must be Rh positive if postpartum dose is given.

fetus, the amount of antibodies is limited. The impact on the fetus is not as severe as Rh incompatibility.

Hyperemesis Gravidarum

Although "morning sickness" is common in the first 12 weeks of pregnancy, excessive vomiting, or **hyperemesis gravidarum**, leads to dehydration and electrolyte imbalance.

Manifestations

The client vomits everything she tries to eat. She may develop tachycardia, hypovolemia, hypotension, and an increase in blood urea nitrogen. Other signs of dehydration include poor skin turgor, dry mucous membranes, dark concentrated urine, and urinary output less than 30 mL/hr. Lack of nutrition leads to protein and vitamin deficiencies. The embryo or fetus can also suffer from lack of water, lack of nutrients, and build up of waste products.

Treatment

The goals of treatment are to regain fluid and electrolyte balance, prevent further emesis, and maintain adequate nutrition. Oral fluids and food are withheld until vomiting stops. Intravenous fluids are given to replace lost fluid and electrolytes. Oral fluids are then introduced in small quantities at a time. If vomiting continues, antiemetics are prescribed. Once fluid balance is restored and further emesis is prevented, the pregnancy usually progresses normally.

Multiple Pregnancy

Multiple pregnancy, the carrying of more than one fetus, is suspected when the fundal height is greater than expected in the first few weeks of pregnancy. Diagnosis is confirmed with an ultrasound. As the uterus enlarges, the discomforts of pregnancy are enhanced.

Preeclampsia, gestational diabetes, and preterm labor are more common with multiple pregnancy, so more frequent prenatal monitoring is indicated. Complications affecting one fetus could ultimately affect the other fetus. For example, by the end of pregnancy, both placentas are close to each other or overlapping. If an abruption develops in one placenta, the other placenta may also detach from the uterus. The umbilical cord from one fetus could become entangled with the other fetus. See Chapter 15 for a discussion of delivery of twins.

MEDICAL CONDITIONS COMPLICATED BY PREGNANCY

Respiratory Disorders

Recall that in the third trimester of pregnancy the uterus pushes upward on the diaphragm, decreasing the mother's ability to breathe deeply and resulting in slight respiratory distress. Respiratory disorders complicate pregnancy by affecting the movement of air through the bronchi, by limiting the exchange of gases in the alveoli, or both. Respiratory disorders decrease the amount of oxygen available to the mother and fetus. When the mother is not breathing well, carbon dioxide builds up in her blood, causing respiratory acidosis in her and the fetus.

Acute respiratory disorders that can affect pregnancy include pneumonia and bronchitis. It is important for the client to report symptoms of respiratory disorders to her primary care provider. These symptoms might include productive or nonproductive cough, painful breathing, wheezing, and shortness of breath. Acute respiratory infections may need to be treated with antibiotics.

Asthma is a chronic respiratory disorder that can affect pregnancy. It is important for the mother to discuss medications used to treat chronic asthma with her primary care provider. Some medications used to treat asthma are also used to treat preterm labor. Dosage adjustments may need to be made.

Cardiac Disorders

Pregnancy puts additional work on the woman's heart. Although the cardiovascular system must be routinely assessed, most young women compensate without undue risk. However, not every young woman has a healthy heart prior to pregnancy. She may have a heart defect or have sustained cardiac damage from a childhood infection or drug abuse. The added workload on the damaged heart may result in congestive heart failure.

clinical ALERT

The following symptoms are indicative of congestive heart failure and must be reported to the primary care provider:

- Frequent cough with or without hemoptysis (bloody sputum)
- Progressive dyspnea with exertion
- Rales in lung bases
- Progressive generalized edema
- Heart murmur
- Fatigue

The client with cardiac disorders may require constant heart monitoring during labor. Signs of worsening heart failure may necessitate a cesarean section delivery.

Urinary Disorders

Pregnancy puts an additional workload on the urinary system. If the pregnant woman has preexisting renal disorders, such as glomerulonephritis, the additional work on the kidneys may result in further renal damage or renal failure.

Signs of worsening renal damage include edema, hypertension, decreased urine output, and increase in serum creatinine and blood urea nitrogen (BUN). The urologist may need to be consulted in the medical management of the pregnant woman with renal complications.

The enlarging uterus can put pressure on the urethra, bladder, and ureters, slowing the flow of urine and increasing the possibility of urinary infection. Signs of urinary infection include burning on urination, cloudy, foul-smelling urine, urinary stasis, and blood in the urine. If the infection progressed into the ureters and kidneys, flank pain and fever are also common symptoms. Urinary infection in the pregnant woman can stimulate uterine contractions and should be treated with antibiotics.

Neurologic Disorders

Preexisting neurologic disorders place the mother at additional risk. Neurologic disorders could cause numbness and muscle weakness, increasing the risk of falls. Some neurologic disorders such as epilepsy can cause loss of consciousness and seizure activity, both of which could result in trauma. At times, stress can increase the likelihood of seizure activity in the epileptic client.

Preexisting neurologic disorders are often controlled by medication. It is important for the primary care provider to be aware of all medication the client is taking. Referral to the neurologist may be needed for medication adjustment.

Hematologic Disorders

ANEMIA

Anemia is a decrease in the number of circulating red blood cells (RBCs), a decrease in hemoglobin, or both. Recall that adequate amounts of iron are necessary for hemoglobin formation. Hemoglobin is the oxygen-carrying compound found inside RBCs. Without an adequate number of RBCs that contain an adequate amount of hemoglobin, the blood is unable to meet the body's need for oxygen.

During pregnancy, an increase in the total red blood cell (RBC) volume is necessary to meet the additional need for oxygen (see Figure 10-2). The RBC volume increases about 30% in women who receive an iron supplement. The RBC volume increases about 18% in women who do not receive an iron supplement. During pregnancy, the plasma volume increases by 50%. Because the plasma increase (50%) is greater than the RBC increase (30%), the hematocrit (concentration of RBCs in the plasma) decreases slightly. This decrease is referred to as **physiologic anemia of pregnancy.**

If the mother is anemic prior to pregnancy or becomes anemic during pregnancy, the fetus may not receive adequate amounts of oxygen. The result is low birth weight, prematurity, and fetal death. See Chapter 11 for more information on maternal nutrition and preventing anemia.

Infections

Any infection during pregnancy should be diagnosed and treated. Although many are not harmful to the fetus, some can cause preterm labor, fetal infections, congenital anomalies, or death. Infections that are particularly dangerous during pregnancy and delivery are mentioned in this section.

STIs

Sexually transmitted infections (STIs) are discussed in Chapter 7 . However, the pregnant woman who has an untreated STI puts her infant at risk (Table 13-4). The intact fetal membranes offer some protection for the fetus, but once they rupture, the fetus will be exposed to the infection. The infecting agent can ascend into the uterus, or the infant can become exposed during the delivery process. Entry sites in the infant include the eyes, nose,

TABLE 13-4
Maternally Transmitted STIs

INFECTION	FREQUENCY/TIMING	MANIFESTATIONS	TREATMENT
Syphilis	Spirochetes cross placenta after 16 to 18 weeks	Rhinitis Fissures on upper lip and corners of mouth Red rash around mouth and anus Copper-colored rash on face, palms, soles Irritability Edema, bone lesions, pain in extremities Jaundice, hepatosplenomegaly Congenital cataracts SGA, failure to thrive	Penicillin Isolation until antibiotics have been given for 48 hours
Gonorrhea	About 1 in 3 newborns delivered vaginally to infected mothers acquire infection	Ophthalmia neonatorum, purulent discharge, corneal ulcers Sepsis Unstable temperature, poor feeding response, hypotonia, jaundice	Ophthalmic antibiotic ointment Follow-up referral to check vision
Herpes simplex type 2	1 in 7,500 births usually	Small cluster vesicular skin lesions	Intravenous vidarabine or acyclovir Follow-up referral for possible microcephaly, spasticity, seizures, deafness, or blindness
Oral *Candida* infection (thrush)	Acquired during vaginal birth Appears 5 to 7 days after birth	White plaques inside mouth Well-demarcated eruptions in diaper area Removal of plaque with cotton-tipped applicator causes raw, bleeding area	Topical gentian violet (1% to 2%) on affected mucosa, oral lesions Topical nystatin
Chlamydia trachomatis	Acquired during vaginal delivery Appears 3 to 4 days after birth Pneumonia may appear 4 to 11 weeks after birth	Pneumonia Conjunctivitis Corneal neovascularization and conjunctival scarring	Ophthalmic erythromycin Follow-up referral for eye complications and late-developing pneumonia
Human immunodeficiency virus (HIV)	Acquired through birth process, during pregnancy, or via breast milk Transmission <2% in women who have been treated with ZDV, who delivered by cesarean section at 38 weeks and prior to rupture of membranes, and who did not breastfeed	Usually asymptomatic, but possible positive antibody titer, indicating passive immunity from the mother Possible SGA and prematurity Failure to thrive, hepatosplenomegaly, recurrent infections Delayed developmental milestones and loss of acquired skills are common	Zidovudine (ZDV), azidothymidine (AZT) Prognosis poor

mouth, and gastrointestinal system. After delivery, antibiotics are routinely administered into the newborn's eyes to prevent bacterial infection (see Figure 17-25 🔗). However, infections from organisms other than bacteria can still infect the baby and can result in blindness. If untreated, some of these infections can cause neurologic damage and death.

TORCH INFECTIONS
The **TORCH group** includes toxoplasmosis, rubella, cytomegalovirus, and herpes virus type 2.

Toxoplasmosis
Toxoplasmosis is caused by a protozoan picked up by eating raw or partially cooked meat; it is also transmitted by cat feces. Individuals with a healthy immune system can naturally destroy toxoplasmosis. Many people are asymptomatic, but others develop flulike symptoms, swollen glands, and muscle aches for a month or more. If the mother contracts toxoplasmosis during pregnancy, there is an increased incidence of stillbirth, preterm labor, and neonatal death. If contracted before the 20th week of pregnancy, fetal anomalies involving the central nervous system may occur.

The best treatment is to prevent the infection by eating fully cooked meat, wearing gloves for activities such as gardening, and avoiding contact with a cat litter box. Infected women may be treated with sulfadiazine (Microsulfon) or pyrimethamine (Daraprim).

Rubella

Rubella, also known as German or 3-day measles, is a highly contagious airborne virus. Symptoms include low fever, swollen glands, and a pink-red rash the size of a pinhead. The rash, appearing shortly after the glands swell, usually starts on the head and ears and progresses to the chest and limbs. Rubella is contagious from 1 week prior to 5 days after the appearance of the rash. Immunizing women and children against rubella would allow them to develop active immunity. Blood testing for hemagglutination inhibition (HAI) will indicate immunity.

A susceptible client should avoid exposure to rubella during pregnancy. The earlier in the pregnancy the mother is infected, the more serious the effects are on the fetus. Congenital rubella syndrome in the fetus is characterized by cataracts (Figure 13-13 ■), deafness, and heart defects. The pregnant client who becomes infected may be counseled about having a therapeutic abortion. Women who are not immune are vaccinated during the postpartum period.

Cytomegalovirus

Cytomegalovirus (CMV), a member of the herpes virus group, is found in saliva, breast milk, urine, cervical mucus, and semen of infected individuals. Antibodies for CMV are found in half of all adults. Symptoms include fever, malaise, and muscle and joint pain. Many people who test positive for CMV antibodies were asymptomatic. A pregnant woman who is infected with CMV can transmit the virus to the fetus. The fetus may have no noticeable defects or a variety of CNS anomalies. There is no treatment for mother or fetus.

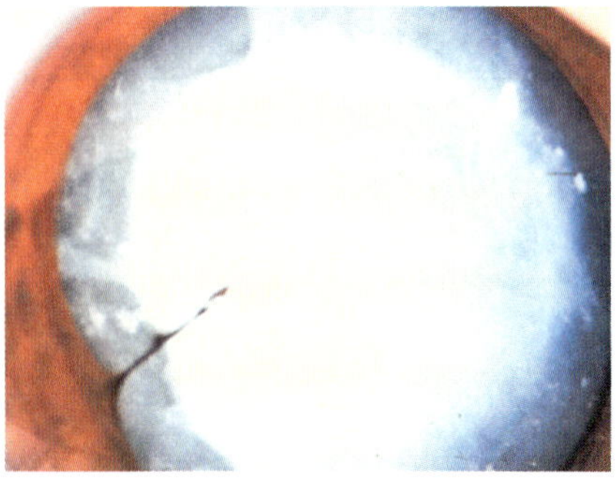

Figure 13-13. ■ Congenital cataract. The cataract reduces or prevents light from reaching the retina. (Source: Vaughan, D., Asbury, T., & Riordan-Eva, P. [1992] General ophthalmology (13th ed., p. 172). New York: McGraw-Hill Companies.)

Herpes Simplex Type 2 or HSV-2 (Herpes Genitalis)

Herpes simplex type 2 or HSV-2 is an STI that is exhibited by painful vesicles on the genitals. The lesions appear several hours to 20 days after exposure. The first episode is usually the most severe. Although recurrence can happen at any time, stress associated with pregnancy can stimulate a new outbreak. There is no cure for HSV-2, but medications like acyclovir (Zovirax) can reduce the time the lesions contain live virus and shorten healing time. If an acute outbreak occurs during the first trimester, there is a 50% chance the pregnancy will end in spontaneous abortion or stillbirth. If no lesions are noted at the beginning of labor, a vaginal delivery may be performed. If active lesions are present at the beginning of labor, there is risk the fetus will be exposed during a vaginal delivery. Therefore, a cesarean section delivery is planned.

AIDS

Acquired immunodeficiency syndrome (AIDS), caused by the human immunodeficiency virus (HIV), is discussed here as it relates to the mother and fetus. Further discussion appears in Chapter 18 ⬮. To understand the transmission, pathophysiology, and treatment of HIV/AIDS, refer to a general medical-surgical textbook.

Although AIDS in the United States remains more prevalent in homosexual and bisexual males, the incidence in women is increasing, and rates among some racial and ethnic groups are significantly higher than others (Box 13-5 ■). The number of pediatric cases is declining, with the majority of reported cases being infants born to HIV-positive mothers. The decline is associated with implementing universal counseling about the risk of transmission from mother to fetus, voluntary testing of pregnant women, and the use of zidovudine (ZDV) therapy for infected women and their infants (Table 13-5 ■).

Many women who are HIV positive actively avoid pregnancy because of the risk to the infant and the probability of their death before the child would be raised. Some women are asymptomatic and may be unaware of HIV exposure until after they become pregnant. Pregnancy is not believed to accelerate the progression of AIDS in the woman who is asymptomatic. However, women with low CD4 counts who are symptomatic have been known to have accelerated progression of AIDS. The administration of ZDV (azidothymidine, AZT) greatly reduces the risk of transmission to the fetus. Most medication used to treat AIDS is safe to administer during pregnancy.

HIV transmission can occur during pregnancy and through breast milk, but most transmission occurs during the birth process. In women who have been treated with ZDV, who delivered by cesarean section at 38 weeks and

Incidence of HIV and AIDS by Ethnic Group

There continues to be an increase in reported cases of HIV/AIDS among heterosexual women in the United States, especially in the regions of the Northeast and the South. A CDC report on AIDS cases in 2003 for females age 13 and older also showed that there were strong racial and ethnic correlations among groups. This study, which encompassed the 50 states and Washington, D.C., documented the actual number of reported cases of AIDS, the percentage of the total number of cases, and the rate per 100,000 population for five groups of women over age 13: White women, Hispanic women, Black women, Asian/Pacific Islanders, and American Indian/Alaska Natives.

The study showed White women as having 1,725 cases of AIDS. This is 15% of all reported cases, and a rate of 2 infected women per 100,000 population.

Hispanic women had almost an equal number of cases of AIDS (1,744), and a similar percentage (16%). However, this number indicates a rate six times greater than that in White women: 12.4 per 100,000 population.

Black women had the highest number of AIDS cases (7,551) and the highest percentage (68%). These figures translate to a rate just over 50 infected women per 100,000 population.

Among Asian/Pacific Islanders, the number of cases of AIDS was 86, representing less than 1% of all cases and the lowest rate (1.6 per 100,000 population).

American Indians/Alaska Natives had the smallest number of reported cases (46) and also less than 1% of all cases of AIDS. However, this number represents a rate three times greater than that of Asian/Pacific Islanders (4.8 per 100,000).

Source: Centers for Disease Control and Prevention. National Center for HIV, STD, and TB Prevention. AIDS Cases and Rates for Female Adults and Adolescents, by Race/Ethnicity 2003—50 States and D.C.

prior to rupture of membranes, and who did not breast feed, the rate of transmission to the infant is less than 2%. Following delivery, infants are usually asymptomatic. They may have a positive antibody titer, which indicates passive immunity from the mother. Many of these infants are small for gestational age and are likely to be premature. However, this could be due to socioeconomic condition and not necessarily HIV. The signs of HIV in infants include failure to thrive, hepatosplenomegaly, and recurrent infections, including Epstein-Barr virus and bacterial infections. Delayed development milestones and loss of acquired skills are common. The prognosis for the infected child is poor.

TUBERCULOSIS

Tuberculosis (TB) is a potentially lethal respiratory infection caused by *Mycobacterium tuberculosis*. It is most prevalent in areas of high poverty, overcrowding, and malnutrition. It may also be seen in refugees or immigrants from countries where TB is prevalent. TB is increasingly associated with HIV infection.

TB is treated with isoniazid and rifampin. When isoniazid is used during pregnancy, the woman should take supplemental pyridoxine (vitamin V_6) and be alert for peripheral neuritis. She will require extra rest and should limit contact with others until the disease becomes inactive.

If the mother's TB tests indicate the disease is inactive, she may breastfeed and care for the infant. If the TB is active, the newborn should not have direct contact with the mother until she in noninfectious. Isoniazid and rifampin cross the placenta and are considered Pregnancy Class C drugs. The possibility of harmful effects is still being studied.

TABLE 13-5

Pharmacology: Drugs for Use in HIV and AIDS

DRUG (GENERIC AND COMMON BRAND NAME)	USUAL ROUTE/DOSE	CLASSIFICATION	SELECTED SIDE EFFECTS	DON'T GIVE IF
Sulfadiazine (Microsulfon)	PO 2–8g/day divided dose q 6 h	Anti-infective	Drug allergy, headache, malaise, anemia	Allergy to sulfa Breast feeding
Pyrimethamine (Daraprim)	PO 50–75 mg/d with sulfadiazine × 1–3 wks, then $\frac{1}{2}$ dose for 1 month	Anti-infective	GI upset, anemia, skin rash, CNS stimulation including seizure	Breast feeding
Acyclovir (Zovirax)	PO 400 mg tid × 7–10 days	Antiviral, anti-infective	Minimal	Breast feeding
Zidovudine (ZDV)	PO 200 mg q 4 h	Antiviral, anti-infective	Headache, dizzy, malaise, bone marrow depression	Hematology indicates toxicity Breast feeding

HEPATITIS B

Hepatitis B, an inflammation of the liver caused by the hepatitis B virus (HBV), is a growing health problem. Usually, it does not affect the course of pregnancy. However, chronic HBV infection can cause liver disease, which might affect the woman's ability to carry a pregnancy.

HBV carriers can infect those who come in contact with blood and body fluids during the birthing process. HBV can be transmitted to the infant at the time of birth. Infants infected at this time are at high risk of becoming chronically infected. The CDC (2002) recommends testing all women, immunizing anyone who is negative for hepatitis B surface antigens (HbsAg), and routinely immunizing all newborns.

Trauma

Even when the pregnant woman is cautious, she may be involved in a traumatic event such as a fall, an automobile crash, or domestic violence. Trauma could cause broken bones, dislocations, lacerations, and soft-tissue injury. All trauma should be considered as placing the pregnancy at risk. Broken bones require calcium and phosphorus to heal, placing additional requirements on the woman's nutritional needs. Splinting and casting of broken or dislocated bones can cause the woman's balance to be altered, increasing her risk for falls. Lacerations increase the risk of hemorrhage and infection. Trauma to the back or the abdomen could cause abruptio placentae or tearing of the delicate fetal tissue.

When the pregnant woman experiences trauma, it is important to monitor her and the fetus until their stability is maintained. At times, the mother will be monitored in the labor and delivery unit until the risk to the fetus is resolved.

The pregnant woman must take precautions to prevent trauma. For example, wearing low-heeled shoes adds stability when she is walking and decreases her risk of falling. Holding the handrail when going up or down stairs also decreases the chance of falling. The pregnant woman should wear the seat belt low across the abdomen to decrease trauma to the abdomen if the driver should stop suddenly. In late pregnancy, if the enlarged abdomen interferes with safe operation of an automobile, the woman may need to stop driving. If there is risk for domestic abuse, the woman may need support to remove herself from the unsafe environment.

Trauma can result in excessive internal or external bleeding. When blood volume declines, the heart is unable to maintain an adequate blood pressure, and hypovolemic shock occurs. The decrease in blood pressure not only impairs circulation to the woman's brain, liver, and kidneys, but also impairs circulation to the fetus. It is critical to stop the bleeding and reestablish the blood volume with IV fluids and blood transfusion. Often the mother will need surgery to repair the tissues. Surgery to the fetus currently can only be accomplished in a few areas of the country; therefore, the fetus may die.

Homelessness

Although being homeless is not a medical condition, it does add risk to the pregnancy. Typically, the homeless mother has little access to quality nutrition, to a clean and restful environment, or to health care. She may be exposed to numerous infections through unprotected sexual intercourse or intravenous drug use. She may place herself and her unborn baby at risk due to illicit drug use. She may be traumatized by the criminal behavior of others. She may have little knowledge about pregnancy, and she may not be familiar with health promotion and illness prevention activities. She may not know what resources are available to her. All of these issues place the homeless mother at risk for life-threatening complications.

Psychosocial Effects of Medical Conditions During Pregnancy

As identified in Chapter 10 🔗, a healthy woman who becomes pregnant is under increased stress due to the pregnancy. If the woman was chronically ill before pregnancy or develops complications during the pregnancy, added stress is placed on her and the family. Additional financial strain on the family is likely when complications arise. For example, if a working woman is required to be on bed rest during the pregnancy, she may be unable to continue her employment, and the family will lose income. If she also must be hospitalized during the pregnancy, additional expense will be incurred. The Nursing Care Plan Chart on pages 291 and 292 addresses the psychosocial effects of premature labor.

RISK FOR IMPAIRED ATTACHMENT

When complications develop during a pregnancy, the parents become fearful that the baby will die. To protect themselves, the couple may emotionally detach from the infant. The nursing diagnosis in this situation would be Risk for Impaired Attachment. It is critical for the mother and father to be emotionally attached to the baby so that a protective, nurturing relationship can develop. The nurse should encourage the expectant parents to talk to the fetus, to feel the fetus move, and to discuss their feelings, fears, and expectations. The nurse can assist the couple to identify community resources that are available to expectant and new parents.

NURSING CARE PLAN CHART

Planning for Mother at Risk for Premature Labor

GOAL	INTERVENTION	RATIONALE	EXPECTED OUTCOME
1. Deficient Knowledge related to preterm labor risk			
The client or couple will obtain information about testing for indicators of preterm labor risk (fetal *fibronectin* level and cervical length evaluation).	Provide written information regarding common risk factors and screening tests.	*Written information allows clients to review information at home, and accommodates clients whose primary learning style may not be auditory.*	Client or couple demonstrates understanding of their own estimated risk for delivering a preterm neonate, by being able to:
	Explain the procedures and rationales for these tests.	*Explanation prepares the client or couple for the procedure and may help to reduce anxiety.*	List at least four common risk factors for preterm labor. State that if fibronectin does *not* appear before week 22 of the pregnancy and if the cervical length is more than 3 cm, preterm labor is not likely to occur within the next 1 to 2 weeks.
	Ensure that vaginal secretions (obtained by swab during pelvic exam) are sent to a laboratory.	*Proper tracking and prompt delivery of specimens are ways of ensuring accurate results.*	
	Reinforce teaching about the fetal fibronectin test and the measure of cervical length.	*Fetal fibronectin is not generally found in vaginal secretions until the 22nd week of gestation. Early presence can be a warning sign of preterm birth, expected to occur within 7 to 14 days. However, a positive result is not a strong indicator of impending birth. Negative results are much more reliable. Cervical length is measured by intravaginal ultrasound. Lengths of 3 cm or more indicate that the risk of delivery within 2 weeks is unlikely.*	Accurately explain their own risk level based on test results.
	Explain need for follow-up appointment to obtain results of testing.	*Reinforcement of teaching is helpful in situations like this, when clients may have anxiety about the outcome of the pregnancy.*	
2. Risk for Ineffective Sexuality Pattern			
Client or couple will alter sexual activity patterns to promote the optimal well-being of the mother and fetus.	Reinforce the need for the client or couple to abstain from or reduce the frequency of sexual intercourse (as determined by the physician).	*Frequent sexual intercourse (5 x per week or more) can increase the risk of preterm labor. Uterine contractions occur during female orgasm. Also, they may be stimulated by prostaglandins absorbed from semen through the vaginal mucosa. Furthermore, bacterial vaginal infections may ascend to the cervix and into the uterus, leading to infection of the amnion.*	Client or couple expresses understanding of the relationship between sexual activity and preterm labor. Client or couple will explore alternate means of having personal intimacy needs met.
	Encourage couple to engage in positive verbal and nonverbal interpersonal communication exchanges daily.	*Frequent affirming comments and gestures to communicate mutual affection enable couples to improve or maintain intimacy.*	The couple will maintain current emotional intimacy level.

(continued)

GOAL	INTERVENTION	RATIONALE	EXPECTED OUTCOME
3. Risk for Caregiver Role Strain			
Client or couple will develop a plan for their life and family that includes new data.	Engage in therapeutic listening and practice "presence" to permit each person to share feelings in an atmosphere of emotional safety.	*Therapeutic listening and compassionate presence promote emotional well-being.*	Client or couple expresses an understanding of the signs and symptoms of ineffective coping as it relates to Caregiver Role Strain.
	Instill hope within realistic boundaries.	*Hope allows people to look forward and to plan.*	
	Evaluate couple's readiness for parenting and their existing support network.	*Delivery of a preterm neonate can be a disruptive event with the potential to impair parent–child bonding and other family processes.*	The client or couple verbalizes their plan for mobilizing their support network.
	Provide other health care referrals as needed, such as to licensed family and marriage therapists or clergy.	*A strong support network can provide the client or couple with practical assistance to reduce personal stressors. Professional counseling may be needed to help the client or couple cope with lifestyle changes.*	The client or couple lists at least 5 self-care strategies to combat psychoemotional stress.
	Teach client or couple the warning signs of and self-care strategies to combat mental distress associated with Caregiver Role Strain.	*Role strain can cause mental distress, which could impair the client or couple's personal functioning and/or relationship.*	The client or couple lists warning signs of mental distress that require intervention by a professional counselor.

ANTEPARTAL LOSS

Fetal Demise

Antepartal loss is usually the death of the fetus. Spontaneous abortion (*miscarriage*) was discussed earlier in this chapter. Intrauterine fetal death (IUFD) after 20 weeks' gestation is often referred to as **stillbirth** or **fetal demise.**

The incidence of fetal death after 20 weeks is 6.8 per 1,000 total births (Magann et al., 2002). Perinatal loss has declined in recent years due to early diagnosis of congenital anomalies and elective termination of pregnancy.

However, some modern technology has increased the incidence of fetal demise. Fetal death occurs more frequently in identical twins and twins conceived by assisted reproductive technologies (Skeie, Foren, Vege, & Stray-Pedersen, 2003). Some invasive procedures such as amniocentesis and chorionic villus sampling also can cause fetal death (Papp & Papp, 2003).

The cause of intrauterine fetal death may be unknown, or it may result from physiologic problems with the mother, the fetus, or the placenta. Bacterial infections, such as *E. coli* and group B streptococci, and viral infections, such as *Toxoplasmosis gondii* and *Listeria monocytogenes*, have been identified as causing fetal demise. Research is being conducted on paternal causes of fetal death. One study identified that paternal exposure to pesticides resulted in a high rate of fetal anomalies and fetal demise (Regidor, Ronda, Garcia, & Dominguez, 2004). Table 13-6 ∎ lists factors that may cause fetal demise.

When the fetal death is sudden, there may be few outward symptoms. The mother may sense "something is wrong." She may seek medical attention because she has noticed a decrease or absence of fetal movement. In this situation, a mother is anxious to have her fears alleviated and to be reassured that the fetus is all right. It is important to determine the presence or absence of FHR as soon as possible and to notify the primary care provider immediately. In some situations, the nurse will perform an ultrasound. In other situations, the primary care provider will perform the examination to determine the status of the fetus. The nurse must be prepared to provide emotional support.

TABLE 13-6

Factors Associated with Antepartal Loss

MATERNAL FACTORS	FETAL FACTORS	PLACENTA FACTORS
Prolonged pregnancy	Chromosomal disorders	Placenta previa
Diabetes	Nonchromosomal birth defects	Abruptio placentae
Preeclampsia and eclampsia	Infections	Cord accident
Advanced maternal age	Complication of multiple pregnancies	Premature rupture of membranes
Rh disease		
Ascending bacteria from the vagina		

When major complications occur, there may be signs of impending fetal death, such as a slowing of the FHR. In these situations, mother and fetus will be monitored continuously. A nurse should be in attendance at all times to offer emotional support should the fetus die. Most fetal monitors have an audible FHR. If fetal death is inevitable, the parents may wish to have the sound or the monitor turned off.

Without medical intervention, spontaneous labor usually begins within 2 weeks of fetal death. Most women are given the choice of waiting a few days for spontaneous labor to begin or inducing labor immediately. Prolonged retention of the dead fetus can result in major maternal complications, including disseminated intravascular coagulation (DIC), a coagulation disorder that can cause life-threatening hemorrhage. Other life-threatening complications are uterine infection, endometritis, and sepsis (see Figure 16-17 ☍). Induction of labor is usually begun within 4 to 48 hours after diagnosis. The mode of induction depends on the gestational age, the readiness of the cervix, and previous deliveries. The birth process, progressing similar to a live birth, may take a few hours to 12 hours or more depending on the gestational age and size of the fetus. The mother may require pain medication.

Physical nursing care of the mother after delivery of a stillborn infant is similar to that of a woman who has had a live birth. She must be observed for bleeding, infection, and adequate voiding. She needs instruction in preventing lactation and in self-care. (See Chapter 16 ☍.) The mother may be discharged within a few hours or remain in the hospital for a few days. If she remains in the hospital, she is usually not placed on an obstetric unit in close proximity to other mothers and infants. Referrals are made for counseling, and active listening is an important nursing intervention. Figure 13-14 ■ provides a comprehensive checklist for the family who has experienced perinatal loss.

Following delivery, the stillborn baby should be examined for obvious anomalies. The placenta, membranes, and cord should be inspected and sent to pathology for examination. Other specific tests may be ordered to determine the cause of fetal death. Depending on the gestational age of the fetus and state law, the fetus may be disposed of by the pathology department, or a burial may be planned by the family.

Maternal Death

In developed areas of the world, it is rare for a mother to die in childbirth. Prenatal, intrapartum, and postpartum care contributes to the survival of the mother.

If the mother dies, it is usually after her condition has deteriorated over a period of time. She (or family members) may express concern about her condition. They may ask questions that are difficult to answer or for which there are no answers. They may seek information about what is happening physiologically, what treatment is being provided, and why it is not working. The nurse, working alone, may not be able to answer questions thoroughly due to the need to assist the physician and to provide treatments and care. In this situation, the nurse should call for additional assistance from the charge nurse, social worker, or clergy.

When the nurse is able to communicate with the family, care must be taken to listen to their questions and respond appropriately. Generally, the family will ask for reassurance that everything possible is being done. At this time of great emotional stress, a detailed explanation of the pathology and treatment being provided is not the best answer. It is the role and responsibility of the physician or primary care provider to answer these questions. The nurse should respond with statements such as:

- "I know this is extremely difficult. As soon as possible, the doctor will answer your questions."
- "Can you tell me your understanding of what is happening? Maybe I can clarify what is going on."
- "I understand your fear and impatience. It seems to take a long time, doesn't it? Can I call someone to sit with you? A family member or clergy?"

When death of the mother does occur, the entire family structure is disrupted. The surviving partner is faced with the care of the newborn (and possibly other children) at a time when emotional resources are low. Each family member needs to work through the grief process as with other death events. Referral to social services can help the family

Parents' names _____
Address _____
Phone _____
Description of loss: _____
_____
Description of previous loss(es) _____
_____

L.M.P. _____ **E.D.C.** _____
Weeks of gestation _____
Sex of baby (if known) _____
Religious affiliation _____

	Office Staff	ER Staff	Labor/Delivery	Postpartum	Neonatal ICU	OR Staff	GYN/Post Op	Community Health	Date(s)
Received pregnancy confirmation									
Lab/amnio results	☐	☐	☐			☐			___
Sonogram photo	☐	☐	☐			☐			___
Acknowledgment of loss/impaired fertility	☐	☐	☐	☐	☐	☐	☐	☐	___
Bring up the subject									
Refer to the baby/expected child									
Call the baby by name									
Anticipatory guidance about normal grief									
Mother	☐	☐	☐	☐	☐	☐	☐		___
Father	☐	☐	☐	☐	☐	☐	☐		___
Family members	☐	☐	☐	☐	☐	☐	☐		___
Postloss options given									
To go home/maternity floor/alternate floor	☐	☐	☐			☐			___
Father to remain with mother/private room			☐	☐			☐		___
Saw/touched/held baby or products of conception	☐	☐	☐		☐	☐	☐		___
If refused, later offers made			☐	☐	☐		☐		___
Family members included in offer	☐	☐	☐		☐		☐		___
Received mementos									
Footprints			☐	☐	☐				___
Bracelet			☐	☐	☐				___
Lock of hair			☐	☐	☐				___
Crib card			☐	☐	☐				___
Blanket			☐	☐	☐				___
Tape measure			☐	☐	☐				___
Certificate of life/remembrance	☐	☐	☐	☐	☐	☐	☐	☐	___
Photographs taken									
Given to parents				☐		☐			___
Filed with chart				☐		☐			___
Bathed/dressed baby			☐		☐				___
Postdeath options discussed	☐	☐	☐	☐	☐		☐		___
Need/desire for funeral director									
Type/location/timing of service									
Burial/cremation/hospital disposal									
Parent involvement									
Choosing burial outfit/mementos									
Announcements—public/personal									
Religious options									
Baby baptized	☐	☐	☐		☐	☐	☐		___
Clergy notified	☐	☐	☐	☐	☐	☐	☐	☐	___
Received information about									
Birth/death certificates	☐	☐		☐	☐		☐	☐	___
Autopsy option discussed	☐	☐	☐	☐	☐		☐		___
Marked chart/room with identifying symbol	☐	☐	☐	☐	☐	☐	☐	☐	___
e.g., butterfly, rainbow, rose									
Received literature/suggested readings	☐	☐	☐	☐	☐	☐	☐	☐	___
Hospital admitting office notified	☐	☐							___
SHARE/support group referral made	☐	☐	☐	☐	☐	☐	☐	☐	___

Figure 13-14. ■ Comprehensive checklist for perinatal loss. (Reproduced, with permission, from Ryan, P.F., et al. [1991]. Facilitating care after perinatal loss: A comprehensive checklist. *Journal of Obstetrics, Gynecologic, & Neonatal Nursing, 20*, 385–389. Oxford: Blackwell.)

mobilize resources such as counseling before potential problems develop.

The death of the mother also takes an emotional toll on nurses and medical staff. Feelings of guilt, anger, fear, sadness, and depression can affect the care of other clients. The nurses and medical staff need to review the situation surrounding the events, the medical record, and what (if anything) could be done differently in the future. A critical incident debriefing helps cope with feelings and emotions that result from a maternal death.

Grief Process

Much research has been done since the mid-1960s about the grief process. Five stages of loss or grief have been identified (Kűbler-Ross, 1969) and described in detail in many nursing textbooks. These stages are reviewed and applied to the real or anticipated loss of a child.

Loss, either real or perceived, is experienced when something is removed from the body or environment. The loss could be tangible such as misplacing a favorite toy, amputation of a limb, or the death of a pet. Loss could be intangible such as the loss of one's job, health, or respect.

Grief is a feeling of extreme sadness resulting from a loss. At times, circumstances are such that we anticipate the loss before it actually occurs. In these cases, the stages of grief will be experienced twice; once when the loss is initially anticipated, and again when the loss actually occurs. It is important to note that individuals move through the stages of grief at different rates. The five stages are shown in Figure 13-15 ■.

STAGE 1: SHOCK AND DISBELIEF

The initial reaction to a loss is one of shock and disbelief. The conscious mind is trying to process what is happening. Sensory perceptions may be altered. Time seems to stand still. It may take several minutes for the parent to understand what is being said. It may be several hours or days

Stages of Grief	
Shock	No! I don't believe it!
Anger	**It's not fair! I don't deserve this!**
Bargaining	If you just make me better, *I promise* I'll. . . .
Depression	*Leave me alone.*
Acceptance	I am ready now.

Figure 13-15. ■ Five stages of grief have been identified, but clients do not always experience all five stages. They may only experience some of the stages, or they may move back and forth from one stage to another.

before the complete impact of the situation has "sunk in." Often parents describe their feelings during this time as being disconnected, in a daze, or "out of it." For most parents, the period of intense shock passes in about 24 hours. During this time, they grope for answers and explanations. They may think that the situation is just a bad dream and that they will wake up. They may make statements such as "this can't be happening" or "this isn't real." Because of their emotional state, information may need to be repeated several times. The nurse must be gentle in explaining and reinforcing the reality of the situation.

Parents display a wide range of behaviors upon hearing bad news. The parent may scream, cry, or collapse to the floor. They may remain in control, strike out at the nearest object, or try to run away. They may yell at the person who is telling them the news. The nurse must anticipate any of these reactions and be ready to provide support. Parents should not be alone at this time. If they try to run away, it is important for someone to go with them. Running away in extreme emotional state puts the parents at risk for injury to themselves and others.

STAGE 2: ANGER

As reality of the situation begins to penetrate the conscious mind, anger begins to surface. The parents may direct the anger at themselves in the form of guilt, or it may be directed toward the spouse, health care providers, other children, others involved in the situation, or God. In their anger, parents frequently make accusing or threatening comments. They may physically try to assault the person they believe is responsible for their child's death. It is important for the nurse to maintain objectivity, defuse the situation, and help the grieving parent work through the anger in a positive manner.

STAGE 3: BARGAINING

To bargain means to make a deal. For example, if I do something for you, then you can do something for me. The bargaining stage of grief is similar. In anticipation of the death of their child, parents may bargain with doctors, nurses, or God. Comments such as "I'll do anything, just save my child's life" indicate the parent is bargaining to prevent the loss. When death has occurred, parents may make statements such as "I would do anything to have just one day with my child." The nurse must understand these comments and support the parents as they come to the realization that there is nothing that can be done to change the inevitability of death.

STAGE 4: DEPRESSION

Depression is a state of persistent sadness. The depressed person lacks energy and enthusiasm to perform all daily activities. They may experience persistent hopelessness, tearfulness, and a sense of worthlessness. The times of sadness seem to come in waves. They are interspersed with times of relative calm as they remember happy experiences. Although this depressed state may last for up to a year, the parents should begin to have longer periods of happiness and shorter periods of extreme sadness. If depression prevents the parent from performing daily activities and interacting socially, professional help may be needed. The nurse can be instrumental in helping the parent explore and understand his or her feelings. Because of the seriousness of depressed states, early recognition and referral is important.

STAGE 5: ACCEPTANCE

The loss of a child is the most difficult experience a parent endures. When the birth of a child is expected, parents begin to dream and plan for the future. When the child dies or has a life-threatening illness or injury, parents not only lose the child, but also lose the dream. Over time, the parents come to accept the loss. They are able to make new dreams and plans for the future. To keep the memory of the lost child alive, parents need to be encouraged to reminisce about the happy times. Keeping some pictures around the house, keeping in contact with the child's friends, or helping other grieving families may help the parents find some good out of their loss.

Family Response to Fetal Loss

The reaction of siblings to the death of a child is as individual as the reaction of adults. Many factors (such as age, development, or birth order) can influence the reaction of siblings. Very young children do not have an understanding of death, so they may not know why their parents are sad over the death of the baby. Siblings need support and compassion. The nurse needs to explain what is occurring in age-appropriate language. Statements such as "the baby's heart stopped beating and it will never start again" will help siblings understand the finality of death. Friends and family members are invaluable to assist with routine household chores and to provide as much stability in the home as possible.

GRANDPARENTS' GRIEF

The grief of grandparents is unique. When a parent becomes a grandparent, a special bond develops with the grandchild. Grandparents develop a feeling of pride in their own children and fulfillment that their family heritage will continue. When a child dies, a part of that family heritage dies, too. The grandparent grieves the loss. When a child dies, the grandparents also feel intense pain for their own child's loss. Having to watch their adult child in pain and being unable to relieve that pain, the grandparents experience helplessness and guilt. As they try to be strong for their child, the grandparents may find that their needs go unrecognized and unmet.

The nurse can offer support by encouraging the grandparents to express their feelings. By acknowledging the grandparents' loss and feelings of helplessness the nurse communicates empathy for them. This opens a therapeutic relationship with the nurse that allows the grandparents to feel comfortable talking about their loss.

CULTURE AND GRIEF

The nurse should work closely with the family. To be most helpful, the nurse must understand the family's culture. There are many culturally influenced rites and rituals surrounding death. Table 13-7 ■ identifies some common cultural traditions regarding mourning and after-death care. A nurse may sometimes work with a family whose culture is not familiar. In this situation, the nurse must ask the family questions. Statements such as "What are your traditions when a child dies?" can be helpful. Box 13-6 ■ provides some insight into cultural approaches to illness and death. The most important aspect is to provide care with compassion and understanding of the extreme stress the family is

TABLE 13-7		
Cultural Traditions in Mourning and After-Death Rites		
RELIGIOUS GROUP	**POSSIBLE RITUALS**	**ORGAN DONATION OR AUTOPSY BELIEFS**
American Indian	Beliefs and practices vary widely Navajo do not touch the deceased or their belongings Mourning is done in private	Varies among tribes
Baha'i	No embalming or cremation; must be buried within an hour's travel distance of place of death Body washed and wrapped in shroud Prayer for the Dead recited	Decision left to individual

TABLE 13-7		
Cultural Traditions in Mourning and After-Death Rites (continued)		
RELIGIOUS GROUP	**POSSIBLE RITUALS**	**ORGAN DONATION OR AUTOPSY BELIEFS**
Buddhism	Last-rite chanting at bedside Cremation common Prayers weekly for 49 days to help soul in its transformation and possible rebirth	Organ donation considered act of mercy, autopsy individual choice
Catholicism	Sacrament of the sick Obligated to take ordinary but not extraordinary means to prolong life Burial preferred (in Catholic cemeteries) Cremation allowed, but remains must be interred, not scattered	Autopsy, organ donation acceptable
Christian Science	Unlikely to seek medical help to prolong life Disposal of body and parts decided by family	Individual decides about organ donation
Hinduism	No restrictions to right-to-die issue Religious prayers chanted before and after death Body washed, wrapped in white cloth, laid in coffin Cremation common Men and women display outward grief, do not take part in any rituals for length of mourning period Thread tied around wrist signifies a blessing; do not remove No embalming	Autopsy, organ donation acceptable
Islam	Attempts to shorten life prohibited Body is washed only by Muslims of same gender, wrapped in a plain cloth (*kafan*) Only burial is permitted by Islamic law (*Shari'ah*) Prayer for forgiveness recited	Organ donation acceptable Autopsy only for medical or legal reasons
Jehovah's Witness	Use of extraordinary means to prolong life is individual choice Burial determined by family preference	Autopsy if required by law Organ donation forbidden
Judaism	If death is inevitable, no new procedure needed, but must continue those ongoing Body ritually washed Burial as soon as possible, all body parts must be buried together Seven-day mourning period	Autopsy permitted if certain circumstances, organ donation is a complex issue
Mennonite	Do not believe life must be continued at all cost	Autopsy, organ donation acceptable
Mormonism	If death inevitable, promote a peaceful and dignified death Burial in temple clothes Burial preferred to cremation ("dust to dust")	Autopsy permitted with permission of next of kin, organ donation is permitted
Protestantism	Burial or cremation is individual decision	Autopsy, organ donation are individual decisions
Seventh-Day Adventist	Follow ethic of prolonging life Disposal of body and burial are individual decisions	Autopsy, organ donation acceptable

Source: Adapted from Spector, R. E. (2000). *Cultural diversity in health and illness* (5th ed., pp. 137–138, 144–149). Upper Saddle River, NJ: Prentice Hall Health; Death and dying. (1997). *Hinduism Today.* Published by Hindu Press International; Funeral rites and customs. (2000). Microsoft Encarta Encyclopedia.

| BOX 13-6 | CULTURAL PULSE POINTS |

Respecting Cultural Practices Related to Illness and Death

At death, cultural practices and patterns generally surface, even if people have drifted from many cultural habits in daily life. Problems may arise if a health care team does not understand behavior that is normal or expected within a culture. For example, a Southeast Asian may use "coining" (rubbing coins) as a way to try to heal a sick person. A person from the Caribbean might look to a witch or *shaman* (medicine man) to help regain health. After death, some American Indians cleanse the body, drum, and then open the window to release the person's spirit. These behaviors might seem bizarre to a nurse who does not understand them or who feels they somehow "break the rules."

When a family presents an idea that is foreign, the nurse should ask questions and try to understand what the practice means to the family in the context of their culture. If possible, a "cultural translator" should be asked to participate, to explain the meaning of the behavior and customs, and to help the staff accommodate these rituals as much as they can.

Source: Adapted from Eby,. L. (2005). *Mental health nursing care.* Upper Saddle River, NJ: Prentice Hall, p. 133.

undergoing. Many times, a gentle touch or sitting quietly with the family is the best intervention at the time.

NURSING CARE

PRIORITIES IN NURSING CARE

Priorities of care for the at-risk pregnancy focus on the following:

- Detecting complications at an early stage
- Assisting with implementation of medial treatment
- Evaluating the response to treatment as evidenced by stability of the specific condition

ASSESSING

The assessment of the high-risk mother and fetus consists of frequent monitoring. The time intervals between data collecting vary, depending on the severity of the symptoms and the stability of the client. The data that can be collected without a physician order include:

- Vital signs: mother's temperature, pulse, respiration and blood pressure, and FHR
- Mother's reflexes and clonus (see Figure 13-10)
- Amount of protein in mother's urine
- Uterine contractions
- Uterine bleeding

- Cervical changes unless contraindicated by uterine bleeding of unknown cause

Data that may be collected with a physician order include:

- Biophysical profile
- Fetal ultrasound

DIAGNOSIS, PLANNING, AND IMPLEMENTING

The plan of care is based on two goals. The first goal is to maintain the pregnancy for as long as possible to allow the fetus time to grow and mature. The second goal is to deliver in the best circumstances for both the mother and the fetus. The nursing diagnosis would be determined by the specific complication the woman is experiencing. For example, if uterine bleeding is present, the nursing diagnosis might include:

- Deficient **F**luid Volume
- Ineffective **T**issue Perfusion
- Deficient **K**nowledge related to high-risk pregnancy

Expected outcomes might include:

- The urine output will be at least 50 mL/hr.
- The FHR will remain within normal limits.
- Client will verbalize an understanding of the high-risk disorder.

Medical and nursing interventions might include:

- Administer intravenous fluids including blood transfusion as ordered. *To maintain fluid volume, IV fluids must be administered. The client should be kept NPO in case surgery is needed. If blood loss is excessive, blood replacement will be needed to maintain tissue perfusion to the placenta.*
- Maintain bed rest with bathroom privileges. *Ambulation could cause increases in uterine bleeding. Activity increases the workload on the cardiovascular systems, which puts additional stress on the maternal heart, decreasing tissue perfusion to the placenta.*
- Administer tocolytic medications (drugs used to inhibit contractions). See Chapter 15 for discussion of drugs that inhibit contractions.
- Administer medication to control blood pressure (Table 13-8) as ordered. *Fluid loss can lead to hypotension. Medication may be needed to maintain blood pressure. When gestational (pregnancy-induced) hypertension is a complication of pregnancy, medication may need to be administered to lower the blood pressure.*
- Provide emotional support. *The mother, her partner, and family members are concerned for the well-being of both the mother and the baby. Hemorrhage or hypertension puts both lives at risk. Being professional, remaining at the bedside, and keeping everyone informed of changes are ways of providing reassurance.*

TABLE 13-8

Pharmacology: Medications Used During High-Risk Pregnancies

CLASSIFICATION	DRUG	USE	SIDE EFFECTS
Uterine relaxants (tocolytics)	Terbutaline (Brethine) Ritodrine (Yutopar)	First-line tocolytic Treatment of preterm labor	Hypotension, cardiac arrhythmia, tachycardia, palpitation, myocardial ischemia, pulmonary edema, maternal hypoglycemia
Macromineral	Magnesium sulfate	Tocolytic, antihypertensive to treat gestational hypertension	Warmth, headache, nystagmus, nausea, dry mouth, dizziness
Oxytoxic	Oxytocin (Pitocin)	Induction or augmentation of labor Treat postpartum hemorrhage	Nausea, vomiting, hypertonicity of uterus, uterus rupture, fetal bradycardia, cardiac arrhythmia
Ergot alkaloids (oxytoxic)	Methylergonovine (Methergine)	Routine management after delivery of placenta Treat uterine atony and hemorrhage	N, V, elevated BP, temporary chest pain, dizzy, headache
Prostaglandin	Dinoprostone Prostaglandin E2	Termination of pregnancy, cervical ripening before induction	Before induction: N, V, D, headache, hypotension, chills
Abortifacients	Carboprost tromethamine Hemabate	Termination of pregnancy, evaluation of uterus following missed abortion, or fetal demise First-line drug for severe post partum hemorrhaging	N, V, D, headache, perforated uterus

- Provide instruction about diagnostic exams, medications, activity, and prognosis. *Providing information about the situation allows the client and family to make informed decisions and reduces anxiety.*

EVALUATING

Evaluating the effectiveness of the treatment for prenatal complications is essential to determine the well-being of both the mother and the fetus. Evaluation consists of a continual process of collecting data and comparing it to older data to determine if the mother and fetus remain stable. If the complication is controlled with treatment, the pregnancy can usually progress to a normal delivery at 38 to 40 weeks. If the complication cannot be controlled, a premature vaginal delivery or cesarean section delivery may need to be performed.

NURSING PROCESS CARE PLAN
Woman with Gestational Diabetes

Victoria, a 33-year-old primigravida, is 26 weeks pregnant. Victoria has had no complications until now. The routine 50-gram glucose tolerance test showed a plasma glucose level of 162 mg/dL. A 3-hour, 100 g glucose tolerance test

confirmed a diagnosis of gestational diabetes. Victoria tells the nurse she wants to do everything she can to have a healthy baby.

Assessment

- 26 weeks' gestation
- 1-hour GTT 162 mg/dL
- Wants to "do everything she can to have a healthy baby"

Nursing Diagnosis.   The following important nursing diagnosis (among others) is established for this client:

- Health Seeking Behavior related to desire to ensure healthy outcome of pregnancy complicated by gestational diabetes

Expected Outcomes

- Client will be compliant with monitoring and treatment plan.
- Client will recognize signs of hypoglycemia and hyperglycemia in early stages for prompt treatment.
- Client will keep in contact with health care provider.
- Client will recognize signs of preeclampsia and report to primary care provider for prompt treatment.

Planning and Implementation

- Educate client about blood glucose monitoring, insulin administration, diet, and activity. *Proper self-monitoring and compliance with treatment plan helps ensure a stable, healthy fetus.*

■ Educate client on signs and symptoms of hypoglycemia and hyperglycemia. *Early detection of hypoglycemia and hyperglycemia will prevent complications and help ensure a healthy fetus.*

■ Schedule prenatal visits according to facility policy for woman with gestational diabetes. *Frequent prenatal checks help ensure stability of gestational diabetes and fetal health.*

■ Educate client on signs of preeclampsia. Monitor for signs of preeclampsia. *Preeclampsia occurs more frequently in diabetic pregnancies.*

Evaluation.   Victoria verbalizes an understanding of the treatment plan and discusses a daily routine for self-care. She states that she will report any signs of hypoglycemia and hyperglycemia. She sets up the next several prenatal visits to monitor maternal and fetal well-being. She expresses understanding of the signs of preeclampsia and says she will report any signs immediately.

Critical Thinking in the Nursing Process

1. Gestational diabetes places the mother at risk for what other complications?

2. What additional monitoring will be done on the fetus of a mother with gestational diabetes?

3. What additional preparation for delivery should be made for a woman with gestational diabetes?

Note: Discussion of Critical Thinking questions appears in Appendix I.

High-Risk Postpartum Care

The postpartum period usually progresses without problems. However, complications that occur during pregnancy or delivery can continue after delivery. For example, the woman who has type I diabetes mellitus will need frequent monitoring of blood sugars and adjustment in insulin dosage until the condition has stabilized. Likewise, the woman who develops gestational diabetes will need frequent blood sugar monitoring until the values remain within normal limits. High-risk postpartum care is discussed in Chapter 16 ⬤⬤.

Note: The reference and resource listings for this and all chapters have been compiled at the back of the book.

Chapter Review

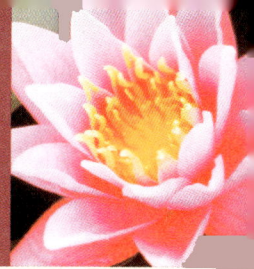

KEY TERMS by Topic

Use the audio glossary feature of either the CD-ROM or the Companion Website to hear the correct pronunciation of the following key terms.

Tests Used to Assess Maternal Well-Being
maternal hemoglobin test, indirect Coombs' test, multiple marker screen, 1-hour glucose screen, vaginal culture for group B streptococcal infection

Complications with Bleeding
miscarriage, incompetent cervix, D & C (dilatation and curettage), cerclage, Shirodkar procedure, ectopic pregnancy, tubal pregnancy, hydatidiform mole, placenta previa, abruptio placentae, disseminated intravascular coagulation

Hypertensive Disorders
chronic hypertension, gestational hypertension, preeclampsia, eclampsia, parietal seizures, generalized seizures, HELLP syndrome

Gestational Diabetes Mellitus
gestational diabetes mellitus, macrosomia

Hemolytic Disorders of Pregnancy
hemolytic disorders, Rh incompatibility, ABO incompatibility

Hyperemesis Gravidarum
hyperemesis gravidarum

Hematologic Disorders
physiologic anemia of pregnancy

Infections
TORCH group, rubella, cytomegalovirus, herpes simplex type 2, tuberculosis, hepatitis B

Fetal Demise
stillbirth, fetal demise

Grief Process
loss, grief

KEY Points

- Complications may occur at any time during pregnancy and can put the mother and fetus at risk.
- Through assessment and monitoring, complications can be identified and treated early.
- The LPN/LVN must be prepared to assist the RN and primary care provider with diagnostic exams, data collection, client teaching, and support.
- Complications can result from problems with the pregnancy or from preexisting medical disorders.
- The LPN/LVN must know the signs of complications and teach them to the mother. The LPN/LVN must report them at once to the RN and primary care provider.
- When the maternal blood and fetal blood are not compatible, the fetal blood can be destroyed.
- Disrupting the placenta not only endangers the fetus but also puts the mother at risk for hemorrhage.
- Hypertensive disorders, including gestational hypertension and preeclampsia, threaten the life of the mother.
- Infections of the mother can pass across the placenta and infect the fetus or infect the infant during the birthing process.
- Preexisting medical conditions place additional stress on the mother during pregnancy and birth.
- The nurse must be prepared to refer the mother and family for counseling and follow-up home care as appropriate.

EXPLORE MediaLink

Additional interactive resources for this chapter can be found on the Companion Website at www.prenhall.com/ towle. Click on Chapter 13 and "Begin" to select the activities for this chapter.

For chapter-related NCLEX®-style questions and an audio glossary, access the accompanying CD-ROM in this book.

Animations

Preeclampsia	Diabetes
Blood pressure	H.I.V.
Evaluating deep tendon reflexes	

FOR FURTHER Study

Sexually transmitted infections (STIs) are discussed in Chapter 7.

Fetal development is discussed in Chapter 8.

Common tests used to evaluate fetal well-being are described in detail in Chapter 9.

See Chapter 10 for a full discussion of prenatal care; Figure 10-2 illustrates a woman's additional need for oxygen during pregnancy; Figure 10-3 illustrates supine hypotensive syndrome.

See Chapter 11 for more information on maternal nutrition and anemia.

For more information on drugs used to inhibit contractions and the delivery of twins, see Chapter 15.

For a full discussion on nursing care of the mother after delivery, see Chapter 16.

For more information on the antibiotics that are routinely administered into the newborn's eyes to prevent bacterial infection, see Figure 17-25.

For more information on acquired immunodeficiency syndrome (AIDS), human immunodeficiency virus (HIV), and hypoglycemia in the high-risk newborn, see Chapter 18.

Critical Thinking Care Map

Woman Presenting with Gestational (Pregnancy-Induced) Hypertension

NCLEX-PN® Focus Area: Physiologic Adaptation

Case Study: Marie, 19 years old, is admitted to the antepartum unit from the clinic following her scheduled prenatal checkup. She is 35 weeks pregnant with her first baby. Marie has gained 4 pounds in the last 2 weeks. Her blood pressure is 162/98. She states she has had a headache and some blurred vision the past 2 to 3 days. She has 2+ edema in her feet, but she has been working all day without a break. States urine output seems less than usual. Urine is 3+ for protein. States she has been able to eat more meat this week.

Nursing Diagnosis: Deficient Fluid Volume related to fluid shift from vascular to subcutaneous tissue

COLLECT DATA

Subjective	Objective
_____	_____
_____	_____
_____	_____
_____	_____
_____	_____
_____	_____
_____	_____

Would you report this? Yes/No

If yes, to: _____

Nursing Care

_____
_____
_____
_____
_____
_____
_____
_____
_____
_____
_____
_____

How would you document this? _____
_____
_____
_____

Data Collected
(use only those that apply)

- 3+ proteinuria
- BP 162/98
- States headache
- High sodium diet
- States blurred vision
- Weight up 4 pounds in 2 weeks
- 2+ edema
- Decreased urine output

Nursing Interventions
(use only those that apply; list in priority order)

- Refer to WIC program.
- Teach need to increase prenatal vitamins.
- Position woman on left side.
- Draw blood to test hemoglobin level.
- Private room with limited visitors.
- Teach need for decreased activity.
- Obtain FHR.
- Assess deep tendon reflexes and clonus.
- Obtain BP every hour.
- Intake and output (I & O)

Compare your documentation to the sample provided in Appendix I.

NCLEX-PN® Exam Preparation

TEST-TAKING TIP Organize the content into small, manageable sections. Put these sections on separate index cards and use them to quiz yourself about the content. Information is more easily retained when you break it into smaller sections.

1 A client is admitted to the emergency department with bright red vaginal bleeding and pelvic cramping. She is 16 weeks pregnant. For which of the following signs should the nurse observe the client?

1. decrease in pulse
2. decrease in FHR
3. decrease in BP
4. increase in urinary output

2 A 21-year-old comes to the clinic for her first prenatal appointment. She is at 9 weeks' gestation, and a blood sample is drawn. Which of the following lab results would indicate the fetus is at risk for erythroblastosis fetalis?

1. low PG
2. B−, antibody positive
3. L:S ratio of 2:1
4. O+, antibody negative

3 A client who is 26 weeks pregnant is admitted to the antepartum unit with gestational hypertension. Which of the following symptoms would indicate her condition is getting worse?

1. epigastric pain
2. blood pressure 138/90
3. deep tendon reflexes of 2+
4. dependent edema of 2+

4 A client who is 32 weeks' gestation is to be admitted with preeclampsia. Her blood pressure ranges from 140s/100s to 160s/110s. She has a headache, generalized edema, and 3+ proteinuria. Which environment would be most appropriate for this client?

1. Semiprivate room, up ad lib, VS and FHR every 8 hours, 2-gram sodium diet.
2. Three-bed ward, ambulation four times a day, VS and FHR twice a day, low sodium diet.
3. Private room, bed rest with bathroom privileges, VS and FHR every 4 hours, regular diet.
4. Labor room, strict bed rest, VS every 15 minutes, FHR continuous, NPO.

5 The client has just been diagnosed with a multifetal pregnancy of monozygotic twins. She asks the nurse to explain what this means. Which of the following statements made by the nurse would be an appropriate response?

1. "The twins occurred from one egg that divided into two embryos; will be identical."

2. "The twins occurred from two eggs fertilized by two sperm; will be fraternal."
3. "The twins occurred from one egg that divided into two embryos; will be dizygotic."
4. "The twins occurred from two eggs fertilized by two sperm; will be monozygotic."

6 A client who has passed the fetus but retained the placenta is said to have which type of abortion?

1. complete abortion
2. incomplete abortion
3. inevitable abortion
4. threatened abortion

7 The LPN/LVN is reviewing the results of a 1-hour glucose screen. A lab value greater than _____ may indicate gestational diabetes.

8 Which of the following instructions would the LPN/LVN recommend to a client who has been discharged following a threatened abortion? Select all that apply.

1. Refrain from strenuous activity.
2. Avoid sexual intercourse.
3. Return to the clinic in 2 days for a D&C.
4. Remain on bed rest for several days.
5. Return tomorrow for a cerclage.

9 The LPN/LVN is caring for a client experiencing a stillbirth. Which of the following statements provides an example of a client who is in the anger stage of the grief process?

1. "If I stay in bed and be still maybe everything will be all right."
2. "We will join a support group."
3. "If my husband had brought me to the hospital yesterday this would not have happened."
4. "Tell me again, I can't believe what is happening."

10 A 34-week pregnant client arrives in the labor room complaining of vaginal bleeding but feels no pain. Which of the following nursing strategies would be contraindicated at this time?

1. Perform a vaginal exam.
2. Place on complete bed rest.
3. Administer betamethasone.
4. Prepare for possible cesarean section.

Answers for NCLEX-PN® Review and Critical Thinking questions appear in Appendix I.

Thinking Strategically About...

You are an LPN/LVN employed in an obstetrician's office. Your responsibilities are to collect and record data on each client, to prepare the client for examination by the obstetrician, and to assist the RN in providing instruction. The following three clients have been taken to examination rooms, and vital signs have been taken.

- Joyce, a 21-year-old married woman, comes for a routine prenatal checkup. She is 18 weeks pregnant with her first child.
- Hilda, a 24-year-old married woman, comes for an unscheduled checkup. She is 34 weeks pregnant with twins. She reports headache, blurred vision, and decreased urine output. She has swelling in her hands and feet that does not resolve at night.
- Anna, a 17-year-old single woman, comes for an initial office visit. She reports a positive at-home pregnancy test. She lives with her parents while she finishes high school. She has not told them about the pregnancy.

CRITICAL THINKING

- What questions should you ask Hilda to add the intellectual standard of *precision* to your assessment of her?
- What questions should you ask Anna to add the intellectual standard of *relevance* to your data about her past health history?

COLLABORATIVE CARE

- What agency should Anna be referred to that will provide support for young single pregnant women?

MANAGEMENT OF CARE AND PRIORITIES IN NURSING CARE

- In what order will you visit these clients?
- What is your rationale for prioritizing care?

DELEGATING

- What part of care of the client in an office or clinic can the LPN/LVN perform?

COMMUNICATION AND CLIENT TEACHING

- What routine teaching should be provided to Joyce at this point of her pregnancy?
- If the obstetrician admits Hilda to the hospital, what information should be communicated to the hospital nurse?

DOCUMENTING AND REPORTING

- What information from Anna's health history should be documented and reported to the RN?

CULTURAL CARE STRATEGIES

- If Hilda is of Hispanic origin, how will her culture impact her care?

Nursing Care During Labor and Birth

UNIT IV

Chapter 14

Care During Normal Labor and Birth

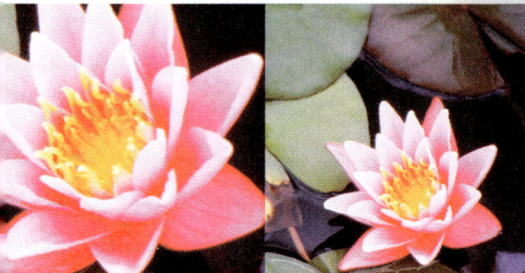

BRIEF Outline

LEARNING Outcomes

After completing this chapter, you will be able to:

1. Define key terms.
2. Describe variables affecting labor and birth.
3. Differentiate the stages of labor.
4. Discuss the mechanisms of labor.
5. Describe delivery room care of the neonate.
6. Identify nursing diagnoses and nursing interventions to assist in the labor process.
7. Provide appropriate care for a client during labor and birth.

Over the past three decades, many changes have been made in birthing practices. At one time, fathers were not allowed in the labor or birthing rooms. They had to stay in a waiting room for hours with little information about the condition of their wives or children. Many women labored in a multiperson ward with curtains separating the clients. Delivery occurred in a cold, white room with a hard table. Anyone entering the room was dressed in surgical attire with hair and shoe covers and masks. Prior to labor women received little instruction in the birth process or in relaxation techniques.

Today, the term *birth* or *childbirth* is used instead of the term *delivery*. Childbirth classes are offered to help the couple prepare for the birth experience. The partner often accompanies the woman through the birthing process. The traditional "delivery room" has given way to a modern, homelike environment. In birthing centers labor, birth, and recovery occur in the same room (Figure 14-1 ■).

This chapter discusses the birthing process and related nursing care. The goal in all instances is to assist in the birth of a healthy infant under the safest conditions possible.

The LPN/LVN usually plays the greatest role in postpartum care, not in labor. Length of postpartum stay will depend on type of delivery, among other variables (Table 14-1 ■). However, you are responsible for knowing what occurs in labor and birth, what complications are possible and how to recognize them, and what is provided to the mother and infant after birth. The material in this chapter not only is important when studying for licensure, but also prepares you to deal with a birth in emergency conditions or if an RN is not available, and advances your knowledge should you pursue further education.

Theories About the Beginning of Labor

Toward the end of pregnancy, the mother and fetus begin preparing for birth. Although researchers are still unsure of the exact trigger of labor, two theories have been developed to answer the question: "Why does labor begin?" Once this question can be answered, preterm labor can be prevented or stopped, and labor can be induced more easily if needed.

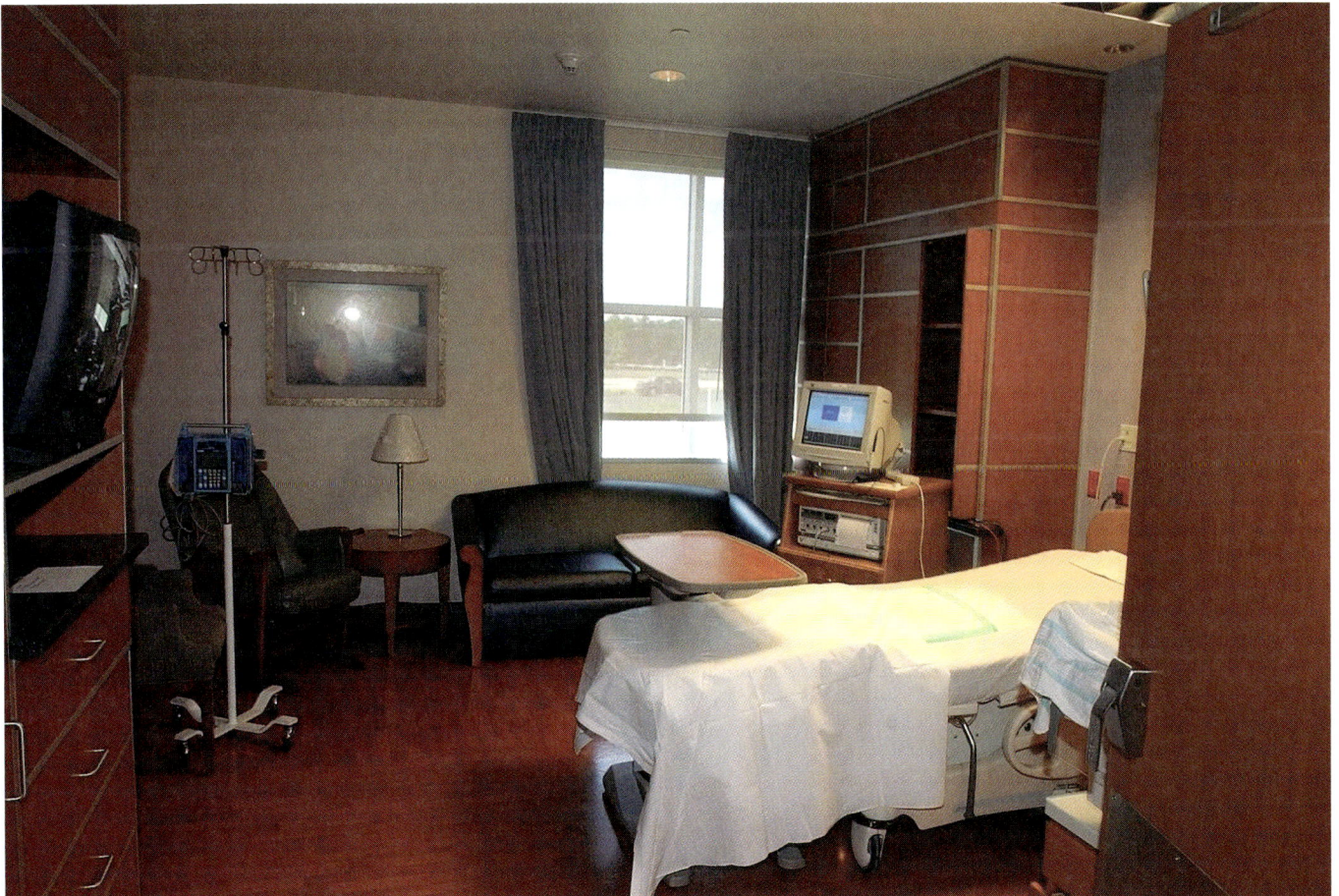

Figure 14-1. ■ Birthing room in a women and babies hospital. (AP Wide World Photos.)

TABLE 14-1

Number of Hospital Stays and Mean Length of Stay by Mode of Delivery

TYPE OF DELIVERY	NUMBER OF HOSPITAL STAYS	MEAN LENGTH OF STAY
All types of delivery	4,052,301	2.6
Vaginal delivery without complication	2,418,100	2.1
Vaginal delivery with complication	328,000	2.7
Vaginal delivery with sterilization and/or dilation and curettage (D&C)	132,700	2.3
Vaginal delivery with operating room procedure except sterilization and/or D&C	3,200	3.3
C-section without complication	893,400	3.4
C-section with complication	277,000	4.6

Note: Hospitalization for childbirth and delivery type identified by diagnosis-related groups (DRGs) 370–375.

Source: AHRQ, Center for Delivery, Organization, and Markets, Healthcare Cost and Utilization Project, Nationwide Inpatient Sample, 2003.

OVERDISTENSION THEORY

One theory to explain the onset of labor is based on the principle that hollow organs tend to empty themselves when overdistended. This theory explains the emptying of the bladder and sigmoid colon. This phenomenon may partially explain the beginning of labor. However, it does not fully explain why labor begins early in some women.

HORMONAL THEORY

The hormonal theory relates to the complex relationship of maternal and fetal hormones (Figure 14-2 ■). Fetal cortisol production increases as the fetus matures. It is believed fetal cortisol decreases the placental production of progesterone and stimulates the precursors of prostaglandin that ripen the cervix. Because progesterone causes the smooth muscles of the uterus to relax, a decrease in progesterone allows those muscles to tighten. Also, as the progesterone level declines, the estrogen level rises. Estrogen increases the sensitivity of the myometrium to oxytocin. *Oxytocin*, a hormone produced by the mother's posterior pituitary gland, causes the uterus to contract.

Signs of Impending Labor

Although several signs indicate the onset of labor is close, the exact time cannot be predicted.

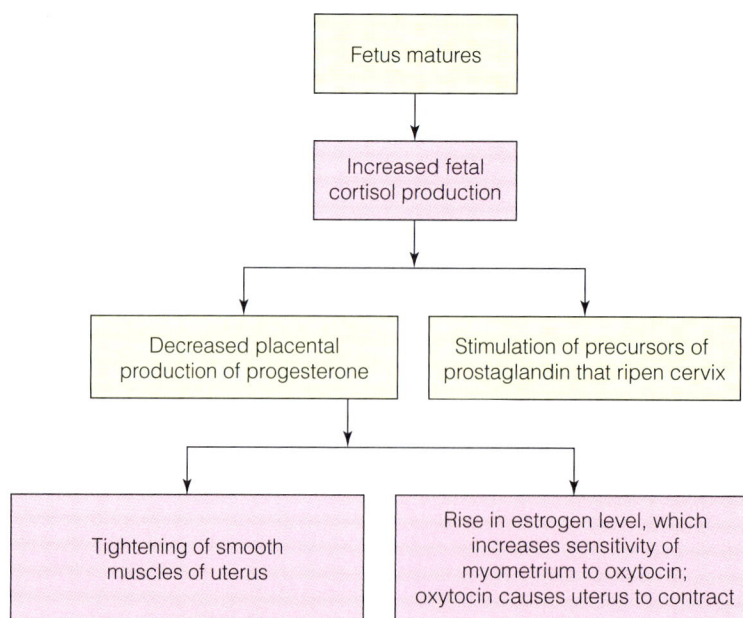

Figure 14-2. ■ Flowsheet showing hormone theory of how labor begins.

LIGHTENING

The descent of the fetus into the pelvis relieves pressure on the diaphragm, allowing the mother to breathe more easily and "feel lighter" (thus the term **lightening**). The descent of the fetus into the pelvis may occur as long as 2 to 4 weeks prior to the onset of labor. In multipara clients, lightening may not occur until labor contractions begin. Although the ease in breathing may make the mother feel lighter, the fetus's entry into the pelvis puts more pressure on the bladder, resulting in urinary frequency. The descent of the fetus also puts pressure on the femoral veins, increasing venous stasis, resulting in lower extremity edema. Low back pain and leg cramps result from pressure on pelvic nerves.

BRAXTON HICKS CONTRACTIONS

Irregular painless contractions occur throughout pregnancy. They become more frequent and more noticeable during the last few weeks. At times, they cause the woman to go to the hospital believing she is in labor. These **Braxton Hicks contractions** squeeze *around* the uterus instead of from the top down, causing no change in the cervix, and so are termed **false labor.** Table 14-2 ■ compares true labor and false labor.

CERVICAL CHANGES

Due to hormonal changes beginning at about 35 weeks of gestation, the cervix begins to mature or "ripen." The cervix becomes softer. **Effacement** (the shortening and thinning of the cervix) and **dilatation** (opening of the cervical opening or *os*) may begin (Figure 14-3 ■).

BLOODY SHOW

Bloody show is the release of the mucus plug from the cervix. The plug may contain a small amount of blood. If the client is not already in labor, it often begins within 48 hours after bloody show. This should not be confused with the small amount of blood-tinged drainage that may be produced during a vaginal examination.

RUPTURED MEMBRANES

Spontaneous Rupture of Membranes

Spontaneous rupture of membranes (SROM) is a tearing or perforation of the amniotic sac releasing amniotic fluid. Spontaneous rupture of membranes usually occurs after labor begins, but in a small percentage of women, the amniotic membranes may rupture before the onset of labor contractions. If spontaneous rupture of membranes occurs outside the medical center, the client should go to the hospital or birthing center for evaluation. If spontaneous rupture of membranes occurs within the medical center, the nurse should obtain fetal heart tones and digitally examine the cervix.

When the amniotic fluid drains out of the uterus, the infant moves closer to the mother's pelvic outlet. If the fetal head is tight against the pelvic bones, there is little risk to the baby. If the fetus is **ballotable** (able to be pushed away from the cervix), the mother is asked to remain in bed until the fetus is no longer ballotable.

If the fetus is ballotable, there is a danger that the umbilical cord may be washed out of the cervix with the amniotic fluid. The infant's body (usually the head) may compress the cord against the pelvis, obstructing blood flow through the umbilical cord. This condition, called a **prolapsed umbilical cord,** results in an obstetric emergency in order to save the life of the infant. Umbilical cord prolapse is discussed in Chapter 15 ⊙.

In most cases of spontaneous rupture of membranes prior to the onset of labor, contractions begin within 24 hours.

TABLE 14-2		
True versus False Labor		
CHARACTERISTIC	**TRUE LABOR**	**FALSE LABOR**
Contractions	• Occur regularly, becoming stronger, lasting longer, occurring closer together. • Increase in intensity with walking. • Are felt in lower back, radiating to lower portion of abdomen. • Continue despite use of comfort measures.	• Occur irregularly, or become regular only temporarily. • Often stop with walking or position change. • Are felt in the back or abdomen above the umbilicus. • Often can be stopped with use of comfort measures.
Cervix	• Shows progressive change, softening, effacement, dilation, passage of bloody show. • Moves in an increasing anterior position. • Requires vaginal exam to detect changes.	• May be soft, but has no significant change in effacement, dilatation, and no bloody show. • Is often in a posterior position. • Requires vaginal examination to determine characteristics.
Fetus	Presenting part becomes engaged in the pelvis.	Presenting part often is not engaged in the pelvis.

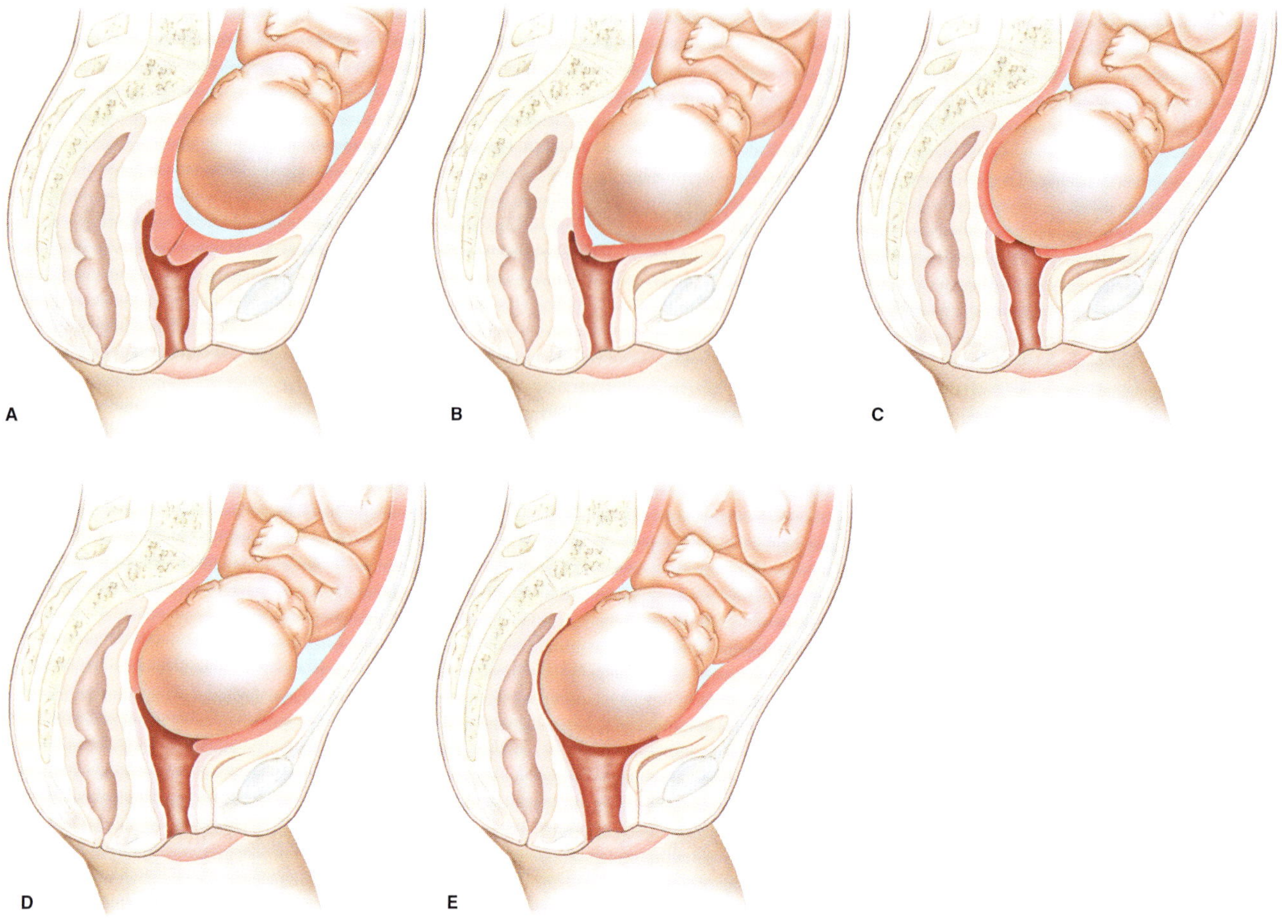

Figure 14-3. ■ Cervical effacement and dilatation of the cervix in a primigravida woman. (**A**) Cervix thick and closed. (**B**) Cervix effaced. (**C**) Cervix effaced and dilated 2–3 centimeters. (**D**) Cervix half open. (**E**) Cervix fully dilated (10 centimeters) and retracted.

Labor may be induced to avoid infection if either of the following applies:

■ Labor does not begin within 24 hours after the membranes rupture.

■ The pregnancy is near term.

Premature Rupture of Membranes

Premature rupture of membranes (PROM) occurs when the membranes rupture before the 38th week of gestation. This condition (also discussed in Chapter 13 ⊕⊕) can indicate the onset of premature labor and needs immediate medical attention. Nursing interventions for a woman with premature rupture of membranes are provided in the Nursing Care Plan Chart below.

SUDDEN INCREASE IN ENERGY

Many women experience a sudden burst of energy a few days before labor begins. The woman feels a need to get the "house in order." This urge is sometimes called the "nesting instinct." The reason for the "nesting" is unknown.

NURSING CARE PLAN CHART

Planning for Client with Premature Rupture of Membranes

GOAL	INTERVENTION	RATIONALE	EXPECTED OUTCOME
1. Deficient Knowledge related to premature rupture of membranes			
The client or couple will obtain information about premature rupture of membranes (PROM) and ensuing delivery.	Provide written information on PROM and term delivery.	*Written information allows clients to review information privately later. Agency literature is a tangible resource for future reference.*	The client or couple will explain the relationship between PROM and term delivery.

GOAL	INTERVENTION	RATIONALE	EXPECTED OUTCOME
	Provide agency literature regarding labor and delivery care services offered to the client. Complete admission assessment under the supervision of the registered nurse. Orient client to the labor and delivery unit/ birthing room. Explain the significance and risks of PROM and estimated time of delivery according to the client's own clinical profile.	*Verbal instructions meet the needs of auditory learners. Clients may not remember details of your discussion due to excitement over the impending birth.* *PROM occurs when membranes rupture before the onset of active labor. Active labor generally begins within 48 hours.* *Clients pregnant at term (37 weeks and beyond) are managed conservatively, by waiting up to 24 hours for normal active labor to begin. Clients with preterm PROM (P-PROM) require specialized treatment to facilitate duration of the pregnancy and fetal maturity.*	Client or couple will list chief components of the birthing plan, which includes PROM treatment measures.

2. Risk for Infection related to PROM

GOAL	INTERVENTION	RATIONALE	EXPECTED OUTCOME
The client or couple will understand risks associated with PROM. Client will avoid infection.	Explain the risk factors associated with PROM: • Upper urinary tract and vaginal infections as well as periodontal disease are associated with the development of PROM, as is sexual intercourse. • PROM may cause maternal and neonatal sepsis, leading to long-term mental deficits in the child. • Sepsis is a leading cause of death. Medication Administration: Oral or Medication Administration: Parenteral–IM Monitor IV delivery system.	*Sepsis is blood infection. Normal flora from the mouth and/or vagina become pathogenic once they enter the blood. Microscopic abrasions of the vagina resulting from sexual activity may introduce pathogens into the blood. Furthermore, vigorous mechanics of sexual intercourse can cause blunt-force puncture of weakened membranes. Prophylactic antibiotic therapy is indicated for clients with delayed onset of labor. Antibiotics may be delivered by IV, as well as by IM or oral route.* *Changes in vital signs may indicate infection and/or fetal distress. Clients less than 34 weeks gestation may receive IM steroids and/or other tocolytic agents to promote fetal lung maturation.*	The client or couple will identify "infection" as the major risk associated with prolonged lack of active labor following PROM. The client's and fetus's vital signs will remain within normal limits. Client will not demonstrate any signs or symptoms of acute infection.

(continued)

GOAL	INTERVENTION	RATIONALE	EXPECTED OUTCOME
3. Effective Therapeutic Regimen Management related to birthing process			
Client will be able to labor effectively to complete the birth process.	Prepare client for *sterile* speculum vaginal examination and explain the procedure.	*Pathogens in the body can be transported via the blood to the uterus, causing infection that weakens the membranes. Sterile examination is necessary to avoid introducing external environmental pathogens into the vagina.*	Client will enter active labor within time frame specified by physician as based on client's own clinical profile.
	Prepare client for ultrasound examination of the uterus.	*Ultrasound and vaginal examination are necessary to facilitate delivery planning. For example, a fetus observed in transverse lie may require cesarean delivery if it has been more than 24 hours since membranes have ruptured and active labor has not yet begun.*	
		Labor may need to be induced for clients of more than 36 weeks (oxytocin) to prevent infection.	
	Monitor vaginal discharge. Medication Administration: Parenteral—IM Monitor IV delivery system.	*Changes in quantity and quality of vaginal discharge may indicate infection and/or hemorrhage.*	

However, the woman should be careful not to tire herself, because she will need energy for labor and for the demands of motherhood after the birth.

Admission to the Birthing Facility

When the client presents at a birthing facility, the staff must carefully assess the woman's condition. The stage of labor, condition of the mother, and condition of the fetus are important concerns.

Answers to some initial questions direct how the nurse proceeds with the rest of the admission process. For example, if the nurse determines that the client is in early labor with the first pregnancy, time is available to establish a nurse–client–family relationship, orient the client to the birthing suite, and provide instruction on relaxation techniques. If it is determined that the client is multipara in the second stage of labor, there may only be time to notify the care provider and to prepare for the birth.

Initially, the nurse will want to learn how long ago contractions began, how far apart they are, and how long they last. The nurse will ask whether the membranes have ruptured and whether this is the woman's first pregnancy. If the woman has been in labor before, the nurse will ask how long the previous labor was.

The nurse will review the prenatal record. Any complications during pregnancy will be noted. If the client has had no prenatal care, a more in-depth assessment will be made if time allows.

The assessment of the client should include:

- Maternal vital signs
- Urine dipstick for glucose and protein
- Fetal heart rate
- Contraction (frequency, duration, and intensity)
- Vaginal examination to determine cervical effacement and dilatation, fetal presentation, position, and station (usually done by the RN or physician).

clinical ALERT

If excessive vaginal bleeding is present, the nurse should consult with the care provider prior to the vaginal exam.

- Nitrazine test of vaginal secretions if the client is uncertain whether the membranes have ruptured. (To perform a nitrazine test, touch the nitrazine paper to vaginal secretions and compare the paper to the color chart provided. The color will indicate whether amniotic fluid is present, and whether the membranes have ruptured.)
- Signs of pregnancy-induced hypertension (PIH), including edema, altered reflexes, and **clonus** (spasms or seizures).

CLIENT WHO IS NOT IN LABOR

If the client is not in labor, she may be sent home. This can be disappointing to the client and family, and emotional support may be needed. If it is questionable whether the client is in labor, she will be asked to walk for an hour and will then be reassessed. Review Table 14-2 for indications of true and false labor.

Variables Affecting Labor

Although the variables affecting labor are many, they can be grouped for easier discussion. These variables, known as the **5 Ps affecting labor,** refer to both maternal and fetal characteristics. The 5 Ps are: passage, passenger, powers, position, and psyche.

PASSAGE

The first P, the **passage,** consists of the maternal structures through which the fetus must travel. The size and shape of the maternal pelvis can vary greatly among different women (Figure 14-4 ■). However, the pelvis must be adequate to accommodate the fetus.

Toward the end of pregnancy, the care provider will take measurements of the maternal pelvis to determine the adequacy of the pelvis. (See important landmarks of the maternal pelvis, illustrated in Figure 14-4.) In **cephalopelvic disproportion** (CPD), the maternal pelvis is smaller than the fetal head. When this occurs, vaginal birth will be impossible. Birth must be by cesarean section. See Chapter 15 🔗 for further discussion on CPD and cesarean birth.

As the due date approaches, the care provider will monitor the station of the fetus. **Station** refers to the relationship between the fetus and the maternal ischial spines. When the fetus reaches 0 station, the head is considered to be fully engaged. Figure 14-5 ■ illustrates stations.

Uterine contractions (discussed under Powers later in this section) push the fetus against the cervix. They cause the cervical mouth (or *os*) to open so the fetus can enter the vagina.

By the end of pregnancy, estrogen has softened the rugae (or folds) of the vagina. These changes allow it to stretch enough for the fetus to pass through it.

The pressure of the fetus against the muscles of the perineum causes the perineal tissue to thin and stretch.

At times, the perineum may tear, or it may need to be surgically cut to lessen trauma to the tissue. In either event, the perineum will be sutured after birth to ensure healing.

PASSENGER

The second of the 5 Ps refers to the **passenger,** or fetus. Two things affect how easily the fetus can be delivered:

- The relationship of fetal parts to the maternal uterus and pelvis
- The size of the fetus

Relationship of Fetal Parts to Maternal Uterus and Pelvis

Three concepts are important in discussing the relationship of fetal parts to maternal structures. These are fetal attitude, fetal lie, and fetal presentation.

FETAL ATTITUDE. **Fetal attitude** is the relationship of fetal body parts to one another. Ideally the fetus assumes a state of flexion (Figure 14-6 ■) with the head flexed onto the chest, the arms flexed over the chest, and the legs flexed over the abdomen. If any part of the fetus is in extension, especially the head and arms, labor will be more difficult and a vaginal birth may not be possible.

FETAL LIE. **Fetal lie** is the relationship of the long axis (head-to-foot or *cephalocaudal* axis) of the fetus to the long axis of the mother. When the long axis of the fetus is parallel to the long axis of the mother, the fetus is in a *longitudinal lie*. If the long axis of the fetus is at a right angle to the long axis of the mother, it is termed a **transverse lie** (Figure 14-7 ■). Obviously, labor with a fetus in transverse lie could be much more difficult than one in which the fetus's body is in line with the mother's. If the fetus does not turn to a longitudinal lie, a vaginal birth will not be possible.

FETAL PRESENTATION. **Fetal presentation,** the body part of the fetus that is closest to the cervix, is determined by the fetal lie. At term, the fetus usually assumes a longitudinal lie with a **cephalic presentation** (head-down position) (Figure 14-8 ■). This position is common because the fetal head is heavy and gravity pulls it into the pelvis. With the fetal head in the pelvis, there is more room in the uterus for the fetus to move the arms and legs. Cephalic presentations fall into further groupings determined by the fetal attitude.

- **Vertex presentation** is the **occiput** (crown of head) presenting first. The fetal head is in complete flexion.
- *Face* (**mentum**) *presentation* is the face presenting first. The head is in full hyperextension.

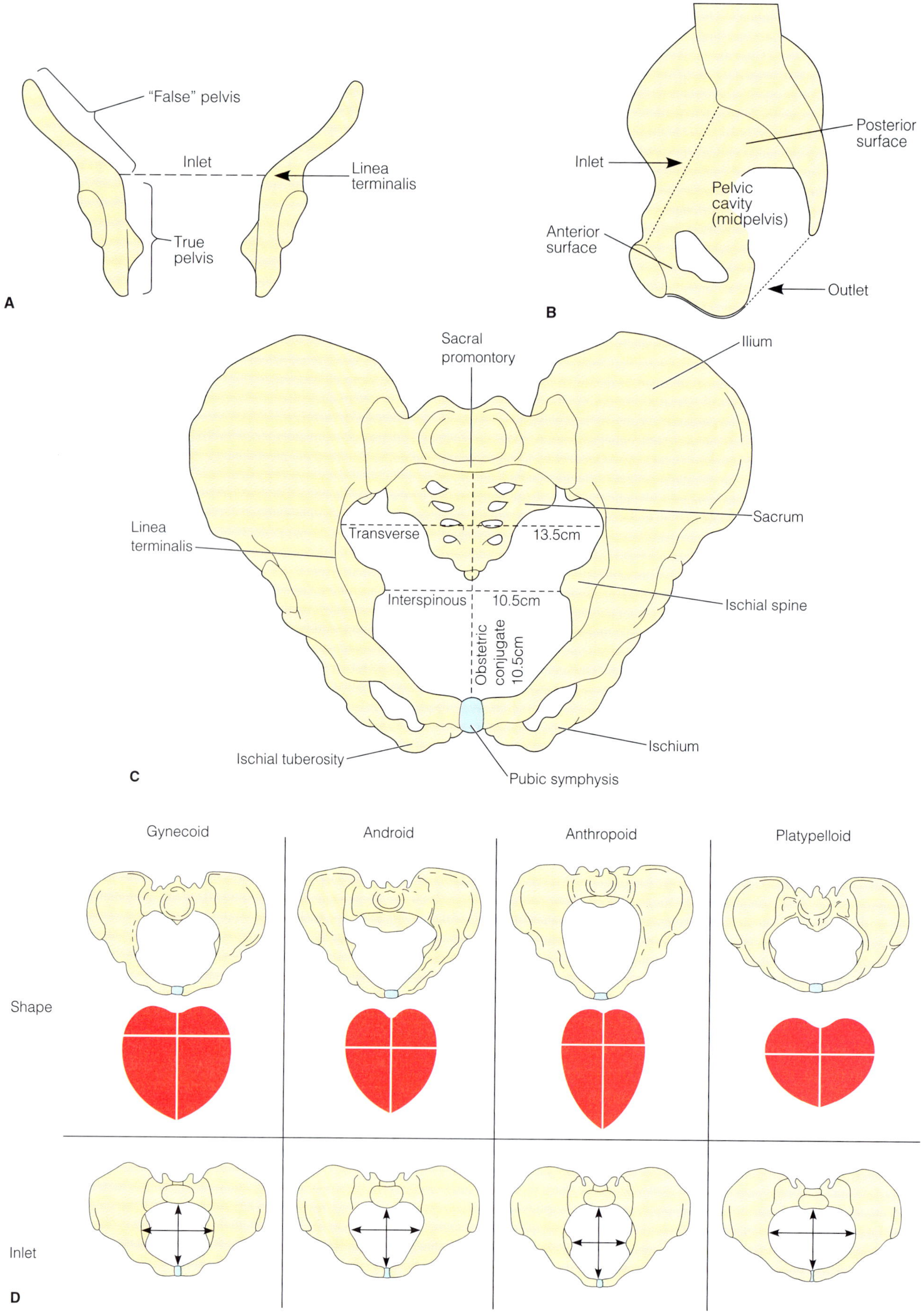

Figure 14-4. ■ Female pelvis. (A) False pelvis is a shallow cavity above the inlet; true pelvis is the deeper portion of the cavity below the inlet. (B) The true pelvis consists of inlet, cavity (midpelvis), and outlet. (C) The pelvic planes: coronal section and common diameters of the bony pelvis. (D) Varying shape of the female pelvis and inlet can affect the passage of the fetus.

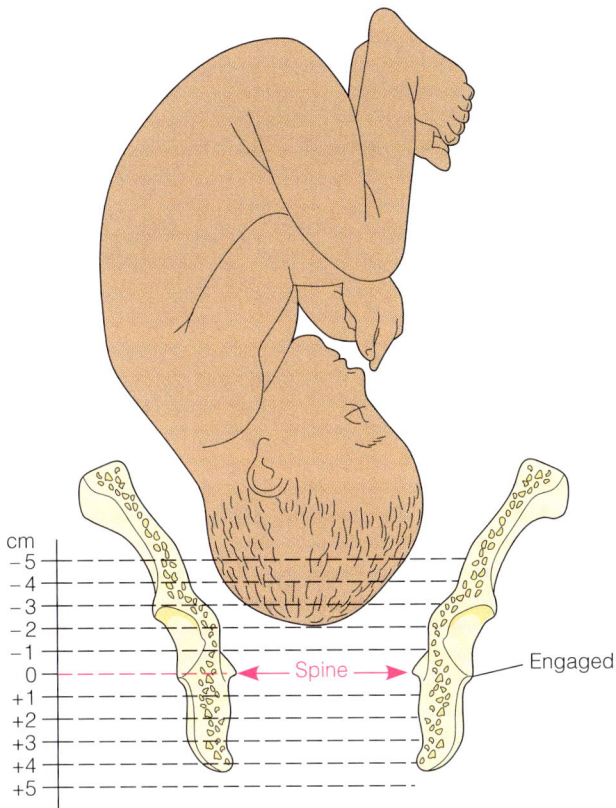

Figure 14-5. ■ Measuring the station of the fetal head while it is descending. In this view, the station is −2/−3.

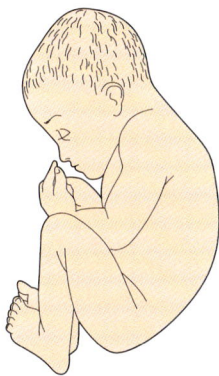

Figure 14-6. ■ Fetal attitude. The relationship of body parts of this fetus is normal. The head is flexed forward, with the chin almost resting on the chest. The arms and legs are flexed.

- *Brow presentation* is the **sinciput** (forehead or brow) presenting first. The fetal head is neither flexed nor hyperextended.

The fetus might assume a longitudinal lie with a **breech** (buttocks) presentation. Figure 14-9 ■ illustrates one type of breech presentation. Breech presentations are further differentiated by the attitude of the fetus's legs:

- *Complete breech*. The hips and knees are flexed on the abdomen. The buttocks present first.

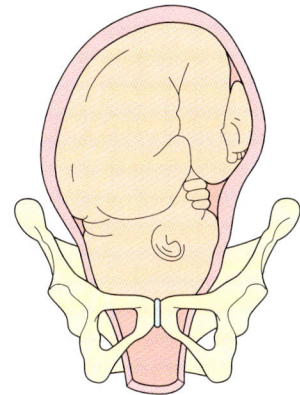

A

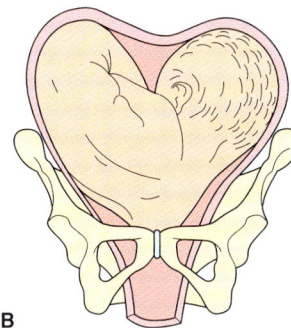

B

Figure 14-7. ■ Fetal lie. (**A**) Longitudinal. (**B**) Transverse.

- *Frank breech*. The hips are flexed, but the knees are extended with the feet close to the head. The buttocks are presenting first.
- *Footling breech*. One or both of the hips and knees are extended, with the foot (feet) being the presenting part.

If the fetus assumes a transverse lie (see Figure 14-7), the presenting part will be the shoulder, arm, back, abdomen, or side. The fetus in a transverse presentation cannot be delivered vaginally. See discussion of cesarean birth in Chapter 15 ⚭.

FETAL POSITION.   **Fetal position** refers to the relationship of the presenting part to the four quadrants of the maternal pelvis. The fetal landmarks are identified in the right or left, anterior or posterior quadrants of the mother's pelvis. Abbreviations are typically used to indicate fetal position.

- The first letter refers to the mother's right or left.
- The second letter refers to the fetal landmark.
- The third letter refers to the mother's anterior or posterior quadrant.

The most ideal position for a vaginal birth is right occiput anterior (ROA) or left occiput anterior (LOA). Table 14-3 ■ and Figure 14-10 ■ describe and illustrate the common fetal presentations.

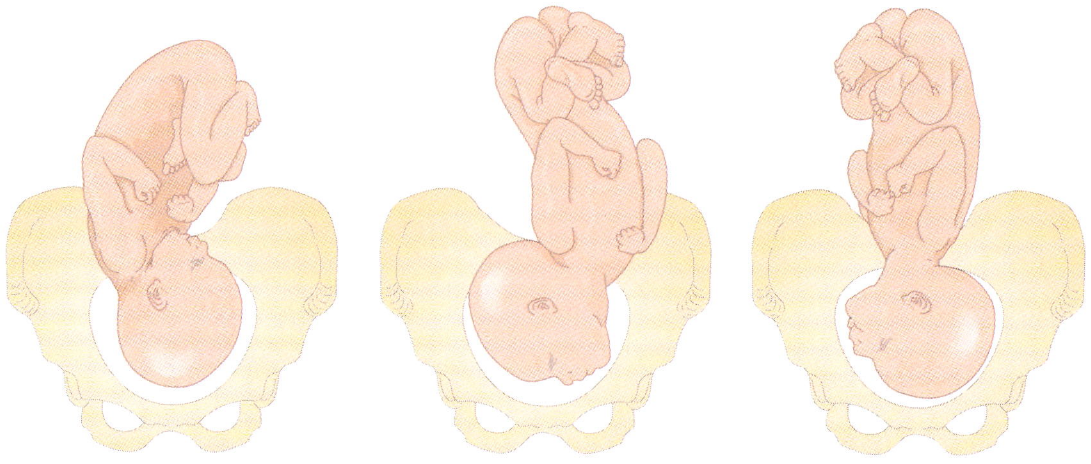

Figure 14-8. ■ Cephalic presentations. (**A**) Vertex/occipital presentation. (**B**) Face (*mentum*) presentation. (**C**) Brow (*sinciput*) presentation.

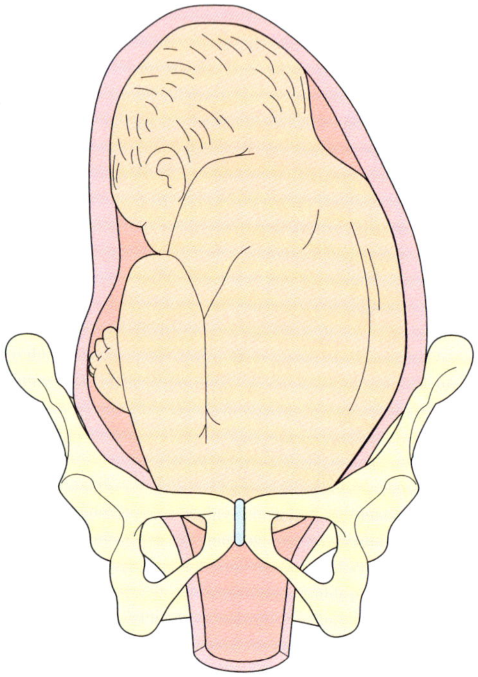

Figure 14-9. ■ Breech presentation. The position illustrated is called complete breech.

Size of the Fetus

The largest part of the fetus is the head. The bones of the fetal skull are not fused but instead are joined by fibrous connective tissue called **sutures.** Large spaces, called **fontanels,** prevent undue pressure on the fetal brain. Figure 14-11 ■ illustrates the position of fontanels and sutures in relation to the position of the fetus within the birth canal. In cephalic presentation, as the fetal head is pushed through the maternal pelvis, the bones of the skull ride over one another, decreasing the diameter of the head. This shaping of the fetal head to the bones of the maternal pelvis is termed **molding** (Figure 14-12 ■). In a breech presentation,

the fetal head moves through the pelvis neck first. This direction of movement prevents pressure on the top of the fetal head, so molding does not occur. The fetal head may be too large to pass through the maternal pelvis, leading to an ominous prognosis.

POWERS

The third of the 5 Ps affecting labor refers to the powers necessary to push the fetus through the passageway. These powers are (1) the power of uterine contractions and (2) the strength of the mother pushing the baby.

Primary Power

The primary power comes from the involuntary muscle contractions of the myometrium. Uterine contractions begin in response to the posterior pituitary hormone, oxytocin. **Contractions,** which begin in the fundus, are the result of shortening of the muscle fibers.

Muscle fibers of the uterus have several unique properties.

1. Uterine muscle fibers contract and relax in a rhythmic pattern. During relaxation, circulation is restored to the placenta, improving oxygenation of the fetus.
2. Contracted uterine muscle fibers remain shortened. This results in a gradual decrease in the size of the uterine cavity. As the uterine muscle fibers shorten, the lower uterine segment is pulled up, and the fetus is pushed down. These actions result in *effacement* (shortening and thinning of the cervix) and *dilatation* (opening of the cervical os). See Figure 14-3 to review effacement and dilatation.

CHARACTERISTICS OF CONTRACTIONS Contractions are described in terms of frequency, duration, and intensity. Figure 14-13 ■ shows contraction patterns in the first, second, and third stages of labor.

TABLE 14-3

Common Fetal Positions

ABBREVIATION OF PRESENTATION	PRESENTING PART	DESCRIPTION OF FETAL POSITION
Figure 14-10. ■ ROA	Occiput	Right side of maternal pelvis, occiput presenting, occiput directed toward anterior (front) of passage
Figure 14-10. ■ ROT	Occiput	Right side of maternal pelvis, occiput presenting, occiput transverse (directed toward side of passage)
Figure 14-10. ■ ROP	Occiput	Right side of maternal pelvis, occiput presenting, occiput directed toward posterior (back) of passage
Figure 14-10. ■ LOA	Occiput	Left side of maternal pelvis, occiput presenting, occiput directed toward anterior (front) of passage

(continued)

TABLE 14-3

Common Fetal Positions (continued)

ABBREVIATION OF PRESENTATION	PRESENTING PART	DESCRIPTION OF FETAL POSITION
Figure 14-10. ■ LOT	Occiput	Left side of maternal pelvis, occiput presenting, occiput transverse (directed toward side of passage)
Figure 14-10. ■ LOP	Occiput	Left side of maternal pelvis, occiput presenting, occiput directed toward posterior (back) of passage
Figure 14-10. ■ RMA	Mentum (chin)	Right side of maternal pelvis, mentum (chin) presenting, mentum directed toward anterior (front) of passage
Figure 14-10. ■ RMP	Mentum	Right side of maternal pelvis, mentum (chin) presenting, mentum directed toward posterior (back) of passage

ABBREVIATION OF PRESENTATION	PRESENTING PART	DESCRIPTION OF FETAL POSITION
TABLE 14-3 Common Fetal Positions		
Figure 14-10. ■ LMA	Mentum	Left side of maternal pelvis, mentum (chin) presenting, mentum directed toward anterior (front) of passage
Figure 14-10. ■ LSA	Sacrum	Left side of maternal pelvis, sacrum presenting, sacrum directed toward anterior (front) of passage
Figure 14-10. ■ LSP	Sacrum	Left side of maternal pelvis, sacrum presenting, sacrum directed toward posterior (back) of passage

- The **frequency** is the time from the onset of one contraction to the onset of the next contraction.
- The **duration** is the time from the onset of a contraction to the end of that contraction.
- The **intensity** is the strength of the contraction at its peak.

As mentioned, blood supply through the uterus to the placenta is decreased during contractions. Ideally, the frequency of contractions should be every 3 to 5 minutes, with a duration of not more than 90 seconds. This allows time, during uterine relaxation, for circulation to be restored and the fetus to recover. To push the fetus through the cervix, contractions must be of moderate to strong intensity.

Secondary Power

The secondary power comes from the mother actively pushing the fetus through the birth canal. Spontaneous urge to push, known as **Ferguson's reflex**, occurs when the presenting part

Figure 14-11. ■ Palpating the sutures in the skull to determine position of the fetus. (A) Left occiput anterior (LOA). The occiput (area over the occipital bone on the posterior part of the fetal head) is in the left anterior quadrant of the woman's pelvis. When the fetus is LOA, the posterior fontanelle (located just above the occipital bone and triangular in shape) is in the upper left quadrant of the maternal pelvis. (B) The left occiput posterior (LOP). The posterior fontanelle is in the lower left quadrant of the maternal pelvis. (C) The right occiput anterior (ROA). The posterior fontanelle is in the upper right quadrant of the maternal pelvis. (D) The right occiput posterior (ROP). The posterior fontanelle is in the lower right quadrant of the maternal pelvis. *Note*: The anterior fontanelle is diamond-shaped. Because of the roundness of the fetal head, only a portion of the anterior fontanelle can be seen in each of the views, so it appears to be triangular in shape.

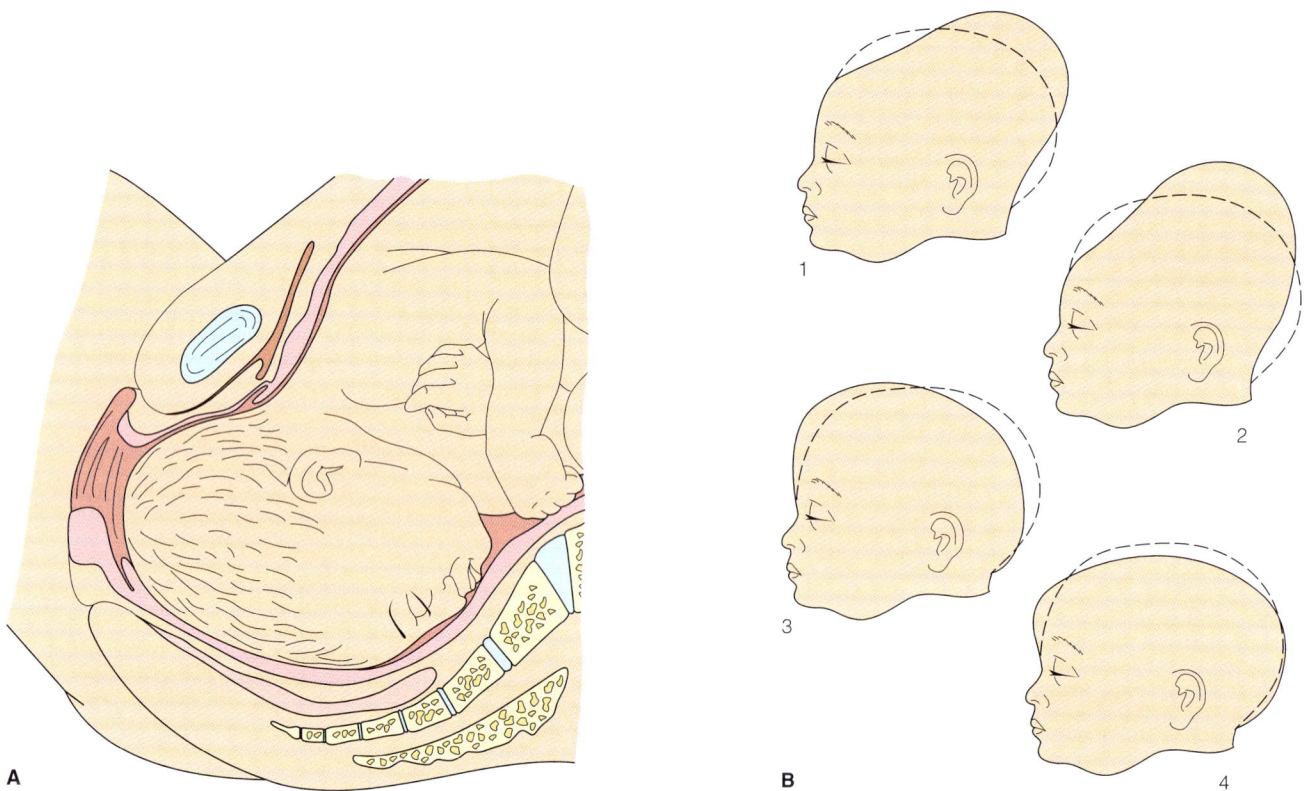

Figure 14-12. ■ Effects of labor on the fetal head. (A) The caput succedaneum formation. The presenting portion of the scalp area is encircled by the cervix during labor, causing swelling of the soft tissue. (B) Molding of the fetal head in cephalic presentations: (1) occiput anterior, (2) occiput posterior, (3) brow, (4) face.

	First stage			Second stage	Third stage
	Early phase	**Active phase**	**Transition phase**		
Frequency	every 5+ min	every 3–5 min	every 2–3 min		
Contraction intensity	Rest / Mild	Rest / Moderate to strong	Rest / Strong to very strong	Rest / Pushing/strong	Very mild to moderate
Contraction duration	30–45 sec	45–60 sec	60–90 sec	60–90 sec	
Contractions that cause dilation and effacement of the cervix				Pushing	Placenta delivered
Dilation (cm) 0 1	2 3	4 5 6 7	8 9 10		
Effacement	50%	75–100%	100%		
Average duration					
First baby Total = 10–16 hr		8–13 hr		1/2–2+ hr	5–30 min
Second, third, and subsequent babies Total = 6–10 hr		5–9 hr		5–60 min	5–30 min

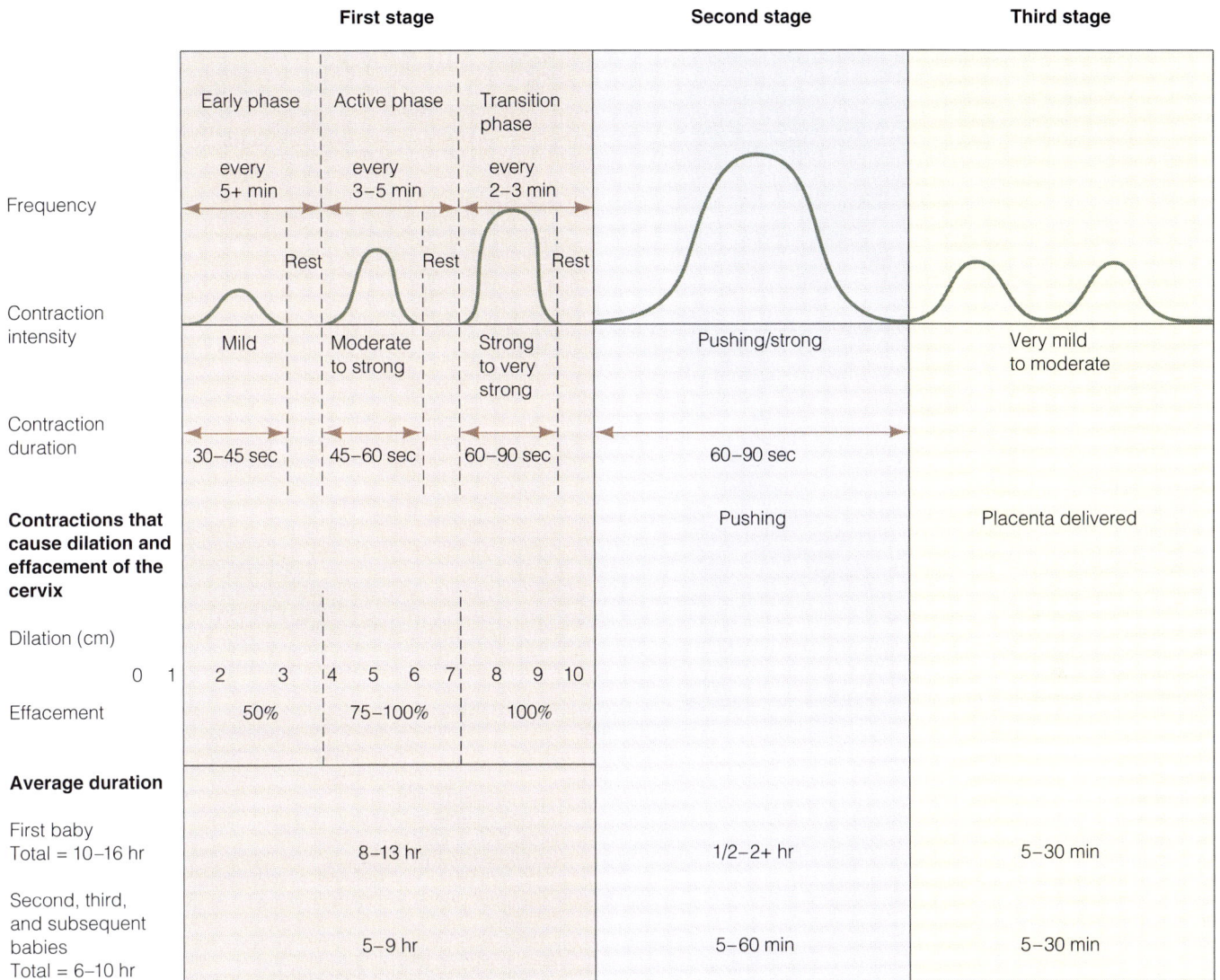

Figure 14-13. ■ Contraction patterns in first, second, and third stages of labor. Primigravidas may be 100% effaced before labor begins.

reaches the pelvic floor. Stretch receptors in the vagina trigger the release of oxytocin, which intensifies contractions. To prevent trauma of the cervix, the woman is discouraged from pushing until the cervix has dilated completely.

POSITION

The fourth P affecting labor is the position of the mother during labor. The mother may need frequent changes in position as labor progresses. Changes in position relieve muscle tension, support different areas of the body, and provide some distraction. Some options are shown in Figure 14-14 ■. It is important for the nurse to assist the client in finding a comfortable position. There is no single "right" position for labor.

If the mother lies on her back, the contractions are more frequent but of lower intensity. When the mother lies on her side, the contractions are less frequent but of greater intensity. Therefore, it may be better to position the mother on

her left side, using pillows to support her back and leg. Side-lying position also prevents supine hypotension syndrome.

PSYCHE

Psyche, the fifth P affecting labor, refers to the mother's emotional status during labor. The mother's emotions while delivering a child are determined by past experiences, expectations, culture, and ideas about how to behave during labor.

Cultures vary considerably in their views and expectations of the labor process. Some differences among cultures are highlighted in Box 14-1 ■.

Fear and anxiety can have a profound effect on the labor experience. If the woman is fearful and anxious, a negative cycle can emerge. Fear and anxiety stimulate the mother's adrenal gland to release additional epinephrine and norepinephrine. These "fight-or-flight" hormones have several effects.

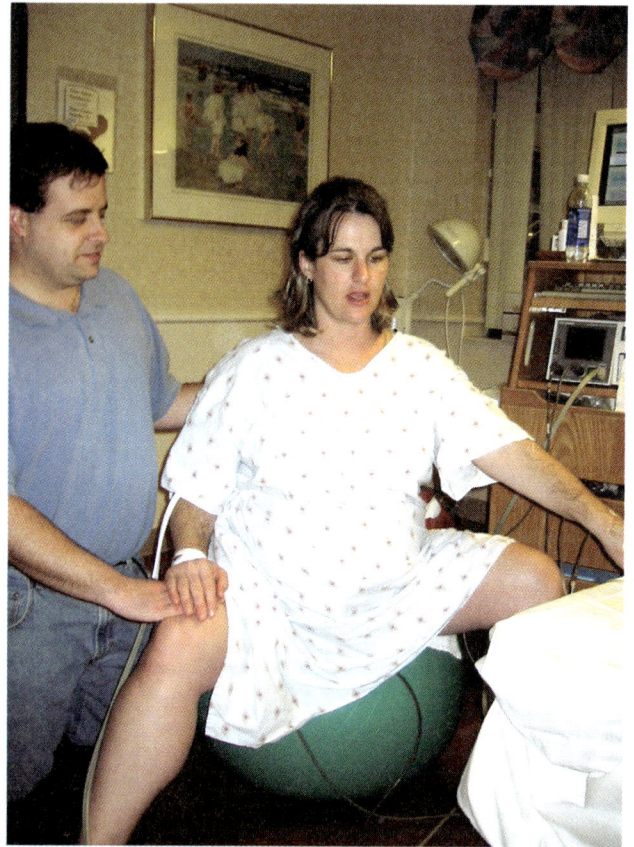

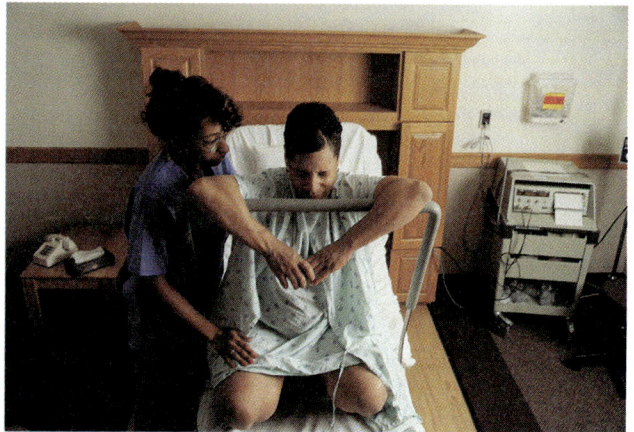

Figure 14-14. ■ (**A**) The nurse helps the client in labor assume a side-lying position to promote efficiency of contractions and maternal comfort. (**B**) Birthing ball facilitates fetal descent and fetal rotation, and helps increase the diameter of the pelvis. (**C**) Birthing bar.

BOX 14-1	CULTURAL PULSE POINTS

Considerations in Birthing Practices

China
Stoic response to pain. Fathers not present during birth. Prefer side lying during labor and delivery because they believe there is less trauma to fetus.

India
Natural childbirth practices preferred. Fathers usually not present. Female relatives usually present.

Iran
Fathers not present. Prefer female support and female caregivers. (If Muslim, may prefer to retain head covering and have body covered; two long-sleeved gowns may be offered.)

Japan
Natural childbirth methods practiced. May labor silently. Father may be present.

Laos
May want to be active and moving about during labor. May use squatting position for birth. Fathers may or may not be present. May prefer not to have amniotomy until right before birth. Prefer female caregivers. Prefer hot food and warm water during labor (St. Hill, Lipson, Ibrahim, & Meleis, 2003).

Mexico
May be stoic about discomfort until second stage, then may request pain relief. Father and female relatives may be present.

South Korea
Stoic during labor. Fathers usually not present.

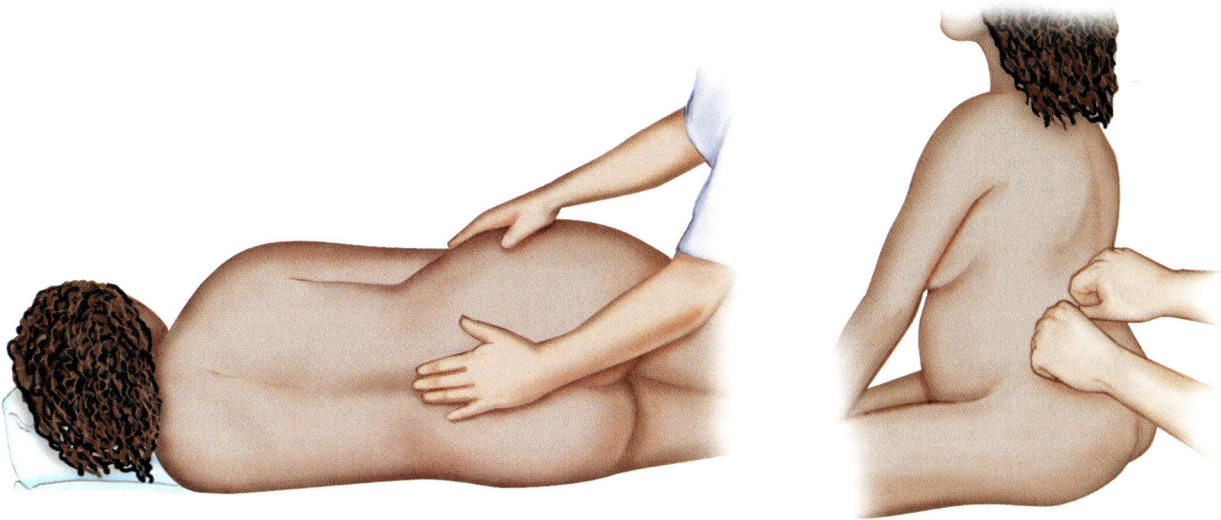

Figure 14-15. ■ Massage techniques for back labor.

- They constrict blood vessels (restricting placental circulation).
- They decrease the effectiveness of contractions.
- They tighten skeletal muscles.

When skeletal muscles of the pelvic floor are tight, they do not stretch easily. To widen them, the uterus needs to contract harder, increasing discomfort. Discomfort increases tension and anxiety. These three factors become a cycle, making the labor a longer and less positive experience. The nurse can provide (or teach a partner to provide) distraction and comfort measures such as a sacral massage for the laboring woman (Figure 14-15 ■).

Pain in Labor

The pain of labor has several unique features. Its focus shifts as labor progresses (Figure 14-16 A–C ■). It may cause anxiety and some level of fear. However, in most instances it is also associated with excitement and anticipation. Although it may begin as a mild ache, it builds to great intensity within a fairly short time. It is relieved abruptly and often very rapidly after birth, especially in women who deliver vaginally.

NONPHARMACOLOGIC PAIN RELIEF

The location of pain in labor relates to the state and phase. Early in labor, a woman may only be aware of a dull, stretching sensation or generalized discomfort. Contractions begin to shorten the uterus and stretch (dilate) the cervical opening. Light activity (walking, changing position, bathing, rocking on hands and knees) may be acceptable during the latent phase to help distract the mother while labor proceeds. Other relaxation techniques, such as guided imagery and light massage, can also be useful. Box 14-2 ■ describes several complementary therapies that may be useful to women in labor.

Childbirth Preparation Classes

In childbirth preparation classes, women are taught relaxation techniques, conditioning exercises, and breathing patterns. Several theories of pain reduction in childbirth are taught in these classes. Women are empowered to make informed choices in their birth experience, to assume responsibility for their health, and to trust in their inner wisdom.

The most common theory is the Lamaze method of relaxation and breathing techniques (Table 14-4 ■ and Figure 14-17 ■), which is useful in decreasing fear and pain. At the beginning of each contraction the woman takes a deep cleansing breath through her nose and exhales though her mouth. She then focuses on controlling her breathing using one of the following breathing patterns:

- First pattern is slow deep breathing of 6 to 9 breaths per minute.
- Second pattern is short, rapid, shallow breathing, inhaling and exhaling through the mouth. The breathing rate is about 4 breaths every 5 seconds.

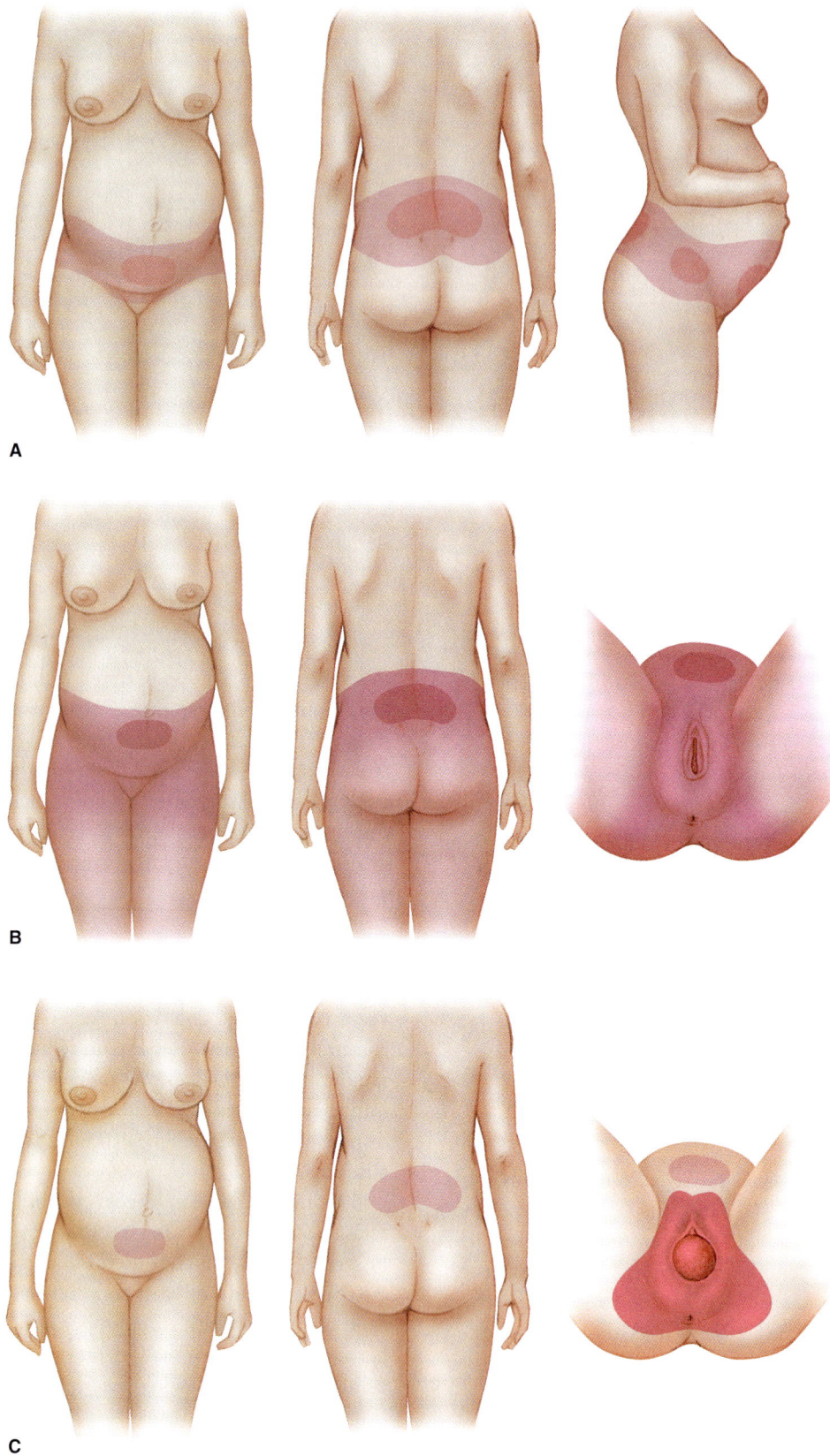

Figure 14-16. ■ Distribution of pain in labor. Graduated shades of color indicate intensity of pain. (**A**) Early phase of Stage one labor. (**B**) Latter phase of Stage one and early Stage two labor. (**C**) Latter phase of Stage two and actual birth. (Adapted, with permission from Bonica, J. J., & McDonald, J. S. [eds.]. [1995]. *Principles and practice of obstetric analgesia and anesthesia* [2nd ed.]. Baltimore: Lea & Febiger.)

BOX 14-2	COMPLEMENTARY THERAPIES

Relaxation Techniques

Labor is a process that may advance slowly or rapidly. It requires great physical energy and puts strain on the musculoskeletal system. It is useful for women as they approach labor to have a variety of methods they can use to provide comfort and/or distraction while the body continues its work. The following options have been found useful and are accessible to all women:

- Hydrotherapy—a warm bath or whirlpool bath
- Application of heat or cold—warm or cold compress directly to an area
- Imagery and visualization—focused, quiet picturing of the uterus opening gently to allow the birth to occur

- Effleurage—(latent and active phases of Stage one labor) rhythmic stroking and massage of the abdomen (see Figure 14-33B)
- Abdominal pressure—(end Stage one labor) deep massage to area of greatest pain intensity
- Biofeedback—response to a painful stimulus with a specific relaxation technique (best if practiced beforehand)
- Comfort measures—rinsing the mouth, gentle cleansing with a warm washcloth, change of clothes if clothing has become damp
- Distractions—soothing or encouraging words, music, watching television, looking out a window, listening to the fetal heartbeat
- Application of childbirth education—using the breathing and other techniques learned in prenatal classes

TABLE 14-4

Patterned-Paced Breathing Techniques During Labor

BREATHING METHOD	GRAPHIC REPRESENTATION
Lamaze Breathing Pattern Levels **First Level (slow paced)** Pattern begins and ends with a cleansing breath (in through the nose and out through pursed lips as if cooling a spoonful of hot food). While inhaling through the nose and exhaling through pursed lips, slow breaths are taken, moving only the chest. The rate should be approximately 6–9/minute or 2 breaths/15 seconds. The coach or nurse may assist by reminding the woman to take a cleansing breath, and then the breaths could be counted out if needed to maintain pacing. The woman inhales as someone counts "one one thousand, two one thousand, three one thousand, four one thousand." Exhalation begins and continues through the same count.	First level for use during uterine contraction (The level begins and ends with a cleansing breath [CB].) CB ... 45 seconds ... CB **Figure 14-17A**
Second Level (modified paced) Pattern begins and ends with a cleansing breath. Breaths are then taken in and out silently through the mouth at approximately 4 breaths/5 seconds. The jaw and entire body need to be relaxed. The rate can be accelerated to 2–2½ breaths/second. The rhythm for the breaths can be counted out as "one and two and one and two and . . ." with the woman exhaling on the numbers and inhaling on "and."	Second level CB ... 60 seconds ... CB **Figure 14-17B**
Third Level (pattern paced) Pattern begins and ends with a cleansing breath. All breaths are rhythmic, in and out through the mouth. Exhalations are accompanied by a "hee" or "hoo" sound in a varying pattern, 2:1, which begins as 3:1 (hee hee hee hoo) and can change to 2:1 (hee hee hoo) or 1:1 (hee hoo) as the intensity of the contraction changes. The rate should not be more rapid than 2-2½ breaths/second. The rhythm of the breaths would match a "one and two and . . ." count.	Third level (darkened spike represents "hoo") CB ... 60–90 seconds ... CB **Figure 14-17C**

(continued)

TABLE 14-4

Patterned-Paced Breathing Techniques During Labor (continued)

BREATHING METHOD	GRAPHIC REPRESENTATION
Abdominal Breathing Pattern Cues The abdomen moves outward during inhalation and downward during exhalation. The rate remains slow, with approximately 6–9 breaths/minute.	Breathing sequence for abdominal breathing $\vert\longleftarrow$ 60 seconds $\longrightarrow\vert$ **Figure 14-17D** ■
Quick Method When the woman has not learned a particular method and is in the active phase of labor, the nurse may teach her a combination of two patterns. Abdominal breathing may be used until labor is more advanced. Then a more rapid pattern consisting of two short blows from the mouth followed by a longer blow can be used. (This pattern is called "pant-pant-blow" even though all exhalations are a blowing motion.)	Pant-pant-blow breathing pattern $\vert\longleftarrow$ 60 seconds $\longrightarrow\vert$ **Figure 14-17E** ■

■ Third pattern (also called pant-blow) is similar to the second pattern, except every few breaths the exhalation is a forceful one through pursed lips.

As labor progresses from the latent to the active phase, the pain and pressure shift (see Figure 14-16B). Nurses can teach partners to provide counterpressure to the continuing contractions. A sacral massage (see Figure 14-15) can provide comfort at this phase.

Some women go into labor wanting to experience **natural childbirth** (labor and birth without medical interventions or pain medication). This approach may motivate a woman to "look beyond the pain" and to use breathing and relaxation techniques to work her way through the stages of labor. Natural childbirth may create a tremendous feeling of empowerment. However, if a woman is encountering difficulties or the labor is progressing very slowly, it may be important for her to safeguard her energy by receiving pharmacologic relief. In such situations, the nurse can help the woman accept the change as necessary for her and her infant's health. It is important to be empathetic but firm in these situations, and to remind the woman that she is handling a difficult situation well. The Health Promotion issue on pages 332 and 333 examines some of the variables that can have a positive effect on the labor experience.

PHARMACOLOGIC PAIN RELIEF

For some women, nonpharmacologic methods of pain relief are not enough, due to the position of the fetus, the length of labor, the level of discomfort the woman can tolerate, and other individual factors. When nonpharmacologic methods are not sufficient, pharmacologic methods of pain relief may be provided. The choice of method depends in part on the phase or stage of labor.

Systemic Medications

Systemic medications administered during labor are narcotic analgesics. These drugs should be administered only when the client's vital signs are stable, the fetus is at term, the FHR is in a normal pattern between 120 and 160, and the client is in active labor. Caution is required when administering systemic medications. Systemic medications can slow or stop contractions if labor is not well established. When given in transition or in the second stage of labor, systemic medications can cause respiratory distress in the newborn. Table 14-5 ■ provides information about medications that may be administered to the client during labor.

Regional Blocks

Regional blocks or regional anesthetics are administered by the physician, anesthesiologist, or nurse anesthetist. Regional blocks chemically stop the nerve conduction of painful stimuli. The effect of the medication is rapid with a gradual return of feeling as the medication is absorbed from the injection site into the blood. It is critical to monitor the mother for hypotension and the fetus for bradycardia following administration of anesthetic agents. Common regional blocks (Figure 14-18 ■) include:

■ *Paracervical block.* The drug is administered around the cervix during active labor to provide anesthesia to the cervix and upper vagina. If the cervix is too thin, the physician may not be able to perform a paracervical

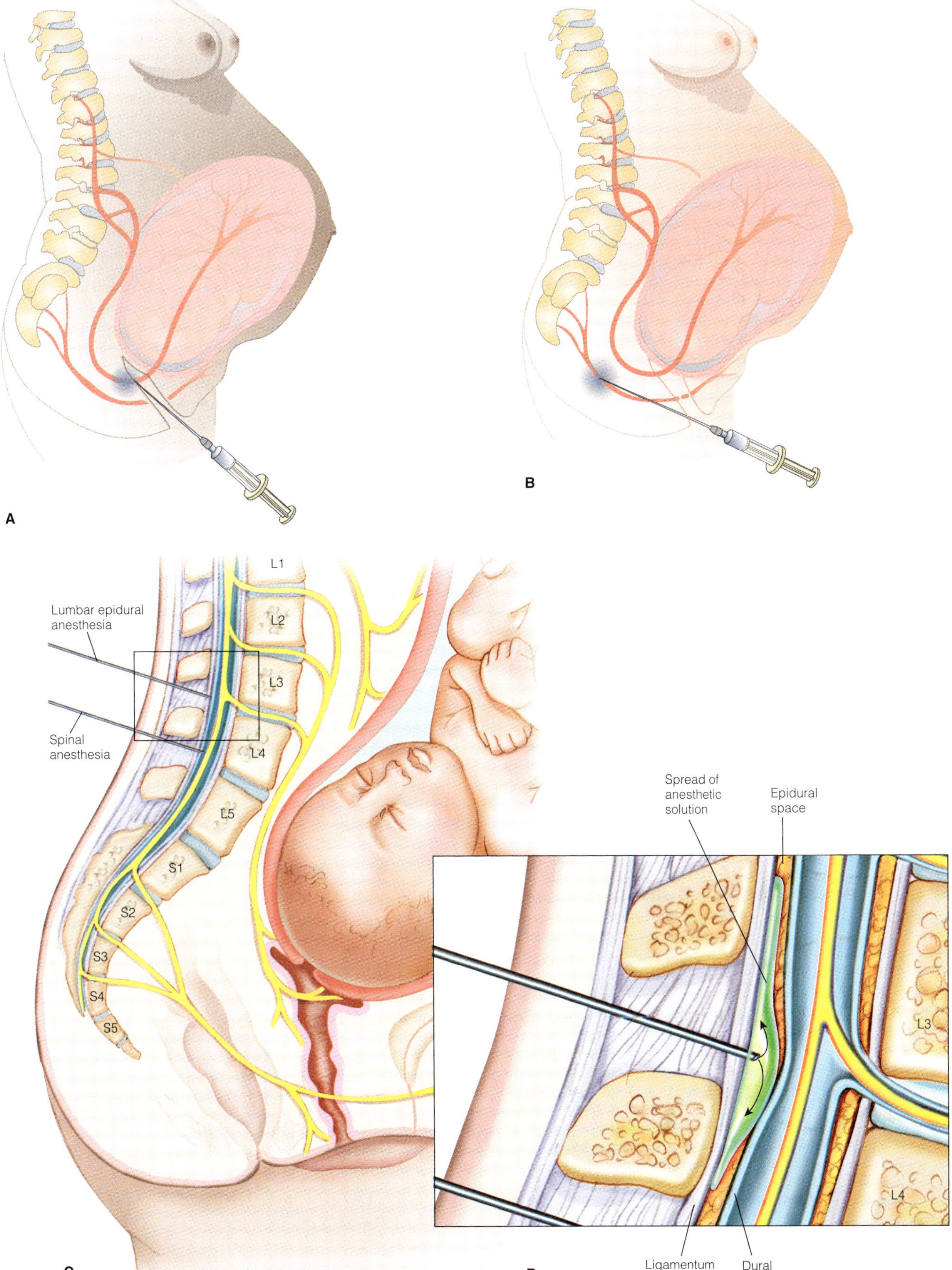

A

B

C

D

Lumbar epidural anesthesia

Spinal anesthesia

L1
L2
L3
L4
L5
S1
S2
S3
S4
S5

Spread of anesthetic solution

Epidural space

L3

L4

Ligamentum flavum

Dural membrane

Figure 14-18. ■ (**A**) Paracervical block (sensory pathways and site of interruption in relation to fetus). (**B**) Pudendal block. (**C**) Placement of epidural and spinal anesthetics. (**D**) Epidural space, located between the dura and the vertebra. The slight bulge illustrates the dura being pushed away from the tip of the needle by the force of the injection.

TABLE 14-5				
Pharmacology: Systemic Pain Medications Used During Labor				
DRUG (GENERIC AND COMMON BRAND NAME)	**USUAL ROUTE/DOSE**	**CLASSIFICATION AND PURPOSE**	**SELECTED SIDE EFFECTS AND NURSING CONSIDERATIONS**	**DON'T GIVE IF**
Butorphanol tartrate (Stadol)	1–2 mg IV every 3–4 hours	Opioid analgesic for pain	Respiratory depression, dizziness, euphoria	In second stage of labor
Meperidine HCL (Demerol)	2.5–15 mg IV every 3–4 hours	Opioid analgesic for pain	Respiratory depression, sedation	In second stage of labor *or* if allergic to drug
Naloxone (Narcan)	0.4–2 mg IV may repeat every 2–3 minutes to total of 10 mg	Narcotic antagonist for relief of respiratory depression in substance abuse	Respiratory depression may recur when Narcan wears off; monitor respiratory status carefully	Total of 10 mg has been given without improvement, *or* if you suspect narcotic overdose

block safely. There is a risk that the paracervical needle could go through the cervix and into the fetal presenting part. Due to the risk to the fetus, many physicians choose not to use this method of anesthesia.

- *Pudendal block.* The drug is administered through the vagina and into the pudendal nerve, resulting in anesthesia of the vagina and perineum. A pudendal block relieves discomfort from stretching of the vagina and perineum during end of the first stage, the second stage and for repair of episiotomy or lacerations. A pudendal block does not relieve discomfort from contractions. There is little risk of maternal hypotension or fetal reactions. Disadvantages of pudendal block include possible hematoma of the pudendal nerve.

- *Epidural block.* The drug is administered through a catheter placed in the epidural space (Figure 14-18C). The drug can be administered intermittently or by continuous infusion. It is important for labor to be well established, usually with at least 4 centimeters cervical dilatation, before a epidural block is administered. If labor is progressing rapidly, there may not be time to administer the medication prior to birth. Anesthesia usually involves the lower abdomen, pelvis, perineum, and lower extremities. Although the client remains fully awake and comfortable, participation in the birth process may be variable. In some clients, a lack of feeling may decrease their ability to push effectively, so the birth may need to be assisted. The client may experience hypotension, bladder distention, and respiratory depression. For this reason, frequent or constant monitoring by the registered nurse is required. Some clinical facilities also require the physician or nurse midwife to be present.

- *Spinal block.* The drug is administered into the cerebrospinal fluid. An advantage of this method of anesthesia is the immediate onset of pain relief. However,

blocking the sympathetic neurons can result in severe hypotension. If the client is not positioned properly, the anesthesia can move upward in the spinal column and suppress respirations. Because of these life-threatening complications, spinal anesthesia is not commonly used.

Local Infiltration

With local infiltration, the drug is injected subcutaneously into the true perineum prior to an episiotomy or repair of a laceration. Figure 14-19 ■ illustrates the technique of local infiltration for episiotomy repair and common episiotomy locations.

General Anesthesia

General anesthesia is rarely used for vaginal deliveries because it causes the client to lose consciousness. However, it may be used for emergency cesarean births (see discussion in Chapter 15 ⬤). Because the drug reaches the fetus in about 2 minutes, there is danger of respiratory depression in the newborn.

Stages of Labor

Labor is a process, or sequence of events, that begins with uterine contractions and ends 1 hour after delivery of the placenta. The labor process is described in four stages.

FIRST STAGE OF LABOR: DILATATION AND EFFACEMENT

The **first stage of labor,** also known as the **dilatation stage,** begins with regular contractions and ends with complete effacement and dilatation of the cervix. This is usually the longest stage and is divided into three phases: latent, active, and transition.

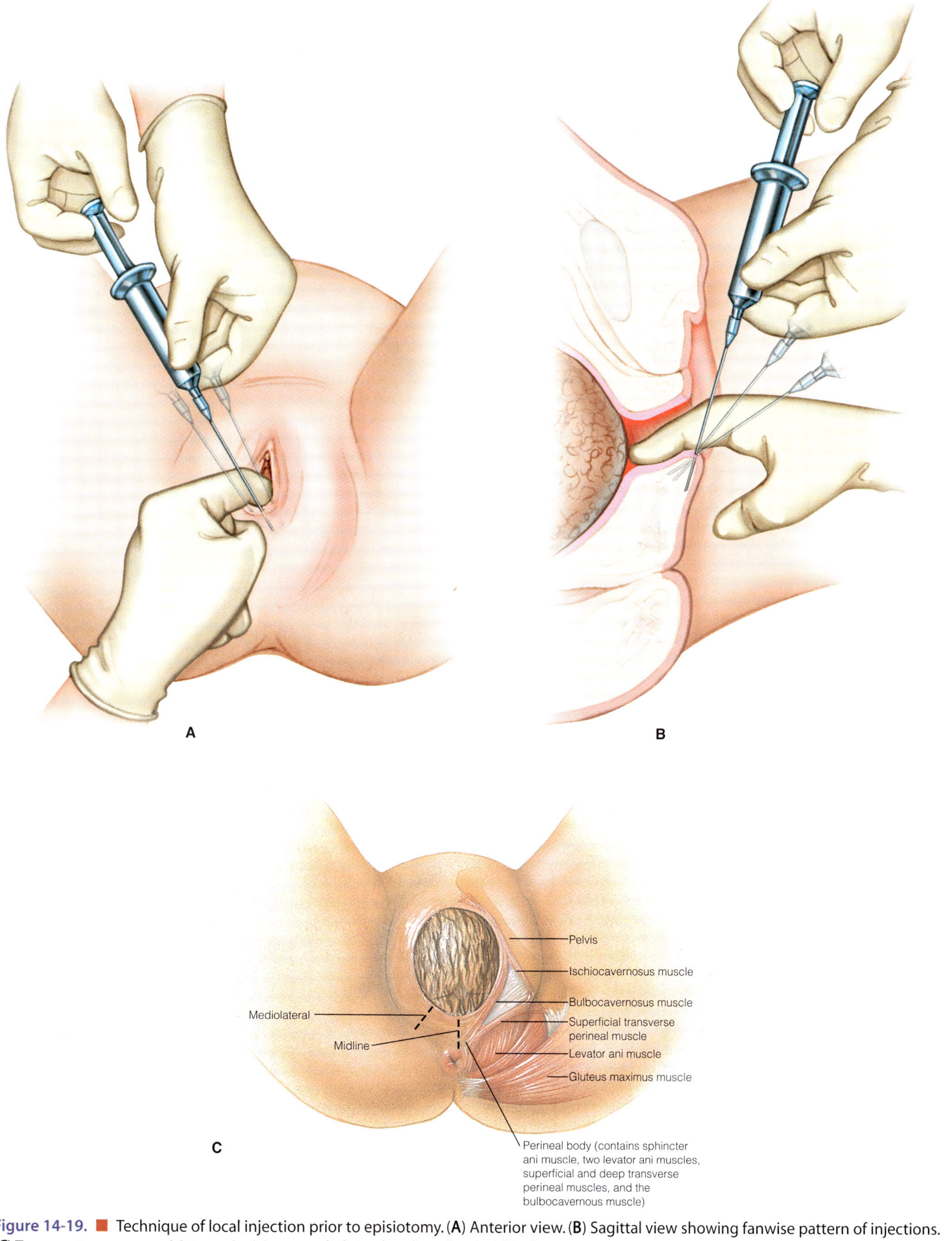

A

B

Mediolateral

Midline

Pelvis

Ischiocavernosus muscle

Bulbocavernosus muscle

Superficial transverse
perineal muscle

Levator ani muscle

Gluteus maximus muscle

Perineal body (contains sphincter
ani muscle, two levator ani muscles,
superficial and deep transverse
perineal muscles, and the
bulbocavernous muscle)

C

Figure 14-19. ■ Technique of local injection prior to episiotomy. (**A**) Anterior view. (**B**) Sagittal view showing fanwise pattern of injections. (**C**) Two most common episiotomy incisions: mediolateral and median (midline).

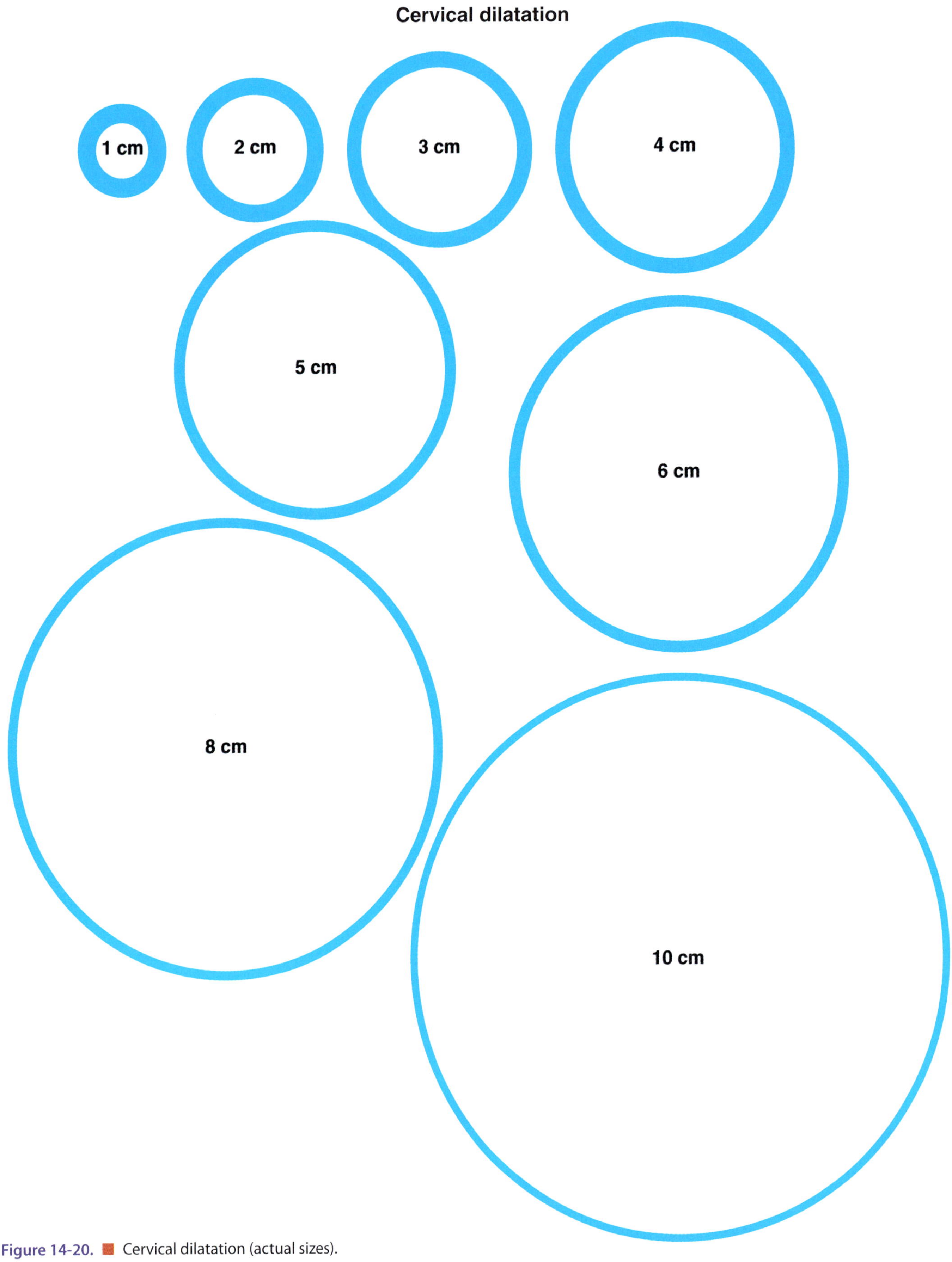

Cervical dilatation

Figure 14-20. ■ Cervical dilatation (actual sizes).

Latent Phase

The **latent phase** of the first stage of labor is from the onset of contractions until the cervix is dilated 4 centimeters (Figure 14-20 ■). Contractions usually occur every 10 to 15 minutes and gradually increase to 5 minutes apart. (To review the pattern of contractions in labor, see Figure 14-13.) Each contraction lasts 30 to 40 seconds and is of mild to moderate intensity.

In the latent phase, the client is aware of the contractions but is relatively comfortable. She is excited that labor has begun, and is often anxious about what lies ahead. If the membranes have not ruptured, the woman is encouraged to walk as long as she does not become tired. This is a good time to reinforce teaching to both mother and partner, especially relaxation methods (see complementary methods in Box 14-2 and review breathing techniques described in Table 14-4).

The latent phase usually lasts 8 to 10 hours with the first pregnancy. With subsequent pregnancies, it usually lasts about 5 hours.

Active Phase

The **active phase** of the first stage of labor begins when the cervix is dilated 4 centimeters and ends with 8 centimeters of dilatation (see Figure 14-20). Contractions occur every 3 to 5 minutes. They last 60 to 90 seconds and are of moderate to strong intensity. Clients perceive an increased amount of discomfort as the fetus descends through the pelvis, stretching muscles and ligaments. During this phase of Stage one, clients seek a position that reduces discomfort. They may need assistance to change position. Some devices that may be useful to women in this phase of labor were shown in Figure 14-14. The client now focuses on relaxation and breathing techniques.

The average length of active labor is 4 to 6 hours for the primigravida client and 3 to 4 hours for the multipara client.

Transition Phase

The transition phase of the first stage of labor is the period during which the cervix widens from 8 to 10 centimeters (see Figure 14-20). The contractions are strong, occurring every 2 to 3 minutes and lasting 90 seconds. (To review the pattern of contractions in labor, see Figure 14-13.) As the fetus descends deeper into the pelvis and Ferguson's reflex is triggered, there is a strong urge to push. The client may need reminding to focus on relaxation and breathing techniques. As mentioned previously, it is important for the client not to push actively until the cervix is completely dilated. If the client pushes too early, the cervix can tear.

Some behaviors are common during the transition phase of labor. The client frequently becomes restless, irritable, and sometimes angry. Statements such as "I can't take anymore" and "Don't touch me!" are common. It is important to help the support person(s) understand that this behavior is part of the labor process.

The average length of the transition phase of Stage one labor is 1 to 2 hours.

AMNIOTOMY.   An **amniotomy** is an artificial rupturing of the fetal membranes (Figure 14-21 ■). The procedure may be performed after cervical dilation has reached at least 2 centimeters. This allows the amnihook to be inserted through the opening in the cervix.

Amniotomy is performed for a variety of reasons.

- It may stimulate the beginning of labor.
- It may shorten the length of labor.
- It allows access to the fetus to apply an internal fetal heart monitoring electrode (see Figure 15-2 ⬭).

There are some disadvantages of amniotomy as well. First, it introduces the possibility of infection because the fetus may be exposed to vaginal and intrauterine microorganisms. Second, it increases the danger of umbilical cord prolapse. Finally, it may lead to increased molding because the amniotic fluid is not present to cushion the fetal head during contractions.

SECOND STAGE OF LABOR: BIRTH

The **second stage of labor** begins when the cervix is completely dilated (see Figure 14-20) and ends with the birth of the baby. Contractions continue every 2 to 3 minutes, lasting 60 to 90 seconds. The client is encouraged to use her abdominal muscles to bear down actively with each contraction.

The second stage of labor could take 1 to 3 hours for the primigravida client. It often takes 15 to 30 minutes for the multipara client.

As the fetal head pushes on the perineum and the client pushes, the tissues of the perineum thin and bulge. The labia open. The fetal head can be seen with contractions, but it recedes into the vagina between contractions. Gradually, more and more of the fetal head appears with contractions. When the largest part of the fetal head is past the vulva and remains visible between contractions, **crowning** has occurred (Figure 14-22 ■). A few more pushes and the fetus will be born.

Episiotomy

In many births, an **episiotomy**, or surgical cutting of the perineal tissue, is performed at this time. An episiotomy may aid birth and prevent tearing of perineal and anal tissue. Figure 14-19C illustrated the position of midline and lateral episiotomies.

CLIENT WANTING SECOND LABOR TO BE BETTER THAN FIRST

Pamela and Cliff are having their second child. With the first pregnancy, Pamela developed pregnancy-induced hypertension and had to be on bed rest for the last 6 weeks of her pregnancy. Her labor was also difficult. She had to be on magnesium sulfate and pitocin. This meant that, due to the need for a Foley catheter and continuous fetal monitoring, she had to stay in bed during the entire labor. The pitocin made her contractions extremely intense and close together. Therefore, she needed an epidural to deal with the pain of contractions. Cliff also felt entirely unprepared to provide her any comfort. He wished he knew more about labor and what a laboring woman needs. When Pamela finally dilated to 10 cm, 14 hours after labor began, the physician had to perform an episiotomy and use forceps to assist with the birth. They did, however, have a healthy, 8-pound baby boy.

Over the last 2 years Pam has been disturbed by thoughts of regret over how her first labor proceeded. For this birth, Pamela and Cliff desire to do things differently. Pamela is showing no signs of gestational hypertension, and the baby seems to be healthy. Pamela and Cliff would like to go into labor naturally, labor without medications, and avoid many of the procedures they encountered last time. During a prenatal visit, they explain their desires to the nurse and ask for assistance.

DISCUSSION

Pain in labor has been defined as "an unpleasant sensory and emotional experience associated with actual or potential tissue damage." During the first stage of labor, the pain experienced is called visceral pain. Uterine contractions cause dilatation and effacement of the cervix as well as tissue ischemia. Visceral pain is felt by the client in her lower abdomen,

back, and thighs. This pain is felt only during contractions. During the second stage of labor, the client experiences somatic pain. Somatic pain is experienced by the client as stretching of the perineal tissues, traction on the perineum and ligaments, and pressure on the bladder, bowel, and pelvis. Pain perception is influenced by past experiences, culture, and the client's emotional well-being. Most women in labor want to avoid or at least reduce the pain of labor. Many desire to manage the pain of labor pharmacologically, whereas others want to avoid medications in an effort to reduce side effects and remain alert and in control.

The nursing literature recognizes four categories of nonpharmacologic pain relief methods or labor support behaviors. These are physical, emotional, advocacy, and instructional/informational. Physical comfort behaviors include touch, massage, personal hygiene, breathing and relaxation techniques, ambulation, positioning, heat or cold application, nutrition, and control of environmental elements. Emotional support behaviors include the continuous presence of caregiver, reassurance, encouragement, praise,

humor, and verbal distraction. Advocacy behaviors include listening, supporting the laboring woman's decisions, negotiating with caregivers about a laboring woman's requests, and respecting privacy. Instructional/informational support consists of role modeling behaviors to the partner and instructing the client and her partner how to breathe, relax, push, etc.

Nonpharmacologic pain relief methods offer many benefits. They can be very effective if applied appropriately. Most have few or no side effects. They are cost effective. Unlike pharmacologic methods of pain relief, the responsibility of pain control can be shared with the family and friends attending the labor and birth. Because there are numerous choices, the laboring woman feels like she has choices or a say so in her pain control.

The nurse can provide these labor support behaviors, but realistically the intrapartum nurses' job also includes technical behaviors that must be attended to such as making maternal and fetal assessment, managing equipment, and performing various procedures. Ideally, each laboring woman could have a private support person with her to provide these labor support behaviors. This labor support person may be her significant other, a family member, or a friend, or she could employ the services of a professional labor support person or a doula. The International Childbirth Education Association defines the doula as a trained professional who recognizes birth as a key life experience. The doula attends to the physical, emotional, and social needs of a woman in labor. The doula may be trained formally or informally. Several organizations provide training and certification.

Research studies have demonstrated the numerous positive patient outcomes related to supportive care provided by doulas. Labors were shorter, cesareans were reduced, oxytocin use was decreased, analgesia/anesthesia use was reduced as was amniotomies, episiotomies, and vacuum extractions.

Some hospitals provide doulas on call for their clients. Other doulas can be hired by the pregnant couple. Some labor and birth nurse managers are also providing training to their intrapartum nurses in labor support behaviors or doula techniques.

PLANNING AND IMPLEMENTATION

There are many ways that an expectant couple can prepare themselves for labor. The nurse should suggest optimal nutrition, regular exercise, adequate rest, resolution of stress factors, and regular prenatal visits. The couple may also explore issues related to labor in books or on websites.

Childbirth education courses offer couples an opportunity to learn more about pregnancy, labor, birth, and parenting. Many agencies offer a variety of courses such as early pregnancy classes, childbirth preparation, breastfeeding, and parenting and sibling classes. These courses are offered in many hospitals or by community organizations. The nurse should encourage the expectant couple to explore options thoroughly. Curriculums vary as do the qualifications and experience of the instructor. Childbirth educators can seek national certification through a number of organizations.

For the couple who desires to attain a more natural birth, the childbirth education course should include a variety of comfort techniques. The course should provide opportunities to practice and perfect these techniques.

The knowledge gained through self-study or childbirth classes can be used by the expectant couple to design a specific plan for their birth. In this plan, the couple can outline their wants, likes, and dislikes related to labor, birth, newborn, and postpartum care. This document should be as detailed as possible. The nurse can be a terrific resource for the expectant couple as they prepare their birth plan. Once this document is drafted, it is important to discuss these issues with the birth attendant as well as the staff at the birth facility. The nurse can assist the expectant couple in approaching the birth attendant. The nurse can become an advocate for the client. The nurse can encourage the expectant couple to become familiar with the birth facility where they will give birth. Much stress can be reduced if the couple has explored the environment where they will give birth. They can meet the staff and begin to develop a relationship with the nurses who may assist them during labor and birth. Touring the birth facility offers them an opportunity to review policies and procedures of the unit and negotiate items on their birth plan. If the client expresses an interest in having additional labor support, the nurse can provide information about the benefits and services of a doula. The nurse can provide referrals if necessary.

SELF-REFLECTION

Think about a time you have been in pain. It may have been a physical injury or after a surgical procedure or simply a trip to the dentist. What nonpharmacological techniques did you use for self-comfort to relieve yourself of pain? What worked? What did not work? Could you teach any of these comfort techniques to a laboring woman? Was there anything you could have done before your encounter with pain that might have assisted you in dealing more effectively with your pain?

SUGGESTED RESOURCES

For the Nurse

Adams, E., & Bianchi, A. (2004). Can a nurse and a doula exist in the same room? *International Journal of Childbirth Education, 19*(4), 12–15.

Bianchi, A., & Adams, E. (2004). Doulas, labor support, and nurses. *International Journal of Childbirth Education, 19*(4), 24–30.

Callister, L.C. (2001). Culturally competent care of women and newborns: Knowledge, attitude and skills. *Journal of Obstetric, Gynecologic, & Neonatal Nursing, 30*, 209–215.

Goetzl, L.M. (2002). ACOG practice bulletin. Obstetric analgesia and anesthesia. *Obstetrics & Gynecology, 100*, 177–191.

Hopper Deglin, J., & Hazard Vallerand, A. (2005). *Davis's drug guide for nurses* (9th ed.). Philadelphia: F.A. Davis Company.

Miltner, R. (2002). More than support: Nursing interventions provided to women in labor. *Journal of Obstetrics, Gynecologic and Neonatal Nursing, 31*(6), 753–761.

Simkin, P., & Bolding, A. (2004). Update on nonpharmacologic approaches to relieve labor pain and prevent suffering. *Journal of Midwifery and Women's Health, 49*(6), 489–504.

For the Client

Dick-Read, G. (2005). *Childbirth without fear.* London: Pinter & Martin, Ltd.

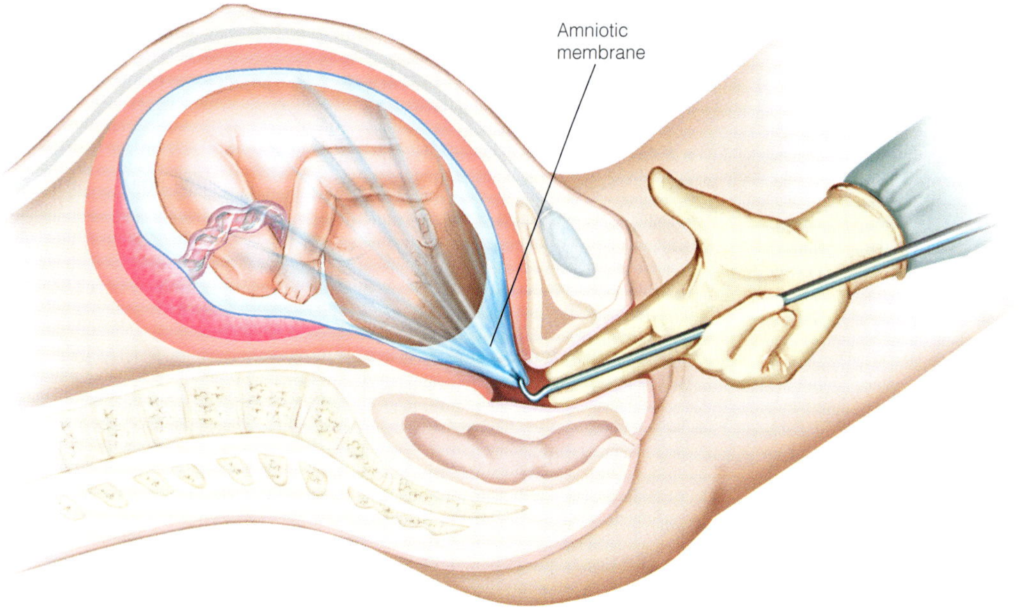

Amniotic membrane

Figure 14-21. ■ Amniotomy is a very common procedure performed during labor.

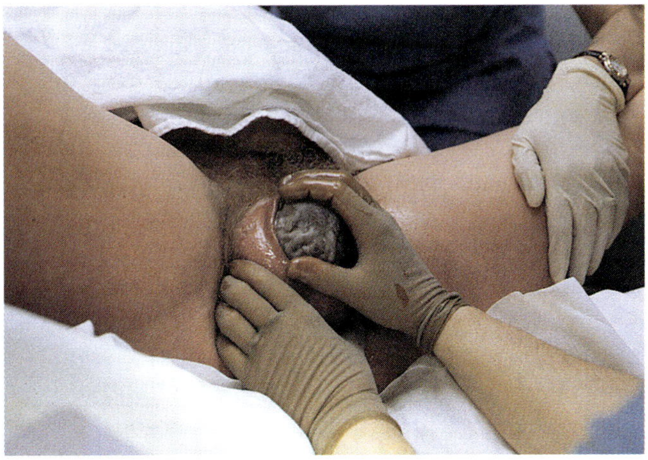

Figure 14-22. ■ Crowning of the fetus.

Mechanisms of Labor

The fetus changes positions as it moves through the pelvis. These movements are called the **mechanisms of labor** or **cardinal movements** (Figure 14-23 ■). The first three movements may occur before the first contractions or during the first stage of labor.

- **Engagement** (Figure 14-23B) is the point at which the presenting part (usually the fetal head) enters the true pelvis. The presenting part is even with or below the ischial spines. The fetus is no longer ballotable.
- **Descent** begins with engagement and continues as the contractions push the fetus through the pelvis.

- **Flexion** (see Figure 14-23C and D) describes the attitude the fetus assumes. Ideal flexion is positive, with head flexed onto the chest, the arms flexed across the chest, and the legs flexed across the abdomen.
- **Internal rotation** may take place prior to labor, but it most commonly occurs during the first or second stages. The fetus turns to an anterior position (OA). The fetal occiput is next to the maternal symphysis pubis.
- **Extension** (see Figure 14-23D and E) occurs when the fetus extends its head, pushing its occiput against the maternal symphysis pubis. This movement causes the fetal head to emerge through the vaginal opening. The health care provider may assist with the birth by applying pressure on the mother's lower perineum, helping the fetus extend its neck by lifting the fetal chin.
- **Restitution** is the turning of the fetal head to be in normal alignment with the shoulders. The fetus then rotates until the shoulders are in an anterior/posterior position (**external rotation**) (see Figure 14-23F).
- **Expulsion** is the birth of the rest of the fetus after restitution. The assisting health care provider applies gentle, downward pressure on the fetal head, allowing the anterior shoulder to emerge under the maternal symphysis pubis. The head is then raised to allow the posterior shoulder to emerge. The rest of the fetus then slides out of the vagina.

Clamping the Umbilical Cord

Clamping the umbilical cord occurs before birth of the placenta, although the exact timing is controversial (Olds, London, Ladewig, & Davidson, 2004). Data show that the

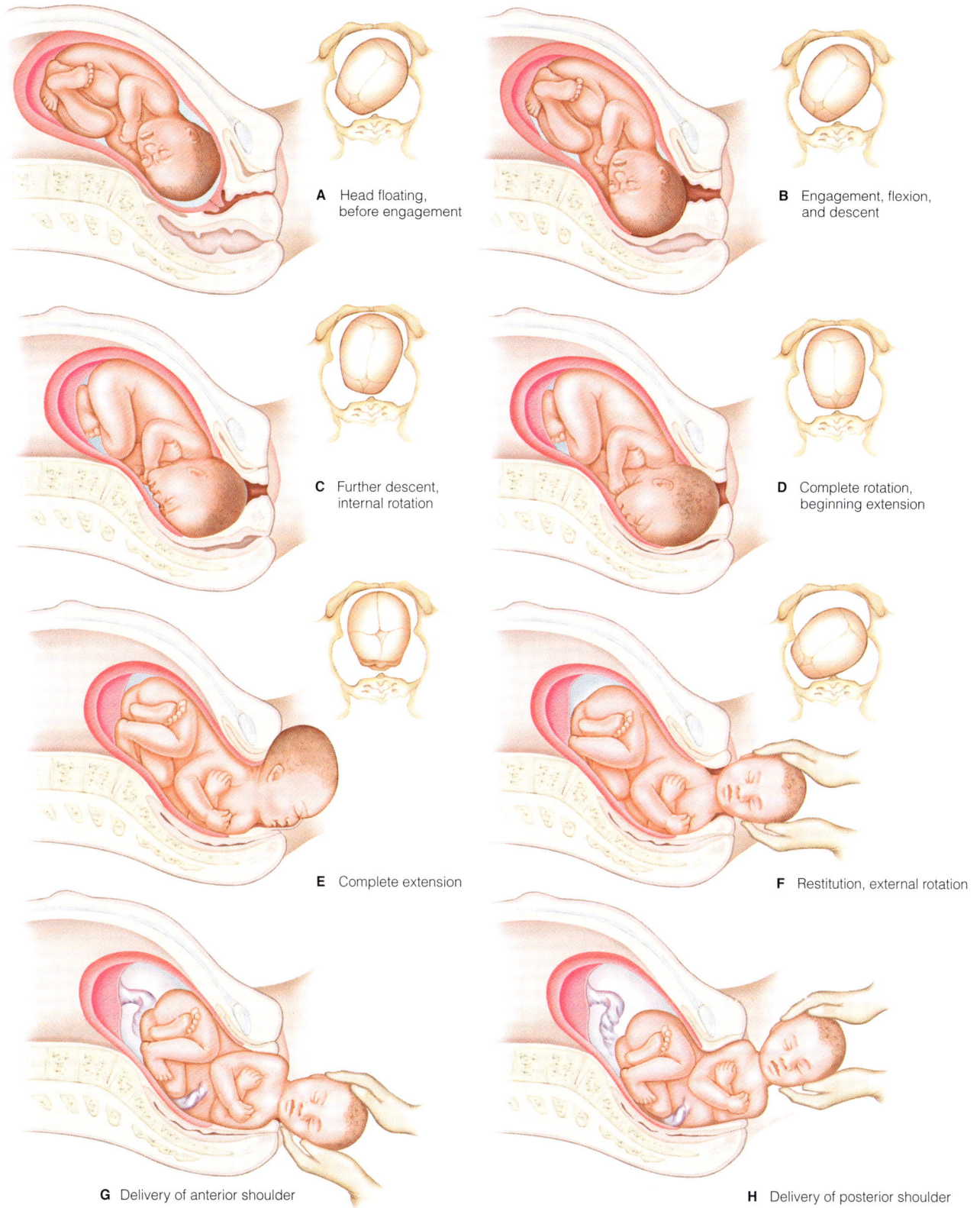

Figure 14-23. ■ Mechanisms of labor: left anterior occiput position. (**A**) Head floating, before engagement. (**B**) Engagement, flexion, and descent. (**C**) Further descent, internal rotation. (**D**) Complete rotation, beginning extension. (**E**) Complete extension. (**F**) Restitution, external rotation. (**G**) Delivery of anterior shoulder. (**H**) Delivery of posterior shoulder. (Adapted, with permission, from McGraw-Hill Companies, Inc. Cunningham, F. G., et al. [Eds.]. [1997]. *Williams obstetrics* [20th ed.]. Stamford, CT: Appleton & Lange, p. 320.)

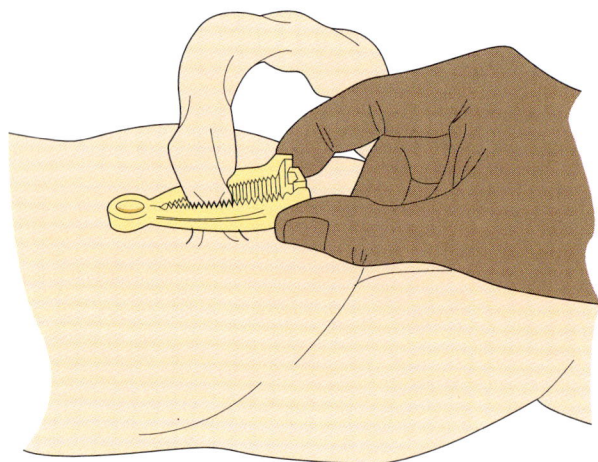

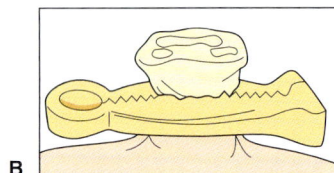

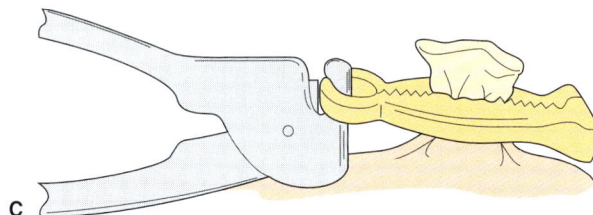

Figure 14-24. ■ Hollister cord clamp. (**A**) Clamp is positioned 1/2 to 1 inch from the abdomen and then secured. (**B**) Cord is cut. One vein and two arteries can be seen. (**C**) Plastic device from removing clamp after cord has dried.

50 to 100 mL of blood from the placenta may increase and help stabilize the neonate's temperature. It may also reduce the incidence of iron-deficiency anemia later in infancy. However, it is possible that the added blood may lead to circulatory overload, with resulting polycythemia and hyperbilirubinemia.

Parents may express specific desires about when the umbilical cord is to be cut. They may also want to assist in cutting the cord. A Hollister cord clamp is illustrated in Figure 14-24 ■.

Once the cord is cut, the end of the cord is observed for the presence of two arteries and one vein. Observations are recorded on the neonatal chart. Presence of only one artery is associated with genitourinary abnormalities (Olds et al., 2004).

Cord Blood

Many parents today arrange for cord blood banking (see Chapter 3 ◯◯) and bring a special container from the cord blood registry with them to the birthing facility. Umbilical cord blood is rich in stem cells, which are increasingly being used in fighting disease. The blood may be stored for later use if the child (or perhaps a family member) needs it. The therapeutic possibilities for umbilical cord blood are still being explored.

After the cord is clamped and before the placenta is expelled, the care provider withdraws blood from the umbilical vein using a large-gauge needle. The nurse labels the blood according to directions and arranges for storage and pickup. Even when cord blood banking is not done, a sample of cord blood will be sent to the lab for blood typing.

THIRD STAGE OF LABOR: PLACENTA EXPULSION

The **third stage of labor** begins with the birth of the fetus and ends with the expulsion of the placenta. The placenta should be delivered within 30 minutes of birth. Continuous contractions following birth cause the placenta to separate from the wall of the uterus. As it separates, there is some bleeding. The membranes are peeled from the uterus as the placenta slides into the vagina. Signs that the placenta is ready to be expelled are a gush of blood from the vagina, a lengthening of the umbilical cord, and a globular shape of the uterus. The client pushes one last time and the placenta is expelled (Figure 14-25 ■).

The placenta may separate in different ways. Expulsion of the placenta with the fetal side out is termed the **Schultze mechanism** (Figure 14-25A). If the maternal side is out when the placenta is expelled, it is called the **Duncan mechanism** (Figure 14-25B). See also Figure 8-4 ◯◯ .

FOURTH STAGE OF LABOR: RECOVERY

The **fourth stage of labor** is the first hour after birth. During this period, the mother's body begins to return to a nonpregnant state. Blood pressure has a moderate decline. The pulse increases and then gradually slows. Normal blood loss is between 250 and 500 mL, mostly at the time of placental separation.

The **fundus** should be located below the umbilicus and in the midline. The uterus should remain firm in order to control bleeding. Saturation of more than one perineal pad with blood during the 1-hour recovery time is considered excessive. (See Figure 16-8 ◯◯ , which shows how to assess perineal pads visually.) The mother may experience uncontrolled

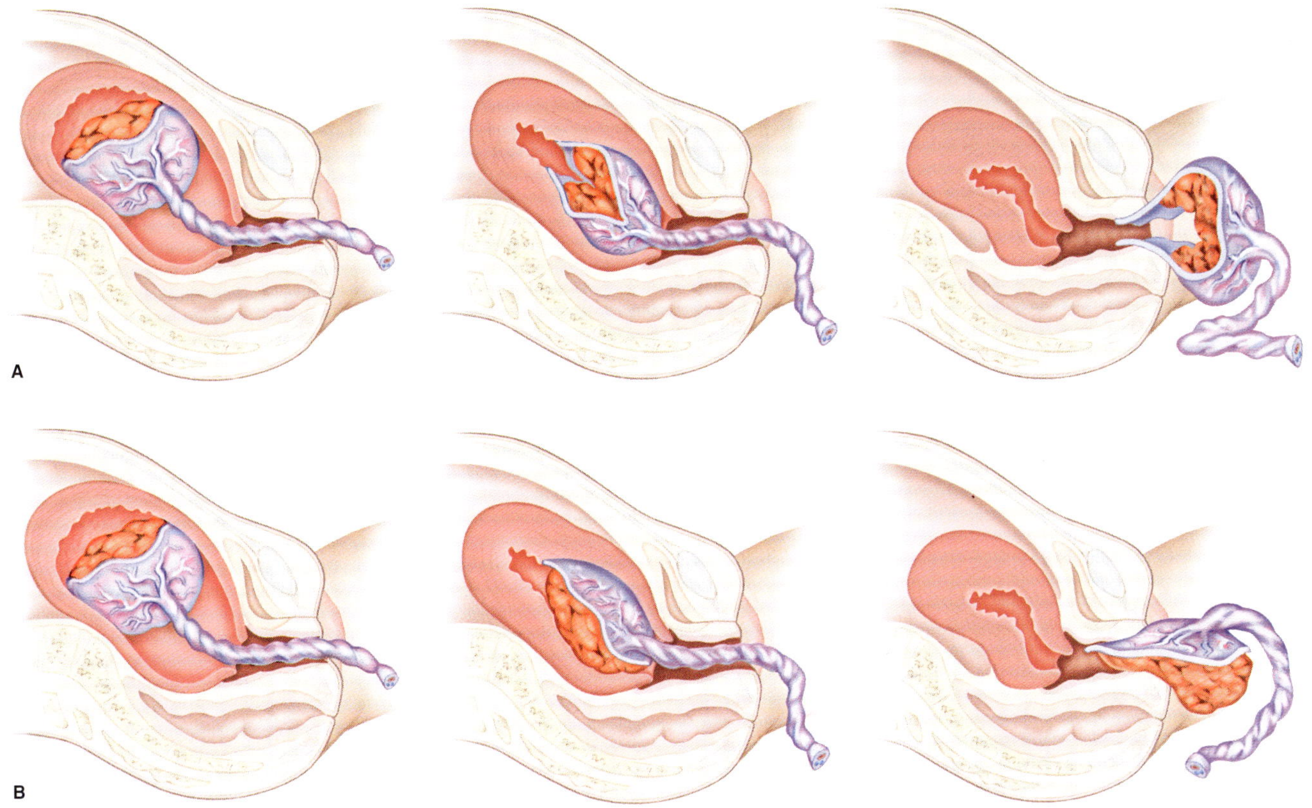

Figure 14-25. ■ Placental separation. (**A**) Schultze ("shiny Schultze") mechanism. (**B**) Duncan ("dirty Duncan") mechanism.

shaking or chills (**postpartal chills**) as a physiologic response to labor and as a result of the rapid weight loss at birth.

Delivery Room Care of the Neonate

AIRWAY
The newborn has needs that must be met immediately after birth. Most important, a patent airway must be established. Prior to and during birth, amniotic fluid, vaginal secretions, and pulmonary mucus can get in the infant's airway. These fluids are often removed with a bulb syringe (see Figure 17-24 ⚭) or suction catheter. The infant's head is placed below its body so that secretions will continue to drain. However, secretions may need to be removed mechanically.

BREATHING
Breathing is initiated because of several factors.
1. As the infant moves through the birth canal, the chest is compressed, increasing the intrathoracic pressure. Once the chest has been delivered, the intrathoracic pressure decreases, sucking a small amount of air into the lungs.
2. When the umbilical cord is clamped, the infant's PCO_2 increases. This stimulates the respiratory center in the medulla of the infant.

3. The intrauterine temperature is approximately 20°F higher than the room temperature following birth. This change in temperature stimulates breathing.
4. The neonate is exposed to sights, sounds, smells, and touch. Sensory, auditory, visual, and tactile stimulation helps encourage breathing as well.

CIRCULATION
Circulatory changes occur as a result of change in thoracic pressure inside the heart and large blood vessels. With breathing, more blood flow is needed through the pulmonary arteries. Initially, an increase in pressure inside the aorta causes a reverse blood flow through the ductus arteriosus, increasing the amount of blood that reaches the lungs.

When this increased amount of blood returns to the left atrium, the pressure in the left atrium increases, closing the foramen ovale within minutes. Within 24 to 48 hours, the ductus arteriosus also begins to close. Permanent closure of the foramen ovale and ductus arteriosus may take 1 to 3 months. See Figure 17-2 ⚭, the newborn circulatory system.

TEMPERATURE
Heat loss in a neonate can be life threatening (see discussion in Chapter 17 ⚭), so it is important to dry the infant as soon as possible. Rubbing the infant with blankets not only

TABLE 14-6

Apgar Score

	SCORE		
SIGN	**0**	**1**	**2**
Heart rate	Absent	Slow—less than100	Over 100
Respiratory rate	Absent	Slow—irregular	Good crying
Muscle tone	Flaccid	Some flexing of extremities	Active motion
Reflex irritability	None	Grimace	Vigorous cry
Color	Pale blue	Body pink, extremities blue	Completely pink (if light skinned); absence of cyanosis (if dark skinned)

dries the skin but also stimulates breathing. The infant can be placed next to the mother's skin and covered with a blanket or placed under a radiant warmer. The infant's head should be covered with a cap to prevent heat loss through the scalp. The infant should not be bathed until the temperature has stabilized. When the infant is bathed, care should be taken to prevent heat loss by keeping as much of the body covered as possible.

APGAR SCORE

At 1 minute and 5 minutes after birth, the newborn will be assessed using the Apgar score (Table 14-6 ■). The **Apgar score** is a rapid evaluation of the infant's adaptation to extrauterine life. The five items are assessed in order of priority. The first is heart rate, followed by respiratory rate, muscle tone, reflex irritability, and color. Each item is assigned a score from 0 to 2. The scores are then totaled.

A score of 8 to 10 requires no special attention. A score between 4 and 7 requires administration of oxygen and rubbing the infant's back to stimulate breathing. If the mother had received a narcotic during labor, naloxone (Narcan) may need to be administered to the infant to reverse respiratory depression. An Apgar score of 0 to 4 indicates that the infant needs immediate resuscitation. Anytime the infant's condition changes, an Apgar score can be a useful evaluation tool. Procedure 14-1 ■ describes the Apgar procedure.

VITAL SIGNS OF THE NEONATE

The neonate's apical pulse rate and respiration rate are counted as part of the Apgar score. Once the neonate has

PROCEDURE 14-1   **Obtaining an Apgar Score**

Purpose

■ To evaluate the physical condition of the newborn at birth
■ To determine the need for resuscitation efforts

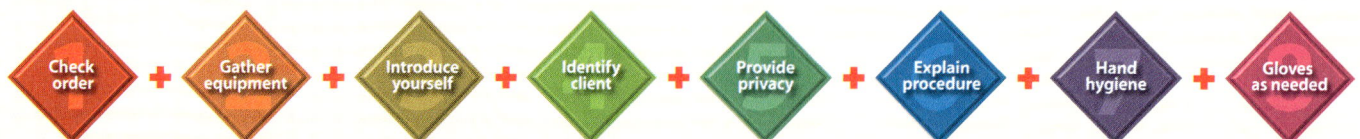

Equipment

■ Neonatal stethoscope
■ Bulb syringe
■ Warm towels

Check order + Gather equipment + Introduce yourself + Identify client + Provide privacy + Explain procedure + Hand hygiene + Gloves as needed

Interventions and Rationales

1. Perform preparatory steps (see icon bar above).

2. Assess the heart rate by auscultation or palpation where the umbilical cord meets the abdomen.

3. Assign a score for heart rate: 0 for absent; 1 for HR less than 100; 2 for HR more than or equal to 100.

4. Assess respiratory effort. Crying indicates good respiratory effort.

5. Assign a score for respiratory effort: 0 for absent; 1 for slow or irregular respirations; 2 for regular respirations or vigorous crying.

6. Assess muscle tone by determining degree of flexion and resistance when straightening the extremity.

7. Assign a score for muscle tone: 0 for flaccidity; 1 for some flexion of extremities; 2 for active motion and good flexion.

8. Assess reflex irritability by physically stimulating the infant during the drying process.

9. Assign a score for reflex irritability: 0 for no response to stimulation; 1 for a notable grimace; 2 for a cry elicited by stimulation.

10. Assess skin color. Observe closely for pallor and cyanosis.

11. Assign a score for skin color: 0 for overall cyanosis and pallor; 1 for acrocyanosis; 2 for pink skin tone over the newborn's entire body.

12. Total the assigned score.

13. Provide appropriate care related to Apgar score. For 8–10: continue with routine newborn care. For 4–7: tactile stimulation and oxygen administration is needed. Scores less than 4: newborn resuscitation is required.

SAMPLE DOCUMENTATION

(date/time) Caucasian male delivered vaginally. Cord clamped and cut by Dr. L. Hogan. Infant transferred to warmer and dried vigorously. Apgar score 7 @ 1 minute. Oxygen administered by mask. Apgar score 9 @ 5 minutes. W. Brown, LVN

stabilized in the first few minutes after birth, a temperature is also taken. It is unusual to take the neonate's blood pressure unless the Apgar score is low and the infant is resuscitated and transported to the newborn intensive care unit. See Chapter 17 ⚭ for detailed care of the newborn.

MEASUREMENTS OF THE NEONATE

The infant's measurements (height, weight, head circumference, chest circumference) are determined at birth.

Height

Length can be difficult to measure (Figure 14-26 ■). The infant is placed flat on the back with the legs extended. Usually, a tape measure is stretched from heel to head to determine length. Weight is taken on a balance or digital scale. Procedures 14-2 ■ and 14-3 ■ describe length and weight measurements for neonates.

Weight

To obtain a weight measurement, lay the neonate supine on a calibrated scale. Place a lightweight absorbent pad between the neonate and the scale to serve as a barrier against cold and moisture. Hold one hand above the neonate to guard against injury.

Head and Chest Circumference

Head and chest circumference are taken to obtain a baseline and are part of follow-up care. Procedures 14-4 ■ and 14-5 ■ describe head and chest circumference measurements for neonates.

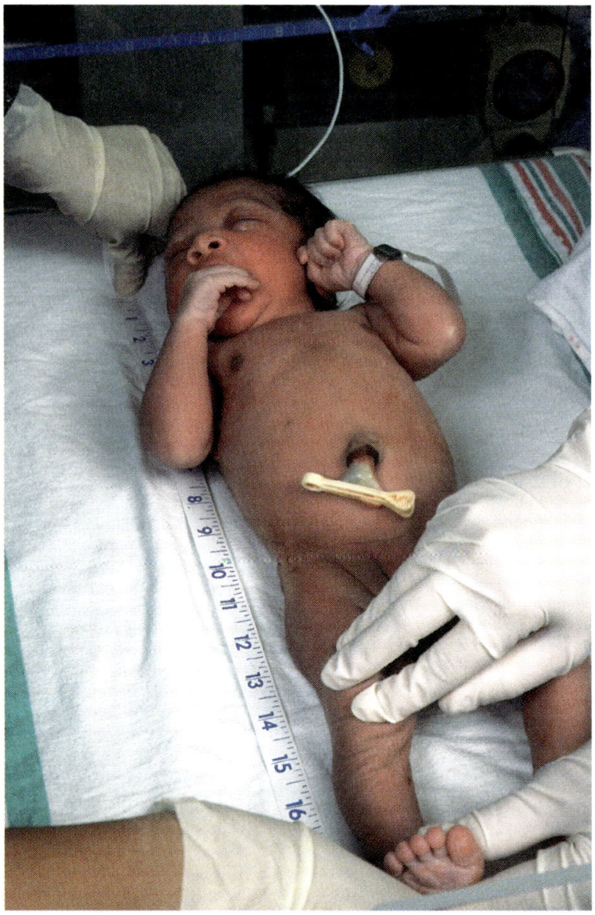

Figure 14-26. ■ Neonatal measurements are taken immediately after birth. For height, it is often helpful to have two staff members work together to ensure the accuracy of the measurement from crown to heel.

PROCEDURE 14-2   Measuring Height and Length

Purpose

■ To obtain an accurate measure of the client's height or length
■ To report baseline measurements that will be used for follow-up

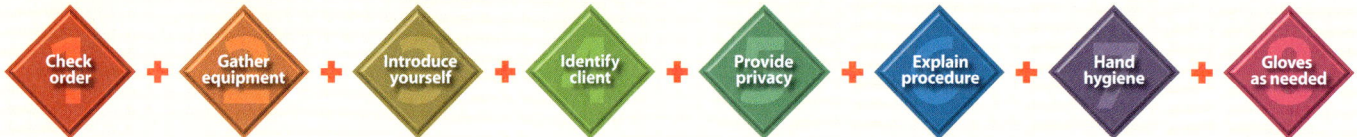

Equipment

■ Tape measure, yard stick, meter stick, or measuring mat

Check order + Gather equipment + Introduce yourself + Identify client + Provide privacy + Explain procedure + Hand hygiene + Gloves as needed

Interventions and Rationales

1. Perform preparatory steps (see icon bar above).

2. Place the infant in a supine position. *This position will provide the greatest opportunity for accurate measurement.*

3. Place the infant's head against a flat surface. Extend legs until the knee is straight. *This defines the full length of the neonate's body.*

4. Use a tape measure, measuring stick, or measuring mat to measure from the crown to the heel (see Figure 14-26). Note the length in inches or centimeters. *Follow facility policy in recording baseline length for future comparison.*

5. Plot the measurement on a standardized growth chart. Note: Appendix II shows growth charts from infancy to age 18.

SAMPLE DOCUMENTATION

(date) 0800 Height recorded on growth chart. T. Tobias, LVN

PROCEDURE 14-3   Obtaining Weight

Purpose

■ To obtain an accurate measure of the client's weight
■ To record a baseline weight for future assessment and follow-up

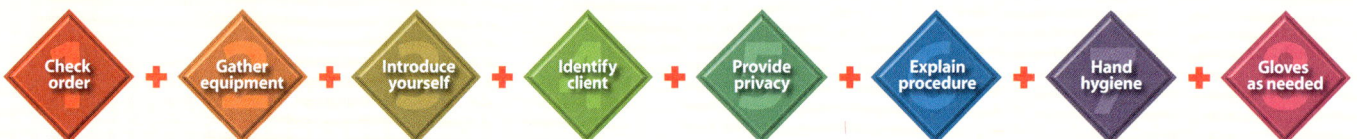

Equipment

■ Infant scale, calibrated

Check order + Gather equipment + Introduce yourself + Identify client + Provide privacy + Explain procedure + Hand hygiene + Gloves as needed

Interventions and Rationales

1. Perform preparatory steps (see icon bar above).

2. Place the neonate in a supine position on the infant scale (Figure 14-27 ■).

3. Stand close with one hand over, but not touching, the infant. *This provides for safety in case the neonate should move.*

4. Read the scale when the neonate is still. *The most accurate measurement will be obtained when the neonate is not moving.*

5. Record the weight.

SAMPLE DOCUMENTATION

(date) 0900 Weight recorded on growth chart.
E. Langlois, LPN

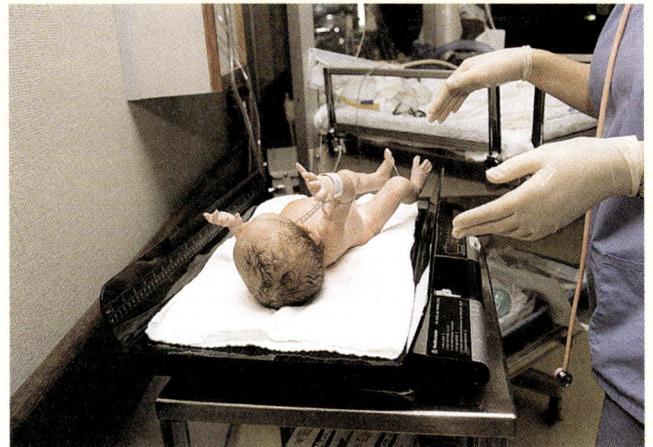

Figure 14-27. ■ To obtain the neonate's weight, place the infant on a platform scale. The caregiver's hands are poised near the newborn as a safety measure. (© Stella Johnson www.stellajohnson.com.)

PROCEDURE 14-4   # Measuring Head Circumference

Purpose
■ To determine normalcy of the infant's head circumference in relation to chest circumference

Equipment
■ Tape measure

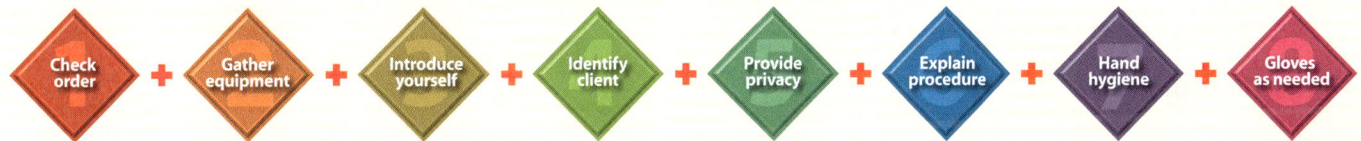

Interventions and Rationales

1. Perform preparatory steps (see icon bar above).

2. Position the infant in a supine position.

3. Place the tape measure slightly above the eyebrows, above the pinna of the ear, and around the occiput (Figure 14-28 ■). *This is the largest diameter of the infant's head.*

4. Document the head circumference in inches or centimeters. The nurse may also document the amount of *molding* (shaping of the head during the birth process). *Documentation provides information for later comparison.*

5. Compare to chest circumference. *Head circumference is equal to or 2 cm greater than chest circumference until age 2.*

6. Plot the measurement on a standardized growth chart.

SAMPLE DOCUMENTATION

(date) 1500 Head circumference recorded on chart. H. Freida, LPN

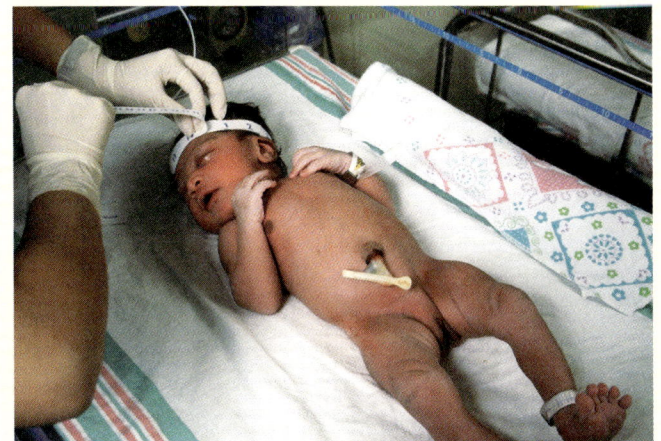

Figure 14-28. ■ Head circumference is usually 33 to 35 centimeters.

PROCEDURE 14-5 ## Measuring Chest Circumference

Purpose

- To determine normalcy of the infant's chest circumference in relation to head circumference

Equipment

- Tape measure

Check order + Gather equipment + Introduce yourself + Identify client + Provide privacy + Explain procedure + Hand hygiene + Gloves as needed

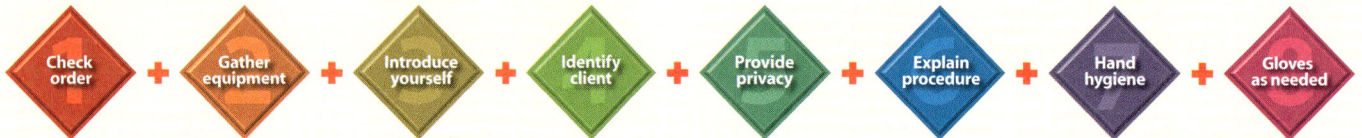

Interventions and Rationales

1. Perform preparatory steps (see icon bar above).

2. Position the infant in a supine position.

3. Encircle the chest with the measuring tape. Place the tape measure against the bare skin of the infant's chest, at the nipple line, under the axillae (Figure 14-29 ■). *This is the largest diameter of the infant's chest.*

4. Document the chest circumference in inches or centimeters.

5. Compare to head circumference. *Head circumference is equal to or 2 cm greater than chest circumference until age 2.*

6. Plot the measurement on a standardized growth chart.

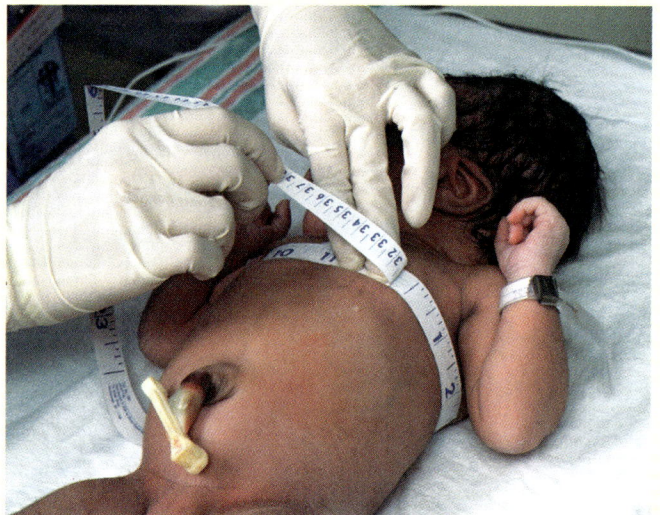

Figure 14-29. ■ Chest circumference is normally the same as the head circumference but should not exceed it.

SAMPLE DOCUMENTATION

(date) 1400 Chest circumference recorded on chart. B. Smartt, LVN

IDENTIFICATION

Proper identification must be made in the birth room before the mother and infant are separated. Identification bands imprinted with the same number, and the mother's name will be placed on the infant and the mother (Figure 14-30 ■). It is important that the infant bands be applied snugly, but not so tightly that they impede circulation.

The identification bands must stay on the infant and mother until both are discharged. Each time the infant is brought to the mother, the identification bands are compared. Some facilities use an identification band equipped with an alarm that would be triggered if the baby were removed from the facility (see Figure 14-30B).

Most hospitals footprint the infant and fingerprint the mother. Vernix must be washed from the infant's feet prior to foot printing. The number on the identification band is also recorded on the footprint sheet. Upon discharge, the mother signs this form as documentation that she has received her infant.

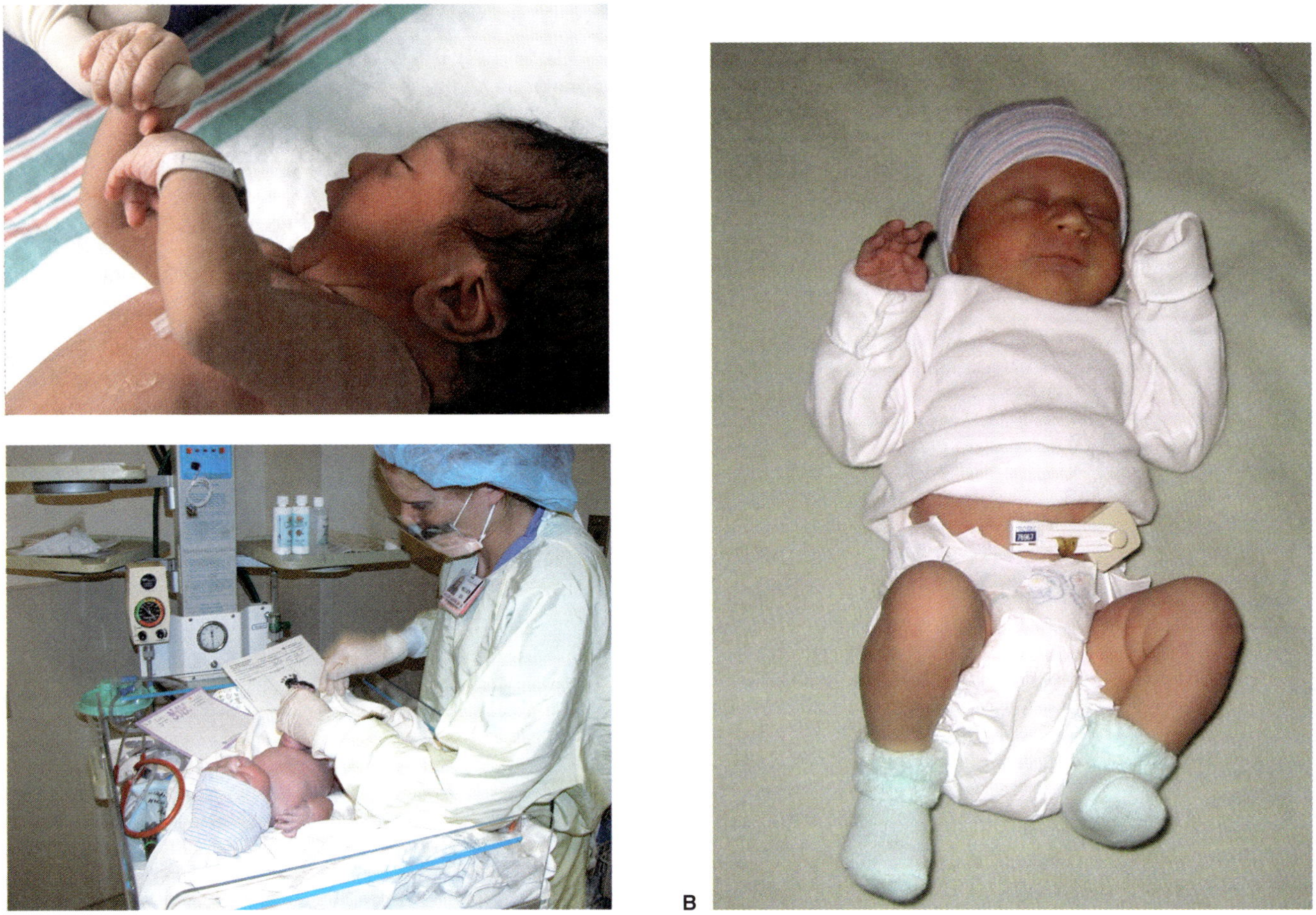

Figure 14-30. ■ (A) Identification band on infant. (B) Umbilical alarm attached to newborn infant. (C) Nurse takes footprint of baby.

NURSING CARE

PRIORITIES IN NURSING CARE

The first priority in nursing care during labor is to assess the mother and fetal well being with the progression of labor. Controlling the mother's discomfort can ease the progression of labor as well as making the birth experience as pleasant as possible. The nurse must monitor the progression of labor and report changes to the primary care provider. And lastly, the nurse must prepare the environment for labor and birth.

ASSESSING

As described previously under Admission to the Birthing Facility, the nurse first determines the condition of the client, the stage of labor, and the status of the fetus. Initial interview questions the nurse would ask are listed in Box 14-3 ■.

Cultural Aspects of Care

The nurse should be aware of his or her own culture and biases in providing care to a client of another culture during labor. The client's cultural background may affect the assessment and her needs during labor. To deliver culturally proficient care, the nurse must be alert to verbal and non-verbal expressions of the client's and family's desires. Box 14-4 ■ identifies some cultural considerations in birth practices as they relate to pain expression.

Initial Data

Assessment data include maternal vital signs and fetal heart rate. Other data to collect are the frequency, duration, and intensity of contractions, and the results of a urine dipstick test for glucose and protein. A vaginal exam is performed by the nurse or care provider to determine the amount of cervical effacement and dilatation, as well as fetal presentation, position, and station.

Admission Questions for the Client

The nurse must make a focused assessment of the stage of labor when a woman presents to the birthing facility. The following questions help determine the stage of labor and how quickly labor is likely to progress.

- When did the contractions begin?
- How far apart are the contractions, and how long do they last?
- Have the membranes ruptured? (Has the water broken?)
- Is this your first pregnancy? How long were previous labors?

Expression of Pain During Labor

Pain response varies from culture to culture, and pain caused by labor and birth is no different. Some women are very stoic and labor quietly; this is frequently true with African American women. Others are notoriously loud. Many cultures feel that women must experience pain and discomfort during labor (e.g., Mexican, Iranian, and Filipinos). In fact, very difficult labor usually results in lavish gifts for Iranian women.

Mexican women are frequently heard repeating "*aye yie yie*" throughout labor. Interestingly, repeating "*aye yie yie*" in succession requires long, slow deep breaths. This has been described as "Mexican Lamaze." This phrase is more than an expression of pain but rather is a culturally accepted method of pain relief.

- A nitrazine test is performed if the client is unsure whether the membranes have ruptured. *Status of the membranes is important. Once they have ruptured, the fetus may be exposed to micro-organisms within the uterus.*
- Any signs of gestational (pregnancy-induced) hypertension—edema, altered reflexes, and clonus (spasms or seizures)—are documented and reported. The procedure for assessing clonus is in Chapter 13, Procedure 13-1 ⚭. *The mother with PIH is at greater risk. Care providers must be alerted to the possibility of complications.*

Review of Prenatal Data

- The nurse reviews the woman's prenatal record to determine the presence of any complications during the pregnancy. If the client has had no prenatal care and labor is not advanced, a more in-depth assessment is performed. *The client who has had no prenatal care may have conditions that could complicate labor or compromise the fetus. Further investigation will help clarify the health status of the woman and fetus.*

Emotional Support for False Labor

Some women present at the birthing facility with false labor or at a very early point in Stage one labor. If it is not clear whether the woman's labor has begun, she is asked to walk for an hour and is then reexamined. If labor has not begun, the nurse must be sensitive to the disappointment the woman may feel.

- The nurse provides encouragement and emotional support, as well as reinforcement of the signs of impending labor. *Therapeutic listening can help the woman overcome her disappointment and embarrassment. Encourage her to discuss any concerns she may have about returning home to wait for labor to begin. Review signs of impending labor and reassure the woman about her ability to recognize these signs.*

Ongoing Data Collection

Once it is determined that the client is in labor, continuous assessment is performed, including frequent vital signs, fetal heart rate, and contraction evaluation. Table 14-7 ■ provides guidelines for assessment of the woman in labor.

- If ordered, the LPN/LVN may set up and attach the electronic fetal monitor (Figure 14-31 ■). The nurse performs Leopold's maneuvers on the client's abdomen to determine fetal position. *Correct placement of the monitor will provide a strong, clear recording of the FHR. Leopold's maneuvers help caregivers determine the position of the fetus; see Procedure 9-4* ⚭ .
- The nurse monitors the client closely. *Most clients will be monitored electronically, either continuously or intermittently. The level of monitoring depends on the stage of labor and the well-being of the client and fetus. In Stage one labor, the nurse's primary roles are to promote comfort, monitor the client's and fetus's status, and report any signs of complications.*
- A vaginal exam will be done at intervals to assess progression of cervical effacement and dilatation, station, and fetal position. Table 14-7 identifies the standard time frame for assessing the progression of labor. *It is not unusual for the fetal heart rate to slow to 100 beats per minute during pushing contractions and then to increase to more than 120 when the uterus relaxes.*

clinical ALERT

If the fetal heart rate does not return to 120 bpm or more between contractions, the care provider should be notified immediately. Oxygen may be given to the mother at this time in order to provide adequate oxygen to the fetus.

TABLE 14-7		
Standards of Assessment in Labor		
ITEM	**ASSESSMENT**	**RATIONALE**
Prenatal data	Review prenatal record to determine EDB, gravida/para, history of previous labors, results of laboratory exams.	Identifies risk (i.e., preterm, rapid labor/ birth, and anticipated complications)
Maternal assessment	• Take vital signs every 1 hour (more frequently if unstable or outside normal limits) • Determine level of comfort and effect of intervention • Monitor fluid balance • Monitor reflexes • Monitor cervical changes • Monitor contractions (frequency, duration, intensity)	Determines mother's tolerance and stability during labor Determines if labor is progressing in a usual pattern
Fetal assessment	• Monitor FHT every 1 hour during early labor, every 30 minutes during active labor, and every 10–15 minutes during transition and birth. Note change in FHT before, during, and after contractions. • Observe amniotic fluid for color (should be clear; green indicates meconium passage by fetus).	Determines fetal tolerance and stability during labor Determines fetal distress during pregnancy and labor

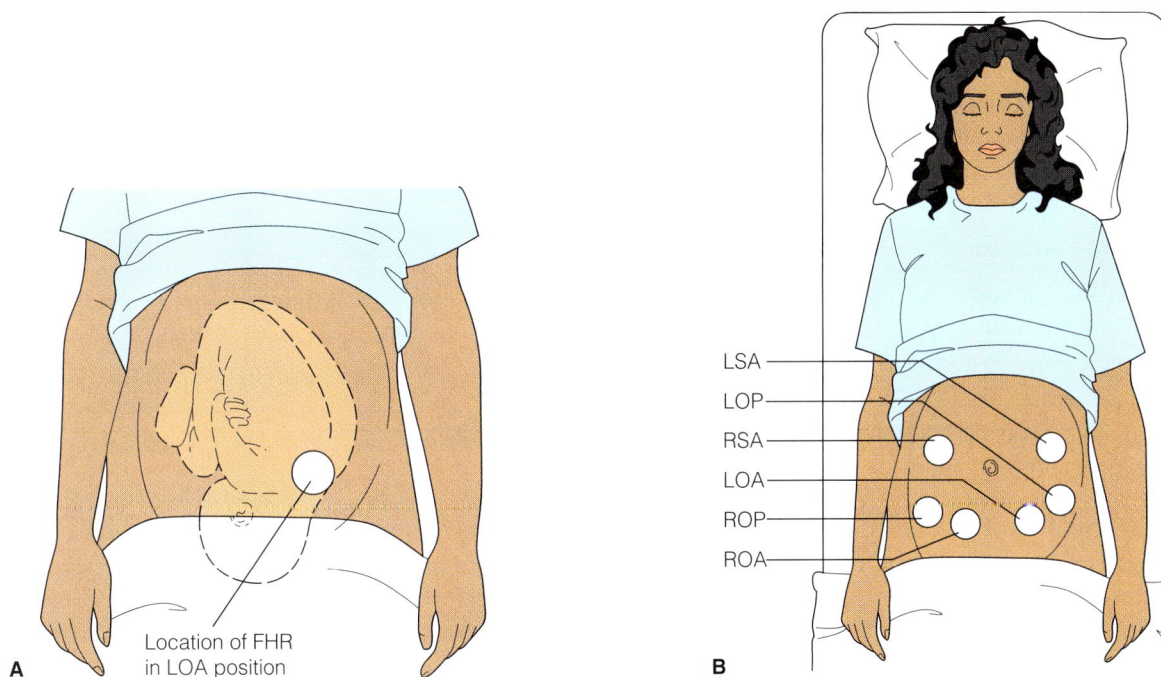

Figure 14-31. ■ (**A**) Location of the fetal heart rate (FHR). (**B**) Other transducer placement locations for FHR monitoring.

■ The nurse needs to be aware of the client's cultural background and how it may affect her assessment and needs during labor (see Box 14-1). *The woman may have some unspoken assumptions about how to move through labor. It is important to clarify desired processes and outcomes so that the nurse can provide appropriate assistance to the laboring woman.*

DIAGNOSING, PLANNING, AND IMPLEMENTING

The following nursing diagnoses may be used in planning nursing care for the laboring client:

■ **P**ain related to the labor process
■ **A**nxiety

- Deficient **K**nowledge
- Risk for Ineffective Individual **C**oping related to fatigue and the birth process
- Altered Urinary **E**limination related to pressure on the urinary bladder
- Deficient **F**luid Volume related to limited oral intake and diaphoresis
- Risk for **I**nfection related to labor process

Typical outcomes for the laboring woman might include these as well as others:

- Pain will be controlled within reasonable limits.
- Client will be able to express feelings and listen to instructions during labor.
- Client will understand how, and will have the necessary energy, to participate in labor and birth.
- Client will void every 2 to 3 hours post birth.
- Client will remain free of infection.

Maintaining Standards of Practice

The goal of nursing interventions is to assist the client and support persons through the labor and birth process. Nonpharmacologic labor support behaviors of nurses fall into four categories: emotional, instructional, physical, and advocacy support behaviors. Box 14-5 ■ describes nonpharmacologic nursing interventions in each of these categories. The nurse also assists with pharmacologic interventions as needed.

- Follow the standards of practice for any client. For example, any client with deficient fluid volume will be given intravenous fluid. Any client with altered urinary elimination would be encouraged to void every 2 hours. If needed, a catheter would be used to drain the bladder. Any client or support person in need would receive emotional support and teaching.

Preparation for the Birth

As labor progresses to Stage two, the nurse prepares the birthing suite. In some areas, the birth takes place in the same room as labor. In other areas, a special birthing room is used.

- Make sure all equipment is in place (Figure 14-32 ■). The equipment should include a warmer, suction, oxygen, and emergency drugs for the infant. Check to be sure all equipment is operational prior to the birth. *It is part of quality care to ensure that there is no unnecessary delay in providing for the needs of the client.*
- Cover a table with sterile drapes. Sterile instruments, sterile drapes, gown and gloves, and bulb syringe are arranged for the care provider's convenience. If birth is imminent, the table can remain uncovered but must

remain sterile. If birth will not occur for some time, the table may be covered with a sterile drape to prevent contamination until it is needed. *Using sterile equipment helps prevent transmission of pathogens to the mother and newborn during the birth process.*

Continuous Monitoring and Support

The role of the nurse during labor is to continue to monitor the client and fetus, assist the physician or nurse midwife, and support the family. Timing of nursing care in the second stage of labor is essential to a smooth birth.

- A reassuring, professional manner helps the client feel the nurse has the situation under control. The nurse should seek additional assistance if necessary. *The laboring woman, especially the primigravida, is undergoing a challenging and potentially frightening experience. The nurse's calm and positive approach allows the mother to remain calm and to focus on the demands of labor.*

Pain Control

- Frequently assess the woman's comfort level and her ability to cope. *Although discomfort is unavoidable, empathy can allow the woman to overcome it and stay focused. The woman's ability to understand directions and to cooperate in the laboring process help guide pain control measures.*
- Evaluate the effectiveness of comfort measures individually, changing methods when needed. *By focusing on individualized care and each woman's responses, the nurse can be sure of providing proficient care.*
- Listen closely to and respect the needs of the client. *Some women prefer to labor and give birth without pharmacologic assistance. Others may prefer to relieve discomfort with medication as soon as possible. There is no "right way" to go through labor. The nurse's role is to provide safety and support to each unique client.*

Because the need for pain control during labor may not be the same as for other clients in pain, more detail will be provided here. There are many comfort measures that may be used for the laboring client. Some work very well for one client but not for another. The nurse must evaluate the effectiveness of comfort measures for each individual and change methods when needed. *By focusing on individualized care and each woman's responses, the nurse can be sure of providing proficient care.*

Nonchemical Comfort Measures

- Teach (if there is time) and encourage nonpharmacologic methods of pain control. *Numerous techniques and methods are available to help the woman manage labor discomfort without medication (see Boxes 14-2 and 14-5).*
- Teach clients to change position often. *Change of position reduces muscle stress.*

Providing Nonpharmacologic Support to the Laboring Woman

Emotional Support

☑ Be present. Give the woman your undivided attention.

☑ Make sure your facial expression and stance are pleasant and convey confidence.

☑ Unless the laboring woman requests otherwise, stay close to her, usually within 2 feet.

☑ Use a reassuring, encouraging tone of voice.

☑ Offer praise for her efforts.

☑ Use humor or verbal distractions as appropriate; use verbal and nonverbal responses from the woman to guide your sense of what is useful.

☑ Rephrase negative thoughts into positive thoughts. (For example, if the woman says, "I don't think I can do it," you could say, "You can do this. Just take it one step at a time.")

Informational Support

☑ Interpret medical jargon or other information from health care providers that the client and partner do not understand.

☑ Use therapeutic communication skills (reflecting, rephrasing, choosing culturally sensitive words, using interpreter if needed).

☑ Role model behaviors for the partner to follow, and encourage participation.

☑ Provide information about procedures and progress.

☑ Remind client about breathing, relaxation, or pushing techniques as needed.

Physical Comfort Behaviors

☑ Remember that a woman's body is made to be able to give birth without pharmacologic assistance.

☑ Adjust the environment (including temperature and lighting) as much as possible for the mother's comfort. Mild, familiar scents may be used; avoid candles and strong scents.

☑ Ensure a nonrestrictive environment that allows freedom of movement.

☑ Offer assistive equipment as appropriate (extra pillows, birthing ball, squatting bar, etc.).

☑ Assist woman with position changes as needed. Positions of comfort vary, depending on the stage of labor:

  ☑ First stage: standing, ambulating, leaning, knee/chest, pelvic rocking, sitting on birthing ball or toilet, rocking chair, squatting, left side lying

  ☑ Second stage: knee/chest, hands/knees with birthing ball, squatting, semi-Fowler's, lateral

☑ Provide comforting touch to convey caring. This can be as simple as stroking the woman's brow. It also includes massage (hand, foot, back), hand-holding, etc.

☑ Provide nourishment. Depending on the stage of labor and level of consciousness, the woman may be offered ice chips, sour candy, Popsicles, oral fluids, or a light meal.

☑ Offer application of heat or cold (warm blanket, cool washcloth, fan, etc.).

☑ Provide equipment for personal hygiene. Assist as needed. A bath or shower may be taken. Ensure safety of the client while transferring and bathing.

☑ Encourage urinary elimination every 2 to 3 hours.

Advocacy Support

☑ Ask about and support the mother's expectations for labor and birth. Understand that the woman's culture may affect her approach to this experience.

☑ Establish a therapeutic relationship in order to protect the woman (provide safety), attend to her needs, and help her make choices related to health care.

☑ Convey respect for the woman's privacy, modesty, relationships, and values. Be professional and nonjudgmental. You do not have to agree with the woman's choices to provide good nursing care.

☑ Provide physical and emotional safety so the woman is able to express both positive and negative emotions.

☑ Encourage problem-solving behavior, and keep the woman at the focus of decision making. Step in if others are trying to interfere.

☑ Support the woman's desires verbally and actively.

Source: Data courtesy of Ellise D. Adams and Ann L. Bianchi. (2005). *50 Ways to comfort a laboring woman.* Presented at The AWHONN 2005 Convention, June 14, 2005, Salt Lake City, Utah.

■ Encourage side-lying or upright positions. A supine position should be discouraged. *A side-lying position supports fewer, stronger contractions. In an upright position, gravity can assist labor progression. A supine position puts pressure on the vena cava.*

■ Provide ice chips and oral care. Clear liquids may be given in early labor but are prohibited as labor becomes more advanced. *Ice chips and oral care provide some moisture and refresh the mouth. Oral liquids are avoided late in labor because of the possibility of vomiting and aspiration.*

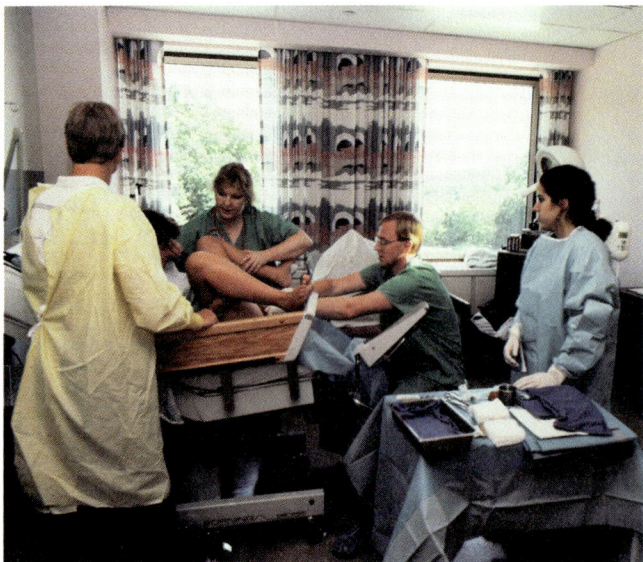

Figure 14-32. ■ The nurse must ensure that all equipment is ready before the birth.

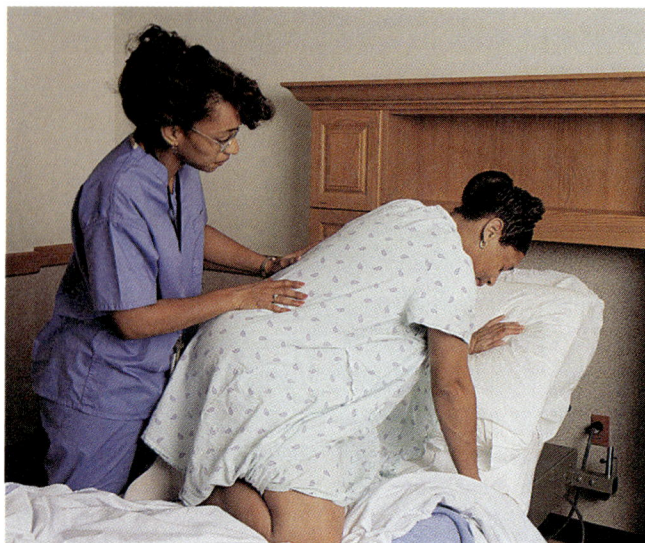

A

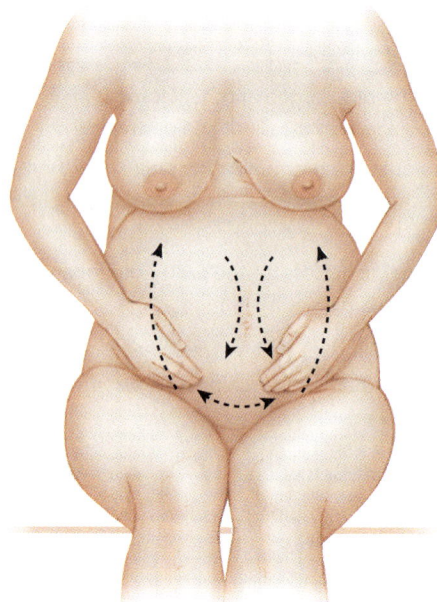

B

- Encourage muscle relaxation, massage (Figure 14-33 A ■) or abdominal **effleurage** (a light stroking with the fingertips in circular motion). Figure 14-33B illustrates abdominal effleurage from the symphysis pubis to the iliac crest. *Relaxation and massage promote overall distraction and relaxation; these help to relieve the discomfort of labor.*
- Promote use of breathing techniques and monitor client. See Table 14-8 ■ for review of specific breathing techniques that are helpful at different stages of labor. *Proper breathing techniques can smooth labor and decrease pain. It is important, though, to monitor the client closely for signs of hyperventilation.*

clinical ALERT

Numbness and tingling of the tip of the nose, lips, or fingers; dizziness; or spots before the eyes are signs of hyperventilation. The nurse should remain with the client and encourage her to take slow shallow breaths. If symptoms become more severe (evidenced by spasms in the hands and feet), have her breathe into a mask or her hands to increase her CO_2 level and alleviate the problem.

Figure 14-33. ■ (**A**) The nurse provides massage to the sacral area. (**B**) Direction of abdominal effleurage for the latent and active phase of the first stage of labor.

Pharmacologic Comfort Measures

- Assist in preparing supplies or equipment for medication administration as ordered. Monitor client closely. *Systemic medications can slow or stop contractions if labor is not well established. Systemic medications given in transition or in the second stage of labor can cause respiratory distress in the newborn.*
- Assist with preparation of equipment for epidural block. Monitor infusion. Be knowledgeable about the side effects

and complications. *With epidural block, clients may not be able to participate fully in the birth process. Lack of feeling may decrease ability to push effectively, so the birth may need to be assisted. The client may experience hypotension, bladder distension, and respiratory depression. For this reason, frequent or constant monitoring by the registered nurse is required. Some clinical facilities require the physician or nurse midwife to be present as well.*

- Provide sterile field and sterile equipment as ordered. *The nurse maintains standards of practice and quality care by preventing the spread of infection.*

TABLE 14-8

Breathing Technique Review for Labor

TECHNIQUE	DESCRIPTION
Cleansing Breath Used at beginning and end of each contraction	Relaxed breath in through nose out through mouth.
Slow-Paced Breathing Used in early and beginning of active labor	Slower than normal breathing: IN 2–3–4/OUT 2–3–4 (not less than $\frac{1}{2}$ normal rate)
Modified-Paced Breathing Used in active and transition	Faster than normal breathing: IN–OUT/IN–OUT/IN–OUT (not more than twice normal rate)
Patterned-Paced Breathing Used in active and transition (Note: A pattern of 5:1 or higher is tiring.)	3:1 Pattern is: IN-OUT/IN-OUT/IN-OUT/IN-BLOW 4:1 Pattern is: IN-OUT/IN-OUT/IN–OUT/IN–OUT/IN–BLOW Pattern with words: may say "Yankee Doodle" or "I think I can" and repeat through contraction Pyramid Pattern such as: 1:1, 2:1, 3:1, 4:1–4:1, 3:1, 2:1, 1:1

■ Be alert for signs of complications and take immediate action. *Even with the best prenatal care and preparation for childbirth, complications can rapidly change the stability of the laboring mother and the fetus. (Chapter 15 ⬭ discusses the most common complications of labor and the related nursing care.)*

Maternal Care for Birth

The client should be positioned according to the physician/nurse midwife preference. Sometimes the client is placed in lithotomy position with a pillow under the right hip to relieve pressure on the large blood vessels. Legs are abducted, with knees bent. Stirrups may be used to support the legs. Other times, the client is placed on her left side with the left leg extended. The right leg is flexed and supported by an assistant. Figure 14-34 ■ demonstrates some common birthing positions.

■ The nurse cleanses the perineum with antiseptic soap immediately prior to the birth. *The antiseptic soap prevents the spread of infection.*
■ The care provider (physician or nurse midwife) then applies sterile drapes. *This provides a clean environment for the newborn.*

Figure 14-35 ■ provides a visual sequence of the birthing process.

■ Once the infant is delivered, the airway will be suctioned. *Suctioning will help open the airway and promote breathing.*
■ A Hollister clamp (see Figure 14-24) or other clamp will be used to clamp the umbilical cord. The umbilical cord can then be cut. The umbilical cord will be examined for two arteries and one vein. Results will be documented. *The presence of two arteries and one vein is normal; the presence of*

only one artery forecasts genitourinary problems. Cord clamping separates the infant from the placenta and promotes stabilization.

The vagina and cervix will be inspected for lacerations. Lacerations and an episiotomy will be sutured. The placenta will be delivered and inspected to be sure it is intact.

■ Following delivery of the placenta, the nurse may be asked to administer Pitocin, either intramuscularly or intravenously. *Pitocin will stimulate uterine contractions and decrease bleeding.*

Box 14-6 ■ describes how to make a single-strength solution of Pitocin. Table 14-9 ■ provides information about the use of Pitocin.

Initial Neonatal Care

Following delivery, the nurse assumes care of the infant, while the care provider (physician or nurse midwife) focuses on preventing the mother from hemorrhaging following the birth.

Several risks exist for the neonate. The most urgent are respiratory distress, circulatory collapse, and hypothermia. These risks require immediate attention. Priorities are for the nurse to maintain the airway, stimulate breathing, and dry the infant.

■ The infant may be placed on the mother's abdomen to begin the bonding process, or the infant may be placed under a warmer. *Both of these locations provide warmth. The infant will lose heat rapidly, so warm, dry blankets should be used. Drying the infant by rubbing its back stimulates crying, which is necessary to expand the lungs.*
■ The airway is suctioned as needed. Procedure 14-6 ■ describes nasopharyngeal suctioning with a DeLee mucus trap. *A patent airway is the first priority in neonates, as in adults.*

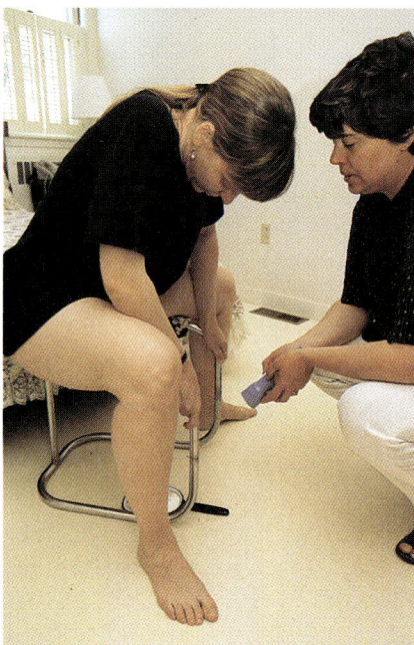

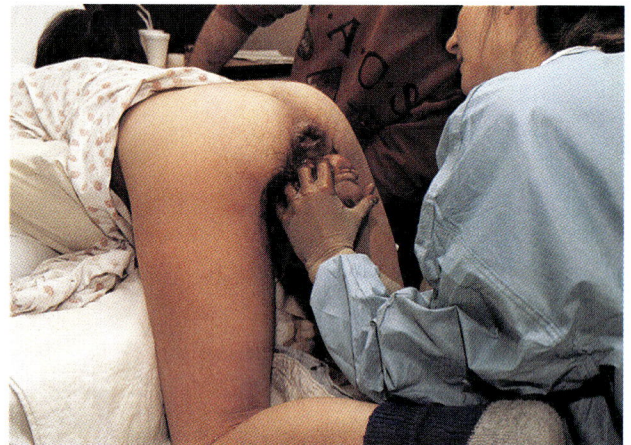

Figure 14-34. ■ Some birthing positions. (**A**) Side-lying (left side) with right leg supported. (**B**) Birthing stool. (**C**) Supine with support from partner. (**D**) Hands-and-knees position (also called knee-chest position), which is used when there is a prolapsed umbilical cord. (B: © Stella Johnson www.stellajohnson.com. C. Margaret Miller/Photo Researchers, Inc.)

■ The Apgar score is taken at 1 minute and at 5 minutes. *The Apgar score creates an objective reading on the neonate's status. It shows that the infant is stabilizing or identifies the need for follow-up care.*

■ Identification (bands, band with alarm, footprint, mother's fingerprint) of the mother and the neonate is performed while still in the delivery room. *Identification (see Figure 14-30) is done before the mother or infant leaves the room in which the birth occurred. This prevents the possibility of misidentification. Follow facility policy closely and make sure the identification bands are neither too loose nor too tight. Loose bands can slip off; tight bands can interfere with circulation.*

■ When the infant is stabilized, he or she will be weighed and measured. If ordered, the nurse will give the infant AquaMEPHYTON (vitamin K) and an antibiotic eye ointment. *The neonate's height and weight are used as a baseline. The infant's liver is immature and vitamin K is needed to*

stimulate the production of blood clotting factors. The eye ointment (often Erythromycin) is used to prevent eye infection. (Chapter 17 ⚭ discusses care of the healthy newborn.)

■ Once the mother and infant are stable, the nurse wraps the infant and allows the mother to hold and, if desired, to breastfeed the infant. The nurse should pick up the delivery room and make the environment presentable for family visitors. *Bonding is important for all members of the family.*

Maternal Care in Stage Four Labor

During the fourth stage of labor/birth, the nurse monitors the mother and newborn.

■ Take maternal vital signs every 15 minutes for 1 hour. *This provides data to track recovery or to recognize complications at an early stage.*

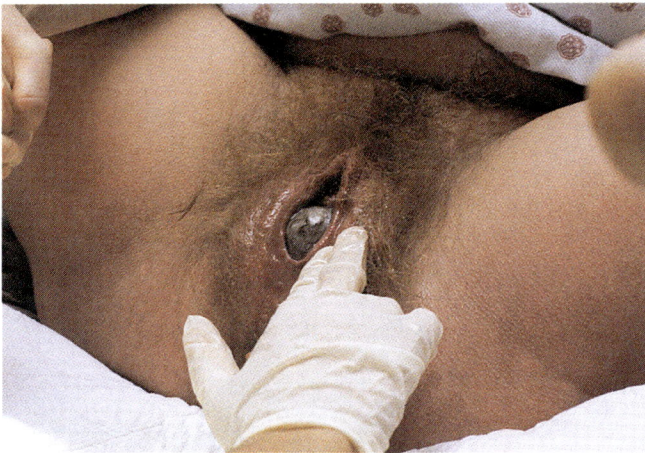

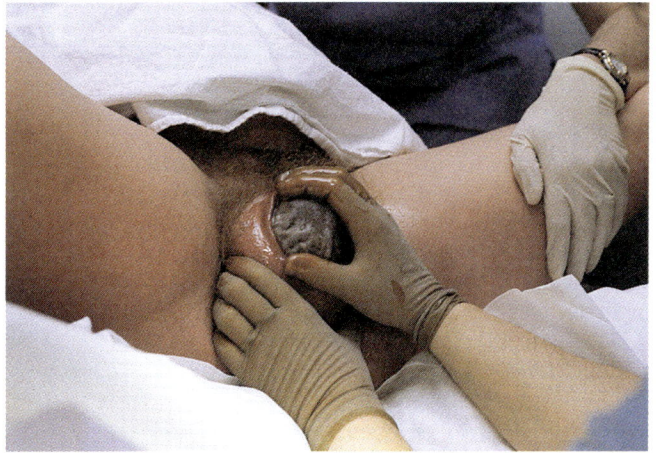

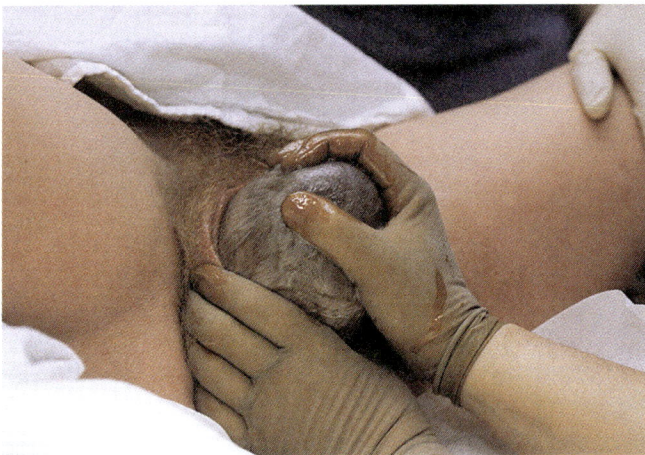

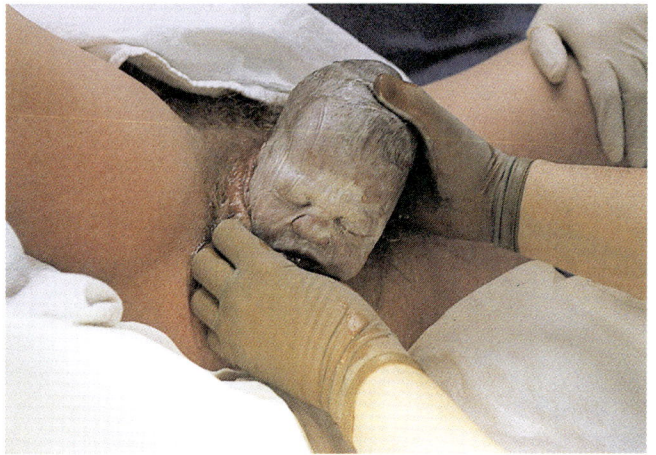

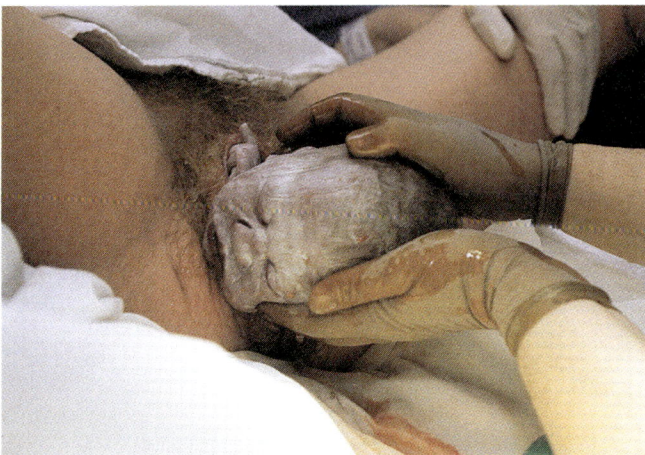

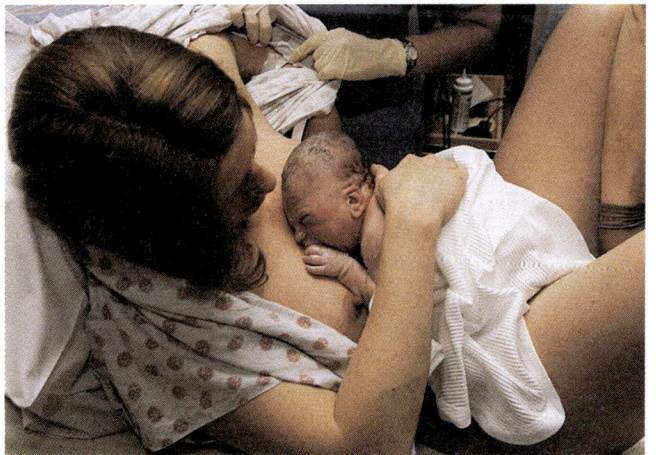

Figure 14-35. ■ Birthing sequence with mother in supine position.

- Provide extra blankets for the mother if needed. *The mother may experience chills after childbirth.*
- Check the fundus for position and firmness, and assess vaginal flow for amount and character. (See Chapter 16 ⌾ for postpartum care.) *The mother's fundus should remain firm, below the umbilicus, and in the midline. Failure of the fundus to remain firm could indicate intrauterine bleeding. If the fundus is not in the proper location, blood clots or a full bladder should be suspected. Vaginal bleeding is assessed by saturation of the perineal pad.* (Text continues on page 353.)

BOX 14-6

Calculations for IV Pitocin Solution

NOTE: 1 Unit = 1,000 milliunits
TO MAKE SINGLE-STRENGTH IV SOLUTION: Add 10 Units of Pitocin to 1 liter of compatible IV fluid (lactated Ringer's, or D_5W).
TO INFUSE: Convert prescribed milliunits/min to mL/hr and set infusion pump. *IV infusion pump MUST be used for client safety.*
AMOUNT ORDERED: 20 milliunits/min
CALCULATIONS: 10 Units/1 L = 10,000 milliunits/1,000 mL OR 10 milliunits/1 mL.

10 milliunits/1 mL = 20 milliunits/X mL
Cross-multiply to get 20 = 10 X
X = 2, so 2 mL/min

Multiply by 60 minutes to get amount infused per hour.
THINK: 20 milliunits = 2 mL/min
2 mL/min $\times$ 60 min/hr = 120 mL/hr (2 $\times$ 60 = 120)

Set the infusion pump for 120 mL/hr.

TABLE 14-9

Pharmacology: Drug Used to Stimulate Labor

DRUG	USUAL ROUTE/DOSE	CLASSIFICATION	SELECTED SIDE EFFECTS	DON'T GIVE IF
Oxytocin (Pitocin)	IV *To stimulate labor*: 0.5–20 milliunits/min *To prevent hemorrhage*: 20–40 milliunits/min	Oxytocic hormone	Prolonged uterine contractions, which can harm fetus Afterpains	Fetal distress is apparent Contractions are more than every 2 minutes, lasting over 90 seconds

---

PROCEDURE 14-6

Nasopharyngeal Suctioning of the Neonate

Purpose

- To remove mucus from the neonate's nose and mouth to allow respiration

Equipment

- DeLee mucus trap or other suction device

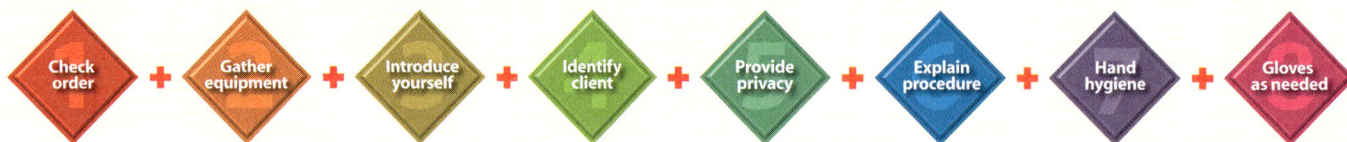

Check order + Gather equipment + Introduce yourself + Identify client + Provide privacy + Explain procedure + Hand hygiene + Gloves as needed

Interventions and Rationales

1. Perform introductory steps (see icon bar above).

2. With gloved hands and without activating suction, insert end of suction device into neonate's nose or mouth (Figure 14-36 ■). *Insertion should be done without suction so the device does not become attached to oral or nasal mucosa.*

3. Place thumb over suction control. Apply suction while removing the tube and rotating it slightly. *The motion of the tube will remove fluids and prevent them from being redeposited in the nasopharynx.*

4. Repeat suctioning as needed. When no fluid is aspirated, stop suctioning. *Excessive suctioning can stimulate the vagus nerve and decrease neonatal heart rate.*

5. If the device is used to suction meconium secretions from the stomach, it should be passed through the newborn's mouth, not the nares. *The neonate's nares are small and delicate. It is quicker and easier to insert the tube through the mouth.*

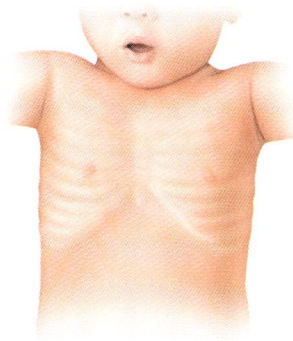

Figure 14-36. ■ A newborn infant being suctioned with a DeLee mucus trap to remove excess secretions from the mouth and nares.

6. Document completion of the procedure and the type and amount of secretions obtained. *Documentation provides information about the neonate at birth and also provides the record of care.*

SAMPLE DOCUMENTATION

(date/time) 5 mL meconium-stained fluid suctioned from nares and throat, reported to nurse midwife. _____ P. Bohlen, LPN

clinical ALERT

Total saturation of a perineal pad in the space of 1 hour is considered heavy bleeding. Report any deviation from normal range to the care provider.

- The fundus may need to be massaged and clots removed. (The procedure for massaging the fundus is provided in Chapter 16 ⬤⬤.) In some facilities and in some states, expelling clots from the uterus is not an LPN/LVN function. *It is important for the LPN/LVN to communicate closely with the RN if the fundus does not remain firm. Always follow facility policy and state nurse practice acts concerning scope of practice.*
- Assess the newborn for signs of respiratory distress. Notify the charge nurse or care provider if the newborn exhibits these signs of respiratory distress: dusky color, grunting respirations, nasal flaring, and sternal retractions (Figure 14-37 ■).
- Ensure that the newborn is kept warm, either by warm blankets or by being placed in a warming bed. The newborn may be kept in the room with the mother or placed in the newborn nursery. (Chapters 11 and 17 ⬤⬤ provide details about newborn care.)

EVALUATING

The client is evaluated for comfort, stability of vital signs, progression of labor, and response of the fetus. The closer the client progresses toward birth, the more frequent the evaluation should be. In many cases the nurse remains at the bedside, caring for only one client at a time. After birth, vital signs are taken and the fundus and vaginal flow are checked often to verify that the mother is stabilizing.

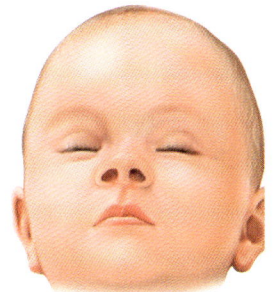

Figure 14-37. ■ Signs of respiratory distress.

NURSING PROCESS CARE PLAN
Woman in Active Stage One Labor

Jane, a 20-year-old primigravida, is admitted to the labor unit in active labor. She states contractions began about 5 hours ago, but she has become uncomfortable with them for about 30 minutes. She appears comfortable between contractions, but is using controlled breathing techniques during contractions.

Assessment. The following data should be collected as soon as possible after admission.
- Vital signs
- Fetal heart tones
- Urine sample for sugar and protein
- The frequency and duration of contractions
- The dilatation and effacement of the cervix
- The presentation, position, and station of the fetus
- The mother's choice for pain control

Nursing Diagnosis. The following important nursing diagnosis (among others) is established for this client.
- Risk for Ineffective Individual Coping related to birthing process and fatigue of labor

Expected Outcome. Mother will actively participate in the birthing process with no evidence of injury to herself or the fetus.

Planning and Implementation
- Constantly monitor events of second and third stages of labor and birth. *This will ensure maternal and fetal well-being.*

- Provide feedback regarding the progression of labor/birth. *Feedback helps relieve anxiety and enhance participation.*
- Provide comfort measures such as positioning, dry linen, oral care, and minimal distractions. *Minimizing distractions can decrease discomfort and aid in focusing on the birth process.*
- Remind mother and support person of breathing techniques, positioning, and bearing down during the birthing process. *These reminders support and encourage participation in the birth process.*

Evaluation
- Labor progresses in a normal pattern.
- Mother verbalizes sufficient comfort.
- Mother remains in control of her behavior.
- Fetal heart rate remains within normal limits.

Critical Thinking in the Nursing Process

1. What are the two top priorities in caring for Jane?
2. Many women in labor are offered a whirlpool bath. Should Jane be offered this method of relaxation? Why or why not?
3. What criteria would the nurse use to determine if Jane should be given a narcotic pain medication that has been ordered PRN?

Note: Discussion of Critical Thinking questions appears in Appendix I.

Note: The reference and resource listings for this and all chapters have been compiled at the back of the book.

Chapter Review

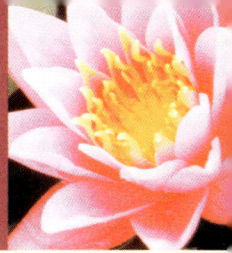

KEY TERMS by Topic

Use the audio glossary feature of either the CD-ROM or the Companion Website to hear the correct pronunciation of the following key terms.

Signs of Impending Labor
lightening, Braxton Hicks contractions, false labor, effacement, dilatation, bloody show, spontaneous rupture of membranes, ballotable, prolapsed umbilical cord, premature rupture of membranes

Admission to the Birthing Facility
clonus

Variables Affecting Labor
5 Ps affecting labor, passage, cephalopelvic disproportion, station, passenger, fetal

attitude, fetal lie, transverse lie, fetal presentation, cephalic presentation, vertex presentation, occiput, mentum, sinciput, breech, fetal position, sutures, fontanels, molding, contractions, frequency, duration, intensity, Ferguson's reflex

Pain in Labor
natural childbirth, regional blocks

Stages of Labor
labor, first stage of labor, dilatation stage, latent phase, active phase, amniotomy, second stage of labor, crowning, episiotomy, mechanisms of labor, cardinal movements, engagement, descent, flexion, internal rotation, extension, restitution, external rotation, expulsion, third stage of labor,

Schultze mechanism, Duncan mechanism, fourth stage of labor, fundus, postpartal chills

Delivery Room Care of the Neonate
Apgar score

Nursing Care
effleurage

KEY Points

- Labor progresses in a planned sequence of events.
- Nursing care during labor involves providing comfort measures for the mother and monitoring the well-being of the infant.
- The mother should be taught relaxation techniques before labor begins.
- The husband or a significant other can be useful in helping the mother relax and remain in control during labor.
- To determine if labor is progressing in a normal pattern, the nurse must understand the stages of labor and the mechanism by which the infant maneuvers its way through the birth canal.
- The nurse must be constantly on the alert to see whether labor is progressing normally. If it is not, the care provider must be notified at once.
- The LPN/LVN assists the RN by attaching monitoring equipment, assisting with relaxation techniques, preparing the delivery room, assisting with the birth, and monitoring client during recovery.

EXPLORE MediaLink

Additional interactive resources for this chapter can be found on the Companion Website at www.prenhall.com/towle. Click on Chapter 14 and "Begin" to select the activities for this chapter.

For chapter-related NCLEX®-style questions and an audio glossary, access the accompanying CD-ROM in this book.

Animations
Second stage labor
Delivery of infant
Leopold's maneuver
Placenta cord blood

FOR FURTHER Study

See Chapter 3 for additional information on cord blood banking.

Figure 8-4 shows the two types of placental expulsion.

A full discussion on breastfeeding and nutrition is found in Chapter 11.

For more about complications of pregnancy, see Chapter 13.

For information about complications of labor and birth, see Chapter 15.

For steps in performing fundal massage, see Procedure 16-1.

See Chapter 17 for care of the normal newborn.

For care of the high-risk newborn, see Chapter 18.

Critical Thinking Care Map

Caring for a Woman in Precipitous Labor

NCLEX-PN® Focus Area: Physiologic Integrity: Basic Care and Comfort

Case Study: 0630 Alyce, a 22-year-old, gravida 2, para 1, is admitted in transition. She states she woke up in labor and her water broke on the way to the hospital. She is obviously uncomfortable and is having difficulty keeping relaxed. States last labor lasted 6 hours.

Nursing Diagnosis: Pain related to increasing frequency and intensity of contractions

COLLECT DATA

Subjective	Objective
_____	_____
_____	_____
_____	_____
_____	_____
_____	_____
_____	_____
_____	_____

Would you report this? Yes/No

If yes, to: _____

Nursing Care

_____
_____
_____
_____
_____
_____
_____
_____
_____
_____
_____

How would you document this?_____
_____
_____
_____

Compare your documentation to the sample provided in Appendix I.

Data Collected
(use only those that apply)

- Cervix 8 cm dilated, 100% effaced
- Station +2
- BP 142/90
- Contractions every 3 minutes, lasting 90 seconds
- Obviously uncomfortable, moaning
- Having difficulty maintaining control
- Fetal heart rate 110
- Clear fluid draining from vagina

Nursing Interventions
(use only those that apply; list in priority order)

- Oxygen at 10 L per mask.
- Administer pain medication IV.
- Encourage to breathe with each contraction.
- Provide popsicles, ice chips, and reading material as distracters.
- Position on left side.
- Prepare sterile field for birth.

NCLEX-PN® Exam Preparation

1 The nurse is preparing an expectant mother for a routine prenatal visit. This client asks you to review the hormonal theory of labor with her. When you are finished reviewing, you will evaluate that she understands the hormonal theory of labor if she says fetal production of which of the following hormones increases as the fetus matures and when sufficient starts a chain of hormonal events that causes labor?

1. cortisol
2. oxytocin
3. progesterone
4. estrogen

2 When gathering data on a client who has experienced "lightening," the client would most likely claim which of the following?

1. "I can breathe much better."
2. "My ankles are less swollen."
3. "I don't have to urinate as often now."
4. "My lower back pain has been relieved."

3 The student nurse observing a birth hears the obstetrician and the circulating nurse talking about the fetus being "a vertex." The student realizes that the fetal part presenting first is which of the following body parts?

1. forehead
2. face
3. buttocks
4. occiput

4 A client in labor complains of feeling faint and the nurse turns her on her side. What effect will the side-lying position have on the laboring client's contractions?

1. little or no effect at all
2. increase in the frequency
3. increase in the intensity
4. will stop the contractions

5 A client is 3 cm dilated, excited about labor, and having contractions every 3 to 5 minutes. This phase is best described as:

1. active phase, second stage.
2. latent phase, first stage.
3. transition phase, second stage.
4. active phase, first stage.

6 The nurse explains the phases and stages of labor to first-time expectant parents. The nurse realizes the client understands when she describes the average length of active phase for a primigravida as lasting which of the following lengths of time?

1. 16–18 hours
2. 12–14 hours
3. 8–10 hours
4. 4–6 hours

7 A client in labor has no family or friends to support her during the labor process so you are supporting her. The physician says the cervix is 8 cm dilated. The client's contractions are strong and she gets irritable with you and tells you not to touch her. Which of the following actions would be appropriate? Choose all that apply.

1. Ask for another nurse to support the client.
2. Tell the client to be cooperative and do as you say.
3. Teach simple relaxation and breathing techniques.
4. Ask the client to actively push with each contraction.
5. Offer the client warm soaks to her lower back.
6. Re-position the client for comfort.

8 You hear the obstetrician, working with a laboring client, say that engagement has occurred. You realize this means which of the following things?

1. The fetus has now become ballotable.
2. Presenting part has entered the true pelvis.
3. Presenting part is just above the ischial spines.
4. There is now observable crowning.

9 You are caring for a client in the fourth stage of labor/birth. At the end of 1 hour, you find the client has saturated two perineal pads. Which of the following actions would be most important?

1. Notify the primary nurse immediately.
2. Assure the client that this is normal.
3. Put the client on the bedpan to void.
4. Start a count of the pads and chart it.

10 The nurse is monitoring a client in the fourth stage of labor. Which of the following are appropriate nursing interventions? (Select all that apply.)

1. Assess vaginal flow for amount and character.
2. Take maternal vital signs every hour for 4 hours.
3. Provide the mother with a cooling bath.
4. Check the fundus for position and firmness.
5. Provide the mother with warm blankets.

Answers for NCLEX-PN® Review and Critical Thinking questions appear in Appendix I.

Chapter 15

Care During High-Risk Labor and Birth

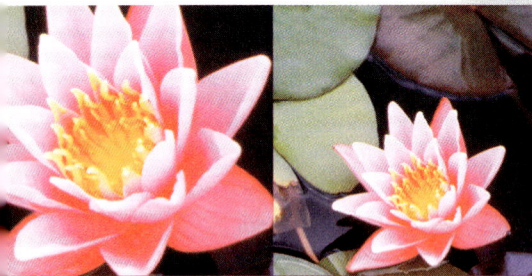

BRIEF Outline

Factors That Create High Risk

Monitoring During High-Risk Labor

Premature Rupture of Membranes

Amnioinfusion

Preterm Labor

Dystocia

Induction of Labor

Assisted Births

Precipitous Birth

Prolapsed Umbilical Cord

Nursing Care

LEARNING Outcomes

After completing this chapter, you will be able to:

1. Define key terms.
2. Describe factors that put a woman at risk for complications during labor and delivery.
3. Describe several tests for monitoring high-risk labor.
4. Describe common complications during labor and delivery, including manifestations, medical interventions, and nursing care.

Although most pregnancies end with a normal labor and delivery, the possibility of anticipated and unanticipated complications exists. The most common complications are discussed in this chapter.

Factors That Create High Risk

By completing an in-depth history, factors that create risk of complications during labor are identified. Complications during pregnancy, such as PIH, gestational diabetes, and vaginal infections, pose additional risk to the mother and fetus during the labor process. Although normal pregnancy should last for 40 weeks, a pregnancy longer than 42 weeks can place the fetus at risk for **postmaturity syndrome** (discussed in Chapter 18 ⚭). Postmaturity syndrome is a condition in infants born after 42 weeks' gestation who exhibit signs of impaired intrauterine oxygenation and nutrition related to placental insufficiency. At times, disorders of the fetus, placenta, or umbilical cord can increase risk during labor or delivery. For example, if the fetal head is larger than the pelvic outlet, a vaginal delivery will be impossible.

Monitoring During High-Risk Labor

ELECTRONIC FETAL MONITORING

Electronic fetal monitoring (EFM) involves a continuous tracing of the fetal heart rate (FHR) and uterine contractions. The FHR can be obtained externally by an ultrasound transducer held in place on the abdomen by a belt (see Procedure 9-2 ⚭). However, external monitoring of the FHR may not be accurate due to fetal movement or the amount of maternal tissue through which the sound must travel. Contractions are determined by a *tocodynamometer* attached by a belt to the woman's abdomen at the level of the fundus. This machine for external monitoring of contractions is accurate in determining the frequency and duration of contractions, but it may not be accurate in determining their strength.

INTRAUTERINE CATHETER

The strength of uterine contractions can be assessed internally. The physician inserts a small plastic catheter through the cervix, past the presenting part (Figure 15-1 ■). The catheter is attached to a monitoring system by an adapter. The strength of contractions is recorded on the labor record. If the contractions are not of an appropriate strength, intravenous Pitocin can be administered to stimulate stronger contractions. If contractions are of sufficient strength, but the cervix fails to dilate and/or the fetus fails to descend, a cesarean delivery will be performed.

FETAL SCALP MONITOR

When labor is not progressing as expected, it is critical to monitor the FHR accurately. Commonly, direct fetal monitoring is used. If fetal membranes have not ruptured, they are artificially ruptured in order for an electrode to be applied to the presenting part (Figure 15-2 ■). A spiral electrode is inserted into the vagina and held firmly against the fetal scalp. The device is rotated until the sharp electrode tip pierces the fetal skin. The applicator is then removed, and the electrode with the attached wires remains. The distal end of the wire is attached to the fetal

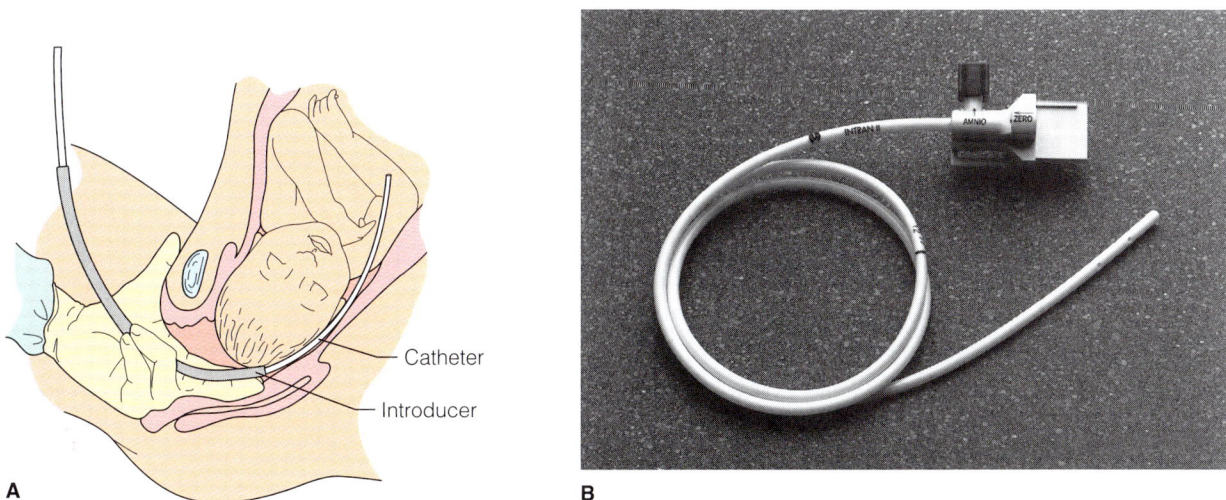

A   **B**

Figure 15-1. ■ (**A**) Technique of inserting a uterine catheter. Note that the introducer (catheter guide) is inserted no farther than beyond the fingertips. (**B**) INTRAN Plus intrauterine pressure catheter. There is a micropressure transducer (electronic sensor) located at the top of the catheter and a port for amnioinfusion at the distal end of the catheter.

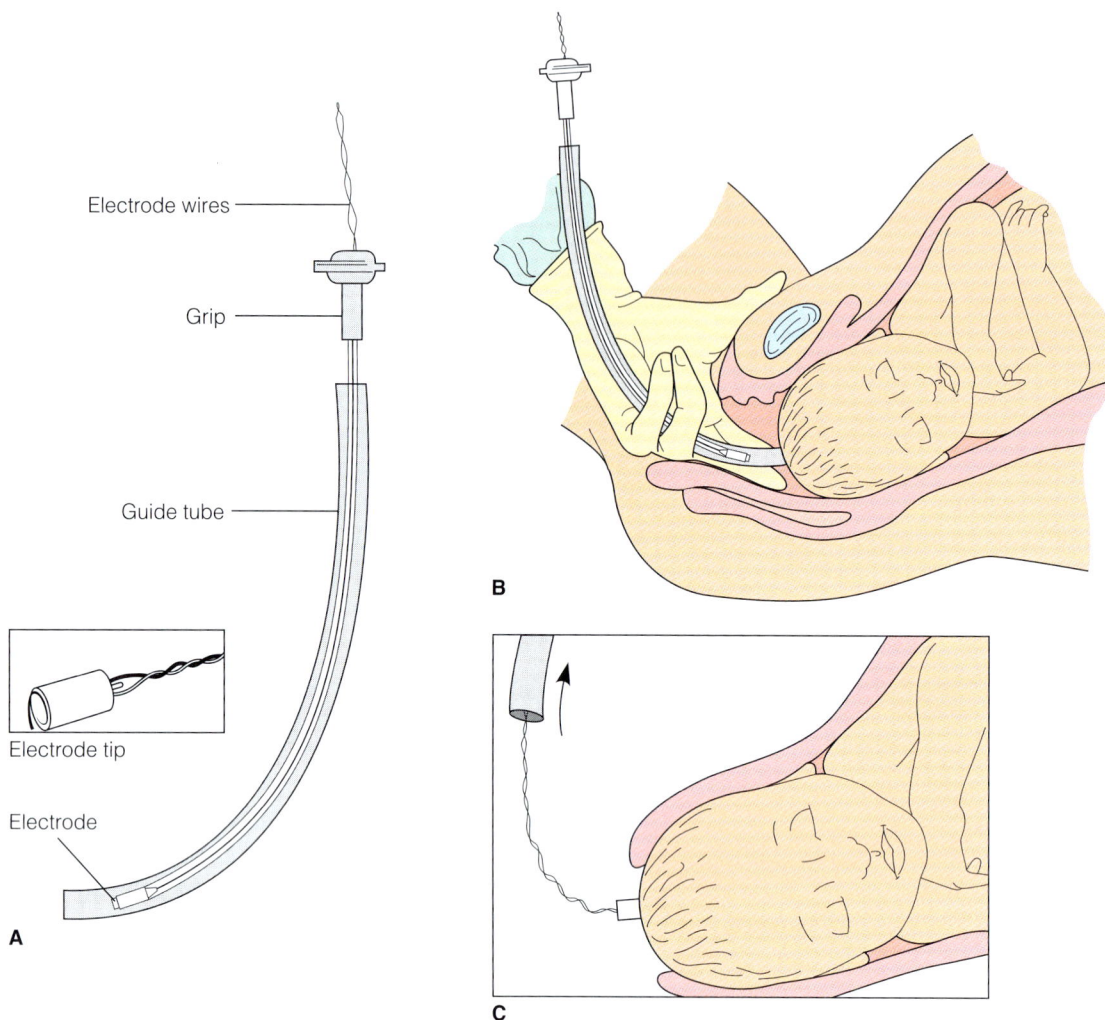

Figure 15-2. ■ Technique for internal direct fetal monitoring. (**A**) Spiral electrode. (**B**) Attaching the spiral electrode to the scalp. (**C**) Attached spiral electrode with the guide tube removed.

monitor. The LPN/LVN assists with the procedure, supporting the client and attaching the wires to the monitor.

The FHR should change in response to the stress of labor. This change is termed **variability.** Monitoring the FHR with the internal electrode allows for viewing short-term variability (STV) or the beat-to-beat change. This is noted as short up and down waves on the monitor tracing (Figure 15-3 ■). Long-term variability (LTV) is a waviness of the FHR that occurs three to five times a minute. If the variability is normal, the fetus is tolerating the labor process.

Accelerations are an increase in the FHR with fetal activity, just as an adult heart rate increases with exercise. At times, the fetus moves in response to contractions. Accelerations in FHR are a sign of fetal well-being.

Decelerations are a decrease in FHR. They are characterized as early, late, and variable, according to where they occur in the contraction cycle. Early decelerations begin before the start of a contraction. They are caused by compression of the

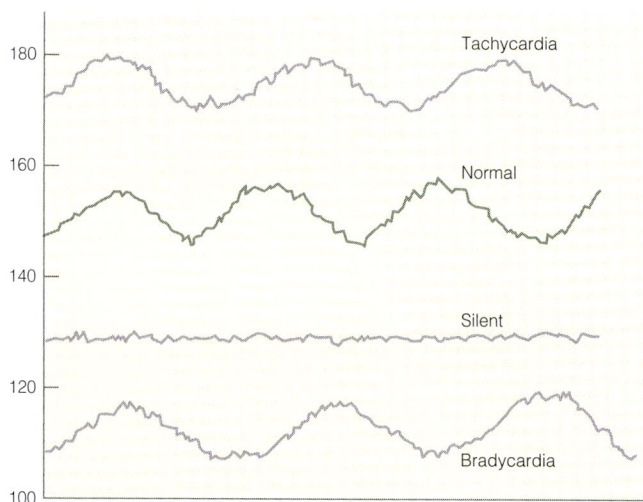

Figure 15-3. ■ Fetal heart rate variability. (Reproduced, with permission, from McGraw-Hill Companies, Inc., from Oxorn, H. (Ed.). (1986). *Oxorn-Foote human labor and birth* (5th ed.). Norwalk, CT: Appleton & Lange, p. 623.)

fetal skull, resulting in central vagal stimulation. Late decelerations result from an insufficient blood flow and oxygen transfer from the uterus to the placenta. Late decelerations begin after the start of the contraction. The nurse should stop IV pitocin infusion, reposition the mother, apply oxygen to the mother, and notify the primary care provider. Variable decelerations occur if the umbilical cord becomes compressed. The waveform is variable in shape and occurrence (Figure 15-4 ■). Generally, there is a sharp decrease in FHR and a rapid return of the FHR. The nurse should reposition the mother until a more reassuring pattern is found, perform a vaginal exam to determine the presence of a prolapsed cord and cervical dilation, and notify the physician. Immediate assisted delivery or cesarean delivery may be indicated.

FETAL BLOOD SAMPLE

If fetal well-being is questionable, the primary care provider may decide to obtain a sample of fetal blood for analysis to determine pH and base deficit. A disposable fetal blood sampling kit is obtained. The woman's vulva and perineum are cleaned and sterile drapes applied. The primary care provider inserts a conical speculum through the vagina and into the cervix to visualize the fetal scalp. The scalp is cleaned. The site is punctured with a 2-maximum microscalpel, and a small amount of blood is collected in two heparinized capillary tubes (Figure 15-5 ■). The sample must be sent STAT to the lab for analysis. Pressure is applied to the site until bleeding stops. Once the results are obtained, a decision regarding the delivery can be made.

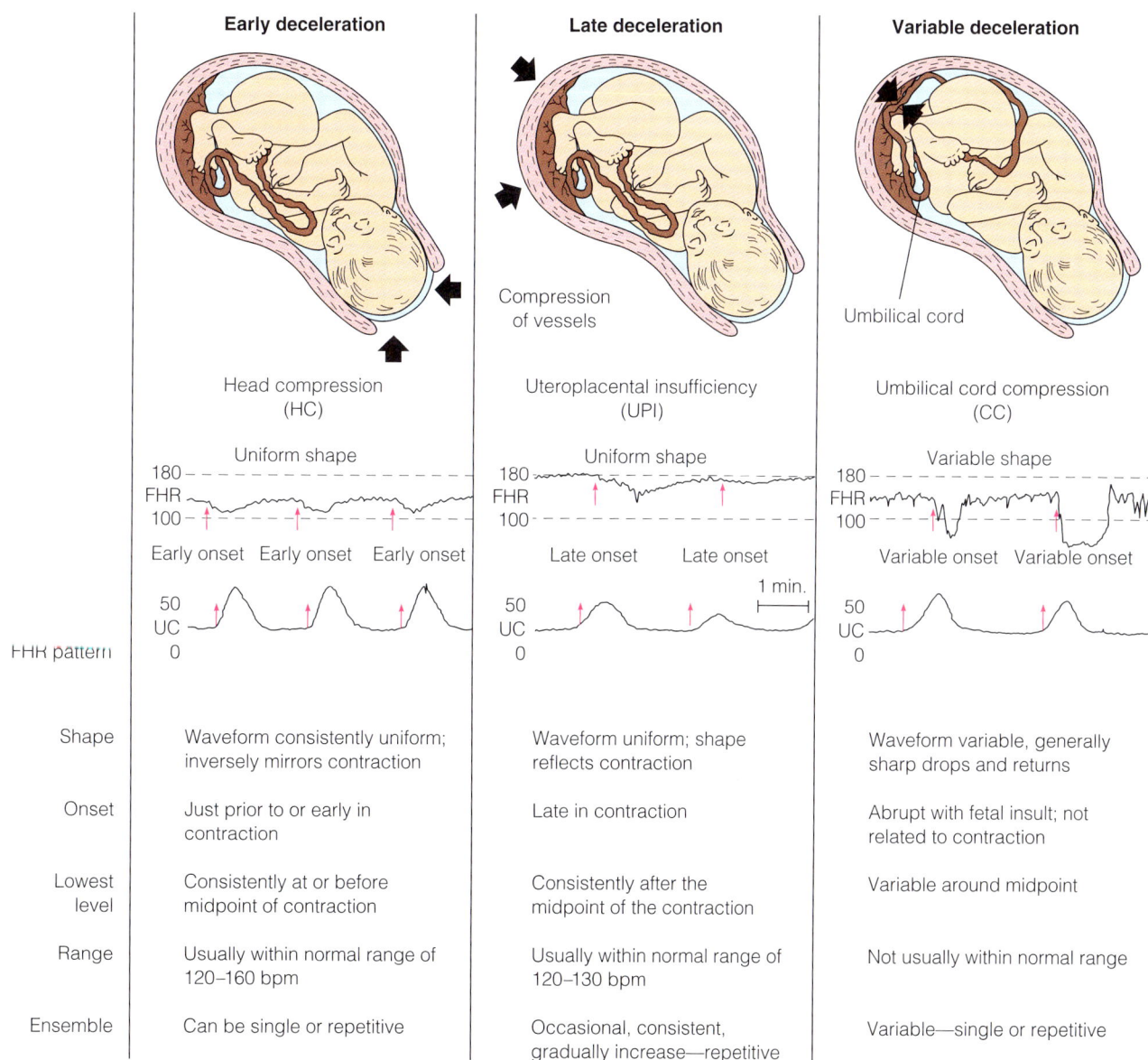

	Early deceleration	Late deceleration	Variable deceleration
	Head compression (HC)	Uteroplacental insufficiency (UPI)	Umbilical cord compression (CC)
Shape	Waveform consistently uniform; inversely mirrors contraction	Waveform uniform; shape reflects contraction	Waveform variable, generally sharp drops and returns
Onset	Just prior to or early in contraction	Late in contraction	Abrupt with fetal insult; not related to contraction
Lowest level	Consistently at or before midpoint of contraction	Consistently after the midpoint of the contraction	Variable around midpoint
Range	Usually within normal range of 120–160 bpm	Usually within normal range of 120–130 bpm	Not usually within normal range
Ensemble	Can be single or repetitive	Occasional, consistent, gradually increase—repetitive	Variable—single or repetitive

Figure 15-4. ■ Types and characteristics of early, late, and variable decelerations. (Data from Hon, E. [1976]. *An introduction to fetal heart rate monitoring,* [2nd ed.]. Los Angeles: University of Southern California School of Medicine, p. 29.)

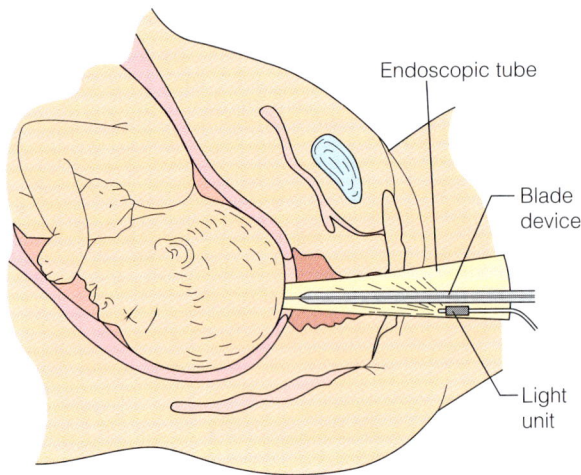

Figure 15-5. ■ Technique of obtaining fetal blood from the scalp during labor. (Reprinted with permission, from McGraw-Hill Companies, Inc. Creasy, R. K., & Parer, J.T. [1977]. *Prenatal care and diagnosis.* In A.M. Rudolph [Ed.], *Pediatrics* [16th ed.]. Englewood Cliffs, NJ: Appleton-Century-Crofts.)

Premature Rupture of Membranes

Manifestations

Premature rupture of membranes (PROM) is spontaneous breaking of the fetal membranes prior to the onset of labor. The woman may experience leaking or a sudden gush of fluid. PROM is associated with infection, trauma, abruptio placentae, hydramnios, multiple pregnancy, placenta previa, bleeding during pregnancy, and incompetent cervix.

There is a high possibility of pathogens ascending from the vagina and infecting the uterus and fetus. At times, the rupturing of the fetal membranes stimulates the placenta to detach (abruptio placentae). The loss of amniotic fluid allows the fetus to descend into the pelvis, which could result in prolapse of the umbilical cord and malpresentation.

Diagnosis

Diagnosis is made by the presence of amniotic fluid in the vagina. A sterile speculum is inserted into the vagina and pooling of amniotic fluid is visualized. If obvious pooling is not witnessed, the diagnosis can be confirmed with nitrazine paper, which turns deep blue when in contact with amniotic fluid. Fetal well-being is assessed by electronic fetal heart rate monitoring or biophysical profile. Gestational age is determined.

Treatment

The treatment of PROM is guided by the condition of the fetus, gestational age of the fetus, and the presence or absence of infection. If the fetus is in distress, a cesarean birth will be performed immediately.

If the mother shows signs of infection, antibiotics are given intravenously and the fetus is born either vaginally or by cesarean regardless of the gestational age. The fetus will be taken to the nursery, assessed for sepsis, and given antibiotics.

In the absence of infection and when the gestational age is less than 37 weeks, the treatment of PROM is usually conservative. The mother is admitted to the hospital and placed on bed rest. Regular complete blood cell counts (CBC) are done to assess for maternal infection. Fetal well-being is assessed by regular fetal heart rate, nonstress test (NST), or biophysical profile. (These tests are discussed in Chapter 9 ⚭.) When the gestational age nears 34 weeks, fetal lung maturity is determined. A single dose of betamethasone may be given to women with PROM prior to the 30th week of gestation. Betamethasone promotes lung maturity in the fetus.

After observation and initial treatment, if leaking fluid has stopped, some women may be sent home. The woman should remain on bed rest, take her temperature and pulse four times a day, and keep a fetal movement chart. She should return to the hospital if leaking fluid increases; if she has a fever, uterine contractions, uterine tenderness, or foul-smelling vaginal discharge; or if there is a decrease in fetal movement.

Nursing Considerations

On admission to the birthing area, the nurse should determine the length of time the membranes have been ruptured. The longer the membranes have been ruptured, the higher the risk of maternal and fetal infection. Maternal blood pressure, temperature, and pulse and fetal heart rate (FHR) are assessed every 4 hours. The nurse generally performs the NST and biophysical profile as ordered. The LPN may be taught to collect the data but does not interpret the findings.

Once a medical plan of care is established, continued nursing care can be planned. If it is determined the pregnancy can continue, the nursing plan of care focuses on preventing infection and maintaining bed rest with bathroom privileges. Daily hygiene is important for infection prevention, but an order of bed rest will require the nurse to bathe the woman in her bed. The nurse should ensure that adequate nutrition and fluids are consumed. The woman may need assistance to disconnect any monitoring equipment so she can walk to the bathroom. Bed rest lasting more than a few days can be emotionally difficult. The woman may worry about her family, the management of her home, and her employment. The nurse can be helpful by providing diversional activities and emotional support.

When preterm birth or cesarean birth is anticipated, the nurse should determine the degree of childbirth preparation and coping ability of the woman and her partner. Consent for induction of labor or cesarean birth is necessary. Induction of labor and cesarean birth are discussed later in this chapter.

Due to the serious nature of PROM, the family will need emotional support and teaching. The LPN/LVN listens empathetically, gives accurate information, and provides teaching as necessary. The couple may need preparation for cesarean birth, a preterm newborn, and the possibility of fetal or newborn death.

Amnioinfusion

Amnioinfusion (AI) is a process of introducing warmed sterile normal saline or Ringer's lactate solution into the uterus. Amnioinfusion increases the volume of intrauterine fluid when low amniotic fluid volume is causing fetal parts to compress the umbilical cord. AI is also used to dilute moderate to heavy meconium in the amniotic fluid. AI results in significant decrease in meconium aspiration in the newborn.

Nursing Considerations

The nurse is often the first to detect the change in fetal heart rate that is associated with cord compression or to observe meconium in the amniotic fluid. When cord compression occurs, the first intervention is to reposition the woman. If this intervention is not successful, amnioinfusion may be considered.

To administer AI, the primary care provider inserts an intrauterine pressure catheter through the vagina and into the uterus. Warmed solution is then infused into the intrauterine pressure catheter. Because the fetal membranes have ruptured prior to inserting the pressure catheter, fluid will continually leak from the vagina. Fluid expulsion of fluid infused into the uterus is important. Fluid expulsion is evaluated by counting sanitary pads and by visual observation during perineal care. The nurse should change the disposable underpads and provide perineal care often.

Preterm Labor

Preterm labor (PTL) is the onset of regular contractions, occurring between the 20th and 37th week, that cause changes in the cervix.

Factors associated with preterm labor include premature rupture of membranes (PROM), multiple pregnancy (Figure 15-6 ■), vaginal bleeding, cervical abnormalities, and infections.

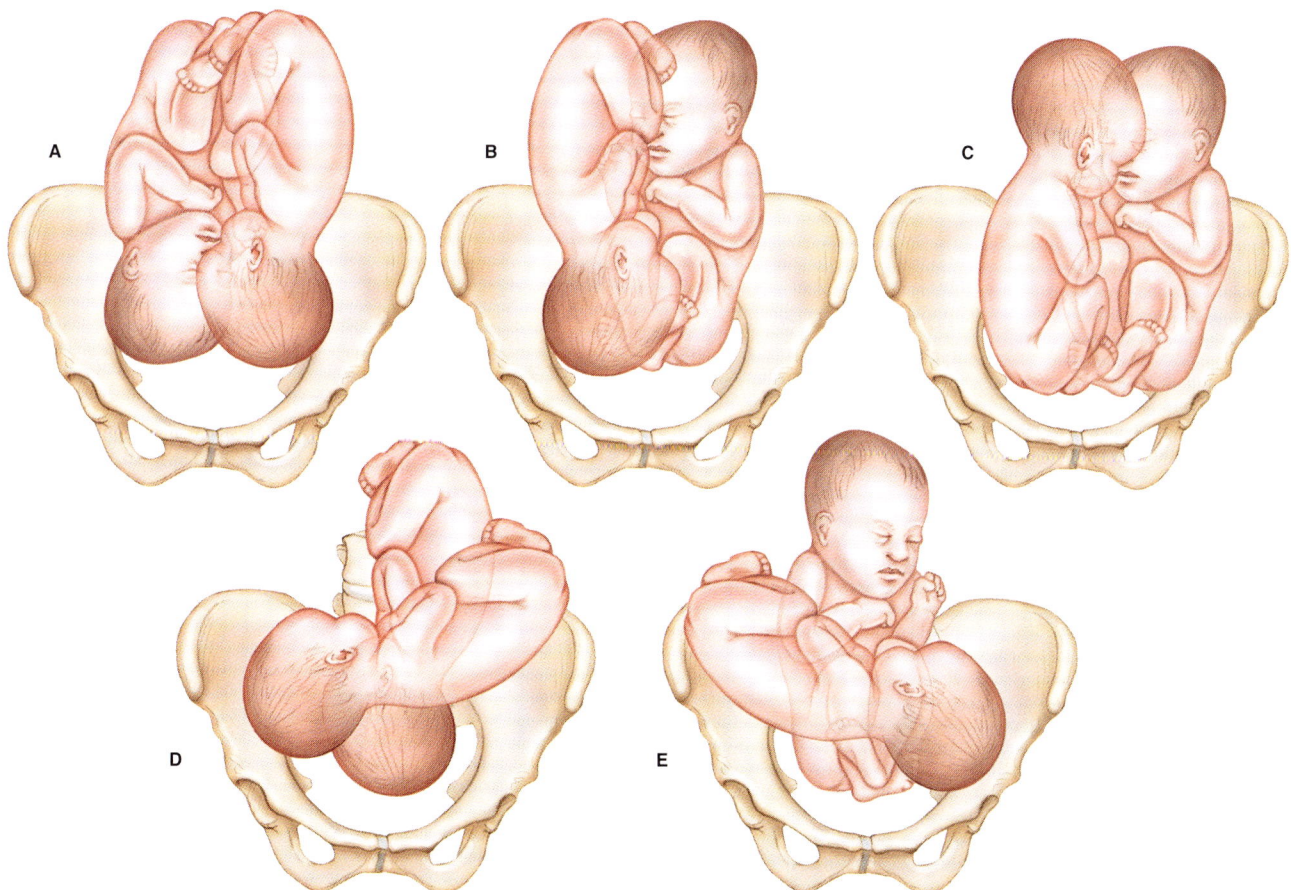

Figure 15-6. ■ Examples of twin presentation. (**A**) Two vertexes. (**B**) One vertex, one breech. (**C**) Two breeches. (**D**) One vertex, one transverse. (**E**) One transverse, one breech. Multiple pregnancy is a major risk factor for preterm labor.

Manifestations

Diagnosis of preterm labor is often difficult because symptoms are similar to those of normal pregnancy. For example, it is common for Braxton Hicks uterine contractions to occur throughout the pregnancy, especially in periods of rapid uterine growth. These may be confused with labor contractions. Pressure from the growing fetus causes the cervix to shorten and dilate in the last few weeks of pregnancy.

Diagnosis

The diagnosis of preterm labor is made if the pregnancy is between 20 and 37 weeks' gestation, and if there are documented uterine contractions (4 in 20 minutes or 8 in an hour), and documented cervical change, cervical dilatation of more than 1 centimeter, or cervical effacement of 80% or more.

Treatment

Most women with preterm labor are admitted to the hospital for assessment and treatment. The primary care provider and parents may decide not to interrupt labor in certain high-risk circumstances. These include severe preeclampsia, hemorrhage, poorly controlled diabetes mellitus, and fetal anomalies that are incompatible with life or fetal maturity.

If a decision is made to attempt to stop labor, tocolytic agents are ordered (Table 15-1 ■). Common tocolytic agents include ritodrine (Yutopar), terbutaline (Brethine), and magnesium sulfate. If labor continues, a corticosteroid, such as betamethasone (Celestone), may be given to accelerate lung maturation in the fetus (see Table 13-1 ⬭). If contractions stop and there is no further change in the cervix, the client may be discharged with instructions to limit activity and take prescribed tocolytic medication. If contractions do not stop, labor continues to the birth of a preterm infant. Preterm infants are usually taken to a neonatal intensive care unit (NICU) for specialized care. See Chapter 18 ⬭ for care of the high-risk newborn.

Nursing Considerations

Preterm labor causes a great deal of emotional stress for the mother and family. If preterm labor occurs after the 35th week of gestation, there is generally a more favorable outcome. By 35 weeks, the fetus has mature lungs and can

---

TABLE 15-1

Pharmacology: Drugs to Stop Contractions in Premature Labor

DRUG (GENERIC AND COMMON BRAND)	USUAL ROUTE/DOSE	CLASSIFICATION	SELECTED SIDE EFFECTS	DON'T GIVE IF
Ritodrine (Yutopar)	IV 50–100 mcg/min PO 10 mg q2h × 24 hr then 10–20 mg q 4–6 hr	Tocolytic (uterine relaxant)	Hypotension, cardiac arrhythmia, tachycardia, pulmonary edema, maternal hypoglycemia	Hypotension or chest pain develops. Stop medication if this happens and report.
Terbutaline (Brethine)	IV 10 mcg/min Increase 5 mcg/min until contractions stop, after 30 min decrease to lowest effective amount	Adrenergic tocolytic (unlabeled use)	Hypotension, cardiac arrhythmia, tachycardia, pulmonary edema, maternal hypoglycemia	Chest pain or hypotension develops. Stop medication if this happens and report.
Magnesium sulfate	Route: IV infusion. Preterm labor: Loading dose 4–6 g over 15–20 min Maintenance dose: 1–4 g/hr via infusion pump PIH: Loading dose 6 g over 20 minutes Maintenance dose: 2g/hr via infusion pump	Tocolytic, antihypertensive to treat PIH	Warmth, headache, nystagmus, nausea, dry mouth, dizziness	Maternal diagnosis of myasthenia gravis. This is the only absolute contraindication to use of drug. Use with caution in mother with history of cardiac and renal disorders.
Betamethasone (Celestone)	12 mg IM daily 2–3 days before delivery (unlabeled use)	Prevent respiratory distress syndrome in newborn	Few with short-term use. Hypertension, adrenal suppression, increase susceptibility of infection	Client is receiving other corticosteroids or if it is contraindicated.

usually breathe without mechanical assistance. Parents are concerned but encouraged that their child has a good chance of survival.

When preterm labor occurs before 35 weeks' gestation, the risk to the fetus is increased. Often, the mother is afraid for the survival of her baby. She may question what has caused the preterm labor. She may believe she did something "wrong" or caused the preterm labor. She might feel guilty or that she is a "bad" mother. The entire family may experience anticipatory grief.

During treatment of preterm labor, the mother is usually asked to remain on bed rest and lie on her side to increase profusion to the placenta. She may be fearful to turn or move in bed. She may be reluctant to get up to the bathroom or ask for assistance with elimination for fear movement will stimulate labor. While she needs a relaxing environment, she also may need distraction to help cope with the emotions she is experiencing.

The nurse should approach the situation in a calm, reassuring manner. The nurse must provide information regarding diagnostic tests and treatments, including the use and side effects of medications. The nurse should encourage the family members to discuss their feelings. Referral may be needed to clergy, social worker, or support groups.

If the mother is discharged prior to delivery, she may be required to remain on bed rest at home. Depending on the family situation, she may need help with household chores including cooking, cleaning, and care of other children. Her spouse, needing to work, may be unable to provide assistance during the day. The family may need assistance from the nurse to locate resources to help with home care.

Dystocia

Dystocia is defined as long, difficult, or abnormal labor pattern.

Dystocia can be caused by a variety of conditions, including ineffective uterine contractions such as hypertonic or hypotonic labor, abnormal fetal presentation or position, or cephalopelvic disproportion (CPD) (a disproportion between large fetus and a small maternal pelvic outlet).

Diagnosis

When labor does not progress in the usual time frame, the nurse should anticipate that further evaluation and intervention may be necessary. The primary care provider may order diagnostic examinations such as ultrasound to determine the fetal position accurately. Intrauterine fetal monitoring is useful in determining the quality of the uterine contractions.

Treatment

Once the cause of dystocia is determined, appropriate interventions can be implemented. Treatment ranges from application of pressure above the mons pubis to cesarean section, and is determined by the particular situation.

HYPERTONIC LABOR

In a normal labor pattern, contractions occur every 3 minutes, last 60 to 70 seconds, and are of moderate to strong intensity (Figure 15-7 ■). At times during the latent phase of labor, *hypertonic labor* occurs. With hypertonic labor, the contractions become ineffective. They increase in rate but have poor quality and an increased resting tone. The myometrium becomes hypoxic, which increases discomfort. The result is a prolonged labor, increased fatigue, and fetal distress.

Diagnosis and Treatment

When a hypertonic labor pattern develops, an evaluation of the size of the maternal pelvis in relation to the size of the fetal head must be made. The fetus should be evaluated for malpresentation or malposition. If these conditions are ruled out, stimulating contractions with oxytocin (Pitocin) may be required to increase the quality of the labor pattern.

HYPOTONIC LABOR

Hypotonic labor, meaning fewer than three contractions in a 10-minute period, occurs after labor has been established. Most commonly, the uterus has been overstretched by a large fetus, multiple pregnancy, **hydramnios** (excessive amniotic fluid), or grand multiparity (many previous births). Hypotonic labor can result in prolonged labor, maternal exhaustion, and fetal distress.

Diagnosis and Treatment

When hypotonic labor develops, the primary care provider should evaluate the size and shape of the maternal pelvis, and the size, maturity, presentation, and position of the fetus. A decision will be made whether to stimulate labor with Pitocin or to deliver the fetus by cesarean.

MALPOSITION OR MALPRESENTATION

Dystocia could occur if the fetus is in a malposition or malpresentation. At times, a fetus in the occiput posterior position may deliver in that position or may be turned to occiput anterior position. The primary care provider can apply lateral pressure to the head by a vaginal exam, causing the fetus to turn in that direction.

The fetus may be in a cephalic presentation (Figure 15-8 ■) but not in a positive degree of flexion, resulting in a face or *mentum* presentation. A face presentation increases the diameter of the presenting part, so that it may not fit through the pelvic outlet. If the face is in the anterior position, there is a higher probability of vaginal delivery than if the face is in the posterior position (Figure 15-9 ■).

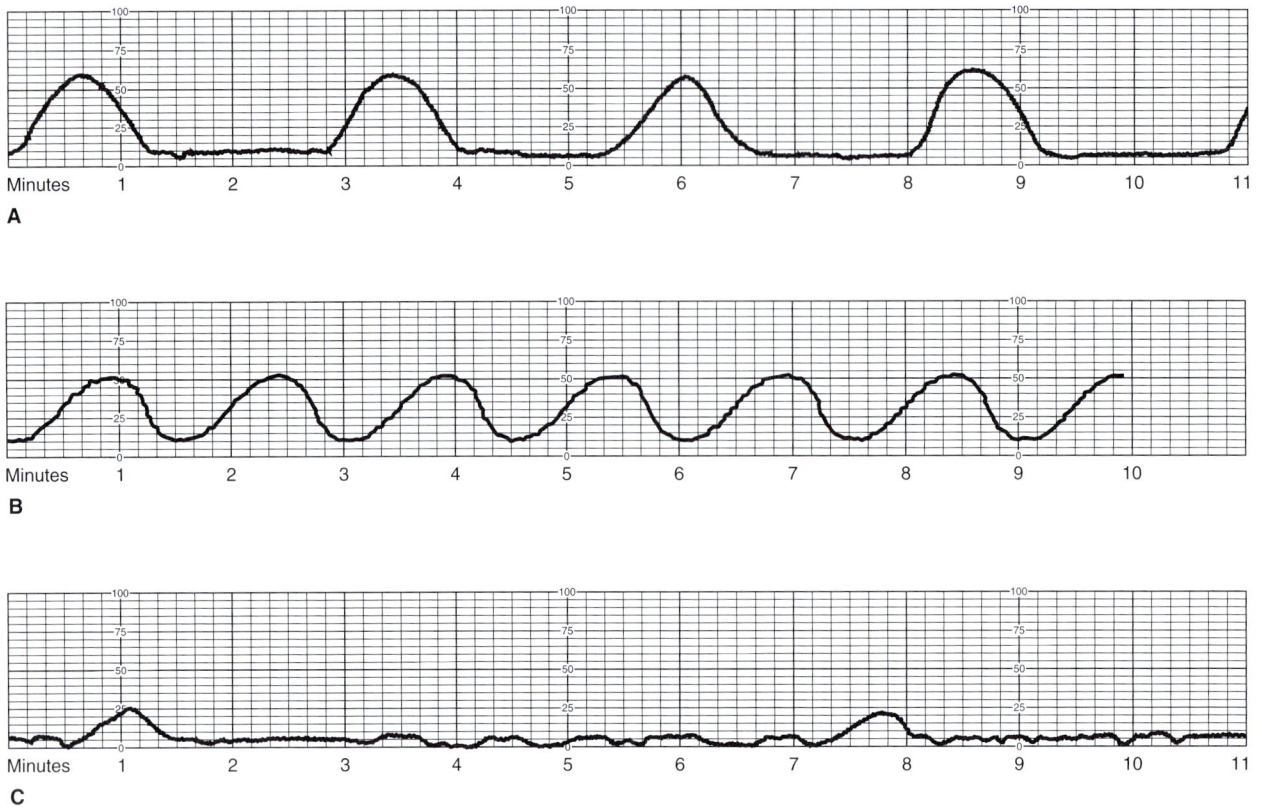

Figure 15-7. ■ Comparison of labor patterns. (**A**) Normal uterine contraction pattern. Note that the contraction frequency is every 3 minutes; duration 60 seconds. The baseline resting tone is below 10 mm Hg. (**B**) Hypertonic uterine contraction pattern. Note that the contraction frequency is every 1½ minutes, duration is 90 seconds. The baseline resting tone is 10 mm Hg. (**C**) Hypotonic uterine contraction pattern. Note in this example that the contraction frequency is every 7 minutes with some uterine activity between contractions, duration is 50 seconds, and intensity increases approximately 25 mm Hg during contractions.

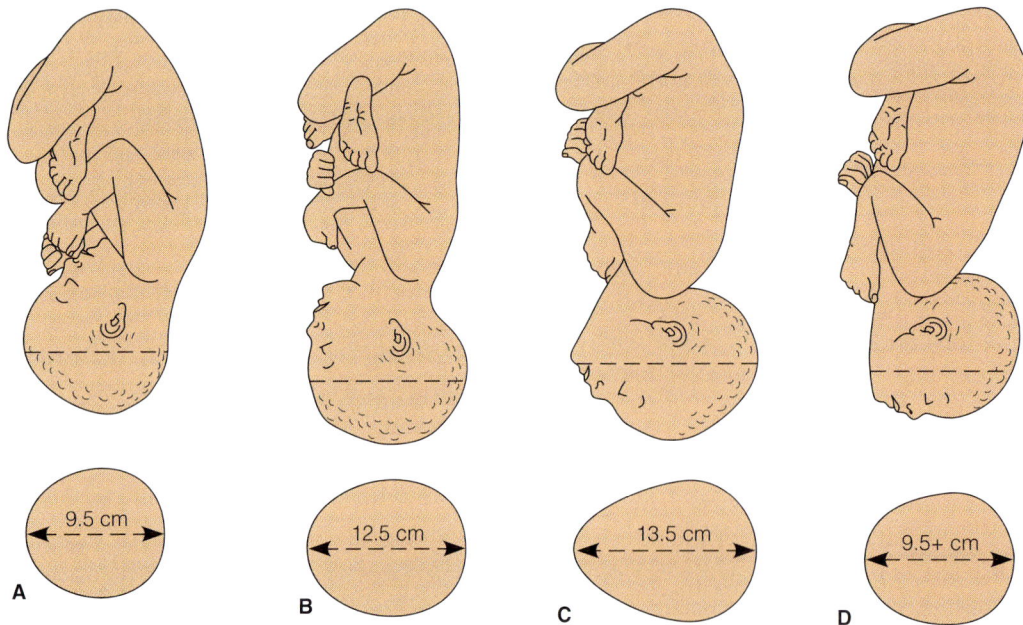

Figure 15-8. ■ Types of cephalic presentations. (**A**) The occiput is the presenting part because the head is flexed and the fetal chin is against the chest. The largest anteroposterior (AP) diameter that presents and passes through the pelvis is approximately 9.5 centimeters. (**B**) Sinciput ("military") presentation. The head is neither flexed nor extended. The presenting AP diameter is approximately 12.5 centimeters. (**C**) Brow presentation. The largest diameter of the fetal head (approximately 13.5 centimeters) presents in this situation. (**D**) Face presentation. The AP diameter is 9.5 centimeters. (*Source:* Danforth, D.N., & Scott, J.R. [Eds.]. [1990]. *Obstetrics and gynecology* [5th ed., p. 170, Fig. 8–9]. New York: Lippincott.)

Figure 15-9. ■ Face presentation. (**A**) Mechanisms of birth in mentoanterior position. (**B**) Mechanisms of birth in mentoposterior position.

The fetus may be in one of several breech or buttock presentations (Figure 15-10 ■). In frank breech presentation, both legs are extended and the feet are near the fetal head. Complete breech presentation occurs when both legs are flexed across the abdomen. At times, the fetus is in the footling breech presentation, with one or both legs extended with the foot (feet) through the cervix.

Possible Complications

If the fetus is in a breech presentation, vaginal delivery may be possible, but at a great risk. Since the buttocks may not fit snuggly against the cervix, or space may occur between the legs, the umbilical cord could pass out of the cervix. The umbilical cord could become compressed against the pelvis. If the umbilical cord extends out of the vagina, air causes the Wharton's jelly to shrink, compressing the umbilical blood vessels.

Another risk to the fetus in breech presentation occurs at time of delivery. As the fetus passes through the pelvis, the umbilical cord, attached to the placenta, will pass between the fetal head and the maternal pelvis.

Treatment

The fetal head must be delivered rapidly because compression of the umbilical cord could result in brain damage or fetal death. If the fetal head does not fit through the pelvis, there is no way to deliver the infant. For this reason, most primary care providers prefer to deliver the fetus in a breech presentation by cesarean.

VERSION. **Version** is the procedure of changing the fetal presentation by abdominal or intrauterine manipulation. The most common type is external cephalic version (ECV) in which the fetal presentation is turned from breech to cephalic. Medication is administered to cause uterine relaxation. Using

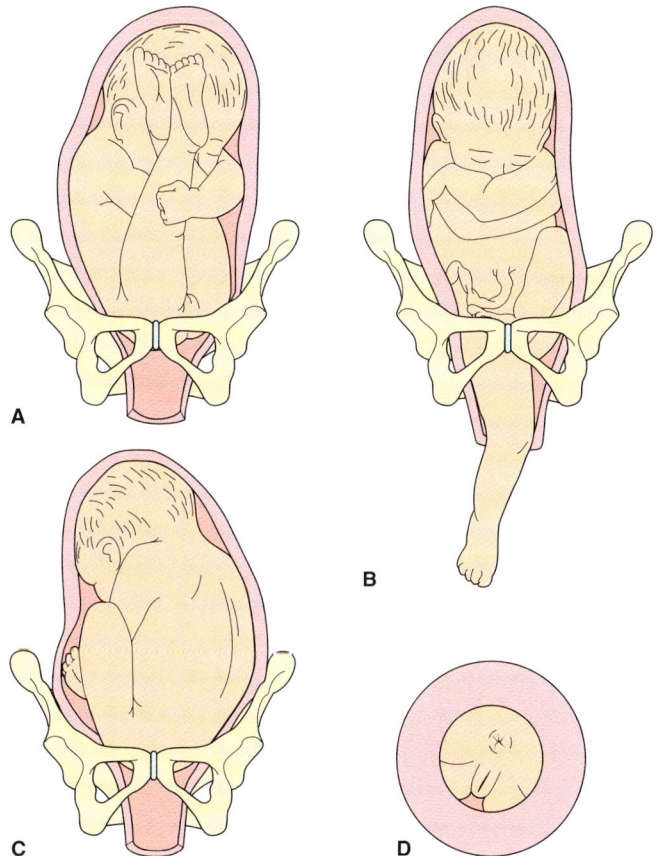

Figure 15-10. ■ Breech presentations. (**A**) Frank breech. (**B**) Incomplete (footling) breech. (**C**) Complete breech. (**D**) Anal sphincter may be felt on examination; buttocks tissue will be soft.

Leopold's maneuver and ultrasound, the primary care provider identifies the fetal head and buttocks. Placing one hand on the fetal head and the other on the fetal buttocks, the primary care provider pushes on the fetus, causing it to make a "backward flip" or a "forward roll" (Figure 15-11 ■).

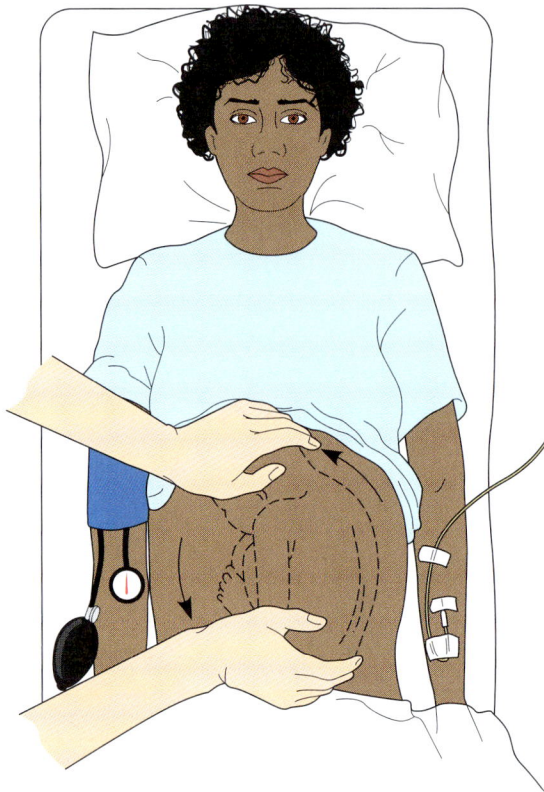

Figure 15-11. ■ External (or cephalic) version of the fetus. A new technique involves applying pressure to the fetal head and buttocks so that the fetus completes a "backward flip" or "roll."

A second, less common method of version, called *podalic version*, is used only if the second fetus in a twin delivery fails to descend readily. Medication is used to relax the uterus. The obstetrician then places a hand up the vagina and into the uterus, grabbing the fetus's feet and drawing them through the cervix. The fetus is then delivered as a breech presentation.

Complications of version include abruptio placentae, fetal distress, umbilical cord compression, and (in the case of podalic version) maternal lacerations. The mother's vital signs and fetal heart rate must be monitored continuously during the procedure. If complications occur, the fetal heart rate drops, or the primary care provider is unable to turn the fetus, the fetus is delivered by cesarean section.

CEPHALOPELVIC DISPROPORTION

A large fetus could cause dystocia. As the fetus moves through the maternal pelvis, the bones of the fetal skull override, decreasing the size of the fetal head. Yet sometimes, even with molding, the fetal head is larger than the maternal pelvis. This condition is known as *cephalopelvic disproportion* (CPD).

Manifestations

Typically, labor contractions will be frequent and strong, but the fetus will not descend through the pelvis.

Treatment

When cephalopelvic disproportion is present, the only way to deliver the fetus safely is by cesarean section.

SHOULDER DYSTOCIA

Another concern with a large fetus is *shoulder dystocia* (Figure 15-12 ■). With this complication, the broad anterior shoulder becomes wedged behind the mother's pubis after the fetal head is delivered.

Treatment

The nurse may need to apply pressure above the mother's pubis to push the shoulder into the pelvic opening. The primary care provider rotates the fetus by turning its head until the shoulder is delivered. This difficult delivery could

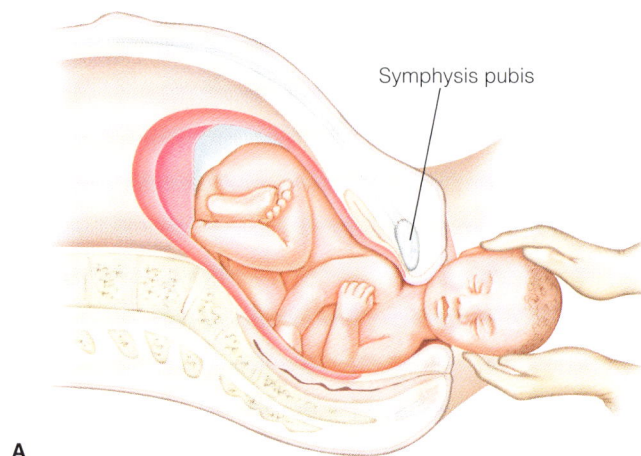

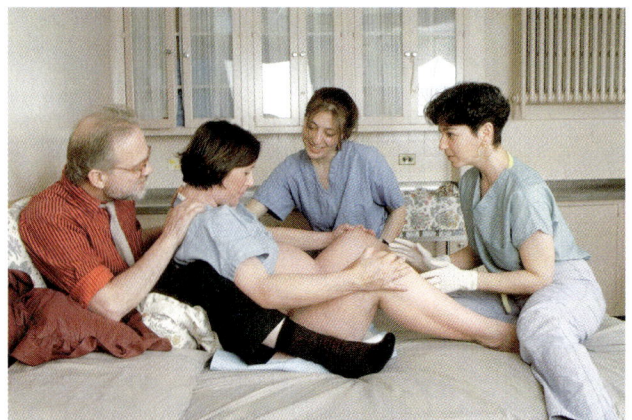

Symphysis pubis

A **B**

Figure 15-12. ■ (**A**) Shoulder dystocia. (**B**) This position with pressure against the mother's knees may be helpful in clients with shoulder dystocia. (**B**: Margaret Miller/Photo Researcher, Inc.)

result in maternal lacerations and a fractured clavicle in the infant. If pressure above the pubis does not allow the shoulder to emerge, fetal death is likely.

Nursing Considerations

Dystocia for any reason places additional emotional stress on the mother. Even with pain relief measures such as epidural anesthesia, long difficult labor is physically tiring. As the woman's energy decreases, she not only loses the reserve to push effectively, but also loses the ability to maintain her own physiological needs to survive.

Long difficult labor is emotionally draining. The woman becomes fearful that something is wrong with her or with the baby. She is fearful for the survival of her baby. Being emotionally drained, the woman may lose the will to fight for her own life should a crisis occur.

It is important for the nurse to recognize the signs of dystocia, to alert the primary care provider, and to encourage and support the woman. The nurse must be aware of the woman's need for energy and provide adequate amount of glucose and fluid through IV infusion. The nurse must anticipate the need for cesarean birth and prepare the woman, both physically and emotionally, for that possibility.

Induction of Labor

Induction of labor is the stimulation of labor by medical or pharmacologic methods. Induction of labor may be necessary if the risk to the mother or infant of continuing the pregnancy is greater than the risk of delivery. Indications for induction of labor include post dates (labor does not begin spontaneously by the 41st week), gestational (pregnancy-induced) hypertension, maternal diabetes, suspected fetal abnormality, history of rapid delivery, and fetal death.

METHODS OF INDUCING LABOR

The methods of induction of labor include:

- *Prostaglandins (PGE$_1$)*. At times, the cervix is ripened (softened) by the insertion of prostaglandin gel into and around the cervix. Labor may begin in a few hours or may be induced 12 to 24 hours later by another method.
- *Artificial rupture of membranes (AROM)*. The physician or nurse midwife inserts an amnihook through the cervix and perforates the amniotic membranes (see Figure 14-21 ⬯). Labor contractions should begin in a few hours.
- *Pitocin (oxytocin) infusion*. A primary intravenous infusion is begun, and a secondary infusion containing Pitocin is

given by piggyback into the primary infusion. If severe side effects of Pitocin occur, the infusion can be easily discontinued and the IV line maintained. The registered nurse increases the dose of Pitocin in small increments until labor is begun. Once labor is begun, it usually progresses like spontaneous labor.

Assisted Births

During the second stage of labor, the mother actively uses her abdominal muscles to push the fetus through the birth canal. For reasons described above, the fetus at times is slow to descend through the pelvis. In the absence of documented cephalopelvic disproportion, the delivery may be assisted with a vacuum or forceps. Because of the risk of fetal and maternal trauma, the use of either appliance should follow strict guidelines and facility policy.

> ### clinical ALERT
>
> Cephalopelvic disproportion (CPD) is an absolute contradiction to assisted vaginal delivery and requires a cesarean delivery.

VACUUM EXTRACTION

Vacuum extraction is used when minimal assistance is expected (Figure 15-13 ■). The vacuum extractor is composed of a soft suction cup attached to a suction hand pump. The primary care provider places the suction cup firmly against the occipital area of the fetal scalp. Care must be taken to avoid the area over a fontanel and maternal tissue. The nurse uses the hand pump to apply the amount of suction determined by the primary care provider. During the next contraction, the primary care provider applies traction. The fetal head should emerge from the vagina with each contraction.

If the suction cup becomes detached from the fetal head, it may be reapplied, and a second attempt at delivery can be made. If the suction cup becomes detached three times, the procedure should be discontinued and another method of delivery should be initiated.

Possible Complications

Fetal complications of vacuum extraction include scalp lacerations, bruising, subdural hematoma, cephalhematoma (see Figure 17-17 ⬯), intracranial hemorrhage, cranial fractures, neurologic injury, and fetal death. Maternal complications include vaginal, rectal, urethral, and perineal lacerations. Nursing care of a client with a hematoma is described in the Nursing Care Plan Chart on pages 370 and 371.

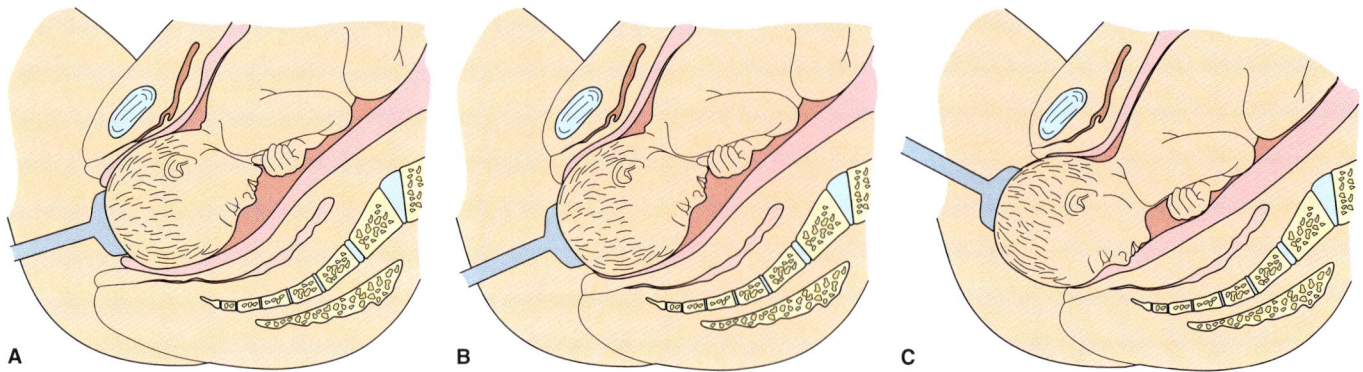

Figure 15-13. ■ Vacuum extractor traction. (**A**) The cup is placed on the fetal occiput creating suction. Traction is applied in a downward and outward direction. (**B**) Traction continues in a downward direction as the fetal head begins to emerge from the vagina. (**C**) Traction is maintained to lift the head out of the vagina.

NURSING CARE PLAN CHART

Planning for Client with Puerperal Hematoma

GOAL	INTERVENTION	RATIONALE	EXPECTED OUTCOME
1. Deficient Knowledge related to puerperal hematoma			
The client or couple will obtain information about puerperal hematoma. Client will consent to plan of emergent treatment, including surgery, as recommended.	Explain that puerperal hematoma is a complication of delivery requiring *emergency* treatment. Explain that a hematoma is a sign of bleeding. The bleeding must be controlled quickly to safeguard the client's health.	*Written reading materials are not provided, given the emergent nature of the client's condition.* *Hematomas develop as the result of hemorrhage from trauma during delivery; blood collects and pools in soft tissue. Continuous blood loss may produce hypovolemic shock and/or death.*	Client and/or couple will understand the urgent need for treatment of the hematoma.
	Provide details on type of hematoma, level of threat, and emergency plan of care specific to the client. Inform client or couple that the size and location of the hematoma determines the level of treatment required and that emergency surgery may be necessary.	*Hematoma that develops after delivery can develop internally (retroperitoneal) or externally (vulvovaginal).* *Puerperal hematomas require treatment. Most require urgent surgical intervention, to stop blood loss and/or to drain the hematoma to prevent infection. Retroperitoneal hematoma (involving branches of the pudendal artery) can be life threatening. The greater the size of the hematoma, the greater the threat.*	Client or couple will explain the rationale behind routine surgical treatment for hematoma. Client will sign surgical consent forms following explanation by attending physician and/or surgeon.
	Repeat and/or clarify preoperative teaching provided by physician or registered nurse. Obtain client's signature on surgical consent form or countersign as witness according to agency policy.	*Clients who are under stress may have difficulty retaining what they have heard. They may need information repeated.* *Follow facility policy in obtaining or witnessing informed consent. Ask questions to be sure the client understands what is occurring.*	

GOAL	INTERVENTION	RATIONALE	EXPECTED OUTCOME
2. Acute Pain related to bleeding in tissue			
Client will achieve pain control.	Medication Administration: Oral Or Medication Administration: Parenteral (Intramuscular injection) Positioning Environmental Management: Comfort	*Constant, severe perineal pain that exceeds the normal level of discomfort expected from episiotomy or indwelling urinary catheter can be a sign of hematoma. Most hematomas occur within 24 hours after delivery.* *Positioning to avoid direct pressure on an external hematoma can reduce pain. Generalized comfort measures are a means to reduce client's pain.*	Client will report a normal postdelivery intermittent pain pattern. Client will achieve pain relief for up to 4 hours following medication administration (pain rated "zero" on a scale of "0 to 10"). Client will report intermittent pain that does not exceed the client's personal rating of "4" on a scale of "0 to 10."
3. Impaired Skin Integrity			
Client will maintain skin integrity of body areas unaffected by therapeutic devices. Client will experience restoration of the integrity of the skin currently impaired by the presence of therapeutic devices.	Provide wound care of intra-venous insertion site(s), surgical site(s), and/ or drain insertion site(s) from hematoma. Monitor vaginal discharge (lochia). Monitor condition/location of "packed" dressings. Provide bathing and post-elimination perineal care: Warm water irrigation via squirt bottle to the perineum after urination and bowel movements.	*Intravenous therapy may be necessary to deliver fluids and/or blood products to restore total blood volume following hemorrhage.* *Drainage of stagnant blood from hematoma reduces the risk of infection.* *Vaginal packing ("pressure" dressing) may be necessary following evacuation of the hematoma to prevent further blood loss and to absorb drainage.* *Changes in lochia (color, quantity, odor) may be signs of infection and/or hemorrhage.* *Wound and skin care measures (dressing changes, etc.) as well as acts of personal hygiene also guard against infection and facilitate comfort.*	Wound sites will remain free of redness, swelling, purulent drainage, and other signs of infection.

FORCEPS EXTRACTION

Forceps are indicated when firmer traction is needed. Only a trained obstetrician is certified in the use of forceps. With the development of the vacuum extractor, the use of forceps has decreased.

Forceps consist of two metal spoon-shaped blades attached to handles that lock together (Figure 15-14 ■). The physician slips one blade into the vagina, along one side of the fetal head, past the ear to the level of the jaw. The second blade is then inserted into the vagina past the other side of the fetal head to the level of the jaw. The handles of the forceps are then locked together. If necessary, the fetal head can be rotated to an occiput anterior position. With the next contraction, the physician applies traction. The fetal head should slowly progress through the pelvis until it emerges from the vagina. The forceps are then removed, and the body of the fetus is delivered unassisted.

Possible Complications

Complications for the fetus and the mother are the same as for vacuum-assisted extraction. However, due to the position of the forceps, facial trauma (including facial

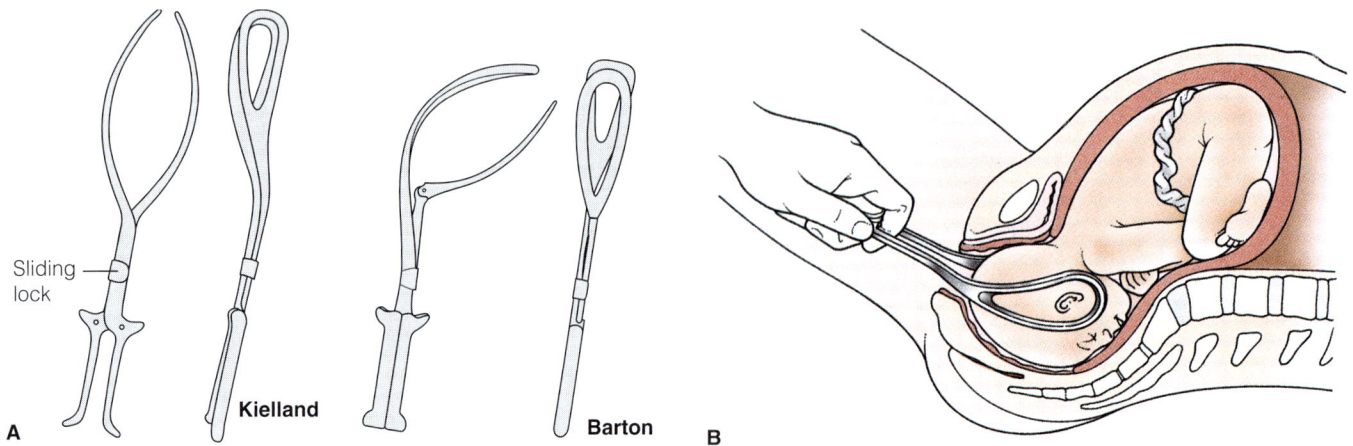

Sliding lock

Kielland   Barton

A   B

Figure 15-14. ■ (**A**) Forceps are composed of a blade, shank, and handle and may have a cephalic and pelvic curve. The blades may be fenestrated (open) or solid. The front and lateral views of these forceps illustrate differences in blades, open and closed shanks, and cephalic and pelvic curves. Kielland and Barton forceps are used for midforceps rotations. (**B**) Pressure marks from forceps used during delivery are usually located on the cheek and jaws. They usually disappear within a day. (Dorling Kindersley Media Library.)

TABLE 15-2

Procedures Commonly Associated with Hospitalizations for Childbirth

ALL LISTED PROCEDURES*	NUMBER OF HOSPITAL STAYS WITH THIS PROCEDURE	PERCENTAGE OF CHILDBIRTHS WITH THIS PROCEDURE
Medical induction, manually assisted delivery, and other procedures to assist delivery	1,946,500	48.0%
Repair of current obstetric laceration	1,260,600	31.1%
Cesarean section	1,171,400	28.9%
Fetal monitoring	912,500	22.5%
Artificial rupture of membranes to assist delivery	808,400	19.9%
Episiotomy	564,500	13.9%
Forceps, vacuum, and breech delivery	311,900	7.7%
Other therapeutic obstetrical procedures	132,400	3.3%
Removal ectopic pregnancy	20,300	0.5%
Diagnostic amniocentesis	17,400	0.4%

*Hospitalization for childbirth determined by DRGs 370–375.

Source: Agency for Healthcare Research and Quality, Center for Delivery, Organization, and Markets. (2003). Healthcare cost and utilization project; Nationwide inpatient sample. Rockville, MD: Author.

paralysis) could also occur. If the forcep blades are not applied correctly, fractures of the fetal skull could occur. Maternal trauma often results in vaginal and perineal lacerations, which may include the rectum and anus. Procedures commonly associated with hospitalizations for childbirth are shown in Table 15-2 ■.

EPISIOTOMY AND LACERATIONS. As described in Chapter 14 ⬅, an **episiotomy** (surgical cutting of the perineal tissue) may be needed to enlarge the vaginal opening and prevent lacerations. An episiotomy is made in the second stage of labor when the fetal head is crowning. Most commonly, the surgical cut is made in the midline of the perineum, but if more space is needed, a lateral episiotomy (see Figure 14-19 ⬭) is made.

Lacerations occur when tissues are unable to stretch any further and tear under pressure. Lacerations can occur in the cervix, vagina, or perineum. Vaginal and perineal lacerations are categorized in terms of degree as follows:

- First-degree laceration is limited to the fourchette (tissue connecting the posterior ends of the labia minora), perineal skin, and vaginal mucous membrane.
- Second-degree laceration involves the perineal skin, vaginal mucous membrane, underlying fascia, and muscles of the perineum. It may extend upward on one or both sides of the vagina.
- Third-degree laceration extends through the perineum and involves the anal sphincter. It may extend up the anterior wall of the rectum.
- Fourth-degree laceration is like third-degree but extends through the rectal wall into the lumen of the rectum.

Following delivery, the episiotomy and lacerations are repaired with absorbable sutures. Frequent perineal care is recommended to prevent infection until healing occurs. In the case of third- and fourth-degree lacerations, stool softeners, increased fiber diet, and increased fluids are recommended to prevent trauma to the rectal tissue from the passage of constipated stool.

SURGICAL BIRTH OR CESAREAN SECTION

Surgical birth or **cesarean section** is performed for a variety of reasons, including placenta previa, abruptio placentae, cephalopelvic disproportion, fetal distress, breech presentation, preeclampsia, multiple pregnancy, and previous cesarean birth. A cesarean birth can be a planned or unscheduled event; it may be an emergency procedure to save the mother and/or fetus. Certain groups are more likely to have cesarean section, as described in Box 15-1 ■. Whether the cesarean is planned or an emergency, the procedures and nursing care are similar.

The Health Promotion Issue on pages 374 and 375 discusses some of the issues involved in birth by cesarean section.

| BOX 15-1 | CULTURAL PULSE POINTS |

Pregnancy Among Older Women

Research funded by the National Institutes of Health for the period from 1995 through 2000 determined that certain data were associated with pregnancy in older women (35 years or older). The researchers compared the mothers' medical risk factors, pregnancy complications, and modes of delivery. Data on three comparison age groups—35 to 39, 40 to 44, and 45 and older—were compared to data collected about mothers age 30 to 34 years old. The study determined the following:

- Between 1980 and 2004, the number of women in the United States giving birth at age 30 or older had doubled and at age 35 and older had tripled. The number of mothers giving birth at age 40 or older had nearly quadrupled.
- Mothers age 35 or older with normal, full-term pregnancies were more likely than younger women to undergo cesarean section.
- Women age 35 or older were more likely than younger women to experience complications during pregnancy, labor, and birth (e.g., diabetes, hypertension). Women giving birth at age 45 or older were the most likely to have high blood pressure and diabetes while pregnant. They were also at greatest risk for excessive bleeding during labor, premature delivery (before 32 weeks), and cesarean birth.
- In relation to their age, women age 45 or older were more likely to experience premature birth, complications during labor and birth, or infant death. Complications included excessive bleeding during labor, prolonged labor lasting more than 20 hours, and dysfunctional labor that did not advance to the next stage.
- The chance of cesarean section in all pregnancies increased with the women's age, even when the mother had carried to term and had no complications due to excessive bleeding or to the baby's positioning. The study was not able to determine whether physician concerns about medical malpractice suits played a role in recommending cesarean birth. Another possible factor in selecting cesarean birth is that women tend to be heavier as they age, and obesity complicates labor and birth.
- The study authors attribute the trend of more women giving birth at an older age, in part, to the increased use of fertility-enhancing therapies. Citing statistics from the U.S. Centers for Disease Control and Prevention, the study authors noted that more than half of all *in-vitro* fertilization (IVF) cycles between 1998 and 2003 were among women 35 years and older.

Source: Data from the National Institutes of Health (NIH). The Nation's Medical Research Agency.

HEALTH PROMOTION ISSUE

CESAREAN DELIVERY ON DEMAND

A pregnant business executive shares with her obstetrician her frustration over not knowing when her baby will be born. She states that she must be able to plan an important meeting and needs control over the date and time of delivery. She feels the uncertainty of when labor will begin and how long it will last is interfering with her personal choices. She requests a scheduled cesarean delivery.

DISCUSSION

Since 1970, the rate of cesarean delivery has increased to 29.1% in 2004 (U.S. Department of Health and Human Services, 2006). Traditionally cesarean delivery was performed for medical reasons such as CPD, placenta previa, or fetal distress. In recent years, more women are choosing cesarean deliveries for a variety of reasons. Many health care providers are questioning the ethics of performing surgery for nonmedical reasons. The risks and benefits of each method of delivery should be explored.

Both methods of delivery carry risk to the mother and to the infant. Quality prenatal care, frequent monitoring during the delivery process, and close observation and treatment following delivery greatly decreases the harmful consequences. The maternal and fetal risks of a vaginal delivery are shown in the table at top right.

Many women fear the pain of delivery. With relaxation and breathing techniques, in combination with medication by the intravenous and epidural route, most discomfort can be alleviated or kept to a tolerable level. While future urinary incontinence is a

MATERNAL RISKS IN VAGINAL DELIVERY	FETAL RISKS IN VAGINAL DELIVERY
Pain	Cranial trauma
Future urinary incontinence	Respiratory distress due to aspiration
Perineal tearing	Hypoxia from umbilical cord compression
Pelvic floor damage causing potential sexual difficulties	

possibility, research published by Rortveit, Daltveit, Hannestad, and Hunskaar (2003) indicates that nearly 16% of women who had a cesarean delivery developed incontinence compared with 21% of women who delivered vaginally. If perineal tearing occurs, the tissue will be sutured and healing should occur in 4 to 6 weeks. As with any wound, infection requiring antibiotic treatment could occur. Pelvic floor muscle strengthening (Kegel exercises) should begin in the prenatal period and continue after delivery. While the pelvic muscle tone may never return to

prepregnancy state, consistent exercises decrease complications.

The risk of vaginal delivery to the fetus may appear great. However, nature has equipped the fetal skull to adapt to the size and shape of the maternal pelvis. In most circumstances, the bones of the fetal skull override and mold to the maternal pelvis. On occasion, the fetal head is too large to adapt to the maternal pelvis or the position or presentation of the fetus is not conducive to vaginal delivery. In these situations, the risk of cerebral trauma increases and a cesarean delivery is

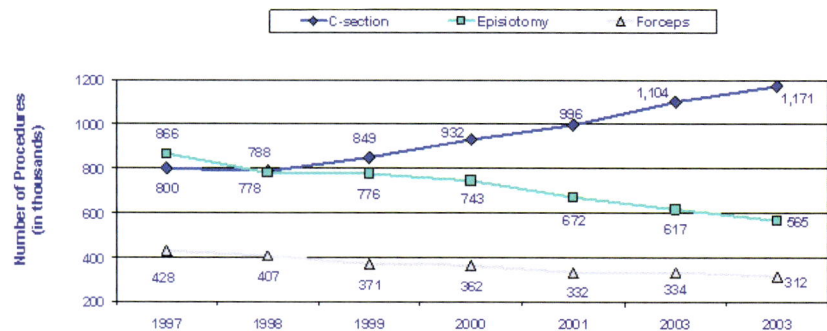

Trend of C-section, episiotomy, and forceps procedures, 1997–2003*

AHRQ Advancing Excellence in Health Care

C-section Episiotomy Forceps

Number of Procedures (in thousands)

C-section: 800 (1997), 778 (1998), 849 (1999), 932 (2000), 996 (2001), 1,104 (2003), 1,171 (2003)
Episiotomy: 866 (1997), 788 (1998), 776 (1999), 743 (2000), 672 (2001), 617 (2003), 565 (2003)
Forceps: 428 (1997), 407 (1998), 371 (1999), 362 (2000), 332 (2001), 334 (2003), 312 (2003)

*Based on all-listed diagnoses and DRGs.

Source: AHRQ, Center for Delivery, Organization, and Markets, Healthcare Cost and Utilization Project, Nationwide Inpatient Sample, 1997–2003.

performed. Anytime the fetus takes a breath prior to airway suctioning, there is a possibility of aspiration and fetal respiratory distress. As the fetus moves through the pelvis, the pressure on the chest stimulates breathing after delivery. Often cord compression during labor can be relieved by close monitoring and changing the mother's position. When signs of fetal distress occur, an emergency cesarean delivery is necessary.

Cesarean delivery also carries a risk to the mother and infant. Maternal and fetal risks of cesarean delivery are shown in the table at top right.

Because of the extent of the abdominal incision, there is an increased loss of blood with a cesarean delivery. As with perineal trauma in a vaginal delivery, infection of the incision requiring antibiotic treatment is a possibility. However, because the abdominal cavity is opened, infection of the entire abdomen is a possibility. When the incision is made, there is an increased risk of damage to other internal organs especially the urinary bladder and uterine blood vessels. If the fetus is large, there is a risk of tearing the uterine incision causing more trauma to uterine tissue. While a vaginal birth after cesarean (VBAC) is a possibility in future pregnancies, there is an increased probability that subsequent pregnancies will require a cesarean delivery. If the surgical incision into the uterus does not heal well, or if the uterus is overdistended as with a large fetus or multiple pregnancy,

MATERNAL RISK IN CESAREAN DELIVERY	FETAL RISK IN CESAREAN DELIVERY
Increased blood loss	Respiratory distress
Infection	Transfer to NICU
Injury to internal organs	Stillbirth
Increased risk of repeat cesarean delivery	
Uterine rupture in future pregnancies	
Increased need for hysterectomy	

there is an increased risk of uterine rupture, resulting in possible death of the fetus and mother. If uterine rupture occurs, a hysterectomy may be required to save the mother's life.

As American women demand more control of their health care, many obstetricians are being pressured to perform cesarean delivery on request for personal instead of medical reasons. Although there are no hard figures for the number of cesarean deliveries on demand, the American College of Nurse-Midwives and the American College of Obstetricians and Gynecologists report that the trend is increasing despite repeated warnings against such practice.

PLANNING AND IMPLEMENTATION

The decision to have children comes with numerous responsibilities, risks, and consequences. Raising children causes parents to change their "usual" way of life. Ideally, the couple will explore and discuss these issues prior

to pregnancy. However, some couples become pregnant before resolving these issues. It is important for the nurse to help the couple explore the risks of childbirth early in the pregnancy. The nurse should provide literature or Internet websites for the couple to explore and increase their knowledge and understanding of the benefits and risks involved. With help from the nurse, the couple can develop a birth plan that includes adjustment in their life schedules.

SELF-REFLECTION

Think about how you would need to adjust your life to "make time" for an unscheduled labor. Could you suggest any of these adjustments to the pregnant woman? What techniques could the couple use to help make an objective birth plan? How will you feel if the couple chooses a different plan than you would?

SUGGESTED RESOURCES

Rortveit, G., Daltveit, A.K., Hannestad, Y., & Hunskaar, S. (2003). Urinary incontinence after vaginal delivery or cesarean section. *New England Journal of Medicine, 348* (10), 900–907.

Scott, J.R. (2006). Cesarean delivery on request: Where do we go from here? *Obstetrics and Gynecology, 107,* 1222–1223.

At times, preoperative procedures for cesarean section must be completed rapidly and under great stress. The client may be tired after hours of labor, worried about the health of her infant, and fearful about her own safety. The nurse must provide teaching and support while performing routine procedures. It will be necessary to have a signed surgical consent. A Foley catheter will be inserted to keep the bladder empty. An intravenous infusion will be started. Hair over the mons pubis is clipped short. In some areas, the father or a significant other may accompany the client to surgery and will need to change into surgical attire.

Anesthesia is usually administered by the epidural or spinal route (Figure 15-15 ■; see also Figure 14-18 ⚭). If an epidural has been used during labor, it will probably be used during surgery. If an epidural has not been used during labor, it will probably be initiated in the surgical suite prior to prepping the abdomen. In the event of an emergency situation, general anesthesia may be used.

Although there are several incisions that can be made to deliver the fetus, the most common is a horizontal incision through the skin at the pubic hair border (Figure 15-16 ■). The bladder is detached from the perimetrium and held out of the way by retractors. A horizontal incision is generally made in the lower uterine segment. The infant is then pulled through the opening. If the infant is large, forceps may be needed to extract the infant's head. Figure 15-17 ■ illustrates a cesarean birth. The infant's airway is suctioned; the infant is dried and evaluated by the Apgar score (see Table 14-6 ⚭).

After the birth, the mother's uterus, fascia, abdominal muscles, and fat are sutured. Skin staples, clips, or Steri-Strips are used to secure the skin. An abdominal dressing may be taped securely in place.

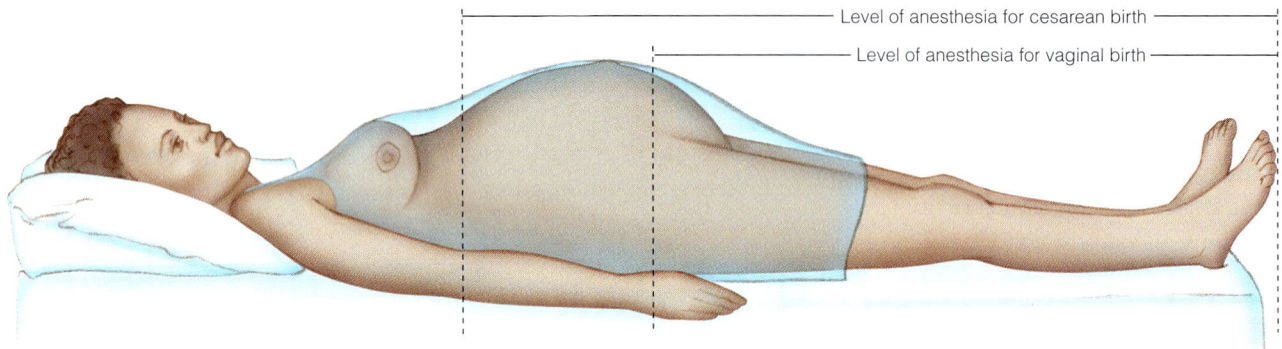

Figure 15-15. ■ Anesthesia levels for a vaginal and cesarean birth. (Data from Ross Products Division, Abbott Laboratories, Columbus, OH 43216 from CEA # 17, Regional.)

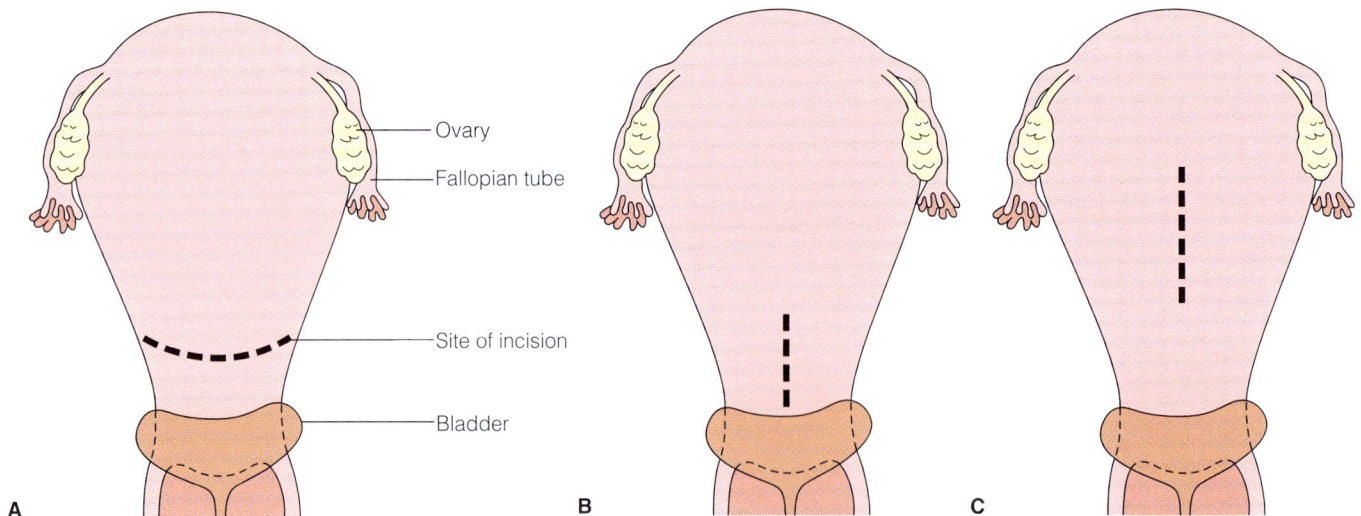

Figure 15-16. ■ The uterine incisions for cesarean birth. (**A**) This transverse incision in the lower uterine segment is called a Kerr incision. (**B**) The Selheim incision is a vertical incision in the lower uterine segment. (**C**) This view illustrates the classic uterine incision that is done in the body corpus of the uterus. The classic incision was commonly used in the past but is associated with increased risk of uterine rupture in subsequent pregnancies and labor.

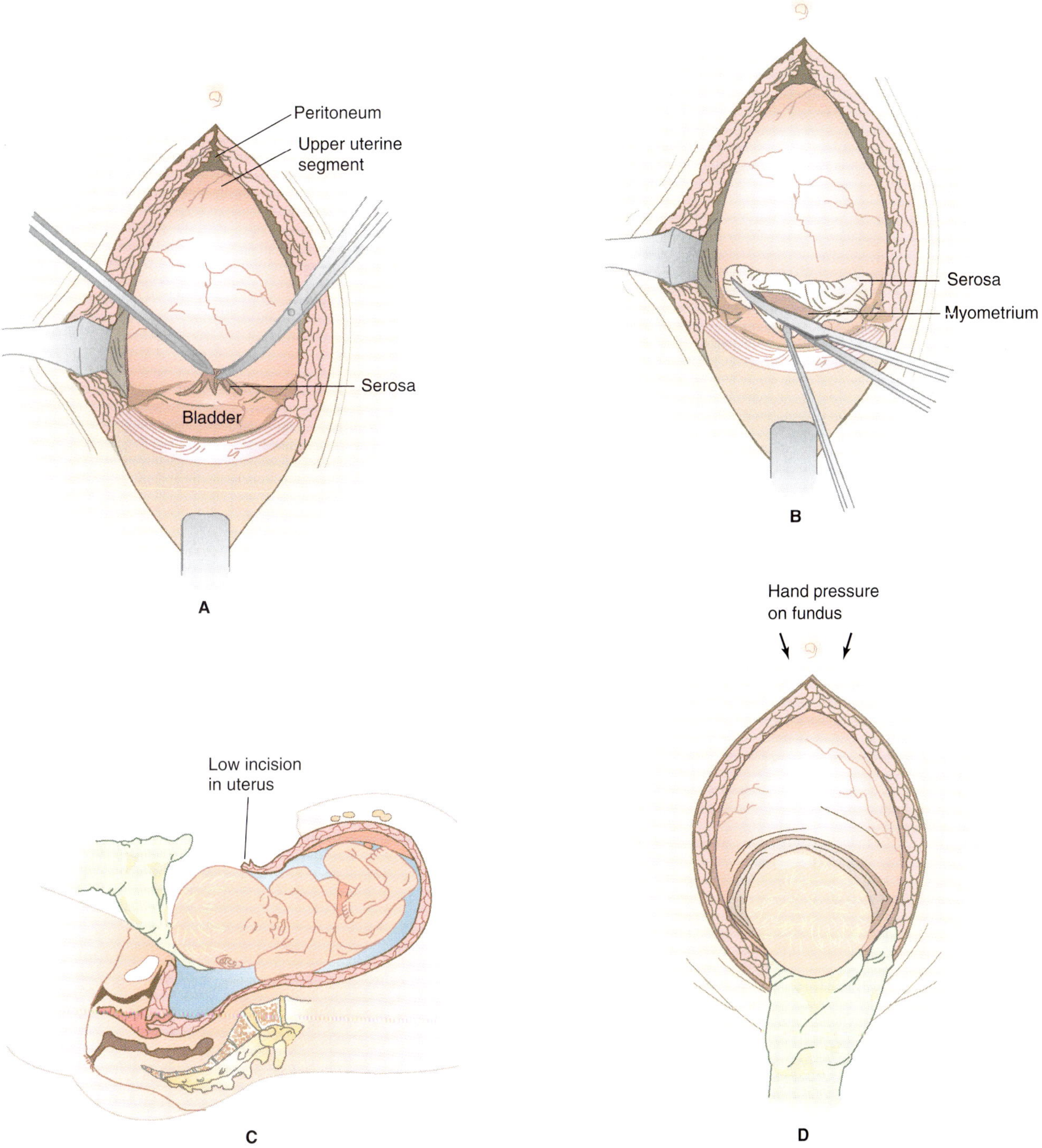

Figure 15-17. ■ Cesarean delivery. (**A**) The loose serosa is held in the forceps. The tip of the hemostat points to the upper margin of the bladder. The retractor is firm against the symphysis. (**B**) Sterile bandage scissors are used to make the incision into the loose serosa. (**C**) and (**D**) After the incisions are made into the uterus and fetal membrane, the physician reaches into the uterus between the symphysis pubis and the fetal head. The head is carefully lifted to bring it from beneath the symphysis forward through the uterine and abdominal wall. (**E**) As the fetal head is lifted through the incision, pressure is usually applied to the uterine fundus through the abdominal wall to help expel the fetus. (**F**) Infant being removed from uterus. (**A, B, C,** and **E**: Adapted, with permission, from McGraw-Hill Companies, Inc. Cunningham, F.G. et al. [1997]. *Williams obstetrics* [20th ed.]. Stamford, CT: Appleton & Lange, pp. 516, 519. **D**: Courtesy of Harriette Hartigan/Artemis. **F**: © M.C. Schlachter Photography.)

(*continued*)

E

F

Figure 15-17. ■ *Continued.*

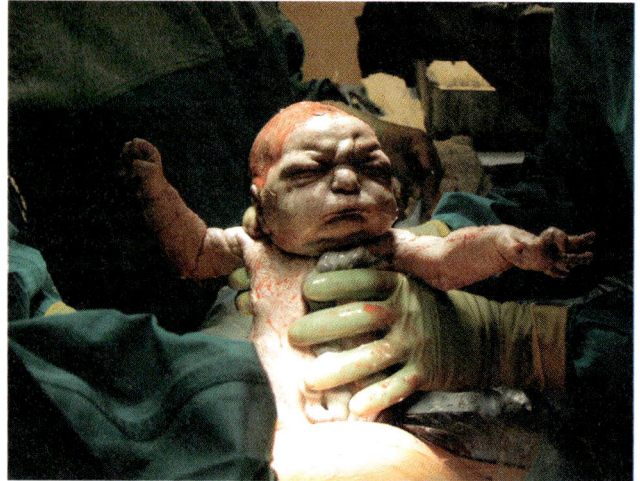

Nursing Considerations

The client will be taken to a recovery area for at least 1 hour. Vital signs will be taken at least every 15 minutes. The fundus, surgical dressing, intravenous infusion, and urinary output are monitored. The airway is maintained until the client is awake and stable. The nurse must remain at the bedside in case an emergency situation develops, requiring immediate action. Once the client is stable, she will be taken to the postpartum unit.

Postpartum care of the woman following cesarean delivery is a combination of routine postpartum care and routine postoperative care. See Chapter 16 for routine postpartum care. The breast, fundus, incision, and vaginal flow will need to be assessed every 4 to 8 hours. The urinary output should be monitored. The Foley catheter is usually removed in 12 to 24 hours. Pain is generally relieved with a patient-controlled analgesia (PCA) pump followed by oral medication within 24 to 36 hours postoperatively. The diet progresses from clear liquid to soft as active bowel sounds return. Activity progresses as tolerated by the woman. The cesarean delivery postpartum mother is usually discharged 3 to 4 days following birth.

VAGINAL BIRTH AFTER CESAREAN

At one time, once a woman had a cesarean birth, she would have a cesarean birth for all subsequent pregnancies. Today, a vaginal birth after cesarean may be possible. Success depends on the reason for the cesarean delivery, the condition of the scar tissue, and the size of the fetus.

If the first cesarean was done because of malposition or malpresentation, a vaginal birth after cesarean is more likely.

If a vertical uterine incision was made in the cesarean delivery, the risk of rupturing the uterus during labor is great. In this case, a repeat cesarean delivery will be performed.

If the first cesarean was needed because of CPD, the size of the fetus would be monitored carefully. The second fetus is often larger than the first, so a repeat cesarean delivery may be needed.

When a vaginal birth after cesarean is attempted, a uterine stimulant (Pitocin) is used with caution, and more frequent monitoring may be needed. The rate of Pitocin infusion should be carefully calculated and labor contractions must be closely monitored. If Pitocin is administered too rapidly, contractions can occur too often and with such force as to rupture the uterus. In this event an emergency cesarean delivery will be required to save the life of both the mother and fetus. When a vaginal birth after cesarean is attempted, a team of anesthesiologist, surgeon, and physician should be available in case emergency cesarean delivery is needed.

Precipitous Birth

Precipitous birth is a birth that occurs rapidly, unexpectedly, and without the attention of a physician or nurse midwife. A precipitous delivery may occur following a **precipitous labor,** one that lasts less than 3 hours.

Precipitous labor and birth increase the risk of ruptured uterus, cervical and vaginal lacerations, hemorrhage, fetal distress, and fetal cerebral trauma. Steps for assisting a

BOX 15-2 **NURSING CARE CHECKLIST**

Assisting a Woman in Precipitous Labor

If the client says "the baby is coming," the nurse should check to see if the fetus is crowning. If the baby is crowning the nurse should:

☑ Stay with the mother.

☑ Call for assistance by putting on the emergency call light. If outside the hospital, have someone call Emergency Medical Services (EMS).

☑ Remain calm and reassure the mother, instruct her to pant.

☑ If time permits, open emergency equipment, wash hands, and put on sterile gloves. If outside the hospital, provide a clean environment and as much privacy as possible.

☑ Provide a sterile or clean area for delivery.

☑ If membranes are intact, tear membranes allowing the amniotic fluid to drain.

☑ Apply gentle pressure to head with one hand to allow it to gradually be delivered. Do not apply firm pressure or try to stop the head from being delivered.

☑ Check the baby's neck for the umbilical cord, known as a **nuchal cord** (Figure 15-18). If there is a nuchal cord, and it is loose enough, slip the cord over the baby's head. If it is too tight, place two clamps on the cord and cut the cord between the clamps. Then unwind the umbilical cord from the baby's neck.

☑ Suction the baby's nose, mouth, and throat.

☑ Gently apply downward pressure to the baby's head to deliver the anterior shoulder. Then, gently lift the baby's head to deliver the posterior shoulder.

☑ Deliver the rest of the body, being careful not to drop the slippery wet baby.

☑ Suction the airway, and dry the baby.

☑ Clamp the umbilical cord in two places and cut it between the clamps, leaving at least 1 inch (2.5 cm) between the baby and the clamp (Figure 15-19). If outside of the hospital, the cord does not need to be clamped and cut until emergency medical personnel arrive. The cord should only be cut under sterile technique.

☑ Deliver the placenta, keeping all tissue for the physician to examine.

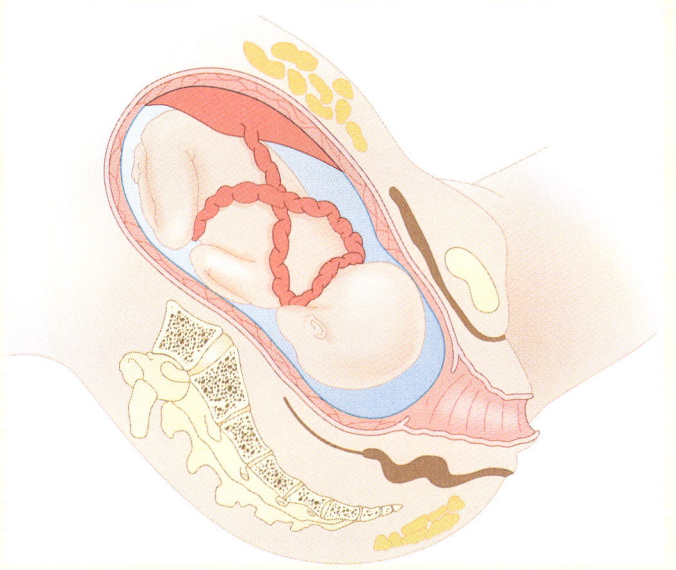

Figure 15-18. ■ Nuchal cord.

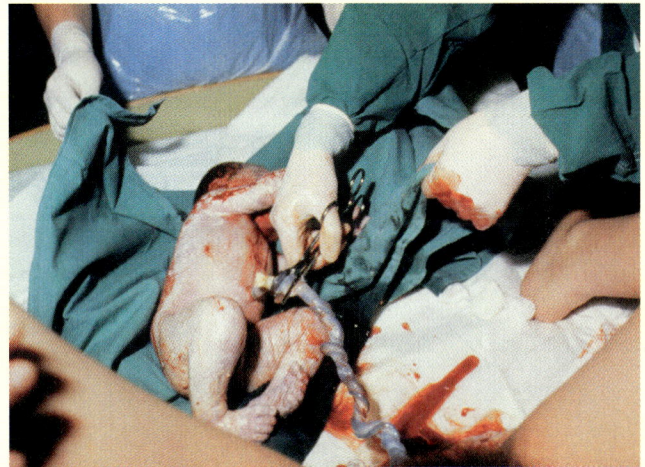

Figure 15-19. ■ Clamp and cut cord, leaving about 1 inch (2.5 cm) between the baby and the first clamp. (Photo Researchers, Inc.)

woman with a precipitous delivery are listed in Box 15-2 ■, which contains Figures 15-18 ■ and 15-19 ■.

Prolapsed Umbilical Cord

Prolapsed umbilical cord occurs when the umbilical cord emerges through the cervix before the presenting fetal part. Although the umbilical cord can become trapped between the presenting part and the pelvis at any time, it more commonly occurs when the fetal membranes rupture before the presenting part is engaged. The umbilical cord can be flushed though the cervix when the fetal membranes rupture. The presenting part then compresses the umbilical cord against the cervix and pelvis (Figure 15-20 ■).

If pressure on the umbilical cord is not relieved, the fetus will develop hypoxia and could die. When a prolapsed umbilical cord is identified, the examiner should insert two

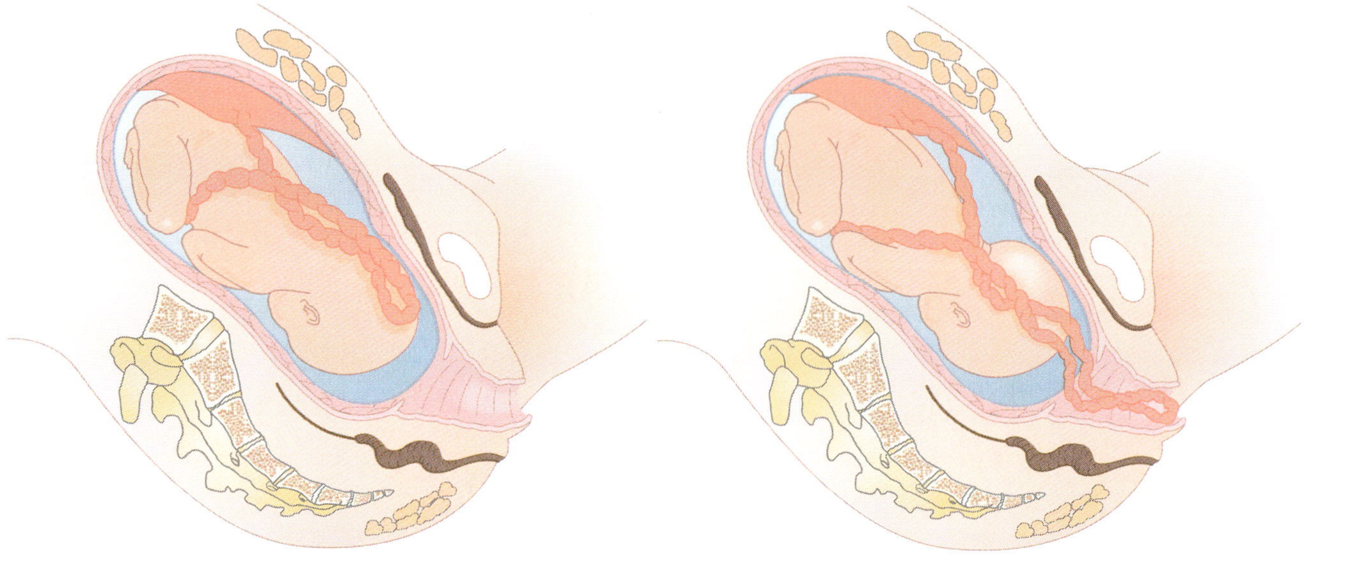

A   **B**

Figure 15-20. ■ Prolapse of the umbilical cord. (**A**) Cord at the inlet. (**B**) Cord prolapsed through the introitus. (Reproduced with permission, from McGraw-Hill Companies, Inc., from Oxorn, H. [Ed.]. [1986]. *Oxorn-Foote human labor and birth* [5th ed.]. Norwalk, CT: Appleton & Lange, p. 285.)

fingers into the vagina and apply upward pressure against the presenting part to relieve pressure on the cord.

Nursing Considerations

While upward pressure on the presenting part is maintained, the client should be turned to a knee-chest position to allow gravity to help keep the fetus away from the pelvis. If the umbilical cord protrudes from the vagina, it should be covered with wet towels to prevent shrinking of the Wharton's jelly and further compression of the umbilical vessels. The physician would be notified, and an emergency cesarean section birth would be performed.

NURSING CARE

PRIORITIES IN NURSING CARE

Priorities of care for the mother and fetus during high-risk labor and delivery include:

- Detecting complications at an early stage.
- Assisting with implementing the medical treatment and preparing for delivery.
- Evaluating the response to treatment.

ASSESSING

Assessing the high-risk mother during labor entails frequent monitoring of vital signs and the progression of labor. At times, medication to augment labor will need to

be given and must be monitored closely. When the mother is at risk, the fetus is also at risk and must be evaluated frequently.

The main method of assessing the progression of labor and well-being of the fetus is by electronic fetal monitoring. The LPN/LVN can assist with application of the monitoring equipment, should recognize normal and abnormal patterns, and should report abnormal patterns immediately to the supervising nurse.

DIAGNOSING, SPLANNING, AND IMPLEMENTING

The plan of care is designed to alleviate the complications, if possible, and to ensure birth of a healthy infant. Possible nursing diagnoses include:

- Ineffective **T**issue Perfusion
- **P**owerlessness
- Anticipatory **G**rieving

The medical and nursing plan of care might include:

- Monitor vital signs carefully. *Maternal vital signs indicate the degree to which the woman is physically coping with the labor. A woman with a preexisting medical condition will be under additional physical stress during labor and should be monitored more frequently (Figure 15-21 ■).*
- Monitor intravenous fluids. *If the woman uses her arms to support her body or legs during delivery, the*

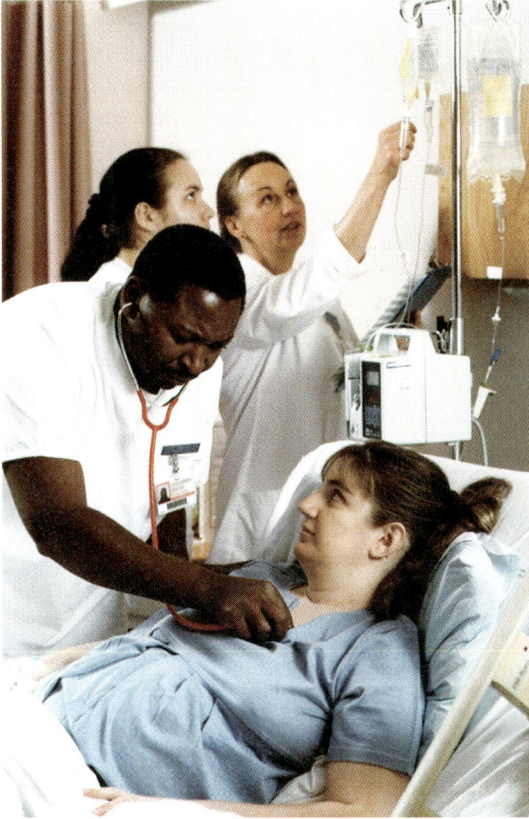

Figure 15-21. ■ When a woman with heart disease begins labor, the caregivers must monitor her closely for signs of congestive heart failure.

intravenous infusion may become dislodged or positional or may stop. Intravenous medication and fluid must be watched carefully.

- Administer medication (e.g., tocolytics or uterine stimulants) (Review Table 15-1.) *The woman must be monitored closely for side effects of medication.*
- Administer oxygen as ordered. *Oxygen may be needed for the mother, for the fetus, or for both.*
- Apply monitoring devices. *The nurse assists by attaching devices properly and efficiently.*
- Prepare for a vaginal delivery with suction extractor or forceps, or a cesarean section delivery. *It is the nurse's role to supply equipment as needed or ordered.*

EVALUATING

Evaluation of the high-risk client in labor is a minute-by-minute comparison of data to normal ranges. Decisions must be made and implemented rapidly in order to maintain the health of the mother and fetus. The role of the LPN/LVN in labor and birth is one of assisting the RN with delegated tasks.

NURSING PROCESS CARE PLAN
Caregiver of Client with Preterm Labor

A 33-week pregnant client has experienced a 10-day hospitalization for preterm labor. The physician has ordered complete bed rest with bathroom privileges only. Her husband has stayed home from work for the past 10 days to care for their 3-year-old child.

Assessment.   The following data were collected:

- Client's husband states he must go back to work.
- Husband exhibits anxiety (paces, skin pale, wrings hands often).
- States he has not slept in 36 hours.
- States he is unable to continue coaching community soccer team.
- States he is afraid his wife will not comply with bed rest if he is not at home.

Nursing Diagnosis.   The following important nursing diagnosis (among others) is established for this client:

- Caregiver Role Strain related to requirement for bed rest of spouse for preterm labor

Expected Outcome.   Husband is able to identify workable options to care adequately for wife with preterm labor.

Planning and Implementation

- Create an environment where the caregiver is comfortable relating his fears and concerns. *A trusting environment allows the client to be honest, and this will in turn allow for resolution to be sought.*
- Assist the caregiver in identifying his strengths. *Promotes a sense of self-confidence.*
- Assist the caregiver in exploring options for support. *Fears, concerns, and tasks required to manage the care of the pregnant client may be handled by persons other than the husband.*
- If other areas of support are unavailable, refer the husband to community resources. *Community resources can relieve the husband's stress.*
- Encourage the husband to choose one diversional activity weekly. *These activities allow the caregiver to retain a sense of self and helps relieve tension.*

Evaluation.   The client's husband is able to set up a weekly rotation with women from his church. He also agreed to referee one soccer game per week.

MediaLink   Delivery of Infant

Critical Thinking in the Nursing Process

1. The client states she is unsure how she will keep from getting bored every day. What suggestions could the nurse give her?
2. The physician orders home tocolytic monitoring daily for the client. Explain this process to the client.
3. What symptoms does the nurse need to teach the client with preterm labor to report immediately?

Note: Discussion of Critical Thinking questions appears in Appendix I.

Note: The reference and resource listings for this and all chapters have been compiled at the back of the book.

Chapter Review

KEY TERMS by Topic

Use the audio glossary feature of either the CD-ROM or the Companion Website to hear the correct pronunciation of the following key terms.

Factors That Create High Risk
postmaturity syndrome

Monitoring During High-Risk Labor
variability, accelerations, decelerations

Premature Rupture of Membranes
premature rupture of membranes

Amnioinfusion
amnioinfusion

Preterm Labor
preterm labor

Dystocia
dystocia, hydramnios, version

Induction of Labor
induction of labor

Assisted Births
episiotomy, lacerations, cesarean section

Precipitous Birth
precipitous birth, precipitous labor, nuchal cord

Prolapsed Umbilical Cord
prolapsed umbilical cord

KEY Points

- Complications occurring during pregnancy often place the mother and infant at risk during the birthing process.
- The mother and fetus must be monitored frequently during labor in order to identify complications early.
- The fetal heart rate must be monitored when the membranes rupture, medication is administered or dosage changed, and before and after any procedure is performed on the mother.
- The nurse must be prepared to implement nursing and medical interventions rapidly should complications develop.
- Women with multiple risk factors must be monitored more frequently during labor and birth.
- The role of the LPN/LVN in the birthing unit is one of assistance to the RN. The LPN/LVN is valuable in collecting and recording data, preparing the room for birth, preparing the surgical suite and assisting in the cesarean birth, and assisting in the recovery area.

EXPLORE MediaLink

Additional interactive resources for this chapter can be found on the Companion Website at www.prenhall.com/towle. Click on Chapter 15 and "Begin" to select the activities for this chapter.

For chapter-related NCLEX®-style questions and an audio glossary, access the accompanying CD-ROM in this book.

Animation
Delivery of infant

FOR FURTHER Study

See Chapter 9 for a complete discussion on fetal well-being.

Table 13-1 discusses a drug for lung maturation.

Normal labor and birth is discussed in Chapter 14.

See Chapter 16 for routine postpartum care.

Apgar score and newborn suctioning are discussed in Chapter 17.

See Chapter 18 for care of the high-risk newborn.

Critical Thinking Care Map

Precipitous Delivery

NCLEX-PN® Focus Area: Physiologic Integrity

Case Study: June, a 34-year-old gravida 8, para 7, was admitted 1 hour ago in labor. A vaginal examination revealed 4 cm dilation with 80% effacement. The monitor shows a contraction every 3 minutes lasting 60 to 70 seconds. She states her last labor, 14 months ago, was 4 hours long. June suddenly puts the call light on, stating "the baby is coming, the baby is coming." Upon entering the room the LPN finds the fetal membranes bulging from the perineum and the top of the fetal head visible.

Nursing Diagnosis: Risk for Trauma related to precipitous delivery

COLLECT DATA

Subjective	Objective
_____	_____
_____	_____
_____	_____
_____	_____
_____	_____
_____	_____
_____	_____

Would you report this? Yes/No

If yes, to: _____

Nursing Care

_____
_____
_____
_____
_____
_____
_____
_____
_____
_____
_____
_____

How would you document this? _____
_____
_____
_____

Compare your documentation to the sample provided in Appendix I.

Data Collected
(use only those that apply)

- Gravida 8, para 7
- 4 cm dilation
- 80% effacement
- Bulging membranes
- Contractions every 3 minutes lasting 60–70 seconds
- Crowning
- States "the baby is coming"
- Last labor 4 hours long

Nursing Interventions
(use only those that apply; list in priority order)

- Instruct June to push with each contraction.
- Leave the room and call the doctor.
- Push firmly on the perineum to prevent delivery.
- Instruct June not to push.
- Put on the emergency call light.
- Deliver baby if necessary.
- Apply gentle pressure to support perineum.
- Instruct June to breathe with each contraction.

NCLEX-PN® Exam Preparation

TEST-TAKING TIP When answering questions about high-risk labor and birth, remember LPN/LVN scope of practice. Look for answers that are both correct and within the scope of practice for LPNs/LVNs in your state.

1 A client at 34 weeks' gestation is admitted to the delivery unit with preterm labor. An amniocentesis is done to determine fetal lung maturity. Which of the following laboratory tests should the nurse monitor?

1. CBC
2. HCG
3. APTT
4. PG

2 A client who is 30 weeks pregnant was admitted 2 days ago with preterm labor. Oral terbutaline 2.5 mg every 3 hours is ordered. Which nursing measure would have the highest priority in her care?

1. Monitor closely for respiratory depression.
2. Check the pulse before each dose of terbutaline.
3. Monitor the FHR continuously.
4. Place the client on strict bed rest.

3 When admitting a client to the OB unit, the nurse notes the client has a history of IV drug use and is positive for hepatitis B (HBV+). When caring for this client, the nurse would be required to wear personal protective equipment at which of the following times? (Select all that apply.)

1. when contacting amniotic fluid
2. when contacting feces
3. when cleaning the tub after the client relaxed in the Jacuzzi
4. when touching the baby during delivery
5. when providing PO liquids for hydration

4 A gravida 3, para 2 client who is at 39 weeks' gestation is admitted to the OB unit with bright red vaginal bleeding. She states she was just walking around the house when it began. She has not had any pain. The nurse's first priority would be to:

1. determine pulse, blood pressure, and FHR.
2. prepare her for an emergency cesarean delivery.
3. inspect the perineal pad to determine the amount of bleeding.
4. position her in lithotomy position for a vaginal delivery.

5 You are a student nurse assisting in the care of a client who is in labor. If the primary nurse examines this client and finds a prolapsed cord, you realize that the nurse will most likely ask for your assistance in which of the following interventions. Choose all that apply.

1. giving medication to hasten a vaginal birth
2. keeping the client in a back lying position

3. positioning client in Trendelenburg position
4. making arrangements for emergency c-section
5. getting the cord back to its original location
6. monitoring fetal heart rate

6 The LPN/LVN is reviewing the past OB history on four clients. Which client would most likely be scheduled for a vaginal birth after cesarean (VBAC)?

1. a client with a previous vertical uterine incision
2. a client who had a previous breech delivery 3 years ago
3. a client who experienced cephalopelvic disproportion (CPD) with the last pregnancy
4. a client carrying a large fetus

7 The LPN/LVN is caring for a client who had a precipitous delivery 2 hours ago. Due to this event, it is most important that the LPN/LVN monitor for:

1. hyperthermia.
2. urinary tract infection.
3. back pain.
4. hemorrhage.

8 The LPN/LVN is caring for a client who is in preterm labor. Which of the following medication orders would be appropriate for the LPN/LVN to administer to promote lung development?

1. magnesium sulfate, 4 grams per hour via IV pump
2. ritodrine PO 10 mg q 2 hr for 24 hr
3. brethine at starting dose of 10 mcg/minute
4. betamethasone 12 mg q 24 hr, 2 to 3 days prior to delivery

9 The LPN/LVN is caring for a laboring client whose fetus is estimated to be over 10 pounds. Which of the following would most likely place the newborn at risk for a broken clavicle?

1. shoulder dystocia
2. forceps delivery
3. vacuum extraction
4. precipitous delivery

10 While caring for a laboring client, you notice decelerations in the fetal heart rate. Which of the following procedures would the LPN/LVN expect to perform?

1. Apply a fetal scalp electrode.
2. Obtain a sample of fetal blood.
3. Position client on the left side.
4. Rupture fetal membranes.

Answers for NCLEX-PN® Review and Critical Thinking questions appear in Appendix I.

Thinking Strategically About...

You are an LPN/LVN employed in a birthing center that has 15 rooms where mothers remain from admission through discharge. There is one operating room for cesarean births. Your responsibilities are to prepare the labor rooms for delivery, take the role of scrub nurse during a cesarean birth, assist with recovery of mothers following vaginal and cesarean birth, and assist with data collection during NST, triage, and early labor.

When you begin work at 3:00 P.M. there are four women and their babies who have completed the recovery period and will be discharged tomorrow morning. There are three women in labor, and a cesarean birth is scheduled for 5:00 P.M. You receive report on the following clients:

- Sitka, gravida 2, para 0, was admitted at 7:30 for an induction of labor. Contractions are every 3 minutes, lasting 50 seconds. She is 8 centimeters dilated and is 100% effaced. She has received morphine for discomfort. Her husband is at her side.

- Joan, gravida 3, para 2, was admitted at 1:30 in active labor. Contractions are every 3 to 4 minutes, lasting 45 seconds. She is 9 centimeters dilated and 90% effaced. She is using controlled breathing techniques and has had no pain medication.

- Margaret, gravida 1, para 0, was admitted 1 week ago in preterm labor with twins. She is now 37 weeks' gestation, and tests have determined the fetuses' lungs are mature. Tocolytic medication has been stopped, labor began, and Margaret is now at 6 centimeters and 80% effaced.

- Katy, a gravida 2, para 1, just arrived for a repeat cesarean birth that is scheduled for 5:00 P.M.

CRITICAL THINKING

- If one of Margaret's twins becomes distressed during labor, what questions should be asked to add the intellectual standard of *significance* to the data being used to determine the need for cesarean birth?

- With only one operating room, what data are significant in determining whether Margaret or Katy should have a cesarean birth first?

COLLABORATIVE CARE

- What nursing specialists should be contacted to assist in planning and providing care for Margaret?

MANAGEMENT OF CARE AND PRIORITIES IN NURSING CARE

- In what order will you perform your duties for the first hour?

- What is your rationale for prioritizing these duties?

DELEGATING

- What part of care for Katy can be delegated to the unit secretary (unit clerk)?

COMMUNICATION AND CLIENT TEACHING

- If Katy's cesarean must be postponed for a few hours due to Margaret's emergency cesarean, what will you tell Katy?

- What teaching and support should Sitka and her husband receive as first-time laboring parents?

DOCUMENTING AND REPORTING

- What information from Joan's labor pattern would indicate a need to get the RN to check her immediately? What would the LPN/LVN chart about Joan's labor?

CULTURAL CARE STRATEGIES

- If Sitka is of Eskimo origin, what will the nurse do differently because of her culture?

Nursing Care During the Postpartum Period

Chapter 16 **Care During the Postpartum Period**

Care During the Postpartum Period

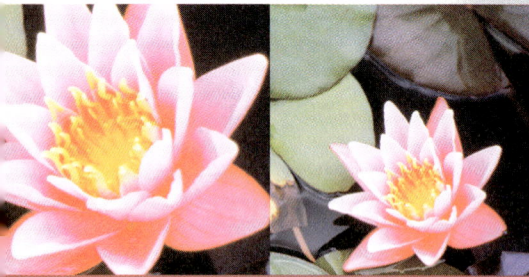

BRIEF Outline

LEARNING Outcomes

After completing this chapter, you will be able to:

1. Define key terms.
2. Describe physical changes in the mother during the postpartum period.
3. Discuss psychological changes in the mother during the postpartum period.
4. Discuss important aspects of postpartum assessment and nursing care.
5. Describe the complications commonly seen during the postpartum period.
6. Discuss client teaching about warning signs in the postpartum period.

The **puerperium** or **postpartum** period begins immediately after the birth of the baby and continues for 6 weeks, or until the woman's body has nearly returned to a prepregnant state. This chapter describes the physiologic and psychological changes that occur during the postpartum period and the nursing care of the new mother.

NORMAL POSTPARTUM CARE

Physical Changes

Every body system undergoes changes during pregnancy. Following birth, the body systems must change again and return to the nonpregnant state. Some of these changes are noticeable, whereas others are subtle.

REPRODUCTIVE SYSTEM
Uterus

The return of the uterus to the nonpregnant state is called **involution.** When the placenta separates from the uterus, the **decidua** (tissue that lines the uterine wall during pregnancy) is irregular in thickness. Over the next 3 weeks, the decidua separates from the innermost layer of the uterus (the *endometrium*; see Figure 5-11) and is expelled through the vagina. This discarded blood, mucus, and tissue is called **lochia.** The placenta attachment site contains large blood vessels. Bleeding from these vessels is controlled by contraction of the *myometrium* (muscle fibers of the uterus). The placenta attachment site heals by **exfoliation** (a shedding of the outer layer) instead of by scar formation, which would prevent uterine attachment of future pregnancies. During exfoliation, the endometrium grows from the margins and from the basal layer under the site. The superficial tissue becomes necrotic and is sloughed off. This sloughing of tissue continues for approximately 4 weeks.

To control bleeding from the large vessels at the placenta site, the uterus must remain contracted, as evidenced by the fundus remaining very firm. If blood pools in the body of the uterus, it will clot, causing the uterus to enlarge, stopping contractions, and causing more bleeding. When the uterus stops contracting, the fundus becomes soft and spongy, which is termed **boggy.** If the fundus is boggy and located above the umbilicus, bleeding is suspected. If the fundus is boggy, the nurse should massage it in a circular manner to stimulate contractions. Clots can be expelled by pushing on the fundus (discussed later in this chapter). In many facilities, expelling clots from the uterus is an RN function. It is important for the LPN/LVN to know facility policy and to communicate closely with the charge nurse if the fundus does not remain firm or if excess bleeding is noted.

The ligaments supporting the uterus in the pelvic cavity stretch during pregnancy. A full bladder can easily push the uterus up and to one side. When the fundus is higher than expected and deviated to the side, a full bladder is suspected. The displaced uterus stops contracting, leading to bleeding. To prevent excess bleeding, the nurse should teach the mother to keep the bladder empty.

The height of the fundus decreases approximately 1 centimeter per day until it is located below the symphysis pubis (Figure 16-1). Factors that enhance involution of the uterus include an uncomplicated labor, complete expulsion of the placenta and membranes, breastfeeding, and early ambulation. **Subinvolution** is the term used to describe failure of the uterus to return to its normal size.

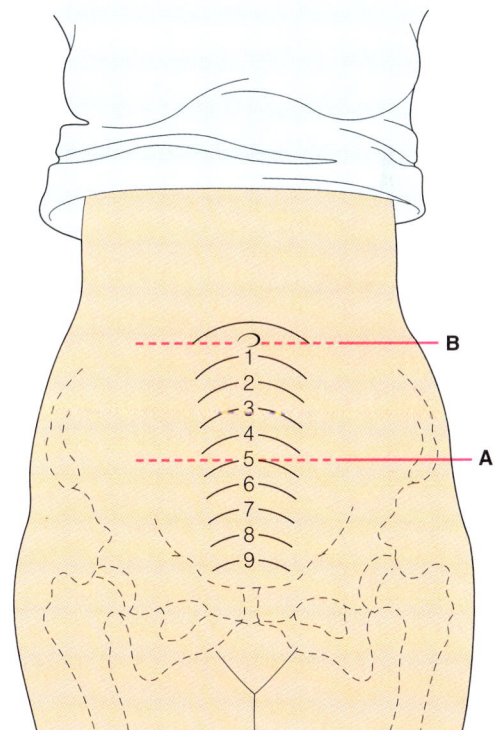

Figure 16-1. ■ Involution of the uterus. **(A)** Immediately after delivery of the placenta, the top of the fundus is in the midline and about halfway between the symphysis pubis and the umbilicus. **(B)** About 6 to 12 hours after birth, the fundus is at the level of the umbilicus. The height of the fundus then decreases about 1 fingerbreadth (about 1 cm) each day.

Factors that slow involution include a full bladder, difficult birth, grand multipara, and retained placenta or membrane fragments.

As previously stated, lochia is the tissue and fluid expelled vaginally after delivery. The total amount of lochia shed from the uterus after birth is 240 to 270 mL.

Lochia is classified by its appearance.

- **Lochia rubra** is dark red and contains epithelial cells, red blood cells, pieces of decidua, and sometimes meconium, lanugo, and vernix caseosa. It may contain small blood clots (quarter size or less), but large clots suggest the possibility of excessive bleeding and should be investigated. Approximately 3 days after delivery, the drainage changes.
- **Lochia serosa** is pinkish in color. Present from days 4 to 10, it contains serous exudate, red blood cells, mucus, and many bacteria. Gradually, the number of red blood cells decreases, again changing the color of the lochia.
- **Lochia alba** is a creamy white or pale yellow. It consists of the last pieces of decidua, white blood cells, mucus, and bacteria. Discharge of lochia alba continues for approximately 2 weeks. Once it stops, the cervix is considered to be closed, and the risk of an infection ascending from the vagina to the uterus is minimal.

It is common for an increase in lochia to be noted during or shortly after breastfeeding. Breast stimulation causes endogenous oxytocin to be released by the pituitary gland, stimulating uterine contractions and causing more lochia to be discharged.

clinical ALERT

Lochia has a slightly musty odor, but it should not be foul smelling. Foul-smelling lochia may signal infection and should be reported to the charge nurse or primary care provider.

Vagina

The vagina, cervix, and perineum appear swollen and bruised for approximately 1 week after delivery. The muscles of the vagina and perineum are flabby for several days but gradually regain tone. Kegel exercises, described in Chapter 10 ⊕, help strengthen these muscles. The edges of an episiotomy or lacerations, sutured under the skin, should be well approximated. Occasionally, a **hematoma,** an accumulation of blood under the skin, is present. A hematoma may look like a bruise, feel like a solid mass in the tissues, and can be extremely painful when touched. The primary care provider should be notified of changes in a hematoma or of any signs of infection.

By 3 weeks, the tissue returns to a nonpregnant state, and lacerations heal.

Breasts

In preparation for lactation, the breasts begin secreting **colostrum** (a thin, yellowish fluid that is high in protein) a few weeks before or shortly after delivery. Even if the mother is not breastfeeding, the mammary glands begin to fill and the breasts become enlarged. After several days without the stimulation of nursing, the milk production stops and the breast tissue becomes soft. If the mother is breastfeeding, the breasts will become engorged within 2 to 3 days. The breasts will cycle between empty and full but will remain firm until breastfeeding stops. (See Breastfeeding section of Chapter 11 ⊕ for more details.)

Ovaries

The return of ovulation and menstruation varies with each individual. For most women, ovulation and menstruation resume in 2 to 3 months, but it may take as long as 6 months. For nursing mothers, this process is usually delayed.

clinical ALERT

Some women may think of breastfeeding as a form of birth control. Teach or remind breastfeeding women that ovulation precedes menstruation. Therefore, breastfeeding is not an effective means of birth control.

MUSCULOSKELETAL SYSTEM

Abdominal Muscles

After delivery, the abdominal muscles appear flabby. It takes several months of exercise for them to regain tone. In the woman who had poor abdominal muscle tone before pregnancy or who had overdistention of the uterus, return of muscle tone may be delayed. The abdomen may remain flabby. Occasionally the abdominal muscle separates during pregnancy, resulting in **diastasis recti abdominis** (Figure 16-2 ■). If diastasis occurs, only skin, fat, and peritoneum support the abdominal contents. Inadequate support results in a pendulous abdomen and backache. Fortunately, diastasis responds well to abdominal exercise.

Pelvis

The cartilage supporting the joints of the pelvis stretches in the last months of pregnancy to allow more flexibility during delivery. The cartilage regains its firmness, but the diameter of the pelvis will never return to the nullipara state. The result is a widening of the hips. A woman who has had an epidural may have decreased sensation in her legs. This puts her at risk for falls.

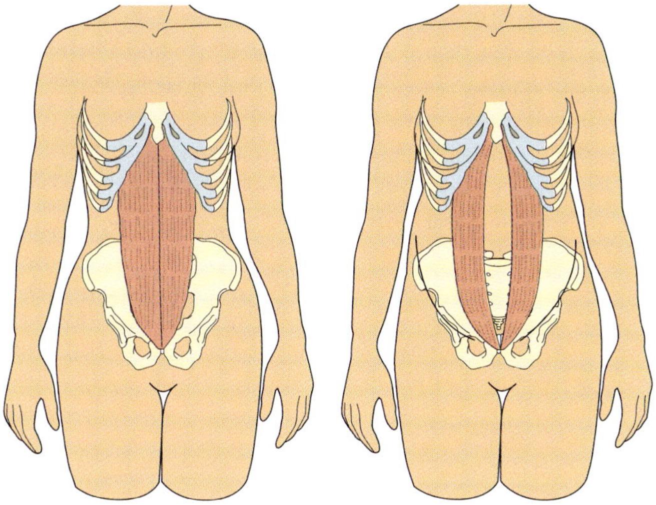

Normal location of rectus muscles of the abdomen

Diastasis recti: separation of the rectus muscles

Figure 16-2. ■ Diastasis recti abdominis, a separation of the abdominal musculature, commonly occurs after pregnancy.

GASTROINTESTINAL SYSTEM

Need to Replenish Energy

Following delivery, the woman may be hungry. She has expended a lot of energy during the birth process, and a light meal can help replace the spent calories. She usually drinks a large amount of fluid to replace what was lost in labor.

Return of Peristalsis

Peristalsis has been sluggish during pregnancy due to the effects of progesterone and the pressure of the enlarged uterus. It will take several days for peristalsis to return to normal. The woman may be reluctant to strain to defecate due to fear of perineal pain or rupturing sutures. The nurse can teach that delaying a bowel movement may increase constipation. Therefore, stool softeners and a diet high in fiber plus adequate fluid may be advised to relieve or to prevent constipation.

Postcesarean Diet

Following a cesarean birth, the woman may be placed on a liquid diet until bowel sounds are present. Her diet will then be advanced quickly. Flatulence, which adds to discomfort, may be relieved with early ambulation, antiflatulence medication, or Harris return flow (HRF) enema, if ordered.

RENAL SYSTEM

Puerperal Diuresis

Following delivery, the woman experiences diuresis (*puerperal diuresis*), which causes rapid filling of the bladder. The urinary bladder, because it is no longer compressed,

will have a greater capacity than it did during the last months of pregnancy.

Difficulty with Urination

Swelling of the perineum, urethral meatus, and surrounding structures may make urination difficult. Also, there may be a decreased sensation of bladder filling due to tissue trauma and swelling. If the woman has had an epidural she may have little or no feeling of a full bladder. There is a possibility of decreased sensation in her legs, making it unsafe for her to try to ambulate to the bathroom. Together, these aspects put the woman at risk for overfilling, incomplete emptying, and urinary retention. As mentioned, a full bladder can increase uterine bleeding as well. Catheterization may be ordered to relieve discomfort and prevent increased uterine bleeding.

If birth was by cesarean, the woman will have a Foley catheter for 12 to 24 hours. Once the catheter is removed, the woman will be encouraged to keep her bladder empty to prevent urinary tract infection and uterine bleeding.

CARDIOVASCULAR SYSTEM

Temperature

Changes in the cardiovascular system following delivery can be seen in alterations in vital signs and blood values (see Table 10-2 ⬭). During labor, the mother's temperature may have risen to 100.4°F (38°C) due to dehydration and physical exertion. Commonly, the mother begins to chill shortly after delivery. The *postpartal chill* is the result of body temperature being higher than the surrounding environment. It also results from neurologic and vasomotor changes during labor. Covering the woman with warm blankets may alleviate the chill and provide comfort. The temperature should return to normal after birth.

> **clinical ALERT**
>
> The postpartal woman should be afebrile 24 hours after delivery. If fever continues, infection should be suspected and the fever should be reported to the primary care provider.

Blood Pressure

The mother's blood pressure should remain stable following delivery. Commonly, the blood pressure rises slightly during labor and returns to the mother's baseline within 1 hour post delivery. Hypotension could indicate a reaction to medication or excessive bleeding. Hypertension, especially accompanied by headache, could indicate gestational hypertension (see Chapter 13 ⬭). If hypertension was a problem prior to labor, the blood pressure must be monitored frequently during the postpartum period.

Blood Values

Blood values should return to normal range during the postpartum period. During pregnancy, coagulation factors have been activated. Delivery trauma or decreased mobility may predispose the mother to **thrombosis** (formation of clots in blood vessels). The white blood cell count may temporarily rise to $25,000/mm^3$, with granulocytes as the predominant cell type. The hemoglobin and hematocrit may be difficult to interpret in the first few days after delivery because of rapid changes in blood volume. Excessive blood loss is not suspected until the hematocrit decreases more than two percentage points from the level on admission to the labor unit.

Many women gain 25 to 30 pounds during the pregnancy. Figure 10-9 shows how this weight gain is distributed. A woman who has gained this amount of weight during pregnancy may be able to return to prepregnancy weight during the postpartum period. She will lose 10 to 12 pounds during the birthing process. Another 5 pounds may be lost in the first few days due to puerperal diuresis. A woman who is physically active will have less difficulty with weight loss than a woman who is sedentary.

ENDOCRINE SYSTEM

Estrogen and Progesterone

Recall that one function of the placenta is to produce estrogen and progesterone to maintain the endometrium and to prevent ovulation during pregnancy. Following delivery of the placenta, the blood levels of estrogen and progesterone decline rapidly (see Table 10-2). The decline of these hormones contributes to the sloughing of the decidua. The return of the menstrual cycle usually occurs 2 to 3 months after delivery. However, because ovulation precedes menstruation, the woman can become pregnant again before the first menses.

Prolactin

Stimulation of the breast increases the production of prolactin by the anterior pituitary gland (see Figure 5-16). Prolactin is responsible for milk production by the lactiferous glands in the breast. Once lactation is well established, prolactin decreases.

Oxytocin

Oxytocin was discussed under changes in the reproductive system earlier in this chapter.

Psychological Changes

The woman needs time to adjust to the role of mother. This adjustment occurs in stages.

TAKING-IN STAGE

During the first day or two, the mother is said to be in the **taking-in stage.** She is "taking in" information about her baby, recalling the experience of delivery, and storing this information in her memory. The mother is tired and may depend on others to help meet her needs. She allows others to care for the baby, participating mainly in feeding the infant. She has a need to talk about her perception of the labor and delivery, and readily shares the experience with visitors.

TAKING-HOLD STAGE

By the third day after birth, the mother is usually ready to resume control. She is moving into the **taking-hold stage.** She is "taking hold" or control of the activities of caring for herself and her newborn (Figure 16-3 ■). She may become preoccupied with her bodily functions, such as elimination. If she is breastfeeding, she begins to be concerned about the quality and quantity of the milk. Although she is ready to meet her physical needs and the infant's needs, she may not be ready to resume responsibility for household activities. It may take several weeks for her to have the physical and mental energy to return to her full activities. In most cases, it takes 3 to 10 months for a woman to be comfortable with the role of mother.

LETTING-GO STAGE

Women and their partners discover that social interactions become increasingly important. The support of family and friends is important at this time. Mothers and fathers must

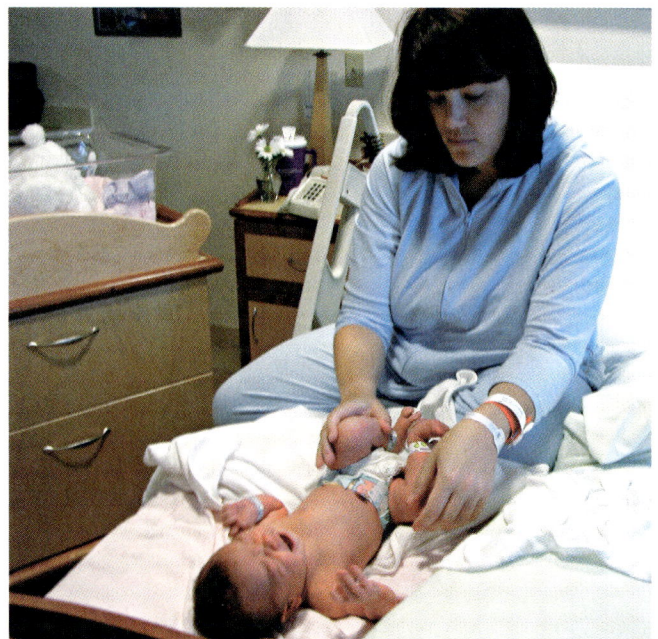

Figure 16-3. ■ As the woman takes hold of her new role, she will begin to perform care activities on the newborn.

learn to care for the infant and to make decisions about meeting the infant's needs. Obtaining information from others who have experienced parenthood is a valuable part of the normal adjustment process. Mothers who have little social interaction and support find the adjustment to motherhood more difficult.

ADOPTION

Emotional care is important for mothers who are giving their babies up for adoption. Even if a woman has decided that she does not want to keep her baby, she may still experience feelings of grief. The Health Promotion Issue on pages 394 and 395 explores this topic further.

POSTPARTUM BLUES

Postpartum blues are a transient period of mild depression that often occurs in the early postpartum period. This state may be manifested by tearfulness, feeling let down, and being unable to sleep. Postpartum blues usually begin on the third or fourth day post delivery and last for a week or two. They may be associated with changing hormone levels and psychological adjustment to motherhood. Fatigue, discomfort, and overstimulation may make postpartum blues worse. If postpartum blues persist or worsen, the woman must be evaluated for postpartum depression and postpartum psychosis, discussed in the High-Risk Postpartum section of this chapter.

Attachment Issues

During pregnancy, the woman begins to develop an emotional attachment to the infant. Personal characteristics of the mother affect the extent of attachment. For example, the woman with a high level of self-esteem enters motherhood with a more positive outlook than the mother who is depressed, angry about her situation, or overly anxious. The mother who has developed a level of trust in her own abilities will be confident in her ability to care for the infant. At the time of birth, each mother has developed an emotional attachment of some kind with the infant.

New mothers generally follow a regular pattern of behavior when meeting their infants for the first time. Touch usually begins with fingertip exploration of the infant's limbs, followed by palmar touch of the torso, and finally enfolding the infant with the entire hand and arms. As the mother spends more time with her infant, she positions the newborn so she can look into its eyes (Figure 16-4 ■). She uses her sense of sight, hearing, and touch to get to know her infant. She responds verbally to the sounds the newborn makes. She may make comments or have questions about the normality of the infant's features, especially if the delivery was difficult or if a previously delivered infant was not healthy. The mother's

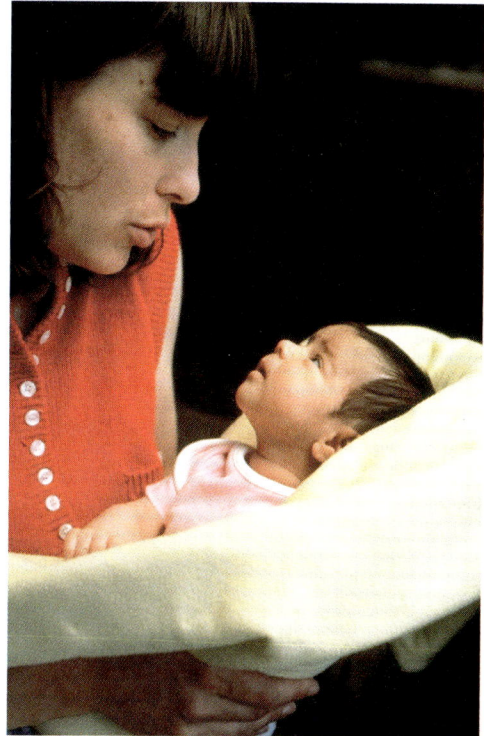

Figure 16-4. ■ Mother–child bonding is strengthened as infant and parent look into each other's eyes. (The Image Works.)

interest in and loving behaviors toward the newborn are part of the bonding process. **Bonding** is the establishment of a strong emotional attachment between two unique individuals.

Negative Feelings

The mother may have negative feelings about the baby. She may be disappointed about the baby's gender or angry that her lifestyle will need to change. Because mothers are "supposed to love their children," the mother may not express these negative feelings. If she does express them, the reaction of friends or family may be, "You don't mean that." The nurse must identify these blocks to therapeutic communication and help the mother and family explore the basis of the negative feelings.

Fathers, Siblings, and Others

Fathers, siblings, grandparents, and others also need time to bond with the infant. The father will express a strong attachment to the infant, similar to that of the mother (Figure 16-5 ■). He will demonstrate **engrossment** (a sense of interest and preoccupation) by holding, maintaining eye contact with, and talking to the infant.

Siblings and grandparents are important members of the family who also need time to develop a bond with the infant. Each family member who has the opportunity to view,

(*Text continues on page 396.*)

HEALTH PROMOTION ISSUE

PREGNANT 15-YEAR-OLD GIVING CHILD UP FOR ADOPTION

A 15-year-old female in your pediatric practice comes to the office with nausea (usually occurring in the morning), amenorrhea for the last 2 months, and breast tenderness. The nurse asks for a clean catch urine specimen and performs a rapid pregnancy test. The test is positive. Her mother asks if they can make an appointment for the following week to discuss her care and her plans for the future. Both mother and daughter are too distraught to discuss the issues today.

When they return the following week, both mother and daughter seem resigned to the pregnancy. They have discussed how they will handle the situation with the client's father, their minister, the father of the baby, and several family members. They want to pursue adoption but have some questions. Do they need to contact anyone during the pregnancy? Can they have some say in who adopts the baby? Will they ever be able to see the baby again or at least find out how the baby is doing? What does it cost to put your baby up for adoption?

DISCUSSION

Types of Adoptions

Adoptions can be confidential or open. A *confidential adoption* is a legal arrangement whereby a child is placed with a family who has been screened by an agency. The adoptive family has background information on the birth mother, but the birth mother does not know the details of the adoptive couple. In an *open adoption*, both the birth mother and the adoptive family will have some degree of exposure to one another. The birth mother can review prospective adoptive families, without knowing their names. She makes a choice from these families and never has a face-to-face meeting. Another degree of exposure between the adoptive parties would be a telephone interview, in which first names are exchanged but, again, no face-to-face meeting occurs. The parties could also meet in the prenatal period or during the selection process. Continuing contact after birth can be arranged for in the open adoption agreement. Some birth mothers desire to see the child on special occasions or just to be allowed to send cards and letters to the child. For the birth mother to have a confidential adoption, an adoption agency must be selected. These agencies can be for profit, nonprofit, or sponsored by certain religions. Some agencies provide counseling to both the birth mother and other family members of her choosing. They may also provide medical and legal assistance.

Open adoptions are more typically handled by an attorney. Open adoptions are not legal in every state. Some states allow the adoptive parents to cover the legal fees for the birth mother. In the states where this is not allowable or if the adoptive parents are not willing to cover these expenses, the birth mother may need to apply for legal aid in her community.

There are several ways a birth mother can find families who want to adopt a child. Some families run advertisements in the newspaper. Local physicians may be able to refer families in their practice who want to adopt. Some communities have prospective adoptive parent support groups who would be able to provide a list of families desiring to adopt. Also the National Adoption Information Clearinghouse provides a matching service for parties interested in adoption.

PLANNING AND IMPLEMENTATION

The nurse should help the birth mother explore her desires for the child's life. The following questions would be appropriate: Is it important to you to have a say in who adopts your child? Will it matter what type of family the child lives with—a single parent, a

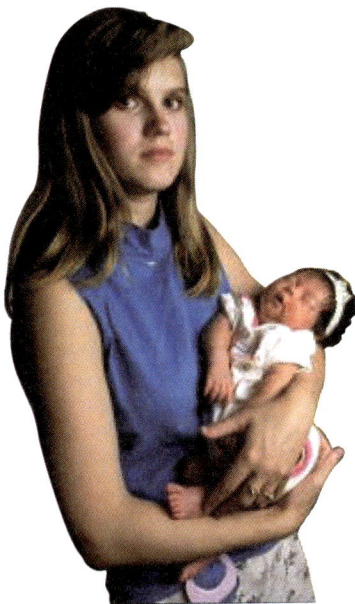

nuclear family? It is okay with you if a homosexual couple adopts your child? Does the race of the family matter? Does the religion of the family matter? Do you think that the family should have substantial amounts of money? Do you desire for the child to have siblings? Would you rather the child live in the city or in the country? Do you have any medical history that it would be important to share with an adoptive family?

It is important for the nurse to determine the birth mother's motivation for deciding to put her child up for adoption. The following questions could assist in this process: Is anyone trying to coerce you, shame you, embarrass you, or provide you with a bribe to adopt your child? Is your decision solely based on your desires? The nurse should ask the birth mother who she has consulted with regarding her decision.

The nurse can assist the birth mother to understand the permanence of adoption. The long-term stability of the adoptive child is partly determined by the birth mother's decision to totally relinquish any control over the child's life. This is not to say that the birth mother may never contact her child later in life. Following a confidential adoption, records are not available to either party. There are, however, several agencies that provide a registry for

birth parents and the adoptee to gain contact information. The registries include Concerned United Birth Parents, American Adoption Congress, and the International Soundex Reunion Registry. For private adoptions, a letter containing contact information for the birth mother can be held by the attorney who handled the adoption. If the adoptee decides that he or she wants to contact the birth mother, the attorney can forward the letter to him or her.

When the birth mother makes a firm decision to put her baby up for adoption, the nurse can be instrumental in providing her with the necessary resources. Contact information for community adoption agencies and/or legal services can be provided. Referrals to support groups for birth mothers would provide emotional support for the teenage girl. If there are no support groups available, a counselor could provide this emotional support. The birth mother will experience a wide range of emotions. She may feel guilt, shame, sorrow, and grief. She may also feel relief. It is important for the nurse to include in the plan of care a mechanism for follow-up visits to monitor her emotional health. The nurse should assess the level of support available to the birth mother. Birth mothers should have someone they can rely on to give them support and encouragement when they experience doubt. The nurse can

encourage activities to assist the birth mother in dealing with her emotions. These activities could include journaling her thoughts, or creating a scrapbook of the pregnancy and birth experience. In 1990, Mary Jean Wolsh-Marsh created Birth Mother's Day to be celebrated on the Saturday before Mother's Day in May. Ms. Wolsh-Marsh wanted a day to commemorate the sacrifice of birth mothers who had lost a child to adoption. Birth mothers may find solace in this type of celebration.

The nurse can also assist the birth mother in making future plans for herself. The birth mother should be encouraged to express her hopes and dreams for the future. The nurse could be instrumental in helping the birth mother take action to make these dreams a reality.

SELF-REFLECTION

What are your feelings about teenage pregnancy? If your teenage daughter were pregnant, what would you counsel her to do? Why? Do you know anyone who grew up in an adoptive home? How would you characterize their life? What are the benefits of adoption to the pregnant woman? To the infant? What do you see as the negative aspects of adoption to the pregnant woman? To the infant?

SUGGESTED RESOURCES

For the Nurse

Narad, C., & Mason, P. (2004). International adoption: Myths and realities. *Pediatric Nursing, 30* (6) 6, 483–487.

Salladay, S. (2004). Ethical problems: Adoption dilemmas. *Nursing, 34* (12), 29.

For the Client

Russell, M. (2004). *Adoption wisdom: A guide to the issues and feelings of adoption.* Santa Monica, CA: Broken Branch Productions.

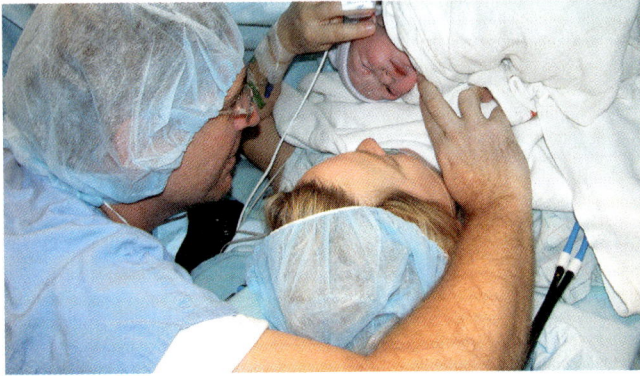

Figure 16-5. ■ The father's intense concentration shows engrossment in his new child.

BOX 16-1   CULTURAL PULSE POINTS

Beliefs and Practices Related to the Postpartum Period
Cultures may have taboos concerning reactions during labor, presence of men, position for delivery, preferred types of health practitioners, and location of the birth. A new mother may need to follow practices of her culture in the postpartum period related to bathing, cord care, exercise, foods, and roles of men. Some cultures even have specific practices related to care and disposal of the placenta.

Source: Ramont, R. P., Niedringhaus, D. M., & Towle, M. A. (2006). *Comprehensive nursing care.* Upper Saddle River, NJ: Prentice Hall, Box 42-1, p. 1117.

hold, and interact with the infant will begin to establish a relationship. With open visiting hours and rooming-in practices, family bonding can begin early.

Cultural Influences in the Postpartum Period

The mother's beliefs about hygiene, food choices, and activity during the postpartum period are influenced by her culture. Western culture places a great deal of emphasis on the birth process itself. Other cultures place more emphasis on postpartum practices. Many women of European heritage want to eat a full meal and drink plenty of cold fluids in the belief that they will replace the nutrients lost during the delivery process. They will want to shower right away, wash their hair, and put on a clean gown.

The women of Mexican, Asian, and African descent often avoid cold, including cold air, food, and drink. They may put off showering to prevent a chill.

Certain cultures teach choices that are meant to help the woman regain harmony or a balance between "hot and cold" within the body. They may avoid heat, including some foods that are considered "hot."

In most Native American cultures, family plays an important role during the postpartum period. The baby's grandmother is the primary helper and teacher for the new mother. She brings experience and knowledge, and allows the new mother time to rest and regain her strength. Some other areas of cultural beliefs and practices related to the postpartum period are provided in Box 16-1 ■.

If the mother's beliefs are different from those of the nurse, the physician, or hospital practices, adjustments may need to be made. It is the nurse's responsibility to advocate for the rights of the mother, father, and family.

NURSING CARE

PRIORITIES IN NURSING CARE

The nurse may use the mnemonic of BUBBLE to help remember important areas of assessment: **B**—breasts, **U**—uterus, **B**—bowel, **B**—bladder, **L**—lochia, **E**—episiotomy/incision.

The first priority for nursing care in the postpartum period is to assess for complications that may slow or prevent the mother from returning to the prepregnant state of health. Some complications may threaten the mother's life if they are not treated promptly.

The second priority is to teach the mother how to care for herself and her infant.

ASSESSING

The postpartum assessment begins by obtaining information about the pregnancy and delivery. This information is used to identify the risk of postpartum complications. Table 16-1 ■ identifies common risk factors and areas that must be included in the assessment. The greater the degree of risk, the more frequently the assessment must be made.

Many parts of the assessment are the same as for any other client. For example, monitoring vital signs and observing for an increase in bloody drainage is the same for the postpartum woman as it is for the postsurgical client. Listening to heart sounds, lung sounds, and bowel sounds is the same as for any other client. The LPN/LVN must know the normal findings in order to report abnormal readings to the charge nurse or physician. Only those parts of the assessment that are particular to the postpartum client will be included here. While performing the assessment, the nurse has an opportunity to teach the

TABLE 16-1

Postpartum Risk Factors and Areas of Assessment

RISK FACTOR	IMPLICATIONS	AREA TO ASSESS
Cesarean section birth	Risk for impaired healing Risk for paralytic ileus Risk for urinary retention	Incision pain every 2–4 hours Incision for infection and healing Bowel sounds, flatus every 2–4 hours Voiding after catheter removed
Prolonged labor	Risk for exhaustion Risk for nutrition and fluid depletion Risk for uterine atony and hemorrhage	Verbalizes adequate rest Intake, output, % of diet consumed Fundus firmness every 1–2 hours Amount of lochia every 1–2 hours Vital signs every 1–2 hours
Precipitous delivery	Risk for uterine atony, hemorrhage Risk for lacerations of birth canal	Fundus firmness every 1–2 hours Amount of lochia every 1–2 hours Vital signs every 1–2 hours
Delivery complications (retained placenta, lacerations)	Risk for lacerations of birth canal Risk for hemorrhage	Fundus firmness every 1–2 hours Amount of lochia every 1–2 hours Vital signs every 1–2 hours
Diabetes	Risk for insulin regulation Risk for periods of hyperglycemia and hypoglycemia Risk for poor wound healing	Obtain blood glucose readings every 2–4 hours Signs of hyper- and hypoglycemia Episiotomy or incision for healing
Gestational hypertension or preeclampsia	Risk for neurologic and cardiovascular damage	Vital signs every 1–2 hours Reflexes and clonus every 1–2 hours Headache and blurred vision
Overdistended uterus (large fetus or multiple gestation)	Risk for uterine atony and hemorrhage	Fundus firmness every 1–2 hours Amount of lochia every 1–2 hours Vital signs every 1–2 hours

new mother about normal body changes and signs of complications.

Vital Signs

The vital signs should be assessed first. Vital signs were assessed every 15 minutes during the first hour after delivery. When the vital signs are stable and within normal range, the time interval between measurements is lengthened. Vital signs should be recorded every 30 minutes for an hour, every hour for 2 hours, every 2 hours for 4 hours, and then every 4 hours. By the second to third postpartum day, the vital signs can be taken once every 8 hours, as long as they have remained stable.

Abnormal findings direct the nurse to pay closer attention to other areas of the assessment. For example, if the temperature is elevated, the nurse should assess for signs of infection. An elevated temperature coupled with premature or prolonged rupture of membranes prior to delivery may indicate a genital infection. Further assessment of the uterus and lochia may be indicated. A slight elevation in pulse is expected in the early postpartum period, but the pulse should return to a normal range within the first 24 hours. Tachycardia after 24 hours can indicate hemorrhage, so further assessment is needed. Tachypnea is also an indication of respiratory stress to the body and should be investigated.

The blood pressure should remain consistent with the baseline blood pressure during pregnancy. As excess body fluids are eliminated during the first few weeks postpartum, the blood pressure should return to the prepregnant state.

clinical ALERT

A marked elevation in blood pressure in the first 24 to 36 hours postpartum could be an indication of gestational hypertension and should be reported. If gestational hypertension occurred prior to delivery, the blood pressure should begin to decrease in the first few days postpartum.

Respiratory System

In the third trimester, the pregnant uterus prevents full expansion of the lungs, trapping secretions in the small airways. Pain medication given during labor also depresses respiration and contributes to the risk of respiratory complications. It is important for the nurse to assess respiratory function, including lung expansion, airway clearance, and gas exchange. An elevated temperature, cough, and abnormal breath sounds indicate mucus buildup in the lungs. To facilitate respiratory function, the woman should be encouraged to deep breathe and cough every 2 hours. An inspiratory spirometer and antibiotics may be ordered.

Pain

Pain should decrease during the postpartum period. Any increases in pain or swelling of incisions or perineal lacerations should be reported promptly. There will be some discomfort as breasts fill. The nurse can teach the mother to know whether discomfort is within a normal range. Breastfeeding mothers, especially multiparas, should be taught that afterpains may be strong during feedings.

New mothers experience pain from engorged breast tissue, the traumatized perineum or abdominal surgical site, and uterine contractions. **Afterpains,** or discomfort from uterine contractions after delivery, occur in most women but are generally more noticeable in multipara mothers. They are stronger during breastfeeding because breast stimulation causes release of oxytocin (see Figure 5-16 🔗), which stimulates contractions. Oral analgesics may be prescribed for discomfort.

Nursing mothers may express concern about the effect of pain medication on the infant. The nurse should explain to the mother that pain can make her tense and anxious, which may decrease milk production. The nurse should also explain that some analgesics may be excreted in breast milk. This medication will not harm the infant but would make the infant sleepy. It is important, therefore, for the mother to feed the infant before she takes the analgesic.

Breasts

The breast assessment begins with checking the bra for design and fit. The postpartum mother should wear a well-fitting bra at all times. The bra should provide support to prevent the weight of the breast from stretching the supporting ligaments and connective tissue. A nursing bra with proper fit provides the needed support and should be used even by nonnursing mothers. The straps should be made of cloth instead of elastic. The back should be wide, with at least three rows of hooks to adjust the fit. The cups of a nursing bra have a supportive inner cup and a partial outer cup that can be unhooked for breastfeeding. Cotton is often recommended instead of synthetic material because it "breathes" and does not hold perspiration inside against the woman's skin.

The bra should be removed so the breasts can be inspected and palpated. The breasts should be inspected for redness and cracked or inverted nipples. The breasts should be palpated for softness, slight firmness associated with filling, or firmness associated with full or engorged glands. Warmth and tenderness should also be noted. Colostrum or milk may drain from the nipple. The mother should be taught to report signs of complications, such as redness, heat, and pain. These may signify mastitis (discussed in the High-Risk Postpartum Care section). She should also report cracked, sore nipples.

Abdomen

To assess the abdomen accurately, the urinary bladder must be empty and the mother should be supine. Placing one hand on the symphysis pubis to support the uterus, the nurse places the middle finger of the other hand on the umbilicus and pushes down on the abdomen to palpate the location of the fundus.

clinical ALERT

Support of the uterus is crucial when palpating the abdomen. Pressure on the fundus without the hand supporting the uterus at the symphysis could lead to uterine prolapse.

The fundus should be firm, in the midline, and between the umbilicus and symphysis. The distance from the umbilicus is measured in finger widths (also called fingerbreadths) and recorded as a number above or below the umbilicus. The following are two methods of documenting the information:

1. For finger widths above the umbilicus, write the number before a capital U (1 finger width above the umbilicus = 1 U). For finger widths below the umbilicus, write the number after a capital U (e.g., 2 finger widths below the umbilicus = U 2). *OR*
2. You may write the number, followed by FB for fingerbreadth(s) and an arrow up, followed by U (for 1 fingerbreadth above the umbilicus, write: 1 FB ↑ U). For fingerbreadths below the umbilicus, write the number, followed by FB, an arrow down, and a capital U (e.g., 2 fingerbreadths below the umbilicus = 2 FB ↓ U).

If the fundus is not firm or in the proper location (Figure 16-6 ■), complications should be suspected. Procedure 16-1 ■ illustrates the proper technique for assessing the fundus.

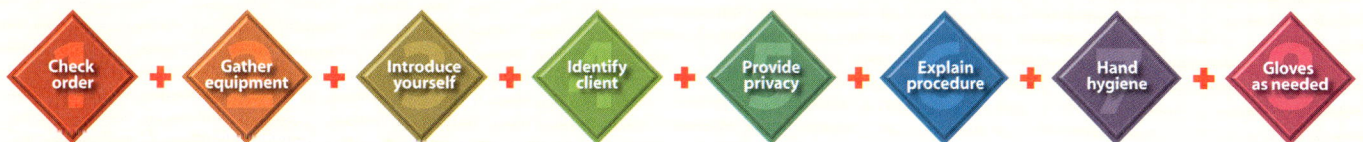

Figure 16-6. ■ The uterine fundus becomes displaced and deviated to the right when the bladder is full.

Fundus

Full bladder

If the fundus is boggy, the LPN should begin to massage the fundus gently in a circular manner. Procedure 16-2 ■ reviews the proper procedure for fundal massage. If the fundus does not regain or maintain firmness within a few minutes, the LPN/LVN should summon assistance. The RN or physician may apply strong pressure on the fundus to remove clots. As mentioned, this is generally not an LPN/LVN function. There is a risk of uterine prolapse if the procedure is not done properly.

The abdomen of the woman who has had a cesarean section delivery should be assessed as for any other abdominal surgical client. The abdomen may be tender, so palpation must be done gently. Bowel sounds should be assessed, and the mother should be asked about the passage of flatus. The abdominal dressing should be assessed for abnormal drainage. The incision should be assessed for signs of infection and healing. Generally, the doctor orders the skin clips, staples, or sutures to be removed several days after surgery.

PROCEDURE 16-1 **Fundal Assessment**

Purpose

■ To assess the fundus for complications following delivery

Equipment

■ Clean exam gloves
■ Clean perineal pad
■ Impervious (leak-proof) bag

Check order + **Gather equipment** + **Introduce yourself** + **Identify client** + **Provide privacy** + **Explain procedure** + **Hand hygiene** + **Gloves as needed**

Interventions and Rationales

1. Perform preparatory steps (see icon bar above).

2. Ask the woman to void. *A full bladder can cause the uterus to deviate from midline and produce uterine atony and hemorrhage.*

3. Position the woman supine with the knees slightly flexed and her head on a pillow. *Flexing the knees relaxes abdominal muscles. The supine position prevents falsely high measurement of the fundal height.*

4. Gently place one hand on the lower uterine segment just above the pubic symphysis. With the other hand, gently palpate the abdomen until the fundus is located (Figure 16-7 ■). The fundus should feel like a hard mass about the size of a large grapefruit. *One hand*

supports and stabilizes the uterus to prevent prolapse, while the other determines the location and condition of the fundus.

5. If the fundus is boggy, gently massage the fundus in a circular motion while continuing to support the lower uterine segment. If the fundus does not become firm within a few minutes, summon assistance by using the call light. *A boggy uterus indicates uterine bleeding that could lead to hemorrhage. Gentle massage stimulates uterine contractions. Do not leave the client when there is risk of hemorrhage.*

6. Measure the height of the fundus in fingerbreadths above, below, or at the umbilicus. *The fundal height is useful in determining the degree of involution.*

7. Determine the location of the fundus in relation to the midline of the body. If the fundus is not in the midline,

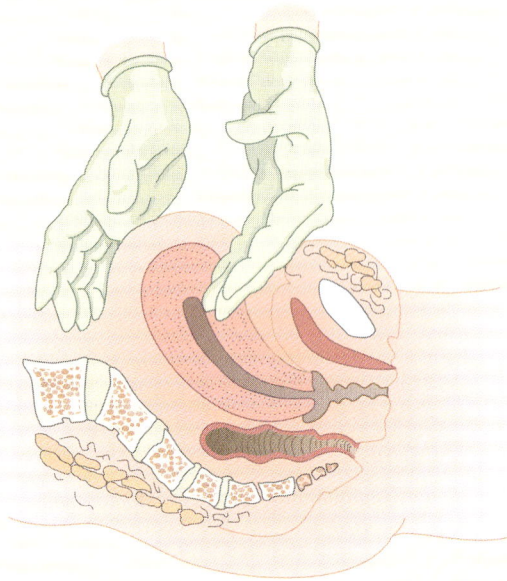

A

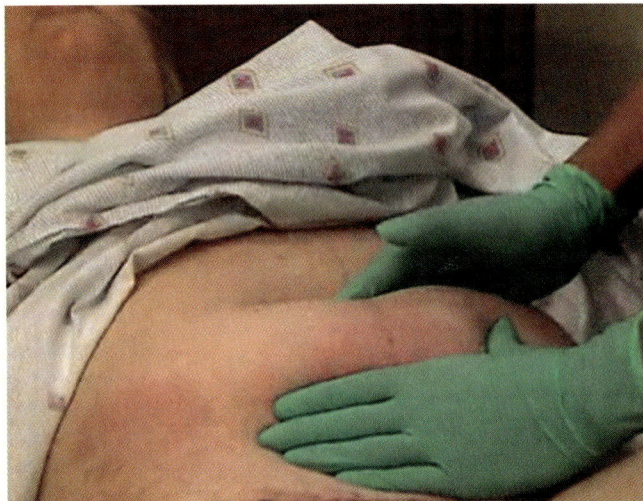

B

Figure 16-7. ■ **(A)** Position of hands to palpate the uterus, assess its firmness, and promote contraction. **(B)** Nurse palpating uterus.

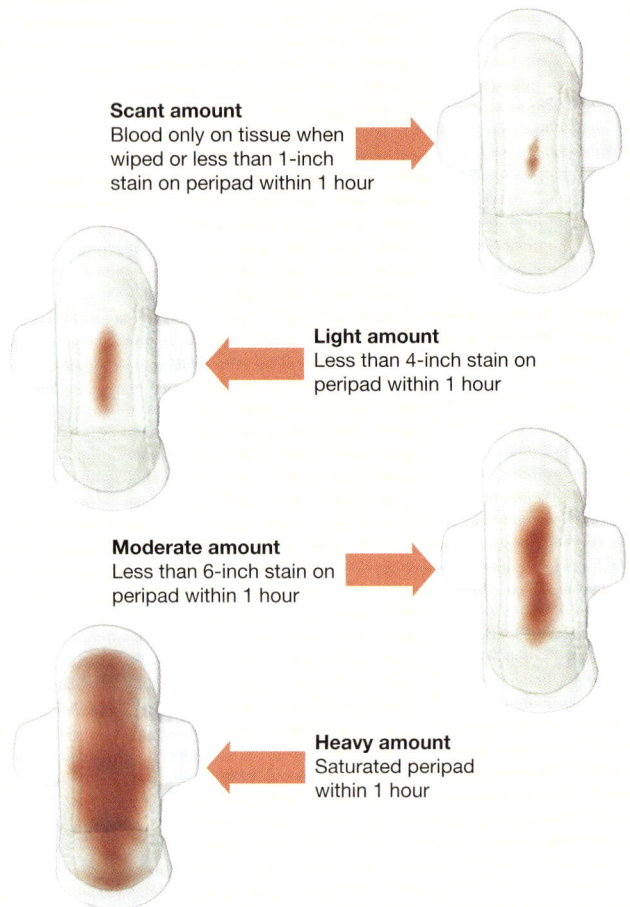

Scant amount
Blood only on tissue when wiped or less than 1-inch stain on peripad within 1 hour

Light amount
Less than 4-inch stain on peripad within 1 hour

Moderate amount
Less than 6-inch stain on peripad within 1 hour

Heavy amount
Saturated peripad within 1 hour

Figure 16-8. ■ Suggested guidelines for assessing lochia volume.

weeks of pregnancy, the uterus may be tipped in that direction.

8. Look at the perineal pad to determine the volume, color, and consistency of lochia (Figure 16-8 ■). *The lochia should be red, of moderate amount, and without clots.*

9. Provide the woman with a clean perineal pad. Dispose of all contaminated articles in the impervious bag following standard precautions. *A clean pad decreases the risk of infection and provides a point from which to assess future blood loss. Standard precautions prevent the spread of infection.*

10. Document the completion and findings of the procedure. *This provides a record of the intervention and data for ongoing assessment of the mother's progress.*

SAMPLE DOCUMENTATION

(date/time)   Fundus in midline, 2 FB ↓ U.
              Moderate amt lochia rubra
              without clots. Peripad
              changed. M. Rodriguez, LVN

evaluate for a full bladder. *A full bladder can push the uterus up and to one side, and may result in uterine atony.*

a. If the woman did not empty her bladder before the procedure and the fundus is not in the midline, the bladder may be full. The client should be asked how long it has been since she has voided. If it has been longer than an hour, the woman should be assisted to the bathroom to void. The mother should then return to bed, and the fundus should be reassessed. *The bladder will fill rapidly in the postpartum period. Assessment with a full bladder does not provide accurate data.*

b. If the bladder is empty and the fundus remains off center, ask the mother about the position of the baby in the last few weeks of pregnancy. *If an infant lies mostly on one side of the uterus during the last few*

Removing Clots from the Uterus

Purpose

■ To remove clots from the uterus in order to evaluate the amount of uterine bleeding and prevent hemorrhage

Equipment

■ Clean exam gloves
■ Clean blue underpad
■ Clean perineal pad
■ Washcloth and warm water
■ Impervious bag

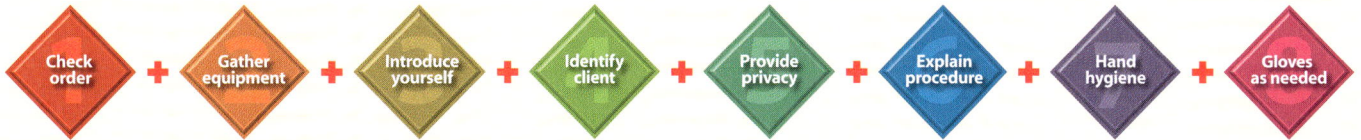

Check order + **Gather equipment** + **Introduce yourself** + **Identify client** + **Provide privacy** + **Explain procedure** + **Hand hygiene** + **Gloves as needed**

Interventions and Rationales

1. Perform preparatory steps (see icon bar above).

2. Assess the fundus as outlined in Procedure 16-1. *Assessment of the fundus determines the need for blood clot removal. If the fundus is boggy and above the umbilicus, blood clots are suspected.*

3. Gently massage the fundus to stimulate contractions. *The fundus must be firm in order to remove clots safely.*

4. Explain to the woman the need to remove clots. The procedure will be uncomfortable but should only last a few minutes. *Explanation should help the woman to relax.*

5. Supporting the lower uterine segment, apply firm pressure from the fundus toward the vagina (Figure 16-9 ■). Observe the perineum for expulsion of blood clots. *Uterine support is necessary to prevent prolapse of the uterus* (Figure 16-10 ■).

6. Reassess the fundus for firmness and location. *The fundus should regain tone once clots are removed.*

7. Remove all bloody pads, provide a wash to the perineum, and apply a clean blue underpad and perineal pad. Follow standard precautions for disposal of contaminated articles. *Cleanliness promotes comfort. All bloody supplies may need to be saved until the amount of blood loss is determined. Following standard precautions prevents the spread of infection.*

8. Assess the fundus every 15 minutes until it remains firm for a minimum of 1 hour. *If the fundus becomes boggy, further bleeding could occur.*

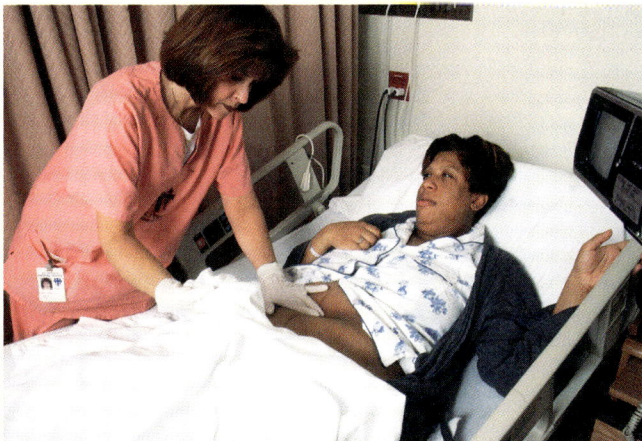

Figure 16-9. ■ Nurse removing clots from uterus. Note that lower hand supports the uterus.

SAMPLE DOCUMENTATION

(date/time)   Fundus boggy and 2 FB ↑ U. Fundus massaged until firm. Manual fundal pressure applied resulting in approximately 10-cm blood clot. Fundus regained tone at U. Dr. Williams notified. K. Chi, RN

(date/time)   Fundus assessed every 15 minutes. Fundus firm at U. Moderate amount red lochia noted on peripad. A. Adams, LPN

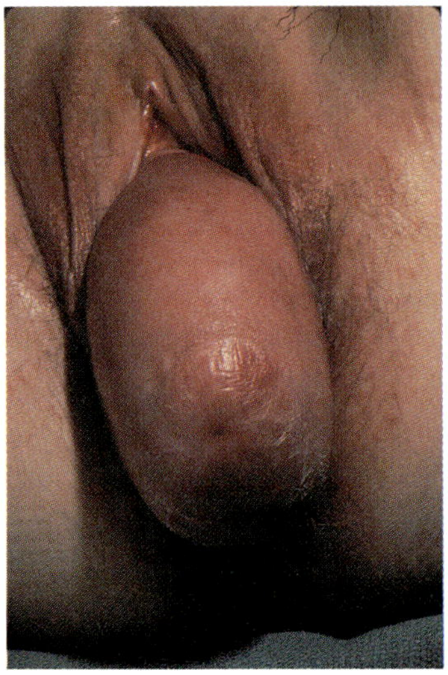

Figure 16-10. ■ Complete uterine prolapse with inversion of the vagina.

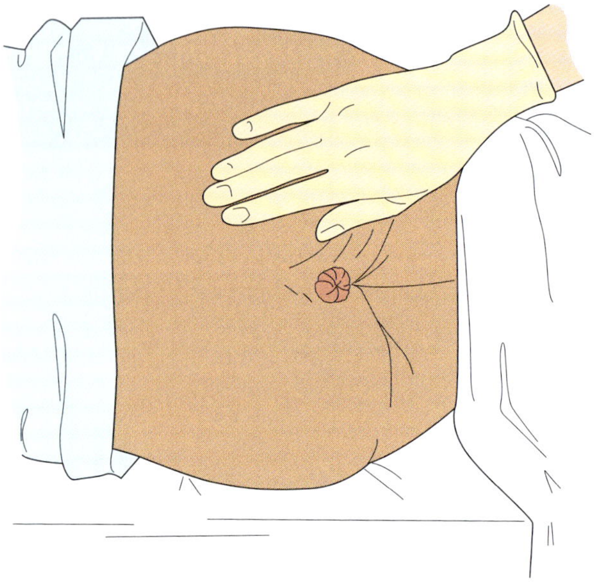

Perineum

The assessment of the perineum includes determining the amount of lochia and inspecting the true perineum. The nurse evaluates the lochia for amount, consistency, color, and odor. During the first 1 to 3 days, the lochia will be red with a few small clots. The passage of many small clots or a large clot is not normal. If this occurs, the cause should be investigated. See Figure 16-8, which illustrates suggested guidelines for assessing the volume of lochia.

There should never be more than a moderate amount of lochia. However, the amount of lochia on the perineal pad is influenced by the length of time the pad is in use and by the woman's activities (e.g., walking). Ask the woman when she changed the pad last, the amount of lochia on the pad, and the presence of any clots. If heavy bleeding is reported or suspected, change the pad, have the woman remain in bed, and reassess in 1 hour. Do not discard the saturated pads, but save them in the bathroom until the bleeding is controlled and the physician has determined the estimated blood loss. In some cases, the physician will ask that the saturated pads, blue underpads, and bloody linen be weighed to determine blood loss.

Assess the odor of lochia. It should be similar to the odor of menstruation and should never be strong or foul. The cause of foul or offensive odor should always be investigated. A specimen may need to be obtained for culture and sensitivity.

To assess the perineum, position the mother in left Sims' position and lift the buttocks to expose the true perineum (Figure 16-11 ■). Observe for discoloration, bruising, and generalized swelling. If an episiotomy or lacerations were repaired, the tissue should be well approximated. Generally, stitches are not visible. Report signs of infection or wound dehiscence to the physician. If hemorrhoids are present, assess for bleeding and tenderness. Generally, the swelling of

Figure 16-11. ■ Intact perineum with hemorrhoids. Note how the nurse's hand raises the upper buttocks.

hemorrhoid tissue resolves in a few weeks. Procedure 16-3 ■ details steps in perineal assessment.

Swelling of the perineum can make voiding difficult. Urinary output should be measured for at least the first two voidings after delivery. The woman should be encouraged to void every 2 to 4 hours. If the bladder can be palpated or urinary retention is suspected, further assessment with a bladder scan may be necessary, and the woman may require urinary catheterization.

It may be several days before bowel elimination occurs due to slowing of peristalsis during pregnancy. If the woman has had a large episiotomy or laceration, the resulting swelling, pain, and fear of tearing the tissue may make defecation difficult. The woman can prevent constipation by increasing her intake of oral fluids, eating a diet high in fiber, and ensuring early ambulation. At times, a stool softener is ordered. Complementary therapy may also be useful (Box 16-2 ■).

BOX 16-2	COMPLEMENTARY THERAPIES

Use of Lysine for Episiotomies

Lysine, an essential amino acid, has been identified as a supplement that decreases the incidence of pain following an episiotomy. Lysine is available as a supplement. The recommended adult dosage is 12 mg/kg of body weight per day. Lysine is also present in dietary sources, including meat, cheese, fish, eggs, soybeans, and nuts.

Source: Ladewig, P., London, M., & Davidson, M. (2006). *Contemporary maternal–newborn nursing care* (6th ed.). Upper Saddle River, NJ: Prentice Hall, p. 801.

Perineal Assessment

Purpose

- To assess the perineum for signs of healing and complications following delivery

Equipment

- Clean exam gloves
- Clean perineal pad
- Small light such as a pen light may be necessary
- Impervious bag

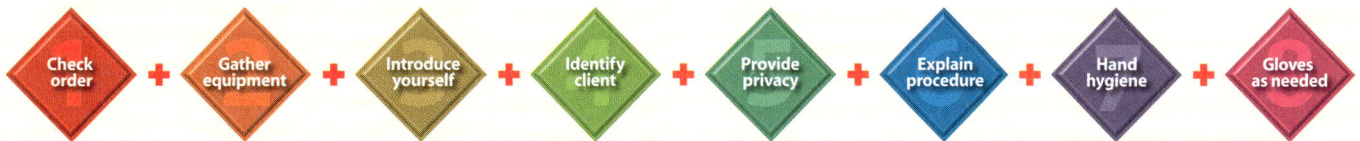

Check order + Gather equipment + Introduce yourself + Identify client + Provide privacy + Explain procedure + Hand hygiene + Gloves as needed

Interventions and Rationales

1. Perform preparatory steps (see icon bar above).

2. Ask the woman about perineal discomfort. "Is it getting better or worse? Is it greater than expected?" *Pain greater than would be expected or that is becoming worse is an indication of complications and must be investigated.*

3. Position the woman in the left Sims' position. *When the woman is supine, the posterior perineum may be difficult to see. Sims' position allows for adequate exposure of the perineum.*

4. Lift the buttocks to expose the perineum (see Figure 16-11). Use a small light to visualize the perineal tissues. *Adequate visualization is necessary for complete assessment.*

5. Assess the perineum in a systematic order. The mnemonic REEDA (redness, edema, ecchymosis, discharge, approximation) may be a helpful reminder.

   - **R** = redness. *Redness is a sign of infection.*
   - **E** = edema. Palpate for softness of tissue. *Some edema is usual following a vaginal delivery. Edematous tissue is soft. A firm mass is a sign of a hematoma and must be reported to the charge nurse.*
   - **E** = ecchymosis. *The tissue may be somewhat bruised, but an increase in bruising or excessive bruising is a sign of a hematoma.*
   - **D** = discharge. Look for drainage from episiotomy or lacerations. *There should be no drainage from repaired episiotomy or lacerations. Purulent or foul-smelling drainage is a sign of infection.*

   - **A** = approximation. The edges of repaired episiotomy or lacerations should be touching. *Within 24 hours, the wound edges should be "glued" together. Sutures are placed under the skin and therefore will not be visible.*

6. Assess the anus for hemorrhoids (Figure 16-11). If hemorrhoids are present, the size, number, and degree of tenderness should be noted. *Hemorrhoids often develop during pregnancy and labor and delivery. Comfort measures may be needed.*

7. Apply a clean perineal pad. Replenish ice pack, if necessary. *Ice packs prevent swelling and may relieve some discomfort.*

8. Dispose of contaminated pads using standard precautions. *Standard precautions prevent the spread of infection.*

SAMPLE DOCUMENTATION

(date/time)   Midline episiotomy edges well approximated. No swelling, ecchymosis, or drainage noted. States comfort measure effective in relieving tenderness. J. Jones, LVN

NURSING CARE PLAN CHART

Planning for Client with Episiotomy

GOAL	INTERVENTION	RATIONALE	EXPECTED OUTCOME
.1. Deficient Knowledge related to episiotomy			
The client or couple will obtain information regarding episiotomy.	Provide written information on episiotomy.	*Written information allows clients to review information at home.*	Client or couple will understand the risks and benefits of episiotomy.
	Explain the rationale for episiotomy. Provide details on the risks and benefits of the procedure.	*Verbal instructions meet the needs of auditory learners.*	The client or couple will demonstrate understanding by listing two primary benefits and two major risks to the mother and/or fetus.
	Inform the client that *routine* episiotomy is topic of clinical debate; encourage client to engage in dialogue with the obstetrical care provider regarding their own opinion and choice in the matter.	*Episiotomy (surgical incision of the vagina) is performed to enlarge the vaginal opening to facilitate delivery. The purpose of the episiotomy is to prevent perineal tears and fetal distress. Benefits to the fetus include cranial protection, reduced asphyxia risk, and reduced risk of shoulder dislocation. Benefits to the mother include faster delivery, avoidance of greater perineal trauma (laceration), and avoidance of complications involving the urinary tract and rectum. Furthermore, irregular tears of the perineum can be more difficult to suture than straight incisions.*	The client or couple will share their preference regarding episiotomy with the care provider.
	Discuss intravaginal massage during the last month of pregnancy as a possible preventive strategy.	*However, recent clinical research indicates that women who have experienced spontaneous tears to the perineum experienced less postpartum pain and an earlier return to normal sexual activity than women who had episiotomy.*	
		Intravaginal massage, performed daily for 5 to 10 minutes beginning in the 34th week has been clinically demonstrated to reduce the likelihood of perineal trauma and the need for episiotomy.	
2. Impaired Tissue Integrity			
Client will experience healing of the perineum.	Discuss any special considerations regarding specific location of the incision.	*There are three basic location types of episiotomy: median (or midline), mediolateral (sometimes called lateral), and modified median, which features two additional half-inch transverse cuts just above the anal sphincter. Median incisions are performed most commonly here in the United States and Canada and are associated with less pain and fewer complications during healing. However, these incisions are more likely to extend into or through the anal sphincter.*	Client will *not* report any of the following signs associated with injury to the surgical site: • Bleeding from the incision • Urinary or fecal drainage from the vagina
	Discuss specific risk factors for clients with a history of *endometriosis.*		
	Teach client to perform routine aspects of episiotomy care: • Apply ice packs • Use warm sitz baths • Do Kegel exercises		
	Medication Administration: Oral (stool softener and analgesic)	*Clients with a history of endometriosis are at increased risk of developing incisional endometriosis (endometrial lesions within the scar tissue).*	
	Dietary Management		
	Monitor vaginal discharge.		

GOAL	INTERVENTION	RATIONALE	EXPECTED OUTCOME
		Ice packs applied within the first 24 hours help to reduce swelling. Local heat (sitz baths, etc.) helps to promote relaxation of the pelvic floor, reducing pain and risk of further injury.	
		Kegel exercises promote natural strengthening of pelvic floor muscles.	
		Dietary management and stool softeners facilitate comfort during bowel movements, so the client may avoid exerting excessive pressure on the perineum while straining to complete a bowel movement.	
3. Risk for Infection related to break in intact skin			
Client will avoid puerperal infection.	Monitor client's fluid intake and output. Monitor client's vital signs. Monitor client's daily elimination patterns. Monitor client's vaginal discharge. Monitor incision site for signs of infection: Excessive swelling, warmth or redness, induration, or purulent drainage.	*Changes in bowel and bladder elimination patterns (especially urination), increased heart rate and body temperature, and changes in lochia can be signs of infection.*	The client's fluid intake and output, vital signs, daily elimination patterns, and lochia flow will remain within normal limits. Incision site will remain free from signs of infection. The client will demonstrate proper use of the "peri" bottle for daily hygiene.
	Instruct client to avoid rubbing with toilet tissue and to use warm water irrigations (via squirt "peri" bottle) for cleansing after urination and bowel movements.	*Toilet tissue is an irritant that can stick to the skin and can sweep bacteria from the rectal area to the vagina. The mechanics of "rubbing" could further harm injured areas, increasing the risk of wound opening and bacterial access to the bloodstream.*	The client or couple will explain the rationale behind the requests to enhance personal hygiene and limit sexual encounters.
		Irrigation of the perineum provides cleansing to remove irritants and/or contaminants such as fecal debris to reduce the risk of infection.	
		Normal intestinal flora become pathogenic when they reach sterile organs, such as the urinary tract or the blood. Trauma to the perineum increases the risk of infection, especially from fecal contamination from ordinary bowel movements.	
	Reinforce teaching on avoidance of sexual activity for 6 weeks.	*Intercourse and/or other sexual activity can cause mechanical injury and/or introduce pathogens into the incisional area.*	

More information about nursing care for a client with an episiotomy is provided in the Nursing Care Plan Chart on pages 404 and 405.

Lower Extremities

The legs should also be assessed for abnormalities caused by pregnancy, including varicose veins and edema (Figure 16-12 ■). If varicose veins are present, care should be taken to protect them from injury. Reassure the woman that edema from pressure on the pelvic veins or PIH should resolve in a few days.

Assess the legs for signs of *thrombophlebitis* (positive Homan's sign: see Figure 16-12B). Note any areas of redness, swelling, or tenderness. With the legs straight and knees slightly flexed, the woman's foot should be sharply dorsiflexed. No discomfort should be present. Pain with dorsiflexion is an

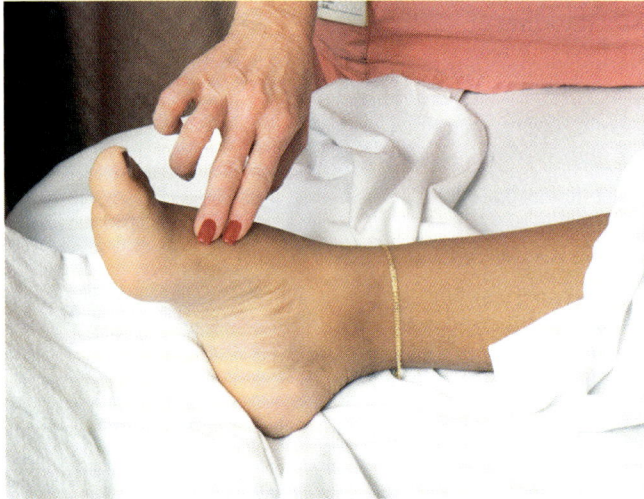

A

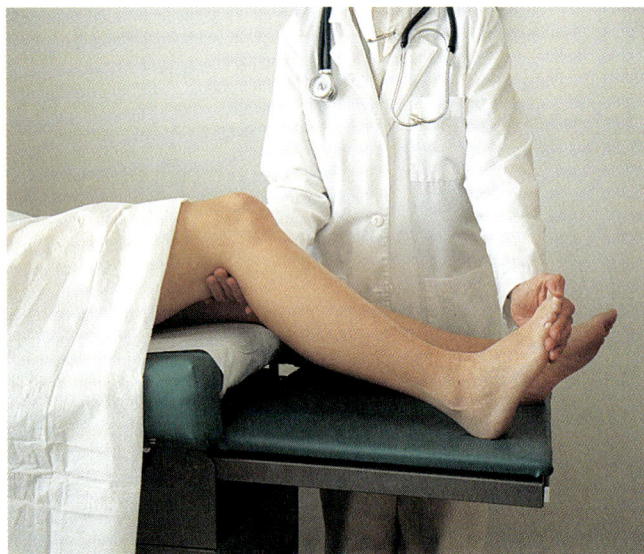

B

Figure 16-12. ■ (A) Nurse assessing client's foot for edema. (B) Assessing for thrombosis. (B: Elena Dorfman.)

indication of an inflamed vessel in the leg. The charge nurse or physician should be notified at once because of the risk of deep vein thrombosis and **thromboembolism** (a blood clot moving within the blood vessels). Figure 16-13 ■ illustrates a postpartum assessment sheet.

Psychological Assessment

Psychological assessment is an important part of postpartum care. The mother's attitude and feelings affect her ability to care for herself and the infant. Fatigue from a long labor makes everything seem more difficult to manage. A tired mother may seem disinterested in the infant and be labeled as a "potential attachment problem." After a nap, the mother is often more receptive to her baby.

Some mothers have little experience caring for a newborn and feel overwhelmed. They may show these feelings by

asking frequent questions and reading all the information that is available. Feeling inadequate may cause others to become passive and quiet. The nurse must help the mother explore these feelings in order to assess the need for further outside support.

To assess for early attachment or bonding with the infant, the nurse needs to observe the mother handling the baby. Through observation, the nurse can answer the following questions:

- To what extent does the mother seek face-to-face interaction with the infant?
- Has she progressed from fingertip touch to enfolding the infant in her arms?
- Is interaction increasing or decreasing?
- Is she sensitive to the newborn's needs?
- Does she seem pleased with her infant? Is she upset by baby's appearance or gender?
- Does she call the baby by name?

Once the nurse has observed the mother–baby interaction, three more questions must be answered: Is there a problem with attachment? What is the problem? What is the source of the problem? The LPN/LVN refers any concerns about attachment to the charge nurse.

DIAGNOSING, PLANNING, AND IMPLEMENTING

Once an assessment is completed, problems must be identified. Generally, new mothers can provide for their own physical needs but may have deficient knowledge about the specifics of postpartum care. Common nursing diagnoses include:

- **P**ain
- Deficient **K**nowledge regarding breast care
- Deficient **K**nowledge regarding perineal care
- Imbalanced **N**utrition: Less than Body Requirements
- **C**onstipation
- Impaired **U**rinary Elimination

Some possible outcomes include the following:

- Client expresses that pain is reduced with medication.
- Client asks for information she can read about breast-feeding and self-care.
- Client states understanding the importance of nutrients to self and infant, and states "maybe I don't have to lose all my pregnancy weight in 2 weeks; maybe I can take a little more time."
- Client asks for dried fruit and extra liquids with meal to assist bowel elimination.
- Client states that pain on urination has lessened from 5 to 2 on scale of 1 to 10.

Client's name _____   Gravida _____ Para _____
                                          Delivery date _____

Physical assessment		
	Remarks	
Vital signs		
Blood pressure		
Pulse		
Respirations		
Temperature		
Fundus		
Condition		
Height and location		
Lochia/vaginal discharge		
Color		
Amount and condition		
Number of pads changed		
Breast		
Breast or bottle feeding		
Breast assessment		
Nipple assessment		
Incision/lacerations (REEDA)		
Perineum		
Episiotomy site		
Lacerations		
Abdominal incision		
Appearance		
Dressing change		
Wound irrigation		
Nutrition		
Diet		
Intake		
Fluids		
Type and amount		
IV solution, rate, site		
Elimination		
Voided		
Amount		
Any discomforts		
Bowel movement		
Number and type		
Constipation		
Treatments		
Comfort measures		
Rest		
Pain (type, location, intensity)		
Interventions		
Sitz bath		
Witch hazel pads		
Surgigator		
Pericare		
Analgesic perineal spray		
Analgesic (name, route, time)		
Other		

Figure 16-13. ■ Postpartum flow sheet of physical assessment of the client.

The plan of care centers on teaching the new mother to meet her needs and the needs of the infant. Teaching care of the infant is addressed in Chapter 17 ⚭.

Pain Management

- Assess the client's level of pain. Pain may be described by various pain rating scales, by location (incision, leg, back, head), and by type (dull, aching, throbbing, radiating, etc.). Box 16-3 ■ provides guidelines for the nurse in assisting the client in pain. *The nurse uses information from the client, plus objective data gained by observing the client, to report the level of pain.*

- Advise the breastfeeding mother with discomfort from engorged breast tissue to take a warm shower or nurse her baby. *These actions will stimulate the let-down reflex and relieve the pressure in the breast.*

- Evaluate breastfeeding technique if the nipples become sore or cracked. *A lanoline ointment may be applied with an order from the primary care provider. This type of ointment is safe for use with breastfeeding infants.*

BOX 16-3	**NURSING CARE CHECKLIST**

Helping a Client in Pain

☑ Ask the client when the pain started. If it is a recurring pain, ask what starts the pain and what causes it to stop.

☑ Ask the client to describe how bad the pain is on a scale of 0 to 10, with 0 being no pain and 10 being the worst imaginable pain.

☑ Ask where the pain is, or have the client show the nurse by pointing to the area of pain. Also, determine if the pain begins in one area and moves to another.

☑ Ask the client to identify what kind of pain exists.

   ☑ Throbbing

   ☑ Shooting

   ☑ Stabbing

   ☑ Sharp

   ☑ Gnawing

   ☑ Burning

   ☑ Dull

   ☑ Tender

   ☑ Radiating

   ☑ Other _____

☑ Provide medication as ordered. Review standing orders for administering pain medications. Consult with charge nurse as needed.

☑ Return to client 20 to 30 minutes after administering pain medication to determine effectiveness of medication.

- A nonnursing mother may express breast discomfort due to beginning lactation. Assist by applying ice and a breast binder to the chest. Administer analgesics as ordered. Teach that it may take several days to suppress lactation and alleviate the problem. *Ice and breast binders can prevent engorgement. Analgesics may be given for discomfort. Knowing that discomfort will subside in several days will usually help the person tolerate it better.*

- Administer analgesics as needed to control perineal discomfort. Provide ice packs and anesthetic spray to the perineum, as ordered by the primary care provider. Recommend other interventions to alleviate perineal discomfort, such as sitting in a reclined position. A sitz bath (discussed in Procedure 16-4 ■) may also be helpful. *The woman will be better able to provide for the needs of herself and her infant if she is comfortable.*

- The woman who has had a cesarean section birth may have epidural analgesia or patient-controlled analgesia (PCA). Follow facility guidelines on the use of these methods of pain relief. Provide information about the prescribed medication, its uses, and side effects. Oral pain medication will be ordered as soon as bowel tones are present and oral intake is tolerated. *As in any situation, medication administration must be carefully carried out. Once peristalsis has ended, oral medications can be tolerated.*

- Provide nonpharmacologic methods of pain relief. *Many women prefer to "forget about" the pain by using alternate methods of pain relief, such as baths, backrubs, distraction, etc.*

Table 16-2 ■ provides information about oral pain medications.

Client Teaching

Client teaching is an important part of the LPN/LVN role. Because many new mothers remain in the hospital for only 24 to 48 hours, the nurse must take every opportunity to teach health-promoting activities.

Hygiene

- Instruct the new mother to bathe daily. Teach that showers are preferable to tub bathing because they can help prevent contamination carried from the feet to the perineum or breast. If a shower is not available, the mother should be taught to clean the tub and rinse the residue away before sitting in the tub. The new mother should be taught to wash the breast without soap and to allow the nipples to air-dry. *Cleanliness is the main technique used to prevent infection. Washing the nipple with soap might cause it to become dry and to crack.*

PROCEDURE 16-4 **Sitz Bath**

Purpose

- To relieve discomfort and promote healing of the perineum

Equipment

- Disposable sitz tub kit, containing disposable basin and plastic bag with tubing
- Clean perineal pad
- Impervious bag
- Towel

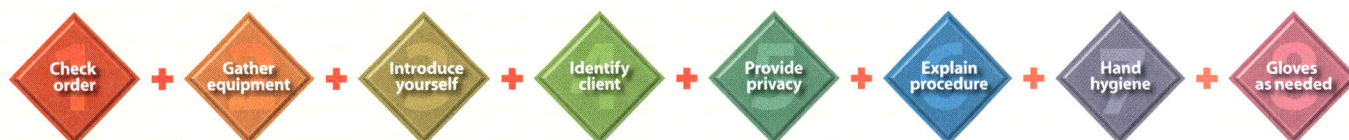

Check order + Gather equipment + Introduce yourself + Identify client + Provide privacy + Explain procedure + Hand hygiene + Gloves as needed

Interventions and Rationales

1. Perform preparatory steps (see icon bar above).

2. Provide client teaching about sitz baths, including the benefits and use of the equipment. *Instructing the client in the use of equipment and the benefits of the sitz bath helps ensure compliance.*

3. Raise the toilet seat, and place the disposable basin on the toilet. *The toilet seat should be raised and basin placed directly on the toilet for maximum support.*

4. Close clamp on tubing. Fill plastic bag with very warm water. Attach tubing to inside bottom of basin in groove provided. *The water in the bag will drain into the basin to keep the water comfortably warm. If the water in the bag is too cool, the water in the basin will cool and not be as effective.*

5. Fill the basin with comfortably warm water. *Warm water will increase circulation to the perineum and promote healing of tissues.*

6. Have the woman remove the perineal pad, dispose of it in the impervious bag, and sit directly on the basin. *Sitting directly on the basin will allow the perineum to be covered by the warm water. If the woman sits on the toilet seat, the perineum would not reach the water.*

7. Instruct the woman to open the tubing clamp periodically to drain the very warm water into the basin, keeping the basin water comfortably warm. As the basin fills, the water will drain into the toilet. *The very warm water should keep the basin water at a comfortable temperature.*

8. Instruct the woman to sit in the warm water for 10 minutes, three to four times a day as ordered. *Sitting in warm water for 10 minutes stimulates circulation without traumatizing the tissues.*

9. Instruct the woman to pat the perineum dry and to apply a clean perineal pad. *Patting the perineum dry prevents further perineal trauma and discomfort.*

10. Assess the perineum following treatment. *The perineum should show signs of healing over time.*

11. Clean the disposable sitz basin, bag, and tubing and store for future use by this client. Equipment should be sent home with client at time of discharge. When healing is complete and treatment is discontinued, dispose of the equipment. *The disposable sitz basin is intended for individual use to prevent cross-contamination between users.*

SAMPLE DOCUMENTATION

(date/time)   Up to bathroom. Sat in sitz bath for 10 minutes. Perineum dried, clean peripad applied. Perineal swelling decreased. Laceration edges well approximated.
B. Abbs, LVN

TABLE 16-2				
Pharmacology: Oral Pain Medications				
DRUG (GENERIC AND COMMON BRAND NAMES)	**USUAL ROUTE/DOSE**	**CLASSIFICATION**	**SELECTED SIDE EFFECTS**	**DON'T GIVE IF**
Ibuprofen (Motrin)	400–800 mg 3–4 times/day	NSAID (nonsteroidal anti-inflammatory drug)	Nausea, dyspepsia, blurred vision, dizziness	Client is allergic to drug
Acetaminophen (Tylenol)	325–650 mg every 4–6 hours	Nonopioid analgesic	Few in usual dose; liver toxicity if dosage guidelines are ignored	Pain is not controlled by usual dose
Oxycodone with acetaminophen (Percocet)	5 mg oxycodone with 325 mg acetaminophen	Opioid agonist/ nonopioid analgesic	Confusion, sedation, respiratory depression	Respiratory rate is less than 10/min
Morphine sulfate (Morphine)	4–10 mg IV every 3–4 hours Patient-controlled analgesia (PCA); dose varies	Opioid agonist	Respiratory depression, confusion, sedation, vomiting, constipation	Respiratory rate is less than 10/min, or client is allergic to drug
Meperidine HCl (Demerol)	50–100 mg IM every 3–4 hours; PCA; dose varies	Opioid agonist	Respiratory depression, confusion, sedation, vomiting, constipation	Respiratory rate is less than 10/min, or client is allergic to drug

If delivery was by cesarean section, instruct the woman to keep the incision clean until healing is complete. Once the dressing is removed, the woman may shower without any special precautions. Instruct her to allow the incision to dry completely after washing and to apply a small dressing if desired. *A small dressing will absorb any drainage from the incision site. If Steri-Strips have been applied to the incision, they will not be harmed by the shower and will come off in about 1 week.*

■ Teach the client to rinse the perineum with clear water after each voiding and bowel movement and to pat it dry. Instruct the new mother to wipe the perineum always from front to back. *Cleansing removes microorganisms. Wiping the perineum from front to back prevents contamination from the anus to the vagina and urethra.*

Sitz Baths

The doctor may order a sitz bath to relieve perineal swelling and discomfort. Some hospitals have porcelain sitz tubs, which must be cleaned between clients. Other facilities use portable individual sitz basins (Figure 16-14 ■) that are sent home with the client.

■ Teach the mother to shower before using the sitz bath. *This will wash away contaminants that could infect the perineum or vagina.*

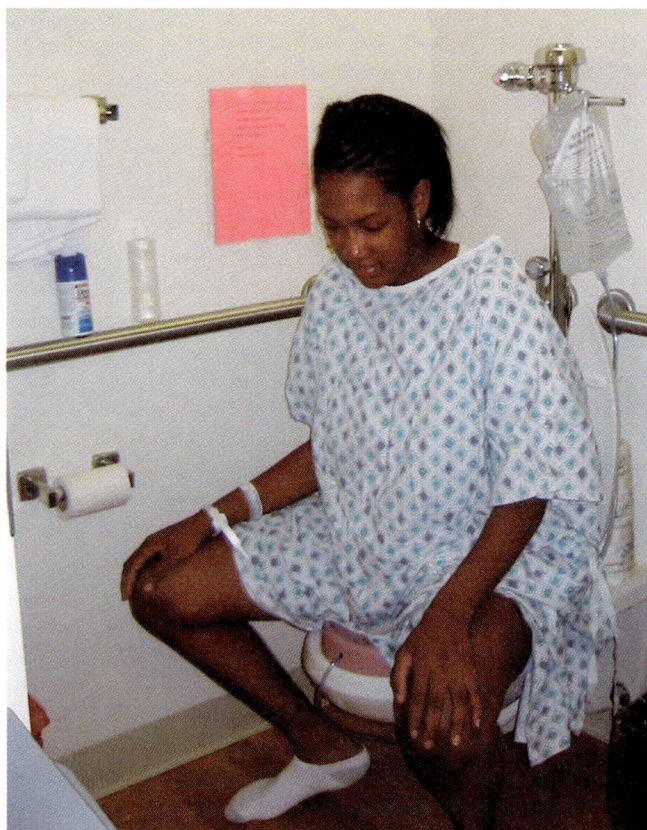

Figure 16-14. ■ A sitz bath promotes healing and provides relief from perineal discomfort during the initial weeks following birth.

Postpartum Nutrition

The new mother needs a balanced diet in order to regain her strength. Most facilities provide written information about proper nutrition after delivery. The hospital dietitian is also a valuable resource.

■ Teach the client that her diet should be high in fiber and fluids. *This diet will prevent constipation.*

■ If the woman has a good understanding of basic nutrition, it may be sufficient to advise her to decrease her daily caloric intake by 300 calories and resume her prepregnancy level of other nutrients. *The 300 calories a day that provided for the needs of the fetus are no longer necessary. The woman will return to her prepregnancy weight more quickly if she reduces the daily intake of calories.*

■ Teach the breastfeeding mother to consume an additional 500 kcal per day, to drink at least 8 glasses of fluid a day (1,000 mL), and to consume 65 g of protein and 1,000 mg of calcium. Most physicians request that the new mother continue to take prenatal vitamins with iron for 3 months (see Breastfeeding section of Chapter 11 ⚭). *These will balance the nutrients used up by milk production and breastfeeding. The prenatal vitamins help ensure that the woman's system is balanced.*

Exercise

■ After delivery, assist the woman to begin activity with ambulation. *Early ambulation promotes healing and prevents complications such as thrombophlebitis.*

■ Encourage the woman to begin with simple postpartal exercises (Figure 16-15 ■). *The new mother may want to engage in abdominal exercises to tighten stretched muscles. Inform the woman that an increase in lochia or pain means she may be overdoing exercise and should decrease her activity. Most agencies provide a booklet describing suggested postpartum exercises.*

Postpartum Immunizations

Two different immunizations are commonly given following delivery, if needed. A **RhoGAM blood stick** (a test to identify incompatibility of mother's and infant's Rh factor) is done within the first hour after birth if Rh status is not known. (Discussion of Rh incompatibility is found in Chapter 13 ⚭.) For the mother who has Rh-negative blood and delivers an infant with Rh-positive blood (see Figure 13-12 ⚭), the doctor usually prescribes an injection of RhoGAM (Rh$_o$ [D] immune globulin) (see Table 13-3 ⚭). This immune globulin can be given as soon as there are test results, but it must be given within 72 hours of delivery (some facilities say within 48 hours). RhoGAM prevents the production of Rh antibodies that could harm a future pregnancy. The purpose of the injection and the usual side effects should be explained to the mother prior to the immunization. Table 16-3 ■ provides information about postpartum immunization.

Exposure to rubella virus can cause congenital malformation in the fetus, so immunization is avoided when pregnancy is possible. If the mother has a negative rubella titer, most physicians recommend an MMR (measles, mumps, rubella) immunization in the postpartum period. If the immunization is given shortly after delivery, there is no chance of exposure to the next fetus. (*Note:* In some facilities, the MMR immunization is given immediately prior to discharge to prevent accidental exposure of other pregnant women to this virus.)

All other adult immunizations can be given in the postpartum period, if necessary.

Building a Support Network and Healthy Patterns

■ Inquire about family and friends who might be available to assist the mother when she returns home. *The mother may need encouragement to realize that people want to help her during this time. It is good to explore specific ways that people can help. Some people do best with a written list.*

■ Discuss and encourage a pattern of good eating, exercise, and rest. *Good nutrition, regular exercise, and periods of rest will help the mother return to her prepregnant state most efficiently.*

■ Respect the mother's rest periods as much as possible, and teach that it is important to listen to her body when a rest is needed. *Many women ignore their own need for rest. Teach the mother that getting rest will benefit not only herself, but also the infant and the family.*

■ Encourage the woman to simplify routines for this period of time and not to make any major changes. *The nurse can reinforce that changes are natural and necessary when an infant is brought home. It will take time to adjust to the new person and new roles. Encourage the mother to keep maintenance tasks simple and to expect energy to return gradually.*

■ Ask the client how she is feeling. *The woman may have anxieties or concerns about parenting. Asking open-ended questions can allow her to raise these issues.*

EVALUATING

The evaluation of nursing care for postpartum clients involves documenting an understanding of the teaching provided. Box 16-4 ■ reviews important aspects of client teaching in the postpartum period. The new mother should be able to demonstrate self-care, including perineal care and suture line care. She should select a balanced diet and consume adequate fluids. She should verbalize an understanding of the use and side effects of medications.

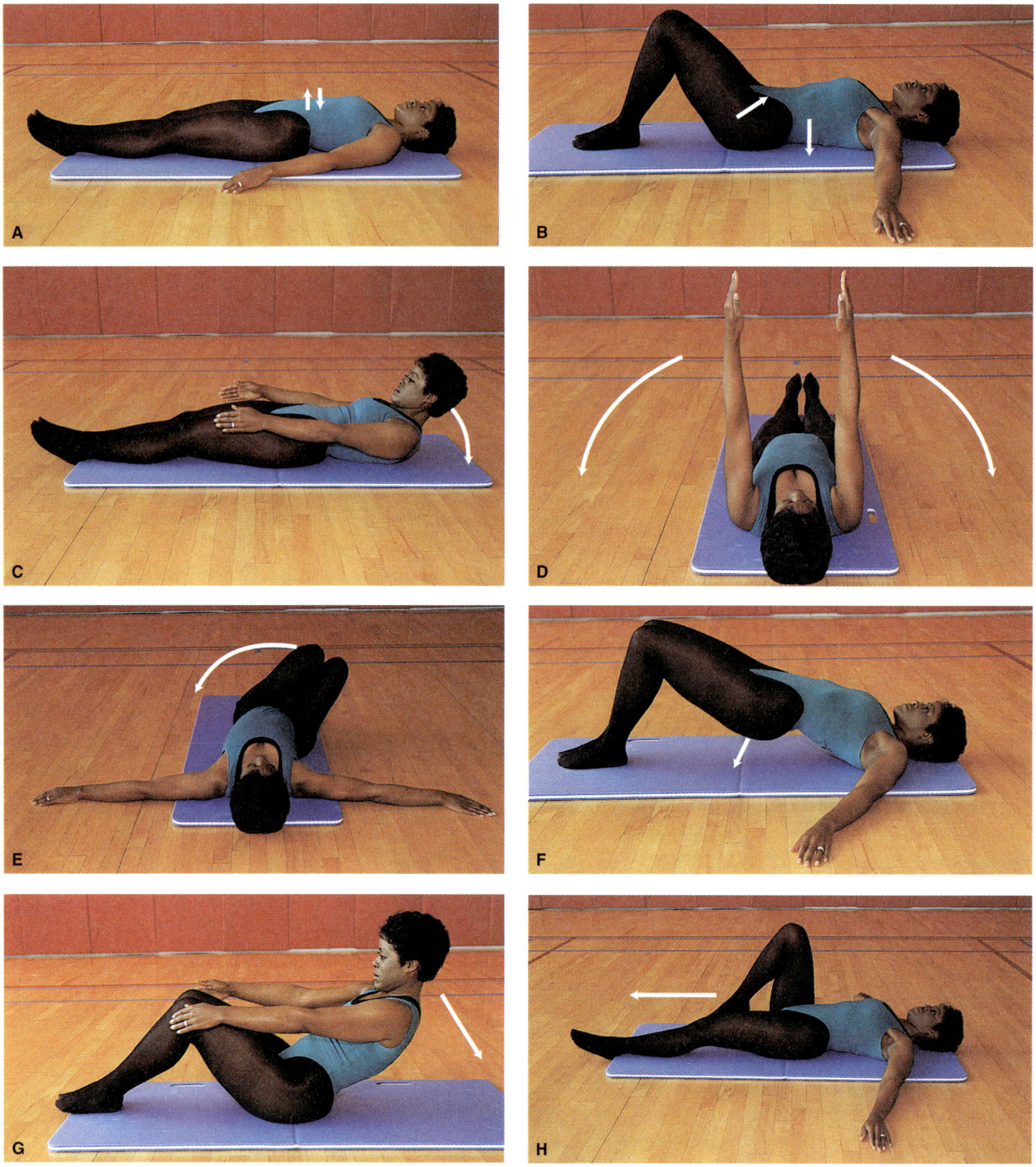

Figure 16-15. ■ Postpartal exercises. Begin with 5 repetitions two or three times daily, and gradually increase to 10 repetitions. First day: (**A**) Abdominal breathing. Lying supine, inhale deeply, using the abdominal muscles. The abdomen should expand. Then exhale slowly through pursed lips, tightening the abdominal muscle. (**B**) Pelvic rocking. Lying supine with arms at sides, knees bent, and feet flat, tighten abdomen and buttocks, and attempt to flatten back on the floor. Hold for a count of 10; then arch the back, causing the pelvis to "rock." On the second day, add (**C**). Chin to chest. Lying supine with legs straight, raise head and attempt to touch chin to chest. Slowly lower head. (**D**) Arm raises. Lying supine, arms extended at a 90-degree angle from body, raise arms so they are perpendicular and hands touch. Lower slowly. On fourth day, add (**E**). Knee rolls. Lying supine with knees bent, feet flat, arms extended to the side, roll knees to one side, keeping shoulders flat. Return to the original position, and roll to opposite side. (**F**) Buttocks lift. Lying supine, arms at side, knees bent, feet flat, slowly raise the buttocks and arch the back. Return slowly to starting position. On sixth day, add (**G**). Abdominal tighteners. Lying supine, knees bent, feet flat, slowly raise head toward knees. Arms should extend along either side of legs. Return slowly to original position. (**H**) Knee to abdomen. Lying supine, arms at sides, bend one knee and thigh until foot touches buttocks. Straighten leg and lower it slowly. Repeat with other leg. After 2 to 3 weeks, more strenuous exercises, such as push-ups and side leg raises, may be added as tolerated. Kegel exercises, begun before birth, should be done many times daily during postpartum to restore vaginal and perineal tone.

TABLE 16-3				
Pharmacology: Immunizations in the Postpartum Period				
DRUG (GENERIC AND COMMON BRAND NAME)	**USUAL ROUTE/DOSE**	**CLASSIFICATION**	**SELECTED SIDE EFFECTS**	**DON'T GIVE IF**
Rh_oD immune globulin (RhoGAM, HypoRho-D)	300 mcg IM	Immunizing agent	Local pain, fever	Client is Rh positive or client has history of hypersensitivity reaction
MMR (measles, mumps, rubella)	1 vial IM	Vaccines	Local pain, fever	Client is allergic to eggs or has history of hypersensitivity reaction

---

BOX 16-4   CLIENT TEACHING

Self-Care After Discharge

Episiotomy/Perineal Laceration Care

Use of the perineal bottle until vaginal bleeding stops can promote healing and prevent infection. Teach the mother always to rinse the perineal area, to cleanse and wipe from front to back, and to change perineal pads after urinating or having a bowel movement. Tell the mother to wait to use tampons until after the follow-up exam.

The doctor or midwife may recommend a sitz bath (see Procedure 16-4) to decrease perineal discomfort. Sitting in a sitz bath 10 to 15 minutes, three times a day, can soothe the perineal tissue. It may be more comfortable to place a bath towel in the tub to sit on. Some hospitals provide a plastic sitz bath to take home.

Vaginal Discharge

Teach the woman that it is normal to have vaginal discharge after delivery. Vaginal discharge may last as long as 5 to 6 weeks, although it should decrease in amount every day. The color will also change from bright red to dark red or brown. After 4 to 5 days, the discharge will become pinkish-red and then change to yellowish or white in color. Excessive activity may cause discharge to become red again with some small clots. If this occurs, the mother should lie down and rest with her feet elevated. If she fills a perineal pad in 1 hour or less, bleeding is excessive. Instruct her to call the doctor or midwife immediately.

Cesarean Birth

The woman who has had a cesarean birth will require the same care as the woman who delivered vaginally, plus routine postoperative care. To prevent respiratory complications, she should turn, cough, and deep breathe every 2 hours. Once the Foley catheter is removed, she should void every 3 to 4 hours. The amount of lochia is generally less than that following a vaginal birth. Therefore, vaginal flow should be small to moderate. Pain control is usually accomplished by oral medication every 4 hours or as needed. Generally pain medication is needed for 7 to 10 days.

Teach the woman who has had a cesarean birth that it is important not to overdo activity for 4 to 6 weeks. Activity should be limited to taking care of oneself and the baby. The woman should avoid lifting anything heavier than the baby. Climbing stairs should be kept to a minimum. The doctor or midwife will determine when normal activities resume, including driving.

Incision Care

Teach that an incision from a C-section does not need special care. Showering should be sufficient to cleanse the area. Scrubbing the incision is not necessary. Paper tape (Steri-Strips) on the incision can be gotten wet. Pat the incision dry after showering, or dry the area with a hairdryer on cool setting. The incision should be inspected in a mirror or by another person. It should be clean, dry, and intact; it should heal without redness, swelling, or foul odor. It is normal to have a small amount of clear fluid ooze from part of the incision. However, teach that bleeding or pearly colored discharge is not normal and should be reported to the doctor or midwife. Instruct the woman to call the doctor or midwife if the incision appears red and feels hot to the touch. Sutures underneath the incision will dissolve. If the staples were not removed in the hospital, it will be necessary to see the doctor or midwife to have them removed.

Hemorrhoids

Hemorrhoids often appear outside the rectum due to the pressure of pushing the baby out during delivery. Often, they will shrink with time. The doctor or midwife may prescribe ointment or suppositories. Teach the woman that ice packs can help decrease pain and swelling, and that some women find that a sitz bath is soothing after the first 24 hours post delivery.

Bowels

Teach the woman to avoid constipation. The mother should drink 6–8 glasses of water a day, and more if breastfeeding. The woman should be instructed to eat a balanced diet, which includes fruits, vegetables, and whole grains. The doctor or midwife may prescribe a stool softener or a laxative.

Menstruation

Instruct the woman that the time before periods begin again varies from woman to woman. Most women start their period within 2 to 3 months after delivery, unless they are breastfeeding. The woman who is breastfeeding may not have a period until after she stops breastfeeding.

Family Planning

Reinforce that the woman should not have sexual intercourse for 4 to 6 weeks after birth. It is recommended to wait until after

(continued)

the follow-up exam to resume intercourse. Birth control methods should be discussed with the doctor or midwife at this appointment. A woman can still become pregnant, even if she does not have a period.

Adjustment to Parenthood

Remind the woman that—although she may feel normal once she goes home—she is still recovering from the delivery of the baby. She needs time to adjust to having a new baby in the home. She should gradually resume activities, but allow time for rest. She should sleep when the baby sleeps. Allow family members and friends to help around the house and to prepare meals. The baby needs the woman to take care of herself.

Remind the woman that many women experience "baby blues." Teach that if weepiness, exhaustion, and anxiety last longer than a couple of weeks, she should see a physician to rule out postpartum depression. Emphasize that symptoms of "baby blues" or postpartum depression do not mean she is a "bad" mother. The period after the birth of the baby is a time of many changes and a whole new type of pressure. It is important not to try to deal with these feelings alone. Teach the mother these ways to ease "baby blues":

- Nap at every opportunity.
- Have small, nutritious, and easy-to-prepare meals throughout the day.
- Express her feelings to nonjudgmental family and friends. Ask for help with cooking and cleaning.
- Make time for herself!

Source: Ramont, R. P., Niedringhaus, D. M., & Towle, M. A. (2006). *Comprehensive nursing care.* Upper Saddle River, NJ: Prentice Hall, Box 42-3, p. 1123.

Discharge Considerations

It is the nurse's responsibility to ensure that client teaching has occurred and that the woman has been given written information about care after discharge. Many parents will be concerned about going home with their new baby. They will worry about what to do if something is wrong. Box 16-5 ■ provides a list of criteria to help parents know when to call care providers for help.

The nurse can also assist by helping the client identify support people for the postpartum period. It may be helpful for the client to list a set of tasks with which she could use help. Only trusted family and friends should be asked to help with child care.

NURSING PROCESS CARE PLAN
Client at Risk for Deep Vein Thrombosis

C. S., a 35-year-old gravida 3, para 2, is transferred from labor and delivery following a primary cesarean section for severe preeclampsia (see Chapter 13 🔗). She is on a PCA pump for postoperative pain. Her husband is at the bedside.

Assessment. The following data should be collected as soon as possible after admission:

- Vital signs and pain
- Lung sounds

BOX 16-5	CLIENT TEACHING

Postpartum Emergencies

Teach the woman/parents to look for these signs in her infant and to call the pediatrician in the following situations:

- An axillary temperature above 100.4°F (38°C) or an axillary temperature below 97.8°F (36.6°C)
- Projectile vomiting or frequent vomiting
- Refusal to feed for 2 feedings or 6 hours
- Listlessness or difficulty in waking baby
- Excessive fussiness during which comfort measures are not effective
- Jaundice increasing and working its way down the baby's trunk
- Two or more loose black or green watery stools
- Fewer than 6 wet diapers in a 24-hour period (after the mother's milk has come in)
- If baby is blue or is not breathing, call 911 or your local emergency number.

Teach the woman to call the obstetrician or midwife if any of the following occurs in herself:

- A temperature above 100.4°F (38°C)
- Sudden bright red bleeding or blood clots that are lemon-size or larger
- Foul-smelling lochia
- Painful urination
- Unexplained, sudden pain
- Hot or reddened area on breast
- If experiencing sudden shortness of breath or chest pain, call 911 immediately.

Provide these special discharge instructions about reasons to call the care provider after a cesarean section:

- Incision not changing for the better; pearly colored, white, or bloody drainage
- Reddened or hot area on incision
- Gaps between edges of incision or opening of incision.

Source: Ramont, R. P., Niedringhaus, D. M., & Towle, M. A. (2006). *Comprehensive nursing care.* Upper Saddle River, NJ: Prentice Hall, Box 42-4, p. 1124.

- Bowel sounds
- Fundus firmness and bleeding
- Deep tendon reflexes
- Response to test for Homan's sign
- Skin on legs—color, moisture, temperature
- Urine output
- Edema
- Capillary refill
- Incision (if woman had cesarean or episiotomy)

Nursing Diagnosis.   The following important nursing diagnoses (among others) are established for this client:

- Risk for Ineffective Peripheral **T**issue Perfusion related to surgical procedure and immobility
- Acute **P**ain related to surgical procedure
- Risk for Respiratory and Incisional **I**nfection related to surgical procedure

Expected Outcomes.   Client will have adequate tissue perfusion in lower extremities as evidenced by lack of symptoms of deep vein thrombosis.

- Client will have adequate pain control as evidenced by verbalizing pain relief.
- Client will have no infection as evidenced by lack of respiratory or incisional symptoms.

Planning and Implementation

- Discuss with client the importance of increasing mobility following surgery. *Compliance may be increased when the client understands the risks of immobility.*
- Increase mobility as tolerated. *Mobility causes calf muscle contraction, which enhances venous return and thus decreases the risk for thrombus formation.*
- As ordered, implement thromboembolic stockings, intermittent pneumatic compression devices, or venous

foot pump compression devices. *These devices work in the same manner as ambulation to prevent thrombus formation.*

- Continue to assess for signs and symptoms of thrombus formation. *Symptom recognition will facilitate prompt treatment.*
- Administer pain medication as ordered. *Pain medication will allow client to rest and will facilitate healing.*
- Encourage use of relaxation techniques such as imagery and massage. *Relaxation decreases muscle spasms and relieves discomfort.*
- Encourage client to do turn, cough, and deep breathe (TCDB) exercises every 2 hours. *Pooling of lung secretions increases risk for respiratory infection. TCDB will help client remove secretions from airways. Repositioning the client also facilitates comfort.*
- Provide dressing changes as ordered. *Changing wet dressings eliminates a reservoir for micro-organisms and decreases the risk of incisional infection.*

Evaluation.   The client verbalizes an understanding of the risks of thrombus formation and implements preventive measures. There will be no development of symptoms of deep vein thrombosis or infection. Client verbalizes comfort.

Critical Thinking in the Nursing Process

1. How can the nurse encourage movement when the client is in pain and states that movement greatly increases her pain?
2. What is the nurse's responsibility when he or she assesses that the client's husband is not allowing his wife to get out of bed in an effort to conserve her energy?
3. Discuss hygiene issues related to *TED* (support) hose.

Note: Discussion of Critical Thinking Questions appears in Appendix I.

HIGH-RISK POSTPARTUM CARE

Postpartum Infections

MASTITIS

Mastitis (infection of the breast) occurs primarily in lactating women. The most common causative organisms are *Staphylococcus aureus, Haemophilus parainfluenzae, Haemophilus influenzae,* and *Streptococcus.* Bacteria invade the breast tissue though fissured or cracked nipples. Overdistention of the breast and milk *stasis* (pooling of milk in the mammary glands) are contributing factors. Transmission of bacteria is generally from the mouth and nose of the newborn, but could also be from dirty hands touching the breast or through the mother's blood.

Preventive Measures

Mastitis may not occur for several weeks after delivery. It is important for the nurse to teach the mother how to prevent mastitis and to teach about its symptoms and treatment. Mastitis can be prevented through good hygiene practices, daily bathing, and hand washing prior to touching the nipple. Wearing a supportive bra, even in bed, will position the breast for proper drainage and prevent pooling of milk. Emptying the breast through nursing or pumping prevents overdistension. Consistently using proper breastfeeding techniques will prevent cracked nipples. If symptoms of mastitis occur, it is important for the client to contact the primary care provider.

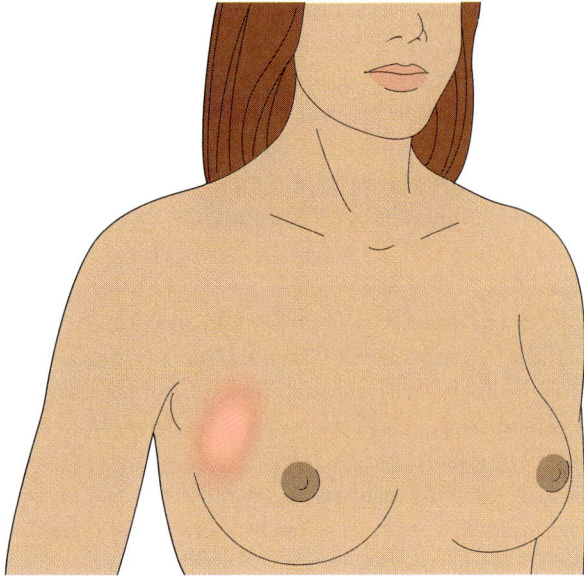

Figure 16-16. ■ Mastitis appears as tenderness, swelling, and erythema (shown here in the outer quadrant of the breast). Axillary lymph nodes may be swollen and tender. Mastitis redness often occurs in a V shape because of the shape of breast segments.

Manifestations

Symptoms of mastitis (Figure 16-16 ■) include redness and swelling of one or more lobes of the breast (often in a V-shaped wedge), fever, headache, breast pain, and flulike symptoms.

Treatment

Medical treatment generally includes antibiotics, moist heat applications, and analgesics. Emptying the breast with frequent breastfeeding or pumping decreases the duration of symptoms and speeds healing. Some mothers are concerned that the baby will become ill from the milk. Generally, this is not the case because of the antibiotic therapy. It is important for the mother to take the antibiotics as ordered.

WOUND INFECTION

In the postpartum period, laceration, episiotomy, or cesarean incision could become infected.

Preventive Measures

Keeping the area clean and dry can prevent wound infection. The client should be taught to shower daily, cover the abdominal incision with a clean dry dressing, rinse the perineum with warm water after each void or stool, and change the perineal pad at least every 2 hours.

Manifestations

Redness, swelling, pain, and purulent drainage are manifestations of a wound infection. An elevated temperature could also indicate an infection. When infection is present,

healing is delayed. If left untreated, *dehiscence* (opening) of the wound would occur. The client needs to be instructed to report any of these manifestations to the care provider without delay.

Treatment

Medical treatment includes antibiotics to prevent or treat an infection. In most cases, the infection clears without further complication. If the tissue is badly infected, it may need to be drained by surgical incision or removal of sutures. If the wound is deep, irrigation and packing may be needed.

POSTPARTUM (PUERPERAL) INFECTION

Postpartum (puerperal) infection is a rare infection of the uterus following childbirth. Strict aseptic technique used in the birthing process prevents this life-threatening complication. Contributing factors are listed in Box 16-6 ■.

Manifestations

Although the contamination occurs during the delivery process, it usually takes several days for the symptoms of infection to begin. The client may have been discharged by this time. It is important to teach the client to watch for the classic symptoms, including a fever of 100.4°F (38°C) or higher, chills, pelvic and abdominal pain, and foul-smelling lochia. If these symptoms occur, the client should contact the primary care provider immediately.

Treatment

Often, antibiotics are ordered if any of the contributing factors occurs during the delivery process. The infection usually begins in the vagina and migrates upward into the uterus **(endometritis),** pelvic lymph nodes, peritoneum

BOX 16-6	ASSESSMENT

Risk Factors for Postpartum (Puerperal) Infection

- Cesarean delivery
- Prolonged rupture of membranes
- Multiple vaginal examinations during labor
- Compromised health status of the mother (due to HIV, anemia, malnutrition, smoking, illicit drug/alcohol use)
- Obstetric trauma (lacerations, episiotomy)
- Intrauterine monitoring equipment
- Instrument-assisted delivery
- Manual removal of placenta
- Preexisting vaginal infections (STIs)

Antibiotics may be ordered for any of these contributing factors.

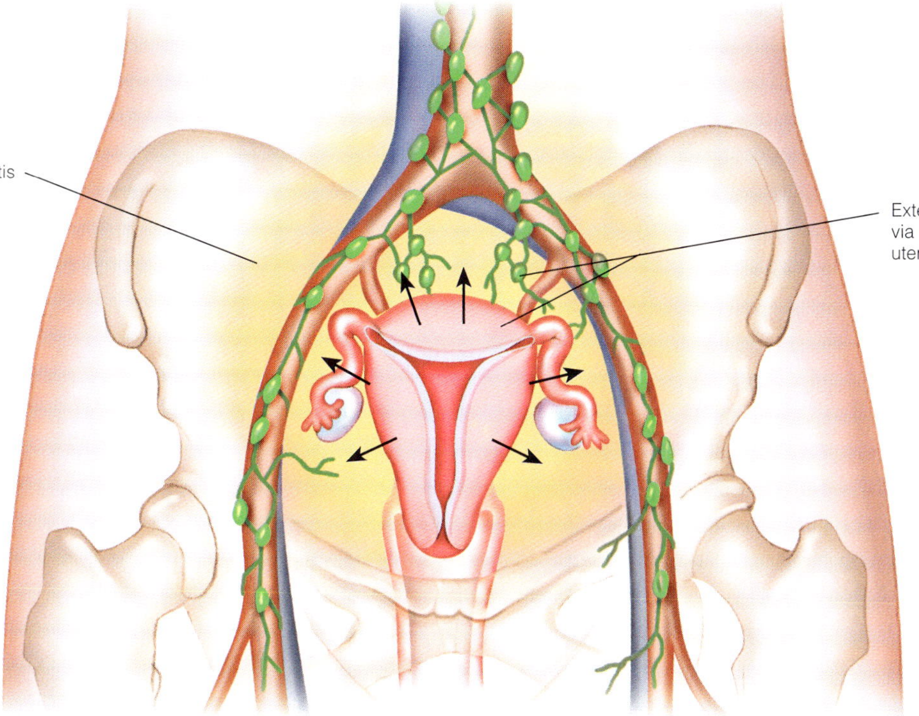

Figure 16-17. ■ Peritonitis may develop. The uterine infection can spread by way of the lymphatics and the uterine wall.

(**peritonitis**) (Figure 16-17 ■), and circulation. Once the organisms are growing in the blood, the disease has progressed to **septicemia.** If antibiotic treatment is not started immediately or if treatment is not effective, death can occur.

Postpartum Depression and Postpartum Psychosis

Postpartum depression, a major mood disorder, most frequently appears 4 weeks post delivery and upon weaning the child from the breast.

Postpartum psychosis is considered an emergency because of the risk of suicide and infanticide. Risk factors for postpartum depression and psychosis are included in Box 16-7 ■.

You will see similarities among postpartum blues, depression, and psychosis. Although postpartum blues are common and to some extent expected, the symptoms can progress to postpartum depression and the more serious postpartum psychosis. Several months after delivery, women have limited contact with their health care providers. Therefore, assessment and diagnosis of postpartum depression and psychosis may go undiagnosed. It is critical for the nurse to identify women at risk, teach them

| BOX 16-7 | ASSESSMENT |

Risk Factors for Postpartum Depression and Psychosis

Postpartum Depression
- Primipara
- Contradictory feelings about the pregnancy
- History of postpartum depression (most significant)
- History of depression or bipolar illness
- Family history of psychiatric disorders
- Lack of stable relationship with partner or parents
- Lack of social support
- Body image disorders, including eating disorders
- History of drug and/or alcohol abuse

Postpartum Psychosis
- Previous puerperal psychosis
- History of bipolar (manic-depressive) disorder
- Prenatal stressors: lack of social support, lack of a partner, low socioeconomic status
- Obsessive personality
- Family history of mood disorders

and their families the signs and symptoms, and encourage them to seek assistance if signs of depression become worse or continue for more than 2 weeks.

Manifestations

The symptoms of postpartum depression are similar to those for other forms of depression. These include sadness, frequent crying, insomnia, or excessive sleeping, appetite change, difficulty concentrating, feelings of worthlessness, lack of interest in usual activities, and lack of concern for appearance.

Postpartum psychosis, a major psychiatric disorder, usually becomes evident in the first 3 months after delivery. The symptoms of postpartum psychosis include agitation, hyperactivity, insomnia, mood *lability* (changeability), confusion, irrational thoughts and behaviors, difficulty remembering or concentrating, poor judgment, delusions, and hallucinations.

Treatment

Postpartum psychosis requires both medical and psychological treatment. Safety of the child is a primary concern. Refer to a mental health textbook for complete information about treatment of this disorder.

The treatment of postpartum depression and psychosis includes a combination of medication, individual and group counseling, and assistance with meeting child care and family needs. The woman needs to be referred to a mental health professional for follow-up treatment. Many of the drugs used to treat depression and psychosis are contraindicated in breastfeeding women.

The role of the LPN/LVN in the care of women with mental health disorders is to:

- Assist the charge nurse and mental health professional in monitoring the symptoms of depression and psychosis.
- Monitor for side effects of medication.
- Be supportive to the family.

The assessment, plan, and evaluation of care of the high-risk postpartum client are similar to the routine care of any postpartum client. The additional treatment of specific complications consists of administering medication and teaching the client and family about this complication.

Note: The reference and resource listings for this and all chapters have been compiled at the back of the book.

Chapter Review

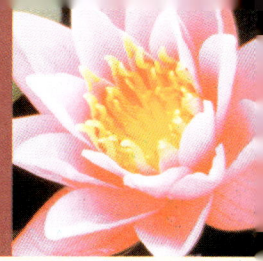

KEY TERMS by Topic

Use the audio glossary feature of either the CD-ROM or the Companion Website to hear the correct pronunciation of the following key terms.

Introduction
puerperium, postpartum

Physical Changes
involution, decidua, lochia, exfoliation, boggy, subinvolution, lochia rubra, lochia

serosa, lochia alba, hematoma, colostrum, diastasis recti abdominis, thrombosis

Psychological Changes
taking-in stage, taking-hold stage, postpartum blues, bonding

Fathers, Siblings, and Others
engrossment

Nursing Care
afterpains, thromboembolism, RhoGAM blood stick

Postpartum Infections
mastitis, postpartum (puerperal) infection, endometritis, peritonitis, septicemia

KEY Points

- Physical changes in the mother during the postpartum period progress in an expected pattern as the body returns to a nonpregnant state.

- The woman experiences psychological changes while adjusting to the role of mother.

- The nurse assesses the postpartum client for signs of healing and adaptation.

- Puerperal complications must be identified early in the postpartum period to prevent serious life-threatening conditions.

- Client teaching about self-care in the postpartum period is a continuous process that occurs with each interaction.

- New mothers must be taught to care for both themselves and their infant.

EXPLORE MediaLink

Additional interactive resources for this chapter can be found on the Companion Website at www.prenhall.com/towle. Click on Chapter 16 and "Begin" to select the activities for this chapter.

For chapter-related NCLEX®-style questions and an audio glossary, access the accompanying CD-ROM in this book.

Animations
Postpartum assessment
Breast, uterus, bladder, bowel, lochia, episiotomy, Homan's sign, emotional status

FOR FURTHER Study

For a full discussion on reproductive anatomy, see Chapter 5.

Kegel exercises are described in Chapter 10 and laboratory values are given in Table 10-2.

See Chapter 11 for additional information on breastfeeding.

High-risk complications, such as preeclampsia and Rh incompatibility, are discussed in Chapter 13.

Chapter 17 addresses teaching of infant care.

Critical Thinking Care Map

Caring for a Postpartum Client at Risk
NCLEX-PN® Focus Area: Coping and Adaptation

Case Study: Mandy, a 19-year-old, G1, P1, is transferred from labor and delivery to the postpartum unit following vaginal birth of a 5-pound, 2-ounce male. Mandy labored for 15 hours and had a second-degree, midline episiotomy. Her history reveals she had no prenatal care, her drug screen was positive for cocaine, and she is unemployed.

Nursing Diagnosis: Risk for Impaired Parent-Infant Attachment related to drug use

COLLECT DATA

Subjective	Objective
_____	_____
_____	_____
_____	_____
_____	_____
_____	_____
_____	_____
_____	_____

Would you report this? Yes/No

If yes, to: _____

Nursing Care

_____
_____
_____
_____
_____
_____
_____
_____
_____
_____
_____

How would you document this? _____
_____
_____
_____

Compare your documentation to the sample provided in Appendix I.

Data Collected
(use only those that apply)

- Positive drug screen
- No prenatal care
- No employment
- States "Leave the child in the nursery."
- "Where can my boyfriend sleep tonight?"
- VS: T 99.0, P 58, R 12, BP 120/70
- Fundus firm, 1 FB above umbilicus
- Scant amount of lochia
- No eye contact made with baby
- Asks "Will the nurses change the baby's diapers? I don't ever want to do that."

Nursing Interventions
(use only those that apply; list in priority order)

- Take the newborn into the client's room, even if she has not requested him.
- Inquire about the child's name.
- Reassess fundal height every 4 hours.
- Report to the charge nurse behaviors that indicate impaired bonding.
- Encourage the client to put the baby up for adoption.
- Teach the client about birth control methods.
- Teach the client about caring for a newborn.
- Continue to assess mother–child interaction.

NCLEX-PN® Exam Preparation

TEST-TAKING TIP What is your learning style? If you need to hear to learn, try to work in study groups and discuss the content. If you learn better by using your hands, rewrite your notes. Use three-dimensional models to understand anatomy or physical assessment. If you need to visualize the content to learn, read a variety of sources on the content; make drawings or schematics related to the content. During the test, recall these experiences when trying to remember content.

1 Which of the following assessment findings are related to uterine atony in the postpartum client? Choose all that apply.

  1. a boggy uterus
  2. increased vaginal bleeding
  3. large amounts of clots expressed
  4. fundus midline
  5. fundus displaced to left or right
  6. scant amount of lochia rubra

2 On the second day postpartum, the nurse palpates the fundus one fingerbreadth below the umbilicus. The fundus was found to be firm. What nursing action is appropriate?

  1. Document the finding.
  2. Call the physician.
  3. Catheterize the client.
  4. Administer Lortab PO.

3 Which client would the nurse expect to be at risk for decreased rate of involution?

  1. primiparous client
  2. precipitous birth
  3. client with indwelling catheter
  4. client nonimmune for rubella

4 The nurse observes a creamy white vaginal discharge at the client's 2-week postpartum clinic visit. Which of the following terms would she use in documenting this finding?

  1. lochia rubra
  2. lochia serosa
  3. lochia alba
  4. lochia nigra

5 The postpartum client plans to breastfeed her newborn. She is concerned about birth control. Which of the following methods would the nurse recommend?

  1. no method necessary; breastfeeding prohibits ovulation
  2. combined oral contraceptives

  3. barrier methods such as a diaphragm
  4. intrauterine device

6 The postpartum client calls the office nurse and states that she is constipated. Which of the following suggestions would the nurse offer? Choose all that apply.

  1. Restrict fluid intake.
  2. Walk 30 minutes per day.
  3. Eat a diet consisting of soft foods.
  4. Increase fluid intake.
  5. Eat a diet consisting of high fiber.

7 Following birth, the nurse encourages a first-generation Asian client to place an ice pack on her episiotomy. What is the expected response from the client?

  1. placing the ice pack on her perineum
  2. requesting to take a shower instead
  3. refusing the ice pack
  4. asking for a chemical cold pack instead

8 On the second day postpartum, the nurse assesses the client's temperature to be 100.6°F. What nursing action is most appropriate?

  1. Assess for further signs of infection.
  2. No action is necessary; this is a normal finding.
  3. Administer Lortab PO.
  4. Encourage the mother to breastfeed.

9 The LPN/LVN understands that which of the following breast assessment findings is considered to be normal for the client who gave birth less than 24 hours ago?

  1. firm, hard to palpation
  2. red streaks surrounding the areola
  3. cracks noted on the nipple
  4. thin yellow drainage noted from the nipple

10 The nurse is to give Colace (docusate sodium) 250 mg PO to a client postpartum. On hand is Colace 100 mg/tablet. The nurse will give _____ tablets.

Answers for NCLEX-PN® Review and Critical Thinking questions appear in Appendix I.

Thinking Strategically About...

You are an LPN/LVN employed on a postpartum unit of a regional medical center. You are working from 7:00 A.M. until 7:00 P.M. (While you are to provide care for new mothers and their infants, the questions here will apply only to the mother's care.) When you go to report, you learn that one nurse has called in ill, resulting in short staffing for the day. The charge nurse has asked for input prior to making client assignments.

- Natasha, gravida 2, para 1, delivered a male infant vaginally 4 hours ago. She had a midline episiotomy and is complaining of "sore hemorrhoids." Her fundus is U1, midline, and firm. She has voided once since delivery. She is planning to bottle-feed her baby.

- Jordan, gravida 3, para 3, delivered a female infant vaginally at noon yesterday. She had a third-degree laceration. Her fundus is U, midline, and firm. She is breastfeeding without difficulty. She plans to go home early this afternoon.

- Yvonne, a gravida 1, para 1 immigrant from Bosnia, delivered a male infant 3 hours ago by cesarean section because the fetus was breech. She has an IV, a Foley catheter to bedside drainage, and an abdominal dressing. Her fundus is firm. She has an IV PCA pump of morphine for pain. She is planning to breastfeed but has not attempted this yet.

CRITICAL THINKING

- What questions should be discussed in making client assignments that would indicate the intellectual standard of *fairness* is being considered?

COLLABORATIVE CARE

- What nursing specialists should be contacted to assist in planning and providing care for Yvonne?

MANAGEMENT OF CARE AND PRIORITIES IN NURSING CARE

- In what order will you perform your care for these three clients?
- What is your rationale for prioritizing these duties?

DELEGATING

- What part of the care for these three clients can be delegated to a CNA?

COMMUNICATION AND CLIENT TEACHING

- What teaching about self-care should be provided to Jordan before she is discharged?
- What teaching should be provided Yvonne about self-care following a cesarean birth?

DOCUMENTING AND REPORTING

- What information regarding these three clients should be reported to the supervising RN?
- What would the LPN/LVN chart about Yvonne's assessment?

CULTURAL CARE STRATEGIES

- Since Yvonne is from Bosnia, what will the nurse do to ensure accurate communication has occurred?

Nursing Care of the Newborn

UNIT VI

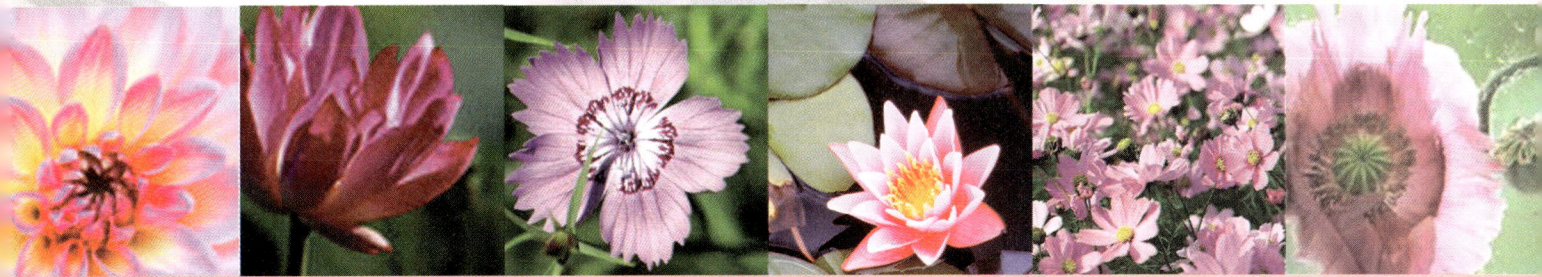

Care of the Normal Newborn

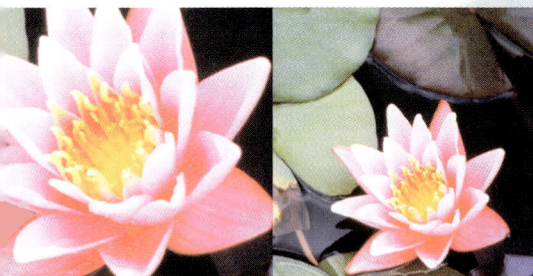

BRIEF Outline

LEARNING Outcomes

After completing this chapter, you will be able to:

1. Define key terms.
2. Discuss physiologic adaptation of the newborn.
3. Discuss Apgar score.
4. Discuss physical characteristics and reflexes of the newborn.
5. Describe nursery care of the newborn.
6. Discuss parent teaching related to care of the newborn.

The **newborn** is the infant from delivery through the first month of life. Initial care revolves around meeting the basic biologic needs and helping the newborn adjust to life outside the womb.

Physiologic Adaptation

An understanding of the physiologic adaptation to life outside the uterus guides the nurse's actions when setting priorities in the care of the newborn. These adaptations are discussed in Delivery Room Care of the Neonate in Chapter 14 ⚭. They are briefly reviewed here in the order of priority (airway, breathing, circulation, and thermoregulation) to set the foundation for newborn care.

RESPIRATORY ADAPTATION

Because the fetus does not breathe inside the uterus, the first priority is to assist the newborn in establishing respirations. Using the bulb syringe or suction catheter, the nurse removes mucus, vaginal secretions, and amniotic fluid from the newborn's airway. Because the infant is positioned with the head down, fluids continue to drain and must be removed.

Breathing usually begins spontaneously (Figure 17-1 ■). However, some newborns need to be stimulated; this is done by rubbing the skin or tapping the feet. If the newborn's respiratory effort is weak or absent, the nurse or respiratory therapist will use an Ambu-bag and mask to breathe for the newborn. Oxygen can be administered by mask to prevent hypoxia.

CARDIOVASCULAR ADAPTATION

The newborn's cardiovascular system (Figure 17-2 ■) must adapt to life outside the uterus. Recall that fetal circulation contains several structures that must close shortly after delivery. For example, when the umbilical cord is clamped, blood can no longer flow through the umbilical arteries and umbilical vein. The branches of these blood vessels that are inside the newborn's abdomen will eventually become connective tissue.

A change in the thoracic pressure causes other circulatory changes to occur. The rhythmic increase and decrease in thoracic pressure not only cause respiration, but also cause the closure of the foramen ovale and ductus arteriosus. Permanent closure of these structures may take several months.

THERMOREGULATORY ADAPTATION

The body temperature of the fetus is regulated by the environment inside the uterus. The mother's body temperature

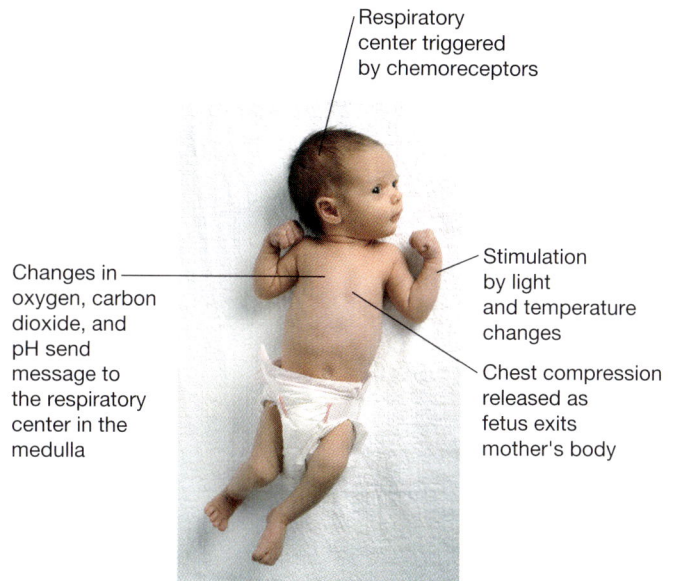

Figure 17-1. ■ Respiratory adaptation of the newborn. The infant's chest is compressed as it moves through the birth canal. Compression is released as it exits the mother's body, allowing air to be drawn into the expanding lungs to replace the amniotic fluid. As blood levels of oxygen and the infant's pH decrease, and as blood levels of carbon dioxide increase, the respiratory center in the medulla triggers changes that cause the diaphragm to contract. Cold air and light further stimulate the respiratory center, causing the newborn to breathe. The newborn's first breaths occur in an irregular pattern, typically at a rate of 30 to 60 breaths per minute. (Dorling Kindersley Media Library.)

maintains the amniotic fluid at 98.6°F (37°C). The wet newborn will immediately begin to lose body heat by evaporation (Figure 17-3 ■). The delivery room is generally kept cool for the comfort of the mother and delivery room staff. However, this cool room will cause the newborn to lose heat by convection, conduction, and radiation. To prevent the rapid loss of body heat, the newborn should be dried with warm blankets, placed next to the warm skin of the mother, and covered with warm dry blankets. A hat will prevent heat loss through the head. If the newborn is exposed for assessment or nursing interventions, or if close observation is needed, the newborn is placed in a bed under a radiant warmer.

In newborns, **cold stress** occurs when excessive heat is lost. Cold stress is temperature change sufficient to cause the newborn to generate heat by **nonshivering thermogenesis.** Newborns are not able to shiver to produce heat. By moving and crying, the newborn increases metabolism and burns stored brown fat (Figure 17-4 ■). The increase in metabolism results in respiratory distress, hypoxia, and a depletion of glycogen stores. If left untreated, it is life threatening.

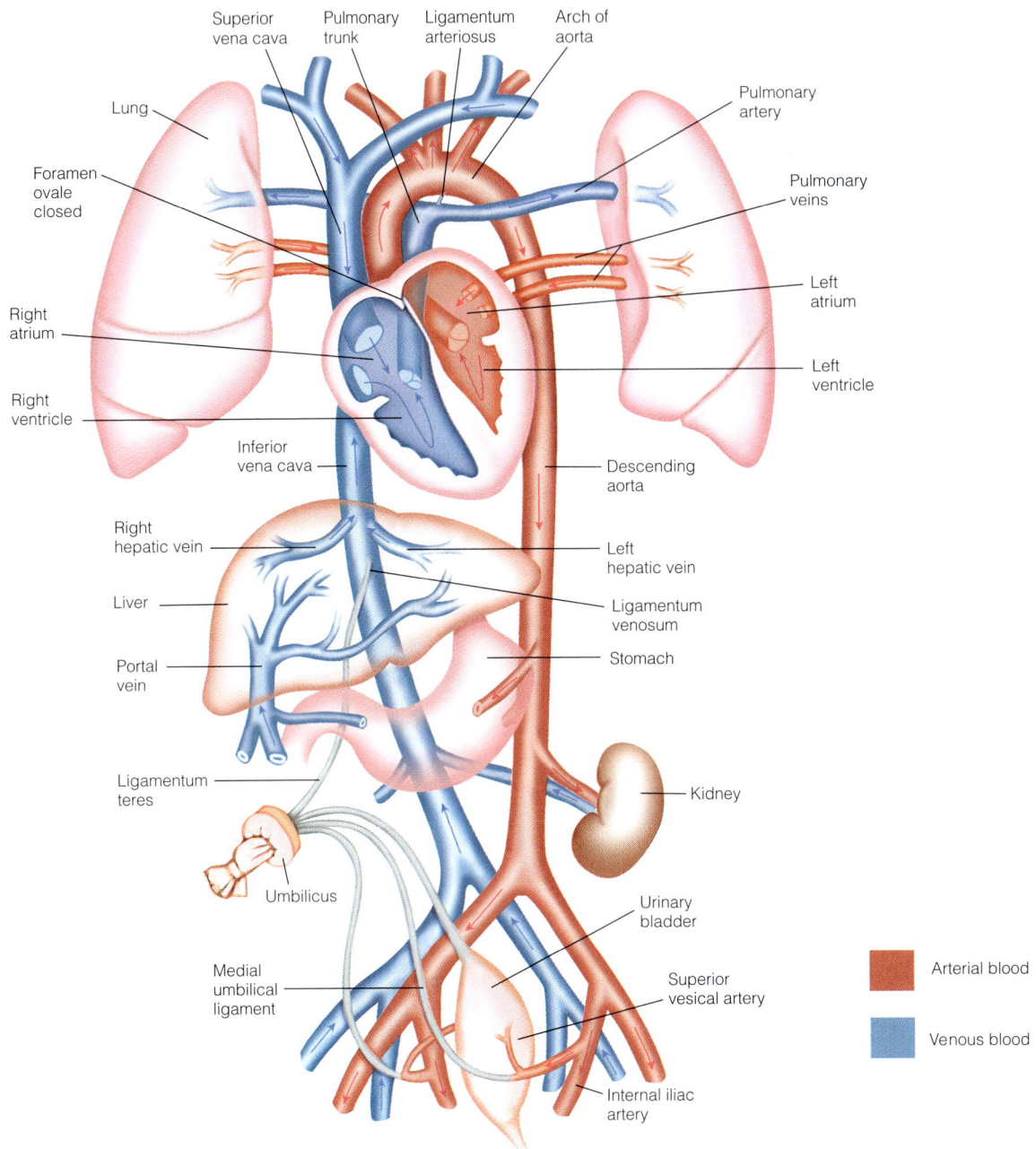

Figure 17-2. ■ The newborn circulatory system.

Apgar Score

The newborn's adaptation to life outside the uterus will be evaluated using an Apgar score (see Table 14-6 and Procedure 14-1 ⬭). This evaluation is typically completed at 1 and 5 minutes, but it can be used anytime the newborn's condition is in question. As you recall from Chapter 14 ⬭, each item—heart rate, respiratory rate, muscle tone, reflex irritability, and color—is assigned a score of 0 to 2, and then totaled. A score of 8 to 10 requires no special attention. A score of 4 to 7 requires the administration of oxygen and stimulation. This level score may be seen if a mother has received a narcotic during labor. Narcotics enter the infant through the placenta and depress the respiratory center, leading to hypoventilation and hypoxia. A narcotic antagonist, such as naloxone (Narcan), may need to be administered to the infant.

A score of 0 to 3 indicates that the infant needs immediate resuscitation. Figure 17-5 ■ shows some of the equipment and techniques that are used for infant

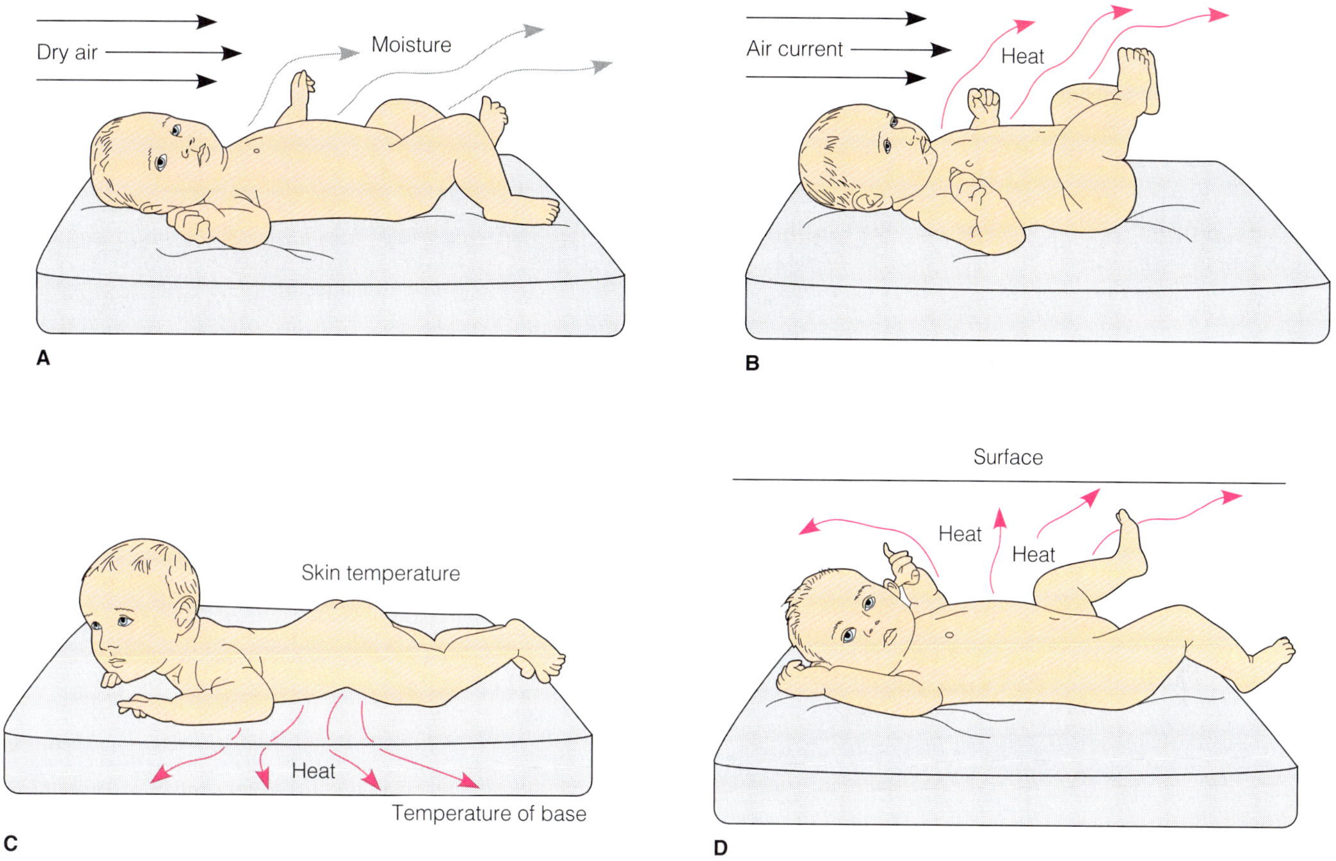

Figure 17-3. ■ Mechanisms of heat loss. (**A**) Evaporation. (**B**) Convection. (**C**) Conduction. (**D**) Radiation.

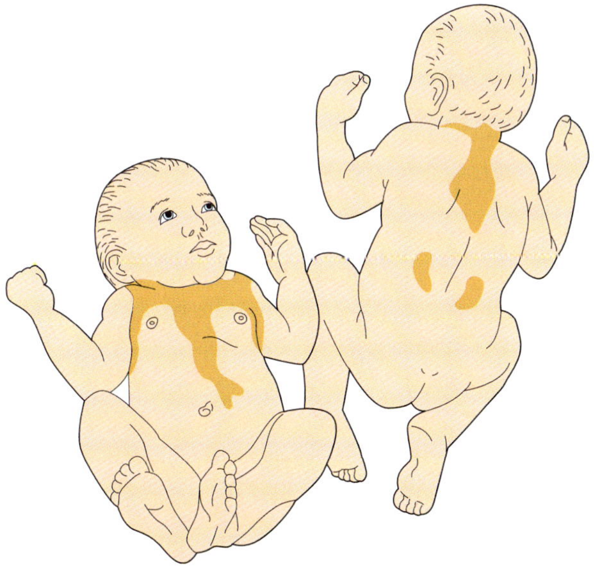

Figure 17-4. ■ The distribution of brown fat (adipose tissue) in the newborn. (Adapted from Davis, V. [1980]. Structure and function of brown adipose tissue in the neonate. *Journal of Obstetrics, Gynecologic and Neonatal Nursing, 9*, 364. Oxford: Blackwell.)

cardiopulmonary resuscitation (CPR). CPR requires special training plus review courses to ensure that the nurse is using up-to-date methods and is following the most current guidelines.

clinical ALERT

CPR can be life threatening if improperly performed on an infant. The nurse performing CPR on a neonate or infant must be qualified in pediatric advanced life support (PALS).

Identification

Before the mother and newborn are separated, identification bands are applied (see Figure 14-30 ⬭). Care must be taken not to constrict circulation or scratch the newborn with the clasp. Identification numbers are compared each time the newborn is brought to the mother and at time of discharge. The mother will be asked to sign documents stating that she has received her newborn.

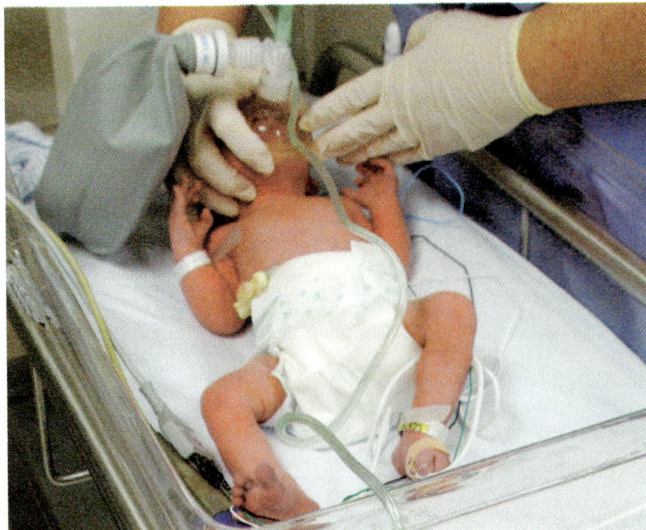

A

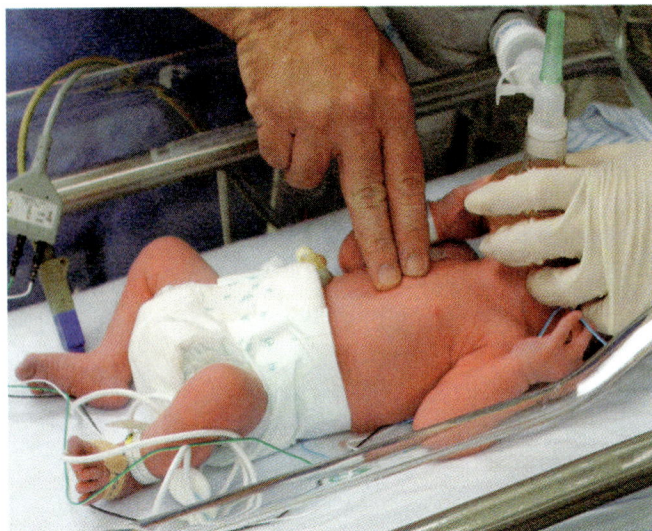

B

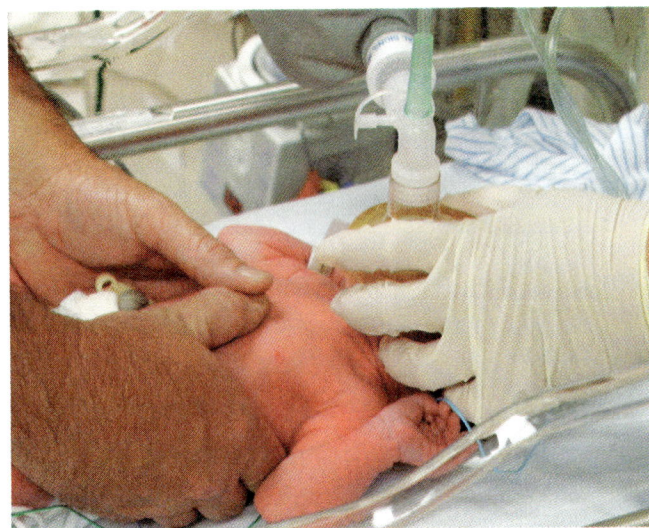

C

Figure 17-5. ■ CPR of an infant. (**A**) Demonstration of resuscitation of a newborn with bag and mask (Ambu-bag). Note that the mask covers the nose and mouth, and the head is in a neutral "sniff" position. The resuscitating bag is placed to the side of the baby so the chest movement can be seen. (**B**) Technique for closed chest cardiac compression (or external cardiac massage) of the neonate. Two fingers of one hand are placed at neonatal nipple line, with the other fingers raised from the surface of the body. In the two-finger method, the tips of two fingers of one hand compress the infant's sternum, and the other hand or a firm surface supports the infant's back. (**C**) Chest compression can also be done using the pads of both thumbs. With either method, the sternum is compressed at a rate of 90 beats per minute.

HEALTHY NEWBORN

The nurse assesses the newborn at the time of delivery to determine the need for resuscitation. The stable newborn can remain with the family. The newborn with complications will be taken to a nursery for further intervention and monitoring. Within the first 1 to 2 hours, the nurse completes a more in-depth assessment to evaluate the newborn's adaptation to life outside the uterus and to identify any complications. The nurse must understand the usual characteristics of the healthy newborn in order to evaluate the newborn's current condition.

Vital Signs

Vital signs for normal newborns are highlighted in Table 17-1 ■. Vital signs continue to change over time.

TEMPERATURE

Temperature is assessed on admission to the nursery and every 30 minutes until the temperature has remained stable for 2 hours. The temperature is then obtained at least once every 8 hours or as specified in facility policy. The newborn's temperature ranges from 97.7 to 99.4°F (36.5 to 37.4°C). The axillary temperature is generally taken using an electronic thermometer (Figure 17-6A ■). When the newborn is placed under radiant heat, a skin thermal sensor is placed over soft tissue such as on the abdomen (Figure 17-6B ■). An alarm will sound if the newborn's temperature rises above the preset value.

HEART RATE

Heart rate should be assessed when the newborn is at rest. An apical pulse should be counted for a full minute. The

TABLE 17-1

Newborn Vital Signs

AGE	TEMPERATURE IN F (C)	PULSE (BEATS/MINUTE)	RESPIRATION (BREATHS/MINUTE)	BLOOD PRESSURE
Birth	97.7–99.5 (36.5–37.4)	90–160 (may be low when sleeping, up to 180 when crying, 220 with fever)	35 (30–60)	80–60/45–40 mm Hg
Day 10	99.0 (37.2)	90–220	30 (28–50)	100/50 mm Hg
1 Month	99.2 (37.4)	85–170	24–45	94–104/50–60

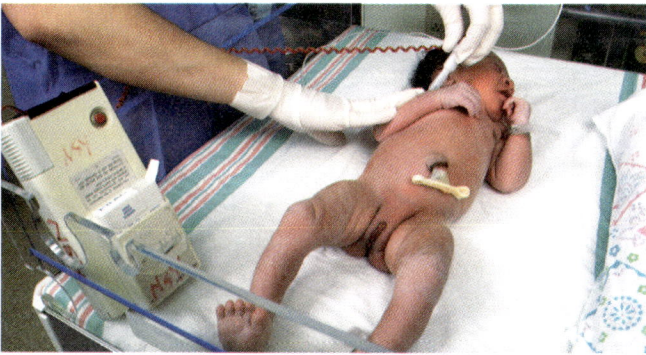
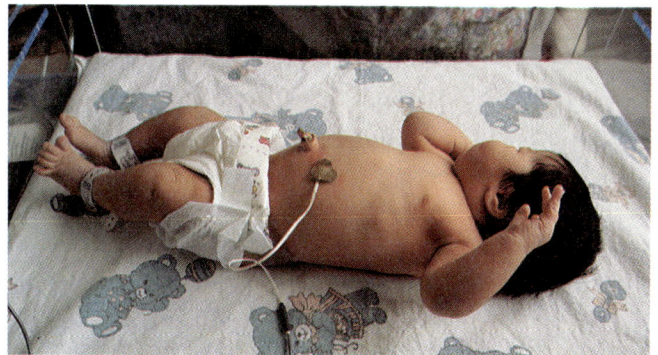

Figure 17-6. ■ Temperature monitoring for the newborn. (**A**) An axillary temperature is measured using an electronic thermometer. (**B**) Skin thermal sensor is placed on the newborn's abdomen, upper thigh, or arm and secured with a porous tape or a foil-covered foam pad.

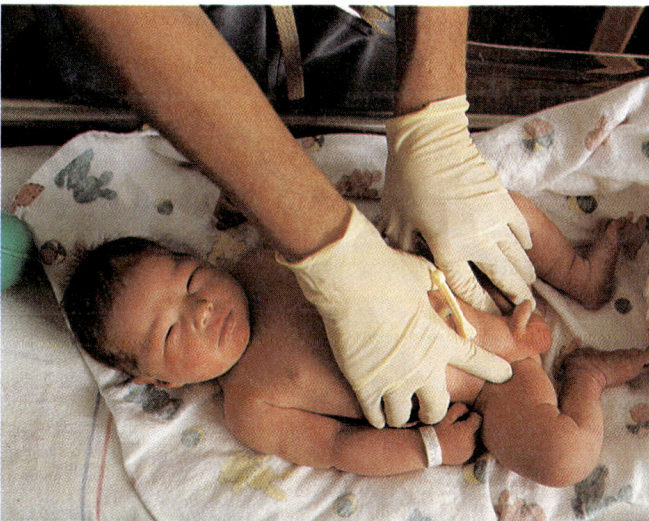
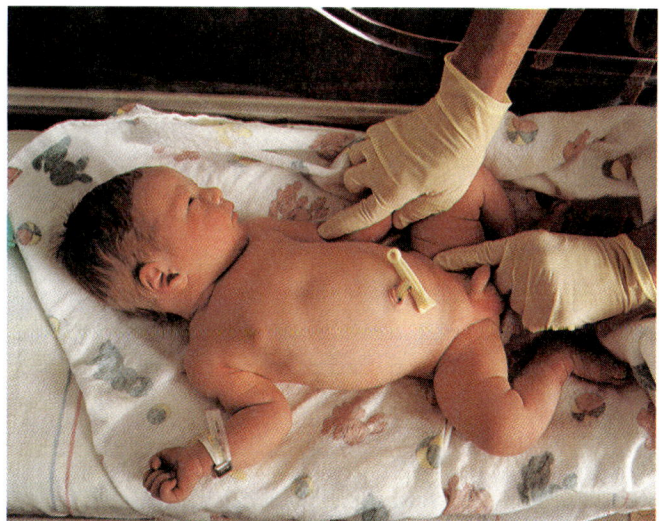

Figure 17-7. ■ (**A**) Bilaterally palpate the femoral arteries for rate and intensity of the pulse. Press fingertip gently at the groin as shown. (**B**) Compare the femoral pulse to the brachial pulse by palpating the pulse simultaneously for comparison of rate and intensity.

normal pulse rate is 120 to 160 beats per minute (bpm), but it may be as high as 180 bpm if the newborn is crying and as low as 90 bpm if the newborn is sleeping. Brachial and femoral pulses should be palpated (Figure 17-7 ■). However, radial pulses are difficult to feel.

RESPIRATORY RATE

The respiratory rate should be assessed when the newborn is quiet. Respirations should be counted for a full minute. The normal respiratory rate is 30 to 60 breaths per minute.

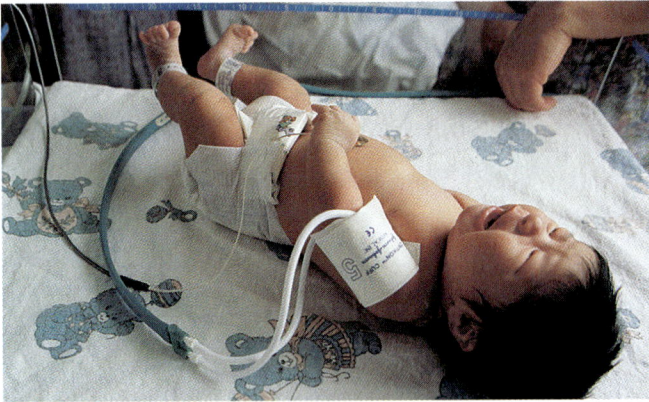

Figure 17-8. ■ Blood pressure measurement using a Doppler device. The cuff can be applied to the upper arm or thigh.

BLOOD PRESSURE

Measurement of blood pressure (BP) in the newborn varies. Some facilities generally do not take newborn BP. Other facilities routinely take it as a baseline in case cardiac issues should arise. If the newborn's condition warrants obtaining a blood pressure measurement, an electronic Doppler device (Figure 17-8 ■) is used. The cuff can be applied to the upper arm or leg. The size of the cuff must be appropriate for the newborn, usually 1 to 2 inches (2.5 to 5 cm) wide.

clinical ALERT

The normal blood pressure for a newborn is 60–80/40–45 mm Hg at birth and 100/50 at day 10. The newborn's extremities must be immobilized during the procedure.

PAIN

Pain is an unpleasant sensation related to actual or potential tissue damage. Pain exists when the client says it does. The newborn is unable to verbalize the pain experience, but it is widely accepted that the newborn does feel pain. Skin sensation is present by 20 weeks' gestation, and the brain centers necessary for pain reception are developed toward the end of pregnancy. The newborn exhibits pain through facial expression and crying. Box 17-1 ■ provides an infant pain rating scale.

BOX 17-1

Infant Pain Scale

S = Sleeping
0 = No pain
1 = Restless
2 = Facial grimacing
3 = Favors body parts (knees at abdomen, pulls at body part)
4 = Crying uncontrollably

Gestational Age

An assessment of gestational age is completed within the first 4 hours after birth. Prenatally, the gestational age was determined from the last menstrual period. This estimation is accurate 75% to 85% of the time. A clinical gestational age assessment tool, the Ballard Newborn Rating Scale (Figure 17-9 ■), was developed to determine gestational age more accurately and consistently. In this assessment tool, points from −1 to 5 are assigned to each characteristic. The points are totaled and referenced to the maturity rating scale to determine the gestational age in weeks.

NEUROMUSCULAR MATURITY

The first area of the gestational age assessment is neuromuscular maturity. Some of the assessments made are illustrated in this section.

Body Position at Rest

At rest, full-term newborns lie in a flexed position, whereas premature newborns lie extended (Figure 17-10 ■).

Wrist Angle

The square window of the wrist or angle of the hand and fingers when compressed by the examiner (Figure 17-11 ■) is 0 to 30 degrees in normal newborns and 90 degrees in the premature newborn.

Arm Recoil

Arm recoil (Figure 17-12 ■) is exhibited when the arms are held in extension next to the body for 5 seconds and then released. In the healthy newborn, the arms recoil to the flexed position.

Popliteal Angle

The popliteal angle is determined by flexing and holding the thigh to the abdomen while extending the leg at the knee. In the healthy newborn this angle is less than 90 degrees, whereas in the premature newborn the angle is 180 degrees (see the Ballard Rating Scale, Figure 17-9).

Scarf Sign

The **scarf sign** is exhibited by moving the arm in front of the neck (Figure 17-13 ■). In the normal newborn, the elbow will not reach the midline. In the premature newborn, the elbow moves past the midline.

PHYSICAL MATURITY

The second area to be assessed is physical maturity. The skin, lanugo, feet, breasts, ears, and genitals are assigned points based on their degree of development.

NEWBORN MATURITY RATING & CLASSIFICATION

ESTIMATION OF GESTATIONAL AGE BY MATURITY RATING
Symbols: X - 1st Exam O - 2nd Exam

NEUROMUSCULAR MATURITY

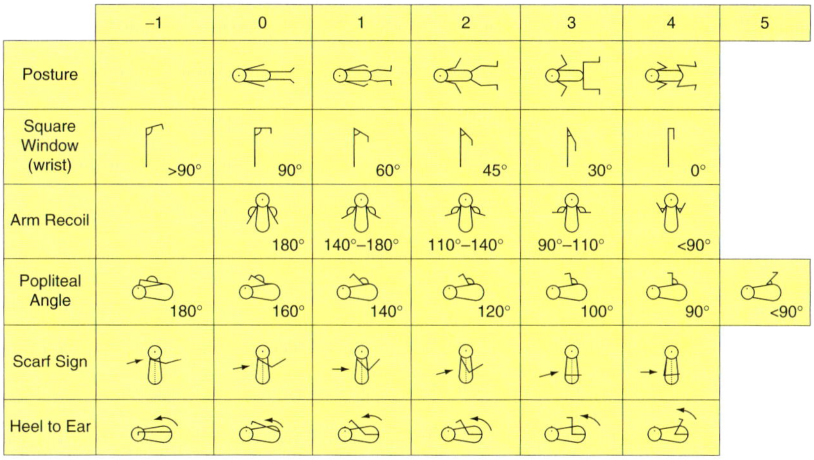

	-1	0	1	2	3	4	5
Posture							
Square Window (wrist)	>90°	90°	60°	45°	30°	0°	
Arm Recoil		180°	140°–180°	110°–140°	90°–110°	<90°	
Popliteal Angle	180°	160°	140°	120°	100°	90°	<90°
Scarf Sign							
Heel to Ear							

Gestation by Dates _____ wks

Birth Date _____ Hour _____ am / pm

APGAR _____ 1 min _____ 5 min

MATURITY RATING

score	weeks
-10	20
-5	22
0	24
5	26
10	28
15	30
20	32
25	34
30	36
35	38
40	40
45	42
50	44

PHYSICAL MATURITY

Skin	sticky friable transparent	gelatinous red, translucent	smooth pink, visible veins	superficial peeling &/or rash, few veins	cracking pale areas rare veins	parchment deep cracking no vessels	leathery cracked wrinkled
Lanugo	none	sparse	abundant	thinning	bald areas	mostly bald	
Plantar Surface	heel-toe 40–50 mm:–1 <40 mm:–2	>50 mm no crease	faint red marks	anterior transverse crease only	creases ant. 2/3	creases over entire sole	
Breast	imperceptible	barely perceptible	flat areola no bud	stippled areola 1–2 mm bud	raised areola 3–4 mm bud	full areola 5–10 mm bud	
Eye/Ear	lids fused loosely:–1 tightly:–2	lids open pinna flat stays folded	sl. curved pinna; soft; slow recoil	well curved pinna; soft but ready recoil	formed & firm instant recoil	thick cartilage ear stiff	
Genitals male	scrotum flat, smooth	scrotum empty faint rugae	testes in upper canal rare rugae	testes descending few rugae	testes down good rugae	testes pendulous deep rugae	
Genitals female	clitoris prominent labia flat	prominent clitoris small labia minora	prominent clitoris enlarging minora	majora & minora equally prominent	majora large minora small	majora cover clitoris & minora	

SCORING SECTION

	1st Exam = X	2nd Exam = O
Estimating Gest Age by Maturity Rating	_____ Weeks	_____ Weeks
Time of Exam	Date _____ Hour_____ am/pm	Date _____ Hour_____ am/pm
Age at Exam	_____ Hours	_____ Hours
Signature of Examiner	_____ M.D./R.N.	_____ M.D./R.N.

Figure 17-9. ■ Ballard Newborn Rating Scale. (Reprinted from Ballard, J. L., Khoury, J. C., Wedig, K., Wang, L., Eilers-Walsman, B. L., & Lipp, R. [1991]. New Ballard score, expanded to include extremely premature infants. *Journal of Pediatrics, 119*, 417. Used with permission from Elsevier, Inc.)

A   **B**   **C**

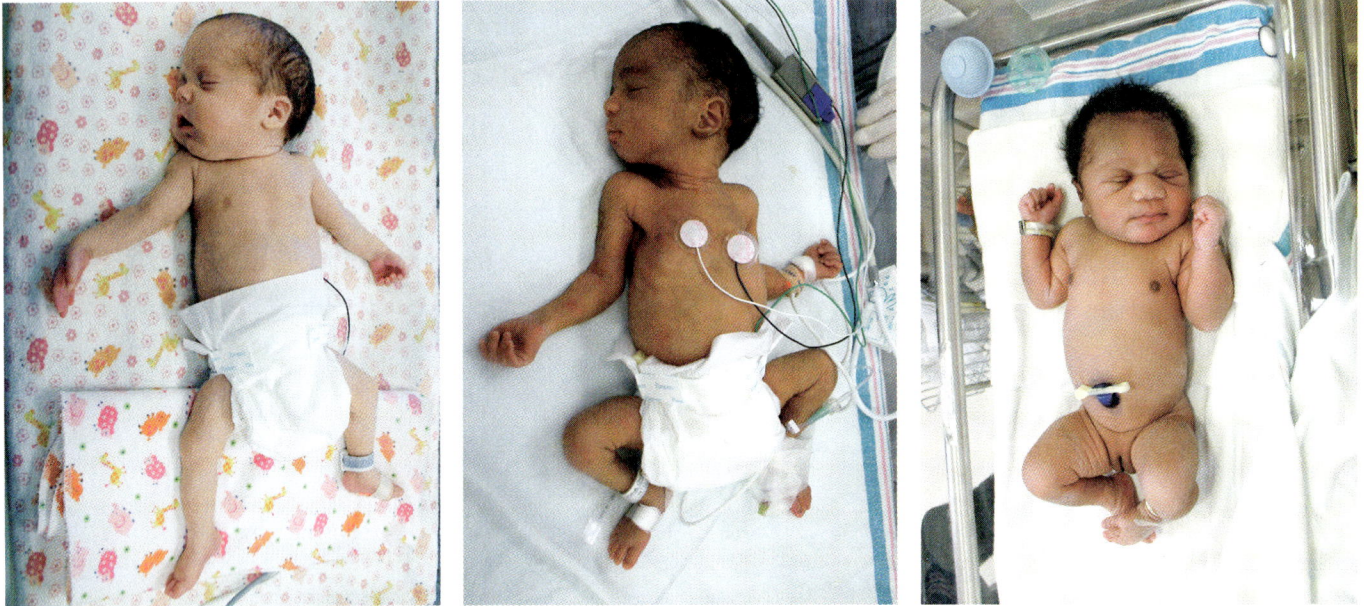

Figure 17-10. ■ Neuromuscular maturity determined by resting posture. (**A**) At a gestational age of approximately 31 weeks, there is extension of the upper extremities and beginning flexion of the thighs. (**B**) At a gestational age of approximately 35 weeks, the newborn shows strong flexion of the arms, hips, and thighs. (**C**) At term, the newborn exhibits hypertonic flexion of all extremities.

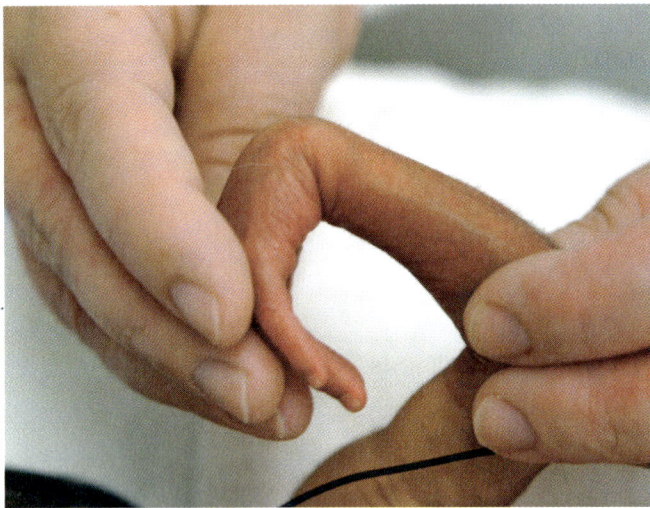

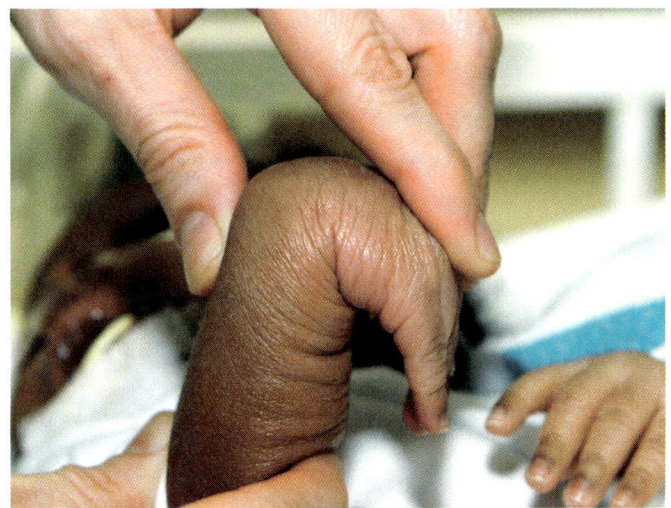

A   **B**

Figure 17-11. ■ Square window sign. (**A**) At about 28 to 32 weeks' gestation, the angle is 90 degrees. (**B**) At about 39 to 40 weeks, the angle is commonly 30 degrees.

Integument

The skin of the premature newborn appears thin and transparent, with numerous blood vessels visible. At term, subcutaneous fat deposits make the skin opaque, with few blood vessels visible. The skin of postmature newborns is dry and peels.

A fine downy hair, lanugo, covers the fetus but disappears from the face by 30 weeks and then from the trunk and extremities.

The creases on the bottom of the foot lengthen and deepen with age. This sign of maturity is accurate for up to 12 hours post delivery. After 12 hours, however, the skin on the soles dries and may peel, becoming an invalid reference of age.

At term, the breast tissue, including the areola, measures 0.5 to 1 cm.

Cartilage gives the ear shape. In the premature newborn this cartilage is not developed, resulting in relatively shapeless pinna. If the pinna is folded over on itself, it remains folded.

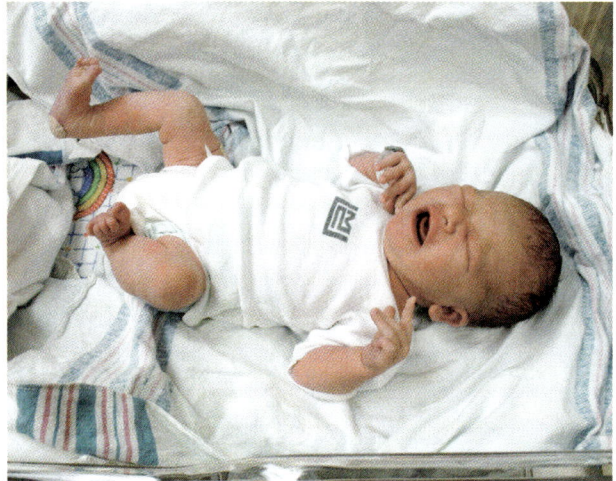

A   **B**

Figure 17-12. ■ To elicit arm recoil reflex, flex the infant's arms to the chest for 5 seconds. (**A**) Then extend the arms at the elbows. (**B**) Release the arms to see the amount of recoil. In healthy newborns, the angle of flexion is usually less than 90 degrees, following rapid recoil to a flexed position. A term infant resists extension and returns briskly to a flexed position. A premature infant exhibits less resistance and less recoil.

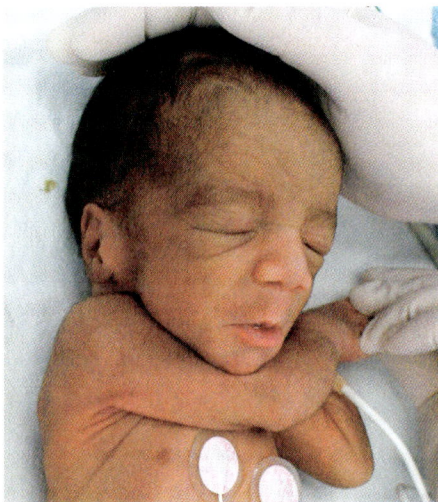
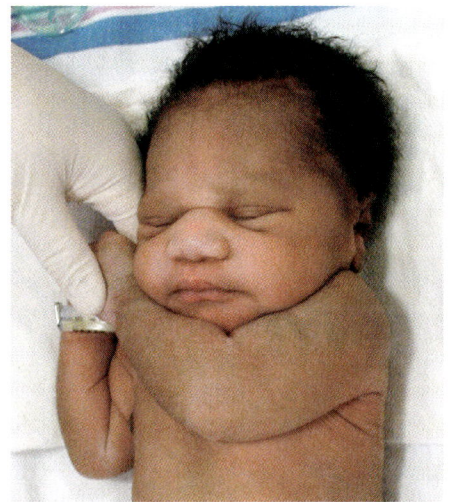

Λ   **B**   **C**

Figure 17-13. ■ Scarf sign. (**A**) Until about 30 weeks' gestation, the elbow moves past midline with no resistance. (**B**) At about 36 to 38 weeks' gestation, the elbow is at midline. (**C**) The elbow will not reach midline after 40 weeks' gestation.

Genitalia

Male genitals are evaluated for the size of the scrotal sac, the presence of rugae, and the descent of the testicles (illustrated later in this chapter). Female genitals are evaluated for size of the labia majora. At term, the labia majora nearly covers the clitoris and labia minora.

Height, Weight, and Head Circumference

The newborn is weighed, and length and head circumference are measured (see Procedures 14-2 through 14-5 and Figure 14-26 ⬭⬭). The healthy newborn weighs between 5 lb. 8 oz and 8 lb. 13 oz (2,500–4,000 g), is 18 to 22 inches (48–52 cm) long, and has a head circumference of 12.5 to 14.5 inches (32–37 cm). These values are recorded on a growth chart for easy reference to national percentile ranges (Figure 17-14 ■). A set of growth charts is provided in Appendix II. Infants whose values are in the 10th to 90th percentile range are considered appropriate for gestational age (AGA). Infants less than 10th percentile are small for gestational age (SGA). Those greater than 90th percentile are large for gestational age (LGA).

CLASSIFICATION OF NEWBORNS—
BASED ON MATURITY AND INTRAUTERINE GROWTH

Symbols: X-1st Exam   O-2nd Exam

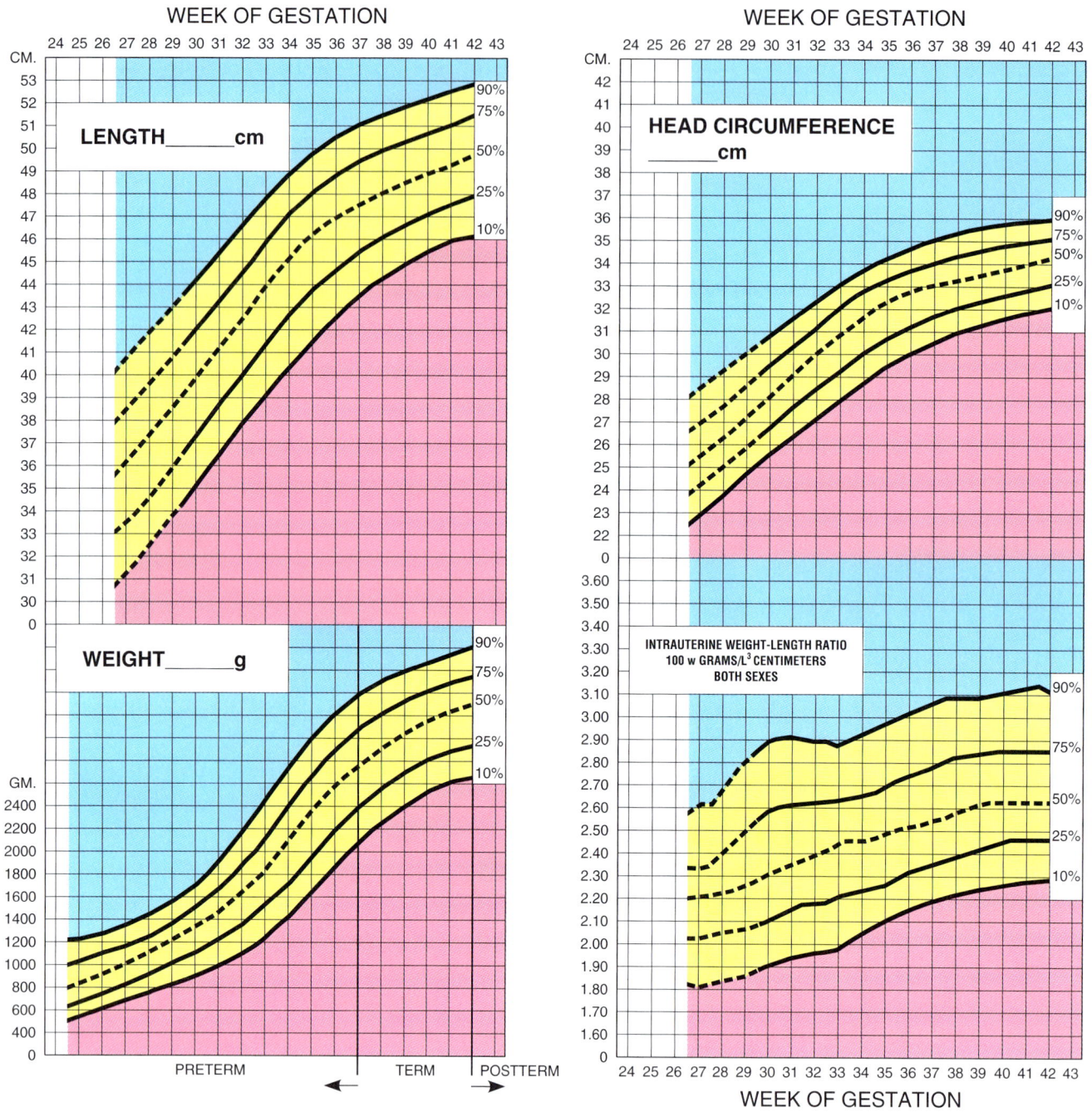

	1st Exam (X)	2nd Exam (O)
LARGE FOR GESTATIONAL AGE (LGA)		
APPROPRIATE FOR GESTATIONAL AGE (AGA)		
SMALL FOR GESTATIONAL AGE (SGA)		
Age at Exam	hrs	hrs
Signature of Examiner	M.D./R.N.	M.D./R.N.

Figure 17-14. ■ The nurse accurately measures the child and then places height, weight, and head circumference on appropriate growth grids for the child's age and gender. (Adapted from Lubchenco, L. O., Hansman, C., & Boyd, E. [1966]. *Pediatrics, 37*, 404, Figure 1. Reprinted, with permission, from the American Academy of Pediatrics; Battaglia, F. C., & Lubchenco, L. O. [1967]. A practical classification of newborn infants by weight and gestational age. *Journal of Pediatrics, 71*, 161, with permission from Elsevier, Inc.)

Characteristics of the Newborn

GENERAL APPEARANCE

The healthy newborn appears plump, pink, and active. The head is disproportionately large for the body. The center of the newborn's body is the umbilicus. The healthy newborn can move all extremities but prefers a flexed position.

SKIN

The skin at birth is red and smooth. **Acrocyanosis** (Figure 17-15A ■), a bluish discoloration of the hands and feet, is common for several hours after delivery. **Ecchymosis** (bruising) and **petechiae** (pinpoint hemorrhages) may be present following a difficult delivery. Some swelling around the eyes is common. The skin may be covered with vernix caseosa, especially in the body folds. The vernix absorbs into the skin, keeping it soft. Lanugo may be present on the face, arms, and back. Within a few days the skin may become dry and peel. A small amount of baby lotion can be used to moisturize the skin. Soap should be avoided.

Jaundice

Physiologic jaundice frequently occurs after the first 24 hours of life. Infants have an increase in red blood cells (RBCs) at birth. With oxygenation through the newborn's lungs, the extra RBCs are no longer needed. **Jaundice** is a condition that occurs because the infant's liver is immature and cannot conjugate the amount of bilirubin released by the destruction of RBCs. The bilirubin remains in the blood, causing a yellow appearance of light skin and a yellowing of the sclera. The jaundice increases for several days. Once the infant passes transitional stools, the jaundice gradually fades.

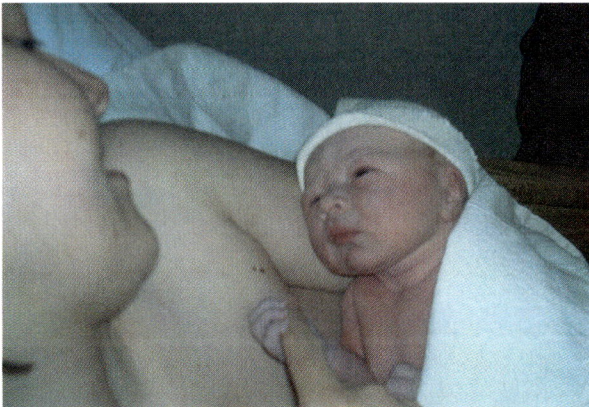

A

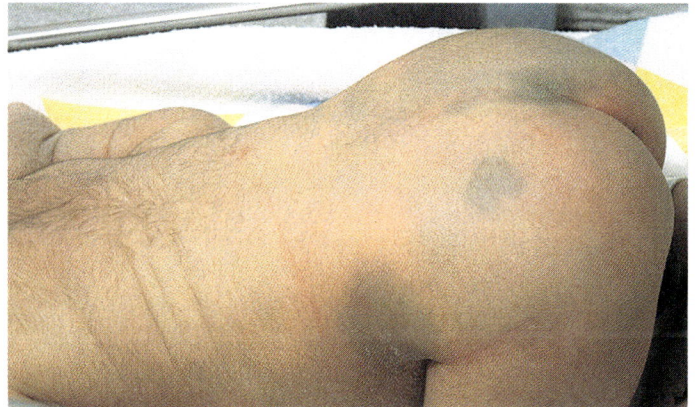

B

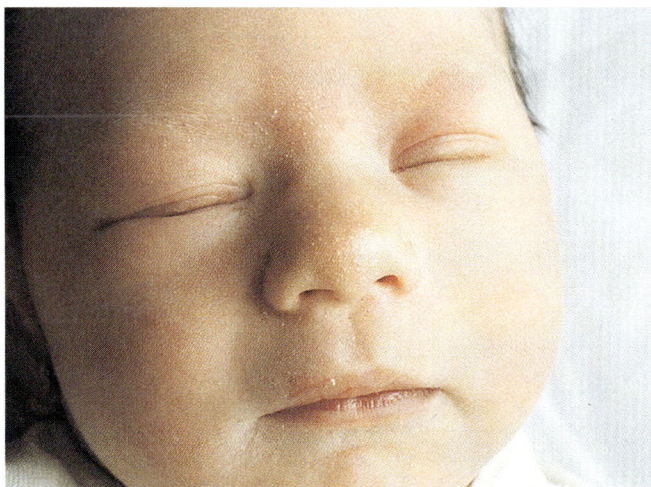

C

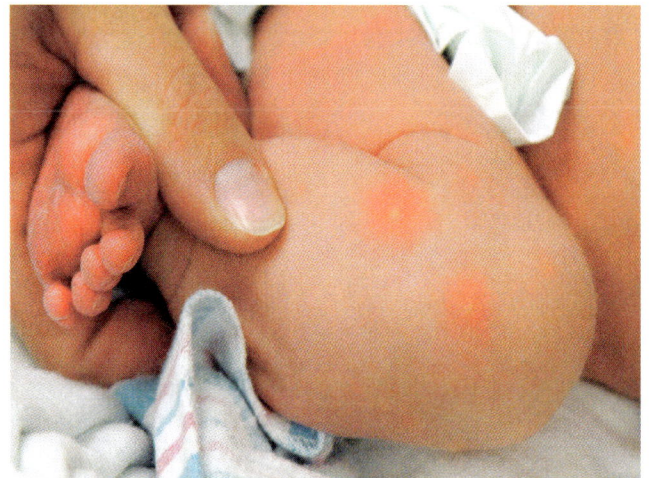

D

Figure 17-15. ■ (**A**) Acrocyanosis. (Courtesy of C. Haggett.) (**B**) Mongolian spots. (**C**) Facial milia. The spots usually disappear spontaneously within a few weeks. (**D**) Erythema toxicum. The condition is noted during the newborn's first 24 hours and may remain for about 1 week, most commonly on the trunk and diaper area. (Reproduced, with permission, of Mead Johnson & Company, Evansville, IN.)

Other Skin Markings

Several discolored areas are commonly found on a newborn's skin. A **Mongolian spot** (see Figure 17-15B ■) is a dark-colored area found over the lower back and sacrum of infants of Black, Hispanic, South Asian, or East Asian descent. Over time, the infant's skin tones darken to become the same color as the Mongolian spot. Some infants are born with dark red spots on the eyelids, forehead, or nape of the neck. These red areas, called **telangiectatic nevi** or **stork bites,** usually fade in time. Parental concern for these and other birthmarks should be discussed with the pediatrician. Consultation with a plastic surgeon may be needed. The sebaceous glands on the face become distended a few days after birth resulting in **milia** (Figure 17-15C ■) or white pinpoint spots resembling whiteheads. A few weeks of bathing cause the sebaceous glands to open and the milia to disappear. **Erythema toxicum neonatorum** is a raised pink papule with a light-colored center resembling a mosquito bite (Figure 17-15D ■). The lesions appear suddenly on the chest, abdomen, and back 24 to 48 hours after birth. They are benign and will disappear without treatment. If other birthmarks are found when assessing the newborn's skin, they should be documented.

HEAD

The head of the newborn may be asymmetric at birth. The anterior and posterior fontanels (Figure 17-16 ■) should be firm and flat. The head is 13 to 14 inches (33–34 cm) in circumference. *Molding*, the shaping of the fetal head to the shape of the mother's pelvis, may take several days to resolve (see Figure 14-12 ⚭). Edema of the scalp, called **caput succedaneum,** may cross the suture lines. **Cephalhematoma,** in contrast, is an accumulation of blood between the periosteum and the skull bone that will not cross the suture lines. Figure 17-17 ■ illustrates caput succedaneum and cephalhematoma. Marks from an internal fetal monitoring electrode, a suction (vacuum) extractor, or forceps may be present if they were used in labor and delivery (see Figure 15-14B ⚭).

The newborn's face should be symmetric. The top of the ears should be in line with the outer canthus of the eye. The pinna may be flat against the head. The eyes of the newborn may show small hemorrhages in the sclera due to the pressure of delivery. The newborn has poor control of the eye muscles resulting in **strabismus** (lack of coordination of the visual axes of the eye; eyes do not stay parallel to each other but may diverge in any direction). This disappears in a few months. The nose may be flattened due to the birth process. The mouth should be midline, with both cheeks moving symmetrically.

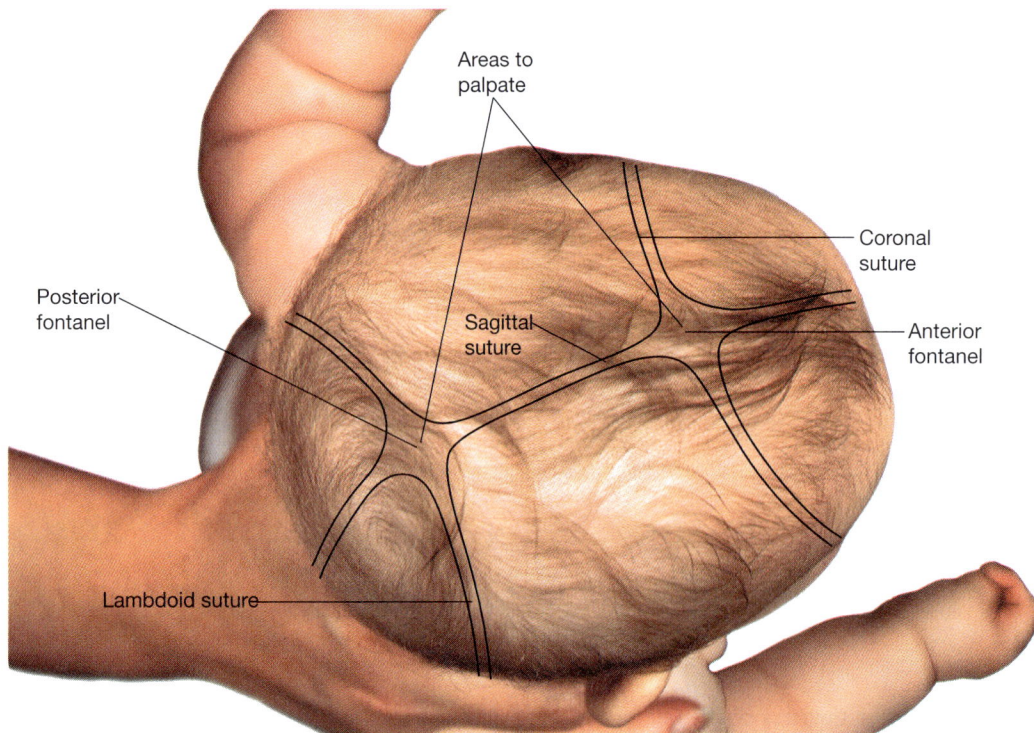

Figure 17-16. ■ Anterior and posterior fontanels. The bones of the skull, showing the fontanel and suture lines.

A

B

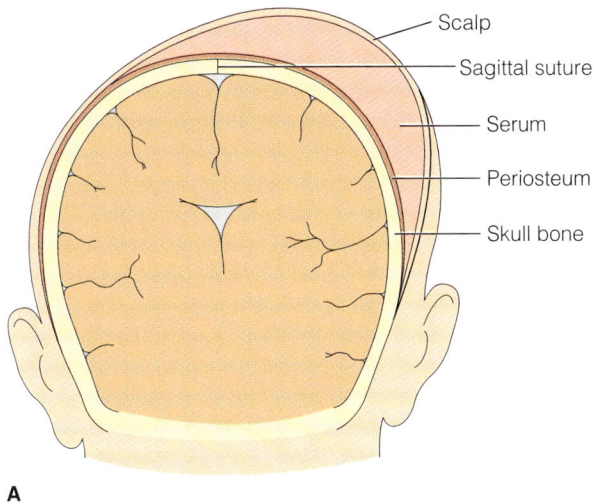

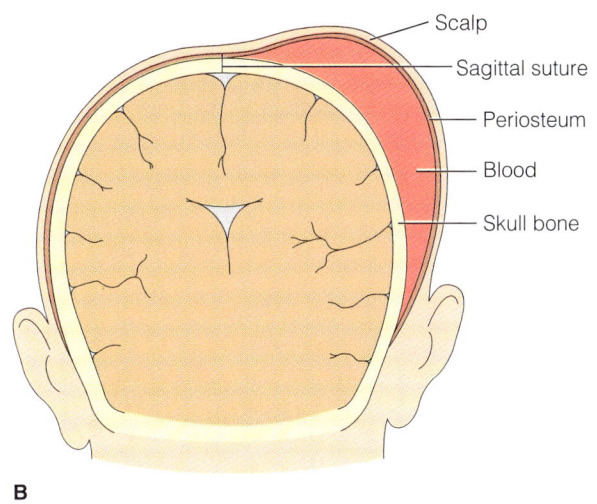

Figure 17-17. ■ (**A**) Caput succedaneum is a collection of fluid under the scalp. (**B**) Cephalhematoma is a collection of blood between the surface of the cranial bone and the periosteal membrane. This is a cephalhematoma over the left parietal bone.

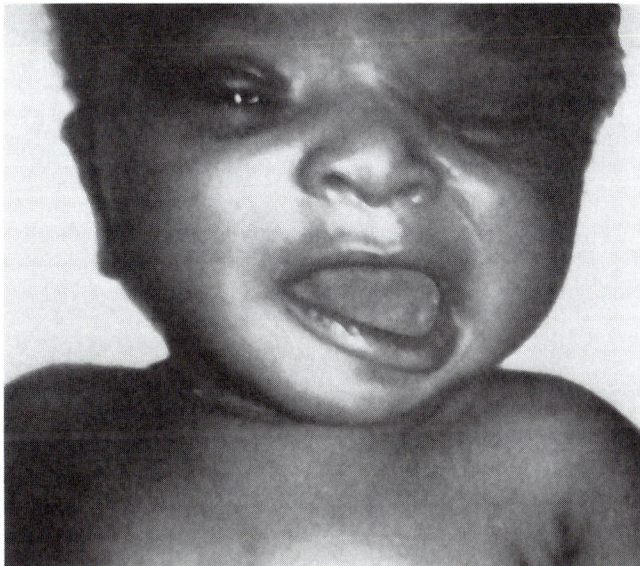

Figure 17-18. ■ Asymmetry of the face indicates facial palsy and should be reported to the primary care provider. (Used with permission from Potter, E. L., & Craig, J. M. [1975]. *Pathology of the fetus and infant* [3rd ed.]. St. Louis, MO: Mosby-Yearbook Medical Publishers. Courtesy of Dr. Ralph Platow.)

Asymmetry of the face indicates facial palsy and should be reported to the primary care provider (Figure 17-18 ■).

The palate and lips should be intact. One or more precocious teeth may be present in the center of the lower gum.

clinical ALERT

If the newborn is born with precocious teeth, they will become loose and fall out. They may need to be removed by the primary care provider to prevent aspiration.

Epstein's pearls, small white cysts, may be present on the palate, but they disappear in a few weeks.

The neck is short with several skin folds. The muscles of the neck are unable to support the weight of the newborn's head. When the newborn is pulled up from a supine position, the head lags behind. However, from a prone position, the newborn can lift the head slightly.

CHEST

The chest should be 12 to 13 inches (30.5–33 cm) in circumference. Two nipples should be identifiable. Some engorgement may be present in both male and female infants due to maternal hormones. The nipple may secrete whitish fluid, called **witch's milk,** for several days.

Heart Sounds

Heart sounds should be assessed when the newborn is in a quiet state. Because of the rapid heart rate, evaluating heart sounds in the newborn takes practice. The normal lub-dub sounds should be heard. A slurring of one sound (usually the lub) may indicate a murmur. Most murmurs are considered normal and disappear within a few months. However, some murmurs indicate an abnormality within the heart. For this reason, the primary care provider should monitor all murmurs.

Lung Sounds and Respiratory Distress

Lung sounds should be assessed when the newborn is quiet. The lungs should be auscultated from both the anterior and the posterior chest. Because heart sounds and bowel sounds are transmitted throughout the chest, localizing abnormal lung sounds may be difficult. Movement of air should be heard in all lung fields. Inspiration may be noisy for the first few hours after birth due to the presence of fluid in the air passages.

Breathing patterns in the newborn are predominantly diaphragmatic, with the chest rising with the abdominal movements. Respirations are usually irregular with brief

MediaLink

Heart and Lung Sounds

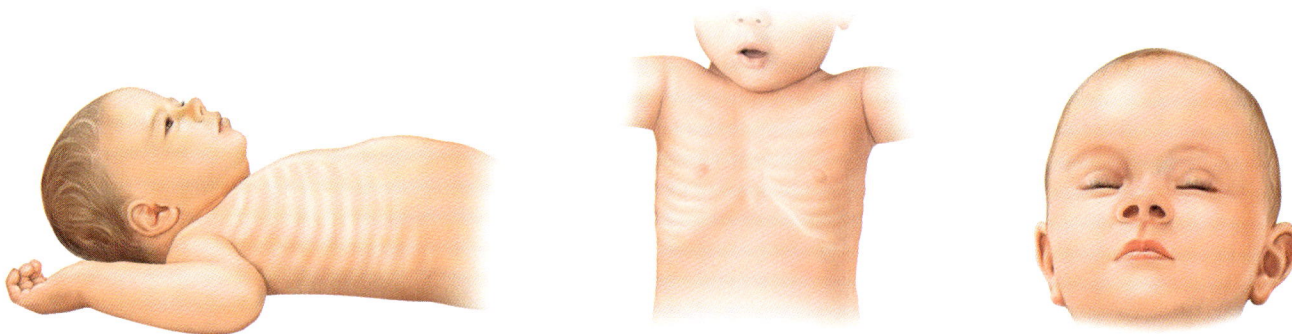

Figure 17-19. ■ Evaluation of respiratory status using the Silverman-Andersen index. The baby's respiratory status is assessed. A grade of 0, 1, or 2 is determined for each area, and a total score is charted in the baby's record or on a copy of this tool and placed in the chart.

periods of apnea. If there are no color or heart rate changes, these brief apneic episodes are considered normal.

The neonate should be observed frequently for signs of respiratory distress. Subtle changes indicate the newborn is having difficulty maintaining gas exchange. The earliest sign is **nasal flaring,** outward movement of the nostrils followed by **expiratory grunting,** and noisy exhalation. If the distress continues, **retractions,** an inward movement of the tissue over the sternum and intercostal muscles) may be seen. Retractions can occur in a variety of locations.

- **Suprasternal** (above the sternum)
- **Substernal** (below the sternum)
- **Supraclavicular** (above the clavicles)
- **Intercostal** (between the ribs)
- **Subcostal** (below the ribs)

Figure 17-19 ■ illustrates areas of retraction in respiratory distress.

Apneic spells (periods without breathing) indicate a worsening of the respiratory distress. Signs of respiratory distress must be reported immediately to the supervising registered nurse and physician.

ABDOMEN

The abdomen should be soft, rounded, and without palpable masses. The LPN/LVN can perform light palpation of the abdomen of the newborn. However, due to the risk of organ damage, the LPN/LVN cannot perform deep palpation of the abdomen. The umbilical cord should be clamped, and three blood vessels should be identifiable. There should be no distention or bulging. If distention is present, the skin becomes tight and blood vessels appear under the skin surface.

clinical ALERT

Abdominal distention is a sign of many abnormalities of the gastrointestinal tract and should be reported to the primary care provider.

Bowel Sounds

Bowel sounds are present in four quadrants within an hour after birth. The stool, or *meconium*, is blackish green and sticky. It is made up of slats, amniotic fluid, mucous, bile, and epithelial cells. Meconium stools may persist for 2 to 3 days until the newborn begins to digest formula and breast milk.

clinical ALERT

If the newborn has not passed meconium stool within the first 24 hours, the primary care provider should be informed. Failure to pass stool could indicate congenital anomalies or other conditions of the gastrointestinal system.

Voiding

The newborn voids five to eight time a day. Fewer than five voids may indicate that the newborn needs more fluids. The newborn passes approximately 30 to 50 mL with each voiding. Using disposable diapers may make it difficult to assess the volume of urinary output because the urine is trapped inside the fibers. If an accurate assessment of urinary output is needed, diapers are weighed before and after use. The difference in weight indicates the amount of urine output.

clinical ALERT

If the newborn has not voided the first 24 hours, the primary care provider should be informed. Failure to void could indicate congenital anomalies or other conditions of the urinary system.

GENITALIA

Genitals should be inspected carefully (Figure 17-20 ■). Some congenital anomalies are discussed in Chapter 18 ◯◯. In the female newborn, the clitoris varies in size and may be so large that it appears similar to a penis. This is generally due to hormone influence and disappears in a few days. Fat deposits in the labia majora cause them

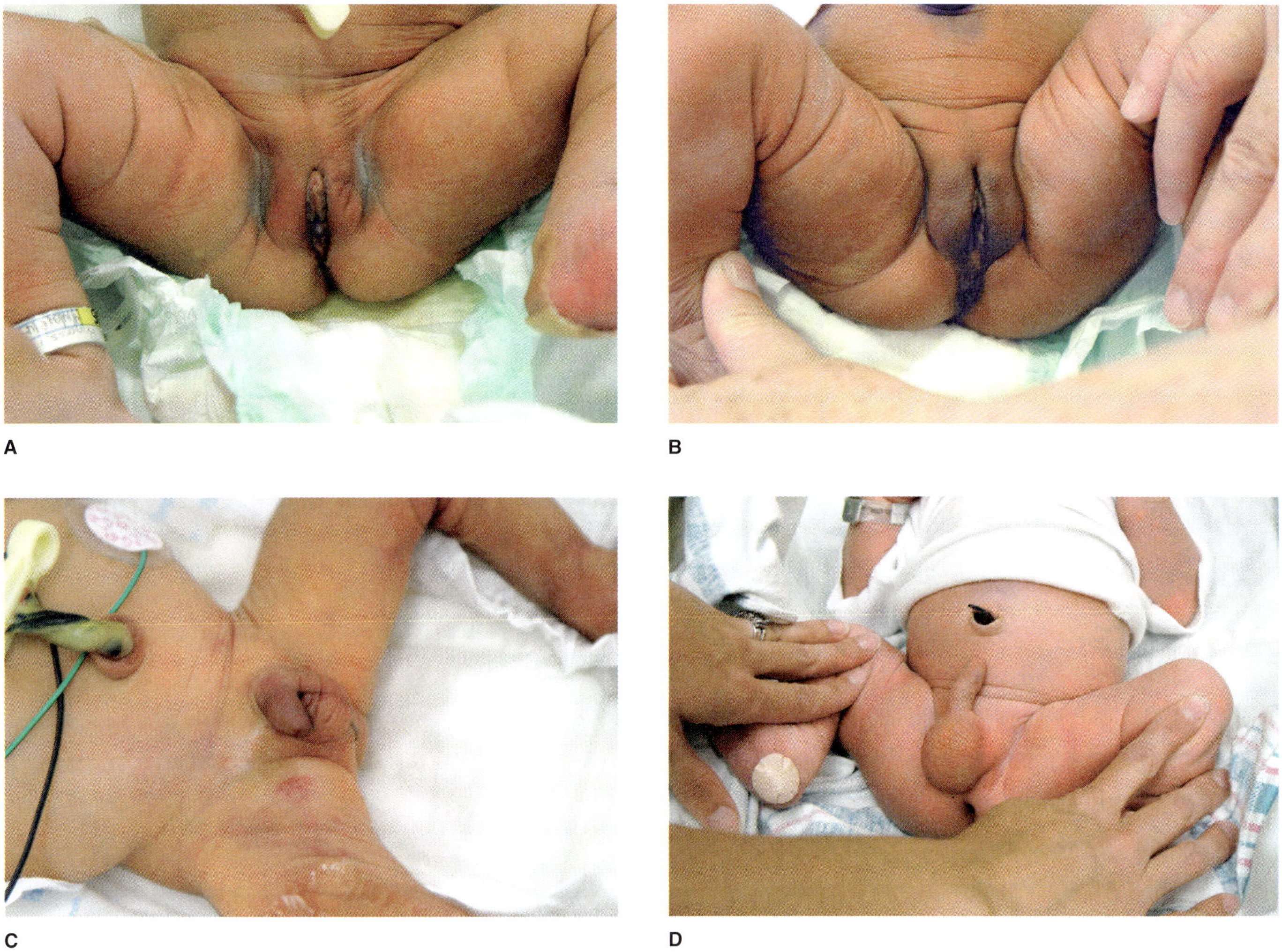

Figure 17-20. ■ (**A**) Female genitals. At a gestational age of 30 to 36 weeks, the newborn has a prominent clitoris, widely separated labia majora, and labia minora protruding beyond the labia majora (when viewed laterally). (**B**) At term, the labia majora are well developed and cover both the clitoris and the labia minora. (**C**) Male genitals. Note the absence of the testicles in the scrotum and a scrotum with few rugae in the preterm newborn. (**D**) In the term newborn, the testicles are descended into the scrotum, and the scrotum is covered by rugae.

to enlarge and cover the labia minora. This generally occurs before birth, but if the newborn is of low birth weight, there may not be enough subcutaneous fat for the labia majora to cover the labia minora. A mucus or slightly bloody vaginal discharge may be present. This **pseudomenstruation** is related to the influence of maternal hormones and disappears in a few days. **Smegma** (the secretion consisting of epithelial cells found around the external genitalia) may be present in the labia folds. Removing it may traumatize the tissue.

In the male newborn, the penis should be inspected to determine the location of the urinary meatus. The urinary meatus should open onto the tip of the glans. If it opens on the ventral surface, the newborn has hypospadias. (Hypospadias is discussed later in this chapter in the Assessment section.) Another condition of the male penis, phimosis, is also discussed later in this chapter.

The anus is inspected for patency. Abnormalities can usually be identified by visual inspection. If a digital examination is necessary, it should be completed by the primary care provider. The passage of stool verifies the functioning of the gastrointestinal tract. Congenital anomalies of the gastrointestinal tract are discussed in Chapter 18 ⊙⊙.

EXTREMITIES

The extremities should be symmetric bilaterally. Each extremity should end with five digits, without **webbing** (skin between two or more digits), **syndactyly** (the fusion of two or more digits), or **polydactyly** (presence of more than five fingers per hand or toes per foot). Muscle tone should be strong, with full range of motion in the *extremities* (arms and legs).

The femur should be well seated in the acetabulum. The registered nurse or physician should assess the hip for displacement or hip click (Figure 17-21 ■). Skin folds of the posterior thigh on the affected side may be noted. The ankle of the newborn appears to turn inward due to the position in the uterus. There should not be resistance when the foot is moved to a normal position. If resistance is

A

B

C

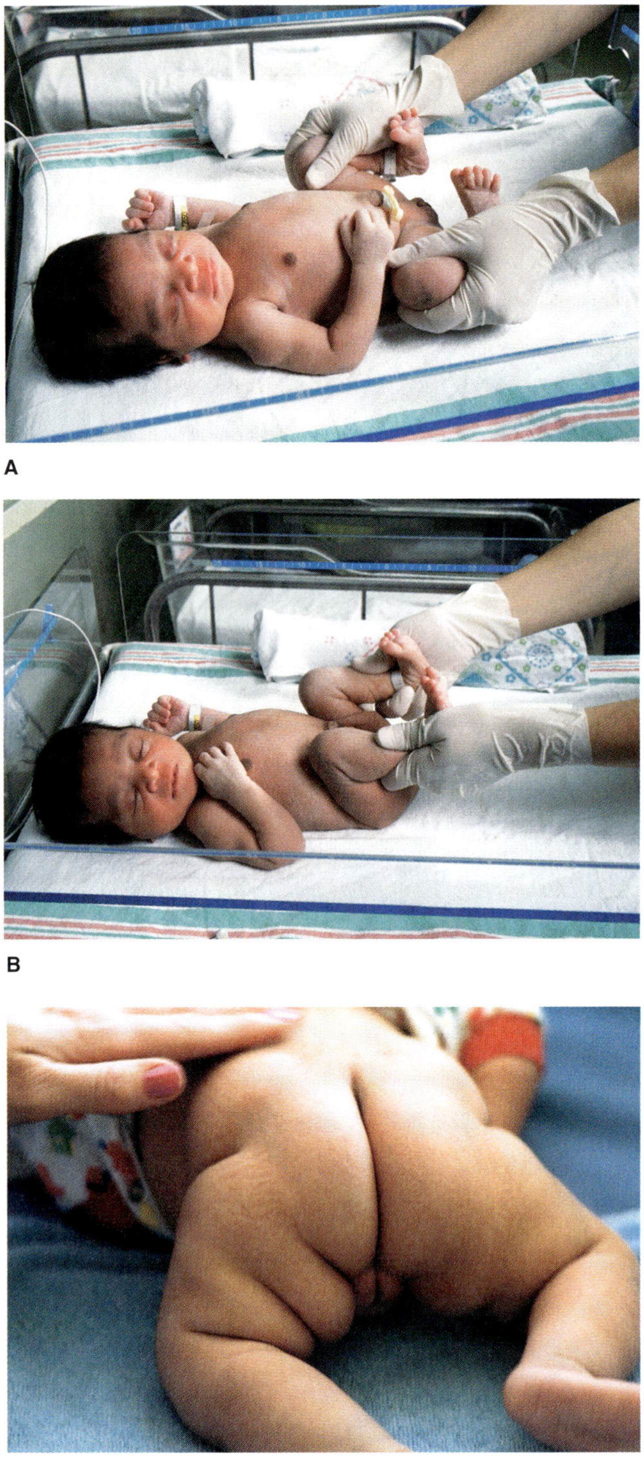

Figure 17-21. ■ (**A** and **B**) Hip integrity is assessed in a newborn by observing and feeling the smoothness of movement in the joint. A "click" is an indication of possible hip dysplasia. (**C**) Posterior skin folds seen on the affected side.

encountered, evaluation for clubfoot needs to be made by the primary care provider.

Reflexes

Reflexes in newborns are signs of neurologic integrity (Figure 17-22 ■). Some reflexes, such as blink, cough, and sneeze, remain intact throughout life. Others disappear by 4 to 6 months. Still others will take 2 years to disappear. Absent or slowed reflexes may indicate prematurity of the infant. They may also result from CNS depressant medications that were transferred to the infant during labor or in breast milk. Reexamination should be done at a later date. Lingering reflexes (those present after the expected time) may indicate neurologic lesions. The child should be referred for further evaluation by the primary care provider.

The **rooting reflex** occurs when the newborn is searching for food. When the newborn's cheek is stroked, the infant will turn his or her head in that direction. The **sucking reflex** is elicited when the newborn's lips are touched. Together these two reflexes are important in feeding. Medications, especially pain medications, can be transferred in breast milk and could depress the sucking reflex. (Breastfeeding is discussed in Chapter 11 ⊘.) The rooting reflex disappears between 3 and 4 months; the sucking reflex disappears by 10 months.

The **palmar grasp reflex** occurs when a finger or small object is placed in the newborn's hand. Newborns grasp the finger tight enough to be lifted from the bed. This reflex lasts 4 months. The **plantar grasp reflex** (Figure 17-22A), lasting 8 months, occurs when the sole of the foot is touched. The toes curl under as if newborns are trying to "grasp" with their feet. This reflex must disappear before infants are able to walk. The **Babinski's reflex** is elicited by stroking the lateral side of the foot from heel to toe. The big toe should dorsiflex and the other toes should flare. This reflex disappears before the infant begins to walk. The **stepping reflex** is obtained by holding newborns with the feet touching the table. Newborns will step as if walking.

The **tonic neck reflex** (Figure 17-22B) is demonstrated by placing newborns supine on a firm surface. When the head is turned to one side, newborns will extend the arm and leg on that side. The opposite arm and leg will flex. The **Moro reflex** or **startle reflex** (Figure 17-22C) occurs when newborns have a sense of falling. This reflex can be elicited by holding the newborn in a sitting position and suddenly lowering the head or by bumping the surface where the newborn is lying. The baby will quickly extend (abduct) the arms with fingers flared, and form a "C with thumbs and first finger." The arms will then adduct in an embracing motion. The lower extremities may extend and then flex. A slight tremor may be noted.

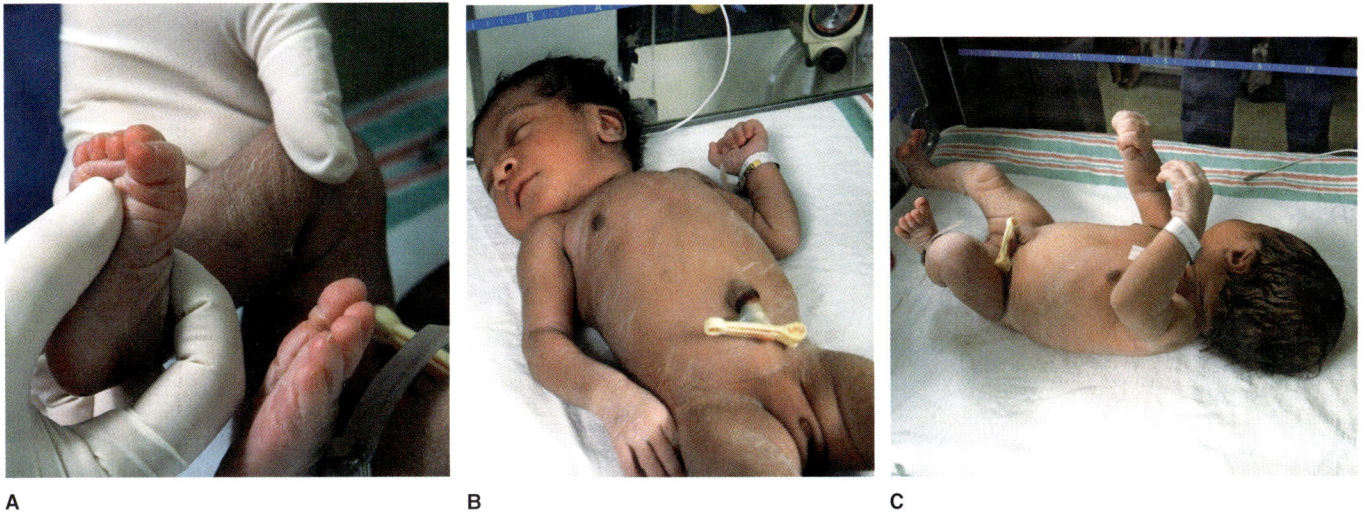

Figure 17-22. ■ (**A**) Newborn exhibiting plantar grasp reflex. (**B**) Newborn exhibiting the tonic neck reflex. (**C**) Newborn exhibiting Moro reflex.

Behavioral State

Three behavioral states have been identified to describe the normal newborn: sleep state, quiet alert state, and crying state (Figure 17-23 ■).

SLEEP STATE

Newborns sleep with their eyes closed for 20 to 22 hours a day. There may be periods of rapid eye movement (REM) sleep. Respirations are regular and slow. There may be startle or jerking movements at times. Environmental stimuli may not change the sleep state.

QUIET ALERT STATE

In the quiet alert state (see Figure 17-23B), newborns lie quietly looking around, experiencing their environment. They appear interested in what is happening around them. They may focus on something within their visual field for several minutes. They may remain in the quiet alert state for a period of time before going back to sleep or crying.

CRYING STATE

The cry should be strong, lusty, and of medium pitch. Crying is a method of communicating for newborns.

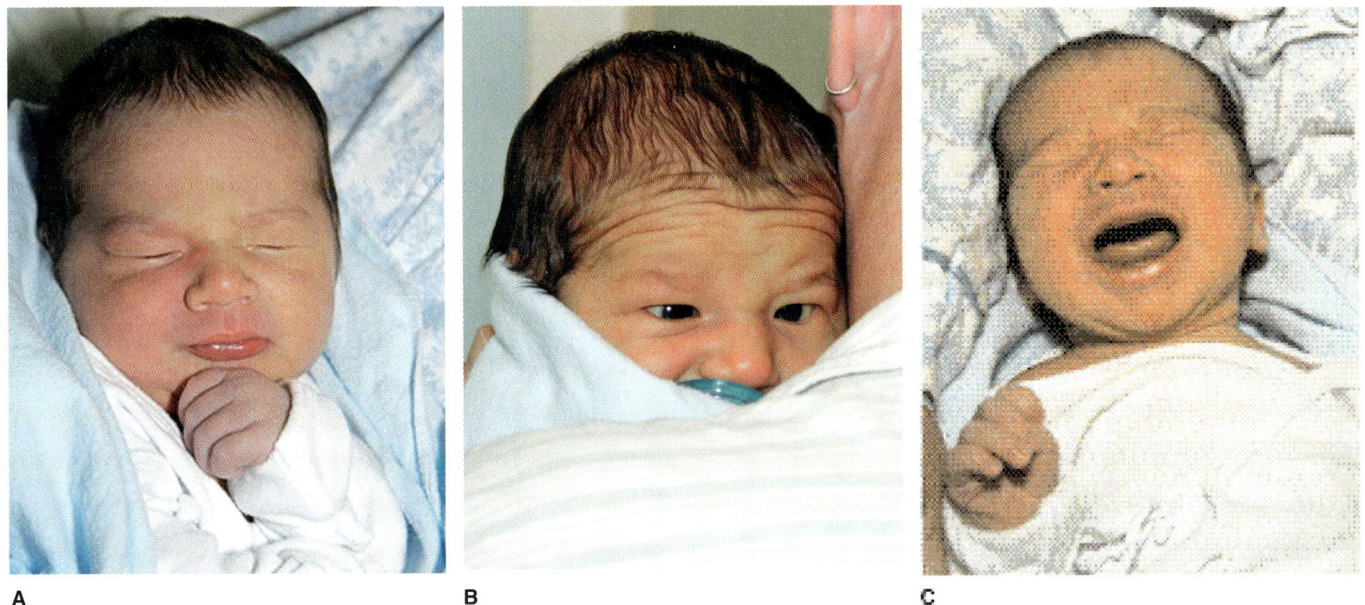

Figure 17-23. ■ Behavioral states. (**A**) Sleeping state. (**B**) Quiet alert state. The infant may make eye contact or focus on one object. (Note the transient strabismus.) (**C**) Crying state.

Crying can be used to increase the metabolism when the infant is cold. Crying can indicate that the infant is hungry, wet, or just needing reassurance. Crying may be accompanied by frequent, jerky movements. A high-pitched cry or one that sounds like a "cat cry" requires further evaluation by a primary care provider.

Nursery Care

If there are no complications, the newborn is usually left with the mother in the delivery area throughout the recovery period. The infant may then be either transferred to the newborn nursery or left with the mother. In any case, the following care will be provided. Anytime care is provided in the presence of the mother or significant others, teaching should be provided and documented.

AIRWAY MAINTENANCE

Maintenance of the airway is always the first priority. It is not unusual for the newborn to spit up mucus and fluid. It is critical that the nurse keep the airway clear to prevent aspiration. The bulb syringe is kept at the head of the bassinette for ready access (Figure 17-24 ■). If necessary, the

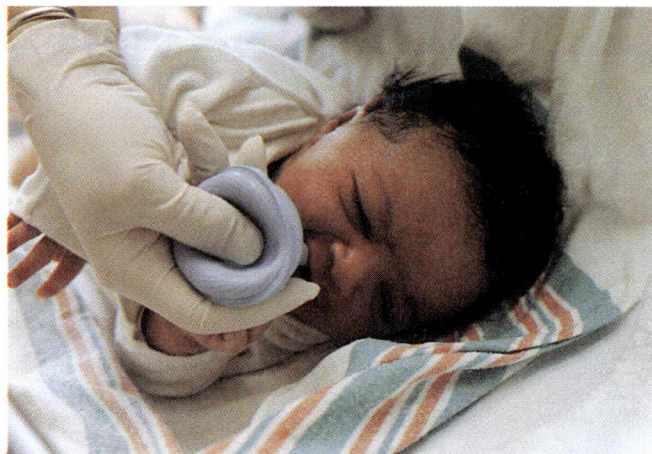

Figure 17-24. ■ Nasal and oral suctioning. The bulb is compressed, the tip is placed in either the mouth or the nose, and the bulb is released. Remember to suction the mouth first, before the nose.

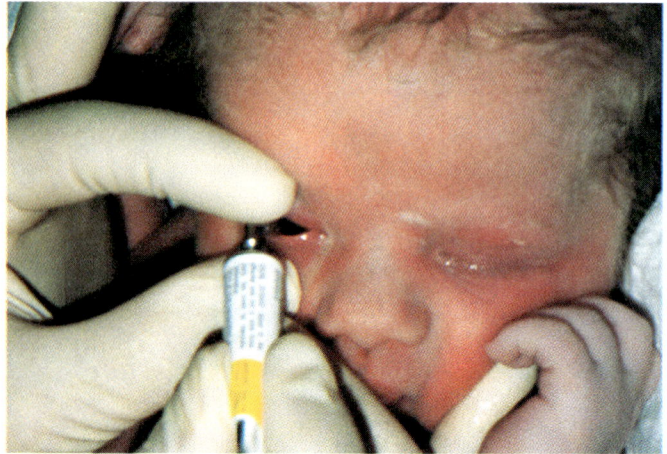

Figure 17-25. ■ Ophthalmic ointment. Retract lower eyelid outward to instill ¼-in-long strand of ointment from a single-dose tube along the lower conjunctival surface.

nurse can pick up the newborn, position the newborn with the head down, and use the bulb syringe to suction the airway.

EYE CARE

Eye care is necessary to prevent **ophthalmia neonatorum** (inflammation of the eyes of the newborn, resulting from contact with gonorrhea or Chlamydia during the birth process). It is mandatory that an antibiotic ointment or solution be placed in the infant's eyes soon after delivery (Figure 17-25 ■).

VITAMIN K ADMINISTRATION

Vitamin K, which is necessary for blood clotting, is normally produced in the intestines from food and intestinal flora. Newborns are unable to produce vitamin K because their intestine is sterile until food is introduced. Within 1 hour after delivery, the newborn is given IM injection of vitamin K (AquaMEPHYTON) to prevent hemorrhagic disorders. Table 17-2 ■ describes the use of this medication. Procedure 17-1 ■ provides steps for performing the procedure.

TABLE 17-2				
Pharmacology: Drug Used to Prevent Hemorrhagic Disorders				
DRUG (GENERIC AND COMMON BRAND NAME)	**USUAL ROUTE/DOSE**	**CLASSIFICATION**	**SELECTED SIDE EFFECTS**	**DON'T GIVE IF**
Phytonadione (AquaMEPHYTON)	Newborn: IM/SC 0.5–1.0 mg immediately after delivery May repeat in 6 hr PRN	Vitamin K	Hypersensitivity, flushing, pain at injection site	None

Administering Intramuscular Injection to the Newborn

Purpose
- To administer medication safely into the muscle of the newborn

Equipment
- Gloves
- Alcohol wipes
- Syringe with medication
- Adhesive bandage

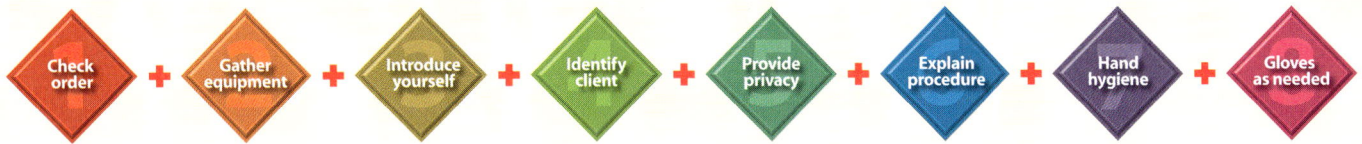

Check order + Gather equipment + Introduce yourself + Identify client + Provide privacy + Explain procedure + Hand hygiene + Gloves as needed

Interventions and Rationales

1. Perform preparatory steps (see icon bar above).

2. Prepare medication for injection. A 1-mL syringe with a ½- or ⅝-inch, 25-gauge needle is used. *A small short needle reaches the muscle but avoids potentially striking the bone.*

3. Put on gloves. *Gloves decrease the possibility of contamination with blood.*

4. Locate the correct site. The middle third of the vastus lateralis muscle is used (see Figure 17-26 ■).

5. Clean the area with an alcohol wipe in a circular motion. *Cleansing the skin prevents infection at the injection site.*

6. Stabilize the leg by placing the palm of your nondominant hand on the baby's knee, grasping the vastus lateralis muscle between your thumb and first finger. *Holding the leg in this manner prevents the baby from moving the leg. Gently squeezing the muscle adds depth to prevent the needle from hitting the bone.*

7. Insert the needle at a 90-degree angle with your dominant hand. *Newborn tissue is soft and requires little force to get the needle into the tissue.*

8. Using your nondominant hand, aspirate observing for a blood return. *Be careful not to move the needle. Aspiration verifies correct placement of the needle.*

9. If no blood returns, slowly inject the medication. *Slow injection of the medication decreases discomfort.*

10. If there is blood in the syringe, remove the needle, dispose of the syringe and prepare a new medication. *Blood in the syringe indicates the needle was in a blood vessel. Injecting the medication at this point would be administering it by the intravenous route.*

Figure 17-26. ■ Injection of vitamin K in a neonate.

11. Following injection of the medication, remove the needle and gently massage the site. *Gentle massage begins medication absorption.*

12. Needles cannot be recapped. Dispose of needle and syringe in the proper container. *The equipment used for an intramuscular injection is considered to be contaminated and poses the threat of transmitting harmful substances.*

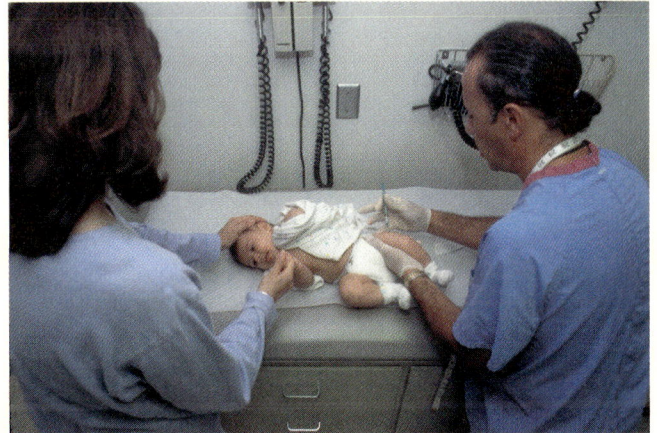

SAMPLE DOCUMENTATION

(date) 0800   1 mg AquaMEPHYTON given IM in right vastus lateralis. Bandage applied. W. Weaver, LVN

UMBILICAL CORD CARE

At delivery, a small plastic or metal clamp is generally placed on the umbilical cord approximately 1 inch from the skin and the cord is cut. The clamp must remain in place until the cord has dried. With each diaper change, the skin at the base of the cord is assessed for redness and drainage. The skin is cleaned with plain water but is not soaked. An aseptic agent such as alcohol, triple blue dye, or Betadine is applied to the cord to aid in drying (Figure 17-27 ■). It is important not to get alcohol on the infant's skin surrounding the cord because it would cause drying and irritation. If the cord is completely dry prior to discharge, the cord clamp can be removed. The core will fall off in approximately 14 days and should not be pulled off, even if it is only partially attached. Until the cord falls off, the newborn should not be submerged in water.

clinical ALERT

Keeping the newborn's cord clean and dry is essential to prevent infection.

BATHING

The newborn has been in contact with maternal body fluids, blood, and amniotic fluid. Following standard precautions, the nurse should not touch the infant without clean exam gloves until the newborn has been bathed (see Procedure 17-2 ■). After the initial bath, daily bathing during the newborn period is discouraged due to the delicate nature of newborn skin. Water-only bath can be alternated with a mild soap bath. When soap is used, it should be a mild cleansing bar or solution with a neutral pH.

SAFETY

Safety in the newborn nursery involves protecting the newborn from injury and abduction. Safety measures must also be taught to the parents.

Most facilities have procedures that must be followed to protect the newborn from abduction. These might include limiting access to the newborn nursery and the obstetric unit. That is, only personnel or parents with proper identification are allowed to enter. Personnel who transport the newborn from the mother's room to the nursery or other areas of the facility must have proper identification. Parents are taught not to give their baby to anyone who does not have identification.

When the newborn is brought to the mother, the identification band (see Figure 14-30A ⬭) is checked to be sure the infant is given to the correct person. The mother is asked to read the number on her identification bracelet, and the nurse checks it with the identification band on the baby.

When a newborn is carried in someone's arms, there is a possibility of dropping the baby. Therefore, transporting the newborn from the room in a bassinette is not only the safest method, but it is also often mandatory.

The baby should not be left unattended on a high surface such as a bed. If the mother is tired, the newborn should be placed in the bassinette instead of having the mother sleep with the baby in her arms.

Common Nursery Procedures

NEWBORN SCREENING TESTS

Hypoglycemia

Newborns who are small for gestational age (SGA) or large for gestational age (LGA) are frequently assessed for hypoglycemia. A small blood sample is obtained from the newborn's

(*Text continues on p. 447.*)

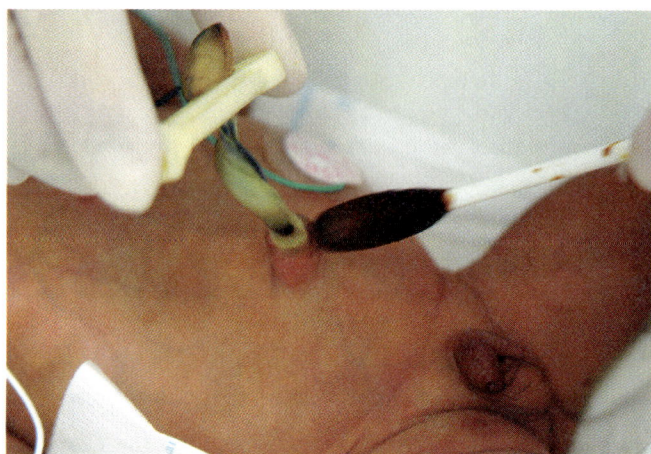
A

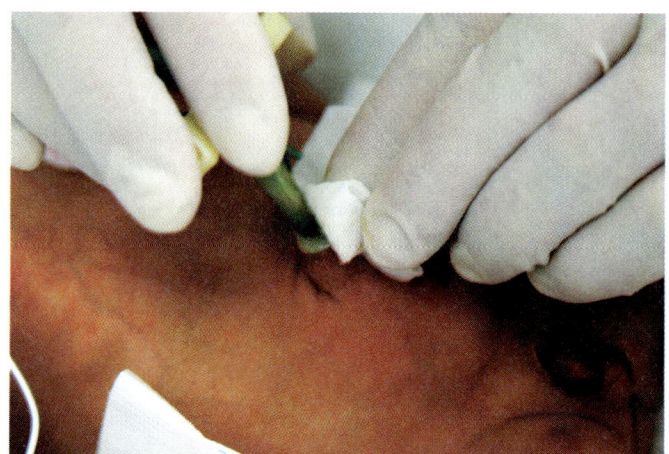
B

Figure 17-27. ■ Two different methods for cord care. (**A**) Betadine cleaning. (**B**) Alcohol cleaning.

Bathing the Newborn

Purpose

- To cleanse the skin of the newborn

Equipment

- Clean t-shirt
- Diaper
- Gloves
- Soft wash cloth
- Soft comb
- Thermometer
- Warm towel
- Warm water
- Warm blankets

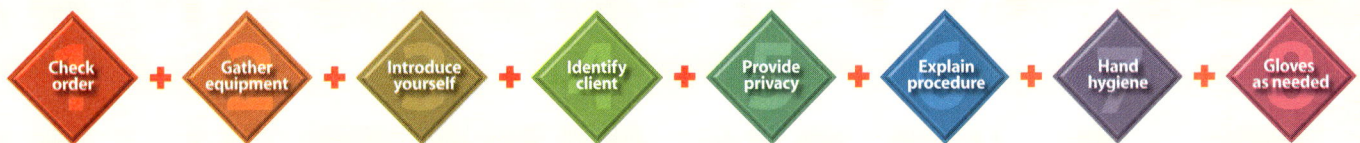

Check order + Gather equipment + Introduce yourself + Identify client + Provide privacy + Explain procedure + Hand hygiene + Gloves as needed

Interventions and Rationales

1. Perform preparatory steps (see icon bar above).

2. Determine that the infant's temperature is stable. *Newborn will lose heat during the bath.*

3. Put on gloves. *Gloves decrease the possibility of contamination with maternal blood and body fluids.*

4. Wet the wash cloth in warm water approximately 98° to 99°F (36.6°–37.2°C). *Warm water decreases body heat loss.*

5. Wash the newborn's face, trunk, extremities, and diaper area in order. *Washing from cleanest to most soiled areas prevents the spread of organisms.*

6. When washing the face, wash the eyes from the inner canthus toward the outer canthus. Wash the ears, taking care to wash behind the ear, and the pinna. Nothing should be inserted into the ear canal or nose. *This technique prevents injury to the newborn's eyes, ears, and nose.*

7. Wash the neck. Insert one hand under the newborn's back to expose the neck and wash all folds. *Blood and amniotic fluid collect in neck folds and should be removed.*

8. Uncover and wash and dry the chest, back, and arms. Avoid rubbing the skin. Provide cord care. *Rubbing the skin might traumatize the delicate tissue. Uncovering only the area to be washed prevents heat loss.*

9. Put a clean warm t-shirt on the baby. Place a blanket over the chest and arms. *Covering the baby prevents heat loss.*

10. Wash the legs, remove the diaper, and clean the perineum. Wash the vulva of the female from front to back to prevent contamination of the vagina and urethra with fecal material. Wash the penis and scrotum of the male, taking care to wash under and in the folds of the scrotum. Do not retract the foreskin in the uncircumcised male. Apply a clean diaper. *The diaper area must be cleaned after each void and stool to prevent skin irritation.*

11. Wrap the baby in a warm towel, leaving the head exposed (Figure 17-28 ■). Hold the baby in one arm using a football hold. Wash the baby's hair, rinse by pouring water over the head, taking care not to get

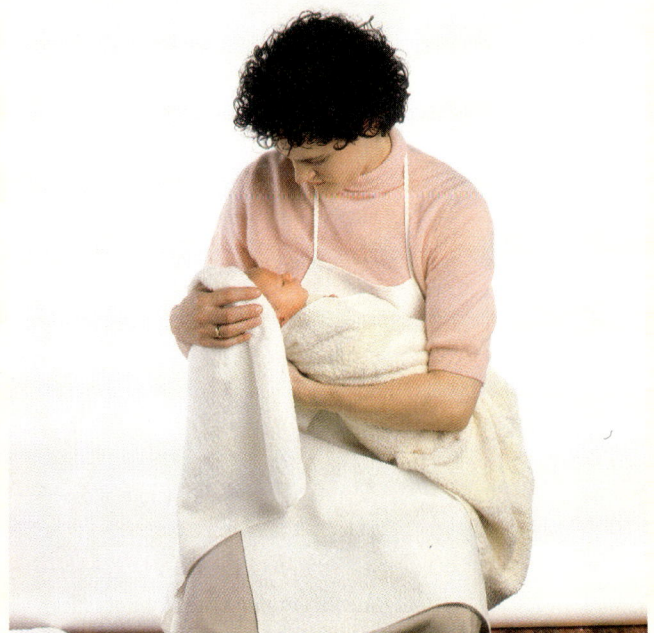

Figure 17-28. ■ When bathing the newborn, cover the areas that are not being washed, and wash the head last.

water into the baby's eyes. Combing the hair while washing it helps to remove dried blood. Dry the head. Apply a cap to decrease heat loss. *Washing the baby's head last conserves body heat.*

12. Wrap the baby in warm blankets or place the baby under a radiant warmer. Take the baby's temperature in 30 minutes to 1 hour. *The temperature reading verifies that the baby has not had excessive heat loss.*

heel to determine the blood glucose level (Figure 17-29 ■). Because of the possibility of damaging the nerves on the bottom of the newborn's foot, correct procedure must be followed. The blood is placed on a reagent strip and the blood glucose level is determined.

The nurse must be familiar with the blood glucose monitor used by the facility. If the standards for the equipment are not closely followed, an inaccurate blood glucose level will be obtained.

Phenylketonuria

Another blood test that is done in the newborn period is screening for phenylketonuria (PKU). This screening test, required by law in all 50 states, determines the presence of an autosomal recessive disorder of amino acid metabolism in which the individual is unable to breakdown

phenylalanine. To meet the legal requirements, facilities obtain the blood sample prior to discharge. For the results of the screening to be most accurate, the test must be done after the baby has received milk (either breast milk or formula). It may take 48 to 72 hours (or more) for the newborn to have an adequate consumption of milk. For this reason, the PKU test may need to be repeated in 1 to 2 weeks. The blood sample is obtained by heel stick. The blood is placed on a PKU specimen card and sent to the laboratory for analysis.

Bilirubin

The primary care provider frequently orders a bilirubin test to monitor the functioning of the newborn's liver. As stated previously, the newborn needs to break down the excess red blood cells. This is accomplished by the spleen and liver.

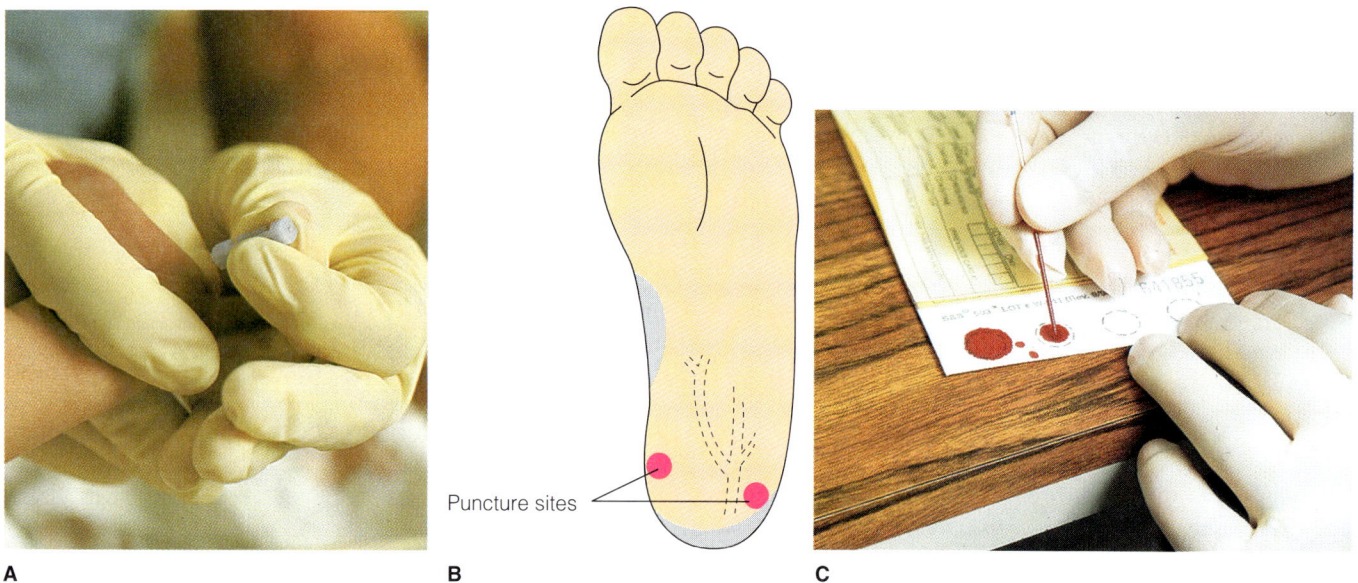

Puncture sites

A   B   C

Figure 17-29. ■ (A) Heel stick. (B) Potential sites for heel sticks. Avoid shaded areas to prevent injury to arteries and nerves in the foot. (C) Collecting a blood sample from the newborn for neonatal metabolic screening. The nurse must be sure to saturate the circle on the test sheet thoroughly.

The excess bilirubin should be broken down by the liver and excreted through the bile. It will take several days for the newborn's liver to be able to complete this process. In the meantime, the bilirubin builds up in the blood, resulting in hyperbilirubinemia. This disorder is discussed in Chapter 18 ⬭. The blood is usually obtained by laboratory personnel. The nurse informs the primary care provider of the results.

NEWBORN PROCEDURES

Circumcision

Circumcision is the surgical removal of the foreskin (*prepuce*) of the penis. Table 17-3 ■ identifies the advantages and disadvantages of circumcision. Parents should make an informed decision prior to signing the consent form. (See Health Promotion Issue in Chapter 1 ⬭.) Only full-term infants should be circumcised. Cultural beliefs must be considered when supporting parents' decisions about circumcision. Box 17-2 ■ identifies common cultural considerations. The Health Promotion Issue on pages 448 and 449 discusses the bioethical issue of circumcision.

Before the procedure begins, an informed consent form must be signed. The infant is kept NPO for several hours. The infant is restrained on a circumcision board, and a blanket should be placed over the infant's chest to prevent heat loss. At this point, the infant frequently begins to cry due to being held in extension. The physician may administer a local anesthetic in the form of an injection or cream. The physician then makes a slit in the prepuce and uses a Yellen (Gomco) clamp or PlastiBell (Figure 17-30 ■) to control bleeding. The prepuce is then cut off. The Gomco clamp will be left in place for 5 minutes to ensure bleeding has stopped; it is then removed. When the Gomco clamp is used, vitamins A and D ointment or petroleum jelly may be applied to the penis

TABLE 17-3	
Advantages and Disadvantages of Circumcision	
ADVANTAGES	**DISADVANTAGES**
Religious conviction	No evidence of medical benefit
Culture	Painful procedure
Social norm	Risk of bleeding
Hygiene	Risk of infection

BOX 17-2	CULTURAL PULSE POINTS

Considerations about Circumcision

- Male Jewish infants may be circumcised on the 8th day of life during a religious ceremony by the *mohel*, a person trained to do circumcision. Parents should be taught home care before leaving the hospital even though the procedure will occur later.

- Muslim parents practice circumcision as a religious rite.

- In European countries, circumcision is infrequently performed except for religious reasons.

to prevent the glans from sticking to the diaper. Ointment is not applied when the PlastiBell is used. The PlastiBell will fall off in 5 to 8 days.

After circumcision, the penis should be checked for bleeding at least every hour for 12 hours. If bleeding occurs, pressure should be applied with sterile 4 × 4 cotton gauze until bleeding stops. If bleeding cannot be controlled, the charge nurse and physician should be notified. The penis should be washed with warm water with each diaper change. Parents should be instructed to be alert for signs of infection until the circumcision has healed, in 7 to 9 days.

The Nursing Care Plan Chart on pages 450 and 451 provides information on nursing care for the family with an infant undergoing circumcision.

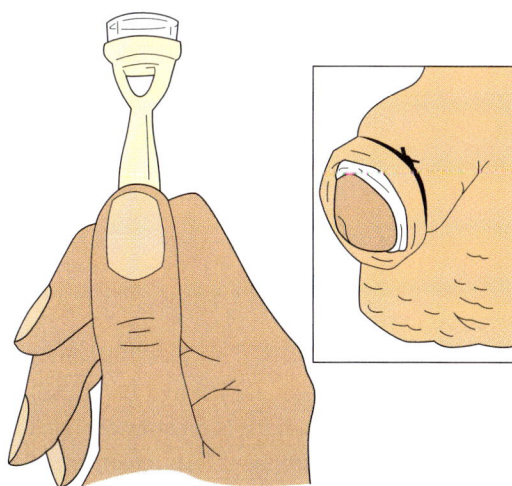

Figure 17-30. ■ Circumcision using the PlastiBell. The bell is fitted over the glans. A suture is tied around the bell's rim, and the excess prepuce is cut away. The plastic rim remains in place for 3 to 4 days until healing occurs. The bell may be allowed to fall off. It is removed if it is still in place after 8 days.

HEALTH PROMOTION ISSUE

BIOETHICS OF NEWBORN MALE CIRCUMCISION

In the United States since the mid-1970s, newborn male circumcision became almost a tradition. Although circumcision is a religious rite in some faiths, most parents circumcised their male newborns for other reasons, including:

- so the son would look like his father.
- so other boys would not tease him in gym classes.
- so it would be easier to keep the penis clean.

Now more parents are choosing not to circumcise their male infants. Most pediatricians agree that in the absence of a documented medical disorder, there is no medical reason to circumcise the newborn male. The bioethics of removing this healthy tissue is under review by national medical groups and the legal community.

DISCUSSION

Circumcision based on religious beliefs or done for medical reasons (including phimosis, hypospadias, and others) is not being questioned. However, the bioethics of removal of healthy foreskin for the cosmetic effect is under review

by medical and legal communities in the United States and other countries around the world. Several questions must be answered in the process of this review.

What are the rights of the child?

Under international law, the child has the right to security and freedom from torture or inhumane and degrading treatment. The child has the right to be consulted when decisions are made regarding his welfare. However, most male circumcisions are done within the first few days of life, when the child is unable to be "consulted" about the decision. Because the nontherapeutic procedure is not essential to the current well-being, it may be in the best interest of the child to postpone the procedure until the child can decide for himself.

What are the rights of the parents?

The parent has the right and responsibility to the child to make decisions based on accurate information and in the best interests of the child. Parents have the right and responsibility to grant permission for the investigation,

diagnosis, and treatment of disease and disorders. In the case of circumcision, it is the psychological well-being of the child in the future that parents are trying to ensure.

What are the benefits of circumcision?

The 1999 American Academy of Pediatrics (AAP) statement (reaffirmed in 2006) does not recommend routine circumcision but acknowledges that some medical benefits exist. The AAP recommends that if circumcision is performed, local analgesic should be administered before the procedure. The circumcised penis is easier to clean. This may prevent urinary tract infections, especially when the boy or man is unable or unwilling to retract the foreskin and clean the glans daily.

Is circumcision harmful?

Removal of the foreskin leaves the remaining skin tight and immovable and eliminates the protection of the glans. This allows for drying of the tissue and lessens the gliding action of the tissue during sexual intercourse. Circumcision puts the newborn at risk for infection and bleeding.

Immunizations

Although immunizations can be given at any age, the Centers for Disease Control and Prevention (CDC) and the American Academy of Pediatrics recommend that immunizations be started in infancy. It is recommended that most immunizations begin in the second month of life. However, hepatitis B can be given in the neonatal period and may be given prior to discharge from the hospital after birth. A parental consent must be signed prior to immunization. See Appendix II for the Recommended Immunization schedule.

Discharge Teaching About Newborn Care

NUTRITION

Nutrition for the newborn is discussed in Chapter 11. Look there for caloric needs of newborns and for teaching about breastfeeding or bottle-feeding.

ELIMINATION

The newborn voids 8 to 10 times a day. The perineal area should be washed with warm water or commercially

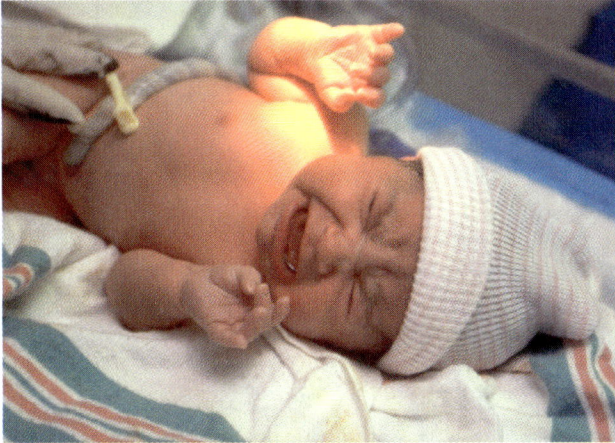

Is circumcision lawful?

Male circumcision is not unlawful. However, in the absence of a medical indication, some suggestions arise that general laws for the protection of children could be applied to the nontherapeutic excision of healthy functional tissue. In most developed countries, female circumcision is regarded as genital mutilation. Could or should this same standard be applied to male circumcision?

PLANNING AND IMPLEMENTATION

The nurse and the primary care provider have the responsibility to inform parents of the benefits, the known risks, and the disadvantages of nontherapeutic circumcision. Similar information must be provided regarding noncircumcision as well. Teaching should begin in the prenatal period, with verification of their understanding prior to the procedure. A consent must be signed prior to the procedure. Circumcision care and teaching must be provided before discharge.

SELF-REFLECTION

Circumcision of the newborn male will continue to be discussed in a variety of settings. The nurse must become informed about the bioethical issues as well as the medical benefits and risks on both sides of the issue. Many times, parents will ask the nurse for advice or "what would you do?" Nurses must be able to put their personal bias aside. They should present information in an objective manner, allowing and encouraging the parents to make an informed decision. Parents should understand that nontherapeutic circumcision is an elective procedure that can wait until they have obtained answers to their questions.

SUGGESTED RESOURCES

For the Nurse

Committee on Bioethics. (1995). Informed consent, parental permission and assent in pediatric practice. *Pediatrics, 95*(2): 314–317.

For the Client

American Academy of Pediatrics. (2006). *Pediatrics, 117*(5), 1846–1847.

prepared wipes following each void. Diapers should be checked and changed frequently to keep the skin dry.

The newborn should pass meconium stool within the first 24 hours after delivery. Holding the infant's legs across the abdomen for a few minutes may help the newborn pass stool. Meconium is sticky, and the newborn's skin should be cleansed thoroughly. Transitional stools are passed after several feedings. Transitional stools are yellowish or greenish-brown, thin, and less sticky (Figure 17-31 ■). Milk curds may be seen. By the fourth day, the stool becomes thicker and pasty. If the infant is breastfed, stools become yellow to golden and have an odor similar to sour milk. Formula-fed newborns pass pale yellow to light brown stool that is firmer and has a stronger odor. The stool will not be brown and formed until the infant is given solid food.

DIAPERING

Most commonly, disposable diapers are used in the hospital nursery. Disposable diapers are made to draw urine inside the fibers and away from the newborn's skin. By keeping the urine away from the skin, rashes and skin breakdown is lessened. Although disposable diapers are better for the newborn's skin, there are also some drawbacks. First, disposable diapers are expensive. The young family may not be able to afford them. Second, disposable diapers are not biodegradable. Some argue that

NURSING CARE PLAN CHART

Planning for Newborn Male Circumcision

GOAL	INTERVENTION	RATIONALE	EXPECTED OUTCOME
1. Deficient Knowledge related to circumcision			
The client or couple will obtain information about circumcision. Client will demonstrate understanding of the procedure.	Provide written materials on circumcision, including postoperative care. Explain the risks, benefits, and controversial nature of circumcision. For newborns undergoing surgery, repeat and/or clarify preoperative teaching to parents provided by physician and/or registered nurse. Obtain surgical consent per agency policy.	*Written information allows clients to review information at home.* *Verbal instructions meet the needs of auditory learners.* *In 2006, the American Academy of Pediatrics reaffirmed its policy on circumcision, which states that benefits of the procedure are not considered significant enough to merit recommendation as a routine procedure. However, families may have overriding cultural and/or religious reasons for choosing this procedure. Risks to the newborn include hemorrhage, penile trauma, and postoperative site infection. Benefits include ease of personal genital hygiene, aesthetic genital appearance, reduced incidence of urinary tract infections, and cultural conformity.*	Client or couple will discuss features of the surgical process. Client or couple will list benefits and risks of the procedure and their rationale for choosing it.
2. Risk for Trauma related to surgical excision of foreskin			
Newborn client will experience postoperative healing of the penis without complications.	Monitor vital signs and examine the genital area q. 15 minutes for the first hour postoperatively and at each diaper change thereafter. Check for any bleeding, swelling, discoloration, odor, or discharge. Report such signs to the registered nurse and/or physician. Review and report the newborn's vitamin K level to the registered nurse. Monitor the newborn's intake and output, including urinary pattern. Report time and characteristics of the first urination after surgery to the registered nurse.	*Swelling and discoloration can be signs of postsurgical trauma. For example, swelling along with a bruised appearance can be a sign of a hematoma as the result of local anesthesia (dorsal penile nerve block).* *Newborns receive vitamin K as a preventive strategy to reduce the risk of bleeding.* *Insufficient urine production and/or difficulty voiding are signs of postoperative complications, including reactions to anesthesia or penile trauma. For example, severe swelling of the glans may cause mechanical obstruction of urine flow.* *Discolored urine may be a sign of bleeding (hematuria), in the urinary tract, from trauma or infection. Odor and discharge are signs of local infection.*	Newborn's vital signs will remain within normal limits following the procedure. Genital area will remain free of excessive redness, swelling, induration, discoloration, odor, or discharge. Newborn will void sufficient quantity of urine (with color in normal range) within 5 hours following the surgery.

GOAL	INTERVENTION	RATIONALE	EXPECTED OUTCOME
3. <u>P</u>ain related to surgical excision of foreskin			
Newborn's sleep and feeding patterns and wake-time activity level will remain within normal limits.	Medication Administration: Oral (Analgesic: Acetaminophen) Comfort measures: Sucrose pacifier Parent cuddling Swaddling Positioning Circumcision site care: Nonstick diaper lining and lubricating ointment per agency policy	*Analgesics block nerve impulses, which produce pain.* *Acetaminophen is a nonsedating analgesic especially recommended for infants and children.* *Excessive irritability is generally a sign of discomfort in a newborn, as is disinterest in or difficulty with feeding.* *Lethargy can be a sign of infection and/or pain.* *Sucrose pacifiers can provide pain relief as a source of distraction. (Offer a pacifier only with parental approval, as some parents choose not to use them.)* *Parent cuddling meets the newborn's need for attachment and security, lessening the baby's anxiety. Anxiety increases pain.* *Swaddling increases the newborn's sense of security, and also limits movement of the legs. Frequent leg movement, especially kicking, may increase pain in the genital area.* *Avoiding the prone position for rest and sleep reduces the risk of hypoxia and prevents pain caused by pressure on the genitals.* *Lining the diaper with a nonstick dressing upon which a lubricating ointment (such as an antibiotic or petrolatum) is placed prevents adhesion of the diaper to the penis. Circular wrapping of the penis with petrolatum gauze is not recommended because the wrap can function as a tourniquet when the penis swells.*	Newborn will demonstrate normal psychomotor activity levels, without signs of severe irritability or agitation, such as "inconsolable" high-pitched crying lasting 15 minutes or more, accompanied by grimacing and tensing of the lower extremities.

disposable diapers are polluting the environment. Parents should not be made to feel guilty if they choose cloth diapers.

Diapers should be changed at least every 2 hours, or as soon as they become soiled. Figure 17-32 ■ illustrates how to apply a diaper. The diaper area should be washed with each diaper change. If a rash appears, commercially prepared ointments may be beneficial. Laying the newborn on

a pad without a diaper fastened exposes the perineum to air and light. This may help prevent or heal skin breakdown.

HYGIENE
Daily hygiene for the newborn includes bathing, umbilical cord care, perineal care, and, if indicated, circumcision care. Until the umbilical cord falls off, the newborn should not be

A

B

C

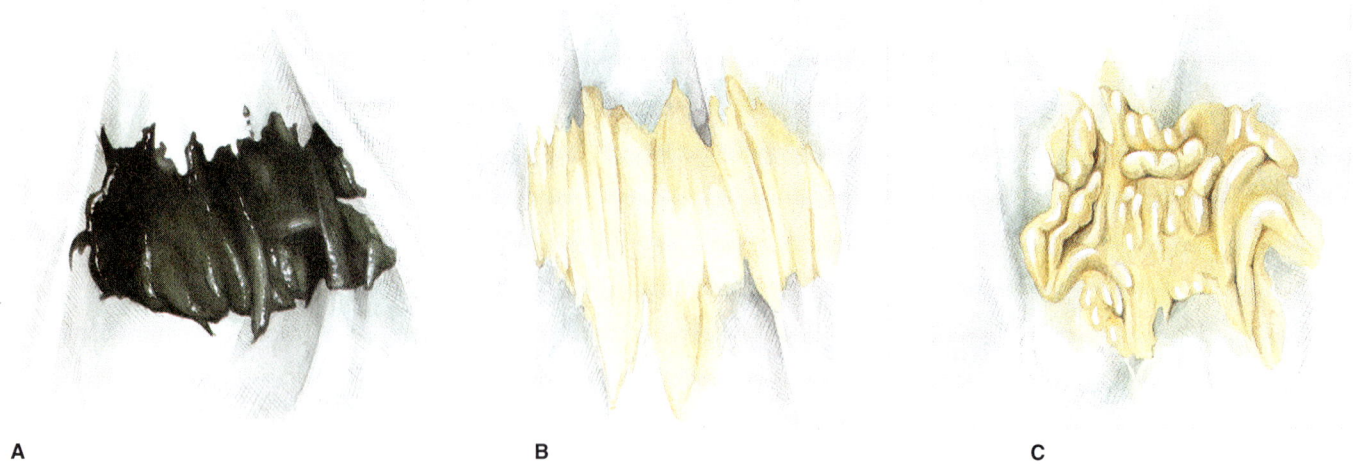

Figure 17-31. ■ Newborn stool samples. (**A**) Meconium stool. (**B**) Breast milk stool. (**C**) Cow's milk stool.

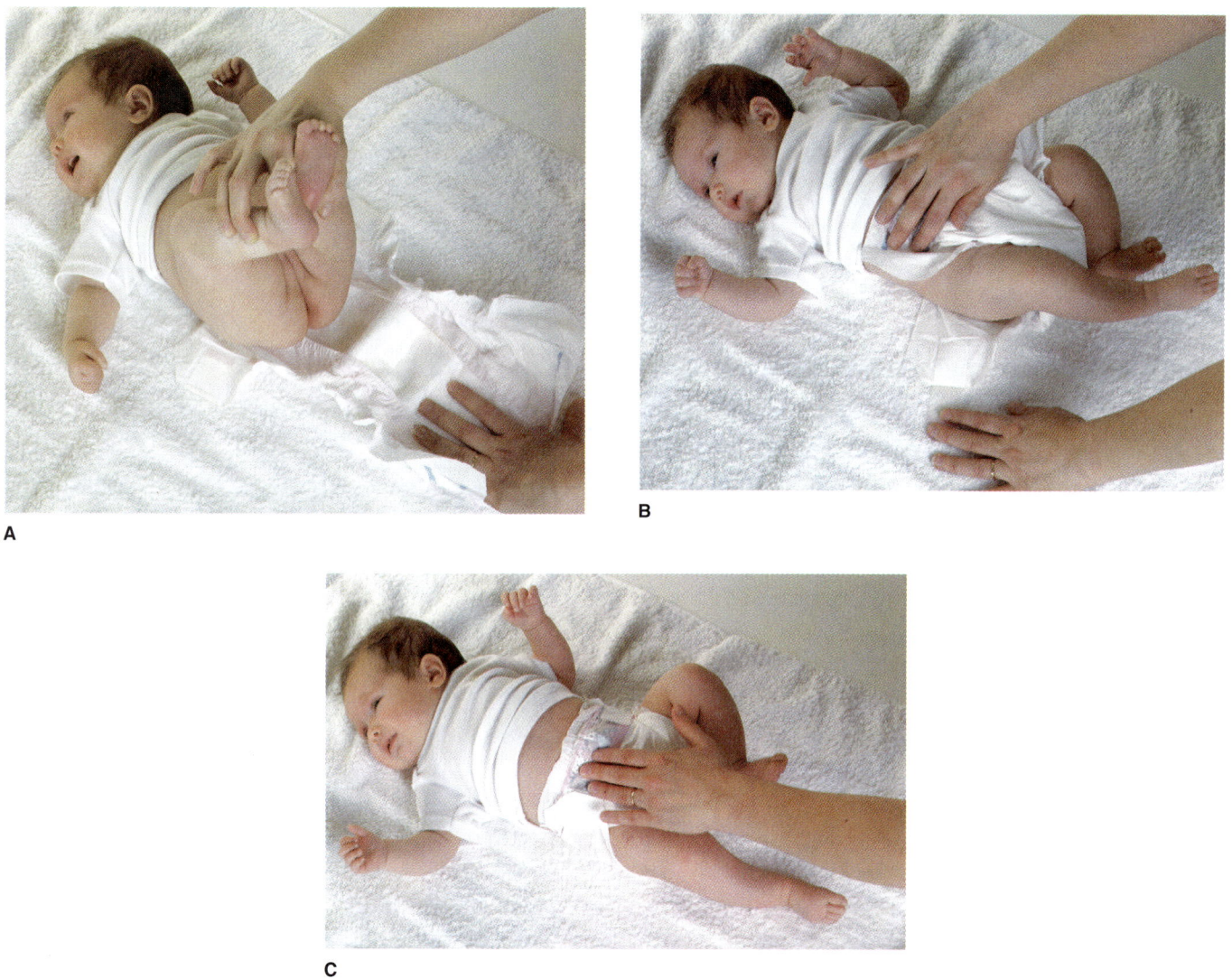

A

B

C

Figure 17-32. ■ Diapering. (**A**) Lift the baby by both legs over diaper. (**B**) Make sure the diaper is fully unfolded across the back and buttocks before securing. (**C**) Fasten the diaper snugly but not tightly. (Dorling Kindersley Media Library.)

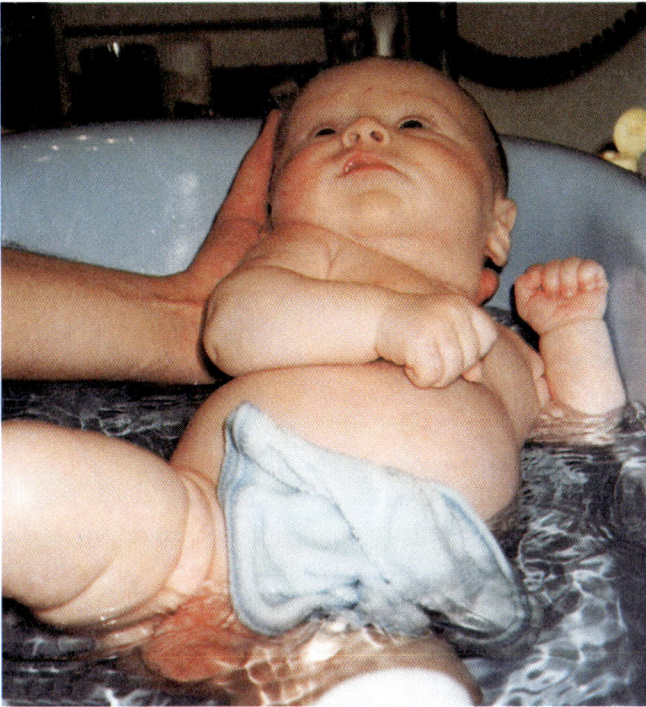

Figure 17-33. ■ When bathing the newborn, the caregiver must support the head and hold the baby carefully. Wet babies are very slippery.

placed in a tub of water. Gentle wiping with a warm, moist washcloth is generally sufficient. The newborn's skin may become dry and peel within a few days. A small amount of lotion or baby oil may be applied to the dry areas. After the umbilical cord falls off, the newborn can be placed in warm water for bathing (Figure 17-33 ■). When wet the newborn is very slick. Care must be taken to prevent the baby from sliding under the water or hitting his or her head on the side of the basin. For this reason, many parents bathe the newborn in the sink or a basin of warm water instead of the bathtub.

Perineal Care

Perineal care should be completed with each diaper change. A warm washcloth or commercially prepared diaper wipe may be used. It is important to remove urine and stool from between the labial folds of female infants. If the male infant is not circumcised, the penis should be cleansed with warm water. The foreskin should not be forced back over the penis. The foreskin will retract normally over time, but it might take 3 to 5 years to do so.

Circumcision Care

If the infant is circumcised, squeeze warm soapy water over the penis, rinse and pat dry. The glans will be sensitive for a few days, so the diaper should be fastened loosely and the baby should not be placed on his abdomen. A small amount of petroleum jelly may be applied (unless a PlastiBell is in place). If excessive bleeding, redness, swelling, and purulent

drainage occurs, the parent should notify the primary care provider.

Umbilical Cord Care

The umbilical cord should remain clean and dry. Care should be taken to prevent infection of the umbilical cord. The skin around the cord may be pink but should not become red or inflamed. A small amount of dark reddish-brown drainage may be present. The cord should be cleaned with warm water three to four times a day or with each diaper change. Applying a small amount of 70% isopropyl alcohol to the cord (but not to the surrounding skin) will facilitate drying and help prevent infection. The diaper should be folded below the umbilical cord to allow for air-drying. If culture demands binding the abdomen, a clean piece of gauze can be recommended. The umbilical cord should fall off in 7 to 14 days. A small drop of blood may appear when the cord comes off. Parents should be taught never to pull on the cord or attempt to loosen it.

SLEEP

The newborn generally sleeps for approximately 20 to 22 hours a day. The newborn likes the security and warmth offered by swaddling (Figure 17-34 ■). To swaddle the baby, place a blanket on a secure surface in the shape of a diamond. Fold the top corner down slightly. Lay the baby on the blanket with the head at the fold. Wrap the right corner around the baby and secure it under the left side. Do not wrap so tightly that the baby is unable to breathe or move. Pull the bottom corner up to the baby's chest. Wrap the left corner around the newborn's right side. Place the newborn on his or her back in the crib. A second blanket can be put over the baby, but the head should remain exposed.

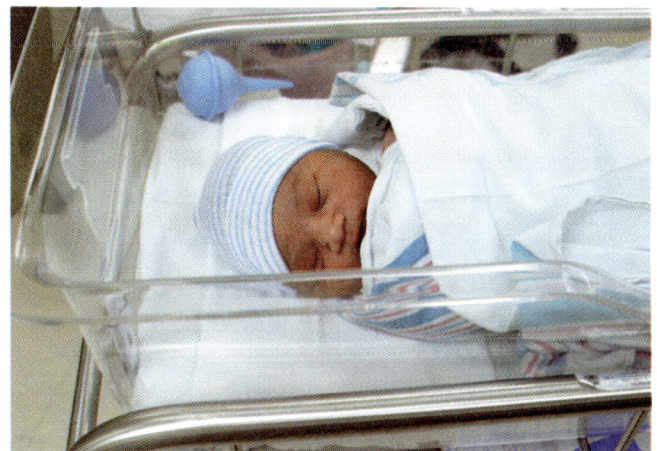

Figure 17-34. ■ It is recommended to position the newborn on the back for sleep. Swaddling maintains warmth and provides security for the infant. (Pearson Education/PH College.)

BOX 17-3 | CLIENT TEACHING

Infant Massage

Infant massage has many benefits. It can soothe a tired infant and minimize distress. It promotes bonding and may boost the infant's immune system. It can help relieve colic and promote sleep.

General Guidelines

Massage is best done when both parent and child are relaxed and calm. It is best to wait about half an hour after the infant's feeding. The room should be warm (78°F). If the room is cold or humid, a light blanket should be used to cover the body parts that are not being massaged. The infant is placed on a soft surface (like a bed).

Baby lotion may be used for the massage. Put lotion on the hands and rub them together so the hands are warm and soft. Depending on the particular infant, it may not be necessary to keep applying lotion.

The time during massage is an optimum time to bond with the infant. Remember to make eye contact and to speak softly while giving the massage.

Always use gentle pressure (no harder than you would use to rub your own eyes).

Massage Process

- Start with the infant lying supine (on the back). With light touch, draw fingertips from the center of the nose up and toward the temples, from the mouth out over the ears and down, and up over the top of the head. Bring the fingertips from the center of the chin up to the tops of the ears.
- Very gently, massage behind the neck and down onto the shoulders. Softly place both hands onto the shoulders. Stroke gently downward from neck to chest.
- Circle the arm at the armpit with the fingers of one hand. Stroke gently down the arm. Be very careful at the elbow because it is a sensitive area. Gently stroke several times from shoulder to wrist and slide fingers down over the hands.
- For the abdomen, trace a clockwise circle below the ribs. Do not include the genitalia in the massage. Stroke lightly around the abdomen and down from the abdomen to the thighs.
- Massage each leg, pressing firmly but gently on the muscles of the thigh and calf. Bend the knees and press the thighs gently against the abdomen.
- Draw the hands along one foot at a time from ankle to toe. Press each toe lightly. Then stroke the whole foot again. Use a circular motion at the heels.
- Turn the infant over onto the stomach. Starting at the head, make long stroking motions that include the head, neck, back, and legs. Gently massage the muscles of the back with small, circular motions. Do not massage the spine; instead, place the hands over the spinal cord for a few seconds to warm the area.
- Massage the backs of the legs from thigh to foot. Then stroke again from head to foot a few times to finish the massage.

A light massage may help the agitated baby to relax before sleep. Box 17-3 ■ provides steps for infant massage.

SAFETY

Safety for the newborn cannot be stressed enough with new parents. All newborns should be placed in a federally approved child safety seat when in an automobile (Figure 17-35 ■). Parents should follow the installation procedure that comes with the car seat. If carrying both supplies and the newborn, parents should secure the newborn in the car before transferring packages.

Parents should be taught that the newborn is at risk of falling if left unattended on a high surface. Even if the newborn is secured in an infant carrier, the baby's motions can tip the carrier over. For example, if the parent places the newborn in a carrier on the kitchen counter while putting away groceries, the baby's motion can cause the carrier to fall from the countertop.

The need to handle infants gently is stressed. Besides teaching parents to support the baby's head when lifting, teaching is also done about the dangers of shaking infants. Some facilities ask parents to view a video about shaken baby syndrome before being discharged home with the neonate.

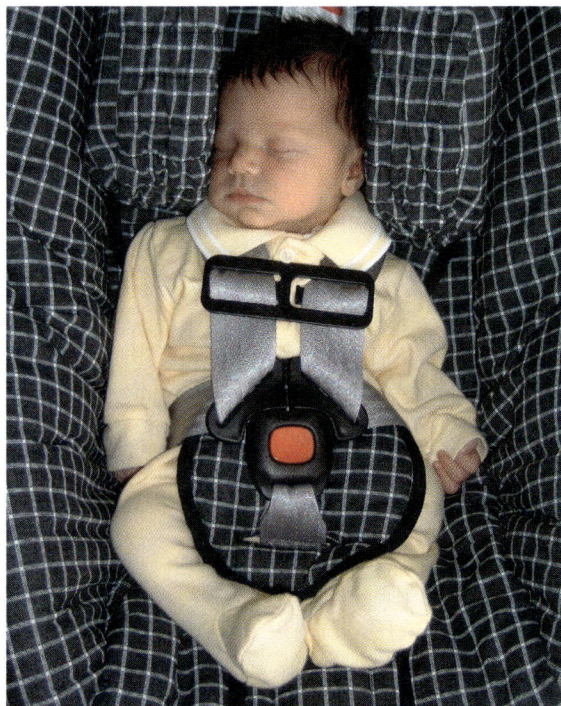

Figure 17-35. ■ Infant safety in motor vehicles must be a part of client teaching.

NURSING CARE

PRIORITIES IN NURSING CARE

The priorities of nursing care for the normal newborn are:

- Maintaining the airway, breathing, and circulation.
- Maintaining body temperature.
- Teaching parents to provide care for their newborn.
- Providing nutrition.
- Ensuring elimination.

ASSESSING

Once the nurse meets the immediate survival needs of the newborn at the time of delivery, the nurse begins the process of preparing the parents to care for their baby. The nurse must assess the learning needs of the parents. If this is the first child, the parents may need more information and support than parents who have had other children. However, the nurse should ensure that experienced parents still have the knowledge and skills they require to provide the necessary care.

The assessment of learning needs is accomplished by asking parents what they already know and by watching them handle the baby. Often, a conversational manner makes parents feel comfortable about asking questions.

DIAGNOSING, PLANNING, AND IMPLEMENTING

A key nursing diagnosis for the new parents might be:

- Deficient **K**nowledge related to feeding, diapering, bathing, safety

Many facilities use prepared teaching plans to provide instruction and documentation of teaching. Nurses often provide and reinforce teaching.

- Teach umbilical and circumcision care. *Keeping the umbilical cord and circumcision clean and dry prevents infection and promotes healing.*
- Demonstrate bathing and stress safety concerns. *Keeping the newborn out of water until the umbilical cord falls off promotes drying of the cord. Once the newborn is bathed in water, safety is a high priority because a wet baby is very slippery.*
- Review client decisions about feeding the baby. Support the client's decision about which method to use. Be sensitive to cultural attitudes about feeding. (For example, a woman of Hispanic culture may want to begin breastfeeding in the privacy of her own home.) Many facilities provide a lactation specialist to discuss breastfeeding methods and concerns. *The newborn needs nutrients every 3 to 4 hours.*

Mothers need to be taught techniques for breastfeeding. Both parents should be taught how to prepare formula for bottle-fed newborns. They should also be given guidelines for bottle care and for positioning infants for feeding (see Chapter 11 🔗 *).*

- Provide information about elimination and about what stools should look like. The appearance will depend on whether the child is breast fed or bottle fed. *Parents should be taught to watch for changes in elimination patterns, including changes in stool color and consistency with feeding.*
- Observe the client and others performing routine care such as dressing or diapering. Ensure that caregivers are practicing good hygiene and safety. *The newborn needs to be handled gently. The head needs to be supported. Parents should be taught to provide perineal care with each diaper change.*
- Review safety concerns, including risk for falls and safety car seats. *New parents may not be aware of possible dangers. Experienced parents may need information about how new equipment is used.*
- Encourage the family to take on some daily chores to support the mother. *Family members can participate in the health and care of the mother and infant by providing time for the mother to recover from labor, rest, and care for the baby.*

EVALUATING

Evaluating is best accomplished by watching the parents give care to the newborn. The nurse should document the teaching and list any printed material that was provided to the parents. Follow-up phone calls or home visits may be needed for parents with limited family support.

NURSING PROCESS CARE PLAN
Care of the Newborn Following Cesarean Birth

Isaiah, 30 minutes old, delivered by cesarean birth, has been transferred from the operating room to the newborn nursery. Isaiah's mother was in labor for 22 hours, received epidural anesthesia, pushed for 3 hours, and required a cesarean birth due to CPD. Apgar scores were 7 and 9 at 1 and 5 minutes. Isaiah is to be monitored and provided with routine care until his mother is stable in the recovery room.

Assessment

- Isaiah's vital signs are within normal limits.
- Head was palpated for caput succedaneum and cephalhematoma.
- All extremities move equally.
- All reflexes are intact.

Nursing Diagnosis. The following important nursing diagnosis (among others) is established for this client:

■ Risk for Ineffective **T**issue Perfusion: Cerebral tissue perfusion related to head trauma from cephalopelvic disproportion (CPD)

Expected Outcomes. The client will have no signs of impaired cerebral perfusion as evidenced by equal movement, intact reflexes, and vital signs within normal limits.

Planning and Implementation

■ Monitor vital signs, movements, and reflexes every 15 to 30 minutes. *CPD can cause cranial trauma resulting in cerebral edema and decreased tissue perfusion. Alterations in vital signs outside normal limits and decreased movement and reflexes are signs of decreased cerebral perfusion in the newborn.*

■ Inform charge nurse and primary care provider of changes. *Alterations in cerebral tissue perfusion require immediate medical attention.*

Evaluation. Client's vital signs, movements, and reflexes remain in normal limits.

Critical Thinking in the Nursing Process

1. What information about cranial trauma with CPD should be shared with the parents?
2. Whose responsibility is it to inform parents of long-term effects of cranial trauma?
3. What are some other signs of decreased cranial tissue perfusion Isaiah may exhibit in the next few months?

Note: Discussion of Critical Thinking questions appears in Appendix I.

Note: The reference and resource listings for this and all chapters have been compiled at the back of the book.

Chapter Review

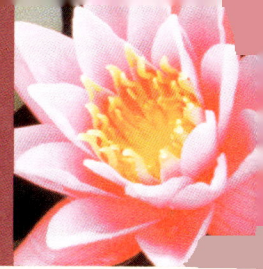

KEY TERMS by Topic

Use the audio glossary feature of either the CD-ROM or the Companion Website to hear the correct pronunciation of the following key terms.

Introduction
newborn

Physiologic Adaptation
cold stress, nonshivering thermogenesis

Gestational Age
scarf sign

Characteristics of the Newborn
acrocyanosis, ecchymosis, petechiae, jaundice, Mongolian spot, telangiectatic nevi, stork bites, milia, erythema toxicum neonatorum, caput succedaneum, cephalhematoma, strabismus, Epstein's pearls, witch's milk, nasal flaring, expiratory grunting, retractions, suprasternal, substernal, supraclavicular, intercostal, subcostal, apneic spells, pseudomenstruation, smegma, webbing, syndactyly, polydactyly

Reflexes
rooting reflex, sucking reflex, palmar grasp reflex, plantar grasp reflex, Babinski's reflex, stepping reflex, tonic neck reflex, Moro reflex, startle reflex

Nursery Care
ophthalmia neonatorum

Common Nursery Procedures
circumcision

KEY Points

- The LPN/LVN must know the normal appearance and reflexes of the newborn and must report deviations to the supervising nurse or physician.

- Most infants are born without complications and require routine care.

- Routine care of the newborn involves sponge baths, feeding, cord care, circumcision care, and diapering, in a warm, calm environment.

- Medications routinely given to the newborn include an antibiotic eye ointment or drops and AquaMEPHYTON IM.

- Hepatitis B immunization may be administered in the newborn nursery with parental consent.

- The LPN/LVN may assist with male circumcision and post procedure care.

EXPLORE MediaLink

Additional interactive resources for this chapter can be found on the Companion Website at www.prenhall.com/towle. Click on Chapter 17 and "Begin" to select the activities for this chapter.

For chapter-related NCLEX®-style questions and an audio glossary, access the accompanying CD-ROM in this book.

Animations

Cord care to a newborn's cord stump

Heart and lung sounds

Circumcision

Hemodynamics

FOR FURTHER Study

For considerations about circumcision without anesthesia, see the Health Promotion Issue in Chapter 1.

Breastfeeding, bottle-feeding, and positioning the infant for feeding are discussed in Chapter 11.

Chapter 13 describes erythroblastosis fetalis, which may cause jaundice that would appear within 24 hours of birth.

Chapter 14 discusses physiologic adaptations to life and care during the first hours after birth; Figure 14-30 illustrates identification bands for mother and newborn in hospital.

Some congenital anomalies and conditions such as hyperbilirubinemia are discussed in Chapter 18.

Critical Thinking Care Map

Caring for Infant with Depressed CNS

NCLEX-PN® Focus Area: Physiologic Adaptation

Case Study: Timothy was born 1½ hours ago following a long difficult labor and delivery. His mother received a total of five doses of morphine sulfate during labor, with the most recent dose 30 minutes before delivery. He has been admitted to the newborn nursery for continued care.

Nursing Diagnosis: Ineffective Breathing Pattern related to mother receiving morphine sulfate

COLLECT DATA

Subjective	Objective
_____	_____
_____	_____
_____	_____
_____	_____
_____	_____
_____	_____
_____	_____

Would you report this? Yes/No

If yes, to: _____

Nursing Care

_____
_____
_____
_____
_____
_____
_____
_____
_____
_____
_____
_____

How would you document this? _____
_____
_____
_____

Compare your documentation to the sample provided in Appendix I.

Data Collected
(use only those that apply)

- Respirations 64/minute
- Mother received morphine sulfate 2 hours ago
- Apgar score 10
- Flaring nostrils
- Color pink
- Temperature 97.2°F (36.2°C)
- Crying
- Grunting respirations
- Passed large meconium stool

Nursing Interventions
(use only those that apply; list in priority order)

- Bathe with antimicrobial soap.
- Start oxygen per nasal catheter.
- Place under radiant warmer.
- Administer Narcan (naloxone hydrochloride).
- Take to mother for feeding.
- Suction airway.
- Apply pulse oximeter.
- Monitor vital signs every hour.
- Place under bilirubin light.

NCLEX-PN® Exam Preparation

1 Routine newborn care includes the administering of antibiotic ointment or drops into the infant's eyes to prevent _____ and _____ infection.

2 The respirations of the normal newborn will be in a(n) _____ pattern at the rate of _____ to _____ breaths per minute.

3 Two days after birth, a newborn in the nursery appears jaundiced. The LPN should:
1. report this to the nurse in charge because it indicates a liver malfunction.
2. document the finding but not report this normal condition.
3. report this to the nurse in charge because it indicates ABO and Rh incompatibility.
4. document the finding but wait another 24 hours before reporting it.

4 A new mother examines her infant and says, "Look, her hands and feet are blue. I know there must be something wrong with her." The best response should be:
1. "Blue hands and feet are normal in newborns. It could last a few days."
2. "You are correct, there must be something wrong. I'll call the doctor right away."
3. "Your baby is cold. We need to wrap her in warm blankets."
4. "This must be birth trauma. I will let the charge nurse know."

5 Shortly after delivery, the mother asks how she will know if the baby is having problems breathing. The best response would be:
1. "He will not cry and will begin to turn blue."
2. "His nostrils will flare out, he will grunt, and the skin over his ribs will sink in."
3. "You won't; he will just stop breathing."
4. "His respirations will become irregular and be more than 30 per minute."

6 A new mother needs further teaching in regard to circumcision care when she states:
1. "I will clean the penis with alcohol three times a day."
2. "If the penis becomes red and swollen, I will call the doctor."
3. "The PlastiBell will fall off by itself, so I don't need to do anything with it."
4. "If I see bleeding, I will apply pressure until it stops."

7 The LPN/LVN is assessing a newborn with an Apgar score of 5. Which of the following nursing actions should the LPN/LVN implement first?
1. measuring head and chest circumference
2. administration of oxygen
3. immediate resuscitation
4. administration of vitamin K

8 The LPN/LVN is performing a gestational age assessment on a 2-hour-old newborn. Which of the following characteristics are more indicative of a mature newborn?
1. extended body position at rest
2. elbow crosses the midline
3. popliteal angle less than 90 degrees
4. transparent skin with numerous blood vessels

9 The LPN/LVN is assisting a new mother to feed her newborn. Which of the following reflexes should the nurse demonstrate to assist with the feedings?
1. rooting reflex
2. palmar grasp reflex
3. tonic neck reflex
4. Moro reflex

10 Which of the following assessment findings should the LPN/LVN report to the nurse?
1. voided times 8 in the past 24 hours
2. high-pitched cry
3. head circumference
4. anterior fontanel firm and flat

Answers for NCLEX-PN® Review and Critical Thinking questions appear in Appendix I.

Chapter 18

Care of the High-Risk Newborn

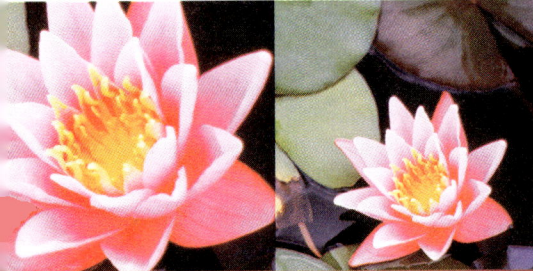

LEARNING Outcomes

After completing this chapter, you will be able to:
1. Define key terms.
2. Discuss the role of the LPN/LVN in caring for the high-risk newborn.
3. Describe general care of the high-risk newborn.
4. Describe common disorders and treatments seen in high-risk newborns.

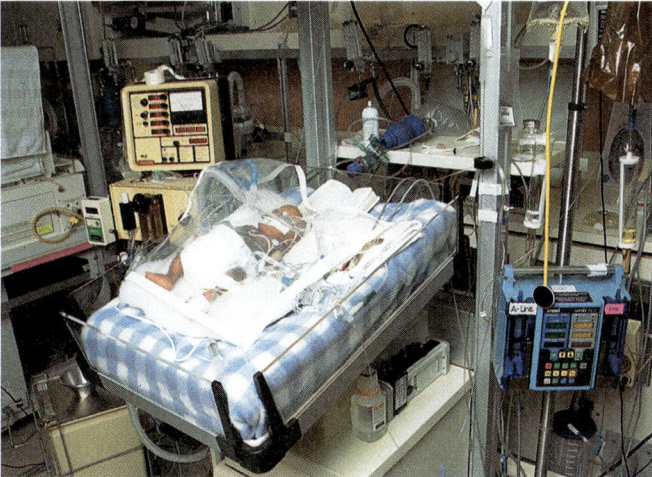

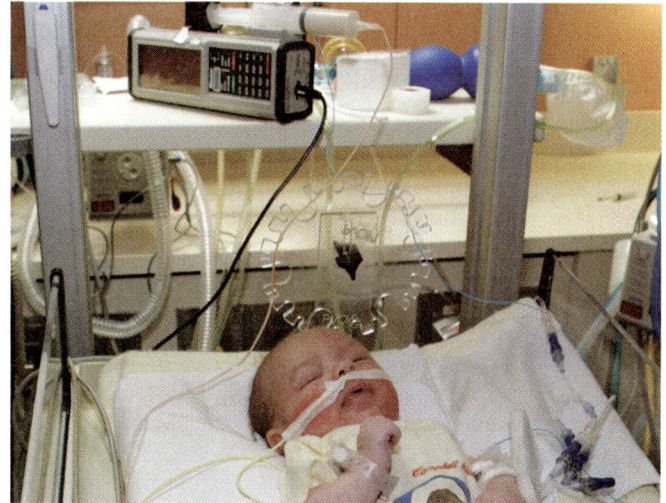

Figure 18-1. ■ (**A**) This premature infant in the neonatal intensive care unit (NICU) is receiving artificial ventilation. (**B**) This premature baby cannot yet coordinate suck and swallow. Gavage feeding is being used until the baby can effectively acquire nutrients.

The high-risk newborn is generally placed in a neonatal intensive care unit (NICU) (Figure 18-1 ■). If an NICU is not available, the neonate is placed in an area of the newborn nursery where the registered nurse can closely observe the baby. The role of the LPN/LVN is one of assisting the RN with collecting data, meeting the basic needs of the newborn, and documenting care. If the facility does not have appropriate accommodations, the newborn may be transferred to another hospital that can meet his or her needs.

Many conditions that place the newborn at risk continue past the first month of life. This chapter addresses the basic nursing care of the high-risk newborn and introduces some congenital anomalies, infections, and disorders that are commonly seen in the high-risk newborn. For more detail on specific disorders, refer to a pediatric nursing textbook.

GENERAL CARE OF THE HIGH-RISK NEWBORN

The **high-risk newborn** is an infant who is born prior to 38 weeks' gestation or after 42 weeks' gestation, who has alterations in intrauterine growth, or who has a medical condition that requires frequent monitoring and treatment. Individualized care is planned and implemented based on the specific needs of each newborn. However, the general care of the high-risk newborn is the same.

Monitoring

VITAL SIGNS
The vital signs of the high-risk newborn must be monitored continuously. Electrodes to record the electrical condition of the heart are placed on the newborn's chest. Respiratory rate and oxygen saturation are also monitored. Blood pressure is monitored electronically. If the newborn's condition warrants, a catheter may be placed through the subclavian or femoral artery to monitor pressure inside the heart.

PAIN
The nurse is responsible to assess pain in the newborn and take measures to prevent, relieve, or control discomfort. Pain pathways and brain structures responsible for long-term memory are developed by 24 weeks' gestation. Untreated pain in the preterm or term newborn can have long-term effects. Assessment tools for use in pain assessment in the newborn have been developed. See Box 17-1 ◷◷ for an example of an infant pain scale.

Unrelieved pain in the newborn can cause irritability, increased metabolism, poor healing, and exhaustion. Nonpharmacologic pain relief can be accomplished by swaddling in warm blankets, touching, holding, and offering a pacifier. Oral glucose solution can be effective in calming the newborn. Pharmacologic pain relief may be accomplished with prescribed morphine or fentanyl for severe pain. Acetaminophen is frequently ordered for mild pain. It is critical for the nurse to calculate the dosage accurately when medicating the newborn to prevent accidental overdose.

BOX 18-1	COMPLEMENTARY THERAPIES

Music as an Aid in the NICU

Premature infants in the neonatal intensive care unit (NICU) are often bombarded with sounds, lights, and other excessive stimuli. This excessive stimuli can have negative effects on the improvement of the infant's condition. Simple positive changes in the environment of the NICU can have positive effects on the premature infant. One of these changes is using music therapy. Music therapy is defined as healing with music, voice, or sound. Several research studies have found music therapy to be effective in the NICU. Infants, after being exposed to calming music, were less likely to experience high arousal states, had shorter hospital stays, and weighed more than infants who were not exposed to music.

Olson (1998) provided six principles essential to the effective use of music therapy:

1. Music is a method of demonstrating caring.
2. Music has emotional and physical effects and can facilitate the healing process.
3. Music can bring a human approach to a clinical environment.
4. Music is a method of individualizing client care.
5. Tone, rhythm, pitch, and volume of music can create a peaceful environment.
6. Music of the child's religious faith provides spiritual care to the client.

Maintaining a calm environment can prevent overstimulation and decrease the newborn's pain response. At times complementary therapies are useful in quieting the infant (Box 18-1 ■).

TEMPERATURE

The premature newborn has less storage of glucose and brown fat than term infants. When the premature newborn gets cold, chilling increases the need for energy, thus the need for glucose. When stored glucose is consumed, hypoglycemia results. To prevent heat loss, temperature is maintained by radiant heat above the bassinette. A sensor is placed over the soft tissue of the abdomen to ensure the newborn does not become too warm. The newborn's axillary temperature may also be taken every 2 to 4 hours.

INTAKE AND OUTPUT

Monitoring intake and output is necessary to ensure adequate fluid balance. Fluids may be given by intravenous infusion, gavage feeding (see Figure 18-1B), or, if the newborn is strong enough, through bottle or cup feeding. Output is monitored by weighing the diaper or, at times, by a suprapubic catheter. Due to the small size of the urethra, a urethral catheter is generally not used.

BLOOD GLUCOSE

Blood glucose levels are frequently used to monitor the metabolic state of the premature or high-risk newborn. Recall from Chapter 17 ⊙ that a small-for-gestational-age (SGA) or large-for-gestational-age (LGA) infant will need frequent blood glucose monitoring until the glucose values have stabilized. Premature newborns may also need frequent blood glucose monitoring until they are obtaining regular feedings. A blood glucose level of 30 mg/dL or less is considered *hypoglycemia* in the newborn and requires treatment as ordered by the physician.

Medical Treatment

Medical treatment is determined by the specific disorder. Common treatments are discussed here. It is important to remember, though, that not every newborn will require all of these treatments.

The premature newborn or newborn in respiratory distress might require mechanical ventilation through an endotracheal tube or, if long-term ventilation is needed, a tracheostomy tube. The nurse or respiratory therapist will maintain an open airway by suctioning mucus from the bronchi. (See Procedure 18-1 ■.) If mechanical ventilation is not needed, oxygen may be administered by an Oxyhood (Figure 18-2 ■) or by nasal cannula or catheter.

> ### clinical ALERT
>
> High amounts of oxygen (over 90 to 100 mm Hg) given to the newborn may cause *retinopathy* (also called *retrolental fibroplasia*). Retrolental fibroplasia can lead to blindness. The newborn who receives high amounts of oxygen will need careful monitoring and periodic eye examinations.

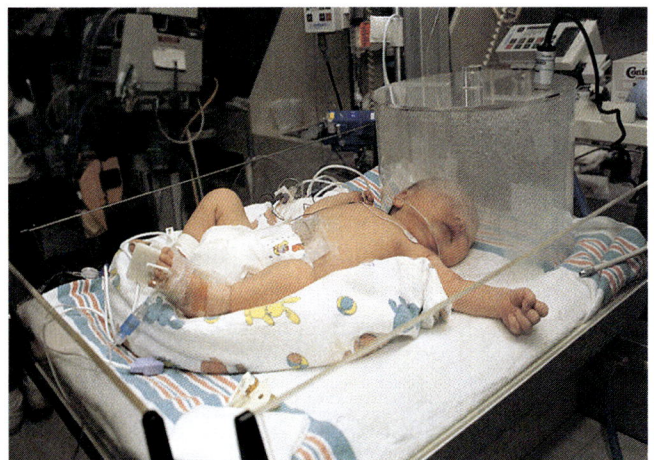

Figure 18-2. ■ An infant under an Oxyhood.

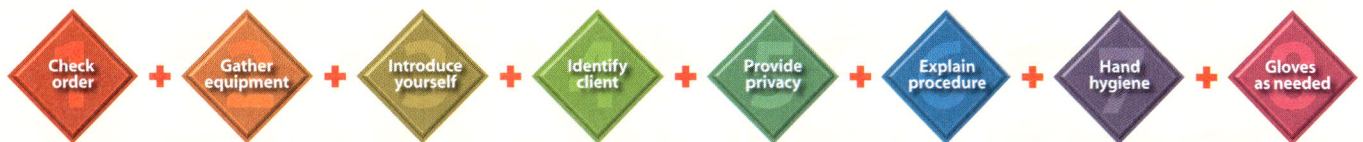

PROCEDURE 18-1 **Suctioning an Infant**

Purpose

- To remove respiratory secretions to assist ventilation
- To obtain a specimen in order to detect harmful bacteria

Equipment

- Bulb syringe
- Normal saline
- Suction catheter, variety of sizes
- Oxygen source, resuscitation bag and mask
- Tracheostomy tubes

Check order + **Gather equipment** + **Introduce yourself** + **Identify client** + **Provide privacy** + **Explain procedure** + **Hand hygiene** + **Gloves as needed**

Interventions and Rationales

1. Perform preparatory steps (see icon bar).
2. Solicit the assistance of a coworker. *This will help prevent injury to the child.*
3. Prior to the procedure, assess the infant's breath sounds, respiratory rate and effort, and patency of airway. *This provides data for evaluating the effectiveness of the procedure.*
4. After suctioning, assess respiratory status.

USING THE BULB SYRINGE

5. Position the infant in a supine position. *This allows ready access to the nares and mouth for suctioning.*
6. Clean the oral cavity by depressing the bulb and inserting the tip of the syringe into the left buccal cavity of the child's mouth. Repeat in the right buccal cavity.

Placing the syringe into the buccal cavity avoids eliciting the gag reflex.

7. Depress the bulb into a tissue or towel. *This clears the bulb syringe.*
8. Depress the bulb and place the tip of the syringe into the nares (Figure 18-3 ■). *If the bulb is not depressed prior to insertion, air could force the secretions into the nasopharynx.*
9. Release the bulb and withdraw secretions.
10. Wipe tip of bulb to remove debris.
11. Rinse the bulb syringe by depressing it into a cup of water and flushing it out. Repeat until clean.

SUCTIONING A CONSCIOUS INFANT

5. Place infant in a semi-Fowler's position with neck hyperextended. Attach suction tubing to source of

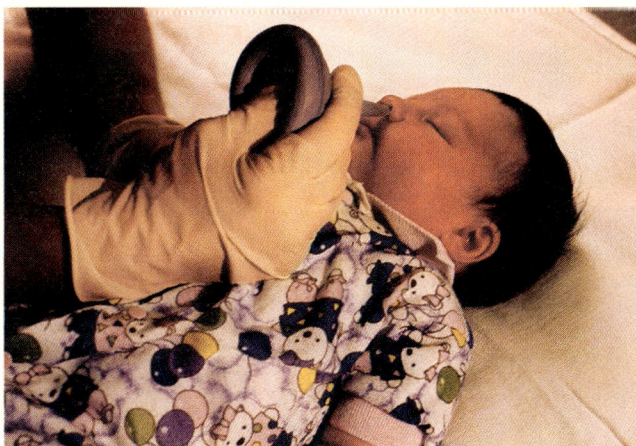

A

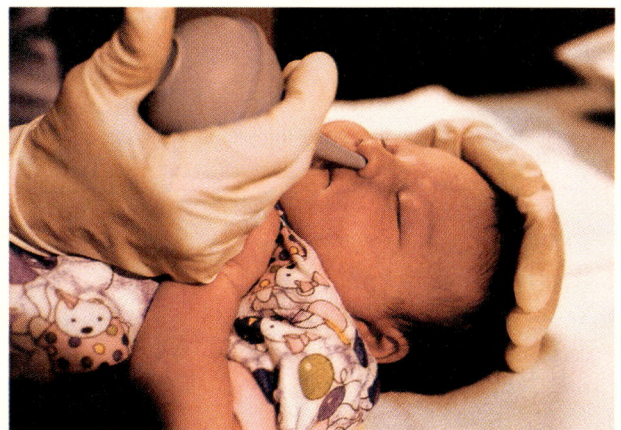

B

Figure 18-3. ■ **(A)** Insertion of a deflated tube bulb syringe. **(B)** Removal of a reinflated bulb syringe.

TABLE 18-1

Suggested Endotracheal Tube and Suction Catheter Size for Children

AGE	ENDOTRACHEAL TUBE SIZE (MM)	SUCTION CATHETER SIZE (FRENCH)
Premature newborn	2.0–2.5	5
Newborn	3.0–3.5	6–8
6 months	3.5	8
12–18 months	4.0	8
3 years	4.5	8
5 years	5.0	10
6 years	5.5	10
8 years	6.0	10
12 years	6.5	10
16 years	7.0–8.0	12

Source: Adapted from Dieckman, R., Brownstein, D., & Gaushe-Hill, M. (eds.) (2nd ed.). (2006). *Pediatric education for prehospital professionals/American Academy of Pediatrics.* Sudbury, MA: Jones and Bartlett Publishers.

suction. Table 18-1 ■ describes selection of the proper sizes of suction catheters and endotracheal tubes. Use settings as ordered by physician or according to agency policy.

6. Apply sterile gloves. *This prevents exposure to and spread of micro-organisms.*

7. Insert the suction catheter into the nares. Close the suction port with the thumb to initiate suction. Limit suctioning to 5 to 10 seconds. Repeat in other nares.

8. Suction the mouth in the same manner.

SUCTIONING AN INFANT WITH DECREASED LEVEL OF CONSCIOUSNESS

5. Administer oxygen by face mask. *Preoxygenating the infant avoids hypoxia during suctioning.*

6. Position the infant in a lateral position. *The lateral position can prevent aspiration because it prevents the tongue from falling back and blocking the oropharynx. It allows gravity to assist in the drainage of secretions.*

7. Apply sterile gloves.

8. Moisten the catheter with water and insert the suction catheter into the nares. *Moistening the catheter eases insertion.*

9. Close suction port with thumb to initiate suction. Limit suctioning to 5 to 10 seconds.

10. Apply oxygen mask. *This improves oxygenation.*

11. Repeat in other nares.

12. Apply oxygen mask.

13. Suction the mouth in the same manner.

14. Apply oxygen mask.

15. To remove secretions beyond the hypopharynx and trachea, advance the catheter further. Apply suction by occluding the suction port. Rotate gently upon withdrawal. *This removes secretions attached to the walls of the trachea. Rotation also prevents suction equipment from adhering to one spot.*

SUCTIONING THE TRACHEOSTOMY TUBE

5. Inform the parent that suctioning may cause coughing and dyspnea.

6. Position the infant in a supine position with the head of bed raised 30 degrees to prevent aspiration.

7. Attach oxygen source to resuscitation bag.

8. Apply sterile gloves.

9. Using the nondominant hand, remove the humidity source from tracheostomy tube.

10. Preoxygenate the infant as ordered.

11. With the dominant hand, insert suction catheter into the tube without suction. Advance the catheter no farther than 0.5 cm below the opening of the tracheostomy tube (Figure 18-4 ■). *This helps prevent transmission of micro-organisms.*

12. Apply intermittent suction, rotating the catheter during withdrawal to remove the maximum amount of secretions. Do not suction for longer than 5 to 10 seconds. *Suctioning for longer could compromise oxygenation.*

13. Withdraw the catheter completely and apply oxygen. *Suction removes both oxygen and secretions.*

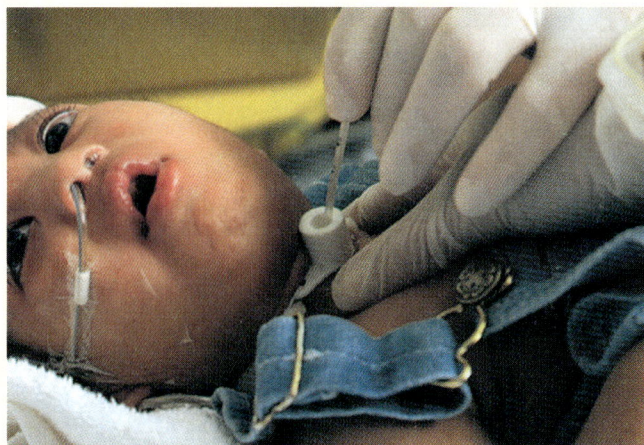

Figure 18-4. ■ Tracheostomy tube suctioning.

SUCTIONING THE ENDOTRACHEAL TUBE

5. Position the infant in a supine position with head of bed raised 30 degrees to prevent aspiration.

6. Attach oxygen source to resuscitation bag.

7. Apply sterile gloves.

8. Have assistant disconnect the ventilator.

9. Preoxygenate the infant as ordered to prevent hypoxia.

10. With the dominant hand, insert the suction catheter into the tube without suction. Advance the catheter no farther than 0.5 cm below the opening of the ET tube.

11. Apply intermittent suction, rotating the catheter during withdrawal. Do not suction for longer than 5 to 10 seconds. *Rotation ensures greater removal of secretions. It also prevents suction from adhering to one spot.*

12. Withdraw the catheter completely and apply oxygen.

13. Reconnect ventilator.

14. Repeat prn.

15. Clear the suction catheter using sterile saline.

SAMPLE DOCUMENTATION

(date) 0845 R 32, uneven and labored. Cough ineffective. Rhonchi auscultated bilaterally. Sterile oral/pharyngeal suctioning performed according to policy. Moderate amount of thick, white secretions obtained. Breathing less labored, R 22. J. Edward, LPN

Medication is usually administered by intravenous infusion. If the need for IV fluids or medications is determined within the first few hours after birth, the doctor may insert a catheter into an umbilical vein. Another site for a central venous catheter is the subclavian vein. The nurse assists with the insertion of the catheter, maintains the infusion, and administers medication as ordered.

Diagnostic examination, such as MRI scan and ultrasound, may be necessary to determine the specific disorder and appropriate treatment. The nurse may need to accompany the newborn to these procedures in order to maintain necessary care. At times, surgery may be needed to correct life-threatening congenital anomalies. Specially trained operating room personnel provide these services. The newborn returns to the NICU following surgery. Drainage tubes (chest tubes, intraventricular catheter, or wound drainage tube) may be in place. The nurse must maintain patency of these tubes.

Nursing Considerations

Besides assisting with medical treatment, the nurse must also provide for the newborn's activities of daily living. The newborn needs nutrients in order to grow. The premature newborn may not have the muscle strength or energy to suck from the breast or bottle. Endotracheal tubes may be inserted through the mouth. In these cases, a small amount of formula or breast milk may be given by gavage feeding every few hours. (See Procedure 18-2 ■.) Sometimes the newborn who lacks strength to suck may be taught to drink from a cup. As the newborn gains strength, bottle-feeding may be used. If the gastrointestinal system is not able to function normally, nutrients

will be given by total parenteral nutrition (TPN). (See Figure 18-1B.)

If the high-risk newborn has adequate fluid intake, he or she should void every few hours. If oral nutrients are administered, the meconium stool should change in a few days to the transitional stools seen in healthy newborns (see Figure 17-31 ⬭). Skin care with each diaper change is important to prevent tissue breakdown.

Activity is necessary to encourage muscle development, to prevent skin breakdown, and to prevent hypostatic pneumonia. The high-risk newborn should be turned and positioned every few hours. The high-risk newborn may be positioned supine, side-lying, or prone with the head of the bed elevated slightly unless contraindicated. Keeping the head elevated prevents the abdominal contents from pushing on the diaphragm and impeding breathing. The extremities should be free to move as much as possible. If any form of restraint is necessary, it should be removed, and active or passive range of motion should be performed every few hours.

The skin of the premature or high-risk newborn is thin and fragile. Care must be taken to protect the skin and tissue and keep them intact. The skin should be kept clean and dry. The linens should be free of wrinkles. The newborn should not be placed on tubes and monitoring wires. A water mattress or sheepskin can be used.

The skin of the postterm infant is also at risk. Because the vernix caseosa is gradually reabsorbed into the skin, postterm babies may have skin that peels, cracks, or even begins to slough off, making them prone to infection. Very few babies today are postterm. Typically, labor is induced to prevent long delays beyond the estimated due date.

PROCEDURE 18-2

Administering a Gavage/Tube Feeding

Purpose

- To provide nutritional support when the infant is unable to obtain adequate calories orally

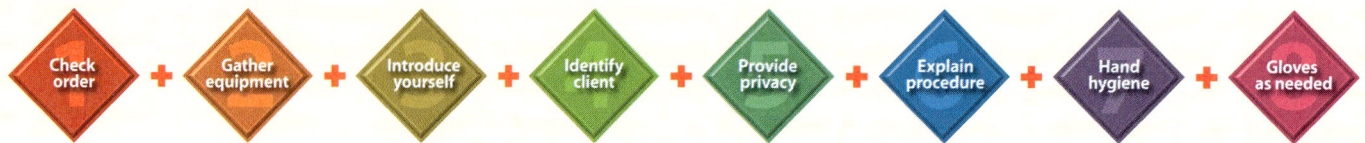

Equipment

- Nutritional supplementation
- Tap water
- 20 mL syringe
- Clean towel

Check order + Gather equipment + Introduce yourself + Identify client + Provide privacy + Explain procedure + Hand hygiene + Gloves as needed

Interventions and Rationales

1. Perform preparatory steps (see icon bar).

2. Allow nutritional supplement to reach room temperature. *This will prevent cramping.*

3. Position the infant in a Fowler's or high Fowler's position. Place a towel across the infant's abdomen. *This position prevents aspiration, and the towel helps keep the infant's clothing free of soiling.*

4. Check placement.

5. Assess residual gastric volume. *The feeding should be withheld if the residual volume is too great because this indicates that digestion may be altered. The agency may designate this volume, and the physician may include the residual volume in the original order.*

6. Flush the tubing with tap water. *This is necessary to clear the tubing of gastric contents.*

7. Clamp the tubing and attach barrel of syringe or primed tubing for continuous feeding.

8. For bolus feeding, raise barrel of syringe no more than 18 in. above the infant's abdomen. Fill the syringe with nutritional supplement. Unclamp the tubing and allow supplement to flow slowly into tube (see Figure 18-1).

9. Watch the infusion carefully and do not allow air into the tube. Clamp the tubing. *Air could cause the infant to have gas.*

10. Maintain the infant in the Fowler's position for 1 to 2 hours. *This will prevent aspiration.*

11. Follow the bolus feeding with a flush of tap water. *The amount of the flush will typically be ordered by the physician.*

12. For continuous feeding, label the bag with date and time. Set the rate as prescribed and monitor it closely.

SAMPLE DOCUMENTATION

(date) 0845 No gastric residual obtained. Orogastric tube flushed with 10 mL tap water. 30 mL Enfamil with iron given bolus via orogastric tube. 30 mL tap water flushed following feeding. HOB at 45 degrees.
A. David, LVN

The newborn needs to be touched and caressed (Figure 18-5 ■). Parents must bond with the newborn. The nurse can promote this bonding process by encouraging the parents to assist with the care of the newborn. It is frightening for parents to see the baby sick, with numerous tubes and monitors attached. They may be frightened to touch or hold their baby. The nurse encourages parents to begin the bonding process by fingertip and palmar touch, followed by stroking, holding, and rocking the newborn as much as possible. Placing the newborn clad only in a clean diaper against the parent's bare chest facilitates bonding. A blanket should be placed over both the baby and the parent to prevent heat loss.

Both the parents and the nurses should call the newborn by name. Parents should be encouraged to talk and sing to the baby. They should be allowed to participate as much as possible in daily care—bathing, diapering, and feeding. The nurse must explain all aspects of care and medical

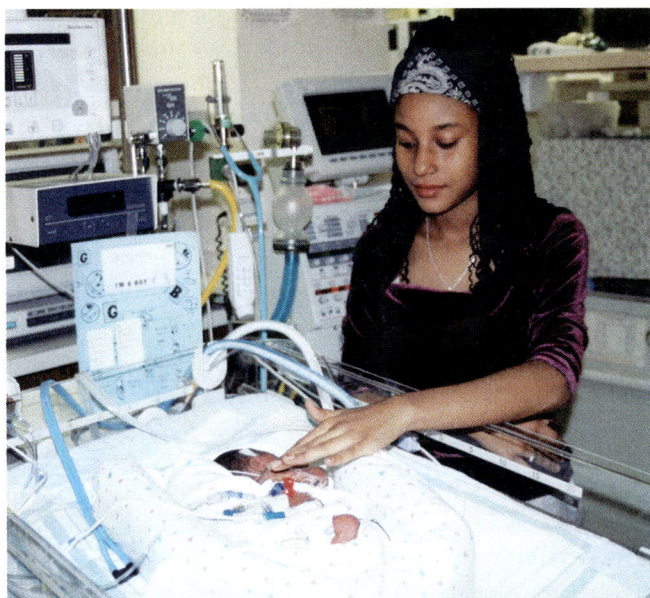

A

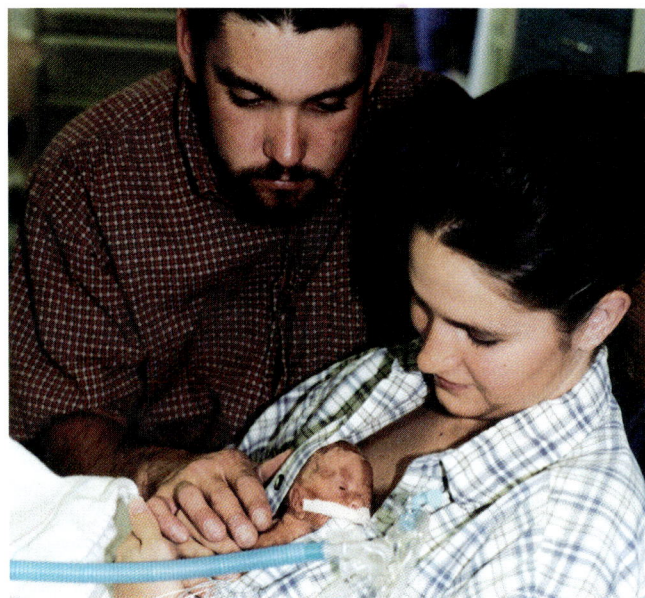

B

Figure 18-5. ■ (**A**) Mother of this 26 weeks' gestational age 600-g baby begins attachment through fingertip touch. (**B**) Kangaroo (skin-to-skin) care facilitates a closeness and attachment between parents and their premature infant. (A: Courtesy of Lisa Smith-Pedersen, RNC, MSN, NNP. B: Courtesy of Carol Harrigan, RNC, MSN, NNP.)

treatment, and teach the parents to provide care. The nurse must be alert for parental comments and behavior that indicate their anxiety or comfort with the situation. Support groups may be useful to help parents of high-risk newborns.

Preterm Newborn

The preterm newborn is one who is born prior to the 38th week of gestation. Although prematurity is one of the leading causes of neonatal death, an infant born before the 38th week can live but may not be equipped to survive unassisted.

Manifestations

The preterm newborn's skin is wrinkled and covered with lanugo. Lacking subcutaneous fat, the premature newborn appears thin with prominent bones including the skull, ribs, and hips. Depending on the gestational age, the premature newborn's cry may be weak and signs of respiratory distress will be evident (see Figure 17-19 ⬭). The limbs are usually extended, exposing more body surface to heat loss.

Diagnosis and Treatment

The nurse should complete a gestational age assessment and compare the data with the mother's reported date of conception. Gestational age determination is discussed in Chapter 17 ⬭. The premature newborn would be placed in the newborn intensive care unit (NICU) under constant observation and monitoring.

Because the organs are immature, treatment is based on the needs of the individual premature newborn. The first priority is supporting respiration and circulation. Body heat is maintained by radiant warmer. Depending on the age and condition of the premature newborn, food and fluids are administered orally or by intravenous infusion. Usually, the premature newborn is cared for in the NICU until vital signs are stable and growth is increasing steadily.

Nursing Considerations

Nursing care of the premature newborn is dependent on the gestational age of the infant. Newborns who are 2 or 3 weeks premature generally do not require the same amount of monitoring and care as the newborn who is 4 or more weeks early. Once premature infants have stabilized, they may be transferred to a less acute unit where they remain until their weight is high enough for them to be discharged (approximately 5.5 lbs or 2,500 g). During this time of growth, the LPN/LVN may be given more responsibility for providing general care of the infant. Families should be encouraged to participate in daily newborn care.

Postterm Newborn

The postterm newborn is born after 42 weeks' gestation. Because the placenta does not function well after the 40th week, the postterm infant is at risk for similar complications as the preterm infant.

Manifestations

The postterm newborn may be large, which increases the probability of a traumatic vaginal birth or cesarean section. Placental insufficiency places the fetus at risk for inadequate oxygen and nutrients. Under stress, the fetus may pass meconium into the amniotic fluid. Limited placental function during labor places the infant at risk for meconium aspiration and hypoxia. Because of resorption of vernix caseosa after 40 weeks, there is little vernix caseosa to protect the skin from the amniotic fluid. Therefore, the skin of the postterm newborn is often dry and cracked, with a parchment-like texture.

Nursing Considerations

Besides routine newborn care, the postterm newborn should be watched closely for respiratory distress and hypoglycemia. Airway maintenance (including suctioning) is critical. The newborn with a low blood glucose will need frequent feeding, either by breast or formula.

The large infant may have birth trauma. This includes but is not limited to fractured clavicle and cephalhematoma. If the clavicle was fractured during birth, the infant will be unable to move the arms equally. The RN and primary care provider should be notified if a fractured clavicle is suspected. A cephalhematoma can put pressure on the underlying brain tissue. Usually a cephalhematoma will absorb over time without neurologic damage. However, the neurologic status of the newborn should be closely monitored and the primary care provider notified of changes.

Newborn with Alteration in Growth

At times the fetus does not grow as expected, resulting in a newborn that is either large or small for the gestational age. In either case, the newborn is at risk for complications and may require close observation and treatment.

LARGE FOR GESTATIONAL AGE

Large for gestational age (LGA) describes a newborn (see Figure 13-11B 🔗) whose birth weight is over the 90th percentile for the gestational age. This condition is called **macrosomia.** The most well-known cause of excessive growth is a mother with diabetes. However, the cause of the majority of LGA newborns is unknown (Rahimian & Varner, 2003).

Manifestations

The LGA newborn is generally proportional. The infant's weight, length, and head circumference are approximately the same percentage above normal. However, the infant of a diabetic mother has an increased weight while remaining within normal limits for length and head circumference.

The excessive weight in the infant born to a diabetic mother (IDM) is caused by high blood glucose levels. Maternal glucose readily crosses the placenta, resulting in an increased production of insulin and hyperplasia of the fetal pancreas. Insulin is an important regulator of metabolism and has a "growth hormone effect" on the fetus. At birth, the maternal supply of glucose is cut off, resulting in *hypoglycemia* in the newborn.

Macrosomic newborns are generally hypoactive at birth and may be hypotonic and difficult to arouse from a sleep state. They may have undergone a long and difficult labor and birth, either vaginally or by cesarean section. They may have respiratory distress and feeding difficulties.

Diagnosis

The diagnosis of LGA is made solely on measurements. However, factors to consider when evaluating the LGA newborn include:

- The size of parents: large parents tend to have large babies.
- The number of pregnancies: multiparous women have two to three times the number of LGA infants.
- The sex of the newborn: male infants tend to be larger than female infants.
- The presence of other disorders: infants with erythroblastosis fetalis or transposition of the great vessels are usually large.
- The presence of maternal disorders such as diabetes.

LGA newborns should be evaluated for complications including but not limited to hypoglycemia, polycythemia, and birth trauma such as fractured clavicle, brachial palsy, facial paralysis, skull fracture, cephalhematoma, and intracranial hemorrhage. Diagnostic exams such as blood tests, x-rays, and ultrasound may be needed.

Treatment

Treatment is directed toward relieving hypoglycemia and polycythemia and correcting birth trauma. LGA newborns need close observation until their condition has stabilized.

Nursing Considerations

Nursing care is directed toward monitoring vital signs and blood sugar levels and observing for signs of birth trauma. Blood glucose levels in the infant of a diabetic mother usually drop within 1 to 3 hours after birth and then return to normal levels between 4 and 6 hours after birth. Therefore, blood glucose levels obtained by heel stick are obtained hourly during the first 4 to 6 hours and then every 4 hours (or by facility policy). Infants whose blood glucose levels fall below 40 mg/dL should be encouraged to breastfeed or be given formula. Infants who are unable to be fed orally will require intravenous administration of glucose solutions. Intravenous access may be through an umbilical vein or a central line.

The nurse must realize that the large newborn is not necessarily a mature newborn. The nurse must assess the LGA newborn frequently for signs of respiratory distress. The airway may need to be suctioned and oxygen administered.

The nurse must be prepared to address parental concerns about the visual effects of birth trauma such as facial or head bruising. Parents may be reluctant to touch the newborn for fear of causing pain. Parents will need instruction regarding all care provided during hospitalization as well as home care after discharge. Following teaching, parents should be able to verbalize understanding of the treatment of their newborn.

SMALL FOR GESTATIONAL AGE

Small for gestational age (SGA) describes infants whose intrauterine growth is below that expected for the gestational age. This condition is also called **intrauterine growth restriction (IUGR)** or intrauterine growth retardation. Causes of SGA can be classified as maternal, environmental, placental, or fetal factors.

- Maternal factors include primiparity, grand multiparity, multiple pregnancy, and low socioeconomic status.
- Maternal disease includes maternal heart disease, substance abuse (with alcohol, nicotine, cocaine, narcotics, or others), maternal anemia, preeclampsia, and disorders that decrease blood flow to the uterus.
- Environmental factors include exposure to x-rays or toxins, high altitude, and excessive exercise. These environmental factors can decrease the oxygen available to the uterus.
- Placental factors include a small placenta, infarcted areas of the placenta, or placenta previa.
- Fetal factors include congenital infections, congenital anomalies, discordant twins (one twin is smaller than the other, possibly due to sharing or overlapping of the placenta).

Manifestations

Intrauterine growth occurs by both an increase in the number of cells and an increase in the size of cells. If a problem develops early in fetal development, fewer new cells are formed and organs will be small and underweight. If a problem develops later in fetal development, only the size of cells is affected, resulting in small organs.

There are two patterns of IUGR:

- *Symmetric (proportional) IUGR* is caused by a long-term maternal disorder such as chronic hypertension, malnutrition, substance abuse, or anemia or fetal genetic abnormalities. In symmetric IUGR there is prolonged restriction of growth of organs, body weight, length, and head circumference. Symmetric IUGR can be seen on ultrasound.
- *Asymmetric (disproportional) IUGR* is caused by a disorder that acutely compromises placenta circulation, such as preeclampsia, placental infarcts, or poor maternal weight gain in pregnancy. Asymmetric IUGR is not apparent until the third trimester of pregnancy. Although the weight is decreased, the total length and head circumference are normal. After 36 weeks' gestation, fetal abdominal circumference should be larger than head circumference. In asymmetric IUGR, the abdominal circumference of the fetus remains smaller than the head circumference. These newborns are at risk for asphyxia, pulmonary hemorrhage, hypocalcemia, and hypoglycemia.

Even though growth is restricted, physical maturity continues according to gestational age. Therefore, the SGA newborn may be physiologically mature.

Diagnosis and Treatment

The diagnosis of SGA is based on prenatal ultrasound birth measurements. A newborn who is slightly underweight but born at term may have few complications and require routine newborn care. Frequent monitoring of blood glucose levels and frequent feeding may be required.

The most common complications occurring in the SGA newborn include:

- Asphyxia: the SGA infant has been hypoxic *in utero* and may have little reserve to undergo labor and vaginal birth.
- Aspiration: hypoxia *in utero* may cause the infant to gasp during birth and aspirate amniotic fluid and vaginal secretions.
- Hypothermia: decrease in subcutaneous fat and depletion of brown fat *in utero* place the SGA newborn at risk for hypothermia.
- Hypoglycemia: an increased metabolic rate, heat loss, and poor glycogen stores in the liver result in hypoglycemia.
- Infection: a decreased reserve and immature immune system potentiates infection in the SGA newborn.

SGA newborns tend to have a poor prognosis, especially if born before 37 weeks' gestation. Diagnosis and treatment during the prenatal period can improve outcomes. SGA newborns require frequent monitoring of complications and individualized medical treatment.

Nursing Considerations

The SGA newborn requires frequent monitoring, including vital signs and blood glucose by heel stick. The first priority is to maintain a clear airway in the SGA newborn. The airway may need frequent suctioning, and oxygen may be administered. Because of the risk of hypothermia, SGA newborns are frequently placed under radiant heat or wrapped in three warm blankets. To prevent or treat hypoglycemia, the newborn is fed (by breast, bottle, or gavage) every 2 to 3 hours.

Parents need teaching about the need for warmth and frequent feeding. Additional assistance may be needed when the newborn is discharged. The nurse should make appropriate referral to home health or other agencies to help monitor the SGA newborn after discharge.

COMMON CONDITIONS AFFECTING THE HIGH-RISK NEWBORN

Many congenital anomalies are identified at birth or within the first few weeks of life. If the anomaly is life threatening, surgery is usually performed immediately to correct the defect. Less threatening anomalies are not repaired until the child is stronger and better able to withstand the surgical procedure. At times, repair is performed in stages, and complete reconstruction may take months or years. Some disorders that place the newborn at risk for long-term health concerns are introduced by body system in this section.

Neonatal Infections and Sepsis

Infections of the newborn usually result from exposure to the mother before or during delivery. Some infections—such as rubella, syphilis, and HIV/AIDS—are transported across the placenta and infect the developing fetus. Other infections—such as gonorrhea and herpes—can be picked up as the fetus moves through the birth canal (see Table 13-4 🔗). (In a woman with active herpes that can be lethal to the baby, delivery is by cesarean section.) The immature immune system of the premature or high-risk newborn makes infections especially dangerous. When the micro-organisms spread to the blood, generalized sepsis occurs. As sepsis becomes more severe, respiratory distress and septic shock may progress rapidly, resulting in death.

Manifestations

Newborn infection may occur within the first month of life. Nonspecific symptoms such as poor feeding, lethargy, and vomiting with or without diarrhea are usually seen first. Later the newborn may become cyanotic, jaundiced, and hypothermic. Due to the instability of the thermoregulatory center in the brain, newborns often have low body temperature with an infection, but may exhibit rapid fluctuation in body temperature.

Diagnosis and Treatment

Diagnosis of newborn infection and sepsis is made by blood and body fluid cultures. The newborn is admitted to the hospital for monitoring, fluid administration, and intravenous antibiotics.

Nursing Considerations

The primary consideration is prevention of infection in the newborn. The mother is screened for sexually transmitted infections prior to birth. Sterile and aseptic techniques are used as appropriate when providing care to limit the transmission of infection to the newborn. Treating the mother with appropriate antibiotics during pregnancy can limit the spread of infection to the fetus.

Parents should be taught to wash their hands before handling the newborn, following diaper change, and prior to handling food, formula, and bottles. Daily hygiene practices limit the transmission of micro-organisms to the newborn.

Cardiovascular Conditions

Cardiovascular conditions include congenital anomalies and hemorrhage and hemolytic disorders.

CONGENITAL HEART DEFECTS

Congenital heart defects are more common when the child has been exposed to rubella, alcohol, or drugs during intrauterine development. Other factors that increase the risk of congenital heart defects include other congenital or genetic defects, advanced maternal age, maternal disorders such as lupus and diabetes, and siblings or parents with congenital defects.

Congenital heart defects can be classified into four groups according to the way the defect affects circulation. These conditions, most of which require surgery and intensive care, are discussed in Table 18-2 ■ (which includes Figure 18-6 ■).

The first defects cause greater than normal flow of blood to the lungs. Defects with *increased pulmonary blood flow* include:

- **patent ductus arteriosus** (PDA), in which the ductus arteriosus is open.
- **atrial septal defect** (ASD), failure of the foramen ovale to close.

(*Text continues on p. 474.*)

TABLE 18-2

Congenital Heart Defects and Their Treatment

TYPE OF HEART DEFECT	ILLUSTRATION OF DEFECT

Patent Ductus Arteriosus (PDA)

Common congenital defect caused by persistent fetal circulation that accounts for 9% to 12% of all congenital heart defects (Driscoll, 1999). When pulmonary circulation is established and systemic vascular resistance increases at birth, pressures in the aorta become greater than in the pulmonary arteries. Blood is then shunted from the aorta to the pulmonary arteries, increasing circulation to the pulmonary system.

Clinical Manifestations

Dyspnea; tachypnea; full, bounding pulses; and poor development occur. Infant is at risk for frequent respiratory infections and infective endocarditis. When a large PDA exists, congestive heart failure, intercostal retractions, hepatomegaly, and growth failure are also seen. A continuous systolic murmur is auscultated, and a thrill may be palpated in the pulmonic area.

Clinical Therapy

When murmur is detected, diagnosis is confirmed by chest x-ray study, electrocardiogram (ECG), and echocardiogram. Chest x-ray film and ECG show left ventricular hypertrophy. PDA can be visualized, and left-to-right shunt can be measured on echocardiogram. Surgical ligation of PDA is the treatment of choice. Intravenous indomethacin often stimulates closure of the ductus arteriosus in premature infants. Transcatheter closure by obstructive device is sometimes attempted in children over 18 months of age.

Prognosis: If PDA is not treated, child's life span is shortened because pulmonary hypertension and vascular obstructive disease develop.

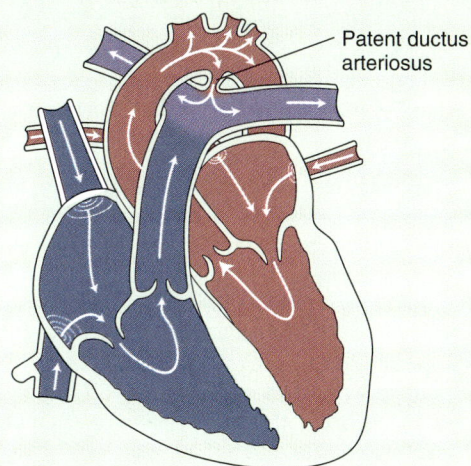

Patent ductus arteriosus

■ Mix of oxygenated and unoxygenated blood

A

Figure 18-6. ■ **(A)** Patent ductus arteriosus (PDA).

Atrial Septal Defect (ASD)

An opening at any point in the atrial septum that permits left-to-right shunting of blood. The opening may be small, as when the foramen ovale fails to close, or large, as when the septum may be completely absent. Of children with congenital heart defects, 6% to 10% have an ASD (Driscoll, 1999).

Clinical Manifestations

Infants and young children usually have no symptoms. Small and moderate-size ASDs are usually not diagnosed until preschool years or later. Congestive heart failure, easy tiring, and poor growth occur with a large ASD. A soft systolic murmur is usually heard in the pulmonic area with wide splitting of S_2.

Clinical Therapy

Diagnosis is made by echocardiogram that identifies right ventricular overload and shunt size. Chest x-ray film and ECG reveal little information unless ASD is large and excessive shunting is present.

Surgery to close or patch ASD is performed to prevent pulmonary vascular obstructive disease. Some ASDs may be closed by transcatheter device (septal occluder) during cardiac catheterization.

Prognosis: Many persons with uncorrected small and moderate-size ASDs have lived to middle age without symptoms. Atrial arrhythmias are common late complications.

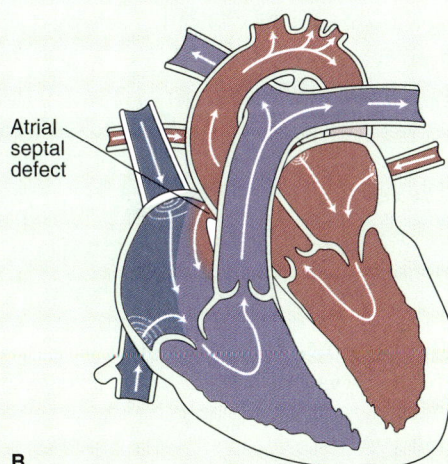

Atrial septal defect

B

Figure 18-6. ■ **(B)** Atrial septal defect (ASD).

Ventricular Septal Defect (VSD)

An opening in the ventricular septum results in increased pulmonary blood flow. Blood is shunted from the left ventricle directly across the open septum into the pulmonary artery. This most common congenital heart defect occurs in approximately 20% of all children with congenital heart disease (Driscoll, 1999).

(continued)

MediaLink ● Congenital Heart Defects

TABLE 18-2

Congenital Heart Defects and Their Treatment (continued)

TYPE OF HEART DEFECT	ILLUSTRATION OF DEFECT

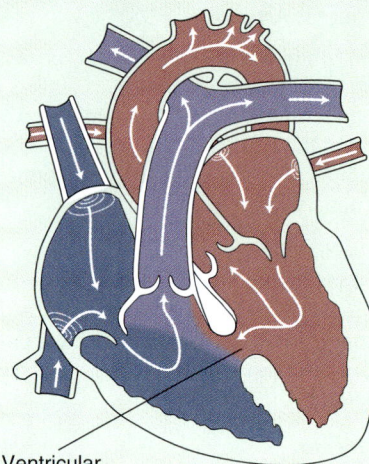

Clinical Manifestations

Only 15% of VSDs are large enough to cause symptoms, such as tachypnea, dyspnea, poor growth, reduced fluid intake, congestive heart failure, and pulmonary hypertension. Systolic murmur is auscultated in lower left sternal border.

Clinical Therapy

Chest x-ray film and ECG reveal few findings in cases of small VSDs. Larger VSDs with shunting are associated with enlarged heart and pulmonary vascular markings on chest x-ray film and left ventricular hypertrophy on ECG. Echocardiogram establishes diagnosis if shunting is present. Cardiac catheterization is used only in preparation for surgery. Most small VSDs close spontaneously. Treatment is conservative when no signs of congestive heart failure or pulmonary hypertension are present. Surgical patching of VSD during infancy is performed when poor growth is evident. Closure of VSD by transcatheter device (i.e., Rashkind device) during cardiac catheterization may be attempted for some defects. Prophylaxis for infective endocarditis is required.

Prognosis: Highest risk associated with surgical repair is in the first few months of life. Children respond well to surgery and experience substantial catch-up growth. Malignant tachyarrhythmias and heart block are a possible complication.

Ventricular septal defect

C

Figure 18-6. ■ (C) Ventricular septal defect (VSD).

Tetralogy of Fallot (TOF)

Combination of four defects: pulmonic stenosis, right ventricular hypertrophy, ventricular septal defect (VSD), and overriding aorta. Some children have a fifth defect: open foramen ovale or atrial septal defect (ASD). About 10% of children with congenital heart defects have tetralogy of Fallot (Park, 1996). This defect is characterized by elevated pressures in right side of heart, causing right-to-left shunt.

Clinical Manifestations

As ductus arteriosus closes, infant becomes hypoxic and cyanotic. The degree of pulmonary stenosis determines severity of symptoms. Polycythemia, hypoxic spells, metabolic acidosis, poor growth, clubbing, and exercise intolerance may develop. Infants have a systolic murmur heard in pulmonic area that is transmitted to suprasternal notch.

Clinical Therapy

Chest x-ray film shows a boot-shaped heart due to the large right ventricle with decreased pulmonary vascular markings. Electrocardiogram (ECG) shows right ventricular hypertrophy. Echocardiogram demonstrates VSD, obstruction of pulmonary outflow, and overriding aorta. Cardiac catheterization is required before surgical correction to completely identify the location of all anatomic structures and any additional defects.

Hypercyanotic spells are managed according to guidelines given in section on nursing management of cyanotic defects. Monitoring child for metabolic acidosis or prolonged unconsciousness is critical. A total repair is performed before 6 months of age when the infant has a hypercyanotic spell. Corrective surgery may be attempted in asymptomatic children by 6 months of age.

Prognosis: Not all children are cured by surgery, but most have improved quality of life and improved longevity. Arrhythmias and right ventricular dysfunction may be residual problems (Waldman & Wernly, 1999). Lifelong infective endocarditis prophylaxis is required.

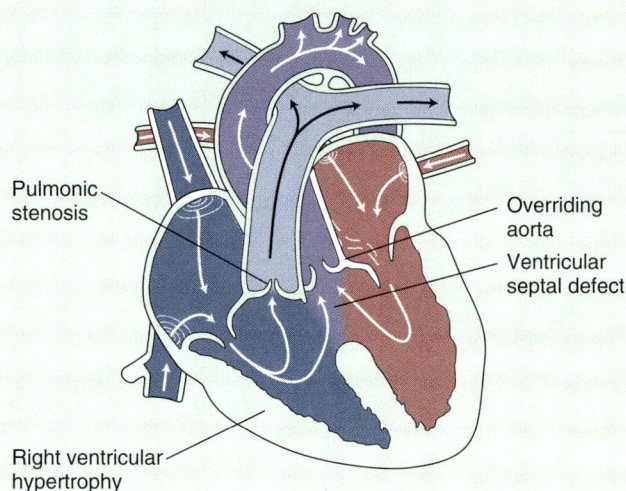

Pulmonic stenosis

Overriding aorta

Ventricular septal defect

Right ventricular hypertrophy

☐ Decreased unoxygenated blood flow

☐ Mixed oxygenated and unoxygenated blood

D

Figure 18-6. ■ (D) Tetralogy of Fallot (TOF).

TABLE 18-2

Congenital Heart Defects and Their Treatment

TYPE OF HEART DEFECT	ILLUSTRATION OF DEFECT

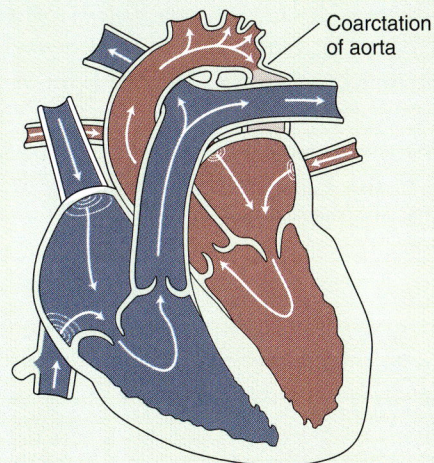

Coarctation of the Aorta (COA)

Narrowing or constriction in the descending aorta, often near the ductus arteriosus, obstructs systemic blood outflow. This defect is common, occurring in 5% to 8% of all children with congenital heart disease (Fedderly, 1999).

Clinical Manifestations
Many children are asymptomatic and grow normally, but constriction is progressive; 20% to 30% of children develop congestive heart failure by 3 months of age. Reduction in blood flow through the descending aorta causes lower blood pressure in legs and higher blood pressure in arms, neck, and head. Brachial and radial pulses are full, but femoral pulses are weak or absent. Older children may complain of weakness and pain in the legs after exercise.

Clinical Therapy
ECG shows left ventricular hypertrophy. Chest x-ray film may reveal enlargement and pulmonary venous congestion, and indentation of descending aorta. Rib notching (change in the smooth contour of the rib apparent on x-ray) is rarely seen before 10 years of age. Magnetic resonance imaging shows coarctation.

   Balloon dilation during cardiac catheterization is recommended for both initial relief and recoarctation. Surgical resection and anastomosis are palliative as coarctation may recur. The subclavian artery can be used as a patch in the infant. Repair in the first year of life is preferred to decrease exposure to hypertension.

Prognosis: Postcoarctectomy syndrome (abdominal pain and distention) occurs in 20% of clients (Walters, 2000). Persistent hypertension in adulthood is common. Infective endocarditis prophylaxis is needed.

☐ Decreased oxygenated blood flow

E

Figure 18-6. ■ **(E)** Coarctation of the aorta (COA).

Transposition of the Great Vessels

Pulmonary artery is the outflow for left ventricle, and aorta is outflow for right ventricle. This condition is life threatening at birth, and survival initially depends on open ductus arteriosus and foramen ovale. This condition occurs in about 5% of children with congenital heart disease (Grifka, 1999). ASD or VSD may also be present with transposition of the great vessels.

Clinical Manifestations
Cyanosis apparent soon after birth, progresses to hypoxia and acidosis. Cyanosis does not improve with oxygen administration. However, cyanosis may be less apparent when a large VSD is also present. Congestive heart failure may develop over days or weeks. Tachypnea (60 respirations/mm) is often present without retractions or other signs of dyspnea. Infants take a long time to feed and need frequent rest periods because of rapid respiratory rate and fatigue. Growth failure may be evident as early as 2 weeks of age if corrective surgery is not performed.

Clinical Therapy
Chest x-ray study may reveal a classic egg-shaped heart on a string (narrow superior mediastinum). Diagnosis is made by echocardiogram when position of arteries arising from ventricles is visible.

   Prostaglandin E_1 is initially ordered to maintain a patent ductus arteriosus until a palliative procedure can be performed. Corrective surgery (arterial switch) is usually performed before 1 week of age. Balloon atrial septostomy may be performed during cardiac catheterization in newborns as a first stage. This may also be corrected surgically.

Prognosis: Survival without surgery is impossible. Arrhythmias, right ventricular failure, and sudden death are long-term complications (8 to 15 years) after the Mustard procedure, so the Mustard or Rastelli procedure are performed only when significant pulmonary valve stenosis is present (Grifka, 1999). Infective endocarditis prophylaxis may be necessary.

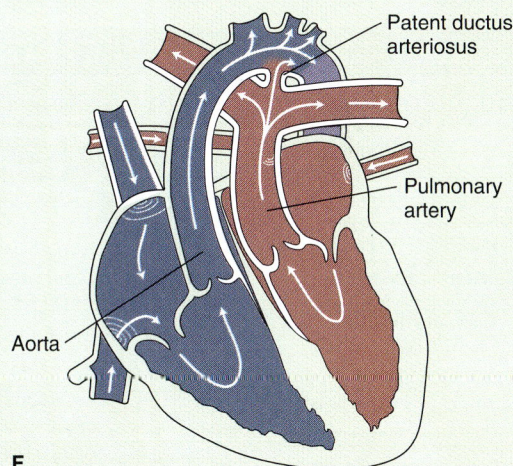

F

Figure 18-6. ■ **(F)** Transposition of the great vessels.

- **ventricular septal defect** (VSD), an opening in the septum between the ventricles.

The second type of defect, with *decreased pulmonary blood flow*, is **tetralogy of Fallot** (TOF). The four characteristics that define TOF are *pulmonary stenosis* (narrowing of the pulmonary valve), ventricular septal defect, right ventricular hypertrophy (enlargement of the right ventricle), and an overriding aortic valve.

The third type of defect involves *obstructed systemic blood flow*. In this type, called **coarctation** (narrowing) of the aorta, overall blood flow is reduced.

The fourth and most immediately life-threatening condition involves *reversed blood flow*. This occurs with **transposition of the great vessels** (the pulmonary artery and aorta are reversed). When the great vessels are reversed, blood flows into the right side of the heart through the vena cava and out of the heart through the aorta. Blood flows into the left side of the heart through the pulmonary veins and out through the pulmonary artery. The result is that unoxygenated blood does not go to the lungs for gas exchange, and oxygenated blood is repeatedly exposed to oxygen. See Table 18-2 for manifestations, diagnosis, and treatment of congenital heart defects.

Manifestations

Newborns with congenital heart defects exhibit signs and symptoms of congestive heart failure. These include, but are not limited to, heart murmurs, cyanosis, respiratory distress, fluid retention, and activity intolerance. Some heart murmurs are loud and easily heard. Others are soft and can only be detected by a trained practitioner. Cyanosis can be either constant, generalized cyanosis, or cyanosis around the mouth **(circumoral)**, seen only when the newborn is active, nursing, or crying. Signs of respiratory distress include tachycardia, orthopnea, grunting, flaring nostrils, and retractions. Fluid retention may be evidenced by bulging fontanels, fewer than six wet diapers per day, moist lung sounds, and generalized tissue edema. Restlessness, crying, and lethargy can be signs of intracranial edema.

Nursing Considerations

Nursing care of the newborn with congenital heart defects is to prepare the infant and parents for surgery. Often the newborn will need to be transferred to a medical center where heart surgery can be performed. There may be little time to prepare the parents for the procedures and transfer. The Nursing Care Plan Chart below describes care of an infant with tetralogy of Fallot.

NURSING CARE PLAN CHART

Planning for Newborn with Tetralogy of Fallot

GOAL	INTERVENTION	RATIONALE	EXPECTED OUTCOME
1. Deficient Knowledge related to Tetralogy of Fallot			
The client or couple will obtain information about tetralogy of Fallot. Client or couple will consent to plan of emergent treatment, including surgery, as recommended.	Provide written materials on normal heart anatomy and physiology and on tetralogy of Fallot. Explain that tetralogy of Fallot is a specific type of congenital heart disease that consists of four separate defects: an opening between the ventricles, an overlapping aorta, narrowed pulmonary artery, and enlargement of the right side of the heart. Explain that treatment for the disorder may include medication and/or surgery.	*Congenital malformations of the heart develop very early in pregnancy, usually by the 5th week.* *These heart defects cause venous blood to enter the arterial circulation, creating chronic hypoxia.* *Enlargement of the heart is caused by an increase in cardiac output necessary to force blood through the narrowed pulmonary artery and to meet the oxygen demands of the tissues.* *Skin color is related to the amount of oxyhemoglobin in the tissues. Hypoxia causes pallor.*	Client or couple will explain the nature of the disorder and the rationale behind treatment for tetralogy of Fallot. Client or couple will sign diagnostic and/or surgical consent forms following explanation by attending physician and/or surgeon.
	For newborns undergoing surgery, repeat and/or clarify preoperative teaching to parents provided by physician and/or registered nurse. Obtain surgical consent per agency policy.	*Limited open heart surgery (Blalock-Taussig procedure) may be performed. (Total corrective surgery is usually reserved for much older children.)*	

GOAL	INTERVENTION	RATIONALE	EXPECTED OUTCOME
2. Impaired <u>G</u>as Exchange related to heart defect			
Parent clients will anticipate *paroxysmal hypercyanotic episodes* ("Tet" spells), and will respond appropriately. Newborn will maintain gaseous exchange level compatible with life. Newborn client will avoid complications of the disorder, including polycythemia, thrombosis, and infection.	Maintain patent airway. Monitor child's vital signs, respiratory status, and self-positioning. Report newborn's condition, especially worsening of respiratory compromise to the registered nurse and/or physician. Explain to the parents that this disorder can cause the baby to have episodes of difficult breathing, during which the baby may look very pale or blue (cyanotic). "Tet spells" may last a few minutes to a few hours and are generally followed by a period of fatigue and sleepiness. Positioning: Placing the child in the "knee-chest" or squatting position. Medication Administration: Oral (Antibiotic prophylaxis) Monitor and/or maintain intravenous access route.	*The aim of treatment is to increase pulmonary blood flow to maintain effective circulatory gas exchange.* *The squatting position facilitates pulmonary circulation and helps to alleviate symptoms as it reduces the work of breathing. Some children will automatically squat when experiencing dyspnea.* *Excessive red blood cell production (polycythemia) is the body's response to chronic hypoxia. Extra blood cells increase the risk of clot formation. Structural abnormalities of the heart increase the risk of bacterial endocarditis.* *Medication for tetralogy of Fallot may include intravenous administration of Prostaglandin-E$_1$ to promote patency of the ductus arteriosus. An open ductus helps to support pulmonary blood flow. Antibiotic therapy helps to reduce the risk of bacterial endocarditis.*	Client will demonstrate effective gas exchange by absence of chronic cyanosis. Client's blood gases will remain within normal limits or in a range as specified by the physician. Parents will demonstrate ability to place the child in the knee-chest position during a "Tet spell."
3. <u>A</u>ctivity Intolerance related to poor tissue oxygenation			
Newborn client will maintain normal activity level. Newborn will respond appropriately to environmental stimuli. Newborn client will avoid complications of the disorder including iron-deficiency anemia and dehydration.	Limit environmental factors that may overstimulate the newborn. Monitor newborn's rest and activity patterns. Maintain adequate nutrition and hydration. Monitor intake and output. Monitor daily weight. Provide comfort measures.	*Environmental stressors (such as anxiety) may increase the baby's motor activity, which increases oxygen consumption.* *Hypoxia causes fatigue, which may result in difficulty feeding.* *Nutritional deficits contribute to iron-deficiency anemia, which in turn contributes to hypoxia. Dehydration increases the heart rate, and also increases the risk of thrombosis.* *Holding, swaddling, and other comfort measures help to reduce the baby's anxiety and thereby reduce oxygen consumption and the work of breathing.*	Newborn's sleep and activity patterns will remain within normal limits. Newborn will not appear lethargic. Newborn client's intake and output will remain within normal limits. Newborn's weight gain and growth pattern will remain within normal limits.

The immediate care of the newborn includes assisting with endotracheal intubation, establishing intravenous access, and administering prescribed medication. Parents will need instruction in the interventions being performed on their baby. They will also need emotional support.

Postoperatively the infant will be monitored in an intensive care unit. All vital signs and blood glucose will be monitored closely. Breathing will be maintained by a mechanical ventilator. Medication will be administered by intravenous infusion. Parents will be encouraged to touch and talk to their baby. As the newborn's condition improves, parents will be encouraged to assume more of the newborn's care.

HEMORRHAGE

Although the newborn can hemorrhage from any trauma site, the most common is **intracranial hemorrhage** (hemorrhage within the cerebral ventricles of the brain), which accompanies premature delivery. Before 35 weeks' gestation, the cerebral ventricles are lined with the germinal matrix. This matrix is susceptible to hypoxia and trauma. If the fetus becomes hypoxic or undergoes labor, hemorrhage from the germinal matrix into the cerebral ventricles is probable. For this reason, premature infants are frequently delivered by cesarean section instead of vaginally.

Manifestations

If intraventricular hemorrhage occurs, the newborn's brain function may be impaired, resulting in mental delay, immobility, or death. The symptoms and condition of the newborn dictate the care required.

HEMOLYTIC DISEASE OF THE NEWBORN (RH INCOMPATIBILITY, ABO INCOMPATIBILITY)

Hemolytic disease of the newborn (discussed briefly in Chapter 13 ⬤⬤) is a general term for several blood disorders that result in red blood cell (RBC) breakdown and an increase in bilirubin **(hyperbilirubinemia)**. The most common cause of hyperbilirubinemia is *physiologic jaundice*, the normal breakdown of RBCs discussed in Chapter 17 ⬤⬤ . A secondary cause of hyperbilirubinemia is *pathologic jaundice*. The most common cause of pathologic jaundice is Rh incompatibility. (You recall that Rh-positive blood contains the Rh protein on the RBC, and Rh-negative blood is missing this protein. If Rh-positive blood and Rh-negative blood are mixed together in the mother, the Rh-negative blood develops antibodies against the Rh-positive protein. During any future pregnancies with an Rh-positive fetus, the mother's Rh-negative blood will destroy the fetal blood.)

Manifestations

The distribution of fetal RBCs results in hyperbilirubinemia and pathologic jaundice. Because the destruction of RBCs occurs before delivery, the newborn exhibits jaundice within the first 24 hours after delivery. The newborn is anemic at birth and has difficulty oxygenating the tissues.

Diagnosis

A cord blood sample is evaluated for bilirubin, which should not exceed 5 mg/dL. Follow-up serum bilirubin levels should not rise more than 5 mg/dL/day. A premature newborn should have therapy instituted when serum bilirubin reaches 10 mg/dL. Any infant with a bilirubin level of 20 mg/dL or higher may need an exchange blood transfusion.

Treatment

Hyperbilirubinemia may be treated with phototherapy (exposure of the newborn to high-intensity light), exchange transfusion, or drug therapy. Figure 18-7 ■ illustrates two types of phototherapy equipment. If pathologic jaundice is left untreated, the newborn may experience mental delays, congestive heart failure, and death. In the NICU, the newborn may be given blood transfusion of compatible blood until the RBC destruction stops. This condition can be prevented by administering RhoGAM to the Rh-negative mother during pregnancy and again following delivery (see Table 13-3 ⬤⬤).

Nursing Considerations

Phototherapy can be provided by a bank of lights, by a fiberoptic blanket attached to a light source wrapped around the newborn's body, by a fiberoptic mattress, or by a combination of these methods. When phototherapy lights are used, the newborn's eyes must be protected from the bright lights. The baby's temperature must be taken frequently to ensure that the infant is not overheated. If the baby's temperature rises, the lights should be turned off for a time. With a fiberoptic blanket, the light stays on at all times. The infant's eyes do not need to be covered. The fiberoptic blanket allows the baby to be more accessible for feeding, for diaper changes, and to bond with parents. Fiberoptic blankets are also available for home care.

Respiratory Conditions

SUDDEN INFANT DEATH SYNDROME

Sudden infant death syndrome (SIDS) is the sudden unexpected death of an infant younger than 1 year. SIDS most often strikes infants between 2 and 4 months of age and is more common in males. Other factors common in SIDS include Native American or African American descent, low birth weight, and multiple births (twins or triplets). SIDS is the

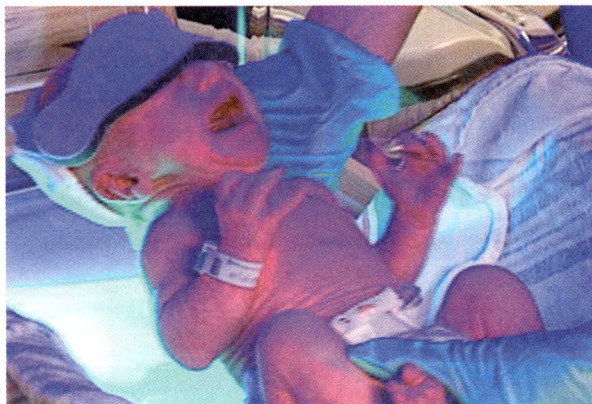

A

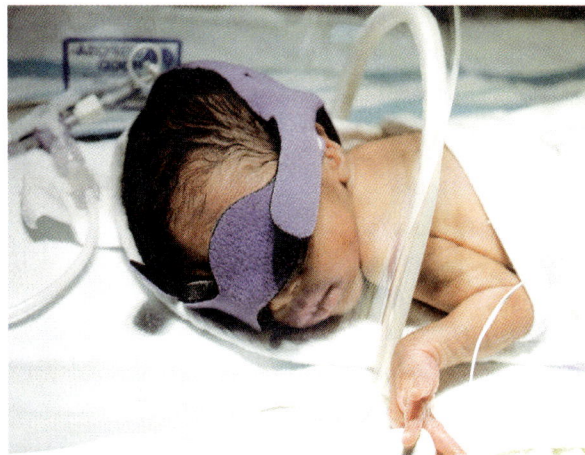

B

Figure 18-7. ■ Phototherapy for hyperbilirubinemia (jaundice). Bilateral eye patches are always used to protect the infant's eyes. (**A**) Newborn on fiberoptic "bili" mattress and under phototherapy lights. A combination of fiberoptic light source mattress and standard phototherapy light source above may also be used. (Note: The color is distorted because of the reflection of the bililight mattress.) (**B**) Infant receiving phototherapy. The phototherapy light is positioned over the incubator. (Courtesy of Lisa Smith-Pedersen, RNC, MSN, NNP.)

leading cause of death in infants between 1 month and 1 year of age. Box 18-2 ■ identifies risk factors associated with SIDS.

Manifestations

When SIDS strikes, the infant is typically found not breathing, and emergency medical help is summoned. The infant is usually in a normal state of nutrition and hydration. In more than 50% of infants, blood-tinged frothy fluids are present in and around the mouth and nose. The diapers are filled with urine and stool. The infant may be clutching a blanket. There is no audible outcry at the time of death. Skin is a white ashen color, not the expected cyanotic blue found with respiratory distress. An autopsy will need to be performed to identify the cause of death.

Prevention and Treatment

Although infants who are at risk can be identified, SIDS remains unpredictable. The main prevention measure is to place infants on their back to sleep. If a child is found in respiratory arrest, CPR must be initiated immediately and emergency medical services called.

Nursing Considerations

The impact of SIDS on the family is one of extreme shock followed by extreme outrage. Family members commonly experience guilt, either self-blaming or projecting blame onto other family members or caregivers (e.g., a babysitter). Older children may fear SIDS will happen to them as well. Siblings may also believe that the infant died because of bad thoughts or desires they had toward their brother or sister.

BOX 18-2	ASSESSMENT

Risk Factors for SIDS

Infant's Risk Factors

- Prematurity
- Low birth weight
- Twin or triplet birth
- Race (in decreasing order of frequency): most common in Native American infants, followed by African American, Hispanic, White, and Asian infants
- Gender: more common in males than females
- Age: most common in infants between 2 and 4 months of age
- Time of year: more prevalent in winter months
- Exposure to passive smoke
- History of cyanosis, respiratory distress, irritability, and poor feeding in the nursery
- Sleeping prone

Maternal and Familial Risk Factors

- Maternal age younger than 20 years
- History of smoking and illicit drug use (increases incidence 10 times)
- Anemia
- Multiple pregnancies, with short intervals between births
- History of sibling with SIDS (increases incidence four to five times)
- Low socioeconomic status; crowding
- Poor prenatal care, low birth weight gain

The nurse has an important role both in supporting the family and in educating the public. Although the need for support of parents and siblings is obvious, grandparents will need additional support. Grandparents will be experiencing grief at the loss of their grandchild, as well as extreme hurt at watching their own children suffer. Family members should be allowed to hold the infant and receive handprints, footprints, and a lock of hair. Provide the family with information about local support groups.

OTHER CAUSES OF RESPIRATORY DISTRESS

Congenital anomalies that affect the respiratory system commonly involve the esophagus. These anomalies are introduced under gastrointestinal conditions.

The premature newborn's lungs are not fully ready to begin the function of breathing and gas exchange. The premature newborn is unable to produce adequate amounts of *surfactant*, the chemical required to maintain the patency of the alveoli. The collapsed alveoli are unable to exchange oxygen and carbon dioxide.

The term newborn should produce an adequate amount of surfactant and breathe independently. However, the newborn may develop respiratory distress for several reasons. During the birth process, the fetus may aspirate amniotic fluid and vaginal secretions. If the mother receives narcotic medication during labor, the fetus may have depressed respiratory effort at birth. Vigorous suctioning of the airway during birth can cause laryngospasm, which obstructs the airway.

The passage of meconium by the fetus is a common occurrence in response to hypoxia or stress during the pregnancy. During delivery, the newborn can inhale the amniotic fluid containing meconium **(meconium aspiration)**. Severe meconium aspiration increases the possibility that the newborn will develop persistent pulmonary hypertension, pneumothorax, and pneumonia.

Manifestations

The newborn becomes hypoxic, breathes faster, depletes the energy stores, and develops respiratory distress. (See Chapter 17 🔗 for signs of respiratory distress in the newborn.) Airway obstruction results in respiratory arrest and death within minutes.

Treatment

To prevent death, the newborn is placed on mechanical ventilation (see Figure 18-1A). However, mechanical ventilation and high oxygen concentration can further damage the alveoli, resulting in permanent lung disease or **bronchopulmonary dysplasia** (BPD).

Nursing Considerations

Establishing and maintaining a patent airway is the highest priority in newborn care. The nurse should suction the airway as needed with a bulb syringe or suction catheter. Oxygen can be administered by nasal catheter or mask. Should mechanical ventilation be needed, a certified respiratory therapist, anesthesiologist, or primary care provider will need to insert an endotracheal tube.

Neurologic Conditions

Neurologic conditions are very serious and require long-term care. They include congenital anomalies, birth trauma, and acquired defects.

CONGENITAL DEFECTS

Two common defects are introduced here. **Spina bifida** is an incomplete closure of the vertebrae and neural tube. Large defects include **meningocele** (a herniation of the meninges through the vertebral defect) or **meningomyelocele** (a herniation of the spinal nerves and the meninges through the vertebral defect). Although the defect can be found anywhere along the spinal column, the most common area is in the lumbosacral region (Figure 18-8 ■).

Manifestations

The outer covering of the defect may be skin or, at times, the transparent, fragile meninges. If the newborn is unable to move the lower extremities, the muscles of the legs will be small and flaccid.

Treatment

Surgery is performed to close the defect. It is critical to protect the tissue until surgical correction can be completed. The meninges may be covered with 4×4 gauze moistened with sterile normal saline.

Nursing Considerations

Postoperatively, the infant is observed closely for signs of infection, bowel and bladder function, and movement of extremities. Prognosis is variable, depending on the location and severity of the defect.

HYDROCEPHALUS

Hydrocephalus results from increased production, decreased absorption, or blockage of the flow of cerebrospinal fluid. Blockage can be caused by a variety of pathologies, including tumor, cysts, or malformation.

Manifestations

At times, hydrocephalus is obvious at birth, but more commonly it develops over time. The classic symptoms include head circumference greater than normal, with the forehead

Sagittal view   Axial view   Sagittal view   Axial view

A   Meningocele   **B**   Meningomyelocele   **C**

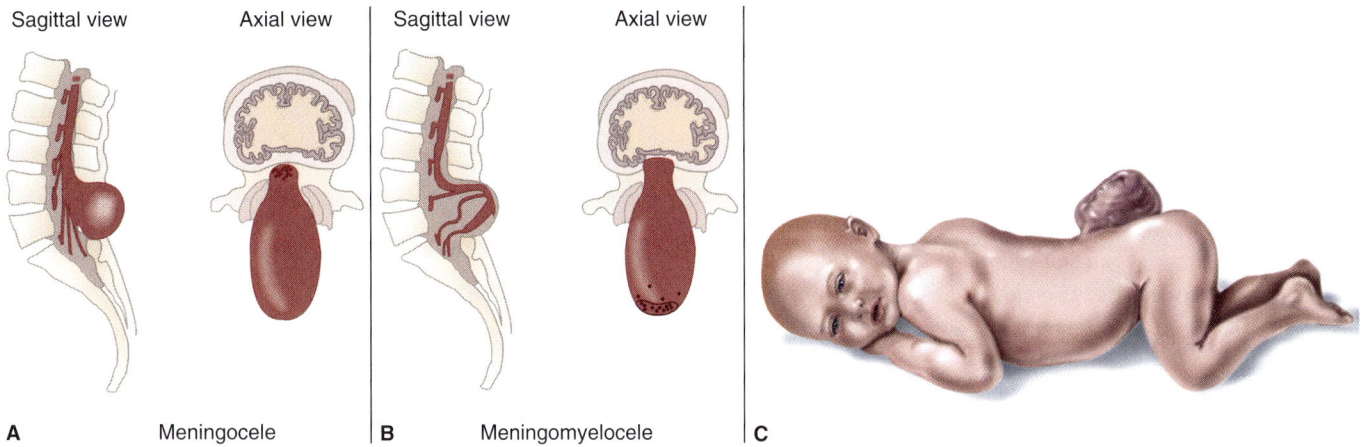

Figure 18-8. ■ (**A**) Meningocele. A saclike protrusion through the bony defect in the spinal column containing meninges and cerebrospinal fluid. Sac may be transparent or membranous. (**B**) Saclike herniation through the defect holding meninges, cerebrospinal fluid, and a portion of spinal cord or nerve root. Fluid leakage may occur, because the lesion may be poorly covered. This defect is more common than the meningocele; 99% of children with this defect are handicapped. (**C**) The infant with a meningomyelocele is placed prone or in a side-lying position, and the exposed sac is protected carefully and kept moist.

and top of the head being out of proportion to the face. The anterior fontanel bulges as intracranial pressure increases.

Treatment

Surgical placement of a ventriculoperitoneal shunt (Figure 18-9 ■) might be necessary to relieve the increasing intracranial pressure.

Nursing Considerations

Nursing responsibilities include routinely measuring the head and completing a neurologic assessment to determine the extent of damage. Postoperatively, the nurse provides routine care, including cleaning the incision sites. Parents should be taught to care for the incision until healing occurs. Parents should know the signs of increased intracranial

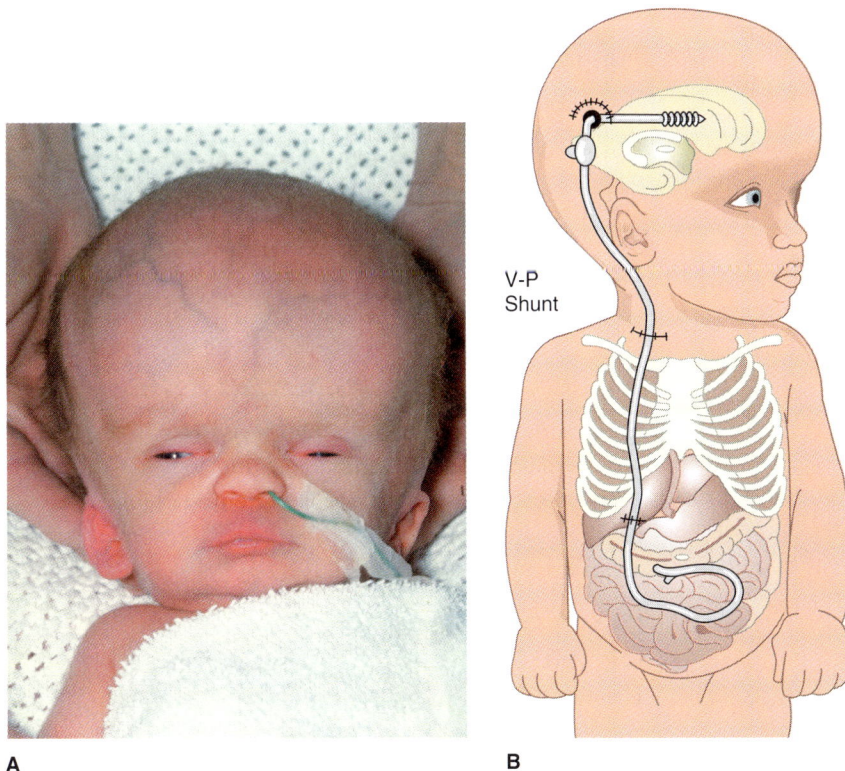

V-P
Shunt

A   **B**

Figure 18-9. ■ (**A**) Infant with hydrocephalus. (**B**) Ventriculoperitoneal shunt, which allows fluid to leave the cranial cavity and so reduces intracranial pressure, is usually placed at 3 to 4 months of age. (**A**: M. A. Ansary/Custom Medical Stock Photo, Inc.)

pressure, including decreased level of consciousness, decreased movement, and pain. Parents may be taught to record the infant's response to pain using a pain scale. As the child grows, the shunt may need to be replaced.

CHROMOSOMAL ABNORMALITIES

Chromosomal abnormalities can result in congenital anomalies, as well as a decrease in mental and physical functioning. **Down syndrome,** the most common chromosomal abnormality, results from **trisomy 21** (three chromosomes at position 21) (see Figure 5-2C ⊙).

Manifestations

Classic signs of Down syndrome include *microcephaly* (small head), wide short neck, epicanthal folds giving the eyes an upward slant, a small nose with a wide nasal bridge, low-set ears, and protruding tongue. The fingers are short and broad, the thumb appears low-set on the hand, and the palm has a single crease (*simian line*). There is an unusually wide space between the first and second toes. There is also an increased incidence of congenital heart defects, diabetes, and hearing loss. The degree of mental retardation is not evident at birth.

Treatment

Down syndrome alone would not necessitate keeping the newborn in the NICU. Unless complications such as prematurity or heart defects are present, the care of the newborn with Down syndrome is the same as for any other newborn.

Nursing Considerations

The newborn with Down syndrome may be hospitalized for some time after birth to allow time for the parents to adjust to the diagnosis and to learn any special care that might be necessary. These newborns may have weak muscle tone resulting in poor sucking reflex. They may have feeding difficulties and be susceptible to aspiration and respiratory infection. Parents will need assistance in feeding, preventing infection, and stimulating the newborn's mental development. Parents should be encouraged to join support groups for parents of children with Down syndrome.

FETAL ALCOHOL SYNDROME

Fetal alcohol syndrome (FAS) is a series of malformations found in infants whose mother drank alcohol during pregnancy. No amount of alcohol intake during pregnancy has been determined safe.

Manifestations

Growth retardation, facial anomalies, microcephaly, CNS dysfunction, mental retardation, and hyperactivity are common with FAS (Figure 18-10 ■).

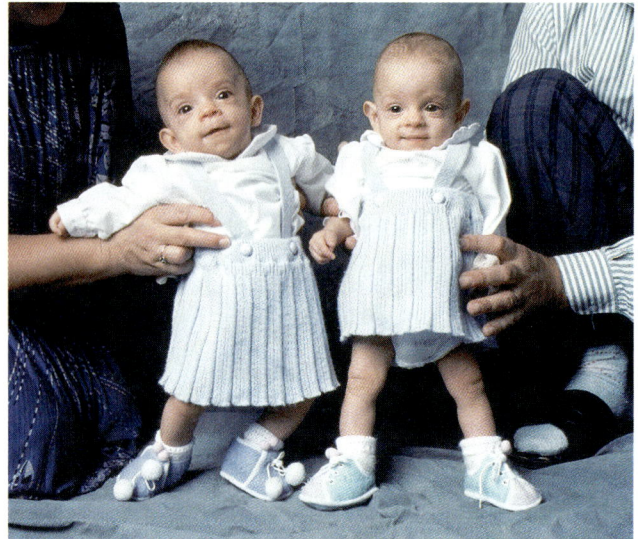

Figure 18-10. ■ Fetal alcohol syndrome is the result of a woman consuming alcohol during pregnancy, and it can have many severe effects on children. Among them are physical malformations, such as those shown here. (George Steinmetz/San Francisco Aids Foundation.)

Nursing Considerations

Immediate care of these newborns will focus on nutritional support. They are often fussy and poor eaters. For the newborn with fetal alcohol syndrome to thrive, the mother must be referred to an alcohol rehabilitation program. The newborn must be closely monitored. Depending on the family situation, the newborn will be placed in foster care until the family is ready to provide total care.

DRUG-ADDICTED NEWBORN

If the mother used illicit drugs during the pregnancy, the infant is at extreme risk to be born addicted to the drugs. The newborn, withdrawing from the addiction, can experience pain, tremors, seizures, lethargy, and failure to thrive. The newborn may have permanent neurologic damage and could die. See Health Promotion Issue on pages 482 to 483 for discussion of this concern.

Musculoskeletal Conditions

Skeletal defects can be minor and easy to correct, or they can be major malformations requiring long-term therapy. These defects are rarely life threatening. However, they require correction, if possible, in order for normal support and movement to take place.

DEVELOPMENTAL DYSPLASIA OF THE HIP

Developmental dysplasia of the hip is a developmental abnormality of the femoral head (ball), acetabulum (socket), or both.

Manifestations

Developmental dysplasia of the hip is displayed by partial or complete dislocation of the hip joint. This results in shortening of the femur, uneven thigh and gluteal folds, and limited abduction on the affected side.

Diagnosis

Developmental dysplasia of the hip is usually diagnosed by physical examination during the newborn assessment, but at times it may be identified later. These assessments include Allis's sign and the Ortolani-Barlow maneuver.

ALLIS'S SIGN.   To evaluate for Allis's sign, the infant's hips and knees are flexed, with the heels placed close to the buttocks (see Figure 17-21). Feet should be placed flat on the examination table. Dislocation of the hip is demonstrated by a lower position of the knee on the affected side. The normal finding is an equal height of the infant's knees.

ORTOLANI-BARLOW MANEUVER.   To perform the Ortolani-Barlow maneuver, the practitioner places the infant on his or her back, flexing the hips and knees at 90-degree angles. The practitioner holds the knees with the thumb over the inner thigh and the first two fingers over the upper femurs. The infant's knees are positioned together, and downward pressure is exerted on the femurs one at a time to determine dislocation. Next the hips are slowly abducted while maintaining pressure on the hip joints. The normal finding is equal hip abduction without resistance. Resistance or a clunking sound or movement indicates hip dislocation. LPNs/LVNs may be trained in this maneuver. If the LPN/LVN notices a hip click, the practitioner should be informed.

Treatment

Treatment of developmental dysplasia of the hip should begin as soon as possible. If only a small amount of abnormality is present, triple diapering is used to support the hip in abduction until ligaments are strong enough to maintain hip alignment permanently. If more support is needed a Pavlik harness (Figure 18-11 ■) is commonly used for 3 to 4 months. If the harness is unsuccessful, surgery followed by a *hip spica cast* (a cast covering the upper thighs and lower torso) may be necessary.

Nursing Considerations

The nursing care of infants with developmental dysplasia of the hip includes maintaining traction through triple diapering, application of Pavlik harness, or providing cast care. Parent should be taught to provide this care prior to discharge.

TALIPES (CLUBFOOT)

Talipes or clubfoot is a congenital, unilateral or bilateral twisting of the foot, usually inward (Figure 18-12 ■).

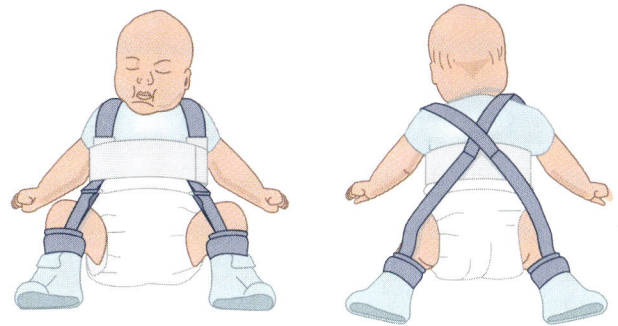

Figure 18-11. ■ Steps for Pavlik harness application. (1) Position the chest halter at nipple line and fasten with Velcro. (2) Position the legs and feet in the stirrups, being sure the hips are flexed and abducted. Fasten with Velcro. (3) Connect the chest halter and leg straps in front. (4) Connect the chest halter and leg straps in back. All straps are marked at the first fitting with indelible ink so they can be reattached easily after the harness is rinsed and dried.

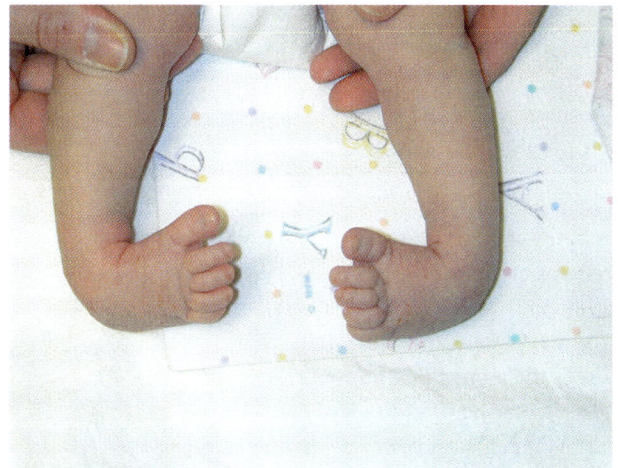

Figure 18-12. ■ Clubfoot, with the midfoot (*equines*) directed downward, the hindfoot (*varus*) turned inward, and the forefoot curled toward the heel and upward. This condition is corrected surgically. (Custom Medical Stock Photo, Inc.)

Manifestations

The foot cannot easily be moved into alignment due to deformity in three areas of the foot:

- The equines or midfoot is directed downward.
- The varus or hindfoot turns inward.
- The forefoot curls toward the heel and upward.

The clubfoot is usually smaller than the other foot, and the child has a shortened Achilles tendon. The muscles of the lower leg are atrophied.

Diagnosis

Talipes is diagnosed by observation of symptoms and confirmed by x-ray.

(*Text continues on page 484.*)

HEALTH PROMOTION ISSUE

ADDICTED NEWBORN

Jason was admitted to the NICU from the newborn nursery. At 39 weeks' gestation, he weighed 5 lbs 4 oz (2,390 g). Jason had Apgar scores of 7 and 8 at 1 and 5 minutes. Over the first 12 hours after birth, Jason became increasingly irritable, developed an inconsolable high-pitched cry, and had tremors. Jason's mother is 20 years old, single, and unemployed. She had no prenatal care and came to the hospital when labor became too painful. She denies use of illicit drugs while pregnant. Jason's meconium tested positive for heroin.

DISCUSSION

Drugs used and abused by the pregnant woman include tobacco, cocaine, methamphetamines, marijuana, heroin, methadone, alcohol, and others. Drugs with low molecular weight (which include the commonly abused drugs) readily cross the placenta and enter the fetus. When the mother habitually uses drugs, the unborn child may become chemically dependent. **Neonatal abstinence syndrome** is the term used to describe the behavior of the infant exposed to chemical substances *in utero*.

The clinical manifestations seen in infants of drug-using mothers vary in timing and degree. Most manifestations are mild, vague, and nonspecific signs characteristic of a variety of conditions that can affect the newborn. Signs of withdrawal are listed here.

Signs of Drug Withdrawal in the Newborn
- Irritability
- Seizures
- Hyperactivity
- High-pitched cry
- Tremors
- Exaggerated Moro reflex
- Hypertonic muscles
- Poor feeding
- Diarrhea
- Dehydration
- Vomiting
- Uncoordinated sucking
- Diaphoresis
- Fever
- Unstable temperature
- Mottled skin
- Nasal stuffiness
- Disrupted sleep patterns

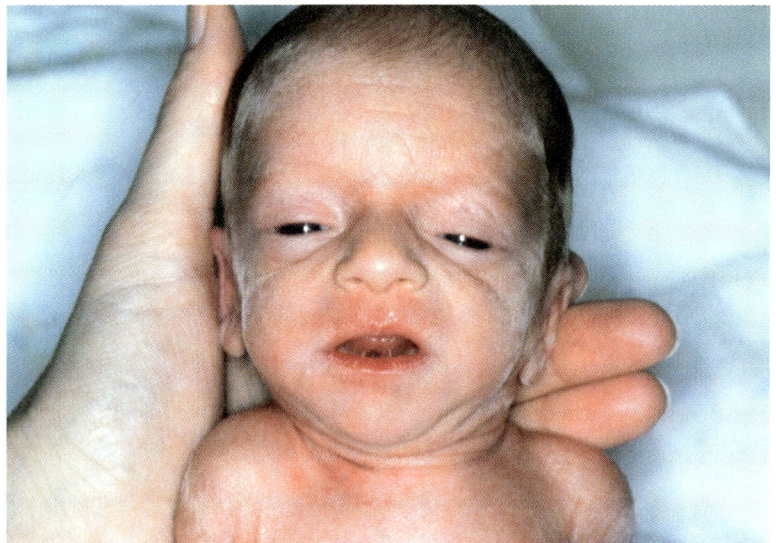

If the mother has taken large quantities of drugs over a long time, symptoms of withdrawal may begin within the first 12 to 24 hours. If the mother consumes the drug just before delivery, it may take 7 to 10 days after delivery for the newborn to exhibit signs of withdrawal. The newborn may be discharged by this time. Symptoms generally become worse over the first few days and then gradually disappear as the drug is eliminated from the infant's body. If the mother continues to use drugs and breastfeeds, the newborn will be reexposed through the breast milk. It is essential that correct diagnosis is made and treatment instituted as soon as possible.

Diagnostic exams for chemical exposure include newborn urine, hair, or meconium sampling. Urine testing will only detect recent substance intake. Meconium and hair testing for drug metabolites are more accurate, identify long-term exposure, and are easy to collect.

PLANNING AND IMPLEMENTATION

Nursing considerations when caring for the infant of a drug-using mother include all the care of the normal newborn plus close observations for life-threatening complications such as respiratory depression. Nursing care is directed toward decreasing stimuli that may increase hyperactivity and irritability. Dimming the lights and lowering the noise level may be beneficial. Comforting measures such as wrapping the infant snuggly, and holding and rocking the infant limits their ability to self-stimulate.

Providing adequate nutrition and hydration is essential. Loose stools, poor intake, and regurgitation after feeding, may result in dehydration. Frequent weighing,

monitoring of intake and output, and additional caloric intake may be necessary. Dehydration and abrasion from the hyperactive infant rubbing against the linen predispose the baby to skin breakdown and infection.

The **Neonatal Abstinence Scoring System** (Kandall, 1999; Finnegan, 1985) is a standardized screening tool used to monitor infants in an objective manner when neonatal abstinence syndrome is suspected or identified. This assessment and documentation tool is used by the RN each time an assessment is indicated.

The relationship of the newborn and mother should be closely monitored and documented. The responsibility of caring for a newborn may be too challenging for the drug-abusing mother. If she is enrolled in a treatment program, and lives in a treatment facility where 24-hour observation and assistance is available, she may be allowed to keep the newborn with her. However, more commonly, the newborn will be placed in foster care until

a safe environment can be provided. Careful evaluation and cooperation among a variety of health care professionals are required in this situation.

SELF-REFLECTION

Substance abuse is a widespread health concern. Some women become prostitutes in order to have money to support their drug habit. Other women have a stable home, employment, and a supportive relationship, but use drugs as a form of recreation. In either situation, babies may be born to these women. The nurse must know what the legal responsibility is to the mother and the newborn. How are you going to feel if you must report the mother to the police? How are you going to feel if the mother and baby are discharged and you find out later that the baby was addicted? Should drug screening be done on every newborn? Does drug screening of the newborn infringe on the rights of the parents?

SUGGESTED RESOURCES

Ballard, J.L., Khoury, J.C., Wedig, K., Eilers-Walsman, B.L., & Lipp, R. (1991). New Ballard score, expanded to include extreme premature infants. *Journal of Pediatrics, 119* (3), 417–423.

Finnegan, L.P. (1985). Neonatal abstinence. In N. M. Nelson (Ed.), *Current therapy in neonatal-perinatal medicine, 1985–1986.* Toronto: B.C. Decker.

Kandall, S.R. (1999). Treatment strategies for drug-exposed neonates. *Clinical Perinatology 25*(1), 231–243.

Treatment

Nonsurgical treatment involves moving the foot into correct alignment and applying a cast to hold the foot in the correct position. The cast is changed every 1 to 2 weeks for about 3 months until alignment is achieved. Failure to achieve alignment could result in the need for surgical correction.

clinical ALERT

Infants can be frightened by the noise of a cast cutter. Thus, the nurse, in consultation with the physician, can suggest that the parents remove the cast prior to the office visit by soaking it in warm water until it disintegrates. If they remove the cast, parents should be encouraged to bathe the skin thoroughly after the cast has been removed. Note that cast removal by parents must be approved by the physician.

Nursing Considerations

The nurse is responsible for assisting with cast application. Proper cast care is taught to the parents. If the infant has surgery, the nurse is also responsible for pain management and observation for drainage and bleeding.

Gastrointestinal Conditions

Gastrointestinal conditions are usually the result of congenital defects or immaturity of the organs and surrounding structures.

Defects of the gastrointestinal system are the most common of the congenital defects. They require surgical correction but are usually not immediately life threatening. However, aspiration, malnutrition, and obstruction could result if detection and correction are not made in a timely manner. For an understanding of these defects, it is important to review normal structure of the entire gastrointestinal system.

CLEFT LIP AND CLEFT PALATE

Cleft palate results from the failure of the medial nasal and maxillary processes to join, leaving an opening between the roof of the mouth and the floor of the nasal passage. **Cleft lip** results from failure of the upper lip to join medially. Cleft lip can be unilateral or bilateral. Clefts could be complete (through the bone and tissue) or partial (involving the bone structures but not the overlying mucous membrane). Cleft lip and cleft palate commonly occur together but can be found separately (Figure 18-13 ■).

Manifestations

The newborn infant will have feeding problems. The infant with a cleft lip will have difficulty making a seal around the nipple. With a cleft palate, the infant will be unable to compress the nipple between the tongue and the palate. The result will be an ineffective suck. With cleft palate, the feeding leaks into the nasal cavity, where it can drain from the nose and not be ingested. Some food can pool in the nasal passage, increasing the risk of sinus and ear infections. Also some of the feeding may drain down the back of the throat without coordinated swallowing, putting the infant at risk for choking.

Treatment

The surgical correction of cleft lip and palate is usually accomplished in the first 3 months of life. For nursing care following surgery, consult a pediatric nursing textbook.

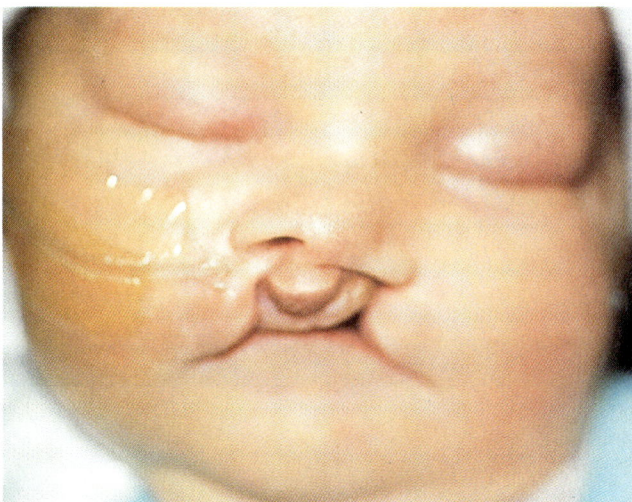
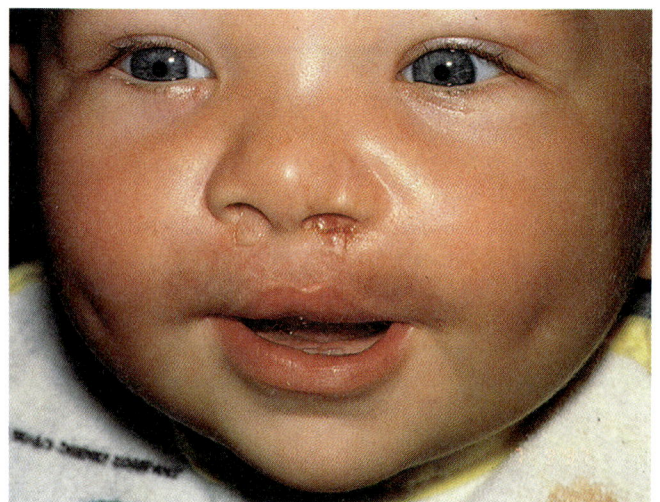

A   **B**

Figure 18-13. ■ (**A**) Bilateral cleft lip. (**B**) Repaired bilateral cleft lip.

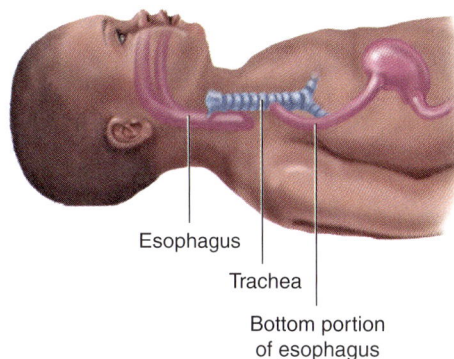

Esophagus

Trachea

Bottom portion of esophagus

Figure 18-14. ■ Esophageal atresia and tracheoesophageal fistula.

Nursing Considerations

Because a cleft palate could be complete or partial, it is important not only to visualize the palate, but also to feel the palate with the little finger to be sure the bones are intact.

The most immediate concern when a baby is born with a cleft lip or palate is providing nutrition. Prior to surgical repair, the infant must be fed using special equipment. A long nipple with enlarged holes or a *Breck feeder* (syringe with a rubber tube) may be used. The woman wishing to breastfeed may pump her breast and then feed the milk to the infant. Parents will need instruction in the use of special equipment as well as encouragement and support to handle the additional responsibilities in the care of their child.

The psychological impact on the family is a concern (Box 18-3 ■). Families naturally anticipate the arrival of a "pretty" baby. When the infant has a cosmetic defect, the family experiences grief. Even after surgical correction of the cleft lip, the child will still have permanent scarring and some degree of cosmetic defect. When the lip and palate are not formed correctly, teeth may not erupt or may erupt out of alignment. A space may be present between the front teeth. The teeth, lips, and palate are used in forming sounds. When these structures are not formed properly, speech therapy is often required.

ESOPHAGEAL ATRESIA AND TRACHEOESOPHAGEAL FISTULA

Esophageal atresia and tracheoesophageal fistula are potentially life-threatening defects. They may be found separately but are most commonly found together. Figure 18-14 ■ shows the areas where the esophagus and trachea may be connected. In **esophageal atresia,** the esophagus ends in a blind pouch before reaching the stomach. **Tracheoesophageal fistula** is a connection between the trachea and esophagus.

Manifestations

The infant with esophageal atresia and tracheoesophageal fistula presents with copious amounts of thin mucus shortly after birth. The secretions clear with suctioning, but they soon reappear. If a tracheoesophageal fistula is present, the stomach may become distended with trapped air. If the defects are not identified prior to feeding, the infant will regurgitate the feeding or the feeding will be aspirated into the lungs. Severe respiratory distress occurs, and aspiration pneumonia may develop.

Diagnosis and Treatment

To diagnose this disorder, an attempt is made to pass a 5 or 8 French nasogastric tube into the stomach. The tube meets resistance and can be advanced only a short distance. X-ray, ultrasound, and echocardiogram are performed to confirm diagnosis.

Treatment is aimed at preventing respiratory complications until the defect can be surgically repaired. In the absence of other anomalies, surgical repair is usually completed in the first few days of life. If other anomalies are present, gastrostomy feedings may be necessary until the infant has stabilized (Figure 18-15 ■).

Nursing Considerations

The nurse should suspect tracheoesophageal fistula any time copious amounts of mucus are suctioned from the newborn's airway shortly after birth. If the infant is unable

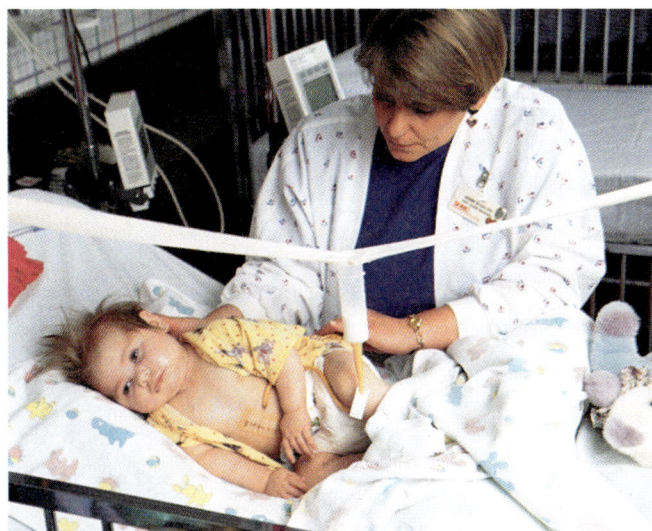

Figure 18-15. ■ Gravity assists the flow of a gavage feeding to this hospitalized infant.

to maintain a clear airway, feeding should be delayed until further evaluation is made. Parents will need teaching and support regarding this potentially life-threatening defect.

IMPERFORATE ANUS

During fetal development, a pit, forming in the perineum, becomes the outer anal opening. The colon forms and gradually approaches the anal pit, and the connecting tissue breaks down, allowing the colon to open to the outside. **Imperforate anus** results when the connecting tissue fails to break down and the opening of the colon does not develop (Figure 18-16 ■).

Manifestations

Most commonly, there is obvious malformation of the perineum. At times, a thin membrane can be seen covering the anus. At other times, the anus is flat or appears as a deep dimple. If meconium is not passed within 24 hours of birth, an imperforate anus should be suspected. Anomalies of the urinary system are commonly present at the same time. If meconium is present in the urine, a fistula has developed.

Treatment

Surgical correction, occurring shortly after birth, is a relatively simple procedure if no other anomaly is present.

Nursing Considerations

The infant should not receive oral intake until the anus is opened surgically. Feeding the infant would stimulate peristalsis and could cause rupture of the colon. If surgery is delayed, IV fluids and nutrition will be necessary.

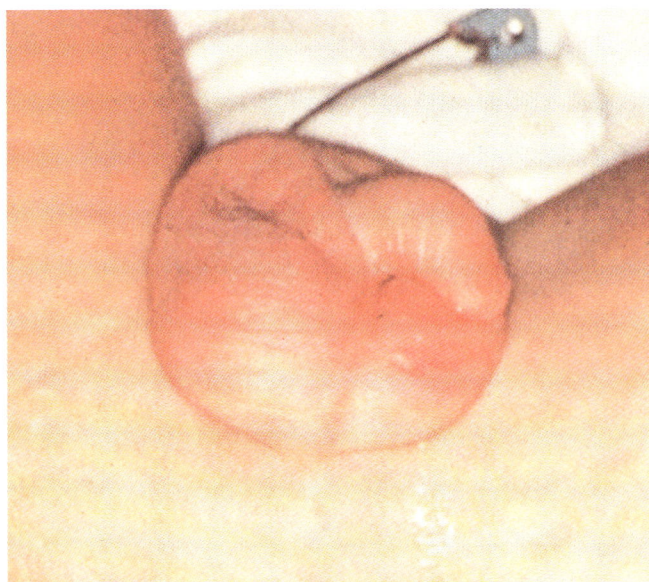

Figure 18-16. ■ Imperforate anus is often obvious at birth. It can range from mild stenosis to a complex syndrome associated with other congenital anomalies.

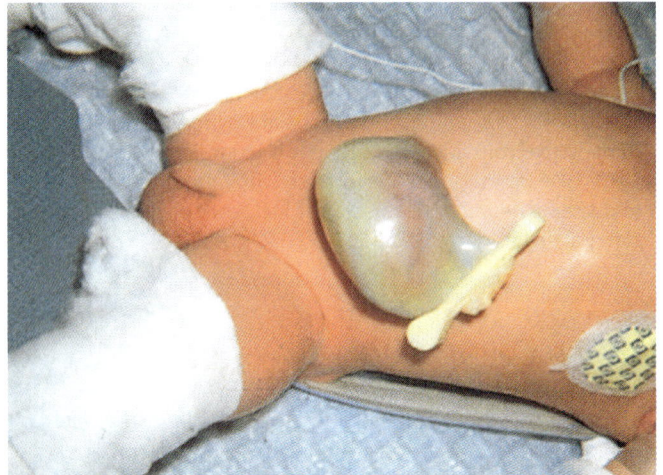

Figure 18-17. ■ In omphalocele, the size of the sack depends on the extent of the protrusion of abdominal contents through the umbilical cord. (Reprinted with permission from McGraw-Hill Companies Inc. from Rudolph, A.M., Hoffman, J.L.E., & Rudolph, C.D. [Eds.]. [1991]. *Rudolph's pediatrics* [19th ed., p. 1040]. Stamford, CT: Appleton & Lange.)

OMPHALOCELE

Omphalocele is a rare congenital malformation of the abdominal wall allowing the abdominal contents to herniate into the umbilical cord (Figure 18-17 ■). There is generally a thin translucent sac (peritoneum) covering the abdominal organs. The size of the sac varies, depending on the degree of defect. Small defects may be repaired with good prognosis. Large defects may result in long-term gastrointestinal disorders.

PYLORIC STENOSIS

Pyloric stenosis is a progressive hypertrophy of the pyloric sphincter resulting in obstruction (Figure 18-18 ■).

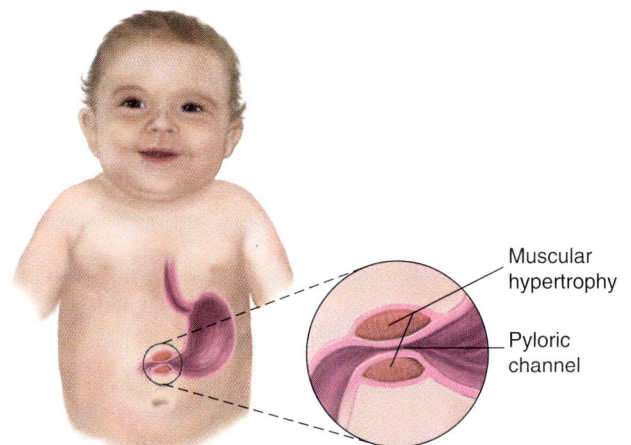

Muscular hypertrophy

Pyloric channel

Figure 18-18. ■ Pyloric stenosis results in projectile vomiting and visible peristalsis.

Manifestations

The infant appears healthy at birth but symptoms usually appear in 2 to 8 weeks. At first, the infant has increased regurgitation after eating. As the obstruction worsens, projectile vomiting ensues, leading to dehydration, weight loss, and electrolyte imbalance.

Treatment

Laparoscopic surgical correction is the treatment of choice. Preoperatively, the infant's condition is stabilized with IV fluids and electrolytes. A nasogastric tube is inserted to decompress the stomach and prevent vomiting and aspiration. The infant is usually taking fluids in 12 to 24 hours and is discharged on a regular newborn diet by 48 hours after surgery.

Nursing Considerations

The newborn with pyloric stenosis appears healthy at birth and is discharged. The office nurse may be the first to suspect a gastrointestinal problem when the parents bring the infant to the clinic for a routine checkup. Parents will need instruction in the postoperative care of their infant. Long-term prognosis is good.

HERNIA

Hernia is a protrusion of the stomach or intestines through a weakness or malformation in the normal musculature. In the infant, three locations are common:

- Umbilical hernia (Figure 18-19 ■) results from protrusion of abdominal contents through a weakened umbilical ring and is most common in African American girls.
- Inguinal hernia, a protrusion of abdominal contents through a weakened inguinal ring, is more common in boys.
- Diaphragmatic hernia, rare but the most life threatening, is a protrusion of the stomach through the diaphragm.

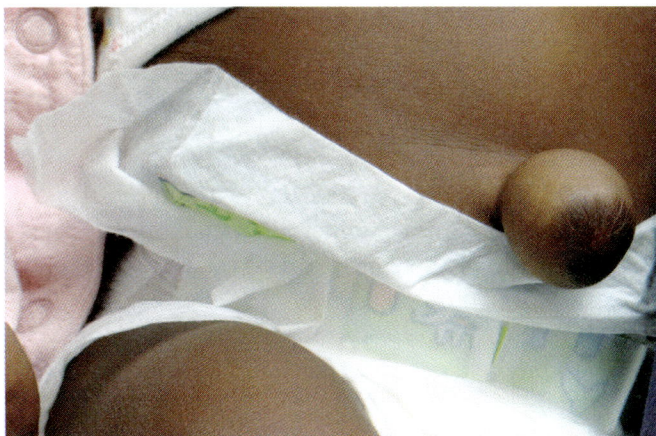

Figure 18-19. ■ Umbilical hernia.

Manifestations

Most hernias appear as a soft swelling below the umbilicus or in the groin. The hernia grows larger with coughing, crying, or straining. Herniation of the stomach through a weakness in the diaphragm results in respiratory distress.

Treatment

Diaphragmatic hernias are considered a surgical emergency in order to reverse the respiratory distress. Some small umbilical or inguinal hernias resolve spontaneously by 3 to 4 years of age. Others are surgically repaired, requiring a short hospital stay.

Nursing Considerations

Parents should be instructed not to push on the hernia or apply tape, straps, or coins. These actions can cause the intestine to strangulate.

NECROTIZING ENTEROCOLITIS

Necrotizing enterocolitis is a potentially life-threatening inflammatory process of the bowel. It occurs primarily in premature infants. Necrotizing enterocolitis has several causes, including intestinal ischemia, viral or bacterial infection, and immaturity of the intestines. The disease is most common in the distal ileum and colon.

Manifestations

The infant initially shows signs of feeding intolerance, including vomiting, irritability, gastric residuals, and abdominal distention. Bloody diarrhea may be present, followed by sepsis and a rapid deterioration of the infant's condition.

Diagnosis

Diagnosis is made based on the infant's symptoms, bowel distension, and bowel wall thickening on x-rays. Blood cultures are positive for the organism, and laboratory results show anemia, elevated white blood cell count, and electrolyte imbalance.

Treatment

Necrotizing enterocolitis requires prompt treatment. All enteral feedings are stopped, an oral gastric tube is inserted to decompress the stomach, and intravenous fluids are started to correct fluid and electrolyte imbalance. Antibiotics are given to treat infection. If perforation or necrosis of the bowel occurs, surgical resection may be required.

Nursing Considerations

Strict enteric precautions are required to prevent the spread of infection to other infants. The nurse is responsible to monitor the infant, administer prescribed intravenous fluids and medication, and relieve the infant's pain. Gradually reintroduce feedings once the bowel function returns.

Only feeding premature infants breast milk has been shown to decrease the incidence of necrotizing enterocolitis. Measuring the abdominal circumference in high-risk newborns every 4 hours can detect the early onset of necrotizing enterocolitis. Parents should be taught all aspects of home care. Once the child is discharged, regular follow-up is needed.

PHENYLKETONURIA

Phenylketonuria (PKU) is an autosomal recessive inherited disorder that affects the body's ability to use protein. Normally, a liver enzyme, phenylalanine hydroxylase, breaks down the amino acid phenylalanine into tyrosine. Children with PKU have a deficiency in this enzyme (Box 18-4 ■).

Manifestations

As phenylalanine builds up in the blood, it causes a musty odor of the body and urine, as well as vomiting, irritability, seizures, hyperactivity, and rash. Over time, elevated levels of phenylalanine result in mental retardation.

Diagnosis

State laws require all infants to be screened for PKU. To ensure accurate results, the infant must receive either breast milk or formula for several days. Tests performed on the infant who leaves the birthing center 24 hours after delivery should be repeated.

Treatment

Special formulas, such as Albumaid XP, Lofenalac, and Minafen, are used in treatment until the child is ready for solid food. Then a diet low in phenylalanine is maintained for life. The diet must also meet the child's requirements for growth. If diet modifications are not followed for at least the first 6 years, there is a significant impact on the child's IQ.

Nursing Considerations

It is important for the hospital nurse to inform parents of the need to repeat the PKU test several days after the newborn has been taking milk or formula. If the test is positive,

---

BOX 18-4	CULTURAL PULSE POINTS

Incidence of Phenylketonuria

Phenylketonuria is more common in communities with numerous intermarriages over several generations. It is rare in African, Jewish, and Japanese populations.

---

parents will need instruction in use of special formulas and adapting the diet as the child grows. Referral to a dietitian is helpful.

GALACTOSEMIA

Galactosemia is an autosomal recessive disorder of carbohydrate metabolism. Galactosemia results from a deficiency in galactose-1-phosphate uridyltransferase (GALT), one of the three enzymes necessary for the conversion of sugar galactose into glucose. High levels of galactose in the blood results in damage to the kidneys, liver, brain, and eyes. Many children develop gram-negative infections.

Manifestations

Within a few days after birth, the baby develops vomiting and diarrhea, does not eat well, becomes hypoglycemic, and develops an enlarged liver. If not diagnosed and treated, the child will become mentally retarded and develop jaundice, ascites, cataracts, seizures, lethargy, and coma. Death usually occurs within 1 month.

Diagnosis

Routine screening of the newborn is done in all but six states. In these six states, diagnosis is made in symptomatic babies from history and laboratory tests.

Treatment

Infants with galactosemia are placed on lactose-free or galactose-free formulas. The child will be on a galactose-free diet (no milk or milk products) for life. Many children who follow a strict diet still develop complications of galactosemia, including learning disabilities, speech defects, visual disturbances, and ovarian failure.

Nursing Considerations

Nursing responsibilities focus on teaching the parents and child about the prescribed diet and referring the family to a nutritionist for counseling. Parents must learn to screen foods and medication for hidden lactose that has been used as a filler. The parents should be referred for genetic counseling.

MAPLE SYRUP URINE DISEASE

Maple syrup urine disease (MSUD) is an autosomal recessive disease that affects amino acid metabolism. A missing or defective enzyme prevents the breakdown of three essential amino acids: leucine, isoleucine, and valine (Box 18-5 ■). The result is alpha ketoacidosis. All three amino acids are necessary for normal hair, skin, and muscle function. Leucine accumulates in the brain, causing cerebral edema, neurologic damage, and death.

Genetic Factors in Maple Syrup Urine Disease

Maple syrup urine disease (MSUD) is rare in the general population. There is a very high rate (1 in 380 live births) among the Pennsylvania Mennonites (a religious group) and in an intermarrying subgroup called the Amish. All newborns in this population should be tested for MSUD (Robinson & Drumm, 2001). Prompt recognition of the condition can allow preventive treatment that vastly increases quality of life.

Manifestations

Within days of birth, the infant becomes lethargic, has variable muscle tone, becomes irritable with a high-pitched cry, and the skin has a sweet smell.

Diagnosis and Treatment

Diagnosis is made by laboratory findings. Specially designed formulas with the three amino acids removed are prescribed. The diet should be rich in other amino acids, vitamins, minerals, and calories. The child needs special low-protein foods that are adequate for growth without causing a catabolic state (tissue breakdown). Daily urine testing for ketones is required to monitor the metabolic state.

Nursing Considerations

Nursing care includes teaching parents to maintain the prescribed diet. This includes mixing the special formula and developing a plan to prevent ketoacidosis on sick days. Referral to a nutritionist is helpful. Support groups can also help families by sharing tips for managing the child's condition.

Genitourinary Conditions

Genitourinary conditions of the newborn are usually caused by congenital defects. Commonly there is a malformation of the lower urinary system, the gastrointestinal system, and the reproductive system. The first concern it to determine whether the infant is able to urinate. If not, intervention is more immediate.

URETHRAL MALPOSITION (HYPOSPADIAS OR EPISPADIAS)

Hypospadias occurs when the urethral opening is on the ventral (lower) surface of the penis. **Epispadias** occurs when the urethra opens on the dorsal (upper) surface of the penis (Figure 18-20 ■). The opening can be found anywhere along the shaft of the penis. If the urethral opening is on the glans, surgical correction may not be needed. If the urethral opening is well down the shaft of the penis, surgical correction may need to be done in stages.

PHIMOSIS

Phimosis occurs when the opening of the foreskin is small and unable to be retracted over the glans. The primary concern is the adequacy of the urinary system. In most cases, circumcision is performed to alleviate the problem.

AMBIGUOUS GENITALIA

Ambiguous genitalia (pseudohermaphroditism) is a rare condition in which determining the gender of the infant is difficult. The most common cause of ambiguous genitalia is adrenal hyperplasia, an autosomal recessive disorder that causes a deficiency in one of the enzymes needed for the production of cortisol and aldosterone. During fetal development, the lack of cortisol triggers the pituitary to overproduce adrenocorticotropic hormone (ACTH). An increase in ACTH stimulates the overproduction of adrenal androgens. An increase in androgens in the 10th week of fetal development stimulates female genitalia to become more male-like. If left untreated, overproduction of androgens cause increased height, early closure of epiphyseal plates, and premature sexual development.

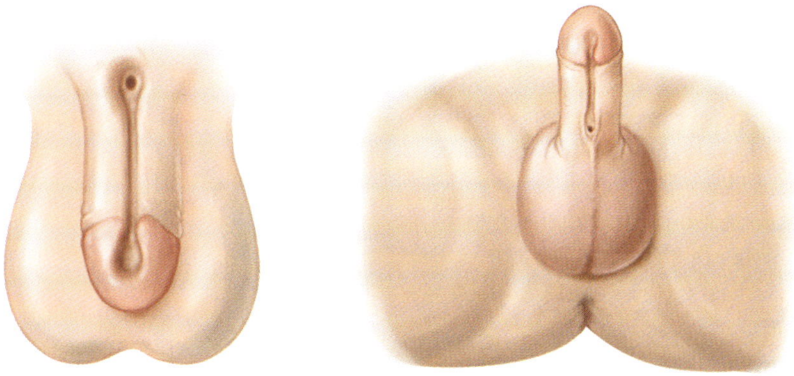

| A | Epispadias | B | Hypospadias |

Figure 18-20. ■ Epispadias and hypospadias. (**A**) In epispadias, the canal is open on the dorsal surface. (**B**) In hypospadias the urethral canal is open on the ventral surface of the penis.

Figure 18-21. ■ Newborn girl with ambiguous genitalia. (Courtesy of Patrick C. Walsh, M.D.)

Manifestations

The female infant is born with an enlarged clitoris and partial or complete fusion of the labia (Figure 18-21 ■). The vagina has a common opening with the urethra. In severe cases, the female infant can be mistaken for male with *cryptorchidism* (undescended testicles), hypospadias, or micropenis.

Diagnosis

In this circumstance, chromosomal analysis may be necessary to determine the gender of the infant. Not only is the reproductive system affected, but in many cases the urinary and intestinal systems are also affected. Ultrasound is helpful in visualizing pelvis structures and may assist with diagnosis pending results of chromosomal studies. Due to the association with adrenal hyperplasia, a complete evaluation of adrenal function should be made.

Treatment

Surgical correction is usually done in stages, with the primary goal being normal functioning of the urinary and intestinal systems. Depending on the degree of defect, reproductive function may be lost. If ambiguous genitalia is caused by adrenal hyperplasia, life-long hormonal therapy will be required. For more information about adrenal hyperplasia, consult a pediatric nursing textbook.

Nursing Considerations

Due to the chronic nature of ambiguous genitalia and the relationship with endocrine function, parents of infants with ambiguous genitalia need a great deal of teaching and emotional support. Explore parent's emotional response to their child and their beliefs about gender roles and sexuality.

Provide instruction in postoperative care as directed by the RN or primary care provider.

EXSTROPHY OF THE BLADDER

Exstrophy of the bladder (Figure 18-22 ■) is a rare condition in which the abdominal wall fails to fuse, allowing the urinary bladder to protrude to the outside. Failure of the abdominal wall to close during fetal development results in separation of the rectus muscles and at times the symphysis pubis. The separation allows the bladder to protrude through the opening. Other genitourinary abnormalities and intestinal herniation are associated with exstrophy of the bladder.

Manifestations

Usually, a defect in the lower abdominal wall is obvious at birth. The skin is open, and underlying tissue is exposed. The bladder appears bright-red and urine continually leaks from the urethra.

Diagnosis and Treatment

Before surgical reconstruction begins, it is important to evaluate the extent of damage to surrounding tissue. Primary closure of the abdominal defect and the return of the bladder to the abdominal cavity is performed in the first 24 to 48 hours of life. Complete surgical reconstruction is accomplished in stages over several years.

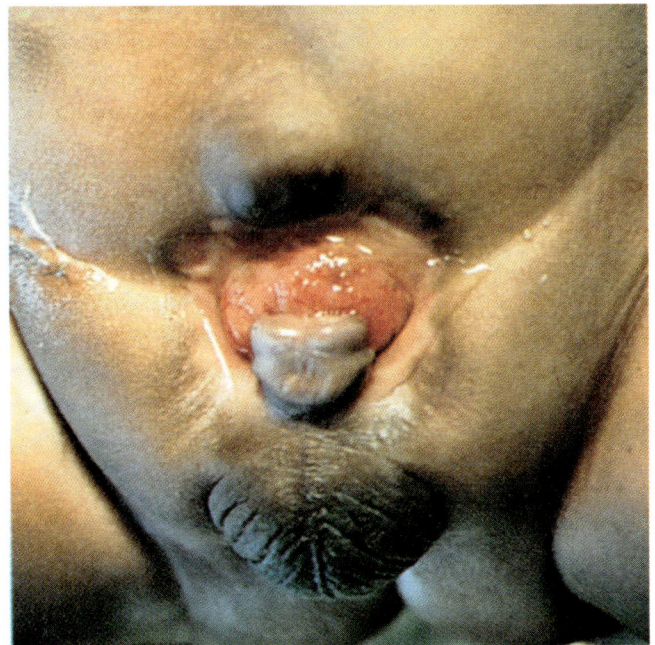

Figure 18-22. ■ This child has bladder exstrophy, noted by extrusion of the posterior bladder wall through the lower abdominal wall. Until surgery can be performed, the bladder mucosa must be protected from trauma and irritation. A sterile, saline-soaked dressing maintains moisture; it is covered with a sterile plastic wrap. The surrounding area must be cleaned daily. Skin sealant is applied to protect surrounding skin from leaking urine.

Nursing Considerations

Nursing responsibilities are to monitor urinary and intestinal function. Initially the defect is covered with dressings saturated in sterile normal saline. Surrounding tissue should be protected with a moisture barrier. Postoperatively, it is critical to follow physician orders regarding skin care and pelvis immobilization to facilitate healing. Monitor drainage tubes to ensure proper functioning.

Parents need emotional support to deal with the disfiguring nature of the defect and the length of time required for complete repair. Encourage parents to participate in infant care to the degree possible. Provide instruction regarding home care.

NURSING CARE

PRIORITIES IN NURSING CARE

The priorities of nursing care for the high-risk newborn are similar to those of the normal newborn. However, the method in which the needs are met may be different.

- Maintaining the airway, breathing, and circulation
- Maintaining body temperature
- Providing nutrition
- Ensuring elimination
- Teaching parents to provide care for their newborn

ASSESSING

The high-risk newborn requires a more frequent and in-depth assessment than the normal newborn. The high-risk newborn may have equipment such as a heart monitor, a mechanical ventilator, or feeding tube. The nurse must ensure that the equipment is functioning properly. The high-risk newborn may have had surgery to correct a congenital anomaly, or he or she may have infection or other contention that requires assessment and monitoring. Parents and family members require assessment information and support in the care of their high-risk newborn.

DIAGNOSING, PLANNING, AND IMPLEMENTING

Nursing diagnoses might include:

- Ineffective **A**irway Clearance
- Risk for **I**nfection
- Risk for Impaired **S**kin Integrity
- Deficient **K**nowledge related to specific disorder, medical equipment, or care of the high-risk newborn

Nursing care might include these and other interventions:

- Suction the airway as needed. *The premature or high-risk newborn may be unable to clear the airway, resulting in hypoxia.*
- Monitor for respiratory distress (Box 18-6 ■). *The high-risk newborn's condition is less stable and can change quickly.*
- Prevent and/or treat infection. *The high-risk newborn may undergo invasive procedures and may have puncture sites or open areas that can become infected. If an infection exists, treatment must be provided to prevent worsening of the condition.*
- Provide skin care, including bathing, turning, and protecting the skin under tape/monitor electrodes, etc. *The skin of the high-risk newborn is thin and fragile. Monitor electrodes, IV lines, and dressings that are taped to the skin. Care must be taken to prevent skin breakdown.*
- Use double diapering as ordered for postoperative urinary care (Figure 18-23 ■). *The double diapering will prevent contamination with feces of the surgical site.*
- Give parents knowledge and support to make the best decisions about care of their newborn. Encourage them to provide care to the newborn to the extent allowable by circumstances and facility policies. *By understanding the specific disorder, the parents can make informed decisions. Parents can provide some of the necessary care in the NICU with instruction and support from the nurse.*
- Model acceptance and loving response of the newborn who appears different. *Parents may be uneasy touching and caring for a baby who is not cosmetically normal or who is*

BOX 18-6   ASSESSMENT

Newborn Distress

In assessing the infant, the nurse would monitor for these manifestations of newborn distress:

- Increased respiratory rate (more than 60 breaths/minute) or difficult respirations
- Sternal retractions
- Nasal flaring
- Grunting
- Excessive mucus
- Facial grimacing
- Cyanosis (central: skin, lips, tongue)
- Abdominal distension or mass
- Vomiting of bile-stained material
- Absence of meconium elimination within 24 hours of birth
- Absence of urine elimination within 24 hours of birth
- Jaundice of the skin within 24 hours of birth or due to hemolytic process
- Temperature instability (hypothermia or hyperthermia)
- Jitteriness or blood glucose less than 40 mg%

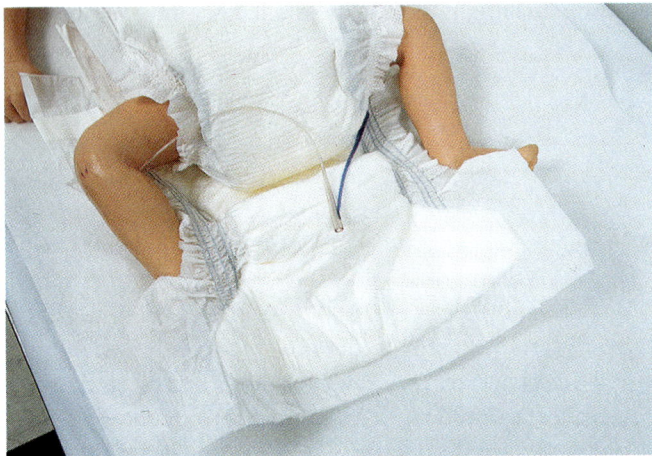

Figure 18-23. ■ A double diapering technique protects the urinary stent after surgery for hypospadias or epispadias repair. The inner diaper collects stool; the outer diaper, urine.

premature. The nurse's modeling of loving behavior and good caring skills will help the parents adjust and begin to cope.

EVALUATING

Parents' reactions to the child should be evaluated on an ongoing basis. Parents will need teaching and support along the way. The infant should be checked at regular intervals for weight gain, signs of infection, and effectiveness of treatment.

NURSING PROCESS CARE PLAN
Care of the Preoperative Newborn with a Congenital Heart Defect

Jeremy, 24 hours old, has been transferred from a small rural hospital to the NICU of a major medical center with a diagnosis of aortic stenosis. Jeremy is breathing room air with minimal respiratory distress. His condition is stable, and he is scheduled for surgery within the next few days. His parents are asking questions regarding his care and prognosis.

Assessment
- Jeremy is breathing on his own.
- There are no signs of respiratory distress.

- Parents are asking questions regarding pre- and postoperative care.

Nursing Diagnosis. The following important nursing diagnosis (among others) is established for this condition:
- Deficient **K**nowledge related to preoperative and postoperative care of the newborn following heart surgery

Expected Outcomes. The parents will have an adequate knowledge base concerning aortic stenosis, as well as the upcoming surgical procedure and care, as evidenced by their ability to state information correctly.

Planning and Implementation
- Reinforce information on aortic stenosis presented by physician. Obtain picture to increase parents' understanding of the condition and possible complications.
- Provide information regarding the expected medical equipment to be used in the postoperative period, including mechanical ventilator, heart monitoring equipment, and chest tubes.
- Correct any misinformation.
- Repeat teaching as needed.

Evaluation
- Parents verbalize understanding of aortic stenosis and related complications.
- Parents verbalize understanding of medical equipment that may be used postoperatively.

Critical Thinking in the Nursing Process
1. What are some other topics that should be discussed with Jeremy's parents before surgery?
2. What topics should the nurse plan to discuss with Jeremy's parents before discharge?
3. What is the role of the LPN/LVN in providing care to the NICU patient and family?

Note: Discussion of Critical Thinking questions appears in Appendix I.

Note: The reference and resource listings for this and all chapters have been compiled at the back of the book.

Chapter Review

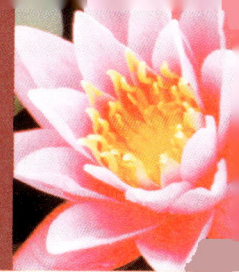

KEY TERMS by Topic

Use the audio glossary feature of either the CD-ROM or the Companion Website to hear the correct pronunciation of the following key terms.

General Care of the High-Risk Newborn
high-risk newborn

Newborn with Alteration in Growth
large for gestational age (LGA), macrosomia, small for gestational age (SGA), intrauterine growth restriction (IUGR)

Cardiovascular Conditions
atrial septal defect, patent ductus arteriosus, ventricular septal defect, tetralogy of Fallot, coarctation, transposition of the great vessels, circumoral, intracranial hemorrhage, hyperbilirubinemia

Respiratory Conditions
meconium aspiration, bronchopulmonary dysplasia

Neurologic Conditions
spina bifida, meningocele, meningomyelocele, hydrocephalus, Down syndrome, trisomy 21, fetal alcohol syndrome, neonatal abstinence syndrome, Neonatal Abstinence Scoring System

Gastrointestinal Conditions
cleft palate, cleft lip, esophageal atresia, tracheoesophageal fistula, imperforate anus, omphalocele, pyloric stenosis, hernia

Genitourinary Conditions
hypospadias, epispadias, phimosis, ambiguous genitalia, exstrophy of the bladder

KEY Points

- The LPN/LVN assists the RN in the care of high-risk newborns.
- The routine care of the newborn follows the same guidelines as for adults including hygiene, nutrition, elimination, and activity.
- Priorities for the care of the high-risk newborn are airway maintenance, promoting tissue profusion, and managing pain.
- Most congenital anomalies require surgical repair beginning in the newborn period. Often surgical repair of anomalies requires several procedures over time to complete the reconstruction.
- The NICU is a frightening place for parents. They need instruction in the NICU routine and equipment.
- Parents need continued support when their infant is facing life-threatening and long-term treatment.

EXPLORE MediaLink

Additional interactive resources for this chapter can be found on the Companion Website at www.prenhall.com/towle. Click on Chapter 18 and "Begin" to select the activities for this chapter.

For chapter-related NCLEX®-style questions and an audio glossary, access the accompanying CD-ROM in this book.

Animations

Congenital heart defects	Heart and lung sounds
Chambers of the human heart	Circumcision
The heart	Down syndrome
Hemodynamics	

FOR FURTHER Study

Chapter 13 briefly discusses hemolytic disease of the newborn.

Normal newborn SGA or LGA infants are also discussed in Chapter 17.

The most common causes of hyperbilirubinemia are discussed in Chapter 17.

Critical Thinking Care Map

Caring for a Preterm Newborn
NCLEX-PN® Focus Area: Physiologic Integrity

Case Study: Olivia, a 38-week-gestation newborn, is brought to the NICU for observation and treatment of a 1-cm meningocele in the lumbar regions of the spinal column. Olivia's mother had no prenatal care. Olivia is moving all extremities and had Apgar scores of 6 and 7.

Nursing Diagnosis: Risk for **I**nfection related to potential rupture of meningocele

COLLECT DATA

Subjective	Objective
_____	_____
_____	_____
_____	_____
_____	_____
_____	_____
_____	_____
_____	_____

Would you report this? Yes/No

If yes, to: _____

Nursing Care

_____
_____
_____
_____
_____
_____
_____
_____
_____
_____
_____

How would you document this? _____
_____
_____
_____

Compare your documentation to the sample provided in Appendix I.

Data Collected
(use only those that apply)

- Respiration: 32 per minute
- Lusty cry
- Apgar: 6 and 7
- Temperature: 99° F
- Lethargic
- Irritable
- No drainage from meningocele
- Flaccid muscle tone
- Moving all extremities
- 1-cm meningocele in lumbar spine

Nursing Interventions
(use only that apply; list in priority order)

- Initial bath
- Oxygen by mask
- Supine position
- Suction airway with suction catheter
- Blood glucose by heel stick
- Wet sterile dressing to meningocele
- Radiant warmer
- Neuro assessment every hour
- Prone position

TEST-TAKING TIP When a question has the key work "avoid," it indicates a "false-response" question. You will need to pick the action that is <u>contraindicated</u>.

1 Seeing his son, who was born with spina bifida, for the first time, a father exclaims, "What is that on his back!" An appropriate response would be:

1. a complete description of the condition, including long-term complications.
2. "That is spina bifida. Your son's spinal column did not fuse completely before birth."
3. conversation that would direct his attention away from the defect.
4. "I don't know. I'll have the doctor call you."

2 Proper technique for suctioning a newborn with a bulb syringe includes which of the following? Select all that apply.

1. placing the newborn on the left side
2. placing the bulb syringe into the buccal cavity
3. suctioning the mouth first
4. suctioning the nares first
5. inserting the bulb into nares, depressing the bulb syringe, and releasing
6. rinsing the bulb with water
7. placing the bulb syringe on the back of the tongue

3 The LPN/LVN is caring for a newborn with fetal alcohol syndrome. Based on this diagnosis, the LPN/LVN knows the immediate care for the newborn will focus on:

1. respiratory support.
2. evaluating elimination patterns.
3. nutritional support.
4. monitoring blood transfusions.

4 Which of the following data reported in the newborn's chart would contribute to persistent pulmonary pneumonia?

1. meconium aspiration during birth
2. low surfactant level
3. high oxygen levels administered following birth
4. mechanical ventilation following birth

5 The LPN/LVN has completed a physical assessment on a 4-hour-old newborn. Which of the following data indicates possible hydrocephalus?

1. bulging anterior fontanel
2. sunken anterior fontanel
3. head circumference of 32 cm
4. herniation of meninges through the vertebral defect

6 The mother of a high-risk newborn in the NICU asks the LPN/LVN why her baby is not wrapped tightly in a blanket like the other newborns. The LPN's/LVN's best response is:

1. "Your newborn gets too hot in a blanket."
2. "It is important for the extremities to move freely to increase muscle development."
3. "There are too many wires attached to the newborn."
4. "Don't worry we are taking good care of your newborn."

7 The LPN/LVN is feeding a newborn and notices the newborn has increased projectile vomiting that has gotten progressively worse over the last week. Which of the following disorders would the LPN/LVN suspect?

1. hernia
2. imperforate anus
3. pyloric stenosis
4. omphalocele

8 The nurse is assessing a newborn and notices the following characteristics. Which of the following are classic signs of Down syndrome? Select all that apply.

1. microcephaly
2. wide short neck
3. facial anomalies
4. simian line on each hand
5. macrocephaly
6. epicanthal folds

9 The nurse is discussing the care of a newborn in the NICU. Which of the following statements made by the parents indicates that they have begun the bonding process?

1. "It must not be good to touch my baby since she is so sick."
2. "My baby likes it when we stroke her arms and legs."
3. "We will schedule our visits after the nurses have completed all treatments."
4. "We do not need to participate in a support group since our baby will recover quickly."

10 The nurse suspects a newborn is exhibiting signs of pathological jaundice. This is based on which of the following data?

1. Jaundice occurring at 12 hours of age.
2. Newborn is Rh negative.
3. Jaundice occurring after 36 hours of age.
4. Newborn's hematocrit level is 44%.

Answers for NCLEX-PN® Review and Critical Thinking questions appear in Appendix I.

Thinking Strategically About...

You are an LPN/LVN employed in a newborn nursery of a regional medical center. The infants in the nursery are either stable newborns or infants who have advanced from the NICU and should be discharged in a short time. You have been working from 7:00 P.M. until 7:00 A.M., and it is time to report to the next nurse and go home.

- John, a male infant, was born vaginally 4 hours ago. Apgar scores were 8 and 9. He nursed well at 6:00 A.M. and is now NPO for a circumcision at 10:00. He has two brothers and a sister waiting for him at home.

- Amanda is a female infant born vaginally at noon yesterday to a 16-year-old mother. The plan is for discharge to adoptive parents early this afternoon. She is bottle-feeding without difficulty. There is an order for PKU, MMR, and hepatitis B immunizations prior to discharge.

- Jeremiah, a Jewish male infant, was born at 34 weeks' gestation. He was on a ventilator for 8 days before his condition stabilized. He has been in the newborn nursery for 3 days and should be discharged in another 48 hours. He is taking formula well every 2 hours, voiding and stooling at regular intervals. His parents arrive around 8 A.M. and spend most of the day with him.

CRITICAL THINKING

- In what order should you present information to the oncoming nurse to demonstrate the intellectual standard of *logic*?

COLLABORATIVE CARE

- What nursing specialists should be contacted to assist in planning and providing care for Amanda?

MANAGEMENT OF CARE AND PRIORITIES IN NURSING CARE

- In what order will you give report on the care for these three infants?
- What is your rationale for prioritizing the report?

DELEGATING

- What follow-up do you need to do on care you delegated to the CNA prior to going home?

COMMUNICATION AND CLIENT TEACHING

- What teaching about newborn care should be provided to Amanda's adoptive parents before she is discharged?
- What communication should be given to Jeremiah's parents about his condition?

DOCUMENTING AND REPORTING

- What information about John's condition should be reported to the supervising RN?
- What would the LPN/LVN chart regarding John's assessment?

CULTURAL CARE STRATEGIES

- Since Jeremiah is from Jewish parents, what aspects of Jewish culture would the nurse need to understand and include in planning?

Appendix I
Answers and Critical Thinking Discussion

Chapter 1

NCLEX-PN® ANSWERS

(1) 1. Outcome 3. Primary nursing care encompasses prevention activities, such as nutritional counseling to prevent gestational diabetes. Magnesium sulfate to treat preterm labor falls under secondary care because the preterm labor is an acute condition. A woman with diabetes has a chronic condition; adapting her management for pregnancy would address an already existing condition and would be tertiary care. Teaching parents about a BiliBlanket for jaundice is secondary as it will affect the elimination of the problem. (2) 4. Outcome 3. Tertiary care is the management of chronic, long-term health care problems such as clients with permanent tracheostomies. Obtaining a urinary sample to evaluate antibiotic therapy is secondary care because the infection was an acute condition. Immunizations are preventive, and so are primary care. Pregnancy is not a chronic condition, so monitoring hematocrit is not tertiary. (3) 1, 2, 3, 4. Outcome 5. While the role of the LPN/LVN varies from state to state, generally administering PO meds, supervising UAP, collecting data, and monitoring lab values are allowable. Developing the nursing diagnosis is an RN role. (4) 4. Outcome 2. The statement "I don't remember too much after they gave me scopolamine" is correct. In 1920 scopolamine was used to induce a twilight sleep to decrease pain and give physicians more control over the birthing process. "Two days after I gave birth I went home to care for my family" is an incorrect statement because it is more reflective of current times. "The birthing suite allowed me to give birth and recover in the same room" is incorrect since it is more reflective of women who gave birth from 1960 to 1980. "I want to continue my career before I have my first child" is incorrect and more reflective of current times. (5) 2. Outcome 2. The LPN/LVN who uses the term *client* believes that this term reflects those who are active participants in their own care. Therefore the statement "My client would like to speak with the doctor now" is correct. "My patient in room 212 would like something for pain" is incorrect because this reflects the belief that the person is ill and in need of others to make decisions. "Don't worry, the doctor will be able to make decisions for you" is incorrect because it does not support the belief that clients are active participants in their own care. The statement "I will help the person in the next

room feed her baby" is incorrect because the term *client* should be used to describe people who are active participants in their own care. (6) 5, 8, 2, 7, 1, 4, 3, 6. Outcome 4. The following steps are the correct order for implementing research into practice. 1. Review current literature. 2. Gather data that provides rationales for a proposed change in practice. 3. Create a presentation presenting the risks and benefits to support a change in practice. 4. Develop clinical practice guidelines and a time frame for possible implementation. 5. Develop a plan to evaluate client outcomes. 6. Invite practitioners and administrators to discuss the proposed new practice guidelines. 7. Document approved changes to the clinical guidelines. 8. Publish positive client outcomes relating to the new clinical practice guidelines. (7) 1. Outcome 5. To function in the role of an LPN/LVN, every LPN/LVN should be knowledgeable of his or her own individual state's nurse practice acts. The Association of Women's Health, Obstetric and Neonatal Nurses is incorrect because it is not a governing body to authorize practice for LPNs/LVNs. The Nurse's Association of the American College of Obstetricians and Gynecologists is incorrect because it does not authorize practice for LPNs/LVNs. The American Nurses Association is incorrect because it is not a governing body to authorize practice for LPNs/LVNs. (8) 3. Outcome 5. Prioritizing care is part of the LPN/LVN role. It is correct for the nurse to place priority on a post C-section client complaining of pain and tenderness behind her knee when walking. This assessment may indicate a blood clot and could be life threatening. Acrocyanosis is quite normal in a 1-hour-old newborn and is not life threatening. A 24-hour-postpartum client needing assistance with newborn care is considered a normal finding. Sore nipples in a 12-hour-postpartum client is not life threatening. (9) 2. Outcome 5. Contacting the nursing supervisor first is correct because the LPN/LVN is responsible for informing the RN if any changes occur in the health status of the client. Contacting the unlicensed assistive personnel is incorrect because UAP do not make decisions for client care. Contacting the breastfeeding mother's significant other first is incorrect; although they may be included, they do not make decisions. The pediatrician may be notified, but not initially. (10) 3. Outcome 5. Teaching the client how to bathe a newborn is correct because health promotion teaching is an important role for the LPN/LVN. Establishing a nursing diagnosis for a client recovering from a C-section is incorrect because LPNs/LVNs do not independently write and update nursing diagnoses. Independently planning care for clients in the home setting is the role of the RN. Only physicians and advanced practice nurses prescribe medications.

CARE PLAN HINTS

1. Parents may object to immunizations due to philosophical or religious reasons. They may also have some concerns about governmental control over their health. They may believe that immunizations are not safe, or they may desire to have an all-natural approach to their health care.

2. In the 1900s polio was epidemic and frequently resulted in paralysis or death. A vaccine for polio was introduced in 1951. By 1967, polio was reduced by 99%, and by 1991 it was eradicated from the Western hemisphere.

3. Once proper teaching has been done, the decision to vaccinate is in the parent's hands. If the family refuses immunizations, the nurse will need to provide additional teaching on disease recognition and reporting. The family should be treated with respect.

Chapter 2

NCLEX-PN® ANSWERS

(1) 3. Outcome 5. Application of a fetal scalp electrode is a clinical skill not taught in a basic nursing education course. In many states, it is not an allowable skill for the LPN. Reporting to the RN is the best response. Response 4 is rude and does not promote collaborative care. (2) 4. Outcome 6. Right supervision includes the tasks of monitoring, evaluating, intervening when necessary, and providing feedback, if appropriate. The decision about the right task is made before delegation occurs. The decision about the right circumstances is made earlier. The decision about the right direction is made before teaching the person the task. (3) 4. Outcome 6. Delegation is transferring to a competent individual the authority to perform a nursing task. Only the CNA with experience meets these criteria. An inexperienced person should not be given this task. An experienced person with diabetes is not the appropriate choice if the person is not on staff. The client's husband probably would know the procedure but is not on staff. (4) 3. Outcome 6. Insulin is a drug that is regulated by some nurse practice acts to be a task designated for the registered nurse. The UAP should never give medications or directly contact the physician without notification of the LPN. The client's husband, in an acute care setting, should not be given the task of administering medication. (5) 2. Outcome 6. The CNA has incorrectly instructed the client regarding

collection of a 24-hour urine specimen. It is the responsibility of the supervising LPN to review the procedure with her to ensure that she can perform it correctly next time. The CNA would not be praised; the first voided specimen is discarded. The CNA needs instruction, not reassignment. The CNA would not receive a raise. (6) 1. Outcome 4. Relevance is correct; it is important for the LPN/LVN to collect as much information about the client to determine what is relevant (such as backache, because it is important to rule out labor). The backache could indicate early labor versus common discomforts of pregnancy during the second and third trimesters. Clarity is incorrect because it is used to eliminate confusion by gathering more information. Accuracy is incorrect since it refers to the correctness of the data being examined. Precision is incorrect since it searches for the exactness of the data to determine precise information. (7) Deductive. Outcome 4. Deductive reasoning allows the nurse to take a statement about a client (postpartum client states she has a full bladder) and to realize that certain conditions may result from a full bladder: boggy uterus, heavy lochia flow, and passage of large clots. Thus, the nurse will encourage the client to empty the bladder often. (8) 3. Outcome 3. Implications of action is correct; the LPN/LVN exercises sound judgment by considering the consequences of the action prior to providing care. Point of view is incorrect; this refers to the LPN/LVN considering different perspectives of a situation vs. the effects of the actions. Assumptions is incorrect. Assumptions refer to ideas that are taken for granted. Concepts is incorrect; this allows the LPN/LVN to use theories and laws from other disciplines to understand nursing problems. (9) 2, 3, and 5. Outcome 4. Statements that reflect the use of clarity as an intellectual standard to assist the nurse in verifying accuracy in order to clarify a problem are: "How would you describe the sensation you feel?" "Give me an example of how it feels." "Tell me more about your pain." The statement "Could you be more specific about the type of pain you have?" is incorrect because it is an example of precision. Precision helps gain scientific exactness for precise information. The statement "Are there any related factors that might contribute to your pain?" strives for depth, not clarity. (10) 2. Outcome 5. Proper training has not been completed by the LPN/LVN is correct. The LPN/LVN must be trained on all new equipment prior to use, and the training must be documented in the LPN's/LVN's file. An unlicensed assistive personnel can hang the fluids is incorrect; only licensed personnel can hang IV fluids. Only RNs can hang IV fluids is incorrect, since LPNs/LVNs are also licensed to hang IV fluids. Certified nursing assistants is incorrect; they are not licensed to hang IV fluids.

CRITICAL THINKING CARE MAP

Subjective Data   Mother states Andrew rarely hungry.

Objective Data   Decreased urine output (four diapers daily when typical should be six to eight); dry mucous membranes; lethargy; intake of 5 oz every 5 to 6 hours.

Report   Yes, to the registered nurse.

Interventions   Obtain vital signs every 1 to 2 hours. Contact the registered nurse to report findings. Teach parents to obtain and record vital signs. Teach parents the importance of adequate fluid intake during the use of the BiliBlanket. Teach parents the symptoms of dehydration. Closely monitor vital signs. Provide fluid replacement per order.

Documentation   (date/time) 1200 4-day-old male infant, lethargic, dry mucous membranes. Mother reports four wet diapers daily. States oral intake 5 oz formula, q 5 to 6 hours. Mother states infant is rarely hungry. T 99, P 150, R 42. Report called to supervising RN. S. Smith, LPN

Chapter 3

NCLEX-PN® ANSWERS

(1) 4. Outcome 4. Reporting possible child abuse is a legal obligation of health care professionals. One cannot assume that the father is telling the truth, or knows the truth. The nurse in charge is required to make the call to the police, not the LPN/LVN. The responsibility is for the child's safety before the stepfather's confidentiality. (2) 3. Outcome 6. It is vital for the nurse to provide nonjudgmental care. Her opinion of the situation cannot affect her nursing care. The nurse cannot side with the mother because he/she agrees with her opinion. Regardless of the nurse's opinion of the household dynamics, he/she cannot side with the father. The care of the newborn in this situation must not be put on hold. (3) 3. Outcome 3. Discussing health care issues with health care personnel involved in the direct care of a client is allowable. Discussing details of any client's condition with a neighbor is a breach of the client's confidentiality. A nurse has the responsibility to keep client charts secure. A health care professional who is not involved in the client's care does not have the right to access a chart, even if the nurse is a friend of the client. (4) 2. Outcome 3. Educating the client in safer sex practices is the correct action in this case. In many states, reproductive rights of minors dictate that they may receive contraceptive information without parental consent. It would breach the client's privacy to contact her parents. The child is not breaking the law, and it is your job to assist her in making informed decisions. The names of her partners is not relevant to your task of assisting the client. (5) 2. Outcome 2. Life and death decisions should be made by the family, with

only support from health care professionals. Deciding to keep information from the infant's mother is not up to the nurse. The news that the hospital only keeps babies on life support for 2 days, if true, does not answer the family's question. The family will deal with preparations in its own way and does not need the hospital staff to decide when it is appropriate. (6) 2. Outcome 2. Informed consent is essential for participation in medical research. The child is not taking part in any experimental drug study, so the mother does not need to know whether you are aware of the drugs and placebos. The mother is not asking for her child to be included in a study, so she will not want to ask the doctor about experiments being conducted. Experimental drugs are used with informed consent, so telling her that only prisoners are used is incorrect. (7) 1, 2, 5. Outcome 6. Health care personnel can expect families and clients to provide adequate information, seek knowledge, and participate actively in treatment. Health care personnel can provide teaching and information, but cannot be held solely responsible for the clients' understanding. Health care personnel can remind clients about appointments, and stress the importance of keeping appointments, but the responsibility for keeping them lies with the client. (8) 1. Outcome 2. Identifying information on the crib card is visible to the public and may compromise client privacy. The mother has a right to access her infant's chart, so giving her access does not endanger privacy. (9) 1. Outcome 5. Questions regarding ethical issues are complicated because decisions regarding these issues may not surface for years. Therefore, ownership of the cord blood is uncertain is correct. Because of the uncertainty of ownership hospitals are unsure of their rights concerning human issues. It is uncertain if the child can claim ownership of the cord blood in order to sell it. It is incorrect to believe that parents can overrule decisions since ownership is uncertain. (10) Emancipated minors. Outcome 5. Emancipated minors are adolescents who are married and have been emancipated by the court, which allows them to make their own health care decisions.

CARE PLAN HINTS

1. Typically most states recognize the rights of parents to make health care decisions for minor children, unless the child is emancipated. Jean would generally be considered emancipated from her parents due to the pregnancy. Jean and the baby's father would have the legal responsibility to make decisions in this case.

2. The nurse should discuss with Jean her right to privacy and only disclose information to family members as Jean directs.

3. Jean and the baby's father should fully understand the issues of delivery of a 24-week preterm infant and possible

treatment as well as prognosis. Spiritual counseling would be helpful if desired by the family. Support groups of families who are experiencing treatment of a preterm infant and loss of a child may be of assistance.

CRITICAL THINKING CARE MAP

Subjective Data   States lack of sleep times 3 days; 24-hour diet recall: six soft drinks; states unable to care for a baby; states family incapable of financially supporting another family member; "My boyfriend says I have to abort the baby or he won't have anything to do with me"; concerned father will be physically abusive if he finds out she is pregnant.

Objective Data   Crying; no eye contact with nurse.

Report   Yes, to the supervising nurse.

Interventions   Encourage client to express feelings and concerns openly. Address client in a nonjudgmental fashion. Explore options available to this client and the pros and cons of each. Encourage client to engage parents in decision-making process. Explore client's past successes in difficult circumstances. Encourage client to explore personal strengths.

Documentation   (date) 0830 G1, 15-year-old white female reported to school health nurse, crying. States 12 weeks pregnant. States parents do not know of pregnancy and she is unsure what to do. Feels there is no solution to this dilemma and has no hope. States fearful of father's reaction to the news of pregnancy, specifically concerned about his physical reaction. States boyfriend is encouraging her to abort the baby. States no sleep times 3 days. 24-hour diet recall: six soft drinks. Data reported to supervising RN. S. Metcalf, LPN

Chapter 4

NCLEX-PN® ANSWERS

(1) 2. Outcome 5. A genogram is used to understand the relationships of family members to each other. The nurse is trying to assess the dynamics of this family, so a genogram is the tool used for this type of assessment. Relationships to the community are described in an ecomap. Genetic links would help in understanding inherited traits, not family dynamics. Physical characteristics do not help in understanding the family dynamics. (2) Ecomap. Outcome 5. An ecomap is a diagram used to demonstrate the interactions of a family within the community. (3) 2. Outcome 4. The mother's behavior of not maintaining eye contact is consistent with her Chinese culture, which demonstrates respect to those in authority. Asking the woman to look at the doctor is counter to her cultural upbringing. Addressing the father only may be important in patriarchal families but is

not the issue here. Avoiding eye contact does not always signify guilt. (4) 1, 2, 5. Outcome 6. The nurse knows that an environmental assessment includes collecting and observing data regarding the physical aspects of the client's environment that would affect the health and well-being of the family. The exterior color of the house does not relate to safety. The number of televisions and their locations do not affect the health and safety of the family. (5) 3. Outcome 4. The nurse respects and supports the client's spiritual beliefs. Talking about medicine directly contradicts the mother's belief. Challenging the request does not show respect for the mother's beliefs and may increase conflict. Response 4 implies that you disagree with the mother. (6) 2. Outcome 4. Cultural and religious beliefs can affect the client's health, and nursing care should be planned with these aspects in mind. The nurse should base the client's care, as much as possible, on the client's culture or religious preferences. Reimbursement is not based on cultural and religious beliefs. Response 4 is a true statement but has nothing to do with care of the client. (7) 2. Outcome 6. Having close, supportive family during a time of loss is an important factor in helping parents deal with their grieving. Parents experiencing the loss of a child do need help with coping mechanisms to help them through their loss. The fact that they mention people have been telling them they need help is an indicator they do need assistance with coping with their loss and response 1 indicates denial. Response 3 is one of blame and anger, indicating intervention is needed. Moving will only prolong the family's grieving process and slow healing. (8) 3. Outcomes 7 and 8. The LPN or LVN should notify the supervising registered nurse about the family's stress so appropriate actions can be taken. The RN would be the appropriate person to meet with the family as a group and determine what steps need to be taken or which referrals need to be made. Based on this assessment, the RN would set up a meeting with a family counselor. Ignoring the problem won't help the family resolve their issues. (9) 2. Outcome 6. The nurse has a responsibility to determine aspects of family functioning that may negatively affect the client's health. The response in option 1 may make the family think they are being compared to other families and may decrease communication between the family and the nurse. Response 3 will upset the family and close the avenues of communication. The nurse is not trained to search out wrongdoing but rather to render client care. (10) 3, 5. Outcomes 6 and 8. Contacting social services and consulting with the registered nurse will produce reliable local resources for the client. Web searches and using the yellow pages may not produce reliable local resources that can be trusted. Surveying other clients may also not be a source of reliable information since circumstances differ from family to family and community to community.

CARE PLAN HINTS

1. The ecomap should include Jean's parents' workplaces, their professional organizations, the families' civic affiliations, their religious affiliations, Jean's school, extended family, and sports activities.
2. With Jean's amputation, access to the home and safety hazards should be assessed.
3. It would be important to assess Jean's school for access. The nurse could also look for a support group of young amputees. Jean's parents may benefit from a support group of others who have experienced traumatic events.

CRITICAL THINKING CARE MAP

Subjective Data Complaint of daily stomachache; refuses to go to school; parents recently divorced; parental relationship strained; some days spent with mother, some spent with father; father has new female relationship.

Objective Data Sam's responses barely audible; dark circles under eyes.

Report Yes, this data should be reported to the registered nurse.

Nursing Interventions Evaluate family strengths and weaknesses. Encourage Sam and his mother to express concerns and fears. Explore negative feelings of anger, worry, sorrow, etc. Encourage each family member to seek to understand the other's feelings. Assist the family in setting realistic goals. Refer to community resources as needed.

Documentation (date) 1000 7-year-old male for office visit accompanied by mother who reports complaints of lack of appetite, excessive sleeping, frequent stomachaches, and refusal to go to school. Mother also reports the family has recently gone through a divorce, there is unrest in the family, and new living arrangements and new caregivers introduced to the child. Dark circles noted under the child's eyes bilaterally. Verbal responses to questions barely audible. D. Adams, LPN

UNIT I Thinking Strategically About ...

CRITICAL THINKING

- How does the Japanese culture exhibit grief? What has she been doing that exhibits her grief?
- What are Jenny's ideas about the safety of her home? What does she think the babies will require in a safe home environment?

- How do you feel when the baby cries? What do you do when the baby cries? If you get frustrated with the baby, what will you do?

COLLABORATIVE CARE

- Marie should be referred to WIC (Women, Infants, and Children), a federal program that provides nutritious foods and education to low-income pregnant, postpartum, and lactating women and to infants and children up to age 5.
- Check local directories for agencies, such as The Compassionate Friends, and support groups from local hospitals and birthing centers.

MANAGEMENT OF CARE AND PRIORITIES IN NURSING CARE

- Visit Marie first, then Jenny, and finally Kumiko.
- Visiting Marie would be the first priority because she is unsure of her ability to care for the infant and could accidentally harm or neglect him. While Jenny was stable when she was discharged, she is at risk for developing preterm labor again and she needs monitoring. Kumiko is three days postpartum and her physical condition should be stable.

DELEGATING

- Family members or CNAs can be taught to take Jenny's blood pressure and apply fetal heart monitoring equipment. Monitor records can be brought to the RN for interpretation. Marie and Kumiko will need to be checked by a licensed nurse.
- To determine that the delegated care has been performed properly, direct supervision is required until the family member or CNA has demonstrated competence in the task being delegated.

COMMUNICATION AND CLIENT TEACHING

- The nurse should watch Marie care for the baby and question her about infant care in specific situations. Through direct observation and questioning, the nurse can determine Marie's knowledge and skill in providing safe care. A teaching plan with supervision can then be implemented to correct any deficiencies.
- Because Jenny is pregnant with twins, she will be more awkward and may need assistance getting into and out of bed. A clear pathway should be provided for her to get to the bathroom. It may be difficult to eat in bed, and care should be taken to avoid spilling hot food. The environment for twins should be the same as for other newborns.

DOCUMENTING AND REPORTING

- If you believe Marie is at a high risk for neglecting the infant, you should stay in the house and call your supervising RN on the telephone.
- The LPN/LVN should document and report findings regarding Kumiko and her family's coping and stages of the grief process.

CULTURAL CARE STRATEGIES

- In Hispanic households, the male is usually the head of the house and would make the decisions regarding health care. Because Marie is unmarried, she may depend on her own father for decisions. Hispanic families should be assessed for the use of *curanderos* (healers), as well as for use of herbs or home remedies that may interfere with medical treatment. The nurse should ask Marie what she plans to do in a variety to situations and reinforce safety and general health teaching.
- In the Japanese culture, the male is the head of the house and the female provides teaching and support for the children. Feelings are often suppressed. The LPN/LVN would need to assess how each family member is expressing their feelings and report findings to the RN for direction. Nonjudgmental therapeutic communication is always appropriate in these situations.

Chapter 5

NCLEX-PN® ANSWERS

(1) 2. Outcome 5. Fertilization could occur anywhere in the female reproductive system, but the most common place is in the distal one-third of the fallopian tube. (2) Outcome 4. An "X" is placed over the testes. (3) 1. Outcome 2. Sperm contain either an X or a Y chromosome. All ova contain an X chromosome. When an X sperm fertilizes an ovum, the result will be a female infant. When a Y sperm fertilizes the ovum, a male infant will develop. (4) 3. Outcome 5. The distal end of the fallopian tube is not attached to the ovary but opens into the pelvic cavity. (5) 3. Outcome 7. Ovulation usually occurs halfway through the menstrual cycle. (6) 1. Outcome 8. Milk is produced on an as-needed basis. When the breast is emptied, more milk will be produced. (7) 2. Outcome 3. Female infants are born with all the ova they will ever produce. (8) 1, 2, 5. Outcome 5. Part of a sexual history involves identifying the client's usual menstrual cycle. Because a yellow odorous discharge could indicate an infection, it is important to determine if she has sexual partners who could also be infected. Although birth control may be important to teach, it does not directly affect the symptoms of this client. Bowel movements and the number of children do not pertain to this client's

problem. (9) 3, 4. Outcome 4. Removing the prostate either destroys or alters the ejaculatory duct, making it difficult for sperm to leave the body. Prostatic fluid is necessary for sperm mobility. Any sperm that may be able to leave the body will be unable to swim through the female system. (10) 3. Outcome 6. Hormones from both the pituitary gland and ovaries are necessary to regulate the menstrual cycle. The uterus does not produce hormones.

CARE PLAN HINTS

1. Ovarian complications are rare following a spontaneous ruptured ovarian cyst or surgery, and the ovary continues to function normally. If the cyst ruptures, blood and other fluid cause inflammation, but this usually resolves in a few days. Sometimes excessive bleeding could cause a surgical emergency.
2. At the beginning of laparoscopic abdominal surgery, carbon dioxide is instilled into the abdominal cavity to allow for visualization of the abdominal/pelvic organs. Following surgery, most of the CO_2 is removed. The remaining CO_2 forms bubbles that rise to the top of the abdominal cavity when the client sits or stands. The pressure of the CO_2 next to the diaphragm causes the pain the client feels in the right upper quadrant and the referred pain in the right shoulder.
3. Because ovarian cysts are caused by improper ovulation and formation of the corpus luteum, some doctors will prescribe birth control pills to prevent ovulation. The pros and cons of this preventive treatment should be discussed thoroughly with the client.

CRITICAL THINKING CARE MAP

Subjective Data States unprotected sexual intercourse with several women over the past few weeks; states "I hope this will not affect my being able to get an erection."

Objective Data Voice shaky; avoids eye contact.

Report Yes, to charge nurse or primary care provider. Client's lack of knowledge regarding sexuality, sexual function, and infection indicates a need for client teaching.

Interventions Encourage client to discuss sexuality; teach client about normal physiology of erection and infection of reproductive system; teach client about the need for protection from infection during sexual intercourse.

Documentation (date/time) Client states concerns over being able to have future erections. Encouraged to express feelings regarding sexuality. Provided instruction of normal physiology of erections and infection of reproductive system. Reported data to J. Smith, Nurse Practitioner. C. Bragg, LPN

Chapter 6

NCLEX-PN® ANSWERS

(1) 1. Outcome 2. Primary prevention addresses activities that protect against disease such as teaching about birth control methods to prevent pregnancy. Secondary prevention is incorrect because it focuses on early identification and treatment of diseases. Health promotion activities will promote well-being. Tertiary prevention is incorrect because it focuses on rehabilitation from disease or injury. (2) 3. Outcome 5. Learning may be impaired in a client who is experiencing moderate anxiety. Asking for more information about crutch walking is incorrect because clients with mild anxiety often are motivated to seek more information. Agitation is experienced when clients have reached the panic level of anxiety. Palpitations are symptoms of clients who have reached the panic level of anxiety. (3) 1. Outcome 4. The nurse should recommend exercising early in the evening. Exercising increases epinephrine, which increases heart rate and may prevent the client from relaxing and falling asleep. Lifting weights right before bedtime is incorrect because it increases the release of epinephrine. Taking a short walk before going to sleep is incorrect because it increases the release of epinephrine. To improve overall health, exercise should be done on most days of the week, not just on weekends. (4) 1, 4, 5. Outcome 6. Drinking herbal tea in the evening, taking a warm bath before bedtime, and using imagery techniques will help promote relaxation and help decrease fatigue. Exercising before bedtime releases epinephrine, which does not promote relaxation. Working on hobbies may be restful and does not need to be avoided. Fluids containing caffeine and high levels of carbohydrates provide energy, which may make it more difficult to relax; herbal teas are a better choice. (5) 3. Outcome 4. Clients should be informed about overconsuming foods containing vitamin A, because too much fat-soluble vitamin A can lead to toxicity. Shopping on a full stomach is a good strategy because people are less likely to make poor food choices when they are full. Selecting foods low in trans fat reflects an understanding of healthy nutrition. Clients who consume eight glasses of water a day demonstrate an understanding of healthy nutrition. (6) 1. Outcomes 3 and 4. Frequent douching is correct, because douching removes the normal vaginal bacteria and increases the risk of vaginal infections. Clients who refrain from douching during menstruation are at a lower risk for developing vaginal infections. Cleansing the perineum with water promotes good hygiene and decreases risk of vaginal infections. Changing tampons every 3 to 4 hours promotes good hygiene and decreases risk of infections. (7) 3, 5, 6. Outcomes 3 and 4. The nurse should teach young adolescents proper use of tampons by instructing them to avoid super-absorbent tampons, wash hands prior to inserting the tampon, and change regular-absorbent tampons every 3 to 4 hours. Holding onto the side of a tampon during insertion increases risk of infection. Douching should be avoided during menses. Tampons are not used for heavy mucus discharge. (8) 4. Outcome 6. Playing music during imagery is correct because it increases the effects of imagery and increases relaxation. Acupuncture is incorrect because nurses do not perform acupuncture. Sleep medication might reduce the effects of imagery by making the client drowsy. Increasing fluid intake is not a nursing strategy during imagery. (9) 1. Outcomes 2 and 4. Screening for osteoporosis is correct because it aids in early detection and treatment, which is the purpose of secondary prevention. Administering a hepatitis B vaccine is incorrect because it is an example of primary prevention to help protect against disease. Providing a list of foods to increase calcium intake is incorrect because it demonstrates primary prevention that will assist clients to help improve nutrition. Teaching proper foot care to a diabetic client will help prevent complications with diabetes and is an example of tertiary care. (10) 3. Outcome 4. Lifting weights is correct because it will help women increase muscle strength. Aerobic activity is incorrect because it aids in improving cardiovascular health. Group sports are incorrect because they are a form of aerobic activity and aid in improving cardiovascular health. Walking is a form of aerobic activity and promotes general health.

CARE PLAN HINTS

1. If Barbara increases her fluid intake, nutrition, and exercise, the effects of tobacco can be eliminated from the body more rapidly.
2. Barbara should be encouraged to try again. It is common for smokers to try to stop several times before they are successful. Barbara needs encouragement for her small successes, not reprimand for her setbacks.
3. Answer is intended for individual discussions.

CRITICAL THINKING CARE MAP

Subjective Data   States she eats too much; little exercise; stressed by work commitments; staying home; reports weight gain of 15 pounds in 3 months.

Objective Data   BP 114/72, T 98.4° F, P 76, R 18; tearful; anxious; no specific physical complaints; establish relationship for health maintenance.

Report   Yes, to the registered nurse.

Interventions   Obtain a health history. Obtain a baseline weight. Identify nutrition needs. Identify learning needs. Provide list of health clubs in the area. Provide information on balanced diet. Provide relaxation techniques. Set up equipment for a complete physical examination.

Documentation (date/time) BP 114/72, T 98.4° F, P 76, R 18. Appears anxious and is crying. States she recently moved to the area for work. States she has no physical complaints, but wishes to establish a relationship for future health concerns. States she has gained 15 lbs. in 3 months. Information on balanced diet, local health clubs, and relaxation techniques provided. J. Moss FNP informed. B. Ross, LPN

Chapter 7

NCLEX-PN® ANSWERS

(1) 2. Outcome 1. Difficulty emptying the bladder is correct because cystocele occurs when the bladder has prolapsed into the vagina making it more difficult to empty during urination. Difficulty defecating is incorrect because it is associated with a rectocele, which causes the anterior rectal wall to protrude into the vagina. Dyspareunia is incorrect because it is associated with a uterine prolapse causing the uterus to protrude into the vagina. Pelvic pressure is incorrect because it is associated with uterine prolapse causing the uterus to protrude into the vagina. (2) 1, 2, 3, 5. Outcome 2. Transmission of HIV can occur through homosexual or heterosexual relationships, and through genital sex, oral sex, or rectal sex. (3) 1, 2, 3, 4. Outcome 3. It is important for the client to validate the presence of the string daily for a week and then following menses thereafter. She must also report promptly any signs of infection or pregnancy. (4) 3. Outcome 4. The client is expressing feelings of anger and resentment that need to be explored further in order to assist her in resolving these feelings. (5) 4. Outcome 1. Fibroid tumor is correct and can cause menorrhagia, which is when the menses is excessive in volume or number of days. Premenstrual syndrome is a collection of symptoms occurring prior to menses and is not associated with fibroid tumors. Endometriosis symptoms include dysmenorrhea with pelvic pain and dyspareunia and is not associated with fibroid tumors. Human papillomavirus may result in cervical cancer not fibroid tumors. (6) 1. Outcome 3. Flagyl is contraindicated during the first trimester of pregnancy is correct because it is considered a teratogen causing harm to fetal development during the first trimester. Flagyl is not prescribed to treat trichomoniasis is incorrect because it is the most common drug for trichomoniasis. Flagyl is not prescribed for repeat infections is incorrect because it is the most common drug for trichomoniasis. Flagyl is contraindicated during the entire pregnancy is incorrect and can be prescribed after the first trimester. (7) 2. Outcome 4. Client uses palm of hand to palpate breast tissue is the correct answer but requires further teaching.

The LPN/LVN should instruct the client to use the finger pads to palpate breast tissue. Client compresses the nipple with the thumb and finger is a correct technique and does not require further teaching. Client palpates tissue from the axilla to the sternum is a correct technique and does not require further teaching. Client inspects breast by lifting arms over her head is a correct technique and does not require further teaching. (8) 4. Outcome 4. The nurse caring for the birth mother should provide emotional support. The birth mother and adoptive mother make decisions about visitation of the infant, not the nurse. (9) 4. Outcome 4. Showering or bathing may wash away vital evidence and should be delayed until such evidence can be gathered in the appropriate manner. (10) 3. Outcome 1. History of human papillomavirus infection is correct because most cervical cancers are a result of the human papillomavirus. History of endometriosis is incorrect and may place the client at risk for infertility. Repeat gonorrhea infections is incorrect and places the client at risk for permanent scarring of the fallopian tubes, which may result in infertility. History of fibroid tumors is incorrect because they are nonmalignant and occur within the uterus.

CARE PLAN HINTS

1. Ms. Kelly should be asked to describe the specific events of the attack. If possible, a law enforcement officer should be present. The nurse should remain nonjudgmental and empathetic. All subjective responses should be documented in the client's precise words.

2. It is important for Ms. Kelly to feel safe. Suggested personal protection devices include extra door locks, burglar alarms, mace or other legal weapons, or hiring a personal bodyguard.

3. Acts of violence can cause long-lasting effects. Professional counseling is recommended for Ms. Kelly and her family. She needs to have opportunities to verbalize her feelings, fears, and anxieties. Support people and professional counselors need to observe closely for signs and symptoms of denial and depression.

CRITICAL THINKING CARE MAP

Subjective Data Headache pain level 4; states vaginal spotting has occurred for 4 days; states has had three sexual partners in 3 months; LMP (record month/day/year).

Objective Data Small amount of dark red vaginal discharge noted; multiple cervical lesions measuring ½ to 1 cm in diameter; labia with diffuse redness.

Report Yes, to MD. Would report vaginal spotting, sexual history, vaginal discharge, lesions, and condition of labia.

Interventions Assess characteristics of the lesion; teach the importance of informing all sexual partners; teach the importance of regular Pap smears; teach the client about cryotherapy treatment.

Documentation (date/time) Client reports headache—pain level 4—and vaginal spotting times 4 days. Small amount of dark, red vaginal discharge noted. LMP (mo/day/yr). States three sexual partners in 3 months. Multiple cervical vesicles measuring ½ to 1 cm in diameter, with diffuse labia redness noted following cervical examination by nurse practitioner. Physician given verbal report. K. Smartt, LPN

UNIT II Thinking Strategically About ...

CRITICAL THINKING

- Roma, I hear you saying that having a hysterectomy did not bother you. Could you elaborate on your feelings?
- Curt, can you rate your pain on a scale of 1 to 10? Can you tell me where the pain is located?

COLLABORATIVE CARE

- Anita should be referred to local cancer treatment centers for local support groups.

MANAGEMENT OF CARE AND PRIORITIES IN NURSING CARE

- Roma should be seen first, then Anita, and finally Curt.
- Roma had the most extensive surgery and is at greatest risk for complications. Because Anita is 1 day postoperative, she should be seen before Curt.

DELEGATING

- After assessing Roma, her hygiene care could be delegated to the CNA, with specific directions for a bed bath or shower. The LPN needs to assess Roma's steadiness during ambulation, so the CNA can help Roma ambulate after the first time she is up.

COMMUNICATION AND CLIENT TEACHING

- Once a general diet is tolerated, Roma should have well-balanced meals, with adequate protein and fresh fruits and vegetables. She should progress her ambulation to several times daily.
- Discharge instruction must include use, action, and side effects of prescribed medication. Activity, diet, pain control, signs of infection, and bleeding should also be included.

DOCUMENTING AND REPORTING

- Curt should void in 2 to 4 hours. If he becomes uncomfortable, or if there are more than 350 mL of urine in the bladder identified on a bladder scan, the RN should be notified. With a doctor order, a straight catheter may be inserted to drain the bladder. All data should be documented.

CULTURAL CARE STRATEGIES

- Anita should be asked if there are any cultural considerations that are important to plan for in her care.

Chapter 8

NCLEX-PN® ANSWERS

(1) 1. Outcome 2. The fertilized egg travels through the fallopian tube and divides rapidly to form a mass that reaches the uterus in 4 to 5 days, at which time it is formed into a two-layered ball. The outer layer develops fingerlike projections called villi to secure the blastocyst to the uterus. These villi begin producing human chorionic gonadotropin 8 to 10 days after fertilization. (2) 3. Outcome 2. The placenta produces estrogen and progesterone to do several things, including prevention of uterine contractions. Relaxin causes softening in the collagen connective tissue of the symphysis pubis and sacroiliac joints. HPL helps the mother's body prepare for lactation. hCG maintains the corpus luteum. (3) 4, 5. Outcome 2. The umbilical cord does contain two arteries and one vein. Maternal and fetal blood does not mix; nutrients and waste is exchanged in the placenta. The fetal respiratory system is not functioning *in utero* because it is not developed. The ductus arteriosus is outside the fetal heart; the blood exchange between placenta and fetus is via the two arteries and one vein. (4) 1. Outcome 3. Fertilization occurs in the outer third of the fallopian tube is correct. Infections in the fallopian tube may cause scarring of tissue therefore decreasing the possibility of the ovum and sperm uniting. Previous infections do not affect hCG levels. Previous infections do not cause delayed ovulation. The ovum is fertile for only 12 to 24 hours; the sperm is fertile for up to 72 hours. (5) 2. Outcome 4. The fetus will require ventilation at birth is correct because at 24 weeks' gestation the fetal lungs are not mature. Breastfeeding is incorrect because at 24 weeks the newborn is unable to suck. Holding the newborn is very limited at this point in care. At 24 weeks the newborn is in the NICU and cord care is done by the nurse. (6) 1, 4, 5. Outcome 3. Clients who are at a higher risk for conceiving a newborn with a chromosomal defect are young teenage girls, women over 30, and couples who have a history of chromosomal abnormalities. Preterm labor, not chromosomal defect, is associated with multiple pregnancy. Smoking during pregnancy is a risk factor for SGA and spontaneous abortion, not for chromosomal defects.

Decreased folic acid intake places pregnant women's fetuses at risk for spina bifida, not for chromosomal defects. (7) 1. Outcome 4. Fetal movement is typically felt between 16 and 20 weeks' gestation is correct. Feeling the baby kick at 12 weeks is too early. Keeping a full bladder is uncomfortable, is not recommended, and will not increase the chances of feeling the baby move. The limbs are beginning to move but are not felt by the mother. (8) 4. Outcome 4. Green leafy vegetables is correct because they are good sources of folic acid. Pregnant women may decrease the risk for spina bifida by increasing foods that contain folic acid. Brown rice does not have folic acid. Dried fruits are good sources of iron, but not of folic acid. Fresh seafood is a good source for vitamin B_{12}, but not of folic acid. (9) 2. Outcome 4. Over-the-counter medications may interfere with pregnancy is correct, because the fetus will receive medications that are passed into maternal blood. The client understands that the placenta does not prevent medication from reaching the fetus. The client understands that increasing folic acid is an appropriate healthy lifestyle choice during pregnancy. Regular exercise is an appropriate healthy lifestyle choice during pregnancy. (10) 1. Outcome 3. The child who receives one dominant gene and one recessive gene is correct; this child will be a carrier of the disorder. When the child receives recessive genes from both parents, the child will have an inherited disorder, not a chromosomal defect. An extra chromosome would lead to a trisomy syndrome, not an inherited disorder. Deletion of one part of a chromosome or an extra would lead to a trisomy syndrome, not to an inherited disorder.

CARE PLAN HINTS

1. The nurse should stress the need for adequate nutrition and the impact on fetal development. The nurse should also stress the need to stop smoking and drinking alcohol due to the impact on fetal development.
2. The size of the uterus is not within normal limits. The fetal heart rate is not within normal limits.
3. The uterus would be larger than normal for the week of gestation. More than one fetal heart rate can usually be heard.

CRITICAL THINKING CARE MAP

Subjective Data   States she does not know what she did wrong; states she does not know how to tell her husband.

Objective Data   Crying.

Report   Yes, to the supervising RN.

Interventions   Provide facial tissue. *She is crying and may need to wipe her eyes and nose.* Place hand on her shoulder. *This nonverbal gesture shows empathy and provides emotional support.* Teach about spina bifida. *Once she has calmed down, she will

need information about spina bifida, its causes, and possible treatment. Provide written information about spina bifida. *She can refer to written information when she is at home. She may be able to send written information to her husband. Written information should contain additional references, including Internet sites.* Provide information about support groups. *Support groups can help her adjust to the diagnosis, share information regarding daily care, and adjust expectations.* Schedule an appointment for 2 weeks. *She will need to be followed closely for the remainder of the pregnancy to determine whether there are other complications and to plan for delivery.*

Documentation   (date/time) Dr. Smith explained results of diagnostic testing. Crying, states "I don't know what I did wrong." States, "I don't know how to tell my husband." Written and verbal information provided regarding spina bifida. Provided information about local spina bifida support groups. Verbalizes understanding of information provided. Appointment scheduled for 2 weeks. J. Chi, LPN

Chapter 9

NCLEX-PN® ANSWERS

(1) 3. Outcome 2. Before 10 weeks the FHT cannot be heard by Doppler. It can be heard at 10 weeks, so 20 weeks is not the earliest it can be heard. (2) 2. Outcome 3. Repositioning the Doppler is correct. If the heart rate heard by the Doppler matches the woman's heart rate, the Doppler should be repositioned in order to pick up the fetal heart rate. Counting the rate for 30 seconds is incorrect because the rate should be assessed for a full minute. Calling the physician is incorrect because the data collected is inaccurate and should be reassessed. Document the rate in the client's chart is incorrect, because the heart rate is the maternal heart rate, not the fetal heart rate. (3) 3. Outcome 3. Drinking 1 quart of water 2 hours before the ultrasound is correct and will allow the bladder to be full so the lower uterine segment of the uterus can be visualized. Eating is not contraindicated prior to the procedure. Emptying your bladder right before the ultrasound will reduce clarity of the ultrasound images. Instructing the client not to drink fluids prior to the ultrasound is incorrect since it is important to have a full bladder for the procedure. (4) 1, 3, 6. Outcome 3. Raising the head of the bed slightly, placing a towel under the right hip, and positioning the client in the supine position are correct nursing interventions for preparing a client for an ultrasound procedure. Beginning intravenous infusion is not part of the procedure for an ultrasound. The supine position, not right side-lying, is necessary for the abdomen to be scanned. Inserting a Foley is not part of the ultrasound procedure. (5) 2. Outcome 3. Monitoring the fetal heart rate for 30 minutes is correct; it

is necessary to monitor for changes in fetal status following the procedure. Remaining on bed rest for 12 hours is incorrect; the client is encouraged to engage in light activity. Fluid intake is needed to replace the amniotic fluid. Encouraging the client to resume normal activity is incorrect because only light activity is recommended to help decrease uterine irritability. (6) 2. Outcome 5. "You may want to ask your husband to come with you" is correct and the most helpful statement by the nurse. Presence of a support person can help decrease anxiety. The statement "You should have read the information we gave you at your last visit" blames the client and blocks communication. The statement "It is not healthy for you to worry" does not offer any means for the client to stop worrying. The nurse's statement "The amniocentesis is a very quick procedure" avoids the client's feelings. (7) 4. Outcome 3. Asking the client to identify any fetal movement is correct and helps the nurse to interpret fetal heart rate pattern in relation to fetal movement. Taking slow deep breaths is not part of the NST procedure. Clients can be positioned in a recliner, in bed in semi-Fowler's, or side-lying during the NST. A full bladder is not necessary for an NST. (8) 1. Outcome 3. Four weeks is correct; this would place the client at 10 weeks' gestation, which is the appropriate time to schedule a chorionic villus procedure. Ten weeks is incorrect; 16 weeks' gestation is too late for a chorionic villus procedure but appropriate timing for an amniocentesis. Sixteen to 18 weeks' gestation is appropriate timing for an amniocentesis. Thirty weeks is incorrect; this would place the client at 36 weeks' gestation, which is appropriate timing for an NST. (9) 1. Outcome 2. A lab report revealing Rh-negative blood should be reported to the nurse so RhoGAM can be given to prevent Rh sensitization. A negative urine protein is a normal finding. Blood glucose of 90 mg/dL is within normal range and does not need to be reported. Hemoglobin level of 14 is within normal range and does not need to be reported to the charge nurse. (10) 2, 3, 5. Outcome 2. Electronic fetal monitor, low frequency vibrator, and ultrasonic gel are correct and essential for the ultrasound and NST, which are part of a biophysical profile. Amber-colored lab tubes are used during an amniocentesis to collect amniotic fluid. One percent lidocaine is used during an amniocentesis. A 2 × 2 gauze dressing and tape are used following an amniocentesis.

CARE PLAN HINTS

1. Other topics that might be discussed include talking to her children about the new baby, encouraging the other children to help with household chores so Jackie can get adequate rest, and how her life might change with a new baby in the house.

2. The LPN/LVN uses therapeutic communication techniques to help the client explore feelings. The LPN/LVN communicates empathy through touch, listening, and a caring attitude.

3. National and state organizations that offer support groups may be accessed through the Internet. Local groups may be accessed through these same sites.

CRITICAL THINKING CARE MAP

Subjective Data States "I don't know anything about all this electronic equipment. Is it safe for the baby?"

Objective Data Weight: 137 pounds (up 4 pounds since last month); blood pressure: 162/94; urine positive for protein; edema in feet and hands

Report Yes, to the supervising RN and primary care provider.

Interventions Place in semi-Fowler's position. *This position is best to obtain FHR and keep the heavy uterus off the vena cava. This position should add to client comfort and relaxation.* Teach about FHR increasing with fetal movement. *Provide information about why the test is being done. Information facilitates relaxation and fosters client participation.* Teach about safety of electronic monitoring equipment. *Information fosters client participation.* Apply belts and monitoring equipment. *Monitoring equipment is held in place by belts. The test may take 20 to 30 minutes and should begin as soon as possible.* Instruct to record fetal movements during NST. *Recording while movements occur ensures accuracy of the test. The client is able to participate in the evaluation of fetus.*

Documentation (date/time) States: "I don't know anything about all this electronic equipment. Is it safe for the baby?" Reassured of safety of NST procedure and equipment. Placed in semi-Fowler's position. Monitor equipment secured with abdominal belts. Instructed to record each fetal movement. NST completed in 20 minutes. Copy of NST placed in chart. Dr. Strong notified. J. Taylor, LPN

Chapter 10

NCLEX-PN® ANSWERS

(1) 4. Outcome 3. The mother should be encouraged to sleep on her side to prevent hypotension, and lying supine can cause supine hypotensive syndrome. Pressure on the bladder is coming from the inside. The womb is taking care of the fetus's comfort. Lying on the left side will not necessarily facilitate sleep. (2) 3. Outcome 2. Naegele's rule involves taking the first day of the last menstrual period, subtracting 3 months and adding 7 days, so the correct date using this rule would be February 13. The rest of the answers are incorrect using this formula. (3) 3. Outcome 4. The nurse should help the client explore options for the

pregnancy. The nurse cannot impose his/her ideas and bias on the client by telling her she "should have thought about that." By telling the client what to do or making decisions (appointment for abortion) for her, therapeutic communication is blocked. (4) 2, 4, 3, 5, 1. Outcome 2. The first priority is to assess the mother's vital signs to establish a baseline. Then assess the fetal heart rate. If they are within normal range, then continue to assess the mother. If you take the FHT first, and it is not normal, the stress will increase the mother's blood pressure and you will not know if the elevation is from the stress, hypertension, or both. All information would be reported to the physician. (5) 2, 4, 5. Outcome 2. Chadwick's sign, ballottement, and a positive pregnancy test are correct and considered probable signs of pregnancy since they could also be linked to other conditions. Uterine soufflé is incorrect since it is a positive sign and diagnostic of pregnancy since it is caused by increased maternal blood flow to the uterus. Abdominal enlargement is incorrect and considered a presumptive sign of pregnancy. Amenorrhea is incorrect since it is a presumptive sign of pregnancy. (6) 2. Outcome 2. 18 cm is correct. During the first 28 weeks of pregnancy appointments are scheduled every 4 weeks. Since fundal height enlarges by 1 cm/wk this would indicate at the next appointment the fundus would measure 18 cm. 16 cm is incorrect because the fundus is expected to enlarge by 4 cm during the next 4 weeks. 20 cm is incorrect because it places the fundal height outside of the normal range of expected growth. 22 cm is incorrect because it places the fundal height outside of the normal range of expected growth. (7) 4. Outcomes 2 and 3. BP of 136/88 is correct for a client in the second trimester. BP decreases slightly during the second trimester and therefore could be assessed as elevated and should be reported to the nurse. Temperature of 98.0 is incorrect since this is within normal range and does not need to be reported. Pulse of 130 bpm is incorrect since this is within normal range and does not need to be reported. Pulse rate can increase by 10 to 15 bpm during pregnancy. Respiration of 14 is incorrect since this is within normal range and does not need to be reported. (8) 1. Outcome 1. G3P2/T2A0 is correct. The client is currently pregnant and has had two previous pregnancies at term, which makes her a gravida 3 and para 2 with the outcome being term for the first two pregnancies. G2P2/T2A0 is incorrect because it does not include the current pregnancy in gravida. G2P1/T1A0 is incorrect because it does not count the current pregnancy in gravida or the second delivery in para or in term. G3P1/T1A0 is incorrect because it does not include the second delivery in para or in term. (9) 1. Outcome 4. "I will decrease intake of foods high in sodium" is correct and requires further teaching because

this applies to ankle edema not varicose veins. "When I am sitting, I will not cross my legs" is incorrect because it does not require further teaching and is an intervention for varicose veins. "I will start wearing support hose" is incorrect because it does not require further teaching and is an intervention for varicose veins. "After work, I will elevate my feet and rest" is incorrect because it does not require further teaching and is an intervention for varicose veins. (10) 3. Outcome 4. Avoiding knee high stockings is correct because this will prevent constriction behind the knee, which may interfere with circulation. Selecting shoes with heels is incorrect since high-heeled shoes create difficulty in maintaining balance, which could lead to falls. Flat shoes should be recommended. Wearing a loose-fitting bra is incorrect because it does not provide support to the breast as they enlarge during pregnancy. A supportive bra should be recommended. Wearing firm-fitting pants is incorrect and could cause constriction and edema in the lower extremities. Loose-fitting clothing should be recommended.

CARE PLAN HINTS

1. By 22 weeks, Mrs. Taylor's abdomen will be enlarging. Safety issues to discuss at this time include walking up and down stairs holding the hand rail, wearing low-heeled shoes, getting in and out of shower/bath tub.

2. At the next visit, Mrs. Taylor will be 26 weeks' pregnant. Signs of preterm labor must be discussed. It is also time to begin discussion regarding pain control during labor and preparation for breastfeeding.

3. The role of the LPN/LVN in providing care in the office is to collect data, answer questions, and support client decisions. The physician should be informed of all signs of complications. The RN or physician should approve all printed material prior to giving them to the client.

CRITICAL THINKING CARE MAP

Subjective Data   States tired, not sleeping all night.

Objective Data   BP 138/76, Resp 24, respiration shallow, slightly labored; lungs sounds clear.

Report   No. These are normal findings for a third trimester pregnancy.

Interventions   Teach need for additional rest in third trimester. Recommend frequent rest periods with feet elevated. Recommend afternoon naps. Discuss the need to get more child care.

Documentation   (date/time) Routine prenatal check. States tired and unable to sleep all night due to needing to void q 2 h. BP 138/76, Resp 24, respiration shallow, slightly labored; lungs sound clear. Discussed need for increased rest with legs elevated. States work responsibilities end in 1 week and will be able to rest more at that time. R. Cooper, LPN.

Chapter 11

NCLEX-PN® ANSWERS

(1) 4. Outcome 6. Although the mother needs instruction on the risk of propping the bottle, the first step is to learn more about the reason for propping the bottle. Propping a bottle deprives the infant of necessary bonding time. It can also be involved in choking. The client will be less likely to comply if the nurse simply tells her what to do. (2) 3. Outcome 6. The baby needs to take the entire areola into the mouth in order to release the milk from the mammary ducts properly and to prevent sore nipples. If only the nipple is taken, milk will not be expressed efficiently. It is a good idea to nurse on both sides at each feeding, though not necessarily for the same amount of time. Some babies may nurse less than 20 minutes per side. (3) 1. Outcome 3. All nutrients are important for a healthy diet but an inadequate amount of folic acid prior to pregnancy can have negative effects on the fetus. Folic acid taken 1 month prior to pregnancy can prevent neural tube defects. Adequate amounts of vitamin A are needed to improve vision. Proteins assist in brain growth and development. Potassium assists with fluid and electrolyte balance. (4) 1, 3, 4, 6, 7. Outcome 2. It is important to include foods high in iron to help increase RBCs. Vitamin C increases the absorption of iron in the intestines. Foods high in vitamin C include oranges, broccoli, and strawberries. Foods high in iron include hamburger, eggs, and green leafy vegetables such as broccoli. Milk is a good supply of protein but does not contain iron or vitamin C. White bread is a good source of carbohydrates but not a good source of vitamin C or iron. (5) 4. Outcome 4. Assessment of physical findings and lab work can identify nutritional deficiencies. Assessment finding of dull hair is an indication of poor nutritional intake. Moist mucous membranes is a healthy sign and indicate good nutrition. Hematocrit level of 34% and a hemoglobin level of 12 g/dL are within normal limits and indicate good nutritional intake. (6) 500. Outcome 4. An extra 500 calories are needed per day while breastfeeding. (7) 4. Outcome 2. Vitamin D helps absorb calcium in the body. If pregnant clients need to increase calcium they also need to increase the intake of vitamin D to aid in absorption of calcium. Vitamin A does not aid in the absorption of calcium. Vitamin B does not aid in the absorption of calcium. Vitamin C aids in the absorption of iron. (8) 2. Outcome 5. Colostrum contains a laxative that aids in the passage of meconium. Newborns sleep more hours than they are awake and are not dependent on the intake of colostrum.

Holding and cuddling during feeding aids in bonding not in digestion. Colostrum does not slow digestion, it is easily digested. (9) 1. Outcome 6. Sliding one finger into the corner of the newborn's mouth to break the suction is correct and prevents irritation and pulling on the nipple tissue. Sucking too long at the breast will cause irritation and sore nipples. Sliding the breast out of the newborn's mouth with two hands without breaking suction pulls on the tissue and causes irritation to the nipples. Pulling the newborn away from the breast without breaking suction pulls the nipples and causes irritation. (10) 3. Outcome 6. All bottles and nipples should be cleaned with a brush in soapy water only and thoroughly rinsed. Bottles and nipples can be boiled especially if there is a question about the safety of the water supply. Placing bottles and nipples in a dishwasher is incorrect. Vinegar is not recommended for washing bottles and nipples.

CARE PLAN HINTS

1. A review of normal nutrition should be discussed. She should receive instruction to increase her calorie intake by 500 calories, increase her fluid intake by 1,000 mL, and continue to take her prenatal vitamins.
2. The LPN should contact the supervising RN or the lactation nurse for assistance.
3. On a follow-up office visit, Maria should be questioned about her nutritional and fluid intake. Her weight should be obtained and compared to her predelivery weight. The baby's weight should be obtained and compared to the delivery weight.

CRITICAL THINKING CARE MAP

Subjective Data Money only for rent and food.

Objective Data Wt. 135 lbs; vital signs WNL, urine negative for protein; pale, thin.

Report Yes, report to the health care provider the information regarding living situation and referral to WIC. Report the pale, thin appearance and nurse's concern regarding nutritional stats.

Interventions Refer to WIC program. *WIC program can provide food vouchers to help ensure proper nutrition during pregnancy and for several years afterward.* Teach need for increased protein, lower carbohydrates in diet. *Eating adequate protein decreases risk of PIH.* Teach need for prenatal vitamins. *Helps ensure adequate nutrition.* Teach need for milk products. *Calcium and phosphorus are important for fetal development.* While a therapist may be needed to treat depression, this intervention does not relate to the nursing diagnosis.

Documentation (date) 0430 17-year-old single female admitted to clinic with 10 wk pregnancy. VS are WNL. Wt 135 lbs. Skin pale. Urine negative for protein. Appears thin.

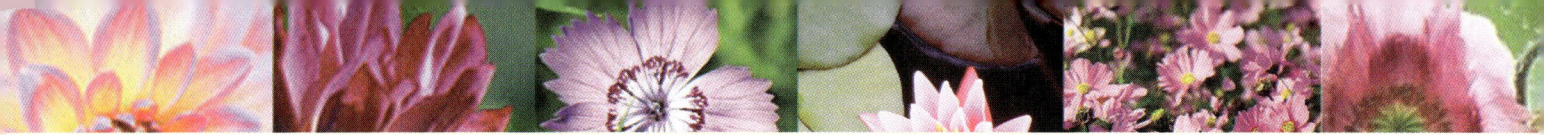

Crying. States she does not know what to do about pregnancy. States she barely has enough money to meet current expenses. Information provided regarding diet, prenatal vitamins, and WIC program. N. Cooper, LPN

Chapter 12

NCLEX-PN® ANSWERS

(1) 2, 3, 5. Outcome 2. Adolescent pregnancies are more typical when the adolescent has less supervision and carries more responsibilities at home. The offspring of adolescent mothers tend to become pregnant at an earlier age. Adolescents who are active in school activities and formulate goals for further education are less likely to become pregnant. (2) 1. Outcome 3. Hemoglobin level of 10 is correct because a level of 10 indicates iron deficiency anemia and is a physical risk for the young pregnant adolescent. Mild contractions at 38 weeks, menarche at age 13, and a blood pressure of 120/84 are normal findings and do not indicate a risk factor for this client. (3) 3. Outcome 6. Protein is correct because it is necessary for tissue growth in the adolescent and the fetus. Since the adolescent's diet is usually lacking in protein, it is important to increase foods high in protein during pregnancy. Fats, sugars, and starches provide less nutritious value than protein. (4) 1, 3. Outcome 6. Grief and guilt are correct because these are normal emotions for the adolescent who decides to terminate the pregnancy. It is unlikely that adolescents who terminate their pregnancies experience disbelief, joy, and doubt. Emotions need to be dealt with early to avoid lifelong mental health issues. (5) 1. Outcome 5. Typically teenagers who are from families that value education and are high achievers themselves will elect to have an abortion. In contrast, teenagers who decide to continue the pregnancy are from families who typically struggle financially, have a history of substance abuse, and whose mother became pregnant at an early age. (6) 2. Outcome 4. Placing the father's name on the birth certificate is correct because it ensures his rights related to paternity and may also encourage the father to accept responsibility for the baby. Having the father attend the birth or visit the baby in the hospital will not ensure his rights to paternity. (7) 1, 2, 5. Outcome 4. Adolescent males who engage in sexual relations earlier than females, have multiple partners, and have less formal education are correct. Usually the partners are at the same emotional level as the pregnant female. (8) 3. Outcome 3. Intrauterine growth retardation is correct because poor nutritional intake puts the adolescent at risk for intrauterine growth retardation. They are also at risk for preterm birth. Prolonged labor and dystocia are related to other factors. (9) 2. Outcome 7. During the early teen years,

providing accurate information about the responsibilities of sexual activity is correct because open communication about sex between the parent and teen decreases the chance for teens to become sexually active. Delaying and avoiding the issue of sex by encouraging teens to attend sex education class or providing reading material does not reduce the risk of teen pregnancy. (10) 4. Outcome 6. It is most important for the nurse to develop a trusting relationship with pregnant adolescents in the beginning. Once this has been established, the adolescent will feel more at ease with procedures and feel safe to problem solve and make decisions. Assessing attitudes toward pregnancy, evaluating socioeconomic situations, and identifying educational goals should be covered once a trusting relationship has been established.

CARE PLAN HINTS

1. Imbalanced **N**utrition: Less than Body Requirements related to low income; Interrupted **F**amily Processes related to being "kicked out" of parents home.
2. Janet should be referred to WIC and education programs for pregnant teens.
3. The nurse should talk with Janet in person or by phone weekly.

CRITICAL THINKING CARE MAP

Subjective Data Nausea and vomiting; missed period for 2 months.

Objective Data Mother requests information regarding options; positive pregnancy test; states does not know what to do.

Report Yes, to primary care provider.

Interventions Tell Maria what to expect during a pelvic exam. *A pelvic exam is part of the initial medical examination and Maria should be told what will happen in it.* Tell Maria what to expect with an ultrasound examination. *An ultrasound is used at the initial obstetric visit to confirm pregnancy. This data is important prior to planning care.* Provide Maria and her mother with information on nutrition. *Maria and her mother should have current information on nutrition to ensure adequate nutrients for Maria's growth and the growth of the fetus. Whether Maria carries the baby to term or chooses to terminate the pregnancy, she needs information about nutrition for her own development.* Give Maria prenatal vitamins. *Prenatal vitamins ensure adequate intake of vitamins for fetal development. Maria is probably around 8 weeks pregnant, and supplemental vitamins are needed at this time.* Provide Maria and her mother with written information about abortion, adoption, and services available for pregnant teens. *Maria and her mother will need to discuss and reach a decision about the pregnancy. Written information that they can take home and study will allow them time to make an informed decision.*

Documentation (date/time) 14-year-old female in with mother for nausea and vomiting every morning for 1 week. States she has not had a menstrual period for 2 months. Mother states she thinks daughter is pregnant. Urine positive for hCG. Instructed in pelvic exam and ultrasound. Instructed in use of prenatal vitamins. Written information provided regarding nutrition during pregnancy, adoption, abortion, and local services available for pregnant teens. Appointment made for 1 month. O. Ames, LPN

Chapter 13

NCLEX-PN® ANSWERS

(1) 3. Outcome 4. A client in shock would experience an increase in pulse and a decrease in blood pressure. The fetus would initially have an increase in pulse. A decrease in FHR would indicate fetal distress, but at 16 weeks' gestation, the health of the mother would have a higher priority. (2) 2. Erythroblastosis fetalis occurs when Rh-negative blood from the mother has been sensitized with Rh-positive blood. The mother's blood attacks the fetal blood. PG and LS ratio indicate fetal lung maturity. (3) 1. Outcome 4. Epigastric pain is a sign of worsening preeclampsia. A blood pressure of 138/90 and some dependent edema are not signs of worsening condition. (4) 4. Outcome 4. This client needs to be evaluated in a quiet, controlled environment. She is experiencing severe preeclampsia and is at risk for further complications and emergency treatment. Other rooms would not provide her with necessary observation. (5) 1. Outcome 2. Monozygotic or identical twins occur from one fertilized egg that divides into separate embryos. (6) 2. Outcome 4. An incomplete abortion is passage of the fetus but not the placenta. (7) 140 mg/dL. Outcome 2. A 1-hour glucose screen lab value of 140 mg/dL indicates possible gestational diabetes. (8) 1, 2, 4. Outcome 4. Discharge instructions for a client following a threatened abortion includes refraining from strenuous activity, avoiding sexual intercourse, and refraining on bed rest for several days. Returning to the clinic for a D & C is incorrect since a D & C is performed when a client experiences a missed abortion. A cerclage is incorrect because a cerclage is performed for habitual abortions caused by an incompetent cervix. (9) 3. Outcome 6. "If my husband had brought me to the hospital yesterday this would not have happened" is an example of a client experiencing the anger stage of the grief process. In the anger stage, clients often direct their anger to their spouse, health care providers, and/or other children. Staying in bed to make everything be all right is incorrect because it is an example of bargaining, trying to make a deal in hopes of preventing the loss. "We will join a support group" is incorrect; this client is experiencing the

acceptance stage by accepting their loss and offering to help others. "Tell me again, I can't believe what is happening" is incorrect because it is an example of a client experiencing the shock and disbelief stage by trying to process the information and needing to hear the information several times. (10) 1. Outcome 4. Performing a vaginal exam is correct because vaginal exams are contraindicated for clients with placenta previa. A vaginal exam poses a risk of dislodging the placenta, causing hemorrhage and possibly fetal death. Placing the client on complete bed rest is not contraindicated because this nursing strategy is necessary to help stop the bleeding. Administering betamethasone not contraindicated because this is the preferred medication to help the lung mature in case of premature birth. Preparing for a possible cesarean section is not contraindicated because this procedure may be necessary if the bleeding continues.

CARE PLAN HINTS

1. Because bacteria thrive in a high glucose environment, the woman with gestational diabetes is at risk for developing infections. She should protect herself from exposure to infectious diseases.

2. Because gestational diabetes increases the risk of preeclampsia and causes the fetus to be large, weekly nonstress tests are frequently ordered to monitor the fetus's well-being.

3. Because the fetus of a woman with gestational diabetes tends to be large, there is an increased risk that a cesarean birth will be required. The woman should be prepared for this possibility.

CRITICAL THINKING CARE MAP

Objective Data   Weight up 4 pounds in 2 weeks, BP 162/98, 2+ edema, 3+ proteinuria.

Subjective Data   States has headache; states vision is blurred; decreased urine output.

Report   Yes, to charge nurse. The LPN/LVN role in high-risk situations is to assist with client care. The RN should validate assessment and contact the primary care provider for orders.

Interventions   Obtain FHR by continuous monitoring. *Fetal assessment is a priority when the mother is experiencing complications.* Obtain BP on admission and every hour. *Frequent monitoring helps identify progression of the disorder and response to medical treatment.* Assess deep tendon reflexes and clonus every hour. *Hyperreflexia indicates CNS involvement and worsening of the disorder.* Position woman on left side. *Lying on left side prevents pressure on vena cava. Blocking the vena cava could decrease blood supply to fetus.* Teach need for decreased activity. *Activity can increase blood pressure leading to a worsening of preeclampsia.* Private room with limited visitors. *Client needs a quiet environment to decrease stimulation to the CNS.*

Documentation (date/time) Admitted to private room from clinic. BP 162/98, T 98.6, P 84, R 18. External fetal monitor applied. FHR 142. No contractions noted on monitor. Reflexes brisk, 1 beat clonus. 2+ pitting edema noted in feet and ankles. Urine 3+ for protein. States headache and blurred vision past 2 to 3 days. States urine output decreased. Instructed in need for rest in left lateral position with limited visitors. RN notified of condition. J. Joseph, LPN

UNIT III Thinking Strategically About …

CRITICAL THINKING

- How would you describe your headache? How would you rate the severity of your headache on a scale of 1 to 10?
- How does living with your parents impact your pregnancy?

COLLABORATIVE CARE

- She should be referred to the WIC program and any local agencies for pregnant single women.

MANAGEMENT OF CARE AND PRIORITIES IN NURSING CARE

- Hilda should be seen first, followed by Anna, and then Joyce.
- Hilda is at greatest risk due to the twin pregnancy and symptoms of preeclampsia. The obstetrician will want information regarding protein in the urine, reflexes, and FHR of both babies. You would need to obtain a health history from Anna. You would also anticipate needing to set her up for a pelvic examination, and possibly an ultrasound. She will need teaching about these procedures. Because Joyce is a routine checkup at 18 weeks, she will require some instruction, but will not require the same amount of care as the other clients.

DELEGATING

- The LPN in the office or clinic can perform routine office procedures and routine client teaching.

COMMUNICATION AND CLIENT TEACHING

- The most important thing to teach Joyce at this point of her pregnancy are the signs of preeclampsia.
- A copy of Hilda's entire prenatal records should be sent to the hospital. A verbal report should be given to the hospital nurse regarding Hilda's blood pressure, protein in the urine, headache, blurred vision, reflexes, and FHRs.

DOCUMENTING AND REPORTING

- Anna's LMP, history of sexually transmitted infections, information regarding anticipated support from Anna's family and the baby's father.

CULTURAL CARE STRATEGIES

- Hispanic women often obtain care from an older female relative instead of seeking professional health care. Praise Hilda for coming for help when she noted signs of complications.

Chapter 14

NCLEX-PN® ANSWERS

(1) 1. Outcome 2. Fetal cortisol production increases as the fetus matures and when sufficient, decreases the placental production of progesterone. As progesterone decreases, the estrogen levels in the placenta rise. Estrogen increases sensitivity of myometrium to oxytocin which is produced by the pituitary gland of the mother, and it is this oxytocin that causes the uterus to contract. (2) 1. Outcome 2. "Lightening" refers to the fetus having descended into the pelvis. The fetus moving downward relieves pressure on the diaphragm allowing the mother to breathe easier and thus feel "lighter"; however, now there is more pressure on the lower pelvis, which causes an increase in venous stasis resulting in lower extremity edema, bladder pressure and urge to void, and increased back pain. (3) 4. Outcome 2. A vertex position is the occiput presenting first. Forehead presentation is also referred to as brow or sinciput. Face presentation is referred to as mentum. Buttocks presentation is also called breech. (4) 3. Outcome 3. When the mother lies on her side, the contractions are less frequent, but of greater intensity. (5) 2. Outcome 3. The latent phase or first stage of labor is from the onset of contraction until the cervix is dilated 4 cm. The active phase is not part of stage two labor. The transition phase is part of stage one, not stage two, labor. The active phase of stage one labor is from 4 to 6 cm dilatation. (6) 4. Outcome 3. The average length of active labor (active phase of first stage) is 4 to 6 hours for the primigravida client. (7) 3, 5, 6. Outcomes 6 and 7. It is normal for the client to become irritable and sometimes angry at this stage of labor. It is important to teach the client simple relaxation and breathing. Warm soaks provide relief via muscle relaxation and diversion from contractions. The lateral position facilitates maternal/fetal circulation and relieves the stress on the back. The client is not to push actively until fully dilated at 10 cm. (8) 2. Outcome 4. Engagement occurs when the presenting part (usually the fetal head) enters the true pelvis. At this time, the presenting part is even with or below the ischial

spines and the fetus is no longer ballotable. **(9)** 1. Outcome 7. Any bleeding in excess of one pad saturated per hour in the fourth stage of labor/birth is considered abnormal. Any deviation from normal range should be reported to the registered nurse and physician. The fundus may need to be massaged and clots removed. **(10)** 1, 4, 5. Outcome 7. Assessing vaginal flow for amount and character, checking the fundus for position and firmness, and providing the mother with warm blankets are all appropriate interventions. Maternal vital signs need to be taken every 15 minutes for 1 hour. The mother is likely to feel chilled because of loss of liquid and hormonal changes; a cooling bath would not help.

CARE PLAN HINTS

1. The first priority is pain control. The second priority is frequent monitoring of labor progression and maternal/fetal well-being. *When the client and fetus are stable, the highest priority is pain control. Fetal heart rate, maternal vital signs, and evaluating contractions should be done every 30 to 60 minutes.*

2. Yes, Jane should be offered a whirlpool bath. *A warm whirlpool bath can help the client relax, easing discomfort and shortening labor. There are no symptoms presented that would indicate complications that would prevent a whirlpool bath.*

3. How rapidly Jane is progressing in labor should be considered before narcotics are administered. Most primigravida mothers can have narcotics when they are 8 to 9 cm dilated. *Narcotic analgesics will have an effect for at least 1 hour and may cause respiratory depression in the newborn. The second stage of labor for most primigravida mothers is 1 to 3 hours. Narcotics therefore can safely be administered at 8 to 9 centimeters.*

CRITICAL THINKING CARE MAP

Subjective Data   Obviously uncomfortable, moaning: having difficulty maintaining control.

Objective Data   Cervix 8 cm dilated, 100% effaced; station +2, BP 142/90; contractions every 3 minutes, lasting 90 seconds. Fetal heart rate 110; clear fluid draining from vagina.

Report   Yes, to supervising nurse. The LPN/LVN needs assistance when birth is near.

Interventions   Position on left side. *Prevents compression of the uterine arteries.* Encourage to breathe with each contraction. *Breathing helps with relaxation and prevents pushing until the cervix is dilated.* Prepare sterile field for delivery. *This is Alyce's second labor and birth. She is in transition and is expected to deliver fairly rapidly. It is best to prepare early.*

Documentation   0630 G2P1 presented by wheelchair to L&D. BP 142/90, FHT 110–120 bpm. Contractions q 3 min,

lasting 90 sec. Sterile vaginal exam done per RN. Cervix 8 cm dilated, 100% effaced. Fetus cephalic, at 2+ station. SROM 0600 clear fluid. Having difficulty keeping relaxed. J. Marshall, LPN

Chapter 15

NCLEX-PN® ANSWERS

(1) 4. Outcome 2. CBC is the number of blood cells of the client. APTT is used to evaluate the coagulation of the blood. The hormone hCG is produced by the embryo. **(2)** 2. Outcome 4. A major side effect of terbutaline is tachycardia. After initial stabilization, constant fetal monitoring and strict bed rest is not necessary. **(3)** 1, 2, 3, 4. Outcome 2. The nurse should use personal protective equipment when contacting any body fluids. Vaginal secretions and amniotic fluid can be present in the bath water. The newborn is considered contaminated with vaginal secretions and amniotic fluid until it is bathed. **(4)** 1. Outcome 4. The first priority is to assess maternal and fetal well-being. The second priority would be to assess the amount of bleeding and then to prepare for medical intervention. **(5)** 3, 4, 6. Outcome 4. A prolapsed cord is an emergency situation and necessitates emergency cesarean section. Trendelenburg position relieves pressure of the fetal head on the umbilical cord. It is important to document fetal heart rate, because fetal oxygenation is compromised. **(6)** 2. Outcome 2. Vaginal birth after cesarean (VBAC) is more likely to occur if the previous cesarean was due to malposition or malpresentation such as breech delivery. A vertical uterine incision with a previous cesarean places the client at risk for uterine rupture, so a cesarean would be necessary. A repeat cesarean will be scheduled for a client who experienced CPD with the previous pregnancy, because typically the second fetus is larger and would place the fetus at risk. If the size of the fetus is estimated to be large, a cesarean avoids problems associated with CPD. **(7)** 4. Outcome 4. The LPN/LVN monitors closely for hemorrhage. A precipitous delivery places the client at risk for hemorrhage due to possible rupture of the uterus or cervical and vaginal lacerations. Hyperthermia does not result from a precipitous delivery but may be associated with an infection. A urinary tract infection is associated with perineal trauma or poor perineal hygiene, not precipitous delivery. Back pain may be associated with the epidural injection site or poor body mechanics. **(8)** 4. Outcome 4. To accelerate fetal lung development, betamethasone 12 mg q 24 hours may be given 2 to 3 days prior to delivery. Magnesium sulfate is a tocolytic to stop preterm labor and to treat PIH. Ritodrine is a tocolytic that helps the uterus to relax. Brethine is a tocolytic to stop contractions associated with preterm labor. (9) 1. Outcome 2. Shoulder dystocia is common when the fetus is large in size, placing the newborn at risk for a broken clavicle. Forceps delivery increases the risk of facial trauma and facial paralysis. Vacuum extraction places the newborn at risk for intracranial hemorrhage and cranial fractures. Precipitous delivery increases the risk for fetal distress and fetal cerebral trauma. (10) 3. Outcome 4. When fetal heart rate decelerations occur, the LPN/LVN may assist by repositioning the mother on her side. Fetal scalp electrodes are applied by the registered nurse. The primary care provider is responsible for obtaining fetal blood samples. Rupture of membranes is the responsibility of the primary care provider.

CARE PLAN HINTS

1. The nurse could suggest reading a novel the client has always wanted to read, working on a self-directed study course for college credit, journaling about the pregnancy experience, writing family and friends, visiting with family or friends over the phone, doing crafts such as embroidery or knitting, or having phone conversations with other pregnant women who are on bed rest.

2. Home tocolytic or uterine monitoring allows the physician to determine if the treatment for preterm labor is successful. This monitoring works the same as uterine monitoring in the hospital. Abdominal belts and monitors detect uterine contractions and translate the data to graph paper. Some home tocolytic companies have the capacity to translate the data via the telephone to the physician.

3. Symptoms of preterm labor that need to be reported include regular uterine contractions, regular backache, ruptured membranes, loss of mucous plug, and decreased fetal movement. Vaginal bleeding and fever (first signs of infection) must also be reported.

CRITICAL THINKING CARE MAP

Subjective Data   States "the baby is coming."

Objective Data   Bulging membranes; crowning.

Report   Yes to supervising RN.

Interventions   Apply gentle pressure to support perineum. Instruct woman to breathe with each contraction. Instruct her not to push. Put on the emergency call light. Deliver baby if necessary.

Documentation   (date/time) Put call light on, stating "the baby is coming." Membranes bulging on perineum. Fetal head crowning. Perineum supported. Instructed to breathe and not push with contractions. RN summoned by emergency call light. Infant girl delivered by J Gilbert, RN. A. Mays, LPN.

UNIT IV Thinking Strategically About ...

CRITICAL THINKING

- What is the degree of distress? Can the distress be alleviated by position, oxygen, or medication? What is the impact of treatment on the other twin?
- Because a cesarean birth takes approximately 1 hour, a decision about a cesarean birth for Margaret should be made before Katy's surgery is started.

COLLABORATIVE CARE

- The nurses from a neonatal intensive care unit should be alerted to the possibility that one or both of the twins might need additional care. A lactation specialist should be contacted if Margaret plans to breastfeed the twins.

MANAGEMENT OF CARE AND PRIORITIES IN NURSING CARE

- Check Joan's room to be sure everything is ready for delivery, including setting up the delivery table if OK by facility policy. Check Sitka's room to be sure everything is in the room for the delivery. Do not set up a sterile field because delivery could be hours away. Assist in admitting and preoperative care of Katy. Prepare the operating room for a cesarean birth.
- This is Joan's third birth, and labor should progress rapidly. She is already 9 centimeters dilated and will be pushing soon. Preparing the room and delivery table now prevents a rush at time of delivery. Sitka is making progress but will probably have several hours of labor left. Making sure everything is in the room early allows time to obtain needed supplies. Assisting with Katy's admission allows the RN the opportunity to assist elsewhere.

DELEGATING

- All of the chart assembly, consents, ordering laboratory exams, and preparing the identification bands can be delegated. The LPN/LVN would need to double-check any orders and the identification bands.

COMMUNICATION AND CLIENT TEACHING

- Katy should be told that an emergency situation has developed with another client and that her surgery will need to be postponed for a short time. The name or exact problem should not be revealed due to confidentiality.
- Sitka and her husband should be told the induction is progressing normally and what to expect in the next few

hours. They should be praised for how well they are doing so far.

DOCUMENTING AND REPORTING

- If Joan suddenly has an uncontrollable urge to push, the LPN/LVN would put on the call light to summon the RN. The LPN/LVN would chart: Date/time "C" q 3 min, lasting 45 sec. Sudden urge to push. Encouraged to breathe through "C". RN notified. J. Prince, LPN.

CULTURAL CARE STRATEGIES

- Because the nurse may not be aware of cultural aspects of care of a pregnant Eskimo, the nurse should ask her if there is anything about her culture that she would like followed during her care.

Chapter 16

NCLEX-PN® ANSWERS

(1) 1, 2, 3, 5. Outcomes 4 and 5. A contracted uterus is firm at midline and there will only be a scant amount of vaginal discharge. When the uterus is not contracted, it will be soft or boggy on palpation and may be displaced to the right or left. Vaginal bleeding will be increased with clots possible. (2) 1. Outcomes 2 and 4. The fundus should decrease about 1 cm per day until it is located below the symphysis pubis. This is a normal finding for the second day postpartum. No further interventions (catheterization, administration of Lortab) need to be done. (3) 2. Outcomes 5 and 7. A precipitous birth generally causes more birth trauma to maternal tissues and delays healing. There is no association between primiparity and decreased rate of involution. An indwelling catheter would be more likely to aid the process of involution. There is no connection between nonimmunity to rubella and lack of involution. (4) 3. Outcome 2. Lochia alba is the term used for the creamy white or pale yellow discharge that occurs 2 to 3 weeks following birth. Rubra means red, serosa means pinkish, and nigra means black. (5) 3. Outcomes 4 and 6. Barrier methods are preferred for breastfeeding mothers. Hormonal methods may interfere with breast milk production. Although ovulation may be altered during breastfeeding, it is not a reliable way to prevent pregnancy. Insertion of an IUD may traumatize the healing uterus. (6) 2, 4, 5. Outcomes 5 and 6. It may take a while for peristalsis to return following birth, resulting in constipation. Exercise, increased fluids, and a diet high in fiber may assist in relieving constipation. Fluid restriction and soft foods might increase the problem. (7) 3. Outcome 3. Asian, Mexican, and African women will often avoid cold following birth;

therefore, the ice pack would be refused. It would not matter whether the cold was an ice pack or a chemical pack. The client might also ask to take a shower, but the refusal is the most likely answer. (8) 1. Outcomes 4, 5, and 7. Temperature over 100.4 F after the first 24-hour period could indicate infection. The nurse should assess the wound for signs of infection. She could assess for abdominal tenderness. These symptoms should be reported. Lortab would reduce pain, not fever. (9) 4. Outcome 3. Before the milk comes in, the breast contains colostrum, which drains from the breast and looks like a thin, yellow fluid. The breasts do not immediately become hard to palpate. Red streaks can be a sign of infection. Cracks are not expected within 24 hours of birth. (10) 2.5. Outcome 4. 250 mg (total dose) divided by 100 mg tablet (dose on hand) = 2.5 tablets.

CARE PLAN HINTS

1. The nurse should first address the client's pain and seek to manage it. Once the pain is effectively managed, the nurse discusses the risks of immobility to seek compliance. Assist the client with movement to minimize discomfort.

2. The nurse should discuss with the client's husband the risks of deep vein thrombosis and how mobility can effectively prevent them.

3. Although it is important for TED hose to remain in place to prevent deep vein thrombosis, the nurse must also assist the client with hygiene. Frequent assessment of the TED is important, especially in the postpartum client due to vaginal discharge. The TED hose should be removed daily and the legs assessed, bathed, and dried thoroughly before replacing them.

CRITICAL THINKING CARE MAP

Subjective Data   No prenatal care; states "leave the child in the nursery." Asks "will the nurses change the baby's diapers, I don't ever want to do that."

Objective Data   Positive drug screen. Did not make eye contact with baby.

Report   Yes, to the RN.

Interventions   Continue to assess mother–child interaction. Inquire about the child's name. Teach the client about caring for a newborn. Report to the charge nurse behaviors that indicate impaired bonding. Take the newborn into the client's room, even if she has not requested him.

Documentation   (date) 1215 19-year-old G1P1 transferred to room 315 via stretcher from labor and delivery following vaginal birth of viable male with second-degree episiotomy @ 1050. States "leave the baby in the nursery" and asks "will the nurses change the baby's diapers? I don't ever want to do that." No eye contact noted between client and newborn.

Newborn transferred to nursery. Charge nurse notified of client's questions and statement. N. Nance, LVN

UNIT V Thinking Strategically About …

CRITICAL THINKING
- How should the clients be divided among the LPNs/LVNs to ensure everyone has approximately the same responsibilities?

COLLABORATIVE CARE
- A lactation specialist who can communicate in Bosnian.

MANAGEMENT OF CARE AND PRIORITIES IN NURSING CARE
- Yvonne should be assessed first, then Natasha, and Jordan last.
- Yvonne is at greatest risk since she delivered most recently and has an IV, Foley catheter, and dressing that must be checked, and because English is her second language. Natasha would be the next priority since she delivered 4 hours ago and this is her first baby. Jordan would be last since she is stable and planning to be discharged in a few hours.

DELEGATING
- Vital signs, assisting with meal trays, helping Jordan to shower, and helping Natasha to the bathroom are tasks that can be delegated. The LPN/LVN should help Yvonne to get up for the first time in order to assess her ability to ambulate.

COMMUNICATION AND CLIENT TEACHING
- Because Jordan has other children, the nurse should review Jordan's knowledge regarding breast care, activity, and nutrition. Because she had a third-degree laceration, Jordan must be instructed in bowel care.
- Because Yvonne is a first-time mother and had an unscheduled cesarean birth, all aspects of self-care will need to be taught. These include personal hygiene, nutrition including adequate fluids, activity, and elimination; she must also be taught about signs of complications.

DOCUMENTING AND REPORTING
- As long as these clients remain stable, the RN only needs to be informed of any pertinent changes in their condition. The RN should be notified of plans to communicate with Yvonne in her native language if possible.

- Yvonne's assessment charting must include heart, lung, and bowel sounds, the location and consistency of the fundus, the condition of the abdominal dressing, the amount and color of vaginal drainage, the amount and color of urine, the condition of the IV site, the type of IV solution and the rate of infusion, and the settings on the PCA pump.

CULTURAL CARE STRATEGIES
- If possible an interpreter should be used when Yvonne is being assessed and when teaching is being provided. If an interpreter is not available, the nurse must use printed instructions to ensure accurate communication.

Chapter 17

NCLEX-PN® ANSWERS
(1) Gonorrhea and chlamydia. Outcome 5. Antibiotic ointment or solution is used to prevent eye infection from gonorrhea and chlamydia. (2) Irregular, 30 to 60. Outcome 4. Normal respirations may be irregular and are 32 to 48 per minute. (3) 2. Outcome 2. Jaundice in the newborn appearing 24 hours after birth is physiologic in origin. It should be documented but does not have to be reported. (4) 1. Outcomes 3 and 4. Newborns frequently have blue hands and feet at birth due to slow circulation. The condition may last a few hours to a few days. (5) 2. Outcome 6. Flaring nostrils, grunting respirations, and retractions are early signs of respiratory distress. Cyanosis indicates hypoxia. (6) 1. Outcome 5. The penis needs to be cleaned with plain water. Alcohol will cause pain and will irritate the incision line. (7) 2. Outcome 3. Priority for this newborn is the administration of oxygen. This score may be due to hypoventilation and hypoxia resulting from the administration of a narcotic agent given to the mother during labor. Measuring head and chest circumference would not be implemented first and is most often assessed in the nursery. Immediate resuscitation is performed on newborns with an Apgar score of 0 to 3. Administration of vitamin K does not take priority over the administration of oxygen but is done after the newborn has stabilized. (8) 3. Outcome 4. A mature newborn has a popliteal angle less than 90 degrees compared to a premature newborn with a popliteal angle of 180 degrees. Extended body position at rest is more characteristic of a premature newborn compared to a mature newborn with flexed body position at rest. The elbow crosses the midline in a preterm newborn when the arm is moved in front of the neck. Due to subcutaneous fat on a mature newborn the elbow will not cross the midline. The skin of a preterm newborn is transparent with numerous blood vessels.

(9) 1. Outcome 4. The rooting reflex allows the newborn to turn his/her head in the direction of the food when the cheek is stroked. The palmer grasp reflex does not assist with feeding but allows the newborn to grasp objects when placed in the hand. The tonic neck reflex does not assist with feeding but allows the newborn to extend the arm and leg on the side in which the head is turned. The Moro reflex does not assist with feeding but occurs when the newborn has a sense of falling at which time the newborn will quickly extend the arms and flare the fingers to form a "C" with the thumbs and first finger. (10) 2. Outcome 2. A high-pitched cry should be reported to the nurse for further investigation. A healthy cry is usually strong, lusty, and medium pitched. A healthy newborn voids 8 to 10 times per day. Head circumference ranges from 32 to 37 cm. An anterior fontanel that is firm and flat is a normal finding in a healthy newborn.

CARE PLAN HINTS

1. The nurse's assessment of stable vital signs, equal extremity movement and intact reflexes should be shared with parents. Parents should be instructed to call the nurse if the assessment changes.

2. It is the primary care provider's responsibility to inform parents of long-term effects of cranial trauma. Unless the newborn exhibits signs of cranial trauma before discharge, the primary care provider may choose not to alarm parents of potential long-term effects.

3. Isaiah will be monitored for normal growth and development milestones at each well-clinic visit. Less than normal growth and development might signal a problem.

CRITICAL THINKING CARE MAP

Subjective Data None. *Subjective data are what the client tells the nurse. The newborn cannot verbalize complaints.*

Objective Data Respiration 64/min, temperature 97.2°F (36.2°C), mother received morphine sulfate 2 hours ago, flaring nostrils, grunting respirations.

Report Yes, report to the charge nurse. If the newborn's condition does not improve within a few minutes or retractions become apparent, the primary care provider should be notified.

Interventions Suction airway. Mucus in the airway can cause respiratory distress. Place under radiant warmer. Hypothermia can cause respiratory distress in the newborn. Administer Narcan (naloxone hydrochloride). *The newborn may have respiratory depression from the morphine sulfate the mother received during labor. The facility policy and doctor's order should be followed.* Apply pulse oximeter. *Data from pulse oximeter is helpful in monitoring the degree of respiratory distress.* Monitor vital signs every hour. *The condition of the newborn should be evaluated at least every hour. More frequent monitoring may be warranted to evaluate the effectiveness of treatment.*

Documentation (date/time) T 97.2, R 64. Nasal flaring and grunting respirations noted. Airway suctioned with bulb syringe. Small amount clear mucus obtained. Placed under radiant warmer, temperature probe applied to abdomen. Pulse oximeter applied to R foot. O$_2$ Sat 93%. Charge nurse notified. O. Shaud, LPN

Chapter 18

NCLEX- PN® ANSWERS

(1) 2. Outcome 3. The father needs some time to adjust to his son's spinal anomaly. Simple answers to questions at this point are the best response. More in-depth information will be given once the doctor has determined the extent of the defect. (2) 2, 3, 6. Outcome 2. Proper technique for suctioning with a bulb syringe includes placing the bulb syringe into the buccal cavity to prevent eliciting the gag reflex, suctioning the mouth first, and rinsing the bulb syringe with water. The newborn is placed in the supine position. The nares are suctioned after the mouth is suctioned. It is important to remember to depress the bulb syringe prior to inserting into the oral cavity or nares. (3) 3. Outcome 3. Newborns diagnosed with fetal alcohol syndrome are poor eaters and often fussy, therefore immediate care will focus on nutritional support. Respiratory problems are not common in newborns with fetal alcohol syndrome. Genitourinary conditions are usually caused by congenital conditions rather than fetal alcohol syndrome. Monitoring blood transfusions are more common in newborns who have hyperbilirubinemia. (4) 1. Outcome 3. Aspiration of meconium during birth places newborns at a risk for developing persistent pulmonary pneumonia. Low surfactant level places the newborn at risk for respiratory problems since surfactant is needed to maintain the patency of the alveoli. High oxygen levels administered following birth places the newborn at risk for retinopathy. Mechanical ventilation places the newborn at risk for bronchopulmonary dysplasia. (5) 1. Outcome 3. Bulging of the anterior fontanel indicates possible hydrocephalus. When the anterior fontanel is sunken in, dehydration is suspected. Normal head circumference is between 32 and 37 cm, typically with hydrocephalus the head circumference is larger than normal. Herniation of the meninges through the vertebral defect indicates a meningocele. (6) 2. Outcome 3. To encourage muscle development in a high-risk newborn, the extremities should be able to move freely as much as possible. Blankets are restrictive and should be removed so active or passive range of motion can be performed. Body temperature can be controlled by radiant heat above the

bassinette not the blanket alone. Too many wires attached to the newborn has nothing to do with wrapping a blanket around a high-risk newborn. Good communication is always an important part of nursing; saying "Don't worry we are taking good care of your newborn" avoids the mother's concerns. (7) 3. Outcome 3. Projectile vomiting is a symptom of pyloric stenosis caused by the hypertrophy of the pyloric sphincter resulting from an obstruction. This is corrected by surgery. A hernia is a protrusion of intestines in the abdominal wall or pelvic muscles and does not cause projectile vomiting. Imperforate anus occurs when the opening of the colon does not develop, causing lower intestinal and oftentimes urinary problems. Omphalocele is not associated with projectile vomiting. (8) 1, 2, 4, 6. Outcome 3. The classic symptoms of Down syndrome include microcephaly, wide short neck, simian line along short broad hands, and epicanthal folds. Facial anomalies are characteristic of newborns with fetal alcohol syndrome. Macrocephaly is common in newborns who have hydrocephalus. (9) 2. Outcome 3. "My baby likes it when we stroke her arms and legs" indicates that the parents are bonding and comfortable touching the newborn. "It must not be good to touch my baby since she is so sick" indicates that the parents may have anxiety about their newborn. "We will schedule our visits after the nurses have completed all treatments" indicates that they have not bonded and are not comfortable being present during the care of their newborn. "We do not need to participate in a support group since our baby will recover quickly" indicates that they may not have accepted the long-term needs for their high-risk newborn. (10) 1. Outcome 3. Pathological jaundice is most commonly caused by Rh incompatibility causing the breakdown of RBC prior to delivery, resulting in jaundice occurring within the first 24 hours after birth. Pathological jaundice due to Rh incompatibility occurs when the newborn is Rh positive and the mother is Rh negative. Physiological jaundice usually occurs around 2 or 3 days after birth and is due to the immature liver being unable to breakdown bilirubin. Normal newborn hematocrit levels range from 44% to 65%.

CARE PLAN HINTS

1. The nurse should provide the same teaching for Jeremy's as for any other new parent including skin care, umbilical cord care, and nutrition. If his mother wants to breastfeed, she may be taught to nurse in the NICU if Jeremy is stable enough. Otherwise, she will be taught to pump her breast for a few days until Jeremy is strong enough to nurse.
2. Besides the routine discharge teaching of a newborn, the parents should be taught to care for his incision and to

administer medications, including actions and side effects.
3. The role of the LPN/LVN in providing care in the NICU is one of assisting the RN and other health care professionals. Because the LPN/LVN may be providing care at the bedside, parent teaching is often informal in nature, answering questions and demonstrating procedures.

CRITICAL THINKING CARE MAP

Subjective Data   None. *Newborn is unable to provide subjective data.*

Objective Data   Temperature 99° F; irritable; no drainage from meningocele; moving all extremities; 1 cm meningocele in lumbar spine.

Report   Yes, to the supervising RN.

Interventions   Prone position; wet sterile dressing to meningocele; radiant warmer; neuro assessment every hour.

Documentation   (date/time) 38 week gestation female admitted to NICU following spontaneous vaginal delivery. Placed under radiant warmer, temperature probe in place on back. 1 cm meningocele noted on lumbar spine. No drainage from meningocele. Moving all extremities. Muscle tone strong. Prone position maintained. Sterile saline saturated 4 × 4's placed over meningocele. RN notified of assessment findings. A. McDonald, LPN

UNIT VI Thinking Strategically About …

CRITICAL THINKING

- When reporting to the next nurse about client condition, begin with the infant's name, gender, age in hours, history of labor/delivery, complications since birth, current assessment findings, and pertinent care needed during the next shift.

COLLABORATIVE CARE

- The discharge planner should be contacted to ensure that all the legal documents have been completed to allow the adoptive parents to remove the infant from the hospital.

MANAGEMENT OF CARE AND PRIORITIES IN NURSING CARE

- Report is usually given in order by room number of the mother. If that is not the routine of the specific unit, report on John, Amanda, and Jeremiah in order.

- John is the greatest risk because of his birth time and the preprocedure care needed. Amanda and Jeremiah are both stable but because Amanda is younger, give report on her first.

DELEGATING
- Be sure the CNA has documented all care provided. For example, check that all voiding and BMs have been recorded.

COMMUNICATION AND CLIENT TEACHING
- The adoptive parents will need teaching about all routine newborn care, including feeding, diapering, bathing, and cord care. Safety teaching should include positioning on back to sleep, use of car seats, and not leaving the infant unattended on high surfaces.

- Parents should be informed of Jeremiah's daily weight gain, feeding, and elimination. They should be encouraged to provide all daily care.

DOCUMENTING AND REPORTING
- The RN should be informed about how well he nursed after the circumcision, the amount of bleeding from the circumcision site, and his voiding and stooling.
- John's assessment must include alert state; cry; heart; lung, and bowel sounds; condition and care of the umbilical cord; condition and care of the circumcision; and elimination.

CULTURAL CARE STRATEGIES
- Circumcision in the Jewish culture is a religious ceremony performed on the 8th day of life. The ceremony may be performed in the hospital or in the home environment.

Newborn Rating Scales, Growth Charts, and Immunization Schedule

NEWBORN MATURITY RATING & CLASSIFICATION

ESTIMATION OF GESTATIONAL AGE BY MATURITY RATING
Symbols: X - 1st Exam O - 2nd Exam

NEUROMUSCULAR MATURITY

	−1	0	1	2	3	4	5
Posture							
Square Window (wrist)	>90°	90°	60°	45°	30°	0°	
Arm Recoil		180°	140°–180°	110°–140°	90°–110°	<90°	
Popliteal Angle	180°	160°	140°	120°	100°	90°	<90°
Scarf Sign							
Heel to Ear							

Gestation by Dates _____ wks

Birth Date _____ Hour _____ am pm

APGAR _____ 1 min _____ 5 min

MATURITY RATING

score	weeks
−10	20
−5	22
0	24
5	26
10	28
15	30
20	32
25	34
30	36
35	38
40	40
45	42
50	44

PHYSICAL MATURITY

Skin	sticky friable transparent	gelatinous red, translucent	smooth pink, visible veins	superficial peeling &/or rash, few veins	cracking pale areas rare veins	parchment deep cracking no vessels	leathery cracked wrinkled
Lanugo	none	sparse	abundant	thinning	bald areas	mostly bald	
Plantar Surface	heel-toe 40–50 mm:−1 <40 mm:−2	>50 mm no crease	faint red marks	anterior transverse crease only	creases ant. 2/3	creases over entire sole	
Breast	imperceptible	barely perceptible	flat areola no bud	stippled areola 1–2 mm bud	raised areola 3–4 mm bud	full areola 5–10 mm bud	
Eye/Ear	lids fused loosely:−1 tightly:−2	lids open pinna flat stays folded	sl. curved pinna; soft; slow recoil	well curved pinna; soft but ready recoil	formed & firm instant recoil	thick cartilage ear stiff	
Genitals male	scrotum flat, smooth	scrotum empty faint rugae	testes in upper canal rare rugae	testes descending few rugae	testes down good rugae	testes pendulous deep rugae	
Genitals female	clitoris prominent labia flat	prominent clitoris small labia minora	prominent clitoris enlarging minora	majora & minora equally prominent	majora large minora small	majora cover clitoris & minora	

SCORING SECTION

	1st Exam = X	2nd Exam = O
Estimating Gest Age by Maturity Rating	_____Weeks	_____Weeks
Time of Exam	Date _____ Hour_____ am pm	Date _____ Hour_____ am pm
Age at Exam	_____ Hours	_____ Hours
Signature of Examiner	_____ M.D./R.N.	_____ M.D./R.N.

Figure A-1. ■ The Ballard Newborn Rating Scale is used to determine gestational age after birth. Reprinted from Ballard, J. L., Khoury, J. C., Wedig, L., Eilers-Walsman, B. L., & Lipp, R. (1991). New Ballard score, expanded to include extremely premature infants. *Journal of Pediatrics, 119*(3), 417–423, with permission from Elsevier Inc.

CLASSIFICATION OF NEWBORNS—
BASED ON MATURITY AND INTRAUTERINE GROWTH

Symbols: X-1st Exam O-2nd Exam

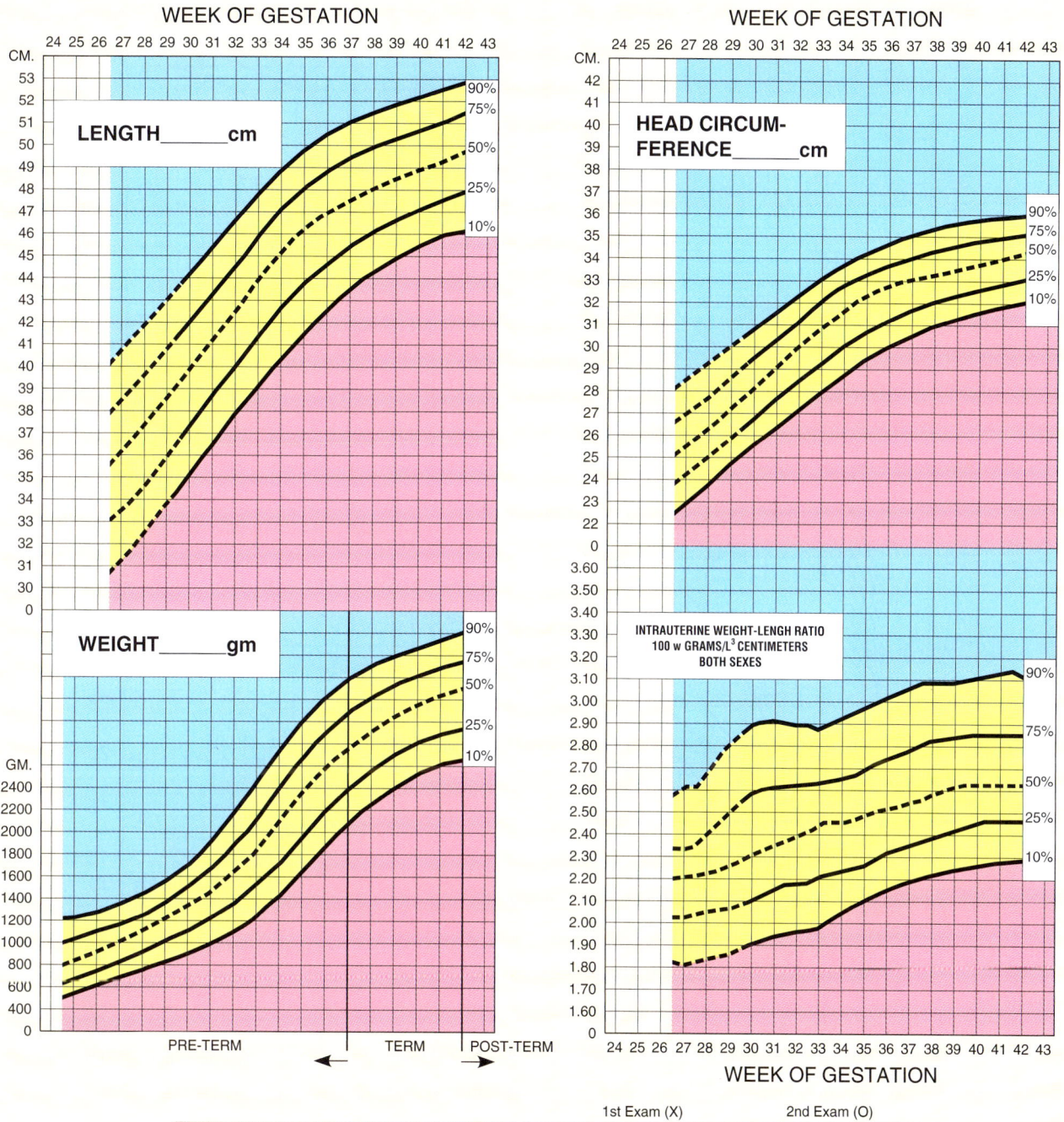

	1st Exam (X)	2nd Exam (O)
LARGE FOR GESTATIONAL AGE (LGA)		
APPROPRIATE FOR GESTATIONAL AGE (AGA)		
SMALL FOR GESTATIONAL AGE (SGA)		
Age at Exam	hrs	hrs
Signature of Examiner	M.D.	M.D.

Figure A-2. ■ Classification of newborns based on maturity and intrauterine growth. *Sources:* Adapted from Lubchenco, L.O., Hansman, C., & Boyd, E. (1966). Intrauterine growth in length and head circumference as estimated from live births at gestational ages from 26 to 42 weeks. *Pediatrics, 37,* 403–408; Battaglia, F.C., & Lubchenco, L.O. (1967). A practical classification of newborn infants by weight and gestational age. *Journal of Pediatrics, 71,* 159.

Birth to 36 months: Boys
Length-for-age and Weight-for-age percentiles

NAME _____

RECORD # _____

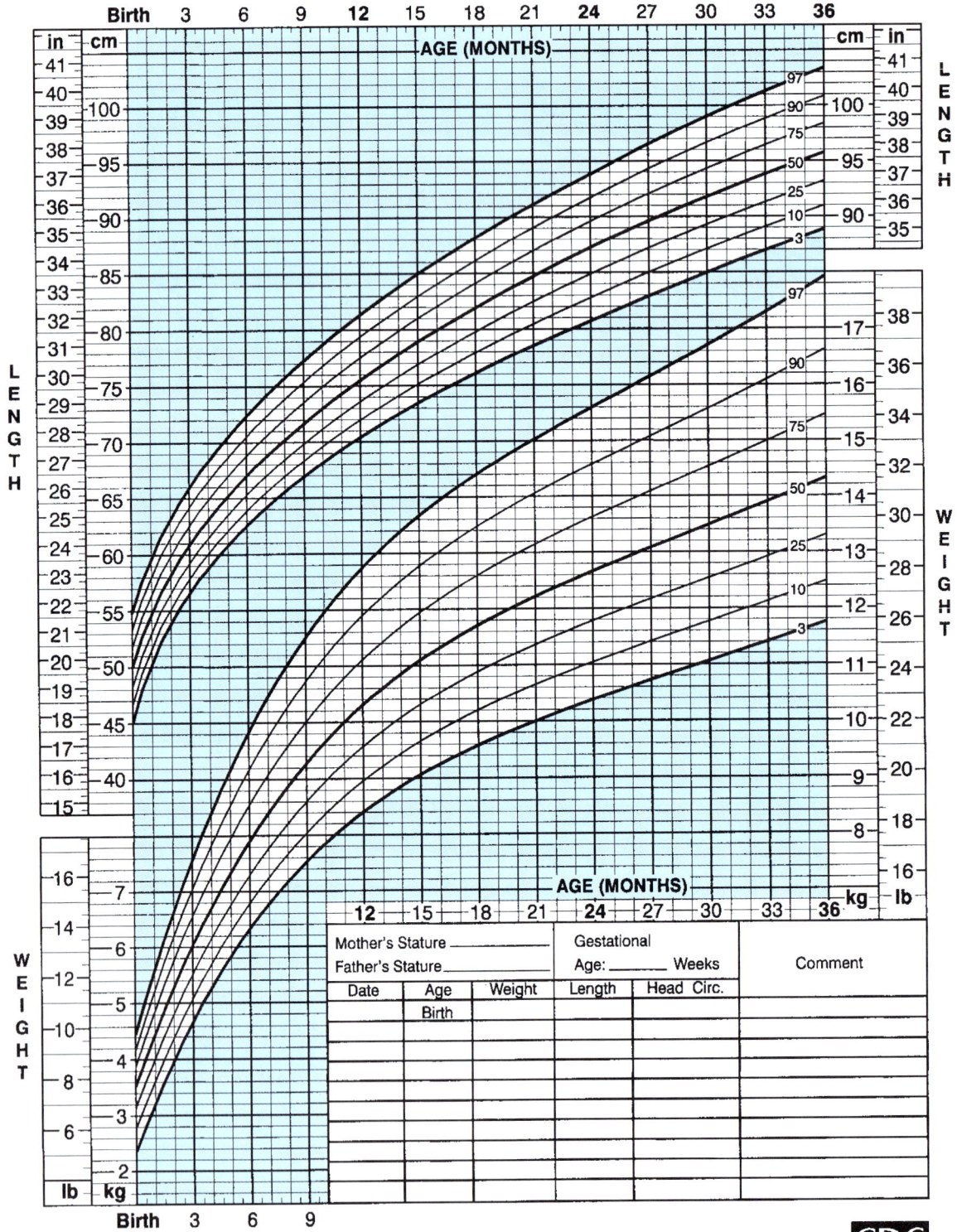

Revised April 20, 2001.
SOURCE: Developed by the National Center for Health Statistics in collaboration with
the National Center for Chronic Disease Prevention and Health Promotion (2000).
http://www.cdc.gov/growthcharts

CDC

Figure A-3. ■ Physical growth percentiles for length and weight—boys: birth to 36 months. From CDC, 2001. www.cdc.gov/growthcharts

Birth to 36 months: Boys
Head circumference-for-age and Weight-for-length percentiles

NAME _____

RECORD # _____

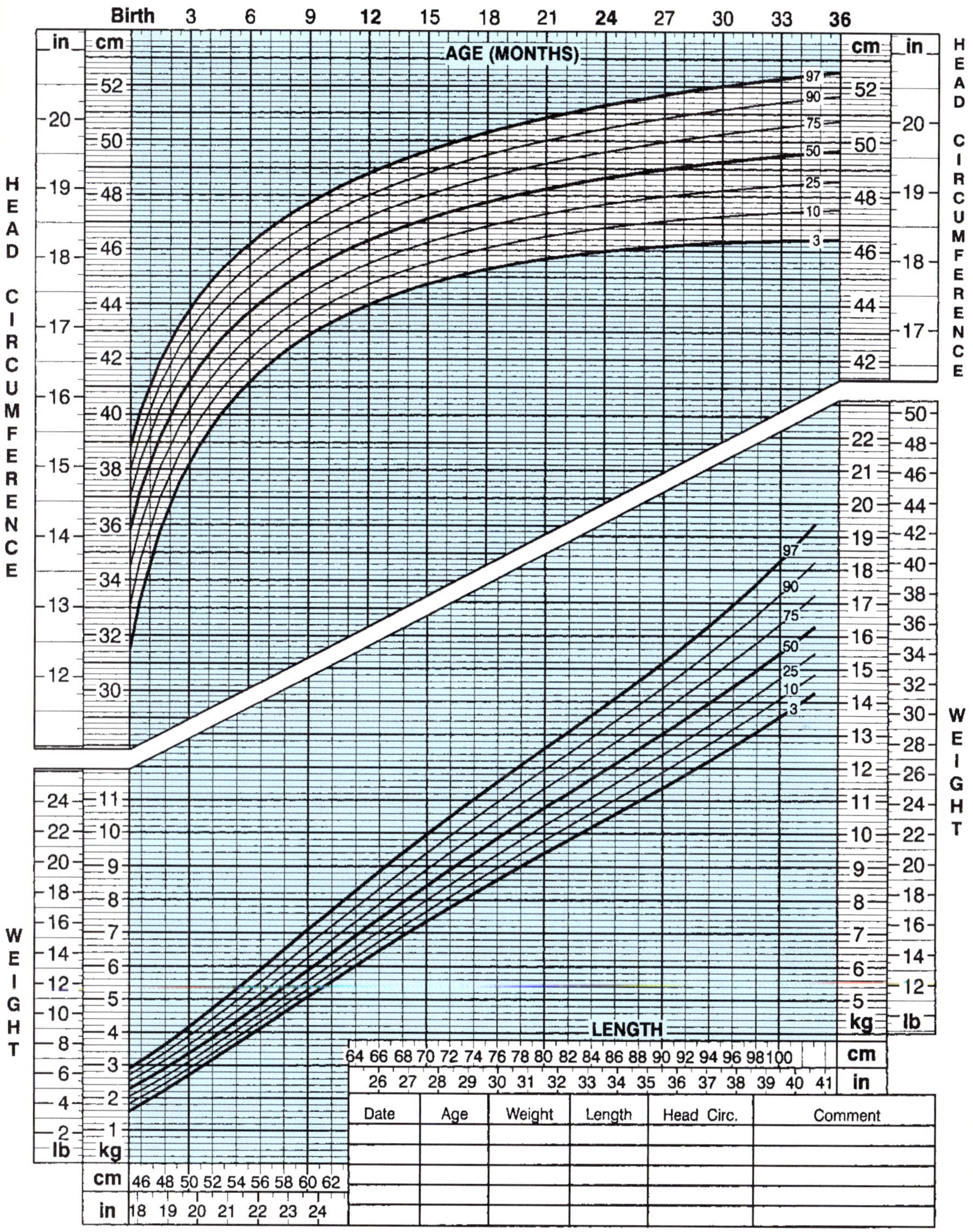

AGE (MONTHS)

Birth 3 6 9 12 15 18 21 24 27 30 33 36

HEAD CIRCUMFERENCE

97
90
75
50
25
10
3

LENGTH

| cm | 64 66 68 70 72 74 76 78 80 82 84 86 88 90 92 94 96 98 100 |
| in | 26 27 28 29 30 31 32 33 34 35 36 37 38 39 40 41 |

Date	Age	Weight	Length	Head Circ.	Comment

WEIGHT

| cm | 46 48 50 52 54 56 58 60 62 |
| in | 18 19 20 21 22 23 24 |

SOURCE: Developed by the National Center for Health Statistics in collaboration with the National Center for Chronic Disease Prevention and Health Promotion (2000).
http://www.cdc.gov/growthcharts

CDC

Figure A-4. ■ Physical growth percentiles for head circumference, weight for length—boys: birth to 36 months. From CDC, 2001. www.cdc.gov/growthcharts

Birth to 36 months: Girls
Length-for-age and Weight-for-age percentiles

NAME _____

RECORD # _____

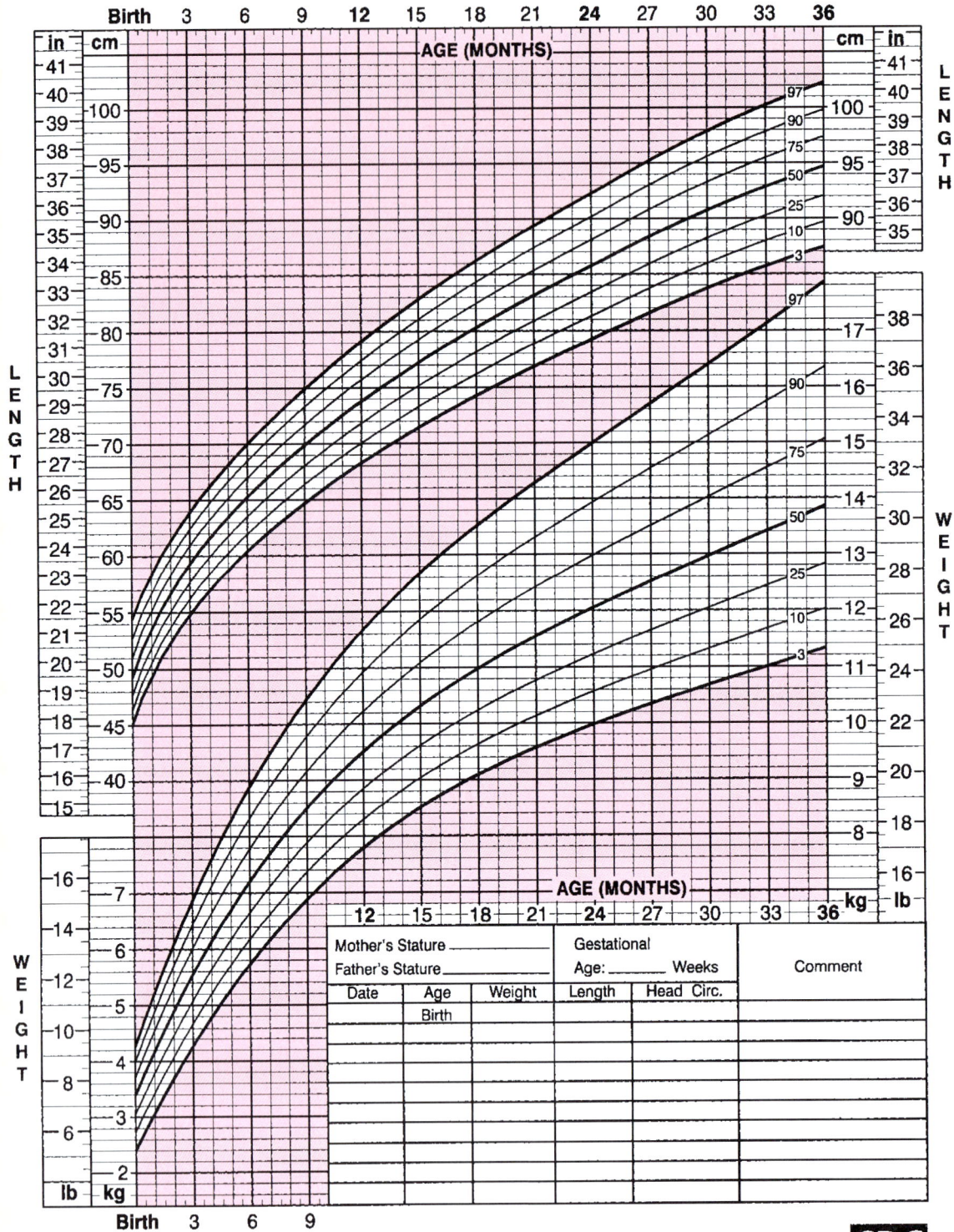

Revised April 20, 2001.
SOURCE: Developed by the National Center for Health Statistics in collaboration with
the National Center for Chronic Disease Prevention and Health Promotion (2000).
http://www.cdc.gov/growthcharts

CDC

Figure A-5. ■ Physical growth percentiles for length and weight—girls: birth to 36 months. From CDC, 2001.
www.cdc.gov/growthcharts

Birth to 36 months: Girls
Head circumference-for-age and
Weight-for-length percentiles

NAME _____

RECORD # _____

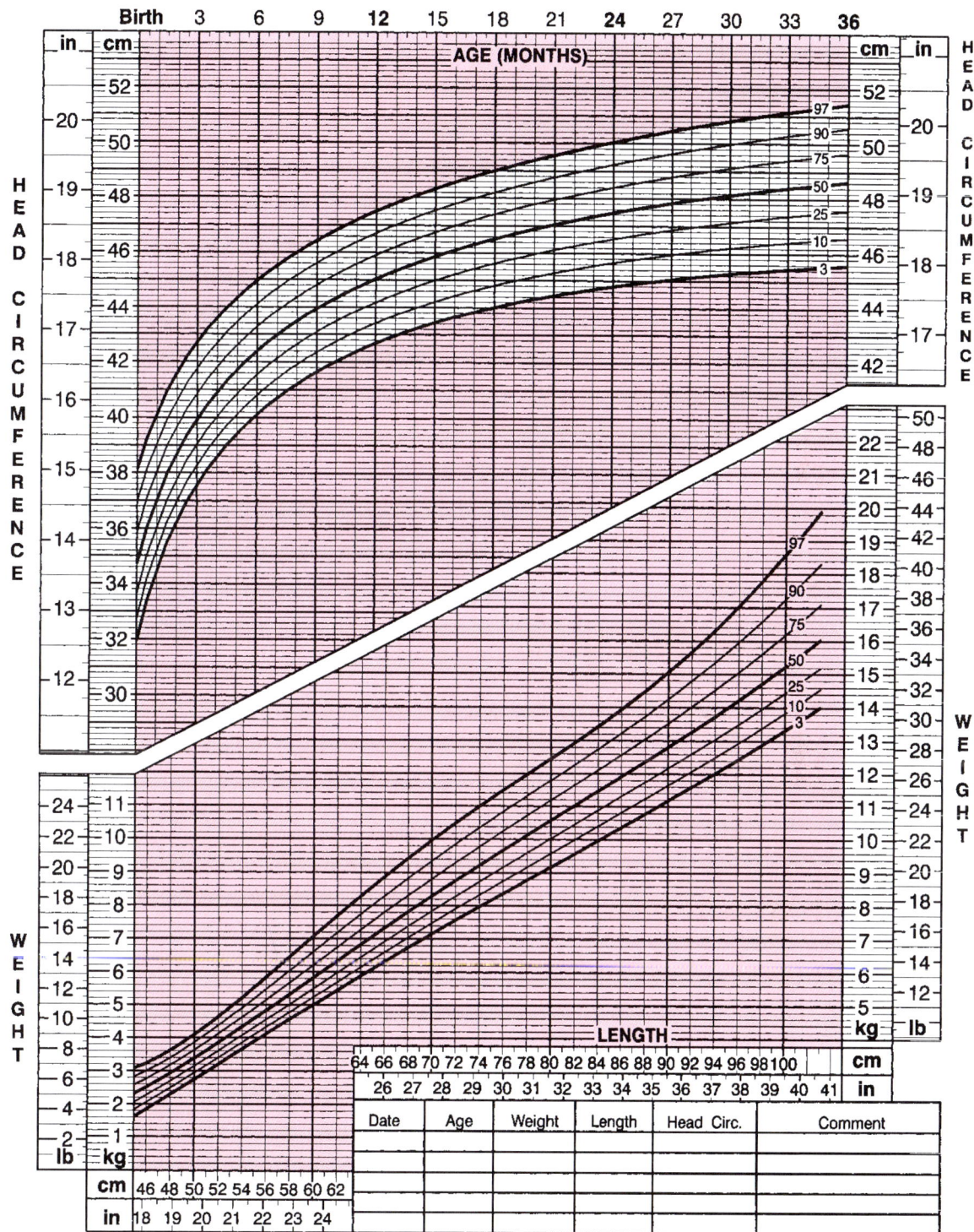

SOURCE: Developed by the National Center for Health Statistics in collaboration with
the National Center for Chronic Disease Prevention and Health Promotion (2000).
http://www.cdc.gov/growthcharts

CDC

Figure A-6. ■ Physical growth percentiles for head circumference, weight for length—girls: birth to 36 months. From CDC, 2001. www.cdc.gov/growthcharts

Recommended Childhood and Adolescent Immunization Schedule UNITED STATES • 2006

Vaccine ▼ / Age ▶	Birth	1 month	2 months	4 months	6 months	12 months	15 months	18 months	24 months	4–6 years	11–12 years	13–14 years	15 years	16–18 years
Hepatitis B[1]	HepB	HepB[1]		HepB[1]		HepB					HepB Series			
Diphtheria, Tetanus, Pertussis[2]			DTaP	DTaP	DTaP		DTaP	DTaP		DTaP	Tdap	Tdap	Tdap	
Haemophilus influenzae type b[3]			Hib	Hib	Hib[3]	Hib	Hib							
Inactivated Poliovirus			IPV	IPV		IPV	IPV			IPV				
Measles, Mumps, Rubella[4]						MMR	MMR			MMR		MMR		
Varicella[5]						Varicella	Varicella				Varicella			
Meningococcal[6]									MPSV4		MCV4		MCV4	MCV4
Pneumococcal[7]			PCV	PCV	PCV	PCV	PCV		PCV	PCV	PPV			
Influenza[8]					Influenza (Yearly)					Influenza (Yearly)				
Hepatitis A[9]										HepA Series				

Vaccines within broken line are for selected populations

■ Range of recommended ages   ■ Catch-up immunization

■ Immunization schedule for infancy through adolescence.   ■ 11–12 year old assessment

This schedule indicates the recommended ages for routine administration of currently licensed childhood vaccines, as of December 1, 2005, for children through age 18 years. Any dose not administered at the recommended age should be administered at any subsequent visit when indicated and feasible. ■ Indicates age groups that warrant special effort to administer those vaccines not previously administered. Additional vaccines may be licensed and recommended during the year. Licensed combination vaccines may be used whenever

any components of the combination are indicated and other components of the vaccine are not contraindicated and if approved by the Food and Drug Administration for that dose of the series. Providers should consult the respective ACIP statement for detailed recommendations. Clinically significant adverse events that follow immunization should be reported to the Vaccine Adverse Event Reporting System (VAERS). Guidance about how to obtain and complete a VAERS form is available at www.vaers.hhs.gov or by telephone, 800-822-7967.

Figure A-7. ■ Immunization schedule for infancy through adolescence.

Appendix III

Common Conversions and Lab Values

Pregnant and Nonpregnant Laboratory Values

TEST	PREGNANT VALUES	NONPREGNANT VALUES
Hematocrit (%)	32–42	37–47
Hemoglobin (g/dL)	10–14	12–16
Platelets (mm³)	Significant increase 3–5 days after birth	150,000–350,000
White blood cells (mm³)	5,000–15,000	4,500–10,000
Fibrinogen (mg/dL)	Up to 600	175–400
Serum glucose (mg/dL)	65 (fasting); less than 140 (2 hours PP)	70–80
Sodium (mEq/L)	135–145	135–145
Potassium (mEq/L)	3.5–5.1	3.5–5.1
Chloride (mEq/L)	100–108	100–108
Bicarbonate (mEq/L)	22–26	22–26
Calcium (mg/dL)	Falls 10% by term	8.5–10.5

Apgar Score

SIGN	SCORE 0	SCORE 1	SCORE 2
Heart rate	Absent	Slow—less than 100	Over 100
Respiratory rate	Absent	Slow— irregular	Good crying
Muscle tone	Flaccid	Some flexing of extremities	Active motion
Reflex irritability	None	Grimace	Vigorous cry
Color	Pale blue	Body pink, extremities blue	Completely pink (if light skinned); absence of cyanosis (if dark skinned)

Score: 0–4 requires resuscitation efforts; 4–7 requires administration of oxygen and rubbing the back to stimulate breathing; 8–10 requires no special attention.

Selected Common Conversions between English and Metric Measurements

1 g = 1 mL (used when weighing diaper to determine fluid output)

1 grain = 60 mg
15 grains = 1 g
1 oz = 30 mL
1.2 lb = 1 kg (used when recording in metric or computing body mass index [BMI])
1 in. = 2.5 cm (used when recording in metric)
39 in. = 1 yd 3 in.
= 1 m (used when recording in metric)

Conversion Formulas for Temperature Readings

CELSIUS TO FAHRENHEIT
From °C up to °F:

$$°F = 1.8 \times °C + 32$$

First **multiply** °C by 1.8; then **add** 32.

FAHRENHEIT TO CELSIUS
From °F down to °C:

$$°C = (°F - 32) \text{ divided by } 1.8$$

First **subtract** 32 from °F; then **divide** by 1.8.

Normal Vital Sign Ranges by Age

AGE	TEMPERATURE IN DEGREES CELSIUS/ FAHRENHEIT	PULSE (AVERAGE AND RANGE)	RESPIRATIONS (AVERAGE AND RANGE)	BLOOD PRESSURE (mm HG)
Newborns	36.8 (axillary)	130 (120–160)	35 (30–60)	60–80/ 40–45
1–3 years	37.7 (rectal)	120 (80–140)	30 (20–40)	90/55
6–8 years	37 (oral)	100 (75–120)	20 (15–25)	95/57
10 years	37 (oral)	70 (50–90)	19 (15–25)	102/62
Teen years	37 (oral)	70 (50–90)	18 (15–20)	120/80
Adult	37 (oral)	80 (60–100)	16 (12–20)	120/80
Older adult (greater than 70 years)	36 (oral)	80 (60–100)	16 (15–20)	Possible increased diastolic

Typical Laboratory Results for Infants and Children

COMPONENT TESTED	NORMAL LABORATORY VALUES
Hematocrit	Newborn: 44–65%; 1–3 years old: 29–40%; 4–10 years old: 31–43%
Urine specific gravity	Newborn: 1.001–1.020; Child: 1.005–1.030
Blood urea nitrogen	Infant: 5–15 mg/dL; Child: 5–20 mg/dL
Potassium	Infant: 3.6–5.8 mEq/L; Child: 3.5–5.5 mEq/L
Sodium	Infant: 134–150 mEq/L; Child: 135–145 mEq/L
Calcium	Newborn: 3.7–7.0 mEq/L or 7.4–14.0 mg/dL; Infant: 5.0–6.0 mEq/L or 10–12 mg/dL; Child: 4.5–5.8 mEq/L or 9–11.5 mg/dL
Blood Gases pH	Child: 7.36–7.44
$Paco_2$	Child: 35–45 mm Hg
HCO_3	Child: 22–26 mEq/L

Note: Lab values may vary. Consult the laboratory at your health care agency.

Lab Values for Urinalysis

CHARACTERISTIC	NORMAL VALUE
Bacteria	None to few organisms present
pH	4.50–8.0
Color	Clear, straw colored, amber
Odor	Slight, nonoffensive odor
Glucose	Negative
Protein	Negative
Red blood cells	Negative on gross examination; 0–5 per high-powered field
White blood cells	Negative; less than 2 per high-powered field
Specific gravity	Newborn: 1.001–1.020; Child: 1.005–1.030
Ketones	Negative

Pediatric Lab Values for Oxygen Saturation

Normal	95–98%
Mild hypoxemia	90–95%
Moderate hypoxemia	85–90%
Severe hypoxemia	85% or lower

Laboratory Values for Cholesterol

TEST	NORMAL	BORDERLINE LEVELS	HIGH LEVELS
Total cholesterol	Less than 170 mg/dL	170–199 mg/dL	More than 200 mg/dL
Low-density lipoproteins	Less than 110 mg/dL	110–129 mg/dL	More than 130 mg/dL
Triglycerides	100 mg/dL	100–150 mg/dL	More than 150 mg/dL
High-density lipoproteins	More than 35 mg/dL	Less than 35 mg/dL	

Lab Values for Children with Renal Failure

LAB	NORMAL	FINDING IN RENAL FAILURE
Blood urea nitrogen	Infant: 5–15 mg/dL	Increased
	Child: 5–20 mg/dL	Increased
Serum creatinine	Newborn: 0.8–1.4 mg/dL	Increased
	Infant: 0.7–1.7 mg/dL	Increased
	2–6 years old: 0.3–0.6 mg/dL	Increased
	Greater than 6 years old: 0.4–1.2 mg/dL	Increased
Serum potassium	Infant: 3.6–5.8 mEq/L	Increased
	Child: 3.5–5.5 mEq/L	Increased
Serum sodium	Infant: 134–150 mEq/L	Increased or decreased
	Child: 135–145 mEq/L	Increased or decreased
Bicarbonate (HCO_3)	24–28 mEq/L	Decreased

Appendix IV

Standard Precautions for Infection Control

Excerpted from *Guideline for Isolation Precautions in Hospitals* (January 1996)

Background

Standard Precautions synthesize Blood/Body Fluid Precautions and guidelines for body substance isolation and apply them to all clients regardless of their diagnosis or presumed infection status. Standard Precautions apply to 1) blood; 2) all body fluids, secretions, and excretions except sweat, regardless of whether or not they contain visible blood; 3) nonintact skin; and 4) mucous membranes. Standard Precautions are designed to reduce the risk of transmission of microorganisms from both recognized and unrecognized sources of infection in hospitals.

II. Standard Precautions

A. *Handwashing*

Wash hands after touching blood, body fluids, secretions, excretions, and contaminated items, whether or not gloves are worn. Wash hands immediately after gloves are removed, between client contacts. Use an antimicrobial agent or a waterless antiseptic agent for specific circumstances (e.g., when hands are not visibly soiled, for control of outbreaks, etc.).

B. *Gloves*

Wear gloves (clean, nonsterile gloves are adequate) when touching blood, body fluids, secretions, excretions, and contaminated items. Put on clean gloves just before touching mucous membranes and nonintact skin. Change gloves between tasks and procedures on the same client after contact with material that may contain a high concentration of microorganisms. Remove gloves promptly after use and wash hands immediately to avoid transfer of microorganisms.

C. *Mask, Eye Protection, Face Shield*

Wear a mask and eye protection or a face shield to protect mucous membranes of the eyes, nose, and mouth during procedures that are likely to generate splashes or sprays of blood, body fluids, secretions, and excretions.

D. *Gown*

Wear a gown (a clean, nonsterile gown is adequate) to protect skin and to prevent soiling of clothing during procedures and client-care activities that are likely to generate splashes or sprays of blood, body fluids, secretions, or excretions.

E. *Client-Care Equipment*

Handle soiled equipment so as to prevent personal contamination of clothing and transfer of microorganisms. Ensure that reusable equipment is not used for the care of another client until it has been cleaned and reprocessed appropriately. Ensure that single-use items are discarded properly.

F. *Environmental Control*

Ensure that hospital procedures for the routine care, cleaning, and disinfection of environmental surfaces, beds, bedrails, bedside equipment, and other frequently touched surfaces are being followed.

G. *Linen*

Handle, transport, and process used linen soiled with blood, body fluids, secretions, and excretions in a manner that prevents skin and mucous membrane exposures and contamination of clothing, and that avoids transfer of microorganisms.

H. *Occupational Health and Bloodborne Pathogens*

1. Take care to prevent injuries when using needles, scalpels, and other sharp instruments or devices. Never recap used needles using both hands, or use any other technique that involves directing the point of a needle toward any part of the body; rather, use either a one-handed "scoop" technique or a mechanical device designed for holding the needle sheath. Do not remove used needles from disposable syringes by hand, and do not bend, break, or manipulate used needles by hand. Place all sharp items in appropriate puncture-resistant containers. Use mouthpieces, resuscitation bags, or other ventilation devices as an alternative to mouth-to-mouth resuscitation methods.

I. *Client Placement*

Place client who contaminates the environment or who does not (or cannot be expected to) assist in maintaining appropriate hygiene or environmental control in a private room.

Date last modified: April 1, 2005

Source: Department of Health and Human Services, Centers for Disease Control and Prevention.

Standard Precautions[†, ‡]

Use Standard Precautions for the care of all patients

Airborne Precautions

In addition to Standard Precautions, use Airborne Precautions for patients known or suspected to have serious illnesses transmitted by airborne droplet nuclei. Examples of such illnesses include:

- Measles
- Varicella (including disseminated zoster)[†]
- Tuberculosis[‡]

Droplet Precautions

In addition to Standard Precautions, use Droplet Precautions for patients known or suspected to have serious illnesses transmitted by large particle droplets. Examples of such illnesses include:

- Invasive *Haemophilus influenzae* type b disease, including meningitis, pneumonia, epiglottitis, and sepsis
- Invasive Neisseria *meningitidis* disease, including meningitis, pneumonia, and sepsis

Other serious bacterial respiratory infections spread by droplet transmission, including:

- Diphtheria (pharyngeal)
- Mycoplasma pneumonia
- Pertussis
- Pneumonic plague
- Streptococcal (group A) pharyngitis, pneumonia, or scarlet fever in infants and young children

Serious viral infections spread by droplet transmission, including:

- Adenovirus[†]
- Influenza

- Mumps
- Parvovirus B19
- Rubella

Contact Precautions

In addition to Standard Precautions, use Contact Precautions for patients known or suspected to have serious illnesses easily transmitted by direct patient contact or by contact with items in the patient's environment. Examples of such illnesses include:

Gastrointestinal, respiratory, skin, or wound infections or colonization with multidrug-resistant bacteria judged by the infection control program, based on current state, regional, or national recommendations, to be of special clinical and epidemiologic significance.

Enteric infections with a low infectious dose or prolonged environmental survival, including:

- Clostridium difficile
- For diapered or incontinent patients: enterohemorrhagic Escherichia coli O157:H7, Shigella, hepatitis A, or rotavirus

Respiratory syncytial virus, parainfluenza virus, or enteroviral infections in infants and young children

Skin infections that are highly contagious or that may occur on dry skin, including:

- Diphtheria (cutaneous)
- Herpes simplex virus (neonatal or mucocutaneous)
- Impetigo
- Major (noncontained) abscesses, cellulitis, or decubiti
- Pediculosis
- Scabies
- Staphylococcal furunculosis in infants and young children
- Zoster (disseminated or in the immunocompromised host)[†]
- Viral/hemorrhagic conjunctivitis
- Viral hemorrhagic infections (Ebola, Lassa, or Marburg)

Source: Centers for Disease Control and Prevention Fundamentals of Isolation Precautions.

[†]Certain infections require more than one type of precaution.

[‡]See CDC *"Guidelines for Preventing the Transmission of Tuberculosis in Health-Care Facilities."* (23)

Contents *These precautions last reviewed and updated by CDC, April 1, 2005.*

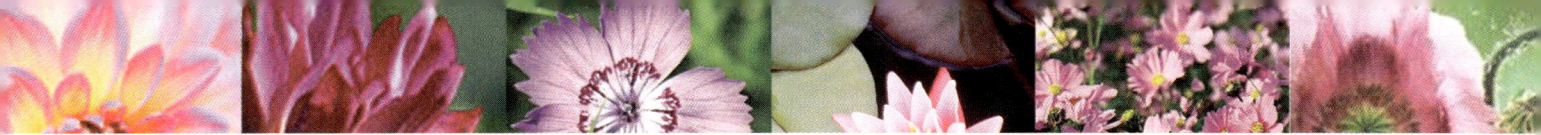

Appendix V

NANDA-Approved Nursing Diagnoses

Note: The initial letter of the key word in each NANDA diagnosis is in boldface.

Activity
  Activity Intolerance
  Risk for **A**ctivity Intolerance
Adaptive Capacity
  Decreased Intracranial **A**daptive Capacity
Airway Clearance
  Ineffective **A**irway Clearance
Allergy Response
  Latex **A**llergy Response
  Risk for Latex **A**llergy Response
Anxiety
  Death **A**nxiety
Aspiration
  Risk for **A**spiration
Attachment
  Risk for Impaired **A**ttachment, Parent
  Risk for Impaired **A**ttachment, Infant
  Risk for Impaired **A**ttachment, Child
Blood Glucose
  Risk for Unstable **B**lood Glucose
Body Image
  Disturbed **B**ody Image
Body Temperature
  Risk for Imbalanced **B**ody Temperature
Bowel
  Bowel Incontinence
Breastfeeding
  Effective **B**reastfeeding
  Ineffective **B**reastfeeding
  Interrupted **B**reastfeeding
Breathing Pattern
  Ineffective **B**reathing Pattern
Cardiac Output
  Decreased **C**ardiac Output
Caregiver Role Strain
  Risk for **C**aregiver Role Strain
Comfort
  Readiness for Enhanced **C**omfort
Communication
  Readiness for Enhanced **C**ommunication
  Impaired Verbal **C**ommunication
Confusion
  Acute **C**onfusion
  Chronic **C**onfusion
  Risk for Acute **C**onfusion

Constipation
  Perceived **C**onstipation
  Risk for **C**onstipation
Contamination
  Risk for **C**ontamination
Coping
  Ineffective Community **C**oping
  Readiness for Enhanced Community **C**oping
  Defensive **C**oping
  Compromised Family **C**oping
  Disabled Family **C**oping
  Readiness for Enhanced Family **C**oping
  Readiness for Enhanced Individual **C**oping
  Ineffective **C**oping
Decision Making
  Readiness for Enhanced **D**ecision Making
  Decisional Conflict (Specify)
Denial
  Ineffective **D**enial
Dentition
  Impaired **D**entition
Development
  Risk for Delayed **D**evelopment
Diarrhea
Disuse Syndrome
  Risk for **D**isuse Syndrome
Diversional Activity
  Deficient **D**iversional Activity
Dysreflexia
  Autonomic **D**ysreflexia
  Risk for Autonomic **D**ysreflexia
Energy Field
  Disturbed **E**nergy Field
Environmental Interpretation Syndrome
  Impaired **E**nvironmental Interpretation Syndrome
Failure to Thrive
  Adult **F**ailure to Thrive
Falls
  Risk for **F**alls
Family Processes
  Dysfunctional **F**amily Processes: Alcoholism
  Interrupted **F**amily Processes
  Readiness for Enhanced **F**amily Processes
Fatigue
Fear

Fluid Balance
  Readiness for Enhanced Fluid Balance
Fluid Volume
  Deficient Fluid Volume
  Risk for Deficient Fluid Volume
  Excess Fluid Volume
  Risk for Imbalanced Fluid Volume
Gas Exchange
  Impaired Gas Exchange
Grieving
  Complicated Grieving
  Risk for Complicated Grieving
Growth
  Risk for Disproportionate Growth
Growth and Development
  Delayed Growth and Development
Health Behavior
  Risk-Prone Health Behavior
  Health Seeking Behaviors (Specify)
Home Maintenance
  Impaired Home Maintenance
Hope
  Readiness for Enhanced Hope
Hopelessness
Human Dignity
  Risk for Compromised Human Dignity
Hyperthermia
Hypothermia
Identity
  Disturbed Personal Identity
Immunization Status
  Readiness for Enhanced Immunization Status
Infant Behavior
  Disorganized Infant Behavior
  Risk for Disorganized Infant Behavior
  Readiness for Enhanced Organized Infant Behavior
Infant Feeding Pattern
  Ineffective Infant Feeding Pattern
Infection
  Risk for Infection
Injury
  Risk for Injury
Insomnia
Knowledge
  Deficient Knowledge (Specify)
  Readiness for Enhanced Knowledge (Specify)
Lifestyle
  Sedentary Lifestyle
Liver Function
  Risk for Impaired Liver Function
Loneliness
  Risk for Loneliness

Memory
  Impaired Memory
Mobility
  Impaired Bed Mobility
  Impaired Physical Mobility
  Impaired Wheelchair Mobility
Moral
  Moral Distress
Nausea
Neglect
  Unilateral Neglect
Neurovascular Dysfunction
  Risk for Peripheral Neurovascular Dysfunction
Noncompliance (Specify)
Nutrition
  Imbalanced Nutrition: Less than Body Requirements
  Imbalanced Nutrition: More than Body Requirements
  Risk for Imbalanced Nutrition: More than Body
    Requirements
  Readiness for Enhanced Nutrition
Oral Mucous Membrane
  Impaired Oral Mucous Membrane
Pain
  Acute Pain
  Chronic Pain
Parenting
  Impaired Parenting
  Readiness for Enhanced Parenting
  Risk for Impaired Parenting
Perioperative Positioning Injury
  Risk for Perioperative Positioning Injury
Poisoning
  Risk for Poisoning
Post-Trauma Syndrome
  Risk for Post-Trauma Syndrome
Power
  Readiness for Enhanced Power
Powerlessness
  Risk for Powerlessness
Protection
  Ineffective Protection
Rape-Trauma Syndrome
  Rape-Trauma Syndrome: Compound Reaction
  Rape-Trauma Syndrome: Silent Reaction
Religiosity
  Impaired Religiosity
  Readiness for Enhanced Religiosity
  Risk for Impaired Religiosity
Relocation Stress Syndrome
  Risk for Relocation Stress Syndrome
Role Conflict
  Parental Role Conflict

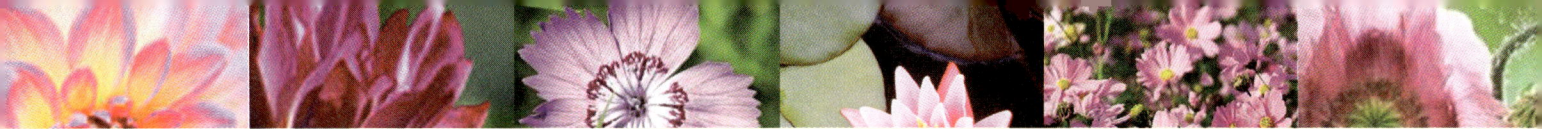

Role Performance
  Ineffective Role Performance
Self-Care
  Readiness for Enhanced Self-Care
Self-Care Deficit
  Bathing/Hygiene Self-Care Deficit
  Dressing/Grooming Self-Care Deficit
  Feeding Self-Care Deficit
  Toileting Self-Care Deficit
Self-Concept
  Readiness for Enhanced Self-Concept
Self-Esteem
  Chronic Low Self-Esteem
  Situational Low Self-Esteem
  Risk for Situational Low Self-Esteem
Self-Mutilation
  Risk for Self-Mutilation
Sensory Perception
  Disturbed Visual Sensory Perception (Specify)
  Disturbed Auditory Sensory Perception (Specify)
  Disturbed Kinesthetic Sensory Perception (Specify)
  Disturbed Gustatory Sensory Perception (Specify)
  Disturbed Tactile Sensory Perception (Specify)
  Disturbed Olfactory Sensory Perception (Specify)
Sexual Dysfunction
Sexuality Pattern
  Ineffective Sexuality Pattern
Skin Integrity
  Impaired Skin Integrity
  Risk for Impaired Skin Integrity
Sleep Deprivation
Sleep
  Readiness for Enhanced Sleep
Social Interaction
  Impaired Social Interaction
Social Isolation
Sorrow
  Chronic Sorrow
Spiritual Distress
  Risk for Spiritual Distress
Spiritual Well-Being
  Readiness for Enhanced Spiritual Well-Being
Stress Overload
Sudden Infant Death Syndrome
  Risk for Sudden Infant Death Syndrome
Suffocation
  Risk for Suffocation
Suicide
  Risk for Suicide

Surgical Recovery
  Delayed Surgical Recovery
Swallowing
  Impaired Swallowing
Therapeutic Regimen Management
  Ineffective Community Therapeutic Regimen Management
  Effective Therapeutic Regimen Management
  Ineffective Family Therapeutic Regimen Management
  Ineffective Therapeutic Regimen Management
  Readiness for Enhanced Therapeutic Regimen Management
Thermoregulation
  Ineffective Thermoregulation
Thought Processes
  Disturbed Thought Processes
Tissue Integrity
  Impaired Tissue Integrity
Tissue Perfusion
  Ineffective Renal Tissue Perfusion (Specify)
  Ineffective Cerebral Tissue Perfusion (Specify)
  Ineffective Cardiopulmonary Tissue Perfusion (Specify)
  Ineffective Gastrointestinal Tissue Perfusion (Specify)
  Ineffective Peripheral Tissue Perfusion (Specify)
Transfer Ability
  Impaired Transfer Ability
Trauma
  Risk for Trauma
Urinary Elimination
  Impaired Urinary Elimination
  Readiness for Enhanced Urinary Elimination
Urinary Incontinence
  Functional Urinary Incontinence
  Overflow Urinary Incontinence
  Reflex Urinary Incontinence
  Stress Urinary Incontinence
  Total Urinary Incontinence
  Urge Urinary Incontinence
  Risk for Urge Urinary Incontinence
Urinary Retention
Ventilation
  Impaired Spontaneous Ventilation
Ventilatory Weaning Response
  Dysfunctional Ventilatory Weaning Response
Violence
  Risk for Other-Directed Violence
  Risk for Self-Directed Violence
Walking
  Impaired Walking
Wandering

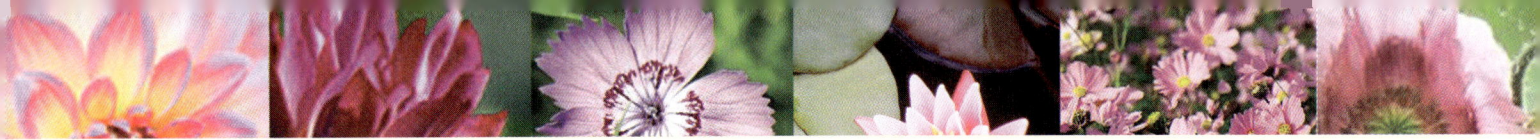

Appendix VI

Spanish Translations of English Phrases*

This appendix includes phrases you might find helpful in working with families during pregnancy, labor, and birth, and after the birth. There are many ways to phrase questions. We have chosen some statements we consider essential and have tried to phrase them in a straightforward way. The phrases are designed to help you in situations in which translation is not possible at the moment.

This list begins with introductory statements, which are presented in a logical conversational flow. The remaining phrases are arranged according to the phases of pregnancy and birth during which they are most applicable.

ESSENTIAL INTRODUCTORY PHRASES

Hello

I am a nurse.
I am a student nurse.
My name is _____.

What is your name?

What name should I call you?

Thank you
Please
Is someone here with you?
Does he (she) speak English?
Goodbye

PHRASES FOR THE ANTEPARTAL PERIOD

Are you taking any medications now?
Show me the medicine bottles please.
Have you ever had trouble with your blood pressure?
When was the first day of your last period?

Have you had any spotting or bleeding since your last period?

Have you been on birth control pills?
When did you stop taking them?
Do you have an intrauterine device (IUD)?
How many times have you been pregnant?
Are you having any problems with your pregnancy?
Is there anything that is worrying you?
I would like to take your blood pressure.
I would like to take your pulse.
I would like to take your temperature.

FRASES INTRODUCTORAS ESENCIALES

Hola

Soy enfermera (enfermero).†
Soy estudiante de enfermería.
Mi nombre es _____.
Me llamo _____.

¿Cuál es su nombre?
¿Cómo se llama?

¿Cómo quiere que la llamemos?
¿Cómo quiere ser llamada?

Gracias
Por favor
¿Hay alguien aquí con usted?
¿Habla él (ella) inglés?
Adiós.

FRASES PARA EL PERIODO PRENATAL

¿Está tomando algunas medicinas ahora?
Por favor, muéstreme los frascos.
¿Ha tenido problemas alguna vez con la presión arterial?
¿Cuál fue el primer día de su última regla?
¿Cuál fue el primer día de su última menstruación?
¿Ha sangrado o ha tenido manchas de sangre desde su última regla?

¿Ha estado tomando píldoras anticonceptivas?
¿Cuándo dejó de tomarlas?
¿Usa un aparato intrauterino?
¿Cuántas veces ha estado usted embarazada?
¿Tiene problemas con su embarazo?
¿Hay algo o alguna cosa que la preocupe?
Quisiera tomarle la presió arterial.
Quisiera tomarle el pulso.
Quisiera tomarle la temperatura.

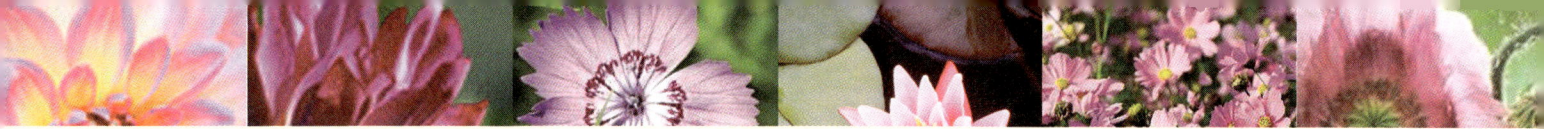

I would like to listen to your heart and lungs.	Quisiera escucharle el corazón y los pulmones.
I would like to check your uterus.	Quisiera examinarle el útero.
Please urinate in this cup and leave it in the bathroom.	Puede orinar en este vaso y dejarlo en el baño.
Please stand up.	Por favor, levántese.
Please sit down.	Por favor, siéntese.
Please lie down.	Por favor, acuéstese.

PHRASES RELATED TO CLIENT SAFETY
FRASES RELACIONADAS CON LA SEGURIDAD DEL CLIENTE

I would like to talk to you alone.	Quisiera hablar a solas con usted.
Are you safe at home?	¿Sufre de peligros en casa?
Are you afraid of your partner?	¿Le tiene miedo a su compañero?
During your pregnancy has your partner hit, slapped, kicked, or punched you?	Durante su embarazo, ¿la ha golpeado?
	¿la ha abofeteado?
	¿la ha pateado?
	¿le ha dado puñetazos?
How many times?	¿Cuántas veces?
Do you have someone for support?	¿Cuénta con alguien que la pueda ayudar?

QUESTIONS THE MOTHER OR FATHER MAY ASK
POSIBLES PREGUNTAS QUE MADRES O PADRES HACEN

How big is my baby?	¿De qué tamaño es el (la) bebé?
How much does the baby weigh now?	¿Cuánto pesa el bebé ahora?
When will I feel my baby move?	¿Cuándo lo (la) voy a sentir moverse?

PHRASES FOR THE INTRAPARTAL PERIOD
FRASES DURANTE EL PARTO

Note: Review the essential introductory phrases for beginning a conversation.	*Nota:* Repase las frases introductoras para comenzar una conversación.
Are you having labor pains?	¿Tiene dolores de parto?
Are you having contractions?	¿Tiene contracciones?
Are you having pain?	¿Tiene dolores?
Do you need medicine for pain?	¿Necesita medicina para el dolor?
Do you need to urinate?	¿Necesita orinar?
This is a bedpan to urinate in.	Aquí tiene el bacín (la chata) (el pato) para orinar.
Can I help you to the bathroom?	¿La ayudo a ir al baño?
Do you need to have a bowel movement?	¿Necesita mover el vientre (obrar)? Necesita "Hacer caca"—coloquial
Has your bag of water broken?	¿Se le ha roto la bolsa de agua(s)?
Have you had any bright-red bleeding during your pregnancy?	¿Ha tenido algún sangramiento de color rojo durante su embarazo?
How many births have you had?	¿Cuántos niños le han nacido?
I need to do a vaginal examination.	Necesito hacerle un examen vaginal.
I will help you.	La voy a ayudar.
I will stay with you.	Me quedaré con usted.
Please pant. I will show you how.	Por favor, jadee. Le voy a mostrar cómo.
Do not push now.	No puje ahora.

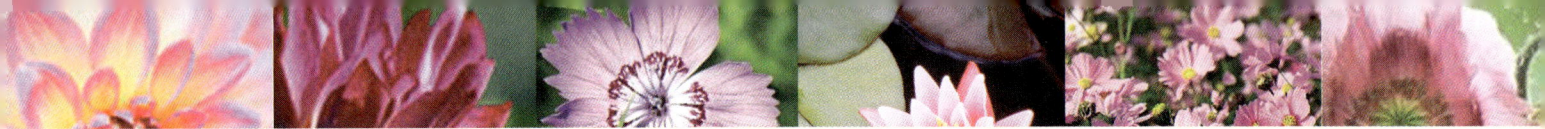

Push now.	Puje ahora.
Stop pushing.	Pare de pujar.
	No puje más.
The doctor needs to do a cesarean birth.	El doctor le va a hacer una operación cesárea.
This is medicine for your pain. You will feel better soon.	Esta medicina es para el dolor. Va a sentirse mejor pronto.
When is your baby supposed to be born?	¿Cuando está supuesto a nacer el bebé?
January	enero
February	febrero
March	marzo
April	abril
May	mayo
June	junio
July	julio
August	agosto
September	septiembre
October	octubre
November	noviembre
December	diciembre
What is your doctor's name?	¿Cuál es el nombre de su doctor?
What is your midwife's name?	¿Cuál es el nombre de su comadrona (partera)?
Your baby is having some trouble now.	El bebé está pasando por algunos problemas.
	El bebé está sufriendo algunas dificultades.
I need to put this oxygen mask on you. It will help your baby. It may smell funny, but it is OK.	Le voy a poner esta máscara de oxígeno. Va a ayudar al bebé. Huele extraño, pero no hay problemas.
Please turn on your left side.	Por favor voltéese al lado izquierdo.
Please turn on your right side.	Por favor voltéese al lado derecho.
Your baby is OK.	El bebé está bien.

PHRASES FOR THE POSTPARTAL PERIOD AND THE NEWBORN AREA

Note: Review the essential introductory phrases for beginning a conversation.

FRASES PARA EL PERIODO DESPUES DEL PARTO Y EL AREA DEL RECIEN NACIDO

Nota: Repase las frases introductoras para comenzar una conversación.

Are you hungry?	¿Tiene hambre?
Are you thirsty?	¿Tiene sed?
Are you cold?	¿Tiene frío?
Are you tired?	¿Está cansada?
I am going to put antibiotic ointment in the baby's eyes.	Le voy a poner al bebé un ungüento antibiótico alrededor de los ojos.
It will help protect your baby from some infections.	Lo (la) va a proteger contra algunos infecciones.
I am going to take some blood from your baby's foot to check the blood sugar and hematocrit.	Le voy a sacar sangre del pie al bebé para determinar el azúcar de la sangre y el hematocrítico.
If your baby begins to spit up, please turn him (her) on his (her) side.	Si el bebé comienza a vomitar, colóquelo (colóquela) de costado.
It may help to position your baby like this.	Lo (la) ayudará—si lo coloca así.
	Lo (la) ayudaría—si lo colocara así.

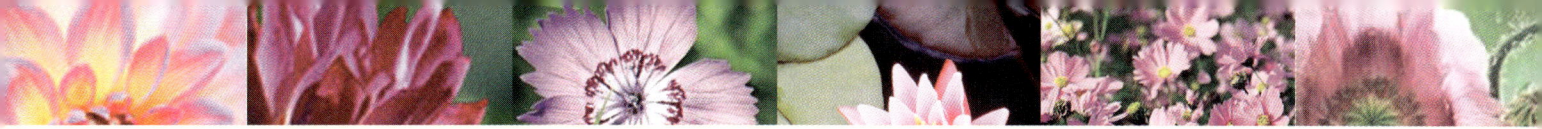

I would like to suggest that you clean your nipples this way before you breastfeed your baby.	Es bueno que se lave los pezones de esta manera antes de darle el pecho al bebé.
It is better that you clean your baby's cord this way.	Es mejor para el bebé que le lave el ombligo de esta manera.
It is better that you bathe your baby this way.	Es mejor que lo (la) bañe de esta manera.
It is better that you clean your baby's penis this way.	Es mejor que le limpie el pene así.
I would like to suggest that you fold the diaper this way.	Le sugiero que doble el pañal así.
I would like to suggest that you fasten the diaper this way.	Le sugiero que asegure el pañal así.
Take the baby's temperature this way.	Tómele la temperatura así.
I need to check (your breasts, your uterus, your flow, your stitches, your legs and feet).	Necesito examinarle (los pechos, el útero, el flujo, los puntos, las piernas y los pies).
I need to feel your uterus.	Necesito examinarle el útero.
I need to massage your uterus.	Necesito darle un masaje en la región del útero.
Place your baby on its side.	Coloque al bebé de costado.
Place the baby's used diapers here.	Coloque aquí los pañales usados.
Please rub your uterus every half hour to keep it firm. I will show you how.	Necesita darse un masaje en la región del útero cada media hora para mantenerlo firme. Le voy a mostrar cómo.
Would you like to see your baby now?	¿Quiere ver a su bebé ahora?
Would you like me to help you feed your baby?	¿Quiere que le ayude a alimentarlo (la)?
Your baby needs a car seat to go home in.	El (la) bebé necesita un asiento para bebé en el automóvil.

SPECIAL NEONATAL NEEDS / NECESIDADES DEL RECIEN NACIDO

We are giving your baby oxygen.	Le vamos a dar oxígeno al (a la) bebé.
Your baby is having problems breathing.	El (la) bebé tiene problemas al respirar.
Your baby needs extra help.	El (la) bebé necesita ayuda especial.
Your baby needs to go to a special care nursery.	El (la) bebé necesita ir a la sala de cuidados especiales para bebés.

*Prepared by Elizabeth Medina, Ph.D. Associate Professor of Spanish, Regis University, Denver, Colorado.
†In Spanish, nouns that end in *a* indicate female gender; nouns that end in *o* indicate male gender.

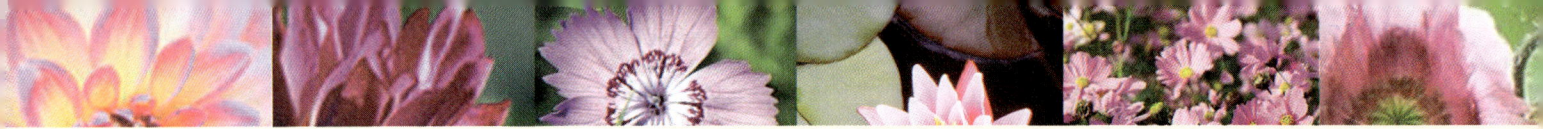

Appendix VII

Sign Language for Health Care Professionals

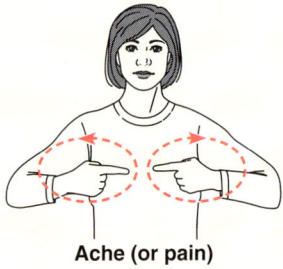

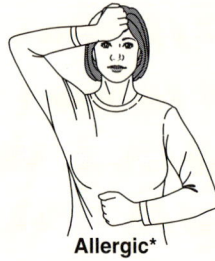

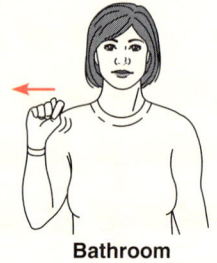

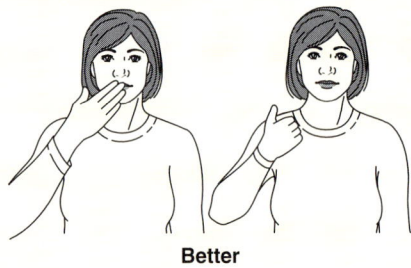

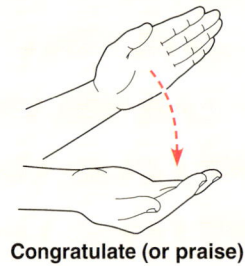

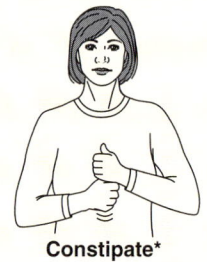

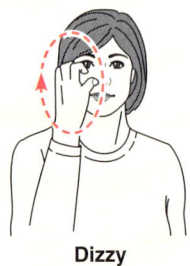

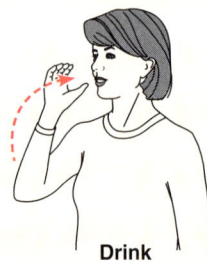

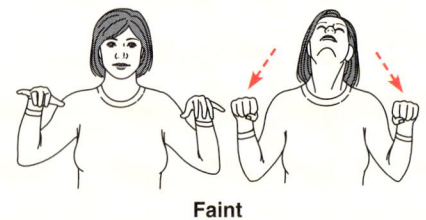

Ache (or pain)

Allergic*

Bathroom

Better

Congratulate (or praise)

Constipate*

Dizzy

Drink

Faint

*Indicates signs that are in manually signed English. Those without an asterisk are American Sign Language.

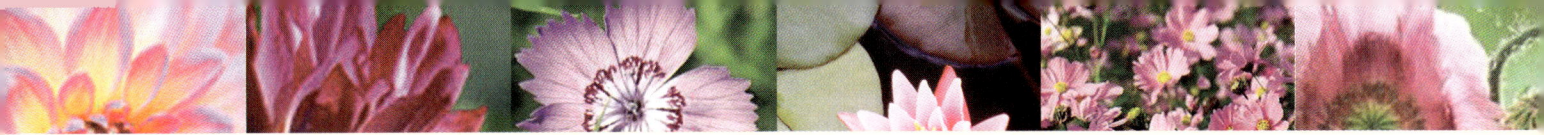

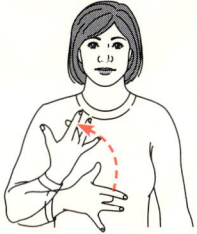

Feel

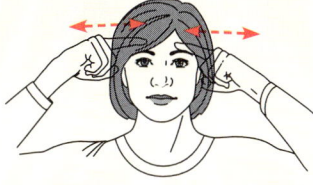

Headache

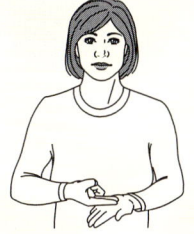

Lie down

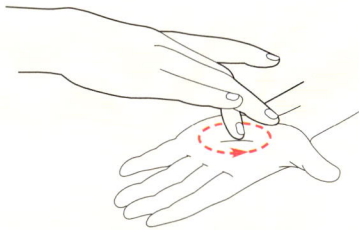

Medicine

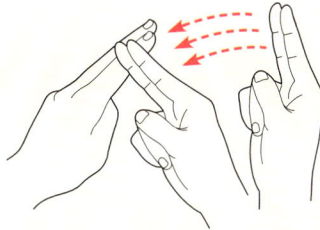

Name

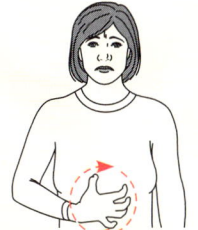

Nauseous

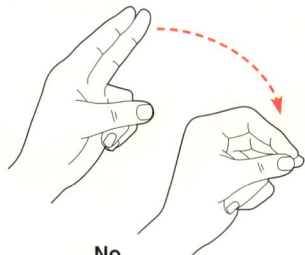

No

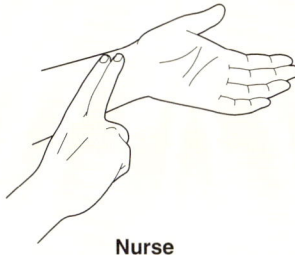

Nurse

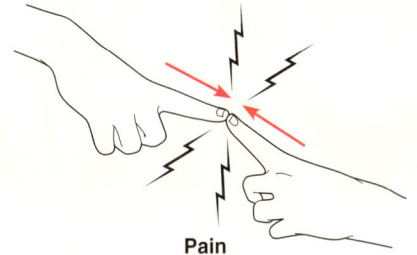

Pain

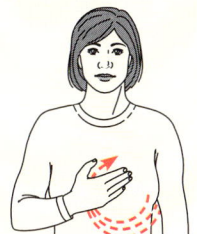

Please

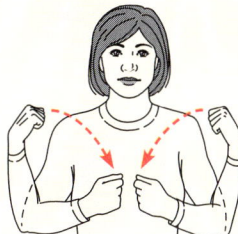

Put on

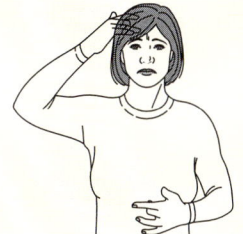

Sick

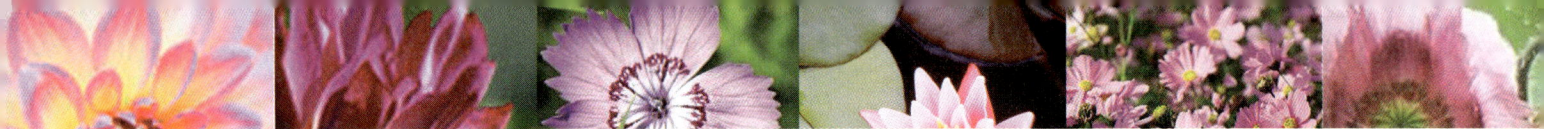

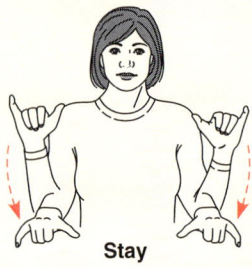

Stay

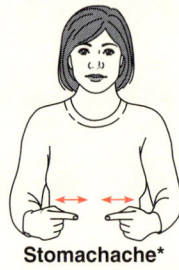

Stomachache*

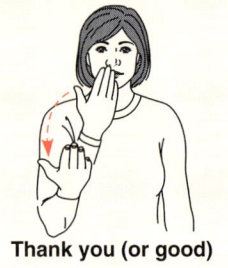

Thank you (or good)

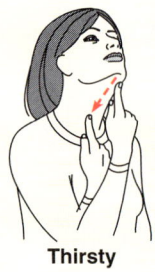

Thirsty

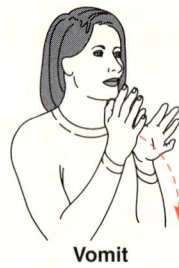

Vomit

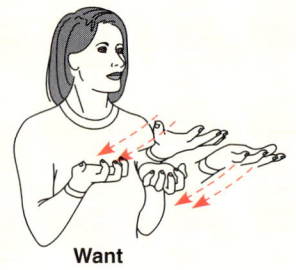

Want

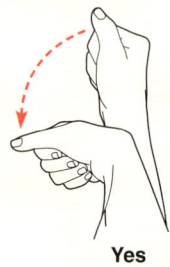

Yes

References and Resources

CHAPTER 1

American Academy of Pediatrics. (2005). The changing concept of sudden infant death syndrome: Diagnostic coding shifts, controversies regarding the sleeping environment, and new variables to consider in reducing risk. *Pediatrics, 116*(5), 1245–1255.

American Nurses Association. (1980). *Nursing: A social policy statement.* Kansas City, MO: Author.

American Nurses Association. (1991). *Nursing's agenda for health care reform.* Washington, DC: Author.

American Nurses Association. (1998). *Standards of clinical practice* (2nd ed.). Washington, DC: Author.

Brady-Fryer, B., Wiebe, N., & Landeer, J. (2004). Pain relief for neonatal circumcision. *The Cochrane Library*, 4.

Clifford, P. A., String, M., Christensen, H., & Mountain, D. (2004). Pain assessment and intervention for term newborns. *Journal of Midwifery and Women's Health, 49*(6), 514–519.

Gennaro, S., Hodnett, E., & Kearney, M. (2001). Making evidence-based practice a reality in your institutions: Evaluating the evidence and using the evidence to change clinical practice. *The American Journal of Maternal/Child Nursing, 26*(5), 236–250.

Henry, P. R., Haubold, K., & Dobrzykowski, T. (2004). Pain in the healthy full-term neonate: Efficacy and safety of interventions. *Newborn Infant Nursing Review, 4*(2), 126–130.

National Council of State Boards of Nursing, Inc. (1995). *Delegation: Concepts and decision-making process.* Chicago: Author.

North American Nursing Diagnosis Association (NANDA). (2008). NANDA *nursing diagnoses: Definitions and classification, 2008–2009.* Philadelphia: Author.

Ramont, R. P., Niedringhaus, D. M., & Towle, M. A. *Comprehensive nursing care.* Upper Saddle River, NJ: Prentice Hall.

Razums, I., Dalton, M., & Wilson, D. (2004). Practice applications of research. Pain management for newborn circumcision. *Pediatric Nursing, 30*(5), 414–417.

U.S. Department of Health and Human Services. (1991). *Healthy People 2000.* Washington DC: U.S. Government Printing Office.

U.S. Department of Health and Human Services. (2000). *Healthy People 2010* (2nd ed.). Washington DC: U.S. Government Printing Office.

Zotti, M. E., Brown, P., & Stotts, C. (1996). Community-based nursing versus community health nursing: What does it all mean? *Nursing Outlook, 44*, 211–217.

CHAPTER 2

Estabrooks, C. (1998). Will evidence-based nursing practice make practice perfect? *Canadian Journal of Nursing Research, 30*(1), 15–36.

National Council of State Boards of Nursing, Inc. (1995). *Delegation: Concepts and decision-making process.* Chicago: Author.

North American Nursing Diagnosis Association (NANDA). (2008). NANDA *nursing diagnoses: Definitions and classification, 2008–2009.* Philadelphia: Author.

Paul, R., & Elder, L. (2006). The miniature guide to critical thinking concepts & tools. Dillon Beach, CA: Foundation for Critical Thinking.

Pravikoff, D., Ranner, A., & Pierce, S. (2005). Readiness of U.S. nurses for evidence-based practice. *American Journal of Nursing, 105*(9), 40–51.

Spratley, E., Johnson, A., Sochalski, J., Fritz, M., & Spencer, W. (2001). *The registered nurse population March 2000: Findings from the National Sample Survey of Registered Nurses.* Rockville, MD: U.S. Department of Health and Human Services.

Wilkinson, J. M. (2007). *Nursing process and critical thinking* (4th ed.). Upper Saddle River, NJ: Prentice Hall.

CHAPTER 3

American Association of Colleges of Nursing. (1999). *Nursing educational agenda for the 21st century.* Washington, DC: Author.

American Nurses Association. (1998). *Standards of clinical nursing practice* (2nd ed.). Silver Spring, MD: Author.

American Nurses Association. (2000). *New position statement adolescent health task force.* Washington, DC: Author.

Anderson, M. A. (2001). *Nursing leadership: Management and professional practice for the LPN/LVN* (2nd ed.). Philadelphia: F.A. Davis.

Centers for Disease Control. (2000). Building data systems for monitoring and responding to violence against women. *Weekly Report on Domestic Violence, 49,* (RR11). Accessed June 28, 2006, at www.cdc.gov.

Coty, E., Davis, J., & Angell, L. (2002). *Documentation: The language of nursing.* Upper Saddle River, NJ: Prentice Hall.

Joint Commission on Accreditation of Healthcare Organizations. (2000). *2000 accreditation manual for hospitals.* Chicago: Author.

Miller, F., Emanuel, E., Rosenstein, D., & Straus, S. (2004). Ethical issues concerning research in complementary and alternative medicine. *Journal of American Medical Association, 291*(5), 599–604.

National Association for Practical Nurse Education and Service. (1998). *Code of ethics for licensed practical/vocational nurses.* Silver Spring, MD: Author.

National Federation of Licensed Practical Nurses. (1998). *Nursing practice standards for the licensed practical/vocational nurse.* Garner, NC: Author.

Richardson, J. (2001). Integrating complementary therapies into health care education: A cautious approach. *Journal of Clinical Nursing, 10*(6), 792.

Simpson, R. L. (1994). Ensuring patient data privacy, confidentiality, and security. *Nursing Management, 25*(7), 18–20.

U.S. Department of Health and Human Services. (1992). *Healthy people 2000.* Rockville, MD: Author.

U.S. Department of Health and Human Services. (2000). *Healthy people 2010.* Rockville, MD: Author.

CHAPTER 4

American Association of Retired People. Help for grandparents raising grandchildren. Accessed April 11, 2007 on the Internet.

Andreasen, K., Andersen, M., & Schantz, A. (2004). Obesity and pregnancy [abstract]. *Acta Obstetricia et Gynecologica Scandinavica, 83*(11), 1022.

Dollberg, S., Seldman, D., Armon, Y., Stevenson, D., & Gale, R. (1996). Adverse perinatal outcome in the older primipara [abstract]. *Journal of Perinatology, 16*(2), 93.

Duvall, E. (1977). *Marriage and family development* (5th ed.). Philadelphia: Lippincott.

Friedman, M. (1992). *Family nursing theory and assessment.* New York: Appleton-Century-Crofts.

Giger, J., & Davidhizar, R. (Eds.). (1995). *Transcultural nursing: Assessment and interventions* (2nd ed.). St. Louis, MO: Mosby.

March of Dimes Birth Defects Foundation. (2007). What you need to know. *During Your Pregnancy: A Mommy After 35.* White Plains, NY: Author. Retrieved April 13, 2007, from https://www.marchofdimes.com/pnhec/159_140008.asp

Moos, M. (2004). Understanding prematurity: Sorting fact from fiction. *Lifelines, 8*(1), 33–37.

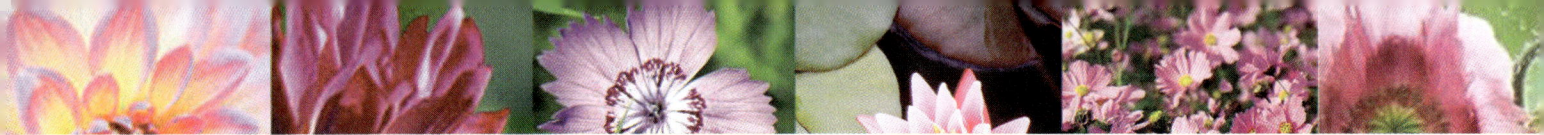

Ramont, R. R., Niedringhaus, D. M., & Towle, M. A. (2006). *Comprehensive nursing care.* Upper Saddle River, NJ: Prentice Hall.

Reddy, U., Ko, C., & Willinger, M. (2006). Maternal age and the risk of stillbirth throughout pregnancy in the United States. *American Journal of Obstetrics and Gynecology, 195,* 764–770.

Simmons, R., & O'Neil, G. (2001). Households and families: 2000. *Census 2000 Brief.* U.S. Census Bureau, U.S. Department of Commerce, Economics and Statistics Administration. Retrieved March 17, 2007, from the Internet.

Simmons, T., & Dye, J. L. (2003). Grandparents living with grandchildren: 2000. *Census 2000. Brief* U.S. Census Bureau, U.S. Department of Commerce, Economics, and Statistics Administration.

Van den Elzen, H., Wladimiroff, J., Cohen-Overbeek, T., de Bruijn, A., & Grobbee, D. (1996). Serum lipids in early pregnancy and risk of pre-eclampsia [abstract]. *BJOG: An International Journal of Obstetrics & Gynaecology, 103*(2), 117 [online]. Retrieved April 13, 2007, from the Internet.

Williams, P., Gumaa, K., Scioscia, M., Redman, C., & Rademacher, T. (2007). Inositol phosphoglycan p-type in preeclampsia: A novel marker? *Hypertension, 49,* 84.

CHAPTER 5

Feigin, R. D. (2005). Prospects for the future of child health through research. *Journal of the American Medical Association, 294,* 1373–1379.

Lea, D. H. (2000). A new world view of genetics service models. *Online Journal of Issues in Nursing, 3*(5).

Masters, W., & Johnson, W. (1966). *Human sexual response.* Philadelphia: Lippincott Williams & Wilkins.

Nathan, D. G., Fontanarosa, P. B., & Wilson, J. D. (2001). Opportunities for medical research in the 21st century. *Journal of the American Medical Association, 285,* 533–534.

National Institutes of Health. (2005). Ethical, legal and social implications (ELSI) research program overview. Available at the NIH website.

Ramont, R. P., Niedringhaus, D. M., & Towle, M. A. (2006). *Comprehensive nursing care.* Upper Saddle River, NJ: Prentice Hall.

Thibodeau, G. A., & Patton, K. T. (1997). *The human body in health and disease* (2nd ed.). St. Louis, MO: Mosby.

U.S. Department of Energy. (2004). *Human Genome Project information: Frequently asked questions.* Available at www.ornl.gov/sci/techresources

U.S. Department of Energy. (2005). *Genomics 101: A primer.* Available at www.mydna.com/genes/genetics/genomics/overview/primer.html

CHAPTER 6

Dailey, R. (1996). Vaginal discharge in the adult: A practice guideline. *The Journal of Emergency Medicine, 14*(2), 227–232.

Johnson, M., Bulechek, G., Dochterman, J., Maas, M., & Moorhead, S. (2001). *Nursing diagnoses, outcomes, & interventions: NANDA, NOC and NIC linkages.* St. Louis, MO: Mosby.

Kumar-Trollope, K. (2001). Cultural and biomedical meanings of the complaint of leukorrhea in South Asian women. *Tropical Medicine and International Health, 6*(4), 260–266.

Leavelle, H. R., & Clark, E. G. (1965). *Preventive medicine for the doctor in the community* (3rd ed.). New York: McGraw-Hill.

Neuman, B. (1982). The Neuman health-care systems model: A total approach to client care. In Neuman, B., *The Neuman systems model: Application to nursing practice.* Norwalk, CT: Appleton-Century-Crofts.

Nyirjesy, P., Peyton, C., Weitz, M., Mathew, L., & Culhane, J. (2006). Causes of chronic vaginitis: Analysis of a prospective database of affected women. *Obstetrics & Gynecology, 108*(5), 1185–1191.

Parse, R. R. (1981). *Man-Living-Health: A theory of nursing.* New York: Wiley.

Pender, N. J., Murdaugh, C. L., & Parsons, M. A. (2002). *Health promotion in nursing practice* (4th ed.). Upper Saddle River, NJ: Prentice Hall.

Watson, J. (1985). *Nursing: The philosophy and science of caring.* Boulder, CO: The University Press of Colorado.

World Health Organization. (1948). *Preamble to the constitution of the World Health Organization as adopted by the International Health Conference,* New York, 19–22 June, 1946; signed on 22 July 1946 by the representatives of 61 States (Official Records of the World Health Organization, no. 2, p. 100) and entered into force on 7 April 1948.

CHAPTER 7

Adams, E., & Bianchi, A. (2004). Can a nurse and a doula exist in the same room? *International Journal of Childbirth Education, 19*(4), 12–15.

Adams, E., & Bianchi, A. (2005). *50 Ways to comfort a laboring woman.* Presented at the AWHONN 2005 convention, June 14, Salt Lake City, Utah.

Bianchi, A., & Adams, E. (2004). Doulas, labor support, and nurses. *International Journal of Childbirth Education, 19*(4), 24–30.

Callister, L. C. (2001). Culturally competent care of women and newborns: Knowledge, attitude and skills. *Journal of Obstetric, Gynecologic, and Neonatal Nursing, 30,* 209–215.

Doulas of North America website. Available at www.dona.org

Goetzl, L. M. (2002). ACOG practice bulletin. Obstetric analgesia and anesthesia. *Obstetrics and Gynecology, 100,* 177–191.

Hopper Deglin, J., & Hazard Vallerand, A. (2005). *Davis's drug guide for nurses* (9th ed.). Philadelphia: F.A. Davis.

International Childbirth Education Association website. Available at www.icea.org

Miltner, R. (2002). More than support: Nursing interventions provided to women in labor. *Journal of Obstetric, Gynecologic, and Neonatal Nursing, 31*(6), 753–761.

Olds, S. B., London, M. L., Ladewig, P. W., & Davidson, M. R. (2004). *Maternal–newborn nursing and women's health care* (7th ed.). Upper Saddle River, NJ: Prentice Hall.

Simkin, P., & Bolding, A. (2004). Update on nonpharmacologic approaches to relieve labor pain and prevent suffering. *Journal of Midwifery and Women's Health, 49*(6), 489–504.

St. Hill, P. F., Lipson, J. G., Ibrahim, A., & Meleis, A. F. (2003). *Nurse's drug guide: 2004.* Upper Saddle River, NJ: Prentice Hall.

CHAPTER 8

Centers for Disease Control and Prevention (CDC), Division of Reproductive Health, National Center for Chronic Disease Prevention and Health Promotion, Division of Vital Statistics, National Center for Health Statistics. Washington, DC: U.S. Government Printing Office. Available at www.access.gpo.gov

DeJonge, C. J. (2000). Egg transport and fertilization. In J. J. Sciarra & T. J. Watkins (Eds.), *Gynecology and Obstetrics* (Vol. 1, p. 127). Philadelphia: Lippincott Williams & Wilkins.

Fowles, E. (2004). Prenatal nutrition and birth outcomes. *Journal of Obstetric, Gynecologic, and Neonatal Nursing, 33*(6), 809–822.

Hood, M. Y., Moore, L. L., Sundarajan-Ramamurti, A., Singer, M., Cupples, L. A., & Ellison, R. C. (2000). Parental eating attitudes and the development of obesity in children. The Framingham Children's Study. *International Journal of Obesity Related Metabolic Disorders, 24*(10), 1319–1325.

London, M. L., Ladewig, P. W., Ball, J. W., & Bindler, R. C. (2007). *Maternal & child nursing care.* Upper Saddle River, NJ: Prentice Hall.

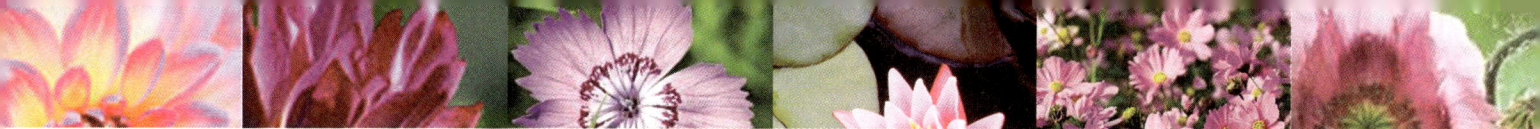

Mattson, S. (1995). Culturally sensitive perinatal care for Southeast Asians. *Journal of Obstetric, Gynecologic, and Neonatal Nursing, 24*(4), 335–341.

Moore, K. L., & Persaud, T. V. N. (2003). *The clinically oriented embryology* (7th ed.). Philadelphia: Saunders.

National Center for Health Statistics. (2005). *National vital statistics reports, 54*(2).

Olds, S. B., London, M. L., Ladewig, P. A. W., & Davidson, M. R. (2004). *Maternal–newborn nursing & women's health care* (7th ed.). Upper Saddle River, NJ: Prentice Hall.

Roach, S. S., & Scherer, J. C. (2000). *Introductory clinical pharmacology* (6th ed.). Buffalo, NY: Lippincott.

Rogers, J., & Davis, B. (1995). How risky are hot tubs and saunas for pregnant women? *MCN, 20*(3), 137–140.

Spector, R. E. (2000). *Cultural diversity in health and illness* (5th ed.). Upper Saddle River, NJ: Prentice-Hall Health.

CHAPTER 9

Berkowitz, R., & Goldstein, D. (2007). Gestational trophoblastic disease. In J. Berek, *Berek & Novak's gynecology* (14th ed., pp. 1581–1603). Philadelphia: Lippincott Williams & Wilkins.

Callister, L. C. (2001). Culturally competent care of women and newborns: Knowledge, attitude and skills. *Journal of Obstetric, Gynecologic, and Neonatal Nursing, 30*, 209–215.

Centers for Disease Control and Prevention (CDC), Division of Reproductive Health, National Center for Chronic Disease Prevention and Health Promotion, Division of Vital Statistics, National Center for Health Statistics. Washington, DC: U.S. Government Printing Office. Available at www.access.gpo.gov

Goetzl, L. M. (2002). ACOG practice bulletin. Obstetric analgesia and anesthesia. *Obstetrics and Gynecology, 100*, 177–191.

Jenkins, T. M., & Wapner, R. J. (2004). Prenatal diagnosis of congenital disorders. In R. K. Creasy & R. Resnik (Eds.), *Maternal–fetal medicine: Principles and practice* (5th ed., pp. 235–280). Philadelphia: Saunders.

Jongen, V., & Koetsier, D. (1997). Pitfalls in the diagnosis of complete hydatidiform mole with coexistent live fetus. *Tropical Medicine & International Health, 2*(3), 289–290.

London, M. L., Ladewig, P. W., Ball, J. W., & Bindler, R. C. (2003). *Maternal–newborn and child nursing*. Upper Saddle River, NJ: Prentice Hall.

Moore, L. (2006). Hydatidiform mole. *e-medicine.* Retrieved April 10, 2007, from www.emedicine.com/med/topic1047.htm

National Library of Medicine. (2007). Hydatid mole: Molar pregnancy. *MedlinePlus Medical Dictionary.* Retrieved April 10, 2007, from the Internet.

Olds, S. B., London, M. L., Ladewig, P. W., & Davidson, M. R. (2004). *Maternal–newborn nursing and women's health care* (7th ed.). Upper Saddle River, NJ: Prentice Hall.

CHAPTER 10

American Pregnancy Association. (2006, August). *Natural herbs & vitamins during pregnancy.* Available on the Internet.

Berek, J. (2007). Cervical & vaginal cancer. In *Berek & Novak's Gynecology* (15th ed., pp. 1437–1438). Philadelphia: Lippincott.

Centers for Disease Control and Prevention (CDC), Division of Reproductive Health, National Center for Chronic Disease Prevention and Health Promotion, Division of Vital Statistics, National Center for Health Statistics. Washington, DC: U.S. Government Printing Office. Available on the Internet.

Choi, E. C. (1995). A contrast of mothering behaviors in women from Korea and the United States. *Journal of Obstetric, Gynecologic, and Neonatal Nursing, 24*(4), 363–369.

DeJonge, C. J. (2000). Egg transport and fertilization. In J. J. Sciarra & T. J. Watkins (Eds.), *Gynecology and obstetrics* (Vol. 1, p. 127). Philadelphia: Lippincott Williams & Wilkins.

Eisenberg, A., Murkoff, H., & Hathaway, S. (1986). *What to eat when you're expecting.* New York: Workman.

Fowles, E. (2004). Prenatal nutrition and birth outcomes. *Journal of Obstetric, Gynecologic, and Neonatal Nursing, 33*(6), 809–822.

Gottlieb, B. (2000). *Alternative cures.* Emmaus, PA: Rodale Press.

Hardy, M. (2000). Herbs of special interest to women. *Journal of the American Pharmaceutical Association, 40*(2), 234–242.

Hood, M. Y., Moore, L. L., Sundarajan-Ramamurti, A., Singer, M., Cupples, L. A., & Ellison, R. C. (2000). Parental eating attitudes and the development of obesity in children. The Framingham Children's Study. *International Journal of Obesity Related Metabolic Disorders, 24*(10), 1319–1325.

Krieger/Elchai, L. (1996–1997). Herbs of special interest to women. *Herbs for a Healthy Balance.* © Creative Minds Unlimited. Available at www.create.org

London, M. L., Ladewig, P. W., Ball, J. W., & Bindler, R. C. (2003). *Maternal–newborn and child nursing*. Upper Saddle River, NJ: Prentice Hall.

Mattson, S. (1995). Culturally sensitive perinatal care for Southeast Asians. *Journal of Obstetric, Gynecologic, and Neonatal Nursing, 24*(4), 335–341.

Moran, R. (1999, Feb. 15). Evaluation and treatment of childhood obesity. *American Family Physician, 59*(4).

Olds, S. B., London, M. L., Ladewig, P. A. W., & Davidson, M. R. (2004). *Maternal–newborn nursing & women's health care* (7th ed.). Upper Saddle River, NJ: Prentice Hall.

Roach, S. S., & Scherer, J. C. (2000). *Introductory clinical pharmacology* (6th ed.). Buffalo, NY: Lippincott.

Rogers, J., & Davis, B. (1995). How risky are hot tubs and saunas for pregnant women? *MCN, 20*(3), 137–140.

Somer, E. (2002). *Nutrition for a healthy pregnancy: The complete guide to eating before, during, and after your pregnancy.* New York: Owl Books.

Spector, R. E. (2000). *Cultural diversity in health and illness* (5th ed.). Upper Saddle River, NJ: Prentice-Hall Health.

U.S. Department of Health and Human Services. (2000). *Healthy People 2010* (2nd ed.). Washington, DC: U.S. Government Printing Office.

CHAPTER 11

American Pregnancy Association. (2006, August). *Natural herbs & vitamins during pregnancy.* Available at www. americanpregnancy.org

Bondok, R., Sharnouby, N., Eid, H., & Elmaksoud, A. (2006). Pulsed steroid therapy is an effective treatment for intractable hyperemesis gravidarum. *Critical Care Medicine, 34*(11), 2781–2783.

Choi, E. C. (1995). A contrast of mothering behaviors in women from Korea and the United States. *Journal of Obstetric, Gynecologic, and Neonatal Nursing, 24*(4), 363–369.

Eiseberg, A., Murkoff, H., & Hathaway, S. (1986). *What to eat when you're expecting.* New York: Workman.

Fowles, E. (2004). Prenatal nutrition and birth outcomes. *Journal of Obstetrics, Gynecologic, and Neonatal Nursing, 33*(6), 809–822.

Johnson, M., Bulechek, G., Dochterman, J., Maas, M., & Moorhead, S. (2001). *Nursing diagnoses, outcomes, & interventions: NANDA, NOC and NIC linkages.* St. Louis, MO: Mosby.

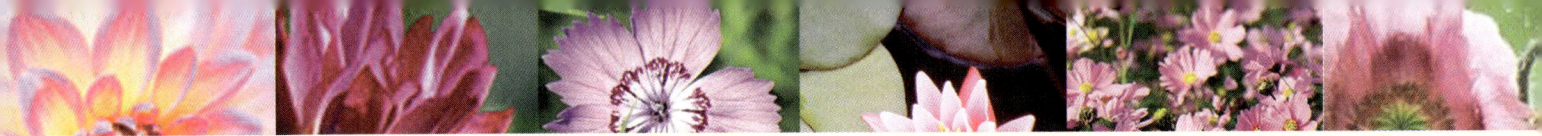

Krieger/Elchai, L. (1996–1997). Herbs of special interest to women. *Herbs for a Healthy Balance*. © Creative Minds Unlimited. Available on the Internet.

Lamondy, A. (2006). Hyperemesis gravidarum and the role of the infusion nurse. *Journal of Infusion Nursing, 29*(2), 89–100.

Somer, E. (2002). *Nutrition for a healthy pregnancy: The complete guide to eating before, during and after your pregnancy.* New York: Owl Books.

Spector, R. E. (2000). *Cultural diversity in health and illness* (5th ed.). Upper Saddle River, NJ: Prentice-Hall Health.

Whitney, E. N., Cataldo, C. B., & Rolfes, S. R. (2002). *Understanding normal and clinical nutrition* (6th ed.). Belmont, CA: Wadsworth Publishing.

CHAPTER 12

Alan Guttmacher Institute. (2002). Sexual and reproductive health: Women and men. *Facts in brief.* Washington, DC. Author.

American Academy of Pediatrics. (2002). Care of adolescent parents and their children. *Pediatrics, 107*(2), 429–434.

Annie E. Casey Foundation. (1998). *Kids count special report: When teens have sex: Issues and trends.* Baltimore, MD: Author.

Annie E. Casey Foundation. (2004). *Kids count 2004.* Baltimore, MD: Author.

Cohen, D.A., Farley, T. A., Taylor, S. N., Martin, D. H., & Schuster, M. A. (2002). When and where do youths have sex? The potential role of adult supervision. *Pediatrics, 110*(6), 66–69.

Doniger, A., Adams, E., Utter, C., & Riley, J. (2001). Impact evaluation of the "not me, not now" abstinence-oriented adolescent pregnancy prevention communication program, Monroe County, New York. *Journal of Health Communication, 6*(1), 45–60.

Goffman, E. (1963). *Stigma: Notes on the management of spoiled identity.* New York: Simon & Schuster.

Johnson, M., Bulechek, G., Dochterman, J., Maas, M., & Moorhead, S. (2001). *Nursing diagnoses, outcomes, & interventions: NANDA, NOC and NIC linkages.* St. Louis, MO: Mosby.

Key, J. D., Barbosa, G. A., & Owens, V. J. (2001). The second chance club: Repeat adolescent pregnancy prevention with a school-based intervention. *Journal of Adolescent Health, 28*(3), 167–169.

Koniak-Griffin, D., Anderson, N., Verzemnieks, I., & Brecht, M. (2000). A public health nursing early intervention program for adolescent mothers: Outcomes from pregnancy through 6 weeks postpartum. *Nursing Research, 49*(3), 130–138.

Manlove, J., Ryan, S., & Franzetta, K. (2003). Patterns of contraceptive use within teenagers' first sexual relationships. *Perspectives on Sexual and Reproductive Health, 35*(6), 246–255.

Martin, J. A., Hamilton, B. E., Sutton, P. D., Ventura, S. J., Menacker, F., & Munson, M. L. (2003). Births: Final data for 2002. *National Vital Statistics Reports, 52*(10), 1–114.

Montgomery, K. S. (2003). Nursing care for pregnant adolescents. *Journal of Obstetric, Gynecologic, and Neonatal Nursing, 32*(2), 249–257.

National Campaign to Prevent Teen Pregnancy. (2000). *Fact sheet report.* Washington, DC: Author.

National Campaign to Prevent Teen Pregnancy. (2006). *Fact sheet report.* Washington, DC: Author.

Nichols, F. H., & Sharron, S. H. (2000). *Childbirth education: Practice, research, and theory* (2nd ed.). Philadelphia: W.B. Saunders, pp. 609–621.

President's New Freedom Commission on Mental Health. (2003). *Achieving the promise: Transforming mental health care in America—Final report.* DHHS Pub. No. SMA-03-3832. Rockville, MD: DHHS, Government Printing Office. Retrieved April 29, 2007, from www.mentalhealthcommission.gov/reports/FinalReport/FullReport.htm

Shelley, J., & Fish, S. (1988). *Spiritual care: The nurse's role* (3rd ed.). Downer's Grove, IL: Intervarsity Press.

Short, M. B., & Rosenthal, S. L. (2003). Helping teenaged girls make wise sexual decisions. *Contemporary OB/GYN, 48*(5), 84–95.

Taylor, D., Chavez, G., Adams, E., Chabra, A., & Shah, R. S. (1999). Demographic characteristics in adult paternity for first births to adolescents under 15 years of age. *Journal of Adolescent Health, 24*(4), 251–258.

World Health Organization. (2002). Chapter three: Child abuse and neglect by parents and other caregivers. *World Report on Violence and Health* [online]. Retrieved April 26, 2007, from www.who.int/violence_injury_prevention/violence/world_report/en/

CHAPTER 13

AWHONN. (2007). Assessing pre-term labor and birth risk. *Lifelines Patient Page.*

Centers for Disease Control and Prevention. (2002). Sexually transmitted diseases treatment guidelines 2002. *Morbidity and Mortality Weekly Report, 51*(RR-6), 1–84.

Jones, D. W., & Hall, J. E. (2002). The National High Blood Pressure Education Program: 30 years and counting. *Hypertension, 39*, 941.

Kübler-Ross, E. (1969). *On death and dying.* New York: Macmillan.

London, M. L., Ladewig, P. W., Ball, J. W., & Bindler, R. C. (2003). *Maternal–newborn and child nursing.* Upper Saddle River, NJ: Prentice Hall.

Magann, E. F., Chauhan, S. P., Bofill, J. A., Waddell, D., Rust, O. A., & Morrison, J. C. (2002). *Maternal morbidity and mortality associated with intrauterine fetal demise: Five year experience at a tertiary referral hospital.* 70th annual meeting, Central Association of Obstetricians and Gynecologists, Maui, HI.

National High Blood Pressure Education Program. (2000). *Hypertension, 35*, 1021–1024.

Papp, C., & Papp, Z. (2003). Chorionic villus sampling and amniocentesis: What are the risks in current practice? *Current Opinion in Obstetrics & Gynecology, 15*(2), 159–165.

Pressinger, R. W. (1998). Cigarette smoking during pregnancy: Links to learning disabilities attention deficit disorder—A.D.D.—hyperactivity and behavior disorders. Special Education Department, University of South Florida, Tampa, FL.

Reed, J., & Klebanoff, M. (1993). Sexual intercourse during pregnancy and preterm delivery: Effects of vaginal microorganisms. *American Journal of Obstetrics & Gynecology, 168*(2).

Regidor, E., Ronda, E., Garcia, A. M., & Dominguez, V. (2004). Paternal exposure to agricultural pesticides. *Occupational & Environmental Medicine, 61*(4), 334–339.

Skeie, A., Foren, J. J., Vege, A., & Stray-Pedersen, B. (2003). Cause and risk of stillbirth in twin pregnancies: A retrospective audit. *Acta Obstetricia et Gynecologica Scandinavica, 82*(11), 1010–1016.

Van Meurs, K. (1999). Cigarette smoking, pregnancy and the developing fetus. Stanford University School of Medicine. *Stanford Medical Review, 1*(1), 14–16.

CHAPTER 14

Adams, E., & Bianchi, A. (2004). Can a nurse and a doula exist in the same room? *International Journal of Childbirth Education, 19*(4), 12–15.

Adams, E., & Bianchi, A. (2005). *50 Ways to comfort a laboring woman.* Presented at the AWHONN 2005 convention, June 14, Salt Lake City, Utah.

Bianchi, A., & Adams, E. (2004). Doulas, labor support, and nurses. *International Journal of Childbirth Education, 19*(4), 24–30.

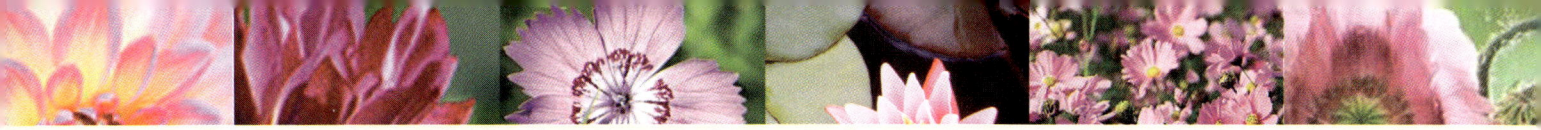

Callister, L. C. (2001). Culturally competent care of women and newborns: Knowledge, attitude and skills. *Journal of Obstetric, Gynecologic, and Neonatal Nursing, 30*, 209–215.

Dick-Read, G. (2005). *Childbirth without fear*. London: Pinter & Martin Publishers.

Doulas of North America website. Available at www.dona.org

Giles, M., Garland, S., & Oats, J. (2005). Management of preterm prelabour rupture of membranes: An audit. How do the results compare with clinical practice guidelines? *Australian and New Zealand Journal of Obstetrics and Gynecology, 45*, 201–206.

Goetzl, L. M. (2002). ACOG practice bulletin. Obstetric analgesia and anesthesia. *Obstetrics and Gynecology, 100*, 177–191.

Greenwald, J. (1993, August). Premature rupture of the membranes: Diagnostic and management strategies. *American Family Physician.*

Hopper Deglin, J., & Hazard Vallerand, A. (2005). *Davis's drug guide for nurses* (9th ed.). Philadelphia: F.A. Davis.

International Childbirth Education Association website. Available at www.icea.org

Johnson, M., Bulechek, G., Dochterman, J., Maas, M., & Moorhead, S. (2001). *Nursing diagnoses, outcomes, & interventions: NANDA, NOC and NIC linkages*. St. Louis, MO: Mosby.

Karat, C., Madhivanan, P., Krupp, K., Poornima, S., Jayanthi, N., Suguna, J., & Mathai, E. (2006). The clinical and microbiological correlates of premature rupture of membranes [abstract]. *Indian Journal of Medical Microbiology, 24*(4), 283–285.

Miltner, R. (2002). More than support: Nursing interventions provided to women in labor. *Journal of Obstetric, Gynecologic, and Neonatal Nursing, 31*(6), 753–761.

Olds, S. B., London, M. L., Ladewig, P. W., & Davidson, M. R. (2004). *Maternal–newborn nursing and women's health care* (7th ed.). Upper Saddle River, NJ: Prentice Hall.

Radnai, M., Gorzo, I., Urban, E., Eller, J., Novak, T., & Pal, A. (2006). Possible association between mother's periodontal status and pre-term delivery [abstract]. *Journal of Clinical Periodontology, 33*(11), 791–796.

Simkin, P., & Bolding, A. (2004). Update on nonpharmacologic approaches to relieve labor pain and prevent suffering. *Journal of Midwifery and Women's Health, 49*(6), 489–504.

St. Hill, P. F., Lipson, J. G., Ibrahim, A., & Meleis, A. F. (2003). *Nurse's drug guide: 2004*. Upper Saddle River, NJ: Prentice Hall.

Verma, U., Goharkhay, N., & Samir, B. (2006). Conservative management of preterm premature rupture of membranes between 18 and 23 weeks of gestation—Maternal and neonatal outcome. *European Journal of Obstetrics & Gynecology and Reproductive Biology, 128*, 119–124.

CHAPTER 15

Cunningham, G., Leveno, K., Bloom, S., Hauth, J., Gilstrap, L., & Wenstrom, K. (Eds.). (2007 [online] 2005 [print]). Chapter 35: Obstetrical hemorrhage. *Williams Obstetrics* (22nd ed.) [online]. Columbus, OH: AccessMedicine/The McGraw-Hill Companies. Retrieved April 15, 2007 from www.accessmedicine.com/content.aspx?aID=731310

Johnson, M., Bulechek, G., Dochterman, J., Maas, M., & Moorhead, S. (2001). *Nursing diagnoses, outcomes, & interventions: NANDA, NOC and NIC linkages*. St. Louis, MO: Mosby.

Ma, R., Lao, T., Feng, Y., Zhao, W., Huang, J., Liang, G., Li, H., & Chen, Z. (2005). Successful treatment of combined vaginal and broad ligament hematoma using pelvic pressure pack and arterial embolization. *Progress in Obstetrics and Gynecology, 14*(6), 523–526.

Placksin, S. (2000). *Mothering the new mother: Women's feelings and needs after childbirth: A support and resource guide*. New York: Newmarket Press.

Rortveit, G., Daltveit, A. K., Hannestad, Y., & Hunskaar, S. (2003). Urinary incontinence after vaginal delivery or cesarean section. *New England Journal of Medicine*, (348)10, 900–907.

Scott, J. R. (2006). Cesarean delivery on request: Where do we go from here? *Obstetrics and Gynecology, 107*, 1222–1223.

U. S. Department of Health and Human Services. (2006). *National Vital Statistics Reports, 50*(15).

Villela, J., Garry, D., Levine, G., Glanz, S., Figueroa, R., & Maulik, D. (2001). Postpartum angiographic embolization for vulvovaginal hematoma: A report of two cases [abstract]. *Journal of Reproductive Medicine, 46*(1), 65–67.

CHAPTER 16

Barclay, L. (2006). Practice guidelines issued for use of episiotomy [online]. *Medscape Medical News* (CME). Retrieved April 19, 2007, from www.medscape.com/viewarticle/529251

Beckmann, M., & Garrett, A. (2007). Antenatal perineal massage for reducing perineal trauma. *Cochrane Database of Systematic Reviews, 1*, 2007.

Cunningham, F. G., Grant, N. F., Laveno, K. J., Gilstrap, L. C. (2001). *Williams obstetrics* (21st ed.). New York: McGraw-Hill.

DeNoon, D. (2006). Massage cuts need for episiotomies [online]. *WebMDHealth*. Retrieved April 19, 2007, from www.medscape.com/viewarticle/522250_print

Eby, L., & Brown, N. J. (2005). *Mental health nursing care*. Upper Saddle River, NJ: Prentice Hall.

Gunes, M., Kayikcioglu, F., Ozturkoglu, E., & Haberal, A. (2005). Incisional endometriosis after cesarean section, episiotomy and other gynecological procedures. *Journal of Obstetrics and Gynaecology Research, 31*(5), 471–475.

Ladewig, P., London, M., & Davidson, M. (2006). *Contemporary maternal–newborn nursing care* (6th ed.). Upper Saddle River, NJ: Prentice Hall.

May, J. (1994). Modified median episiotomy minimizes the risk of third-degree tears [abstract]. *Obstetrics & Gynecology, 83*(1), 156.

Narad, C., & Mason, P. (2004). International adoption: Myths and realities. *Pediatric Nursing, 30*(6), 483–487.

Ramont, R. P., Niedringhaus, D. M., & Towle, M. A. (2006). *Comprehensive nursing care*. Upper Saddle River, NJ: Prentice Hall.

Russel, M. (2004). *Adoption wisdom: A guide to the issues and feelings of adoption*. Lawrenceville, NJ: Tapestry Press.

Sallday, S. (2004). Ethical problems: Adoption dilemmas. *Nursing, 34*(12), 29.

Simpson, K., & Thorman, K. (2005). Obstetric "conveniences": Elective induction of labor, cesarean birth on demand, and other potentially unnecessary interventions. *Journal of Perinatal and Neonatal Nursing, 19*(2), 134–144.

Youngkin, E., & Davis, M. S. (1998). *Women's health: A primary care clinical guide* (2nd ed.). Upper Saddle River, NJ: Prentice Hall.

CHAPTER 17

American Academy of Pediatrics. (2006). Policy statements of the American Academy of Pediatrics. *Pediatrics, 117*(5), 1846–1847.

Ball, J., & Bindler, R. (2006). *Child health nursing*. Upper Saddle River, NJ: Prentice Hall.

Ballard, J. L., Khoury, J. C., Wedig, K., Eilers-Walsman, B. L., & Lipp, R. (1991). New Ballard score, expanded to include extremely premature infants. *Journal of Pediatrics, 119*(3), 417–423.

Blackburn, S. T. (2003). *Maternal fetal and neonatal physiology: A clinical perspective* (2nd ed.). St. Louis, MO: Saunders.

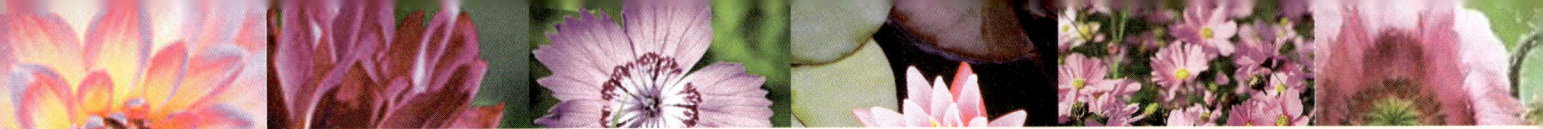

Committee on Bioethics. (1995). Informed consent, parental permission, and assent in pediatric practice. *Pediatrics, 95*(2), 314–317.

Dougherty, G. (1998). When should a child be hospitalized? *Pediatrics, 101*(1), 6.

Greenberg, M. (2004). *Infant circumcision* [online]. Retrieved April 30, 2007, from www.drgreenberg.ca

Johnson, M., Bulechek, G., Dochterman, J., Maas, M., & Moorhead, S. (2001). *Nursing diagnoses, outcomes, & interventions: NANDA, NOC and NIC linkages*. St. Louis, MO: Mosby.

National Organization of Circumcision Information Resource Centers website. Available at www.nocirc.org

Olds, S. B., London, M. L., Ladewig, P. W., & Davidson, M. R. (2004). *Maternal–newborn nursing and women's health care* (7th ed.). Upper Saddle River, NJ: Prentice Hall.

Orshan, S. (2008). Chapter 20: The Healthy Newborn. *Maternity, Newborn and Women's Health Nursing: Comprehensive Care Across the Lifespan*. Philadelphia: Wolters Kluwer/Lippincott Williams & Wilkins.

Seidel, J. M., Ball, J. W., Dains, J., & Benedict, G. W. (2003). *Mosby's guide to physical examination* (5th ed.). St. Louis, MO: Mosby.

Tappero, E. P., & Honeyfield, M. E. (1996). *Physical assessment of the newborn* (2nd ed.). Petaluma, CA: NICU Ink.

CHAPTER 18

Ballard, J. L., Khoury, J. C., Wedig, K., Eilers-Walsman, B. L., & Lipp, R. (1991). New Ballard score, expanded to include extreme premature infants. *Journal of Pediatrics 119*(3), 417–423.

Driscoll, D. J. (1999). Left-to-right shunt lesions. *Pediatric Clinics of North America, 46*(2), 355–368.

Fedderly, R. T. (1999). Left ventricular outflow obstruction. *Pediatric Clinics of North America. 46*(2), 369–384.

Finnegan, L. P. (1985). Neonatal abstinence. In N. Nelson, (Ed.), *Current therapy in neonatal perinatal medicine*. Toronto: B.C. Decker.

Grifka, R. G. (1999). Cyanotic congenital heart disease with increased blood flow. *Pediatric Clinics of North America, 46*(2), 405–425.

Johnson, M., Bulechek, G., Dochterman, J., Maas, M., & Moorhead, S. (2001). *Nursing diagnoses, outcomes, & interventions: NANDA, NOC and NIC linkages*. St. Louis, MO: Mosby.

Kandall, S. R. (1999). Treatment strategies for drug-exposed neonates. *Clinical Perinatology 25*(1), 231–243.

Olson, S. (1998). Bedside musical care: Applications in pregnancy, childbirth, and neonatal care. *Journal of Obstetric, Gyneocologic, & Neonatal Nursing, 27*(5), 569–575.

Orshan, S. (2008). *Maternity, newborn and women's health nursing: Comprehensive care across the lifespan*. Philadelphia: Wolters Kluwer/Lippincott Williams & Wilkins.

Park, M. K. (2002). *Pediatric cardiology for practitioners* (4th ed.). St. Louis, MO: Mosby.

Rahimian, J., & Varner, M. W. (2003). Disproportionate fetal growth. In A. H. DeCherney & L. Nathan (Eds.), *Current obstetric & gynecologic diagnosis & treatment* (9th ed., pp. 301–314). New York: Lang Medical Books/McGraw-Hill.

Robinson, D., & Drumm, L. (2001). Maple syrup urine disease: A standard of nursing care. *Pediatric Nursing, 27*(3), 256–264, 270.

Walters, H. L. (2000). Congenital cardiac surgical strategies and outcomes: HEARTS. *Pediatric Annals, 29*(8), 489–498.

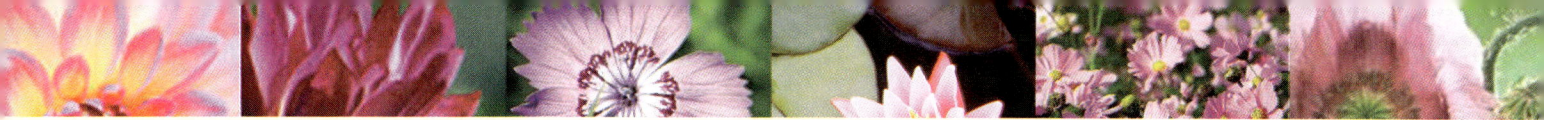

Glossary

(Note: Glossary terms may appear in more than one chapter. Boldface numbers after the glossary term indicate the chapter(s) in which the term is defined. Other words or terms that may require definitions are italicized in the text and are defined there.)

1-hour glucose screen: test done at 24 to 28 weeks' gestation in which values above 140 mg/dL indicate gestational diabetes **(13)**

5 Ps affecting labor: variables affecting labor grouped for easier discussion, referring to both maternal and fetal characteristics: passage, passenger, powers, position, and psyche **(14)**

A

ABO incompatibility: a clash between the mother's type O and the fetus's type A, B, or AB blood **(13)**

Abortifacients: abortion-inducing herbs that induce menstruation **(10)**

Abortion: termination of pregnancy before the fetus is able to live outside the mother; the loss of pregnancy before the 20th week **(3, 7, 10)**

Abruptio placentae: separation of the placenta that may occur in late pregnancy or during labor **(13)**

Accelerations: an increase in the fetal heart rate with fetal activity **(15)**

Accuracy: correctness **(2)**

Acquired immunodeficiency syndrome (AIDS): a life-threatening, end-stage infection with HIV **(7)**

Acrocyanosis: a bluish discoloration of the hands and feet that is common for several hours after delivery **(17)**

Acrosome: a specialized structure covering the head of the sperm and containing enzymes that can break down the covering of the ovum **(5)**

Active phase: phase of the first stage of labor begins when the cervix is dilated 4 centimeters and ends with 8 centimeters of dilatation **(14)**

Acupressure: a form of healing in which the therapist uses finger or thumb pressure over specific pressure points **(6)**

Adaptability: how well the family changes when faced with problems **(4)**

Adoption: the legal transfer of the responsibility for raising a child from the birth mother to the adoptive parent(s) **(7)**

Afterpains: discomfort from uterine contractions after delivery, occurring in most women but generally more noticeable in multipara mothers **(16)**

Alveoli: glandular cells that are arranged in grape-like clusters **(5)**

Ambiguous genitalia: (also called *pseudohermaphroditism*) a rare condition in which determining the gender of the infant is difficult **(18)**

Amenorrhea: the absence of menses **(7, 10)**

Amniocentesis: the withdrawal of amniotic fluid through a needle inserted into the abdomen and the uterus **(9)**

Amnioinfusion: a process of introducing warmed sterile normal saline or Ringer's lactate solution into the uterus to increase the volume of intrauterine fluid when low amniotic fluid volume is causing fetal parts to compress the umbilical cord; also used to dilute moderate to heavy meconium in the amniotic fluid **(15)**

Amnion: the inner layer of the placenta **(8)**

Amniotic fluid: formed by the amnion; consists of abut 98% water; also contains glucose, proteins, urea, lanugo, and vernix caseosa **(8)**

Amniotomy: an artificial rupturing of the fetal membranes **(14)**

Anencephaly: absence of neural tissue in the cranium **(8, 11)**

Anomalies: developments of abnormal organs or structures **(8)**

Antrum: the cavity of a hollow organ or a sinus, as the *antrum* of the graafian follicle **(5)**

Anxiety: a common reaction to stress, a state of mental uneasiness, apprehension, or dread or a feeling of helplessness related to actual or unidentified threat to self or significant relationships **(6)**

Apgar score: a rapid evaluation of the infant's adaptation to extrauterine life; five items are assessed in order of priority: heart rate, respiratory rate, muscle tone, reflex irritability, and color; each item is assigned a score from 0 to 2, and the scores are then totaled **(14)**

Apneic spells: periods without breathing **(17)**

Areola: the colored ring around the nipple **(5)**

Artificial insemination: process of artificially instilling sperm into the vagina or uterus **(7)**

Assumptions: ideas taken for granted **(2)**

Ataxia: staggering gait **(6)**

Atrial septal defect: failure of the foramen ovale to close after birth **(18)**

Autosomal: found on chromosomes 1 through 22 **(8)**

Autosomes: chromosomes that are alike in males and females **(5)**

B

Babinski's reflex: reflex in infants elicited by stroking the lateral side of the foot from heel to toe; the big toe should dorsiflex and the other toes should flare; reflex disappears before the infant begins to walk **(17)**

Bag of waters: fetal membranes **(8)**

Ballotable: able to be pushed away from the cervix **(14)**

Ballottement: a test for pregnancy in which the examiner puts two fingers into the vagina and pushes upward on the uterus; if the woman is pregnant, the fetus will rebound against the fingers **(10)**

Barriers: including male and female condoms, vaginal diaphragms, and cervical caps; devices placed in the vagina or over the penis to prevent sperm from entering the cervix **(7)**

Bartholin's glands: (also known as *greater vestibular glands*) glands whose ducts open onto the vestibule and secrete a thin mucus-like substance that provides lubrication during sexual intercourse **(5)**

Basal body temperature: body temperature in the morning before rising or moving about or eating anything **(7)**

Benign prostatic hyperplasia: a prostate disorder where the prostate gland enlarges in the center, compressing surrounding tissue and narrowing the urethra **(7)**

Beriberi: condition resulting from thiamin deficiency; a disease that damages the nervous system, heart, and other muscles **(11)**

Beta-carotene: the orange pigment in plants; the carotenoid with the greatest vitamin A activity **(11)**

Binuclear family: both parents sharing custody of the children, resulting in the children moving between the two households **(4)**

Biophysical profile: a test that assesses five variables: fetal breathing, fetal movement, fetal tone, amniotic fluid volume, and fetal reaction **(9)**

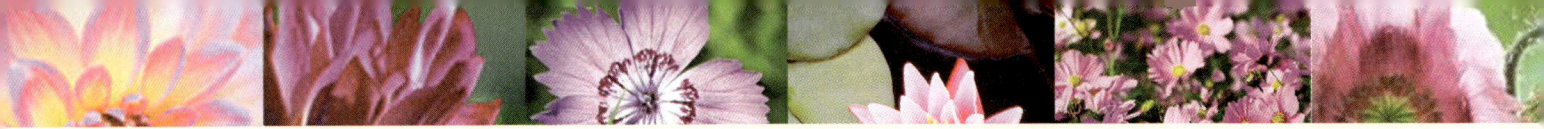

Biotin: a coenzyme in metabolism, crucial in the synthesis of glucose from noncarbohydrate sources (such as amino acids and glycerol), in the synthesis of fatty acids, and in the breakdown of some amino acids (11)

Blastocyst: a two-layer ball formed by the cells of the morula in the uterus (8)

Blended family: a family situation in which one or both spouses have had a previous marriage and children from that marriage (4)

Bloody show: the release of the mucus plug from the cervix (14)

Body: the upper portion of the uterus (5)

Boggy: soft and spongy (16)

Bonding: the establishment of a strong emotional attachment between two unique individuals (16)

Boundary: an imaginary border where the members of the system come in contact with others outside the system (4)

Braxton Hicks contractions: painless contractions occurring throughout the pregnancy, and becoming more noticeable after the 20th week during periods of rapid fetal growth (10, 14)

Breadth: scope (2)

Breech: describing buttocks presentation of the fetus (14)

Bronchopulmonary dysplasia: chronic lung disease that affects infants with respiratory distress syndrome, congenital heart defects, meconium aspiration, or other conditions that result from assisted mechanical ventilation (18)

Bulbourethral glands: (also known as *Cowper's glands*) glands located below the prostate that secrete a mucus-like fluid into the penile section of the urethra that helps neutralize the acid environment of the urethra and lubricate the end of the penis (5)

C

Candidiasis: (also called *monilia* or *yeast infection*) a common organism causing vaginitis (7)

Caput succedaneum: edema of the scalp (17)

Carbohydrates: compounds needed for energy and made up of both simple and complex molecules of carbon, hydrogen, and oxygen (6)

Cardinal movements: the movements that occur when the fetus changes positions as it moves through the pelvis, also called mechanisms of labor (14)

Care plan: an organized and prioritized plan that addresses the nursing diagnoses and helps the client reach measurable, identified outcomes or goals (1)

Carrier: a person who has one dominant gene and one recessive gene (8)

Cephalhematoma: an accumulation of blood between the periosteum and the skull bone that will not cross the suture lines (17)

Cephalic presentation: head-down position (14)

Cephalocaudal: occurring from head to toe (8)

Cephalopelvic disproportion: condition in which the maternal pelvis is smaller than the fetal head (14)

Cerclage: (also called *Shirodkar procedure*) procedure done at 16 weeks' gestation; involves surgically placing a suture in the cervix in a purse-string design to hold the cervix closed (13)

Cervical dysplasia: abnormal changes in the tissue of the cervix (7)

Cervix: the lower region of the uterus (5)

Cesarean section: surgical birth (15)

Chadwick's sign: a bluish purple discoloration of the cervix and vagina (10)

Chancre: painless open sore (7)

Chlamydia: a sexually transmitted infection caused by *Chlamydia trachomatis* (7)

Chloasma: "mask of pregnancy," a darkening of the forehead, cheeks, and area around the eyes (10)

Chorion: the outer layer of the membranes (8)

Chorionic villi: finger-like projections on the outermost fetal membrane (8)

Chorionic villus sampling: obtaining a small piece of the outermost fetal membrane from the placenta (9)

Chromosomes: structures made of DNA and protein that govern development of an organism (5)

Chronic hypertension: occurrence when the blood pressure is 140/90 or higher before pregnancy and continues for more than 12 weeks after delivery (13)

Cilia: minute hairlike structures (5)

Circumcision: the surgical removal of the foreskin (*prepuce*) of the penis (5, 17)

Circumoral: around the mouth (18)

Clarity: clearness (2)

Cleft lip: condition that results from failure of the upper lip to join medially; can be unilateral or bilateral (18)

Cleft palate: condition that results from failure of the medial nasal and maxillary processes to join, leaving an opening between the roof of the mouth and the floor of the nasal passage (18)

Clients: active participants in a process who obtain assistance from specialists (1)

Climacteric: menopause (7)

Clitoris: erectile tissue located just behind the junction of the labiae that provides for sexual arousal and pleasure (5)

Clonus: spasms or seizures (14)

Closed adoptions: adoptions in which the birth parents and adoptive parent do not communicate (12)

Coarctation: narrowing or constricting, especially of the aorta or of a blood vessel (18)

Cohabitating family: Unmarried partners with or without children (4)

Cold stress: condition that occurs when excessive heat is lost (17)

Colostrum: a translucent yellow fluid rich in protein, antibodies, and other substances to meet the needs of the newborn (5, 10, 16)

Communal family: a family that includes several adults and children, who may or may not be related, who live in the same household where family decisions and responsibilities are shared (4)

Community-based nursing: a response to the changes in health care that brings nursing to people where they work, play, and live (1)

Competent individual: a person who has received training, including instruction and clinical practice, to perform certain tasks and can demonstrate safe performance (2)

Complementary and alternative medicine: those practices that do not form part of the dominant system of health management in the area (6)

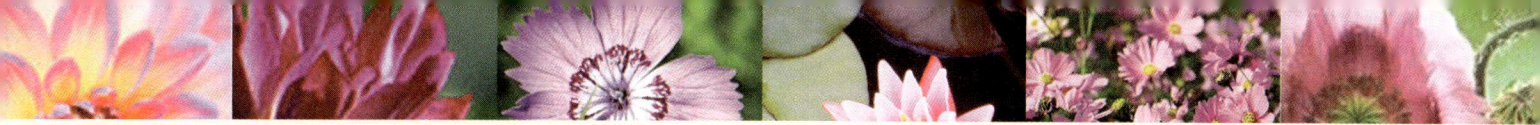

Conception: the uniting of ovum and sperm **(8)**

Concepts: ideas; theories, laws, and principles **(2)**

Conclusions: decisions based upon prior thought **(2)**

Conditionally essential amino acids: amino acids that are normally not essential but that cannot be supplied by the body or by the diet **(11)**

Confidence in reason: trust in the outcome of logical thought **(2)**

Confidentiality: keeping secret any privileged information **(3)**

Conization: removal of a cone-shaped wedge of cervical tissue **(7)**

Consumers: purchasers of a service **(1)**

Contraception: the prevention of pregnancy **(7)**

Contractions: shortening of muscle fibers that begins in response to the posterior pituitary hormone, oxytocin, in the uterine fundus **(14)**

Coping mechanisms: response to a stressor (*coping response*) **(6)**

Coping response: response to a stressor (*coping mechanism*) **(6)**

Corpus luteum: a glandular structure formed by the ruptured ovarian follicle; also called "yellow body," describing its yellow appearance **(5)**

Cotyledons: the irregular sections of the maternal side of the placenta **(8)**

Cowper's glands: (also known as *bulbourethral glands*) glands located below the prostate; these glands secrete a mucus-like fluid into the penile section of the urethra that helps neutralize *the acid environment* of the urethra and lubricate the end of the penis **(5)**

Craniofacial: pertaining to the head and face **(8)**

Critical thinking: self-directed, self-disciplined, self-monitored, and self-corrective thinking **(2)**

Crowning: occurrence when the largest part of the fetal head is past the vulva and remains visible between contractions **(14)**

Cryopreservation: process used to freeze ova that have been fertilized **(8)**

Cult family: a group in which a leader makes all decisions and controls the actions of those who live there **(4)**

Cultural competence: a set of skills, knowledge, and attitudes that include awareness and acceptance of differences, awareness of one's own cultural values, understanding of the dynamics of difference, development of cultural knowledge, and the ability to adapt practice skills to fit the cultural context of the client **(1)**

Cultural proficiency: when the components of cultural competence become second nature to the nurse **(1)**

Culture: a style of behavior patterns, beliefs, and *products of human work* (e.g., art, music, literature, architecture) within a given community or population **(4)**

Culture theory: framework for describing factors of culture that should be considered when working with families including communication, space, time, and role **(4)**

Cystocele: prolapse of the urinary bladder into the vagina **(7)**

Cysts: fluid-filled sacs **(7)**

Cytomegalovirus: a member of the herpes virus group, is found in saliva, breast milk, urine, cervical mucus, and semen of infected individuals **(13)**

D

D & C (dilatation and curettage): procedure in which the cervix is dilated, a curette is inserted into the uterus, and the endometrium is scraped, removing all products of conception **(13)**

Decelerations: a decrease in the fetal heart rate **(15)**

Decidua: tissue that lines the uterine wall during pregnancy **(16)**

Deductive reasoning: the process of making specific statements from a generalized concept **(2)**

Delegation: transferring to a competent individual the authority or right to perform selected nursing tasks in selected situations **(1, 2)**

Demandingness: relating to the demands that parents make on the children, their expectations for mature behavior, the discipline and supervision they provide, and their willingness to confront behavioral problems **(4)**

Depth: complexity **(2)**

Descent: movement during labor that begins with engagement and continues as the contractions push the fetus through the pelvis **(14)**

Diastasis recti abdominis: the result of the abdominal muscle separating during pregnancy **(16)**

Dilatation: opening of the cervical opening or *os* **(14)**

Dilatation stage: (also known as *first stage of labor*) begins with regular contractions and ends with complete effacement and dilatation of the cervix **(14)**

Disaccharides: sugar composed of pairs of monosaccharides **(11)**

Disseminated intravascular coagulation: a life-threatening pathologic process of the blood clotting mechanism **(13)**

Dominant: exerting a controlling influence **(8)**

Douche: vaginal irrigation **(6)**

Doula: a supportive companion who accompanies the woman through birth, providing physical and emotional support and information, and advocating for the woman and the family **(10)**

Down syndrome: most common chromosomal abnormality, resulting from trisomy 21 (three chromosomes at position 21) **(18)**

Ductus arteriosus: the connection from the main pulmonary artery to the aorta outside the fetal heart **(8)**

Ductus deferens: a duct that carries spermatozoa from the epididymis to the ejaculatory duct **(5)**

Ductus venosus: branch of the umbilical vein that carries blood to the inferior vena cava **(8)**

Duncan mechanism: expulsion of the placenta with the maternal side out **(14)**

Duration: the time from the onset of a contraction to the end of that contraction **(14)**

Dysmenorrhea: painful menses **(7)**

Dyspareunia: painful intercourse **(5, 7)**

Dystocia: long, difficult, or abnormal labor pattern **(15)**

E

Ecchymosis: bruising **(17)**

Eclampsia: once called *toxemia*; a common, complex condition that develops after 20 weeks' gestation **(13)**

Ecomap: a diagram of family member interactions with the immediate environment **(4)**

Ectopic: outside the normal location **(7)**

Ectopic pregnancy: implantation of the blastocyst outside the uterine cavity **(13)**

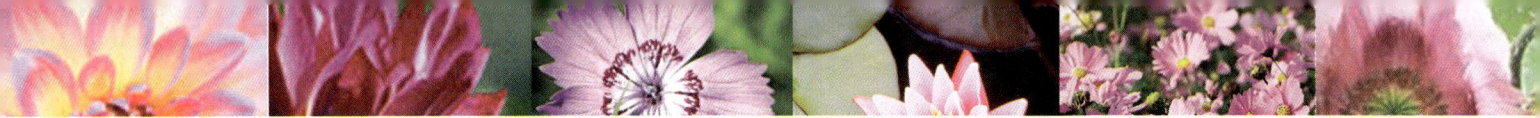

Effacement: the shortening and thinning of the cervix **(14)**

Effleurage: a light stroking with the fingertips in circular motion **(14)**

Ejaculatory duct: passes through the substance of the prostate gland, allowing sperm to empty into the urethra and pass through the penis to the exterior at the external urinary meatus **(5)**

Elective abortion: abortion performed at the request of the mother but not for reason of maternal risk or fetal disease **(7)**

Emancipated minors: self-supporting adolescents who are emancipated by court decision including minors who marry; minors who are responsible for their own health care decisions and expenses **(3)**

Embryo: the developing baby from weeks 3 through 8 **(8)**

Embryonic disc: the inner layer of the blastocyst that will become the embryo **(8)**

Embryonic stage: Stage II of fetal development from weeks 3 through 8 during which all body systems are formed **(8)**

Endometriosis: occurs when endometrial tissue grows outside the uterine cavity **(7)**

Endometritis: infection in the uterus **(16)**

Endometrium: the inner lining of the uterus **(5)**

Engagement: the point during labor at which the presenting part (usually the fetal head) enters the true pelvis **(14)**

Engorgement: swelling of the breast tissue caused by an increase in blood and lymph preceding true lactation **(11)**

Engrossment: a sense of interest and preoccupation **(16)**

Epididymis: structure located on top of each testis that consists of a single tightly coiled tube approximately 20 feet long where the sperm mature and develop the ability to move **(5)**

Epididymitis: inflammation of the epididymis **(7)**

Episiotomy: surgical cutting of the perineal tissue **(14, 15)**

Epispadias: condition that occurs when the urethra opens on the dorsal (upper) surface of the penis **(18)**

Epstein's pearls: small white cysts that may be present on the newborn's palate, but that disappear in a few weeks **(17)**

Erectile dysfunction: (ED, or impotence); the inability to achieve or maintain an erection that allows for satisfactory sexual intercourse **(7)**

Erythema toxicum neonatorum: a raised pink papule with a light-colored center resembling a mosquito bite **(17)**

Erythroblastosis fetalis: a serious anemia, usually resulting from maternal antibodies to Rh-positive fetal blood **(9)**

Erythrocyte hemolysis: condition resulting from vitamin E deficiency; seen in premature infants because the transfer of vitamin E from the mother takes place in the last few weeks of pregnancy **(11)**

Esophageal atresia: a life-threatening defect in which the esophagus ends in a blind pouch before reaching the stomach **(18)**

Essential amino acids: nine amino acids that the body cannot make or cannot make in sufficient quantities; must be included in the diet **(11)**

Estrogen: the hormone responsible for the development and maintenance of the secondary sex characteristics and growth of the endometrium **(5)**

Ethical: having values and ideas that shape a sense of right and wrong **(3)**

Ethnicity: identity based on common ancestry, race, religion, and culture **(4)**

Exfoliation: shedding of the outer layer **(16)**

Expiratory grunting: noisy exhalation **(17)**

Expulsion: the birth of the rest of the fetus after restitution **(14)**

Exstrophy of the bladder: rare condition in which the abdominal wall fails to fuse, allowing the urinary bladder to protrude to the outside **(18)**

Extended family: a network of relatives including grandparents, aunts, uncles, and cousins who live within a 50-mile radius and take an active role in the emotional support of the family; currently, individuals including close friends and even pets **(4)**

Extension: movement during labor that occurs when the fetus extends its head, pushing its occiput against the maternal symphysis pubis; this movement causes the fetal head to emerge through the vaginal opening **(14)**

External rotation: the rotation of the fetus until the shoulders are in an anterior/posterior position **(14)**

F

Fair-mindedness: the consciousness to treat all points of view equally, without reference to one's own points of view **(2)**

Fairness: impartiality **(2)**

Fallopian tubes: (also called *uterine tubes* or *oviducts*) tubes or ducts that serve to transport the ovum from the ovary toward the uterus **(5)**

False labor: irregular contractions of the uterus prior to actual labor and without accompanying dilatation of the cervix **(14)**

Family: two or more individuals who come together for the purpose of nurturing; traditionally linked to the relationship between parent and child, between spouses, or both **(4)**

Family assessment: an ongoing process of examining the relationships and functioning of family members **(4)**

Family development theory: theory that describes the changes the family undergoes over time **(4)**

Family role: expectations or behaviors associated with position in the family, e.g., mother, father, grandparent, child **(4)**

Family system: a group of individuals (as defined by its members) who establish a relationship for the benefit of the nurturing, supporting, educating, and providing for the needs of each individual **(4)**

Family systems theory: a set of concepts to describe the functioning of families in the larger society **(4)**

Family-centered care: treatment to a designated client with recognition that the family system or unit may also need intervention **(4)**

Fat-soluble vitamins: vitamins A, D, E, and K; require bile for their absorption from the small intestine and are transported through the lymphatic system before entering the blood stream **(6, 11)**

Female circumcision: a partial or complete removal of the clitoris, generally performed before puberty, resulting in a loss of pleasure during sexual intercourse **(5)**

Ferguson's reflex: the spontaneous urge to push during childbirth that occurs when the presenting part reaches the pelvic floor **(14)**

Fertility awareness: based on the assumption that ovulation occurs at the same time each month **(7)**

Fertilization: the process of uniting two sex cells **(8)**

Fetal alcohol syndrome: series of malformations found in an infant whose mother drank large quantities of alcohol during pregnancy **(18)**

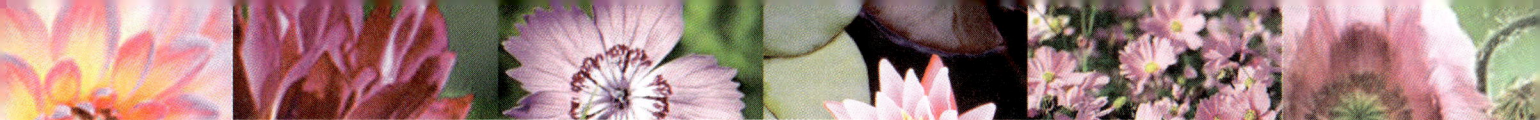

Fetal attitude: the relationship of fetal body parts to one another **(14)**

Fetal demise: intrauterine fetal death (IUFD) **(13)**

Fetal heart tones: the fetal heartbeat **(10)**

Fetal lie: the relationship of the long axis (head-to-foot or *cephalocaudal* axis) of the fetus to the long axis of the mother **(14)**

Fetal membranes: (also called the *bag of waters*) membranes formed by the chorion and the amnion **(8)**

Fetal position: the relationship of the presenting part to the four quadrants of the maternal pelvis **(14)**

Fetal presentation: body part of the fetus that is closest to the cervix, is determined by the fetal lie **(14)**

Fetal stage: Stage III of fetal development from weeks 9 through 38 to 40 during which all body systems are refined and begin to function **(8)**

Fetoscope: an older assessment tool similar to a stethoscope **(9)**

Fetus: the developing baby from week 9 until delivery **(8)**

Fibroadenoma: a freely movable, rounded mass with well-defined borders and a solid rubbery texture **(7)**

Fibrocyst: fluid-filled mass **(7)**

Fibrosis: the replacement of inflamed or damaged tissue with connective or scar tissue **(7)**

Fimbriae: finger-like projections along the edge of each fallopian tube **(5)**

First stage of labor: (also known as the *dilatation stage*) begins with regular contractions and ends with complete effacement and dilatation of the cervix **(14)**

Flexion: the attitude the fetus assumes during labor **(14)**

Folic acid: helps synthesize DNA required for all rapidly growing cells **(11)**

Follicle-stimulating hormone: hormone released by the anterior pituitary gland when a child enters puberty **(5)**

Fontanels: large spaces between the bones of the fetal skull that prevent undue pressure on the fetal brain **(14)**

Foramen ovale: an opening in the septum between the right atrium and left atrium inside the fetal heart **(8)**

Foreskin: loose-fitting, retractable skin encasing the glans **(5)**

Fourth stage of labor: the first hour after birth **(14)**

Fraternal twins: twins that occur when two ova are fertilized by two sperm; dizygotic twins **(8)**

Free radicals: highly unstable molecules; radicals lack an atomic particle called an electron **(11)**

Frequency: the time from the onset of one contraction to the onset of the next contraction **(14)**

Fructose: found naturally in fruits and honey; the sweetest of the simple sugars **(11)**

Fundus: upper portion of the uterus; a round dome just above the attachment of the fallopian tubes **(5, 14)**

Funic soufflé: the sound occurring at the FHR; caused by fetal blood flowing through the umbilical cord **(10)**

G

Galactose: a simple sugar found in lactose **(11)**

Gamete: sex cell **(5)**

Gamete intrafallopian transfer (GIFT): procedure in which the ova are placed in a catheter with motile sperm and inserted into the fimbriated end of the fallopian tube where fertilization occurs **(8)**

Gametogenesis: sex cell formation **(5)**

Generalized seizure: loud cry (called an epileptic cry), loss of consciousness, tonic (back arching) contractions, any cyanosis, followed by clonic (jerking, contracting, and relaxing) contractions, possible frothing, tongue biting, and incontinence **(13)**

Genital warts (condylomata acuminata): a sexually transmitted infection **(7)**

Genogram: a diagram of relationships among family members **(4)**

Genome: our organism's complete set of DNA **(5)**

Gestation: fetal development **(8)**

Gestational diabetes mellitus: an abnormal glucose metabolism caused by the additional requirement for insulin, appearing only during pregnancy **(13)**

Gestational hypertension: a transient disorder characterized by an increased blood pressure of 140/90 or higher **(13)**

Glans: distal end of the penis **(5)**

Glucose: commonly known as blood sugar; serves as the major source of energy for all body activities; the basis of the common disaccharides and the polysaccharides **(11)**

Gonorrhea: a sexually transmitted infection caused by *Neisseria gonorrhoeae* **(7)**

Goodell's sign: a softening of the cervix **(10)**

GP/TPAL: initials used to describe a woman in relation to pregnancies and births; the initials stand for gravida, para/term, preterm, abortion, live birth **(10)**

Graafian follicles: mature follicles **(5)**

Granulosa cells: a layer of cells surrounding the oocyte that thickens, forming an antrum **(5)**

Gravida: number of pregnancies **(10)**

Greater vestibular glands: (also known as *Bartholin's glands*) the ducts of these glands, opening onto the vestibule, secrete a thin mucus-like substance that provides lubrication during sexual intercourse **(5)**

Grief: feeling of extreme sadness resulting from a loss **(13)**

H

Hegar's sign: a softening of the lower uterine segment **(10)**

HELLP syndrome: a condition characterized by hemolysis, elevated liver enzymes, and low platelet count **(13)**

Hematoma: an accumulation of blood under the skin **(16)**

Hemolytic disorders: conditions that cause fetal red blood cells to break during pregnancy, during labor, or immediately following delivery **(13)**

Hemoptysis: bloody sputum **(7)**

Hepatitis B: an inflammation of the liver caused by the hepatitis B virus **(13)**

Hernia: protrusion of intestines through a weakness in the abdominal or pelvic muscles **(18)**

Herpes simplex type 2: an STI that is exhibited by painful vesicles on the genitals **(13)**

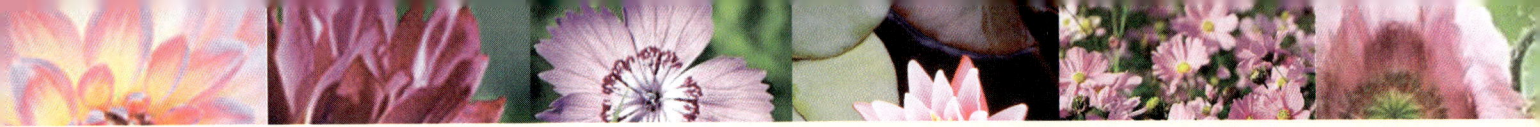

High-risk newborn: an infant who is born prior to 38 weeks' gestation or after 42 weeks' gestation, who has alterations in intrauterine growth, or who has a medical condition that requires frequent monitoring and treatment **(18)**

Hirsutism: excessive hair growth **(7)**

Holistic: inclusive of the physical, psychological, and spiritual aspects of the person **(1)**

Homeostasis: state of balance **(6)**

Hormonal contraceptives: available in a variety of forms, usually a combination of estrogen and progestin **(7)**

Human chorionic gonadotropin: the chemical produced by the chorionic villi; it can be used to determine the likelihood of pregnancy and as a marker for Down syndrome **(8, 9)**

Human immunodeficiency virus (HIV): a retrovirus that attacks and destroys the body's immune system **(7)**

Human placental lactogen: a hormone that stimulates changes in the maternal metabolism **(8)**

Hydatidiform mole: a rare condition in which the chorionic tissue increases abnormally and forms sacs (vesicles) that resemble drops of water **(13)**

Hydramnios: excessive amniotic fluid **(15)**

Hydrocele: fluid in the scrotal sac **(7)**

Hydrocephalus: defect that results from increased production, decreased absorption, or blockage of the flow of cerebrospinal fluid **(18)**

Hymen: thin membrane partially covering the vaginal orifice **(5)**

Hyperbilirubinemia: abnormally high concentration of bilirubin in the blood **(18)**

Hyperemesis gravidarum: excessive vomiting during pregnancy **(10, 13)**

Hyperplasia: excessive proliferation of normal cells **(7)**

Hypospadias: condition that occurs when the urethra opens on the ventral (lower) surface of the penis **(18)**

Hysterectomy: removal of the uterus **(7)**

I

Identical twins: twins that develop from one fertilized ovum; monozygotic twins **(8)**

Imagery: the use of the imagination with the intent of stimulating mind, body, and spiritual healing **(6)**

Imperforate anus: condition that results when the connecting tissue fails to break down and the opening of the colon does not develop **(18)**

Implantation: the embedding of the blastocyst into the endometrium **(8)**

Implications: consequences **(2)**

Incest: sexual intercourse between close blood relatives that may or may not be consensual **(7)**

Incompetent cervix: condition indicated by a weak cervix that dilates in the second trimester, expelling the fetus **(13)**

Indirect Coombs' test: test done at 28 weeks on Rh-negative woman; a change from a normal negative value to a positive value indicates that the woman's blood has been sensitized by fetal Rh-positive blood **(13)**

Induction of labor: the stimulation of labor by medical or pharmacologic methods **(15)**

Inductive reasoning: the process of making generalized statements from a limited set of facts **(2)**

Inferences: deductions **(2)**

Infertility: the inability to achieve pregnancy after 1 year or more of unprotected intercourse **(7)**

Infibulation: the removal of the labia majora and labia minora **(5)**

Information: knowledge gained through research or observation **(2)**

Informed consent: written approval for a treatment or procedure, following explanation of pros and cons by the physician or other professional who is performing the procedure **(3)**

Inhibin-A: blood marker that may be used to determine the likelihood of Down syndrome **(9)**

Intellectual autonomy: having a rational control over one's ideas and beliefs **(2)**

Intellectual courage: the consciousness to be fair in facing and addressing ideas, beliefs, or viewpoints that might, on a superficial level, seem absurd, false, or unappealing **(2)**

Intellectual empathy: imagining oneself in the place of others in order to understand them better **(2)**

Intellectual humility: having a consciousness that one's knowledge base, prejudices, biases, and point of view have limitations implying the lack of boastfulness, arrogance, and conceit **(2)**

Intellectual integrity: being true and consistent with intellectual standards, holding oneself to the same standards of proof as one holds those with opposing views, and honestly admitting when one is inconsistent in one's thoughts and actions **(2)**

Intellectual perseverance: persistence in the attempt to understand despite distractions, obstacles, or confusion over unsettled questions **(2)**

Intellectual standards: concepts that guide the critical thinker to better and better reasoning **(2)**

Intensity: the strength of the contraction at its peak **(14)**

Intercostal: between the ribs **(17)**

Internal rotation: the movement during labor or prior to labor when the fetus turns to an anterior position (OA); the fetal occiput is next to the maternal symphysis pubis **(14)**

Interpretations: ways of clarifying the meaning **(2)**

Interventions: nursing actions to assist the client toward an improvement in health, including administration of prescribed analgesics and nonpharmacologic comfort measures **(1)**

Intracranial hemorrhage: hemorrhage within the cerebral ventricles of the brain **(18)**

Intracytoplasmic sperm injection: technique in which the mature ovum is held in a pipette and a needle containing a single sperm is gently inserted into the cytoplasm of the ovum; the fertilized ovum is allowed to incubate for several days and then is placed into the uterus **(8)**

Intraductal papillomas: tumors growing in a mammary duct **(7)**

Intrauterine device: a small T-shaped piece of metal covered with copper or levonorgestrel **(7)**

Intrauterine growth restriction: (also known as *small for gestational age*) condition of a fetus whose growth is below that expected for the gestational age; formerly called intrauterine growth retardation **(18)**

In-vitro fertilization: uniting ova and sperm in a laboratory setting **(7, 8)**

Involution: the return of the uterus to the nonpregnant state **(16)**

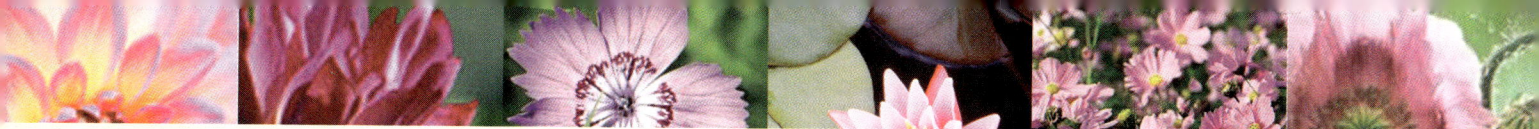

J

Jaundice: a condition that occurs because the infant's liver is immature and cannot conjugate the amount of bilirubin released by the destruction of RBCs **(17)**

K

Karyotype: a picture analysis of the chromosomes **(8)**

L

Labia majora: two large folds of skin extended downward from the mons pubis **(5)**

Labia minora: small folds of tissue located inside the labia majora that join anteriorly at the midline **(5)**

Labor: a process, or sequence of events, that begins with uterine contractions and ends 1 hour after delivery of the placenta **(14)**

Lacerations: condition that occurs when tissues are unable to stretch any further and tear under pressure; can occur in the cervix, vagina, or perineum **(15)**

Lactation: milk production **(5)**

Lactiferous ducts: the milk-carrying ducts of the mammary gland that open on the nipple **(5)**

Lactogenesis: milk production **(5)**

Lactose: the principal sugar in milk; made from glucose and galactose **(11)**

Lanugo: fine fetal hair **(8)**

Large for gestational age: (also called *macrosomia*) condition of a newborn whose birth weight is over the 90th percentile for the gestational age **(18)**

Latent phase: phase of the first stage of labor from the onset of contractions until the cervix is dilated 4 centimeters **(14)**

Legal: required by law **(3)**

Let-down reflex: release of milk after delivery **(10)**

Leukorrhea: a white mucous discharge from the vagina that may or may not be pathological **(6)**

Libido: the sexual drive **(7)**

Lightening: the descent of the fetus into the pelvis relieves pressure on the diaphragm, allowing the mother to breathe more easily and "feel lighter" **(14)**

Linea nigra: a dark line on the abdomen from the umbilicus to the pubis **(10)**

Lipids: fatty acids; fats made up of triglycerides (fats and oils), phospholipids, and sterols **(6, 11)**

Lochia: the discarded blood, mucus, and tissue of the decidua separated from the innermost layer of the uterus that is expelled through the vagina **(16)**

Lochia alba: lochia that is creamy white or pale yellow, consisting of the last pieces of decidua, white blood cells, mucus, and bacteria; continues for approximately 2 weeks **(16)**

Lochia rubra: lochia that is dark red and contains epithelial cells, red blood cells, pieces of decidua, and sometimes meconium, lanugo, and vernix caseosa; it may contain small blood clots (quarter size or less), presenting approximately 3 days after delivery **(16)**

Lochia serosa: lochia that is pinkish in color; presenting from days 4 to 10, contains serous exudates, red blood cells, mucus, and many bacteria **(16)**

Logical: reasonable **(2)**

Loss: either real or perceived, the experience when something is removed from the body or environment **(13)**

Lumpectomy: removal of a lump **(7)**

M

Macrosomia: (also known as *large for gestational age*) excessive growth in the fetus; condition of a newborn whose birth weight is over the 90th percentile for the gestational age **(13, 18)**

Maltose: a disaccharide formed in the hydrolysis of starch, resulting from the combination of two units of glucose; the result of the fermentation process that yields alcohol **(11)**

Mammography: diagnostic x-ray of the breast **(7)**

Mammoplasty: breast reconstruction **(7)**

Massage: the rubbing of the skin and underlying muscles to improve circulation and promote relaxation **(6)**

Mastectomy: removal of the breast **(7)**

Mastitis: infection of the breast **(16)**

Maternal hemoglobin test: test repeated at 7 months to assess for anemia **(13)**

Maternal serum alpha-fetoprotein: a blood marker that is elevated when the fetus has an open neural tube defect, anencephaly, omphalocele, or gastroschisis; the marker is also elevated in multiple gestations; a low MSAFP is associated with Down syndrome **(9)**

Maternal–newborn nursing: the care of women during pregnancy, childbirth, and postpartum and the care of the child from birth through the first 6 weeks of life **(1)**

Mature minor act: an act that permits adolescents age 14 or 15 to make decisions about their treatment **(3)**

Mechanisms of labor: (also called *cardinal movements*) the movements that occur when the fetus changes positions as it moves through the pelvis **(14)**

Meconium: the first fetal stool **(8)**

Meconium aspiration: inhalation by a fetus of amniotic fluid contaminated with meconium **(18)**

Medical diagnoses: statements about a disease process or disorder **(1)**

Menarche: the first menstrual period, usually during puberty **(5)**

Meningocele: herniation of the meninges through a vertebral defect **(18)**

Meningomyelocele: herniation of the spinal nerves and the meninges through a defect in the spinal column **(8, 18)**

Menopause: the period marked by the natural and permanent cessation of menstruation, occurring between the ages of 35 and 58 **(5)**

Menorrhagia: excessive menstruation in volume or number of days **(7)**

Menorrhalgia: (also known as *dysmenorrhea*) painful menses **(7)**

Menses: the sloughing off of the endometrium caused by a decrease in progesterone **(5)**

Mentum: face **(14)**

Metrorrhagia: bleeding between periods **(7)**

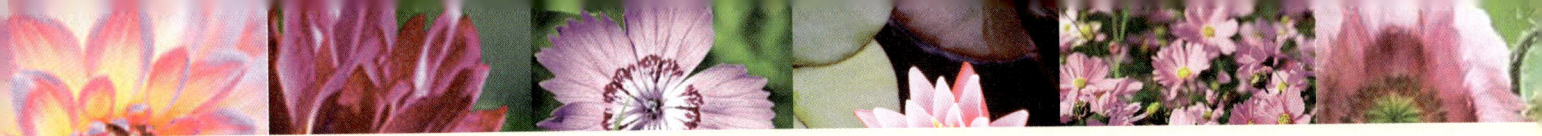

Milia: white pinpoint spots resembling whiteheads **(17)**

Mind–body therapies: techniques that utilize mental processes to bring about healing **(6)**

Minerals: compounds necessary for fluid balance, clot formation, strong bones and teeth, and nerve muscle coordination; include sodium, chloride, potassium, calcium, phosphorus, magnesium, iron, and iodine **(6)**

Miscarriage: spontaneous occurrence of the termination of pregnancy **(3, 10, 13)**

Mittelschmerz: abdominal pain with ovulation **(7)**

Molding: the shaping of the fetal head to the bones of the maternal pelvis **(14)**

Mongolian spot: a dark-colored area over the lower back and sacrum of Black, Hispanic, South Asian, or East Asian infants **(17)**

Monilia: (also called *candidiasis* or *yeast infection*) a common organism causing vaginitis **(7)**

Monosaccharides: simple sugars **(11)**

Monounsaturated: type of fatty acid that has only one double carbon bond **(11)**

Mons pubis: the skin-covered fat pad over the symphysis pubis **(5)**

Morbidity: the prevalence of a specific disease or disorder in the population at a specific period of time **(1)**

Moro reflex: (also called *startle reflex*) reflex that occurs when newborns have a sense of falling; can be elicited by holding the newborn in a sitting position and suddenly lowering the head or by bumping the surface were the newborn is lying; baby will quickly extend the arms with fingers flared and form a "C with thumbs and first finger," arms will then adduct in an embracing motion, and lower extremities may extend and then flex; a slight tremor may be noted **(17)**

Mortality: the number of deaths over a given period of time for a given population **(1)**

Morula: a many-celled, mulberry-shaped mass **(8)**

Multifetal pregnancy: a pregnancy with more than one fetus such as twins, triplets, or quadruplets **(7, 8)**

Multigravida: woman who has been pregnant two or more times **(10)**

Multipara: woman who has delivered two or more times after 24 weeks' gestation **(10)**

Multiple gestation: a pregnancy with more than one fetus such as twins, triplets, or quadruplets **(8)**

Multiple marker screen: test done at 16 weeks to evaluate maternal serum alpha-fetoprotein, estriol, and hCG levels **(13)**

Myomectomy: removal of tumor and surrounding myometrium **(7)**

Myometrium: the smooth muscle forming the wall of the uterus **(5)**

N

Naegele's rule: the most common method for determining the due date of a pregnancy; to apply the rule, take the first day of the LMP, subtract 3 months, and add 7 days **(10)**

Nasal flaring: outward movement of the nostrils **(17)**

Natural childbirth: labor and birth without medical interventions or pain medication **(14)**

NCLEX-PN® focus area: 1 of 11 areas of client needs around which the NCLEX-PN® test is constructed **(2)**

Neonatal Abstinence Scoring System: a standardized screening tool used to monitor infants in an objective manner when neonatal abstinence syndrome is suspected or identified **(18)**

Neonatal abstinence syndrome: behavior of a newborn who was exposed to chemical substances *in utero* **(18)**

Newborn: the infant from delivery through the first month of life **(17)**

Niacin: vitamin found in coenzymes that are needed to metabolize glucose, fat, and alcohol **(11)**

Nocturia: the need to void frequently at night **(7)**

Nonessential amino acids: amino acids that do not need to be included in the diet because the body can create them **(11)**

Nonshivering thermogenesis: generation of heat by moving to increase metabolism and burning stored brown fat in infants **(17)**

Nonstress test: diagnostic test used to assess fetal movement and FHR **(9)**

Nuchal cord: umbilical cord that is wound around the neck of the fetus during labor and birth **(15)**

Nuclear family: traditional family type consisting of parents and biologic offspring **(4)**

Nulligravida: never been pregnant **(10)**

Nullipara: never delivered an infant after 24 weeks' gestation **(10)**

Nursing diagnoses: names for client conditions that nurses are qualified and trained to treat independently **(1)**

O

Objective data: data that can be observed and measured by the senses or by mechanical instruments **(1)**

Occiput: crown of head **(14)**

Omphalocele: congenital malformation of the abdominal wall allowing the abdominal contents to herniate into the umbilical cord **(18)**

Oocyte: immature sex cell **(5)**

Oogenesis: the development of the female gamete or ovum, resulting from the process of meiosis **(5)**

Oophorectomy: surgical removal of the ovaries **(7)**

Open adoptions: adoptions in which the birth mother and adoptive parents can meet and communicate about the child **(12)**

Ophthalmia neonatorum: inflammation of the eyes of the newborn, resulting from contact with gonorrhea or chlamydia during the birth process **(17)**

Orchiectomy: removal of one testis and spermatic cord **(7)**

Orchitis: inflammation of the testes **(7)**

Ossification: formation of bone **(8)**

Osteomalacia: softening of the bones in adults, most often in young women who had low intake of vitamin D and calcium and who had repeated pregnancies and lactation **(11)**

Osteoporosis: a disorder in which the bones become brittle and break easily; occurring especially in women following menopause **(6, 11)**

Outcome: the client goal that relates to a specific nursing diagnosis **(1)**

Ovarian cancer: the most lethal of female reproductive cancers, remains asymptomatic until the cancer has spread to surrounding tissue or has been transported by the lymphatic system to other parts of the body **(7)**

Ovarian follicles: cavities in the ovary containing a maturing ovum surrounded by its encasing cells **(5)**

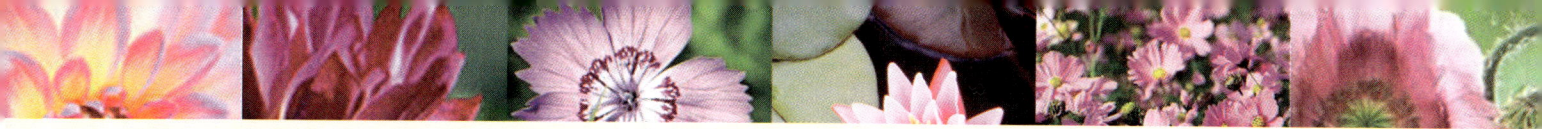

Oviducts: (also called *uterine tubes* or *fallopian tubes*) tubes or ducts that serve to transport the ovum from the ovary toward the uterus **(5)**

Ovum: egg **(5)**

Oxidative stress: a condition of increased oxidant production characterized by the release of free radicals and resulting in cellular degeneration **(11)**

Oxytocin: a hormone produced by the posterior pituitary gland that stimulates uterine contractions **(10)**

P

Palmar grasp reflex: reflex in infants that occurs when a finger or small object is placed in the newborn's hand; newborns grasp the finger tight enough to be lifted from the bed; reflex lasts 4 months **(17)**

Para: number of deliveries after 24 weeks' gestation **(10)**

Parietal seizure: brief change in consciousness with blank stare, blinking of the eyes, fluttering eyelids, or lip smacking **(13)**

Passage: the maternal structures through which the fetus must travel **(14)**

Passenger: fetus **(14)**

Patent ductus arteriosus: a defect in which the ductus arteriosus remains open after birth **(18)**

Patients: people who are ill, need care, and who may have others make decisions for them **(1)**

Pellagra: niacin deficiency; causes diarrhea, dermatitis, dementia, and death **(11)**

Penis: the male organ of copulation or sexual intercourse **(5)**

Percutaneous umbilical cord sampling: the removal of umbilical cord blood through a needle inserted into the uterus **(9)**

Peritonitis: infection in the peritoneum **(16)**

Petechiae: pinpoint hemorrhage **(17)**

Phimosis: condition that occurs when the opening of the foreskin is small and unable to be retracted over the glans **(18)**

Physiologic anemia of pregnancy: condition occurring between 26 to 32 weeks' gestation resulting from hemodilution, as evidenced by a hematocrit of 34% to 40% **(10, 13)**

Placenta: a highly vascular organ connecting the mother and the fetus **(8)**

Placenta previa: result from the blastocyst implanting low in the uterus, allowing the placenta to grow partially or totally across the cervical opening **(13)**

Plantar grasp reflex: reflex in infants lasting 8 months; occurs when the sole of the foot is touched, the toes curl under as if newborns are trying to "grasp" with their feet; reflex must disappear before infants are able to walk **(17)**

Points of view: perspectives **(2)**

Polar bodies: small cells that are produced during the development of an oocyte and ultimately degenerate **(5)**

Polycystic ovary syndrome: results from numerous follicular cysts **(7)**

Polydactyly: presence of more than five fingers per hand or toes per foot **(17)**

Polysaccharides: complex carbohydrates or large compounds composed of chains of monosaccharides **(11)**

Polyunsaturated: type of fatty acid that has two or more double carbon bonds **(11)**

Postmaturity syndrome: a condition in infants born after 42 weeks' gestation who exhibit signs of impaired intrauterine oxygenation and nutrition related to placental insufficiency **(15)**

Postpartal chills: uncontrolled shaking or chills as a physiologic response to labor and as a result of the rapid weight loss at birth experienced by the mother **(14)**

Postpartum: period that begins immediately after the birth of the baby and continues for 6 weeks or until the woman's body has returned to a prepregnant state **(16)**

Postpartum blues: a transient period of mild depression that often occurs in the early postpartum period **(16)**

Postpartum (puerperal) infection: a rare infection of the uterus following childbirth **(16)**

Postterm delivery: delivery after 42 weeks' gestation **(10)**

Precipitous birth: a birth that occurs rapidly, unexpectedly, and without the attention of a physician or nurse midwife **(15)**

Precipitous labor: labor that lasts less than 3 hours **(15)**

Precision: scientific exactness **(2)**

Preeclampsia: a common, complex condition that develops after 20 weeks' gestation; once called toxemia **(13)**

Preembryonic stage: Stage I of fetal development from fertilization through 14 days when the fertilized ovum travels through the fallopian tube, differentiates into trophoblast and embryonic disc, and attaches to the endometrium **(8)**

Pregnancy: the carrying of the resulting offspring in the uterus **(8)**

Premature rupture of membranes: condition that occurs when the membranes rupture before the 38th week of gestation; can indicate the onset of premature labor and needs immediate medical attention **(14, 15)**

Premenstrual syndrome: a group of symptoms resulting from an imbalance of estrogen and progesterone, as well as increased prolactin and aldosterone levels **(7)**

Prepuce: loose-fitting, retractable skin encasing the glans **(5)**

Presumptive signs: the subjective signs the mother experiences during pregnancy **(10)**

Preterm delivery: delivery after the 24th week but before the 38th week **(10)**

Preterm labor: the onset of regular contractions, occurring between the 20th and 37th week, that cause changes in the cervix **(15)**

Primary care: care that is specific to maintaining health and preventing illness or injury from occurring **(1)**

Primary spermatocyte: a diploid spermatocyte that has not yet undergone meiosis **(5)**

Primigravida: woman in her first pregnancy **(10)**

Primipara: woman with first delivery after 24 weeks' gestation **(10)**

Progesterone: the hormone that stimulates thickening and vascularization of the endometrium **(5)**

Prolapsed umbilical cord: condition that results when the infant's body (usually the head) compresses the cord against the pelvis, obstructing blood flow through the umbilical cord **(14, 15)**

Proliferative phase: portion of the menstrual cycle that begins around day 3 when follicle-stimulating hormone (FSH) secretion from the anterior pituitary gland begins to increase **(5)**

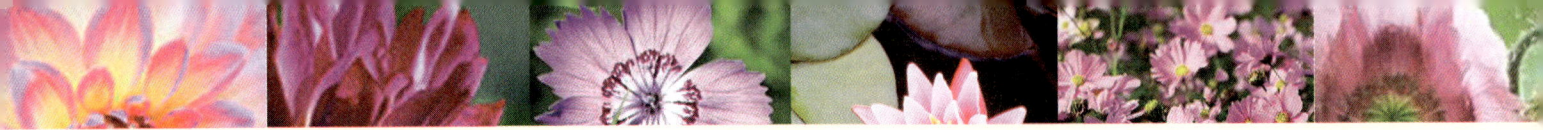

Prostate: a doughnut-shaped gland located just below the urinary bladder that produces a thin milky fluid that helps activate the sperm and maintain their motility **(5)**

Prostate cancer: leading type of cancer in men that rarely occurs before the age of 40; usually begins in the posterior region of the prostate and may spread into the seminiferous tubules or bladder **(7)**

Prostatitis: inflammation of the prostate **(7)**

Proteins: compounds made up of amino acids, a combination of carbon, hydrogen, oxygen and nitrogen; they are required for cell growth and repair **(6, 11)**

Pseudomenstruation: a mucous or slightly bloody vaginal discharge that may be present in female newborns, related to the influence of maternal hormones, and disappearing in a few days **(17)**

Pseudopregnancy: false pregnancy **(10)**

Puberty: a period of transition and sexual maturation **(5)**

Puerperium: period that begins immediately after the birth of the baby and continues for 6 weeks or until the woman's body has returned to a prepregnant state **(16)**

Purpose: an end, aim, or result **(2)**

Pyloric stenosis: progressive hypertrophy of the pyloric sphincter resulting in obstruction **(18)**

Q

Quickening: the first fetal movements felt by the mother **(8, 10)**

R

Race: biologic deviations shown in physical features, such as skin color, hair texture, and facial features **(4)**

Rape: forced sexual intercourse that involves vaginal, anal, or oral penetration **(7)**

Reasoning: process of forming conclusions, judgments, or inferences from facts or assumptions **(2)**

Recessive: incapable of expressing control **(8)**

Rectocele: develops when the anterior rectal wall protrudes into the vagina **(7)**

Reduction mammoplasty: when the size of the breast is reduced by removing fat tissue with an attempt to leave the mammary glands intact **(7)**

Reflexology: a system of massaging based on work by William H. Fitzgerald **(6)**

Regional blocks: regional anesthetics administered by the physician, anesthesiologist, or nurse anesthetist that chemically stop the nerve conduction of painful stimuli **(14)**

Reiki: (pronounced RAY-key) Japanese energy healing that employs a light laying on of hands from heart to throat, heart, abdomen, knees, and feet; often used with people who have cancer or chronic health problems **(6)**

Relaxin: a hormone produced by the corpus luteum, and placenta that decreases uterine activity, decreases the strength of uterine contractions, softens the cervix, and causes softening of the collagen connective tissue of the symphysis pubis and sacroiliac joints **(8)**

Relevance: connection to the matter in hand **(2)**

Religion: the belief in a superhuman power recognized as creator or governor of the universe **(4)**

Reportable disease: a disease that poses a public health hazard **(3)**

Reportable STIs: sexually transmitted infections that must be reported to the public health department and Center for Disease Control **(7)**

Responsiveness: relating to how much parents foster individuality, self-assertion, and self-regulation, and how responsive they are to special needs and demands **(4)**

Rest: a state of calmness and relaxation without emotional stress or anxiety **(6)**

Restitution: the turning of the fetal head to be in normal alignment with the shoulders **(14)**

Retractions: an inward movement of the tissue over the sternum and intercostal muscles **(17)**

Rh incompatibility: a condition in which antibodies in the mother's Rh negative blood react to Rh positive fetal blood as a foreign substance **(13)**

RhoGAM blood stick: a test to identify incompatibility of mother's and infant's Rh factor **(16)**

Riboflavin: vitamin that serves as a coenzyme in many chemical reactions, especially the release of energy from nutrients inside cells **(11)**

Rickets: disease resulting from vitamin D deficiency; the bones fail to calcify properly leading to soft, easily bendable bones **(11)**

Rooting reflex: reflex that occurs when the newborn is searching for food; when the newborn's cheek is stroked, the infant will turn his or her head in that direction **(17)**

Rubella: also known as German or 3-day measles; a highly contagious airborne virus **(13)**

Rugae: folds in the mucous membrane that allow for stretching of the vagina during labor **(5)**

S

Salpingitis: infection of the fallopian tubes **(8)**

Salpingo-oophorectomy: removal of the uterus and both ovaries **(7)**

Saturated: type of fatty acid carrying the maximum amount of hydrogen **(11)**

Scarf sign: indication of newborn maturity exhibited by moving the arm in front of the neck **(17)**

Schultze mechanism: expulsion of the placenta with the fetal side out **(14)**

Scrotum: a skin-covered pouch suspended from the groin that contains the testes, epididymis, and lower end of the vas deferens at the beginning of the spermatic cord **(5)**

Second stage of labor: begins when the cervix is completely dilated and ends with the birth of the baby **(14)**

Secondary care: care that is specific to helping the client return to health after an acute disorder or disease **(1)**

Secretory phase: the second half of the menstrual cycle after ovulation; the corpus luteum secretes progesterone, which prepares the endometrium for the implantation of an embryo; if fertilization does not occur, then menstrual flow begins **(5)**

Semen: the mixture of sperm and fluid from the reproductive glands **(5)**

Seminal fluid: the mixture of sperm and fluid from the reproductive glands **(5)**

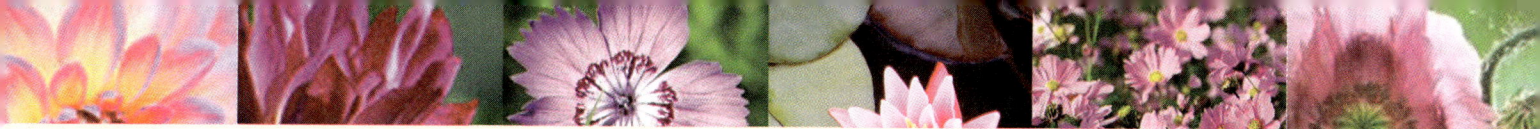

Seminal vesicles: sacs located under and behind the urinary bladder; produces a thick, yellowish fluid rich in fructose that helps provide a source of energy for the highly mobile sperm **(5)**

Seminiferous tubules: long narrow coiled tubes where sperm are produced **(5)**

Septicemia: the progression of disease once pathogens are growing in the blood **(16)**

Sequelae: conditions that occur because of another condition **(12)**

Sex-linked: found on the X or Y chromosome **(8)**

Shirodkar procedure: (also called *cerclage*) procedure done at 16 weeks' gestation that involves surgically placing a suture in the cervix in a purse-string design to hold the cervix closed **(13)**

Significance: importance **(2)**

Sinciput: forehead or brow **(14)**

Single-parent family: either a mother or a father raising the children alone **(4)**

Sleep: a state of altered consciousness, in which the person's perception and reaction to the environment are decreased; characterized by decreased activity, variable levels of consciousness, changes in the body's physiological state, and a decreased response to stimuli **(6)**

Small for gestational age: (also called *intrauterine growth restriction*) growth below that expected for gestational age **(18)**

Smegma: the secretion consisting of epithelial cells found around the external genitalia **(17)**

Spermatic cord: comprises the vas deferens, blood vessels, and nerves; passes out of the scrotum, through the inguinal canal, and into the abdominal cavity circling the urinary bladder to join the duct from the seminal vesicle to form the ejaculatory duct **(5)**

Spermatids: the result of the meiotic division that will develop into sperm **(5)**

Spermatogenesis: sperm production **(5)**

Spermatogonia: sperm precursor or stem cells **(5)**

Spermatozoa: sperm cells **(5)**

Spermicides: chemicals in the form of creams, foams, jellies, or suppositories that are inserted into the vagina prior to sexual intercourse **(7)**

Spina bifida: defect with incomplete closure of the vertebra and neural tube **(8, 11, 18)**

Spinnbarkeit: the stringy, elastic character of cervical mucus during the ovulatory period **(7)**

Spontaneous rupture of membranes: a tearing or perforation of the amniotic sac releasing amniotic fluid **(14)**

Startle reflex: (also called *Moro reflex*) reflex that occurs when newborns have a sense of falling; can be elicited by holding the newborn in a sitting position and suddenly lowering the head or by bumping the surface were the newborn is lying; baby will quickly extend the arms with fingers flared and form a "C with thumbs and first finger," arms will then adduct in an embracing motion, and lower extremities may extend and then flex; a slight tremor may be noted **(17)**

Station: the relationship between the fetus and the maternal ischial spines **(14)**

Stepfamily: family unit that occurs when parents remarry **(4)**

Stepping reflex: reflex in infants obtained by holding newborns with the feet touching the table; newborns will step as if walking **(17)**

Stereotyping: expectation that all members of a group will think and behave the same **(4)**

Stillbirth: intrauterine fetal death (IUFD) or fetal demise **(13)**

Stork bites: (also known as *telangiectatic nevi*) dark red spots on the eyelids, forehead, or nape of the neck that usually fade in time **(17)**

Strabismus: lack of coordination of the visual axes of the eye; eyes do not stay parallel to each other but may diverge in any direction **(17)**

Stress: a response to internal or external changes in the client's state of balance **(6)**

Stressor: any event that results in stress **(6)**

Striae gravidarum: "stretch marks" that occur when the underlying connective tissue separates during periods of rapid growth **(10)**

Subcostal: below the ribs **(17)**

Subinvolution: the failure of the uterus to return to its normal size **(16)**

Subjective data: knowledge gained from an understanding of the client or group's personal experience **(1)**

Substernal: below the sternum **(17)**

Sucking reflex: reflex in infants elicited when the newborn's lips are touched **(17)**

Sucrose: a combination of glucose and fructose **(11)**

Supine hypotensive syndrome: condition that occurs after the 20th week when the mother lies supine and the heavy uterus presses on the inferior vena cava, resulting in reduced blood flow back to the right atrium; it may cause low blood pressure, dizziness, and pale skin **(10)**

Supraclavicular: above the clavicles **(17)**

Suprasternal: above the sternum **(17)**

Surfactant: substance produced by fetal lungs and composed of phospholipids, decreases the surface tension of fluid inside the alveoli allowing the lungs to expand **(8)**

Surgical sterilization: the tying and cutting of the vas deferens or fallopian tubes **(7)**

Sutures: the fibrous connective tissue joining the bones of the fetal skull **(14)**

Syndactyly: the fusion of two or more digits **(17)**

Syphilis: a sexually transmitted infection caused by the bacteria *Treponema pallidum* **(7)**

System: an organized group of entities that can perform a particular function in the face of change from within or without **(4)**

T

Taking-hold stage: time (usually by the third day after childbirth) when the mother is taking control of the activities of caring for herself and her newborn **(16)**

Taking-in stage: the first day or two after childbirth, when the mother is "taking in" information about her baby, recalling the experience of delivery, and storing this information in her memory **(16)**

Telangiectatic nevi: (also known as *stork bites*) dark red spots on the eyelids, forehead, or nape of the neck that usually fade in time **(17)**

Tenesmus: painful straining to defecate **(7)**

Teratogen: a chemical that can cause abnormal fetal development; agent that causes defects in a developing embryo **(7, 8)**

Term delivery: delivery between 38 and 42 weeks **(10)**

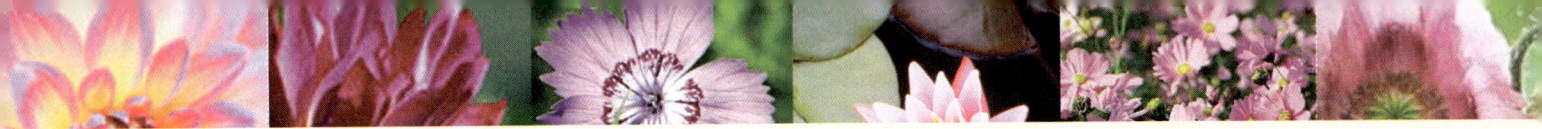

Tertiary care: the management of chronic, terminal, complicated, long-term health care problems to help the client return to or maintain the highest possible level of functioning and to adapt as necessary to the changes the condition requires **(1)**

Testes: pair of gonads **(5)**

Testicular cancer: cancer that grows within the testicle, eventually replacing all normal tissue **(7)**

Testosterone: hormone produced in the interstitial cells that causes the development of male accessory organs, muscle mass and strength, and masculine characteristics such as a deep voice and body hair **(5)**

Tetralogy of Fallot: congenital condition that combines pulmonary stenosis (narrowing of the pulmonary valve), ventricular septal defect, right ventricular hypertrophy (enlargement), and an overriding aortic valve **(18)**

Therapeutic abortion: the termination of the pregnancy to save the life and preserve the health of the mother or when the fetus has a serious developmental or hereditary disorder **(7)**

Third stage of labor: begins with the birth of the fetus and ends with the expulsion of the placenta **(14)**

Thromboembolism: a blood clot moving within the blood vessels **(16)**

Thrombosis: formation of clots in blood vessels **(16)**

Tonic neck reflex: reflex in infants demonstrated by placing newborns supine on a firm surface; when the head is turned to one side, newborns will extend the arm and leg on that side, the opposite arm and leg will flex **(17)**

TORCH group: **t**oxoplasmosis, **r**ubella, **c**ytomegalovirus, and **h**erpes virus type 2 **(13)**

Tracheoesophageal fistula: potentially life-threatening defect in which a connection between the trachea and esophagus is present **(18)**

Trans fats: hydrogenated fats that do not metabolize well in the body and that may lead to conditions such as atherosclerosis **(6, 11)**

Transabdominal ultrasound: imaging with high-frequency radio waves obtained through the abdominal wall **(9)**

Transposition of the great vessels: congenital condition in which the pulmonary artery and aorta are reversed, causing the blood to be insufficiently oxygenated **(18)**

Transposons: jumping DNA; DNA fragments that move around and between chromosomes **(5)**

Transvaginal ultrasound: an imaging test using high-frequency sound waves, obtained after inserting a small probe into the vagina **(9)**

Transverse lie: the long axis of the fetus is at a right angle to the long axis of the mother **(14)**

Trichomoniasis: an infection caused by the protozoa *Trichomonas vaginalis*; most commonly transmitted through sexual contact **(7)**

Trimester: 3-month block of time to describe the progression of pregnancy **(10)**

Trisomy: chromosomal defect resulting from existence of three chromosomes where a pair should be **(8)**

Trisomy 21: (also known as Down syndrome) three chromosomes at position 21 **(18)**

Trophoblast: the outer layer of the blastocyst that will become the fetal membranes **(8)**

True perineum: the area between the vaginal opening and the anus **(5)**

Tubal embryo transfer: procedure similar to gamete intrafallopian transfer; ova are placed into the fallopian tube at an earlier stage of development **(8)**

Tubal pregnancy: pregnancy in the fallopian tube **(13)**

Tuberculosis: a potentially lethal respiratory infection caused by *Mycobacterium tuberculosis* **(13)**

Tunica albuginea: covering on the outside of the testes that forms the septum between the many sections or lobules **(5)**

Tunica vaginalis testis: covering on the front and sides of the testes and epididymis **(5)**

U

Ultrasound: a diagnostic test used to outline the shape and determine the consistency of various organs and diagnose pregnancy; it can also be used to determine the exact position, size, and gender of the fetus and to identify some developmental anomalies **(9)**

Umbilical arteries: arteries that connect the internal iliac arteries in the fetus to the placenta **(8)**

Umbilical cord: cord that connects the fetus to the placenta **(8)**

Umbilical vein: vein through which the fetal blood flows back to the fetus **(8)**

Unconjugated estriol: one of the blood markers that can be used to determine the likelihood of Down syndrome **(9)**

Unsaturated: type of fatty acid that does not carry the maximum amount of hydrogen, resulting in a double bond between two carbon atoms **(11)**

Urethra: the canal through which urine is discharged from the bladder and through which semen is discharged in the male **(5)**

Urinary meatus: opening onto the vestibule **(5)**

Uterine prolapse: condition that develops when the ligaments supporting the uterus in the pelvic cavity are stretched or damaged **(7)**

Uterine soufflé: the sound occurring at the same rate as the maternal pulse; caused by increased maternal blood flow to the uterus **(10)**

Uterine tubes: (also called *fallopian tubes* or *oviducts*) tubes or ducts that serve to transport the ovum from the ovary toward the uterus **(5)**

Uterus: a small organ about the size of a pear that consists almost entirely of muscle with a small cavity in the center **(5)**

V

Vagina: a 4-inch-long tube that connects the cervix to the vaginal opening, composed mainly of smooth muscle, the vagina is lined with mucous membrane **(5)**

Vaginal culture for group B streptococcal infection: a test obtained at 35 to 37 weeks that specifically looks for streptococcal infection in the mother because of its potentially adverse effect on the fetus **(13)**

Variability: change in the fetal heart rate in response to the stress of labor **(15)**

Vas deferens: the duct that transports the sperm from the epididymis to the penis **(5)**

Ventricular septal defect: opening in the septum between the ventricles **(18)**

Vernix caseosa: white, cheesy covering of the fetus's skin **(8)**

Version: the procedure of changing the fetal presentation by abdominal or intrauterine manipulation **(15)**

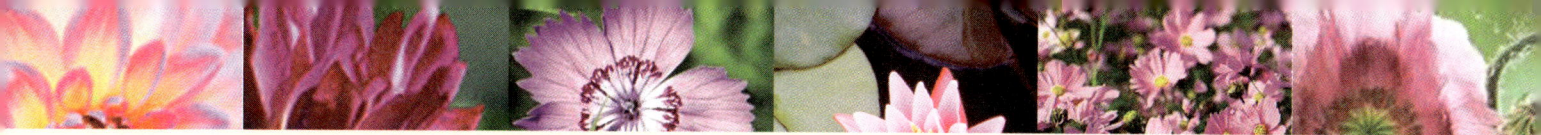

Vertex presentation: the crown of head presenting first **(14)**

Vestibule: the area between the labia minora **(5)**

Viability: the ability to live outside the uterus **(8)**

Vitamins: organic compounds that cannot be manufactured in the body **(6)**

W

Water-soluble vitamins: vitamins that dissolve in and are transported in water; can be found in all water-filled compartments within the body **(6, 11)**

Webbing: skin between two or more digits **(17)**

Wharton's jelly: white gelatinous tissue that protects and supports the two umbilical arteries and one umbilical vein **(8)**

Witch's milk: whitish fluid that may be secreted by a neonate's nipples shortly after birth **(17)**

Y

Yeast infection: (also called *candidiasis* or *monilia*) a common organism causing vaginitis **(7)**

Yolk sac: a structure inside the ovum in which the fetal blood is initially formed **(8)**

Z

Zygote: the fertilized egg **(8)**

Zygote intrafallopian transfer: procedure similar to gamete intrafallopian transfer; ova are placed into the fallopian tube at an early stage of development **(8)**

Index

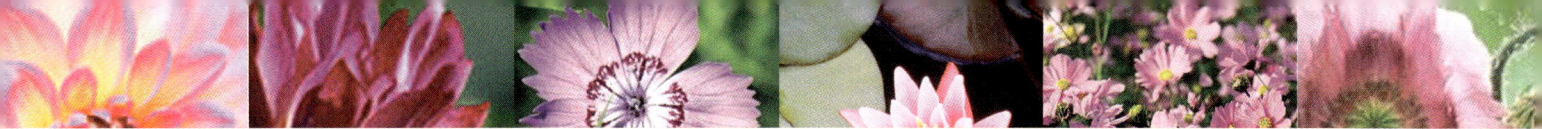

Antrum of the follicle, 85
Anxiety, 113
Aorta, coarctation of, 473f, 473t, 474
Apgar score
    normal newborns, 426–427, 428f
    procedure for obtaining, 338–339, 338t
Apnea, 438
Appearance, general, of newborns, 435
Appropriate (size) for gestational age, 433, 434f
AquaMEPHYTON. See Vitamin K (AquaMEPHY-
        TON, phytonadione)
Arab heritage, people with, 177
Areola, breast, 88, 88f
Arm recoil of newborns, 430, 431f, 433f
Aromatherapy, 16
Artificial insemination, 5t, 148
Artificial rupture of fetal membranes, 331, 334f,
        369, 372t
Ascorbic acid. See Vitamin C (ascorbic acid)
Ashkenazi Jews, 177
Asian diet pyramid, 105
Asian heritage, people with
    cleft lip and palate, incidence of, 485
    genetic testing, 177
    HIV and AIDS in women, 289
    illness and death, practices respecting, 298
    maternal mortality rates, 10t
    postpartum period, 396
    pregnancy, activities during, 222t
Asian Pacific group, major cultural traits of, 62
Assessing, in nursing care
    adolescent pregnancy, 262
    families, 70
    fetal development, 179
    labor and birth, high-risk, 380
    labor and birth, normal, 343–345, 345f, 345t
    legal and ethical issues, 45
    newborns, high-risk, 491
    newborns, normal, 455
    nutrition, prenatal, postpartum, and neonatal, 247
    postpartum period, 396–406, 397t, 399f, 400f,
        401f, 402f, 406f, 407f
    pregnancy, high-risk, 298
    pregnancy, normal, 221–223, 222t
    prenatal fetal assessment, 197
    reproductive anatomy and physiology, 91, 94f
    reproductive and health issues, 154
    women's health, 117
Assessing, nursing process, 7, 7f
Assessment
    abuse, potential for, 67
    admission of client in labor, 344
    breast cancer risk factors, 126
    health risks, data collection about, 117
    high-risk pregnancy, risk factors for, 270
    newborn distress, 491
    postpartum depression and psychosis, risk factors
        for, 417
    postpartum (puerperal) infection, risk factors
        for, 416
    preeclampsia and eclampsia, 282
    SIDS, risk factors for, 477
    unhealthy families, signs of, 67
Assessment, in nursing process care plans
    client at risk for deep vein thrombosis, 414–415
    client wanting to breastfeed, 248

client with ovarian cyst, 95
client with preterm labor, 48, 381
client with rape trauma syndrome, 155
client with situational low self-esteem, 263
family desiring alternative therapies, 8
newborn care following cesarean birth, 455
newborn with congenital heart defect, preopera-
        tive care of, 492
pregnancy, first, 180
pregnant woman who wants to travel, 226
stressful family situation, 71
woman in active stage one labor, 354
woman undergoing chorionic villus sampling, 199
woman who wants to stop smoking, 118
woman with gestational diabetes, 299
Assessment of clients
    families, tools and techniques for, 64–67, 64f,
        65f, 66f
    fetal, general, 186–187, 187f
    preconception planning, 177–178, 179f, 180
Assisted births
    cesarean section, 372t, 373–378, 376f, 377–378f
    episiotomy, 372–373, 372t
    forceps extraction, 371–372, 372f, 372t
    vacuum extraction, 369–371, 370f, 372t
    vaginal birth after cesarean, 378
Assisted reproduction, 37, 40
    See also In vitro fertilization
Association of Women's Health, Obstetric and
        Neonatal Nurses, 5
Assumptions, making, 24
Asymmetric (disproportional) intrauterine growth
        restriction, 469
Ataxia, 114
Atrial septal defects, 470, 471f, 471t
Attachment and bonding, postpartum, 290, 393,
        393f, 394f
Authoritarian parenting, 63t
Authoritative parenting, 63t
Autopsies, 296–297t
Autosomal chromosomal abnormalities, 173
Autosomes, 83
Azidothymidine (AZT, Retrovir, ZDV, zidovudine),
        287t, 288, 289t
AZT (azidothymidine, Retrovir, ZDV, zidovudine),
        287t, 288, 289t

B

Babinski reflex, 440
Backache during pregnancy, 213t
"Bag of waters," 165
    See also Fetal membranes
Baha'i faith, 296t
Ballard Newborn Rating Scale, 430, 431f
Ballotable fetus, 309
Ballottement as sign of pregnancy, 205–206
Bard, Samuel, 3t
Bargaining, in grief process, 295, 295f
Barrier methods of contraception, 144f, 145, 145t,
        147f, 148f, 149f
Bartholin's gland, 86, 87f
Basal body temperature, 144, 146f
Bathing newborns, 444, 445–446, 445f
Battered women, characteristics of, 134
Batterers, characteristics of, 134
Beginning families, 59t

Behavioral state of newborns, 441–442, 441f
Benign prostatic hyperplasia (BPH), 140–141, 141f
Benzathine penicillin G, 142t
Beriberi, 235
Best Pharmaceutical for Children Act (2002), 5t
Beta-carotene, 236
Betamethasone (Celestone), 277, 277t, 362,
        364, 364t
Bicarbonate level, 211t
Biliblanket, 33
Bilirubin
    hyperbilirubinemia, 33, 476, 477f
    newborn screening tests, 446–447
Binuclear families, 56
Biofeedback, 325
Biophysical profile
    fetal assessment, 195
    high-risk pregnancy, risk factors for, 270
Biotin, 104, 235
Birth
    See also Labor and birth; Labor and birth,
        high-risk
    adolescent birth rates and pregnancy in U.S.,
        253, 254f
    increased use of term, 307
    partners of adolescent mothers, 259
    preparation of facility for, 346
Birth control. See Contraception
Birthing balls, 322f
Birthing bars, 322f
Birthing facilities
    admission to, 312–313
    birthing facilities and staff, 221
    modern birthing rooms, 307, 307f
Black cohosh (Cimicifuga racemosa), 130, 212
Black people. See African heritage, people with
Bladder exstrophy, 490–491, 490f
Blastocysts, 163, 164f, 165f, 167f
Bleeding
    excessive during labor, 312
    hemorrhage in high-risk newborns, 68, 476
    high-risk pregnancy, 274–278, 274f, 275f, 276f,
        277t, 278f
    postpartum, excessive, 353
Blended families, 56, 56f
Blindness. See Visual impairment
Blood
    cord blood, banking, 41, 336
    fetal samples, obtaining, 361, 362f
    heel sticks samples, 446, 446f
    percutaneous umbilical cord sampling, 190, 190f,
        191–192
    volume of, postpartum, 392
Blood pressure
    normal newborns, 429t, 430, 430f
    postpartum changes, 391
    postpartum elevation, 397
    pregnancy, increase during, 207
Blood tests. See Laboratory tests
Bloody show as sign of labor, 309
Body building, 107
Body of the uterus, 85f, 86
Body position of newborns at rest, 430, 431f,
        432f
Body systems, fetal, 169–171, 169t, 170f,
        171f, 172f

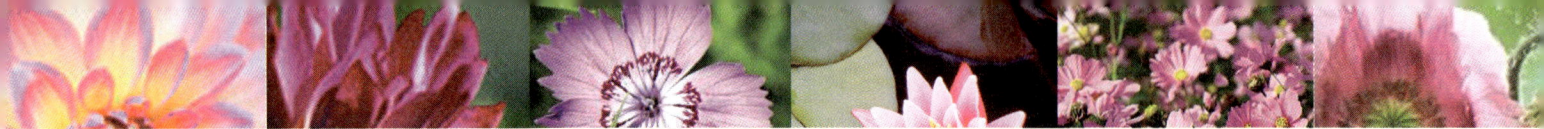

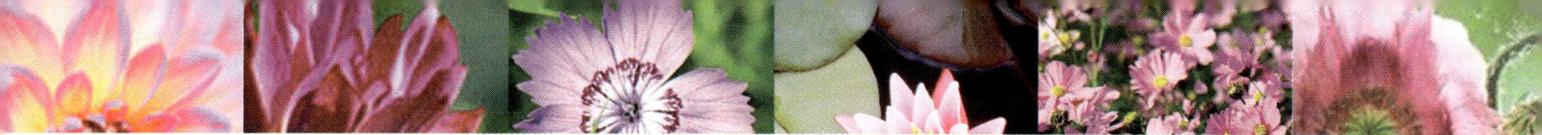

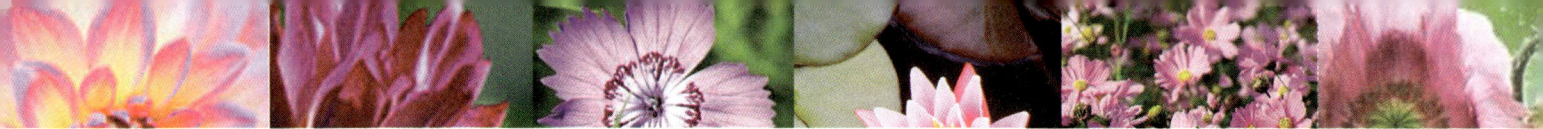

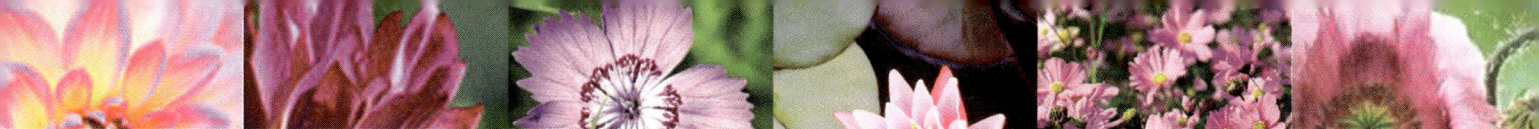

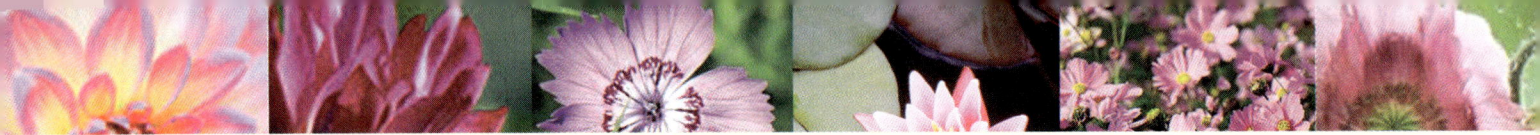

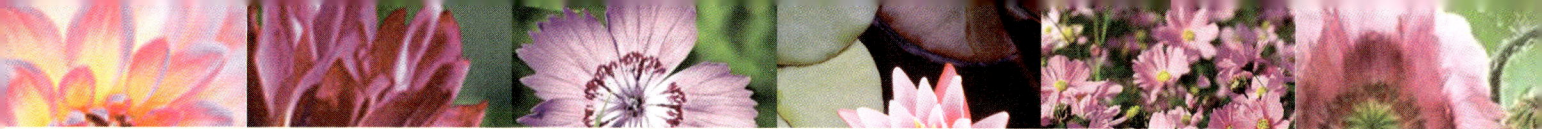

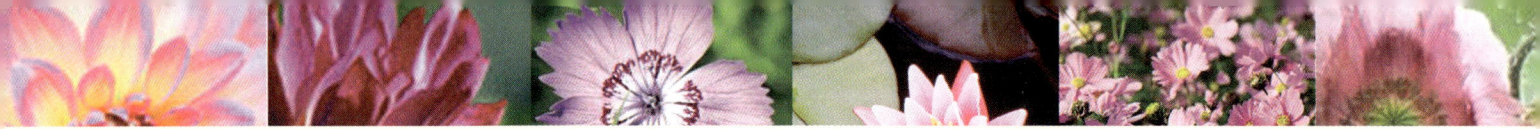

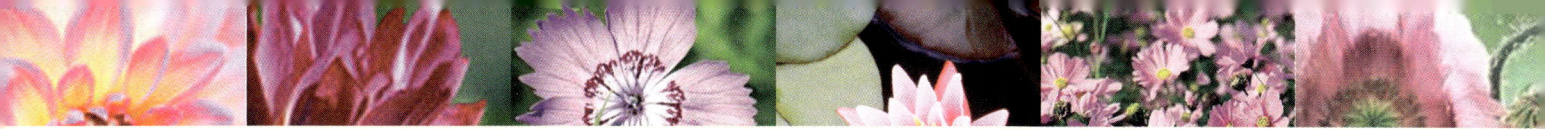

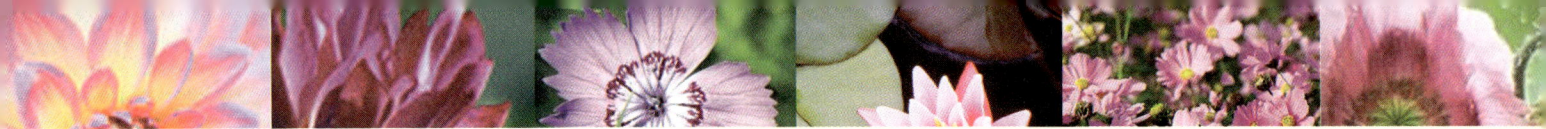

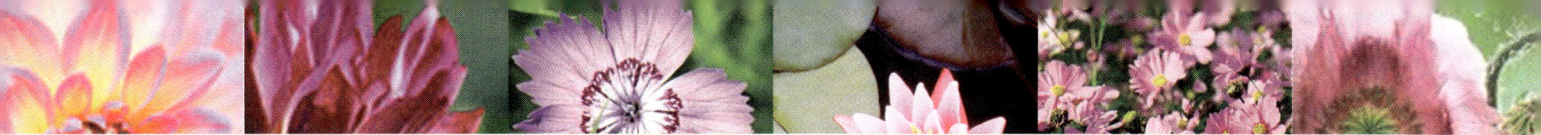

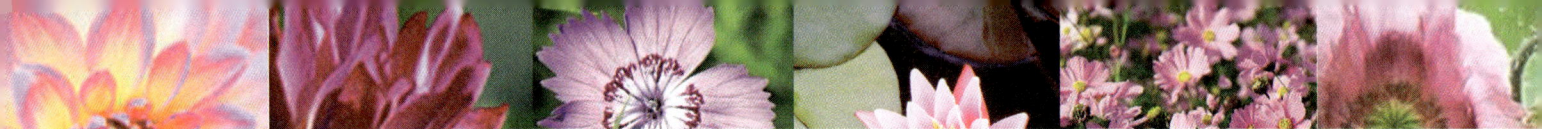

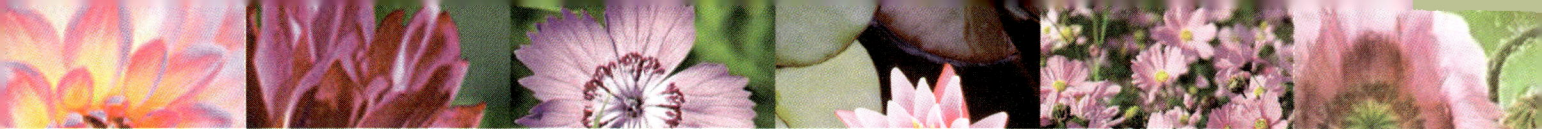

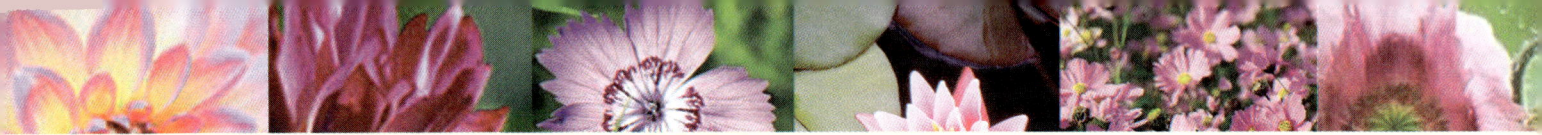

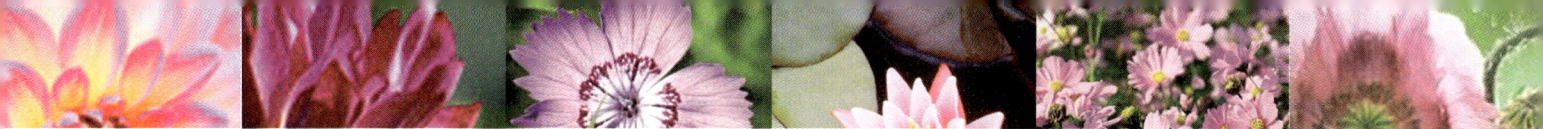

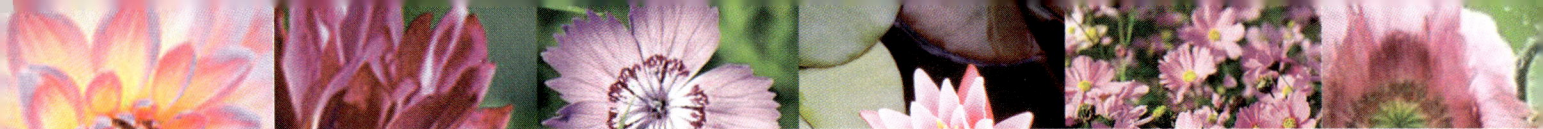

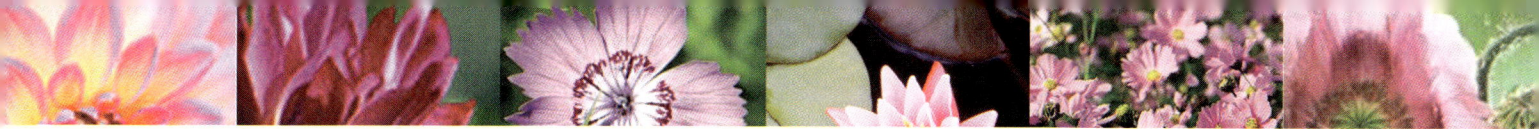

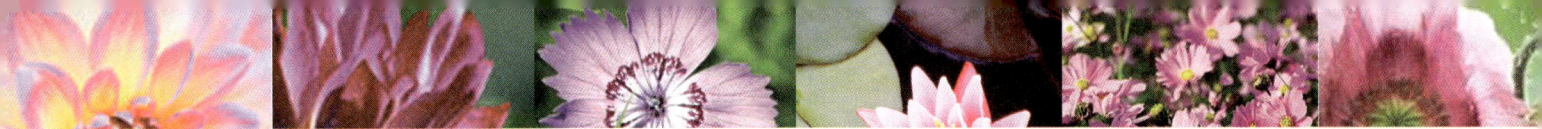

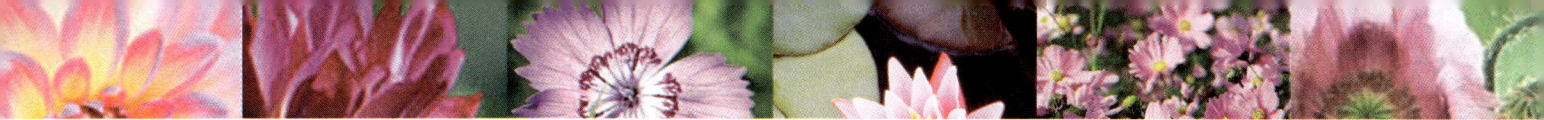

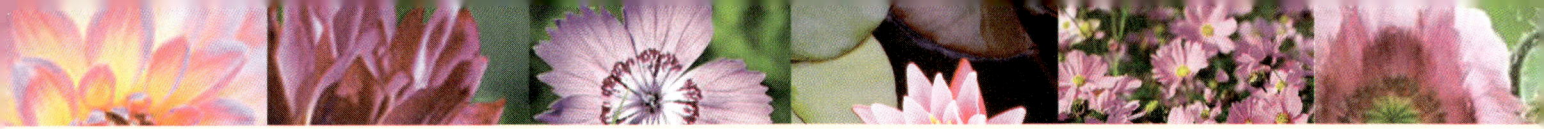

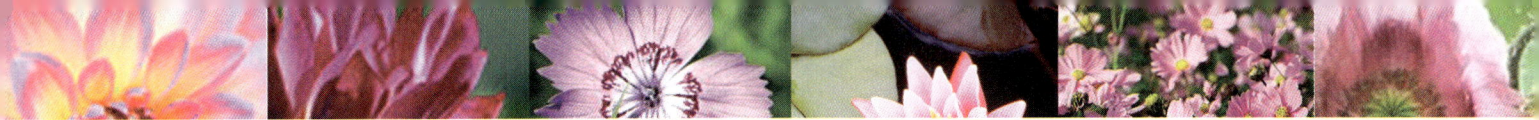

SINGLE PC LICENSE AGREEMENT AND LIMITED WARRANTY

Guide to Special Features

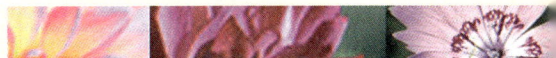

Guide to Special Features

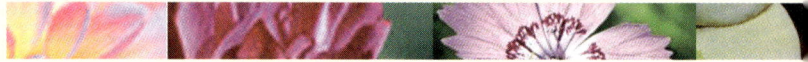

NURSING PROCESS CARE PLANS

PROCEDURES

THINKING STRATEGICALLY ABOUT . . .